Stedman's

CARDIOVASCULAR & PULMONARY WORDS
INCLUDES RESPIRATORY

FOURTH EDITION

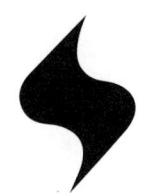

Stedman's

CARDIOVASCULAR & PULMONARY WORDS INCLUDES RESPIRATORY

FOURTH EDITION

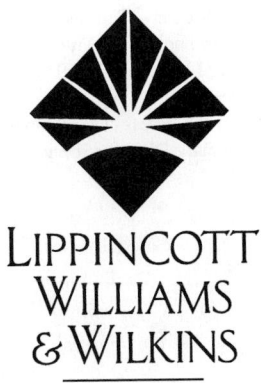

LIPPINCOTT
WILLIAMS
& WILKINS

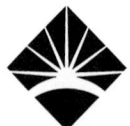

Publisher: Julie K. Stegman
Series Managing Editor: Trista A. DiPaula
Associate Managing Editor: Steve Lichtenstein
Production Coordinator: Jason Delaney
Typesetter: Peirce Graphic Services, LLC.
Printer & Binder: Malloy Litho, Inc.

Copyright © 2004 Lippincott Williams & Wilkins
351 West Camden Street
Baltimore, Maryland 21201-2436

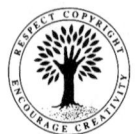

Printed in the United States of America

2004

Library of Congress Cataloging-in-Publication Data

Stedman's cardiovascular and pulmonary words.— 4th ed.
    p. ; cm.— (Stedman's word books)
Rev. ed. of: Stedman's cardiovascular & pulmonary words. 3rd ed. 2001.
Includes bibliographical references.
  ISBN 0–7817-5429–1
  1. Cardiopulmonary system—Diseases—Terminology. 2. Cardiopulmonary system—Terminology. 3. Cardiology—Terminology. I. Title: Cardiovascular and pulmonary words. II. Title: Stedman, Thomas Lathrop, 1853–1938. III. Stedman's cardiovascular and pulmonary words. IV. Series.
  [DNLM: 1. Cardiovascular Diseases—Terminology—English. 2. Cardiology—Terminology—English. 3. Pulmonary Disease (Specialty)—Terminology—English. WG 15 S8124 2004]
RC702.S74 2004
616.1'001'4—dc22

2004001409
01
2 3 4 5 6 7 8 9 10

Contents

Acknowledgments

An important part of our editorial process is the involvement of medical transcriptionists—as advisors, reviewers, and/or editors.

We extend special thanks to Ellen Atwood and Nicole Peck, CMT, for editing the manuscript, helping resolve many difficult questions, and remaining dedicated to this project. We are grateful to our Editorial Advisory Board members, including Kathy Hess, CMT; Velta Jo Reider; Diana Rezac; Suzanne Taubert, CMT; and Tina Whitecotton, MT, who were instrumental in the development of this reference. They recommended sources and shared their valuable judgment, insight, and perspective.

We also extend thanks to Jeanne Bock, CSR, MT, and R. Jo-Ann Clarke for their exemplary work in researching and compiling the appendix. Additional thanks to Helen Littrell for performing the final prepublication review. Other important contributors to this edition include Sue Bartolucci; Susan Caldwell; Marty Cantu, CMT; Janice Deal, RN, BSN; Shemah Fletcher; Beverly S. Oberline, CMT; and Mary Chiara Zaratakiewicz.

Special thanks to Lisa Fahnestock for her exact and diligent work in keeping the manuscript correct and current. And, as always, Barb Ferretti played an integral role in the process by serving as quality control contact for the content.

As with all our *Stedman's* word references, this resource incorporates the suggestions and expertise of our many contacts in the medical transcriptionist community. Thanks to all of our advisory board participants, reviewers, and editors; AAMT meeting attendees; and others who have written us with requests and comments—keep talking, and we'll keep listening.

Editor's Preface

My dad used to tell this tale about himself. The class laggard wanted help with an English assignment, so dad slyly told him to write: "Don't use ain't 'cause ain't ain't a word." Just today, I chanced upon two coined terms, one of which had two forms. In *Geriatrics* (2003;58:5), an editorial on syncope in the aging revealed "syncop-aging," and later introduced "syncopizing." A news brief regarding the United States' first mad cow's offspring spoke of having to "depopulate" that group of calves. Although it is unlikely that "depopulate" will enter mainstream medical terminology, the *Geriatrics* article points out a basic flaw in how new words enter the realm of common usage.

Basic medical research and writing draws upon "The Literature." Each presentation or variation of an illness, condition, or procedure cites previous experts who have been published. When a new term enters "The Literature," it also enters a new realm of existence allowing that term to be extracted, quoted, and relied upon. Errors, or novel coinages, from those publications' spelling and grammar are duplicated, and thus unfortunately form a basis for validity of usage. Errors in resource materials contribute further.

Enter the Internet, which has contributed to this process exponentially. Although positively affecting the ability to quickly and accurately extract previously arcane information only contained in expensive print sources, a few clicks of the mouse can bring up endless hits to verify, or condemn, terminology. Sometimes the wrong spelling has more hits than the right one.

Additionally, most sophisticated word processors have grammar checkers that would make most English teachers cringe, and which are woefully inadequate, not to mention confusing, for evaluating the technical language and style of medical reports. Relying on the suggestions of grammar checkers is a sure-fire way to perpetuate error.

To complicate matters further, the American and British English-speaking countries have long been identified as being "separated by a common language." English has replaced French and German for technical writing. The country of origin of a medical article determines how many errors, or differences, in spelling and context appear. This extends even to names of diseases and anatomical terms. Once published, these also enter the chain of citations.

Medical research, development of new methods, drugs, equipment, and even new diseases such as SARS, all provide an unprecedented proliferation of new terms. People today receive more information in an hour, it is said, than our forebears did in an entire lifetime.

Adding to all this complexity are various style guides, nationally and internationally recognized, as well as the ones that the various institutions and organizations adopt, which may or may not agree with each other on standards and styles.

What does all this mean to medical transcriptionists and others who rely on *Stedman's* Word Books? It is no longer quite so easy to simply state: "Ain't ain't a word."

Moving through the above list backwards, two things stand out. First and foremost, a transcriptionist must develop individual expertise, understanding the nature of the report, the anatomy, processes, drugs, and the equipment involved. Next, sifting through various preferred styles and knowing which to apply can be made easier by answering a simple question: Who is the boss, who is the client, who pays the bills? Some physicians insist on certain abbreviations and terms that may not adhere to what is found in *Stedman's* books or style guides. It is still possible to produce high-quality, accurate products by applying a style to the satisfaction of the person who has hired the work. Personally, I draw the line at misspelled words, usually the ones that the dictator has spelled out.

One thing transcriptionists have always had to do, and which continues to be a critical skill, is to—let me coin my own word—"transterpolate." (Please don't think this is a valid term or should be in common usage, though I would not be surprised to see it turn up on Google in a few months.) To transterpolate, one must not only translate a written word from the spoken, but also simultaneously interpolate by listening to a dictation, hearing those ineffable bits beyond the actual sound waves producing the word, place in an anatomical or procedural context, add a dash of common sense, and finally produce correctly spelled, pertinent text. This skill cannot be learned from a book. This process is similar to the vast difference of learning a foreign language in school, then realizing you understand nothing when encountering the idiomatic speech of that country. Transcriptionists must accrue expertise by doing. After doing enough, it seems that the unclear or previously unknown words can almost bypass the brain and leap directly to the keyboard through the fingertips. Reliable references enhance this ability.

How can you be sure that the words in this reference are accurate? This is basically a spelling book; it's not a style guide, not a manual, not a dictionary, and not a thesaurus. Beyond ensuring that words are spelled correctly, *Stedman's* continues to refine the process by which words are included in specialty books such as *Stedman's Cardiovascular & Pulmonary Words, Fourth Edition.* Some of these steps are to:

- Recognize that preferences and usage vary among geographical regions
- Include valid variants
- Carefully examine the new terms from "The Literature" between editions
- Determine which are accurate and pertinent to the specialty
- Use teams of people to perform specific overlapping tasks

Since the last edition, many new checks, balances, and quality control steps have been implemented by *Stedman's*. The various freelance editors have gained experience and knowledge. Dr. John Dirckx has provided wonderfully erudite reasoning as to why medical terms are the way they are. And finally, you, the user of *Stedman's* Word Books, have kept us on our toes by questioning inclusions, providing new terms for consideration, and spotting those pesky errors that slip in despite all our care.

My thanks to all those team members who have contributed to a great new edition. Special thanks to Nicole Peck, CMT, and Jeanne Bock,

CSR, MT, both of whom went the extra mile and then some. My profound gratitude to R. Jo-Ann Clarke for her special attention to the trials in the appendix, and to all the new abbreviations found in this edition.

By the way, the real point of dad's story was that later the laggard proudly displayed his A, while dad's scholarly paper only received a B.

Ellen Atwood
January, 2004

Publisher's Preface

Stedman's Cardiovascular & Pulmonary Words, Fourth Edition, offers an authoritative assurance of quality and exactness to the wordsmiths of the healthcare professions—medical transcriptionists, medical editors and copyeditors, health information management personnel, court reporters, and the many other users and producers of medical documentation.

In *Stedman's Cardiovascular & Pulmonary Words, Fourth Edition,* users will find protocols, diagnoses, therapeutic procedures, new techniques, lab tests, and clinical research terms, as well as abbreviations with their expansions pertinent to cardiology, pulmonary, and respiratory medicine. The appendix sections, substantially enhanced over the previous edition, provide anatomical illustrations with useful captions and labels; normal lab values; pulmonary function terms; ventilator terms; sample reports; common terms by procedure; drugs by indication; and an exhaustive listing of cardiology-related trial and study names.

This new edition, including more than 95,000 entries, includes the *Stedman's* Word Book Series trademarks: fully cross-indexed terms by first and last word, an A-Z format with main entries and subentries, and appendix material for additional comprehension and application of the terminology.

We at Lippincott Williams & Wilkins strive to provide you with the most up-to-date and accurate word references available. Your use of this Word Book will prompt new editions, which we will publish as often as updates and revisions justify. We welcome your suggestions for improvements, changes, corrections, and additions—whatever will make this *Stedman's* product more useful to you. Please complete the postage-paid card in this book for future suggestions and recommendations, or visit us online at www.stedmans.com.

Explanatory Notes

Medical transcription is an art as well as a science. Both approaches are needed to correctly interpret the dictation of a physician, whose language is a product of education, training, and experience. This variety in medical language means that there are several acceptable ways to express certain terms, including jargon. *Stedman's Cardiovascular & Pulmonary Words, Fourth Edition,* provides variant spellings and phrasings for many terms. These elements, in addition to complete cross-indexing, make *Stedman's Cardiovascular & Pulmonary Words, Fourth Edition,* a valuable resource for determining the validity of terms as they are encountered.

Alphabetical Organization

Alphabetization of main entries is letter by letter as spelled, ignoring punctuation, spaces, prefixed numbers, or other characters. For example:

VSG 2/3F graphic card
V-slit lamp
VSR

Terms beginning or ending with Greek letters show the Greek letters spelled out and listed alphabetically. For example:

alpha, α
> a. agonist
> a. blocking agent
> estrogen receptor a. (ERα)

In subentry alphabetization, the abbreviated singular form or the spelled-out plural form of the noun main entry word is ignored.

Format and Style

All main entries are in boldface to expedite locating a sought-after term, to enhance distinction between main entries and subentries, and to relieve the textual density of the pages.

Irregular plurals and variant spellings are shown on the same line as the singular or preferred form of the word. For example:

pharynx, pl. **pharynges,** gen. **pharyngis**

glycocalix, glycocalyx

Hyphenation

As a rule of style, multiple eponyms (e.g., Virchow-Robin space) are hyphenated. Some eponyms are actually first and last names, thus not hyphenated: Pierre Robin syndrome. Also, hyphens have been added between a manufacturer and one or more eponyms (e.g., Storz-Duredge steel cataract knife). Please note that in many cases, hyphenation is a question of style, not of accuracy, and thus is a matter of choice.

Possessives

Possessive forms have been dropped in this reference for the sake of consistency and conformance with the guidelines of the American Association for Medical Transcription (AAMT) and other groups. Please note, however, that in many cases, retaining the possessive, like hyphenating, is a question of style, not of accuracy, and thus is a matter of choice. To form the possessive of a word, simply add the apostrophe or apostrophe "s" to the end of the word.

Cross-indexing

The word list is in an index-like main entry-subentry format that contains two combined alphabetical listings:

(1) A *noun* main entry-subentry organization, which is typical of the A-Z section of medical dictionaries like *Stedman's*:

airways
  anatomic a.
  lower a.
  upstream a.

parasystole
  atrial p.
  junctional p.
  pure p.

(2) An *adjective* main entry-subentry organization, which lists words and phrases as you hear them. The main entries are the adjectives or modifiers in a multiword term. The subentries are the nouns around which the terms are constructed and to which the adjectives or modifiers pertain:

cardiac
  c. insult
  c. stress test
  c. waist

cholesterol
  c. cleft
  c. pericarditis
  c. thorax

This format provides the user with more than one way to locate and identify a multiword term. For example:

circus
  c. movement

movement
  circus m.

cough
  c. threshold

threshold
  cough t.

It also allows the user to see together all terms that contain a particular descriptor, as well as all types, kinds, or variations of a noun entity. For example:

murmur
  accidental m.
  bellows m.
  decrescendo m.

breath
  b. excretion test
  shortness of b.
  b. sound

Wherever possible, abbreviations are separately defined and cross-referenced. For example:

BRAT
Baylor rapid autologous infusion

Baylor
B. rapid autologous infusion (BRAT)

infusion
Baylor rapid autologous i. (BRAT)

For this edition, we have also included longer abbreviations, frequently used by themselves as slang, but which actually are short forms for valid clinical language. These follow the regular abbreviation format with the short form in bold and the expansion indented:

sed rate   **V tach**
sedimentation rate   ventricular tachycardia

They are further cross-referenced by first and last word of the expansion:

sedimentation   **ventricular**
s. rate (sed rate)   v. tachycardia (V tach)

rate   **tachycardia**
sedimentation r.   ventricular t. (V tach)
(sed rate)

References

In addition to the manufacturers' literature we gather at various medical meetings, scientific reports from hospitals, and the lists created by our MT Editorial Advisory Board members from their daily transcription work, we used the following sources for new terms in *Stedman's Cardiovascular & Pulmonary Words, Fourth Edition*:

Books

Alpert JS, Ewy GA. Manual of Cardiovascular Diagnosis and Therapy, 5th Edition. Philadelphia: Lippincott Williams & Wilkins, 2002.

Drake E. Sloane's Medical Word Book, 4th Edition. Philadelphia: Elsevier, 2002.

Hillis LD. Manual of Clinical Problems in Cardiology, 6th Edition. Philadelphia: Lippincott Williams & Wilkins, 2003.

Hoekstra JW, ed. Handbook of Cardiovascular Emergencies, 2nd Edition. Philadelphia: Lippincott Williams & Wilkins, 2001.

Jablonski S. Cardiology Acronyms & Abbreviations, 4th Edition. Philadelphia: Lippincott Williams & Wilkins, 2003.

Lance LL. Quick Look Drug Book 2003. Baltimore: Lippincott Williams & Wilkins, 2004.

Rao PS, Kern MJ, eds. Catheter Based Device: for the Treatment of Non-Coronary Cardiovascular Disease in Adults and Children. Philadelphia: Lippincott Williams & Wilkins, 2003.

Rhodes SB, David M, eds. Dorland's Cardiology Word Book for Medical Transcriptionists. Philadelphia: Elsevier, 2001.

Sharis PJ, Cannon CP, ed. Evidence-Based Cardiology, 2nd Edition. Philadelphia: Lippincott Williams & Wilkins, 2003.

Stedman's Medical Dictionary, 27th Edition. Baltimore: Lippincott Williams & Wilkins, 2000.

Topol EJ. Textbook of Cardiovascular Medicine, 2nd Edition. Philadelphia: Lippincott Williams & Wilkins, 2002.

Vera Pyle's Current Medical Terminology, 9th Edition. Modesto, CA: Health Professions Institute, 2003.

Images

Agur, AMR, Lee, MJ. Grant's Atlas of Anatomy, 10th Edition. Baltimore: Lippincott Williams & Wilkins, 1999.

Anatomical Chart Company. Atlas of Pathophysiology. Philadelphia: Lippincott Williams & Wilkins, 2001.

Caldwell S. Pikesville, MD. Stedman's Medical Dictionary, 27th edition. Baltimore: Lippincott Williams & Wilkins, 2000.

Cohen BJ. Medical Terminology, 4th Ed. Philadelphia. Lippincott Williams & Wilkins 2003.

Hardy NO. Westport, CT. Stedman's Medical Dictionary, 27th Edition. Baltimore: Lippincott Williams & Wilkins, 2000.

LifeART Super Anatomy Collection 1, CD-ROM. Baltimore, Lippincott Williams & Wilkins.

LifeART Super Anatomy Collection 2, CD-ROM. Baltimore, Lippincott Williams & Wilkins.

LifeART Super Anatomy Collection 5, CD-ROM. Baltimore, Lippincott Williams & Wilkins.

LifeART Super Anatomy Collection 7, CD-ROM. Baltimore, Lippincott Williams & Wilkins.

MediClip Clinical Cardiopulmonary Images, CD-ROM. Baltimore: Lippincott Williams & Wilkins.

Moore KL, PhD, FRSM, FIAC & Dalley AF II, PhD. Clinical Oriented Anatomy, 4th Ed. Baltimore: Lippincott Williams & Wilkins, 1999.

Nettina, Sandra M. The Lippincott Manual of Nursing Practice, 7th Ed. Lippincott, Williams & Wilkins, 2001.

Smeltzer SC, Bare BG. Textbook of Medical-Surgical Nursing, 9th Ed. Philadelphia: Lippincott Williams & Wilkins, 2000.

Journals

The American Journal of Cardiology. Belle Mead, NJ: Excerpta Medica, 2002-2003.

Cardiology in Review. Baltimore: Lippincott Williams & Wilkins, 2002-2003.

Chest. Northbrook, IL: American College of Chest Physicians, 2002-2003.

Clinical Pulmonary Medicine. Baltimore: Lippincott Williams & Wilkins, 2002-2003.

Journal of the American College of Cardiology. New York: Elsevier Science, 2002-2003.

The Latest Word. Philadelphia: Elsevier, 2001-2004.

Websites

http://health.ucsd.edu/labref/
http://www.acc.org/
http://www.cardiologyonline.com/
http://www.cardiologytoday.com/
http://www.cardiosource.com/

http://www.escardio.org/

http://www.healthcentral.com/mhc/top/003371.cfm#Normal%20values:

http://www.medscape.com/cardiologyhome?LID=5762837

http://www.nhlbi.nih.gov/

A
   apical
   atrium
      A band
      biochanin A
      A 67 lead
      A mode
      A wave
A1
   angiotensin I
   aortic first sound
A2
   angiotensin II
      A2 multipurpose catheter
a
   arterial
   arterial blood
   artery
      a dip
      a wave
A-I
   angiotensin I
A-II
   angiotensin II
      A-II receptor
A$_2$
      A$_2$ incisural interval
      A$_2$ to opening snap interval
      thromboxane A$_2$
A$_4$
      leukotriene A$_4$
AA
   abdominal aorta
   African American
   alveoloarterial
   amino acid
   aortic arch
   arteries
   ascending aorta
      AA atheroma
      AA cascade
A-a
   alveolar-arterial
   alveolar-atrial
      A-a gradient
A-a 02
   alveolar-arterial oxygen gradient
   alveolar-arterial oxygen tension
aa
   arteries
AAA
   abdominal aortic aneurysm
   aneurysm of ascending aorta
   angiography of abdominal aorta
   arrest after arrival

   aneurysm of ascending aorta
      (AAA)
AACD
   abdominal aortic counterpulsation device
Aachener Aphasie Test
AACVPR
   American Association of Cardiovascular
      and Pulmonary Rehabilitation
AAD
   acute aortic dissection
   antiarrhythmic drug
A$_{2A}$ adenosine receptor
AAE
   annuloaortic ectasia
   anuloaortic ectasia
AAF
   aortic arch flush
AAG
   alveolar arterial gradient
AAI
   activating adjusting instrument
   atrial demand inhibited
   atrial inhibited
      AAI pacemaker
      AAI pacing
      AAI rate-responsive mode
AAI/AAIR pacemaker
A$_1$-A$_2$ interval
A-A interval
AAI-RR pacing
AAL
   anterior axillary line
AAO
   ascending aorta
AAPF
   antiarteriosclerosis polysaccharide factor
AaPO$_2$
   alveolar-arterial PO$_2$ difference
AARC
   American Association for Respiratory
      Care
AAS
   aneurysm of atrial septum
   aortic arch syndrome
AASP
   ascending aorta synchronized pulsation
AAST
   American Association for the Surgery of
      Trauma
AAT
   alpha-1 antitrypsin
   atrial demand triggered
   automatic atrial tachycardia
      human pooled AAT
      AAT mode

AAT (*continued*)
    AAT pacemaker
    AAT pacing
AAV
    adeno-associated virus
AAV-CF therapy
AAVNRT
    atypical atrioventricular nodal reentrant
    tachycardia
AAW
    anterior aortic wall
AB
    apex beat
A&B
    apnea and bradycardia
ABA
    arrest before arrival
ABAb
    anti-beta 1 adrenoreceptor antibody
abacavir
abacterial
    a. thrombosis
    a. thrombotic endocarditis
Abbe
    A. flap
    A. operation
Abbokinase
    A. injection
    A. Open-Cath
Abbott infusion pump
Abbreviated Injury Scale (AIS)
ABC
    airway, breathing, circulation
    aspiration biopsy cytology
    ABC lead
    ABC protocol
ABCD
    airway, breathing, circulation, defibrillate
ABCDE
    airway, breathing, circulation, disability,
    exposure
    ABCDE in trauma patient
ABCIC
    airway, breathing, circulation,
    intravenous, crystalloid
abciximab (ABX)
ABD
    automated border detection
    automatic boundary detection
abdominal
    a. angina
    a. aorta (AA, AO)
    a. aortic aneurysm (AAA)
    a. aortic aneurysmectomy
    a. aortic counterpulsation device
    (AACD)
    a. aortic endarterectomy
    a. aortography
    a. asthma

    a. belt
    a. bruit
    a. compartment syndrome (ACS)
    a. heart
    a. jugular test
    a. left ventricular assist device
    (ALVAD)
    a. paradox breathing pattern
    a. part of esophagus
    a. pocket
    a. pulse
    a. respiration
    a. vascular retractor
abdominalis
    aorta a.
    ectopia cordis a.
abdominocardiac reflex
abdominojugular reflux
abdominothoracic
    a. arch
    a. pump
ABE
    acute bacterial endocarditis
ABECB
    acute bacterial exacerbation of chronic
    bronchitis
Abee support
Abelcet
Abell-Kendall equivalent
Abelson cannula
aberrancy
    acceleration-dependent a.
    atrial trigeminy with a.
    bradycardia-dependent a.
    deceleration-dependent a.
    paradoxical a.
    paroxysmal atrial tachycardia
    with a.
    postextrasystolic a.
    tachycardia-dependent a.
aberrant
    a. QRS complex
    a. subclavian artery
    a. thyroid
    a. ventricular conduction (AVC)
aberrantly conducted beat
aberration
    intraventricular a.
    nonspecific T-wave a.
    ventricular a.
abetalipoproteinemia
    Bassen-Kornzweig a.
    familial a.
ABF
    aortic blood flow
    aortobifemoral
ABG
    arterial blood gas
    ABG point-of-care test

ABG PCT
  arterial blood gas point-of-care test
abhesive
ABI
  ankle-brachial index
  atherothrombotic brain infarction
    ABI Vest Airway Clearance system
ability
  torquing a.
Abiomed
    A. biventricular support system
    A. implantable heart-replacement
      device
ABL
    ABL 555 analyzer
    ABL 520 blood gas measurement
      system
    ABL 625 system
ablation
  Ablatr temperature control
    device a.
  accessory conduction a. (ACA)
  alcohol a.
  atrial isthmus a.
  atrioventricular junctional a.
  atrioventricular nodal a.
  A-V junction a.
  a. catheter
  catheter a.
  catheter-induced a.
  chemical a.
  continuous-wave laser a.
  coronary rotational a.
  direct-current shock a.
  electrical catheter a.
  endocardial catheter a.
  endovascular radiofrequency
    catheter a.
  epicardial radiofrequency catheter a.
  fast-pathway radiofrequency
    catheter a.
  fluoroscopic isthmus a.
  His bundle a.
  irrigated catheter a.
  Kent bundle a.
  laser a.
  linear a.
  linear-phased radiofrequency
    catheter a.
  maze a.
  percutaneous radiofrequency
    catheter a.

  percutaneous transluminal coronary
    rotational a. (PTCRA)
  percutaneous transluminal septal
    myocardial a. (PTSMA)
  pulsed laser a.
  radiofrequency a. (RFA)
  radiofrequency catheter a.
  Revelation Tx microcatheter for
    RF a.
  RF catheter a.
  rotational a.
  septal a.
  slow-pathway a.
  superior pulmonary vein a.
  surgical a.
  tissue a.
  transcatheter a.
  transcoronary alcohol a. (TAA)
  transcoronary chemical a.
  transvenous a.
ablative
    a. cardiac surgery
    a. device
    a. laser angioplasty
    a. technique
ablator
  radiofrequency a.
Ablatr
    A. temperature control device
    A. temperature control device
      ablation
Ablaza-Blanco aortic wall retractor
ABLC
  amphotericin B lipid complex
abnormal
    a. cleavage of cardiac valve
    a. coronary artery (ACA)
    a. left axis deviation (ALAD)
    a. right axis deviation (ARAD)
    a. ST segment
    a. vasopressin (AVP)
    a. wall motion (AWM)
abnormality
  angiographically occult a.
  atrioventricular conduction a.
  baseline ST-segment a.
  brisk wall motion a.
  clotting a.
  coloboma, heart anomaly,
    ichthyosis, mental retardation,
    ear a. (CHIME)
  conotruncal a.

NOTES

abnormality *(continued)*
    electrical activation a.
    familial congenital cardiac a.
      (FCCA)
    fibrinolytic a.
    figure-of-eight a.
    focal motion a.
    functional pacing a.
    hemodynamic a.
    high-risk repolarization a.
    immunochemical a.
    left atrial a.
    left ventricular wall motion a.
    lusitropic a.
    neurogenic a.
    nonspecific T-wave a.
    pleuroparenchymal a.
    regional wall motion a. (RWMA)
    sinus node/AV conduction a.
    snowman a.
    transient wall motion a.
    ventricular depolarization a.
    wall motion a. (WMA)

aborted
    a. sudden death
    a. systole

abortive pneumonia

abouchement

ABP
    ambulatory blood pressure
    arterial blood pressure
    automated boundary protection
    automatic systolic blood pressure
      measurement

aBP
    arterial blood pressure

ABPA
    allergic bronchopulmonary aspergillosis

ABPM
    ambulatory blood pressure monitoring

ABR
    arterial baroreflex

Abrahams sign

Abrams
    A. heart reflex
    A. needle
    A. pleural biopsy punch

Abrams-Lucas flap heart valve

abrasion
    pleural a.

abreugraphy

abrupt pulse

ABS
    acrylonitrile-butadiene-styrene

AB-SAAP
    autologous blood selective aortic arch
      perfusion

abscess
    anular a.

    aortic root a.
    apical a.
    Brodie a.
    caseous a.
    cold a.
    embolic a.
    lung a.
    myocardial a.
    papillary muscle a.
    periaortic a.
    periprosthetic valve a.
    retropharyngeal a.
    ring a.
    subphrenic a.

abscessus
    Mycobacterium a.

absent
    a. breath sounds
    a. pericardium
    a. pulmonary valve
    a. respiration

Absidia

absolute
    a. alcohol
    atmosphere a. (ata)
    a. cardiac dullness (ACD)
    a. dullness (M3)
    a. humidity
    a. pressure
    a. refractory period (ARP)
    a. risk reduction (ARR)

absorbable
    a. gelatin
    a. gelatin film
    a. gelatin sponge
    a. suture

absorbance
    time of flight and a. (TOFA)

absorbent vessel

absorption
    a. atelectasis
    a., distribution, metabolism, and
      excretion (ADME)
    fluorescent treponemal antibody a.
      (FTA-ABS)
    net a.

abuse
    alcohol a.
    cocaine a.
    drug a.

ABX
    abciximab

ABx, ABX, abx
    antibiotic

AC
    adenylyl cyclase
    alternating current
    ante cibum
    anterior chamber

anterior circulation
anticoagulant
aortic closure
aortic compliance
aortocoronary
atriocarotid
Mytussin AC
Robafen AC

A-C
aortocoronary bypass
A-C interval
Robitussin A-C

AC137
human analog amylin AC137

ac
anterior chamber
atrial contraction

ACA
abnormal coronary artery
accessory conduction ablation
anterior cerebral artery
anterior communicating aneurysm
anterior communicating artery
anticentromere antibody
arrhythmic cardiac arrest
asthma care algorithm

acacia
gum a.

A2C, A4C view

ACAD
asymptomatic coronary artery disease
atherosclerotic coronary artery disease

acadesine

Acanthamoeba
A. astronyxis
A. castellanii
A. culbertsoni
A. glebae
A. hatchetti
A. palestinensis
A. polyphaga
A. rhysodes

acanthocytosis
acapella chest physical therapy device
acapnia
acarbia
acarbose
acardiotrophia
acarian asthma
acaricidal chemical
Acarosan dust mite powder
acaryote

Acat 1 intraaortic balloon pump
ACB
albumin cobalt binding
aortocoronary bypass
arterialized capillary blood
asymptomatic carotid bruit
ACB test

ACBG
aortocoronary bypass graft

ACC
American College of Cardiology

ACCA
American College of Cardiovascular
Administrators

ACC/AHA
American College of
Cardiology/American Heart Association
ACC/AHA pacemaker implantation
guidelines

accelerated
a. atrioventricular junctional rhythm
a. A-V junctional rhythm
a. A-V node conduction
a. hypertension
a. idioventricular rhythm (AIVR)
a. idioventricular tachycardia
a. respiration
a. ventricular rhythm (AVR)

acceleration
flow a.
a. time

acceleration-dependent aberrancy
acceleration-guided activity pacing
accelerator
a. globin (AcG)
a. globin blood coagulation factor
a. nerve
proconvertin prothrombin
conversion a.
serum prothrombin conversion a.
(SPCA)
serum thrombotic a. (STA)

accelerometer
Caltrac a.
intracardiac a.
Koelner Vitaport a.
multiaxis a.
triaxial a.
TriTrac-R3D a.
uniaxial a.

Accent balloon angioplasty catheter
Accent-DG balloon

NOTES

accentuated antagonism

access

    A. AccuTnI troponin I test
A-Port vascular a.
Check-Flo performer introducer set for radial artery a.
echo record a. (ERA)
Low Profile Port vascular a.
A. MV system
a. by radial artery multilink stent (ARMS)
Rapidpoint a.
side-entry a. (SEA)
venous a.
venovenous a.

Access-9 large bore hemostasis valve

accessory

    a. arteriovenous connection
a. atrium
a. conduction ablation (ACA)
a. cusp
a. inspiratory muscle
a. muscles of respiration
N95-Companion a.
a. obturator artery
a. pathway (AP)
a. pathway effective refractory period (APERP)
a. pathway mediated tachycardia
a. pulmonary blood flow (APBF)
a. saphenous vein
a. thyroid

accident

    cardiac a.
cardiovascular a. (CVA)
cerebrovascular a. (CVA)
right cerebrovascular a. (RCVA)

accidental murmur

Accolate

accommodation

    period of a.

accompanying

    a. artery of ischiadic nerve
a. artery of median nerve

ACCP

    American College of Chest Physicians

accretio cordis

accrochage

Accucap CO$_2$/O$_2$ monitor

Accu-Chek II Freedom

Accucom cardiac output monitor

Accudynamic adjustable damping

Accufix

    A. II DEC pacing lead
A. pacemaker
A. pacemaker lead

AccuGage vessel calipers

Accuhaler

Acculink self-expanding stent

AccuMark calibrated infant feeding tube

AccuMeter theophylline test

accumulation

    lipid a.
phytanic acid a.

AccuNet embolic protection system

Accupril

Accurbron

Accuretic

Accurox mask

Accustaple

AccuTnI troponin I test

Accutorr

    A. multiparameter monitor
A. oscillometric device

Accutracker

    A. blood pressure device
A. II ambulatory blood pressure monitor

ACD

    absolute cardiac dullness
active compression-decompression
area of cardiac dullness
arrhythmia control device

ACD-CPR

    active compression-decompression cardiopulmonary resuscitation

ACE

    acute coronary event
Adriamycin, cyclophosphamide, etoposide
aerosol cloud enhancer
angiotensin-converting enzyme
    ACE antisense gene therapy
    ACE deletion/insertion polymorphism
    ACE detachable mask
    ACE fixed-wire balloon catheter
    ACE inhibitor
    ACE kit
    ACE MDI spacer
    universal ACE

ACE-II

    angiotensin-converting enzyme II
    ACE-II genotype

ACE-ID

    angiotensin-converting enzyme ID
    ACE-ID genotype

acebutolol hydrochloride

acecainide hydrochloride

acedapsone

ACE-DD

    angiotensin-converting enzyme DD
    ACE-DD genotype

ACEI, ACEi

    angiotensin-converting enzyme inhibitor

Acel-Imune

acenocoumarol

Aceon
acepifylline
ace of spades sign
acetabular artery
acetaldehyde
acetaminophen
    a. and dextromethorphan
    a., dextromethorphan,
      pseudoephedrine
    hydrocodone and a.
acetate
    anaritide a.
    carbon-11 a.
    caspofungin a.
    cortisone a.
    Cortone A.
    desmopressin a.
    Florinef A.
    fludrocortisone a.
    guanabenz a.
    guanfacine a.
    Hydrocortone A.
    leuprolide a.
    medroxyprogesterone a. (MPA)
    megestrol a.
    methylprednisolone a.
    paramethasone a.
    PET with C-11 a.
    pirbuterol a.
    polymyxin, lysome, EDTA,
      thallous a. (PLET)
    sodium a.
acetazolamide
acetic acid
acetohexamide
acetonide
    triamcinolone a. (TAA)
acetoorcein stain
acetylcarnitine
acetylcholinesterase deficiency
acetylcholine test
acetyl-CoA
***N*-acetylcysteine**
acetyldigitoxin
acetyldigoxin
acetylglucosaminyltransferase
acetylhydrolase
***N*-acetylprocainamide**
acetylsalicylate
    lysine a.
acetylsalicylic acid (ASA)
acetylstrophanthidin (AcS)

acetyltransferase
ACG
    angiocardiogram
    angiocardiography
    aortocoronary graft
    apexcardiogram
    apexcardiography
AcG
    accelerator globin
      AcG blood coagulation factor
AChA
    anterior choroidal artery
achalasia
    esophageal a.
Aches-N-Pain
Achieve Off-Pump system
Achiever
    A. balloon dilatation catheter
    A. balloon dilator
Acholeplasma laidlawii
achromatic mass
achromatin, achromin
achromatolysis
Achromobacter xylosoxidans
Achromycin V Oral
ACI
    acute cardiac ischemia
    acute coronary infarction
    acute coronary insufficiency
    asymptomatic cardiac ischemia
acid
    acetic a.
    N-acetylneuraminic a.
    acetylsalicylic a. (ASA)
    amino a. (AA)
    aminocaproic a.
    5-aminolevulinic a.
    aminosalicylic a.
    p-aminosalicylic a.
    amoxicillin and clavulanic a.
    arachidonic a.
    ascorbic a.
    aspartic a.
    betamethyliodophenyl
      pentadecanoic a.
    carbon-11-labeled fatty a.'s
    clavulanic a.
    cystidine monophospho-*N*-
      acetylneuraminic a. (CMP-NANA)
    deoxyribonucleic a. (DNA)
    diethylenetriamine pentaacetic a.
      (DPTA, DTPA)

NOTES

acid *(continued)*
  docosahexaenoic a.
  EET a.
  eicosapentaenoic a. (EPA)
  enalaprilic a.
  endomethylene tetrahydrophthalic a.
    (EMTA)
  epoxyeicosatrienoic a.
  ethacrynic a.
  ethylenediaminetetraacetic a.
    (EDTA)
  fatty a.
  ferrous salt and ascorbic a.
  ferrous sulfate, ascorbic a., vitamin
    B-complex, and folic a.
  fibric a.
  folic a.
  fosinoprilic a.
  free fatty a.'s (FFA)
  fusidic a.
  gadolinium-diethylenetriamine
    pentaacetic a. (Gd-DTPA)
  gamma-aminobutyric a. (GABA)
  glycyrrhizinic a.
  5-HPETE a.
  hyaluronic a.
  hydrobromic a.
  hydrochloric a.
  hydrocyanic a.
  hydrofluoric a.
  20-hydroxyeicosatetraenoic a. (20-
    HETE)
  hydroxyethyl piperazine-
    ethanesulfonic a. (HEPES)
  hydroxyethyl piperazine-
    ethenesulfonic a.
  a. infusion test
  inorganic a.
  iodophenylpentadecanoic a.
  lactic a.
  linoleic a.
  lysophosphatidic a.
  a. maltase deficiency
  mefenamic a.
  messenger ribonucleic a. (mRNA)
  mevalonate a.
  monosaturated fatty a.
  monounsaturated fatty a.'s (MUFA)
  a. mucopolysaccharide (AMP)
  nalidixic a.
  n-3 fatty a.
  n-6 fatty a.
  nicotinic a.
  nonesterified fatty a.
  omega-3 unsaturated fatty a.'s
  osteopontin messenger
    ribonucleic a.
  palmitic a.
  paraaminobenzoic a.

  paraaminosalicylic a. (PAS, PASA)
  perchloric a.
  a. phosphatase
  phosphinic a.
  polyglycolic a.
  poly-L-lactic a. (PLLA)
  polyunsaturated fatty a. (PUFA)
  potassium citrate and citric a.
  pyruvic a.
  recombinant deoxyribonucleic a.
    (rDNA)
  retinoic a.
  ribonucleic a. (RNA)
  saturated fatty a. (SFA)
  sialic a.
  sulfosalicylic a.
  Tc-diethylenetriamine pentaacetic a.
  ticarcillin and clavulanic a.
  tranexamic a.
  trans fatty a.'s (TFA)
  triglyceride fatty a. (TGFA)
  unesterified fatty a. (UFA)
  uric a.
  urocanic a.
  very long-chain fatty a. (VLCFA)
  volatile fatty a. (VFA)
  zofenoprilic a.
acid-base
  a.-b. determination
  a.-b. disorder
  a.-b. imbalance
acidemia
acid-fast bacillus
acidic fibroblast growth factor (aFGF)
acidity
  total a.
acidosis
  acute respiratory a.
  hypercapnic a.
  hyperchloremic a.
  ischemia-induced intracellular a.
  lactic a.
  metabolic a.
  respiratory a.
acid-reactive
  thiobarbituric a.-r.
aciduria
acinar
  a. adenocarcinoma
  a. nodule
  a. rosette
Acinetobacter
  A. anitratus
  A. baumannii
  A. calcoaceticus
  A. calcoaceticus-baumannii complex
  A. lwoffi
acinus, pl. **acini**

lung a.
pulmonary a.
acipimox
ACIST injection system
acitretin
ACLA, aCLa
anticardiolipin antibody
ACLA IgG
ACLA IgM
Acland-Banis arteriotomy set
Acland-Buncke counterpressor
acleistocardia
ACLS
advanced cardiac life support
ACM
anticardiac myosin
automated cardiac flow measurement
ACMT
artificial circus movement tachycardia
acnes
Propionibacterium a.
ACO
acute coronary occlusion
ACoA, AcoA
anterior communicating artery
ACOM, AcomA
automated cardiac output measurement
aconitine
acorn
A. CorCap cardiac support device
A. II nebulizer
Acosta disease
Acoustascope esophageal stethoscope
acoustic
a. densitometry
a. imaging
a. impedance
a. impedance probe
a. microscope
a. quantification (AQ)
a. shadow
a. shadowing
a. window
ACPE
acute cardiogenic pulmonary edema
acquired
a. atelectasis
a. immunodeficiency syndrome (AIDS)
a. pulmonary hypertension
a. valvular heart disease (AVHD)

a. valvular heart syndrome (AVHS)
a. ventricular septal defect (AVSD)
acquisition
a. gate
gated equilibrium ventriculography, frame-mode a.
gated equilibrium ventriculography, list-mode a.
multiple gated a. (MUGA)
tagged a.
a. time
a. zoom (AZ)
a. zoom technology
Acra-Cut Spiral craniotome blade
Acremonium
acridinium ester labeled nucleic acid probe
acrivastine and pseudoephedrine
acroasphyxia
acrocephalopolysyndactyly
acrocyanosis
Acrodisc unit
acrohypothermy
acromegalic heart disease
acromegaloid facial appearance (AFA)
acromegaly
acromelalgia
acromial
a. articular facies of clavicle
a. articular surface of clavicle
acrosclerosis
acrotic
acrotism
acrylate
Acrylon
acrylonitrile-butadiene-styrene (ABS)
ACS
abdominal compartment syndrome
acute chest syndrome
acute confusional state
acute coronary syndrome
Advanced Cardiovascular Systems
American Cancer Society
anodal closure sound
ACS Alpha balloon
ACS Amplatz guidewire
ACS anchor exchange device
ACS Concorde over-the-wire catheter system
ACS Endura coronary dilation catheter

NOTES

ACS *(continued)*

ACS Enhanced Torque 8/7.5-F Taper Tip catheter
ACS exchange guidewire
ACS extra-support guidewire
ACS Hi-Torque Balance middleweight guidewire
ACS LIMA guide
ACS LIMA guidewire
ACS Mini catheter
ACS Monorail catheter
ACS Multi-Link coronary stent
ACS Multi-Link coronary system
ACS Multi-Link Duet stent
ACS Multi-Link RX Ultra coronary stent system
ACS Multi-Link RX Ultra stent
ACS Multi-Link Tristar stent
ACS OTW Lifestream coronary dilatation catheter
ACS OTW Photon coronary dilatation catheter
ACS OTW Photon coronary dilation catheter
ACS OTW Solaris coronary dilatation catheter
ACS OTW Solaris coronary dilation catheter
ACS Photon coronary dilatation catheter
ACS RX Comet angioplasty catheter
ACS RX Comet coronary dilatation catheter
ACS RX Comet VP coronary dilatation catheter
ACS RX Lifestream coronary dilation catheter
ACS RX Multi-Link stent
ACS RX perfusion balloon catheter
ACS RX Solaris coronary dilatation catheter

AcS

acetylstrophanthidin

ACS Ao

ascending aorta

ACSM

American College of Sports Medicine
ACSM regression equation

ACST Tx2000 coronary dilatation catheter

ACSV

aortocoronary saphenous vein

ACSVBG

aortocoronary saphenous vein bypass graft

ACT

activated clotting time
activated coagulation time
adaptive current tomography
anticoagulant therapy
axial computed tomography
ACT MicroCoil delivery system

act

emergency medical treatment and active labor a. (EMTALA)
Prescription Drug User Fee A. (PDUFA)

ACTA

American Cardiology Technologists Association

Actagen-C

ACTe

anodal closure tetanus

ACTH

adrenocorticotropic hormone

Acthar

ActHIB vaccine

Actigraph

Mini-Motionlogger A.

Actilyse

Actimmune

actin

alpha-cardiac a.
a. cytoskeleton
a. fiber
filamentous a. (F-actin)
a. gene
a. monomer
smooth muscle a. (SMA)

actin-myosin crossbridge

Actinobacillus

A. actinomycetemcomitans
A. equuli
A. hominis
A. suis
A. ureae

Actinomadura

Actinomyces

A. bovis
A. israelii

actinomycetemcomitans

Actinobacillus a.

actinomycetoma

actinomycosis

pulmonary a.
thoracic a.

action

catecholamine a.
girdle-like a.
mechanism of a.
a. potential
a. potential duration (APD)
purinergic a.
A. Research Arm Test
respiratory depressant a.
thoracic expanding a.

Actiq Oral Transmucosal

Actis VFC
Activase
    Cathflo A.
    A. injection
activated
    a. balloon expandable intravascular stent
    a. clotting time (ACT)
    a. coagulation time (ACT)
    eptacog alfa a.
    a. factor VII (FVIIa)
    a. graft
    a. partial thromboplastin time (APTT, aPTT)
activating
    a. adjusting instrument (AAI)
    a. transcription factor (ATF)
activation
    complement a.
    eccentric atrial a.
    endothelial cell a.
    granulocyte a.
    heparin-induced platelet a. (HIPA)
    length-dependent a.
    a. map-guided surgical resection
    myofilament contractile a.
    platelet a.
    right ventricle a. (RVA)
    a. sequence
    a. sequence mapping
    thrombosis a.
activator
    plasminogen a.
    a. protein (AP)
    recombinant tissue plasminogen a. (rt-PA)
    recombinant tissue-type plasminogen a.
    single chain urokinase-type plasminogen a.
    tissue plasminogen a. (tPA)
    tissue-type plasminogen a.
    two-chain urokinase plasminogen a. (tcu-PA)
    urokinase plasminogen a. (uPA)
    vampire bat salivary plasminogen a. (DSPA)
active
    A. Can defibrillator lead system
    a. compression-decompression (ACD)

    a. compression-decompression cardiopulmonary resuscitation (ACD-CPR)
    a. compression-decompression resuscitator
    a. congestion
    a. dynamic stiffness
    a. fixation pacemaker lead
    a. hyperemia
    a. pressure (AP)
    a. transport
    a. tuberculosis
active-site inhibited factor VIIa
Activitrax
    A. II pacemaker
    A. single-chamber responsive pacemaker
    A. variable rate pacemaker
activity
    antifactor Xa a.
    cholesterol-esterifying a. (CEA)
    coagulation a.
    a.'s of daily living (ADL)
    dehydrogenase a.
    early return to normal a.'s (ERNA)
    heparin neutralizing a. (HNA)
    hyperadrenergic a.
    intrinsic sympathomimetic a.
    leisure time physical a. (LTPA)
    lipoprotein lipase a. (LPLA)
    melanoma inhibitory a. (MIA)
    membrane-stabilizing a.
    Motor Club Assessment test of motor a.
    muscle sympathetic nerve a. (MSNA)
    myocyte metabolic a.
    plasma renin a. (PRA)
    platelet a.
    postheparin lipolytic a. (PHLA)
    prothrombin a. (PTA)
    pulseless electrical a. (PEA)
    respiratory a.
    a. scale
    a. sensor
    sinoaortic baroreflex a.
    snooze-induced excitation of sympathetic triggered a. (SIESTA)
    spike a.
    sympathetic nerve a. (SNA)

NOTES

activity *(continued)*
> sympathetic nervous system a.
> triggered a.
> ventricular ectopic a. (VEA)

activity-guided
> a.-g. pacemaker
> a.-g. pacing

activity-sensing pacemaker

ACT-ONE stent

Actron

Actros pacemaker

actuarial survival curve

actuation
> direct mechanical ventricular a.
> (DMVA)

actuator
> dry-powder a.

AcuNav ultrasound catheter

acupuncture

Acuseal cardiovascular patch

Acuson
> A. cardiovascular system
> A. computed sonography
> A. echocardiograph
> A. V5M multiplane transesophageal echocardiographic transducer
> A. V5M transesophageal echocardiographic monitor
> A. XP-128 echocardiographic system
> A. XP-5,-10,-128 ultrasonoscope

acute
> a. allograft rejection
> a. aortic dissection (AAD)
> a. bacterial endocarditis (ABE)
> a. bacterial exacerbation of chronic bronchitis (ABECB)
> a. brain syndrome
> a. cardiac ischemia (ACI)
> a. cardiogenic pulmonary edema (ACPE)
> a. cardiovascular (ACV)
> a. cardiovascular disease (ACVD)
> a. caudate stroke
> a. cellular xenograft rejection
> a. chemical injury
> a. chest syndrome (ACS)
> a. compression triad
> a. confusional state (ACS)
> a. congestive heart failure
> a. coronary care unit
> a. coronary event (ACE)
> a. coronary infarction (ACI)
> a. coronary insufficiency (ACI)
> a. coronary occlusion (ACO)
> a. coronary syndrome (ACS)
> a. cor pulmonale
> a. diaphragmatic myocardial infarction

> a. dissecting aneurysm
> a. endothelial dysfunction
> a. exacerbation of chronic bronchitis
> a. exacerbation of chronic obstructive pulmonary disease
> a. fibrinous pericarditis
> a. glomerulonephritis (AGN)
> a. heart disease (AHD)
> a. heart failure
> a. hemispheric stroke
> a. hemorrhagic bronchopneumonia
> a. idiopathic pericarditis (AIP)
> a. infective endocarditis (AIE)
> a. intermittent porphyria (AIP)
> a. interstitial pneumonia (AIP)
> a. interstitial pneumonitis (AIP)
> a. ischemic coronary syndrome (AICS)
> a. ischemic stroke (AIS)
> a. isolated myocarditis
> a. laryngotracheal bronchitis
> a. left ventricular failure (ALVF)
> a. lower respiratory tract infection (ALRI)
> a. lung injury (ALI)
> a. lung rejection
> a. lupus pericarditis (ALP)
> a. lupus pneumonitis (ALP)
> a. lymphocytic leukemia (ALL)
> a. margin of heart
> a. mediastinitis
> a. miliary tuberculosis
> a. mitral stenosis (AMS)
> a. multiple brain infarcts (AMBI)
> a. myelocytic leukemia (AML)
> a. noncardiogenic pulmonary edema
> a. obliterating bronchiolitis
> a. occlusive thrombosis (AOT)
> a. occlusive thrombus (AOT)
> a. pharyngitis
> A. Physiology, Age, Chronic Health Evaluation (APACHE)
> a. pleurisy
> a. preload alteration
> a. pulmonary alveolitis
> a. pulmonary edema (APE)
> a. pulmonary embolism
> a. radiation pneumonitis
> a. rejection (AR)
> a. renal failure
> a. respiratory acidosis
> a. respiratory distress syndrome (ARDS)
> a. respiratory failure (ARF)
> a. response
> a. retroviral syndrome
> a. rheumatic arthritis
> a. rheumatic fever (ARF)

a. right heart syndrome (ARHS)
a. severe hypotension
a. sickle cell chest syndrome
a. sickle chest syndrome (ASCS)
a. tamponade
a. thrombosis (AT)
a. ventricular assist device (AVAD)

acutely
a. decompensated congestive heart failure (AD-CHF)
a. decompensated cor pulmonale

acute-on-chronic status
Acutrim Precision Release
ACV
acute cardiovascular
assist/control ventilation
atrial carotid ventricular
ACV disease

ACVB
aortocoronary venous bypass

ACVD
acute cardiovascular disease
atherosclerotic cardiovascular disease

ACX
ACX balloon
ACX II balloon catheter

ACx
anomalous circumflex
ACx coronary artery

acyanotic heart disease
acyclovir
acylcarnitine
acyl-CoA
acyl-coenzyme A

acyl-CoA:cholesterol acyltransferase inhibitor
acyl-coenzyme A (acyl-CoA)
acyltransferase
lecithin cholesterol a. (LCAT)

AD
aerodynamic mass diameter
aerosol bolus dispersion
anodal duration
autogenic drainage

Ad
adenovirus

Ad5FGF-4 gene therapy product
ADA
adenosine deaminase
anterior descending artery
ADA deficiency

ADAC
ADAC Cirrus single-headed SPECT camera
ADAC Vertex dual-headed SPECT camera

Adagen
Adalat
A. CC
A. PA

ADAM
aerosol-derived airway morphometry

Adamkiewicz artery
Adams-DeWeese
A.-D. device
A.-D. vena caval serrated clip

Adams disease
Adams-Stokes (AS)
A.-S. attack
A.-S. disease
A.-S. syncope
A.-S. syndrome

Adante monorail catheter shaft
adaptation
microcirculatory a.

adapter
Biolase laser a.
Bodai a.
catheter a.
Harris a.
large bore Tuohy-Borst side-arm a.
Passy-Muir O2 A.
Protex swivel a.
side arm a.
Tuohy-Borst a.
Venturi jet a.

adaptive
a. current tomography (ACT)
a. support ventilation (ASV)

adaptive-rate pacemaker
ADC
anodal duration contraction
apparent diffusion coefficient
ADC imaging

AD-CHF
acutely decompensated congestive heart failure

Adcon-C resorbable liquid patch
Addison
A. disease
A. maneuver
A. plane
A. point

NOTES

adducin polymorphism
Addvent atrioventricular pacemaker
adefovir
A, D, E, J, Z point
adenine nucleotide translocator
adeno-associated
    a.-a. viral vector
    a.-a. virus (AAV)
    a.-a. virus for cystic fibrosis
adenocarcinoma
    acinar a.
    adenosquamous a.
    bronchiolar a.
    bronchioloalveolar a.
    bronchogenic a.
    mucinous a.
    papillary a.
    pneumonic-type a.
Adenocard injection
adenochondroma
adenoid
    a. cystic carcinoma
    hypertrophic a.
adenoma
    adrenal a.
    bronchial a.
adenomatoid tumor
adenomatosis
    pulmonary a.
adenopathy
    hilar a.
    mediastinal a.
    perihilar a.
    retrocrural a.
Adenoscan
    A. contrast medium
    A. infusion
adenosine
    a. airways responsiveness
    a. deaminase (ADA)
    a. deaminase deficiency
    a. diphosphate (ADP)
    a. echocardiography
    a. monophosphate (AMP)
    a. nuclear perfusion imaging
    a. nucleotide translocator (ANT)
    a. radionuclide perfusion imaging
    a. stress
    a. ^{99m}Tc sestamibi SPECT
    a. thallium test
    a. triphosphatase (ATPase)
    a. triphosphate (AT, ATP)
    a. triphosphate disodium
    a. triphosphate-sensitive potassium
    channel opener
    a. triphosphate single-photon
    emission computed tomography
    (ATP-SPECT)
adenosine-induced hyperemia

adenosine-supplemented blood
  cardioplegia
adenosquamous
    a. adenocarcinoma
    a. carcinoma
adenotonsillar hypertrophy
adenotriphosphatase
    sodium-potassium a. (NaK-ATPase)
adenoviral
    a. pneumonia
    a. type 40/41 infection
    a. vector
Adenoviridae
adenovirus (Ad)
adenovirus-based phospholamban-
  antisense expression
adenovirus-mediated gene transfer
adenylate
    a. cyclase
    a. cyclase stimulator forskolin
    a. cyclase toxin
adenylyl cyclase (AC)
adequate
    a. blood flow
    a. blood supply
    a. collateral
    a. hemostasis maintained
ADG
    atrial diastolic gallop
ADH
    antidiuretic hormone
adherence assay
adherens junction
adherent
    a. leaflet
    a. mobile thrombus
    a. mural thrombus
    a. pericardium
adhesin
adhesin-receptor interaction
adhesiolysis
adhesion
    band of a.
    chest wall a.
    fibrinous a.
    freeing up of a.
    heterotypic a.
    homotypic a.
    inflammatory a.
    pleural a.
adhesive
    Biobrane a.
    BioGlue protein-based surgical a.
    Histocryl Blue tissue a.
    a. inflammation
    a. pericarditis
    a. phlebitis
    a. pleurisy
adhesiveness

ad hoc procedure
adiabatic fast passage
adiastole
adiemorrhysis
adipocyte
adipose
    a. folds of pleura
    a. tissue
adiposis
    a. cardiaca
    a. universalis
adipositas cordis
adiposum
    cor a.
adjunctive
    a. balloon angioplasty
    a. measure
ADL
    activities of daily living
    ADL scale
ADMA
    asymmetric dimethylarginine
ADME
    absorption, distribution, metabolism, and
    excretion
administration
    bronchodilator a.
    closed-loop sedative a.
    sedative a.
    viability identification with
      dipyridamole-dobutamine a.
      (VIDA)
administrators
    American College of
      Cardiovascular 1.'s (ACCA)
admixture
    venous a.
ADN
    aortic depressor nerve
ADOPT-like software
ADP
    adenosine diphosphate
    area diastolic pressure
ADR
    adrenergic receptor
    ADR Ultramark 4 ultrasound
ADRA1A
    alpha 1A adrenergic receptor
ADRA1B
    beta-1B adrenergic receptor
ADRA2C
    alpha 2C adrenergic receptor

ADRAR
    alpha-2-adrenergic receptor
adrenal
    a. adenoma
    a. cortex
    a. gland
    a. hyperplasia
    a. hypertension
    a. medulla
    a. medullary implant
Adrenalin Chloride
adrenaline
adrenergic
    alpha-a.
    a. antagonist
    a. nervous system
    a. receptor (ADR, AR)
    a. receptor kinase (ARK)
    a. receptor kinase 1 (ARK-1)
    a. stimulant
adrenoceptor
    alpha a.
    beta a.
    a. blocker
adrenocorticotropic hormone (ACTH)
adrenogenital syndrome
adrenomedullary triad
adrenomedullin (AM)
    a. infusion
    a. peptide
adrenoreceptor
Adriamycin
    A. cardiotoxicity
    A., cyclophosphamide, etoposide
      (ACE)
    A. PFS
    A. RDF
Adrucil injection
Adson
    A. aneurysm needle
    A. hook
    A. maneuver
    A. retractor
    A. test
Adson-Coffey scalenotomy
adult
    a. respiratory distress syndrome
      (ARDS)
    A. Star 1010, 2000 ultra-high-
      frequency ventilator
    a. tuberculosis
adult-onset asthma

NOTES

adultorum
　　scleredema a.
Advair Diskus
advanced
　　a. cardiac life support (ACLS)
　　a. cardiac mapping
　　A. Cardiovascular Systems (ACS)
　　A. Care cholesterol test
　　a. heart failure
　　a. heart failure shared clinical
　　　experience network (AHF SCENE)
　　a. life support (ALS)
　　a. sleep phase syndrome
　　a. trauma life support (ATLS)
　　a. venous access device
advancement
　　elastic mandibular a. (EMA)
　　genioglossal a.
　　maxillomandibular a. (MMA)
**Advantx LC+ cardiovascular imaging
　system**
adventitial
　　a. bed
　　a. cell
　　a. fibroblast
　　a. layer
adventitious
　　a. breath sounds
　　a. heart sounds
　　a. membrane
adverse
　　a. event
　　a. ventricular remodeling
Advicor
Advil Cold & Sinus Caplets
AE
　air embolism
　atrial ectopic
　　AE heartbeat
**AE-60-I-2 implantable pronged unipolar
　electrode**
**AE-60-K-10 implantable unipolar
　endocardial electrode**
**AE-60-KB implantable unipolar
　endocardial electrode**
**AE-60-KS-10 implantable unipolar
　endocardial electrode**
**AE-85-I-2 implantable pronged unipolar
　electrode**
**AE-85-K-10 implantable unipolar
　endocardial electrode**
**AE-85-KB implantable unipolar
　endocardial electrode**
**AE-85-KS-10 implantable unipolar
　endocardial electrode**
AECD
　　automatic external cardioverter-
　　　defibrillator
　　Powerheart AECD

AECG
　　ambulatory electrocardiogram
AED
　　automatic external defibrillator
AEF
　　aortoenteric fistula
AEG
　　atrial electrogram
Aegis
　　A. aortic cannula
　　A. ICD system
AEI
　　atrial emptying index
AEM
　　ambulatory electrocardiographic
　　monitoring
Aequitron
　　A. pacemaker
　　A. ventilator
aequorin
AER
　　agranular endoplasmic reticulum
aerated lung
aeremia
aerendocardia
aeroallergen
Aerobacter
aerobic
　　a. capacity (VO$_2$)
　　a. exercise (AEX, AEx)
　　a. exercise stress test
　　a. metabolism
　　a. respiration
　　a. threshold
AerobiCycle
AeroBid-M
AeroBid Oral Aerosol Inhaler
AeroChamber
　　A. mask
　　A. Plus valved holding chamber
　　A. spacing device
　　A. VHC
Aerodose insulin inhaler
aerodynamic
　　a. mass diameter (AD)
　　a. size
Aerodyne stationary bicycle
AeroEclipse breath actuated nebulizer
aeroembolism
aeroemphysema
AeroGear
　　A. asthma action kit
　　A. fanny pack
aerogenes
　　Pasteurella a.
aerogenic tuberculosis
aerogenosum
　　sputum a.
aerogenous

aeroirritant
Aerolate
    A. III
    A. JR, SR
Aerolizer
    Foradil A.
Aeromonas
    A. caviae
    A. hydrophila biovar sobria
    A. sobria
    A. veronii
AeroNOx
    A. nitric oxide delivery and
      analysis system
    A. nitric oxide transport system
Aeropent
aerophagia
aerosol
    albuterol sulfate inhalation a.
    a. bolus dispersion (AD)
    Brethaire Inhalation A.
    a. challenge test
    a. cloud enhancer (ACE)
    a. deposition
    Duo-Medihaler a.
    Flovent a.
    a. inhalation monitor (AIM)
    Maxair Inhalation A.
    Nasalide Nasal A.
    a. nebulizer
    pirbuterol acetate inhalation a.
    respirable a.
    Sclerosol intrapleural a.
    steroid a.
    Tilade Inhalation A.
    Virazole A.
aerosol-derived airway morphometry
  (ADAM)
aerosolization
aerosolized
    a. antibiotic
    a. bronchodilator
    a. pentamidine
    a. pentamidine isethionate
    a. surfactant
Aerosomes drug delivery device
AeroSonic personal ultrasonic nebulizer
Aerospan
AeroTech II nebulizer
aerotherapy
aerothorax
AeroView optical intubation system

AERP
    atrial effective refractory period
aeruginosa
    Pseudomonas a.
AERx
    AERx drug delivery device
    AERx inhaler
AES
    aortic ejection sound
Aescula
    A. left ventricular lead
    A. LV lead
AET
    atrial ectopic tachycardia
AEX
    aerobic exercise
AEx
    aerobic exercise
AF
    aortic flow
    atrial fibrillation
    atrial flutter
    atrial fusion
      nonrheumatic AF
      rheumatic AF
AF0150 contrast agent
AFA
    acromegaloid facial appearance
    AFA syndrome
AFB
    aortofemoral bypass
AFBG
    aortofemoral bypass graft
AFCL
    atrial fibrillation cycle length
AFE
    amnionic fluid embolism
    amniotic fluid embolism
AfeCTA immunoassay
AFF
    atrial fibrillation-flutter
    atrial filling fraction
afferent
    a. arteriole
    a. artery
    a. impulse
    a. nerve fiber
afferentia
    vasa a.
affinity
    A. blood pump
    a. chromatography

NOTES

affinity *(continued)*
    a. maturation
    A. oxygenator
    A. pacemaker
afflux, affluxion
aFGF
    acidic fibroblast growth factor
AFib
    atrial fibrillation
AFL
    atrial flutter
AFO
    ankle-foot orthosis
AFocus steerable diagnostic catheter
AFORMED
    alternating failure of response,
      mechanical, to electrical depolarization
      AFORMED phenomenon
AFP
    alpha-fetoprotein
    doxorubicin, 5-fluorouracil, cisplatin
    AFP II pacemaker
AFR
    atrial flutter response
    AFR algorithm
African
    A. American (AA)
    A. Burkitt lymphoma
    A. cardiomyopathy
    A. endomyocardial
    A. endomyocardial fibrosis
    A. histoplasmosis
    A. sleeping sickness
    A. tick typhus
africanum
    Mycobacterium a.
Afrin Tablet
afterdepolarization
    delayed a. (DAD)
    early a. (EAD)
    late a.
    monophasic action potential
      early a. (mEAD)
afterload
    increased a.
    a. matching
    a. mismatching
    reduced a.
    a. reduction
    a. resistance
    right-ventricle a.
    ventricular a.
afterloading catheter
afterpotential
    depolarizing a. (DAP)
    diastolic a.
    oscillatory a.
    a. oversensing
    pacemaker a.

    positive a.
    a. sensing
afterspike hyperpolarization (AHP)
AFV
    aortic flow velocity
AG
    angular gyrus
Ag
    silver
Ag-AgCl$_2$ electrode bipolar catheter
agalactiae
    Streptococcus a.
agammaglobulinemia
agar
    brain-heart infusion a. (BHIA)
    brain-heart infusion blood a.
      (BHIBA)
    a. diffusion assay
agarose
    a. gel
    a. gel electrophoresis
    MetaPhor a.
Agatston score
AGE
    arterial gas embolism
age-dependent apnea
Agency for Health Care Policy and Research (AHCPR)
Agenerase
agenesis
    pulmonary a.
AGENT
    angiogenic gene therapy agent
agent
    AF0150 contrast a.
    Albunex contrast a.
    alpha-1-adrenergic blocking a.
    alpha blocking a.
    AlphaNine clotting a.
    Angimark contrast a.
    angiogenic a.
    angiogenic gene therapy a.
      (AGENT)
    Angiomark contrast a.
    antianginal a.
    antiarrhythmic a.
    anticholinergic a.
    antidiabetic a.
    antihypertensive a.
    antiinflammatory a.
    antiplatelet a.
    bacteriostatic a.
    beta-adrenergic blocking a.
    beta-adrenoreceptor blocking a.
    beta blocking a.
    blood-borne infectious a.
    bronchodilating a.
    calcium channel blocking a.
    chemoattracting a.

chemoattracting a.
chemotherapeutic a.
cholinergic a.
contrast a.
cytoprotective a.
diuretic a.
dopaminergic a.
Eaton a.
Fibrimage diagnostic imaging a.
fibrinolytic a.
FS-069 contrast a.
histocompatibility a. B27
hydrophilic a.
hypertensive a.
hypoglycemic a.
hypotensive a.
Imagent contrast a.
imaging a.
inhalation a.
inotropic a.
Levovist echocontrast a.
lipid-lowering a.
macrolide antimicrobial a.
mucoregulatory a.
neuromuscular blocking a. (NMBA)
neuroprotective a.
nonglycoside inotropic a.
nonsteroidal antiinflammatory a.
Norwalk a.
Optison contrast a.
Pittsburgh pneumonia a.
progestational a.
prothrombin time fixing a. (PTFA)
provoking a.
psychotropic a.
Quantison contrast a.
saluretic a.
sclerosing a.
sonicated contrast a.
steroid-sparing a.
thrombolytic a.
toxic a.
TWAR a.
type III antiarrhythmic a.
ultrasound contrast a. (UCA)
vagolytic a.
vasodilator a. (VA)
age-related
a.-r. apnea
a.-r. bone loss
a.-r. endothelial dysfunction
age-undetermined myocardial infarction

agger valvae venae
agglutinating antibody
agglutination
agglutinative thrombus
agglutinin
cold a.
a. febrile
Aggrastat
aggregate
intravascular a.
aggregation
platelet a.
aggregometer
Chrono-log optical a.
Chrono-log platelet a.
aggregometry
Born a.
impedance a.
Aggrenox
aggrephore
aggressive platelet blockade
aging
agitated saline solution
agitation
echocardiogram with saline a.
a. syndrome
aglycon
AGN
acute glomerulonephritis
agonal
a. clot
a. respiration
a. rhythm
a. thrombosis
a. thrombus
agonist
alpha a.
alpha-adrenoreceptor a.
beta a.
beta-adrenergic a.
beta-adrenoreceptor a.
calcium channel a.
imidazoline receptor a.
muscarinic a.
PD 123319 AT receptor a.
agony clot
agranular endoplasmic reticulum (AER)
agranulocytosis
A greater than E
agricultural anthrax
Agrobacterium
Agrylin

NOTES

A-H
> atrio-His

AH
> arterial hypertension
> artificial heart
> ataxic hemiparesis
> atrium-His bundle
>> AH bundle
>> AH conduction time
>> AH curve
>> AH interval

AHA
> American Heart Association
> antiheart antibody
>> AHA type I diet

AHA.SOC
> American Heart Association Stroke
> Outcome Classification

AHCPR
> Agency for Health Care Policy and
> Research

AHD
> acute heart disease
> arteriosclerotic heart disease
> atherosclerotic heart disease

AHES
> artificial heart energy system

AHF SCENE
> advanced heart failure shared clinical
> experience network

AH:HA ratio

AHI
> apnea-hypopnea index

AHM
> ambulatory Holter monitoring

AHMA
> antiheart muscle autoantibody

Ahn thrombectomy catheter

AHP
> afterspike hyperpolarization

AHR
> airways hyperreactivity
> airways hyperresponsiveness
> atrial heart rate

A-hydroCort Injection

3a-hydroxy-dihydroprogesterone

AI
> aortic incompetence
> apical impulse
> apnea index
> atherogenic index
> atrial insufficiency

AIA
> aspirin-induced asthma

AICA
> anterior inferior cerebellar artery
> anterior inferior communicating artery
>> AICA riboside

AICD, A-ICD
> atrial implantable cardioverter-
> defibrillator
> automatic implantable cardioverter-
> defibrillator
> automatic internal cardioverter-
> defibrillator
>> Guardian AICD
>> Ventak AICD

AICS
> acute ischemic coronary syndrome

AID
> automatic implantable defibrillator

AID-Check monitor

AIDS
> acquired immunodeficiency syndrome

AIDS-related
>> AIDS-r. lymphoma (ARL)
>> AIDS-r. lymphoma of the lung
>> (ARLL)

AIE
> acute infective endocarditis

AIH
> aortic intramural hematoma
> aortic intramural hemorrhage

AIM
> aerosol inhalation monitor

AIMO
> anterior inferior mandibular osteotomy

AIOD
> aortoiliac obstructive disease

AIP
> acute idiopathic pericarditis
> acute intermittent porphyria
> acute interstitial pneumonia
> acute interstitial pneumonitis

air
> alveolar a.
> a. bronchogram
> a. bronchogram sign
> a. cell
> a. clamp inflatable vessel occluder
> complemental a.
> complementary a.
> a. crescent sign
> a. embolism (AE)
> a. embolization
> a. embolus
> a. entry
> a. exchange
> expiratory trapping of a.
> extrapleural a.
> functional residual a.
> high-efficiency particulate a.
> (HEPA)
> a. hunger
> a. medical transportation (AMT)
> a. movement
> a. pollution

a. pulmonary embolism
reserve a.
residual a.
a. sac
a. space
supplemental a.
A. Supply wearable air purifier
tidal a.
a. trapping
a. tube
a. vesicle
vitiated a.
A. Viva
A. Wise program
airborne
a. allergen
a. transmission
air-conditioner lung
air-driven artificial heart
Aire-Cuf tracheostomy tube
Airet
airflow
a. cessation
expiratory a.
inspiratory a.
a. limitation
a. obstruction
a. velocity
air-fluid level
Airlie House criteria
Air-Lon tracheal tube brush
AirMed
A. mask
A. ventilator
air-powered nebulizer
air-puff tonometer
AirSep
A. CPAP
A. OxiScan Oximetry recording,
reporting, and archiving system
A. Ultimate nasal seal gel insert
airspace
a. consolidation
a. disease
peripheral a.
airspace-filling pattern
air-trapping
airway
a. bacterial colonization
Berman a.
a. branching
a., breathing, circulation (ABC)

a., breathing, circulation, defibrillate
(ABCD)
a. breathing, circulation, differential
diagnosis
a., breathing, circulation, disability,
exposure (ABCDE)
a., breathing, circulation,
intravenous, crystalloid (ABCIC)
a. clearance
a. closure
Combitube a.
Connell a.
a. edema
esophageal obturator a. (EOA)
esophagogastric tube a. (EGTA)
a. hypersecretion
a. hysteresis
laryngeal mask a. (LMA)
a. lumen
a. morphometry
a. mucosa
a. occlusion technique
a. pattern
a. permeability
pharyngotracheal lumen a. (PTL,
PTLA)
a. pressure disconnect (APD)
a. pressure release ventilation
(APRV)
a. protection
PtL a.
a. remodeling
a. secretion
a. stenosis
a. stenting
a. submucosa
a. tapering
airway-esophageal balloon pressure
airway-parenchymal dysanapsis
airways
anatomic a.
conducting a.
flabby a.
a. hyperreactivity (AHR)
hyperresponsive a.
a. hyperresponsiveness (AHR)
lower a.
nasal a.
a. obstruction (AO)
reactive a. disease (RAD)
a. reactivity index (ARI)
a. resistance (Raw)

NOTES

airways *(continued)*
    respiratory a.
    retropalatal a.
    a. smooth muscle (ASM)
    upper a.
    upstream a.
AirZone peak flowmeter
AIS
    Abbreviated Injury Scale
    acute ischemic stroke
    analyzer of interrated sequences
        AIS model of a beating ventricle
AITD
    autoimmune thyroid disease
AIVR
    accelerated idioventricular rhythm
Ajellomyces dermatitidis
ajmaline test
Akaike information criteria
A-K diamond knife
A-kinase
akinesia
    distal a.
    psychic a.
    septal a.
akinesic
akinesis
    inferobasilar a.
akinetic segment
AK-Mycin
Akron tilt table
Akt gene transfer
Akutsu III total artificial heart
AL
    angiographic area of lateral projection
    anterior leaflet
        AL I, II guiding catheter
Al
    aluminum
ALAD
    abnormal left axis deviation
Aladdin
    A. Infant Flow system
    A. nasal CPAP system
Aladdin^II NCPAP
ala nasi
alanine
    a. aminotransferase (ALT)
    a. exchange
alanine/valine (A/V)
ALAO
    angiographic area of left anterior oblique
    projection
alar
    a. chest
    a. flaring
A larger than V wave
alaryngeal speech
AlaSTAT latex allergy test

Alatest Latex-specific IgE allergen test kit
alatrofloxacin
alba
    pneumonia a.
albendazole sulfoxide
Albert
    A. Grass Heritage digital PSG system
    A. Grass Heritage EEG system
    A. Grass neurodata system
Albertini treatment
albicans
    Candida a.
    Monilia a.
albida
    macula a.
albidus
    Cryptococcus a.
Albini nodule
Albright syndrome
albumin
    a. cobalt binding (ACB)
    a. cobalt binding test
    macroaggregated a. (MAA)
    perfluorocarbon-exposed sonicated dextrose a. (PESDA)
    radioactive iodinated serum a. (RISA)
    a. resuscitation
    serum a.
    sonicated dextrose a.
albumin-coated vascular graft
albuminoid sputum
albuminuria
Albunex contrast agent
albuterol
    ipratropium and a.
    a. nebulizer updraft
    A. Spiros inhaler
    a. sulfate inhalation aerosol
    a. sulfate inhalation solution
    a. sulfate syrup
ALCA
    anomalous left coronary artery
Alcaligenes
    A. bookeri
    A. dentrificans
    A. faecalis
    A. odorans
    A. piechaudii
    A. xylosoxidans
ALCAPA
    anomalous origin of left coronary artery from pulmonary artery
    ALCAPA syndrome
Alcatel pacemaker
Alcian blue-PAS stain

alcohol
  a. ablation
  absolute a.
  a. abuse
  ethyl a.
  a. intoxication
  polyvinyl a. (PVA)
  a. septal reduction
alcoholic
  a. cardiomyopathy
  a. heart muscle disease
  a. malnutrition
  a. myocardiopathy
  a. pneumonia
alcoholism, leukopenia, pneumococcal sepsis (ALPS)
Alcon Closure System
Aldactazide
Aldactone
aldehyde-tanned bovine carotid artery graft
aldesleukin
Aldoclor
Aldomet
Aldoril
aldosterone
  a. antagonist
  a. depression
aldosterone-receptor blocker
aldosteronism
aldosteronoma
Aldrete needle
Aldrich ST elevation score
ALEC
  artificial lung-expanding compound
AlereNet system
Alert catheter
alertness test
aleuronoid granule
Alexander-Farabeuf periosteotome
Alexander rib stripper
alexandrite laser
alexithymia
  A. Provoked Response Interview
alexithymic personality features
alfa
  dornase a.
alfa-2a
alfa-2b
alfentanil hydrochloride

Alfieri
  A. method
  A. repair
algiovascular
alglucerase
algorithm
  AFR a.
  AMS a.
  Artrek automated edge-detection a.
  asthma care a. (ACA)
  atrial flutter response a.
  atrial tachycardic response a.
  automatic mode conversion a.
  automatic mode-switching a.
  closed loop a. (CLA)
  detection a.
  Levenberg-Marquardt a.
  lossy a.
  MAR a.
  mean atrial rate a.
  trilinear cylindric interpolation a.
algovascular
ALI
  acute lung injury
aliasing
  a. artifact
  a. flow
  image a.
Alice4
  A. RESP-EZ respiratory effort belt
  A. Sleep Diagnostic system
alignment
  a. catheter
  a. mark
alimentary habits
alimentation
  coronarography and a. (CORALI)
Alimta
A-line
  arterial line
alinidine
aliphatic amines asthma
aliquot
Alkaban-AQ
alkaline
  a. phosphatase (AP)
  a. phosphatase antialkaline phosphatase (APAAP)
alkaloid
  ergot a.
  Rauwolfia a.
alkaloidal cocaine

NOTES

alkalosis
    altitude a.
    hypochloremic metabolic a.
    metabolic a.
    respiratory a.
alkaptonuria
Alka-Seltzer Plus Flu & Body Aches Non-Drowsy Liqui-Gels
Alkeran
alkylxanthine
ALL
    acute lymphocytic leukemia
    antihypertensive and lipid lowering
all
    a. or none law
    a. track wire (ATW)
Allain method
allantoic
    a. circulation
    a. vein
Allegiance nasal prongs
Allegra
allele
    AT1 receptor C a.
    mutant a.
    prothrombin G20210A mutated a.
    S2 a.
allelic deletion
Allen
    A. and Davis classification
    A. test
Allen-Brown
    A.-B. criteria
    A.-B. shunt
Allerbiocid
Aller-Chlor Oral
Allerdryl
Allerest Maximum Strength
allergen
    airborne a.
    environmental a.
    a. exposure
    HDM a.
    house dust mite a.
    Rattus norvegicus a.
allergen-induced
    a.-i. asthma
    a.-i. mediator release
allergic
    a. alveolitis
    a. angiitis and granulomatosis
    a. asthma
    a. bronchopulmonary aspergillosis (ABPA)
    a. bronchospasm
    a. diathesis
    a. granulomatous angiitis
    a. reaction
    a. rhinitis

    a. salute
    a. shiner
    a. vasculitis
allergy
    bronchial a.
    a. purpura
    seasonal a.
AllerMax Oral
Allernix
Allerphed Syrup
allescheriosis
allethrin
allethrolone
alligator clip
Allis clamp
Allison
    A. hiatal hernia repair
    A. lung retractor
Alliston procedure
alloantibody
allogeneic transplant
allograft
    a. arteriosclerosis
    cardiac a.
    cryopreserved heart valve a.
    cryopreserved human aortic a.
    cryopreserved valved a.
    a. rejection
    a. vasculopathy
allometric
allorhythmia
allorhythmic
allosteric modification of enzyme
Allport-Babcock searcher
ALMCA
    anomalous left main coronary artery
ALMI
    anterior lateral myocardial infarct
almitrine bismesylate
almokalant
ALMV
    anterior leaflet of the mitral valve
Aloka
    A. color Doppler
    A. color Doppler system for blood flow imaging
    A. model SSD-830 2.5- and 3.5-MHz transducer
    A. ultrasound
Alond
ALP
    acute lupus pericarditis
    acute lupus pneumonitis
alpha
    a. 1A adrenergic receptor (ADRA1A)
    a.-actinin
    a.-adrenergic
    a. adrenoceptor

a. agonist
a. blocking agent
a. 2C adrenergic receptor
  (ADRA2C)
estrogen receptor a. (ER alpha)
a.-fetoprotein (AFP)
a. Gal antibody
heavy chain cardiac myosin a.
  (MYHCA)
lecithin cholesterol
  acetyltransferase a. (LCATA)
a. lipoprotein
a.-methyldopa
a.-myosin heavy chain (alpha-MHC)
a. receptor
A.-Tamoxifen
a.-tocopherol
alpha-1
a.-1 adrenoceptor blockade
a.-1 antitrypsin (AAT)
a.-1 antitrypsin deficiency
a.-1 proteinase inhibitor
alpha-2
alpha-2 macroglobulin
alpha-2-plasmin inhibitor
alpha-adrenergic
a.-a. blocker
a.-a. stimulation
alpha-1-adrenergic
a.-1-a. blocking agent
a.-1-a. receptor
alpha-2-adrenergic receptor (ADRAR)
alpha-adrenoreceptor
a.-a. agonist
a.-a. blocker
alpha-alpha homodimer
alpha-B-crystallin protein
alpha-cardiac actin
alpha-hydroxybutyrate dehydrogenase
alpha-MHC
alpha-myosin heavy chain
AlphaNine clotting agent
Alphavirus
Alport syndrome
alprazolam
alprenolol
alprostadil
ALPS
alcoholism, leukopenia, pneumococcal
  sepsis
  ALPS syndrome

ALRI
acute lower respiratory tract infection
ALS
advanced life support
amyotrophic lateral sclerosis
Alstrom syndrome
ALT
alanine aminotransferase
Altace Oral
ALTE
apparent life-threatening event
alteplase (TPA)
recombinant a.
alteration
acute preload a.
coexistent cardiac a.'s
ST a.
altered airway secretion
alternans
auditory a.
auscultatory a.
concordant a.
cycle length a.
discordant a.
electrical a.
microvolt T-wave a.
pulsus a.
QRS a.
respiratory a.
ST segment a.
systole a.
a. test
total a.
T wave a. (TWA)
U wave a.
Alternaria tenuis
alternating
a. bidirectional tachycardia
a. current (AC)
a. failure of response, mechanical,
  to electrical depolarization
  (AFORMED)
a. pulse
alternation
cardiac a.
concordant a.
cycle length a.
discordant a.
electrical a. of heart
mechanical a.

NOTES

alternative
 Cardia Salt a.
 Citrol Smoking a.
alternobaric exposure
altitude
 a. alkalosis
 a. hypoxia
Altocor
altretamine
aluminum (Al)
 a. carbide
 a. hydroxide gel
 a. lung
 a. oxygen regulator
 a. potroom asthma
Alupent
ALVAD
 abdominal left ventricular assist device
 ALVAD artificial heart
Alvarez prosthesis
alvei
 Bacillus a.
alveobronchiolitis
Alveofact
alveolar
 a. air
 a.-arterial (A-a)
 a. arterial gradient (AAG)
 a.-arterial PO_2 difference ($AaPO_2$)
 a. asthma
 a. bronchiole
 a. capillary
 a.-capillary block
 a. capillary intravascular pressure
 a.-capillary membrane
 a. carbon dioxide pressure
 a. carbon dioxide tension
 a. cell
 a. cell carcinoma
 a. dead space
 a. destruction
 a. duct emphysema
 a. ectasia
 a. edema
 a. flooding
 a. gas
 a. hyaline membrane
 a. hypertension
 a. hyperventilation
 a. hypoventilation
 a. hypoxia
 a. infiltrate
 a. leak
 a. macrophage
 a. opacification
 a. overdistention
 a. oxygen partial pressure (PAO_2)
 a. oxygen tension

 a. pattern
 a. period
 a. permeability (AP)
 a. phospholipidosis
 a. pressure (Palv)
 a. proteinosis
 a. recruitment
 a. sac
 a. ventilation
 a. ventilation/perfusion (Va/Q)
 a. ventilation per minute (V_A)
 a. volume (VA)
alveolar-air equation
alveolar-arterial (A-a)
 a.-a. oxygen gradient (A-a 02)
 a.-a. oxygen tension (A-a 02)
 a.-a. PO_2 difference ($AaPO_2$)
alveolar-atrial (A-a)
alveolar-capillary
 a.-c. block
 a.-c. membrane
alveolares
 sacculus a.
alveolar-filling pattern
alveolaris
 sacculus a.
alveolarization
alveolar-septal amyloidosis
alveoli (*pl. of* alveolus)
alveolitis
 acute pulmonary a.
 allergic a.
 cryptogenic fibrosing a. (CFA)
 desquamative a.
 diffuse sclerosing a.
 extrinsic allergic a.
 fibrosing a.
 lymphoid a.
alveoloarterial (AA)
alveolocapillary
 a. membrane
 a. partial pressure gradient
alveoloclasia
alveolus, pl. **alveoli**
 pulmonary a.
 alveoli pulmonis
 A. stent technology system
 ventilated alveoli
ALVF
 acute left ventricular failure
ALVT
 aortic and left ventricular tunnel
ALWMI
 anterolateral wall myocardial infarct
AM
 adrenomedullin
AM-50 portable air compressor

A

AMA-Fab
    antimyosin monoclonal antibody with
    Fab fragment
    AMA-Fab scintigraphy
amalonatica
    Citrobacter a.
amantadine hydrochloride
Amapari virus
amaurosis partialis fugax
amaurotic
amazon thorax
Amazr catheter
Amba
ambasilide
Ambenyl Cough Syrup
Amberlite particles
AMBI
    acute multiple brain infarcts
Ambien
ambient pressure
ambiguus
    situs a.
    visceroatrial situs a.
AmBisome
Amblyomma americanum
Ambrose
    A. classification
    A. plaque type
ambroxol
Ambu
    A. bag
    A. CardioPump
    A. Spur disposable resuscitator
ambulance
    basic life support a.
ambulatory
    a. blood pressure (ABP)
    a. blood pressure monitoring
        (ABPM)
    a. blood pressure monitoring and
        treatment of hypertension (APTH)
    a. electrocardiogram (AECG)
    a. electrocardiographic monitoring
        (AEM)
    a. electrocardiography
    a. Holter monitor
    a. Holter monitoring (AHM)
    a. monitoring
    a. nuclear detector
    a. O_2
    a. oximetry monitoring (AOM)

    a. venous pressure (AVP)
    a. ventricular function probe
ambuphylline
Amcath catheter
amdinocillin
A.M.E.
    Austin Medical Equipment
    A.M.E. tongue retaining device
amebiasis
    pulmonary a.
amebic
    a. pericarditis
    a. pneumonia
ameboid
    a. cell
    a. movement
ameboma
America
    Heart Failure Society of A.
        (HFSA)
Americaine
American
    African A. (AA)
    A. Association of Cardiovascular
        and Pulmonary Rehabilitation
        (AACVPR)
    A. Association for Respiratory
        Care (AARC)
    A. Association for the Surgery of
        Trauma (AAST)
    A. Cancer Society (ACS)
    A. Cardiology Technologists
        Association (ACTA)
    A. College of Cardiology (ACC)
    A. College of Cardiology/American
        Heart Association (ACC/AHA)
    A. College of Cardiology/American
        Heart Association Task Force on
        Practice guidelines
    A. College of Cardiovascular
        Administrators (ACCA)
    A. College of Chest Physicians
        (ACCP)
    A. College of Sports Medicine
        (ACSM)
    A. College of Sports Medicine
        regression equation
    A. Heart Association (AHA)
    A. Heart Association classification
    A. Heart Association guidelines

NOTES

American *(continued)*
    A. Heart Association Stroke
    Outcome Classification
    (AHA.SOC)
    A. Heart Association type I diet
    Hispanic A. (HA)
    A. Pacemaker Corporation lead
    A. Roentgen Ray Society
    A. Sleep Disorders Association
    (ASDA)
    A. Society of Electrocardiography
    (ASE)
    A. Thoracic Society classification
    of dyspnea
    A. tracheotomy tube
    A. trypanosomiasis
americanum
    Amblyomma a.
americanus
    Necator a.
Amesec
A-methaPred injection
Amgenal Cough Syrup
Amicar
Amidate
amifloxacin
AMI infant apnea monitor
amikacin sulfate
Amikin injection
amiloride
    a. hydrochloride
    a. and hydrochlorothiazide
amine
    sympathomimetic a.
amino acid (AA)
aminocaproic acid
aminoethyl ethanolamine
aminoglutethimide
aminoglycoside
aminoguanidine
5-aminolevulinic acid
aminopenicillin
aminophylline, amobarbital, and
  ephedrine
Aminorex
aminosalicylate
    phenyl a.
    potassium a.
    a. sodium
    sodium a.
aminosalicylic
    a. acid
    a. acid hypersensitivity
aminoterminal propeptide
aminotransferase
    alanine a. (ALT)
    aspartate a. (AST)
amiodarone
    desethyl a.

    a. hydrochloride
    a. pulmonary fibrosis
    a. therapy
amiodarone-induced hyperthyroidism
Amipaque contrast medium
Amiscan
Amis 2000 respiratory mass
  spectrometer
Ami-Tex LA
amitriptyline
AML
    acute myelocytic leukemia
    anterior mitral leaflet
amlodipine
    a. and benazepril
    a. besylate
AMM
    antibody to murine cardiac myosin
ammonia
    anhydrous a.
    aromatic a. spirit
    N-13 a.
    nitrogen-13 a.
ammonium chloride
ammunition
    beanbag shotgun round a.
amnesia
    global a.
    verbal a.
    visual a.
amniocentesis
amnionic fluid embolism (AFE)
amniotic
    a. fluid embolism (AFE)
    a. fluid syndrome
A-mode
    A-m. echocardiography
    A-m. echo-tracking device
Amorolfine
amorphous
    a. hydrogenated silicon carbide (a-
    SiC:H)
    a. parenchymal opacification
amount of use (AOU)
amoxapine
amoxicillin
    a. and clavulanate potassium
    a. and clavulanic acid
    a. and potassium clavulanate
Amoxil
AMP
    acid mucopolysaccharide
    adenosine monophosphate
    average mean pressure
    CAR AMP
        carotid pulse amplitude
ampere

amphetamine
- a. sulfate
- a. toxicity

amphipathic helix

Amphojel

amphoric
- a. echo
- a. murmur
- a. rale
- a. respiration
- a. voice

amphoriloquy

Amphotec

amphotericin
- a. B
- a. B cholesteryl sulfate complex
- a. B (conventional)
- a. B lipid complex (ABLC)
- a. B (liposomal)

ampicillin and sulbactam

Ampicin

Amplatz
- A. dilator
- A. gooseneck microsnare
- A. left I, II catheter
- A. right coronary catheter
- A. right I, II catheter
- A. Super Stiff guidewire
- A. tapered extra stiff wire guide
- A. tapered movable core wire
- A. technique
- A. thrombectomy device (ATD)
- A. torque wire
- A. tube guide
- A. ultra stiff wire guide
- A. ventricular septal defect device

Amplatzer duct occluder

Amplex guidewire

Amplicor
- A. assay for *Mycobacterium tuberculosis*
- A. *Mycobacterium tuberculosis* test

amplified *Mycobacterium tuberculosis* direct test (AMTDT)

amplifier
- endocardiographic a. (EA)

amplifying myocyte

amplitude
- apical interventricular septal a.
- atrial pulse a.
- carotid pulse a. (CAR AMP)
- contractile a.

C-to-E a.
D-to-E a.
- a. image
- a. linearity
pulse a.
- a. of pulse
P wave a.
R wave a.
signal a.
ventricular pulse a.
wall a.
wave a.
- a. zone time epoch coding (AZTEC)

amprenavir

amprolium hydrochloride

ampulla, pl. **ampullae**
- Bryant a.
- Thoma a.

ampullary aneurysm

amrinone lactate

AMS
- acute mitral stenosis
- automatic mode switching
  - AMS algorithm

amsacrine

AMT
- air medical transportation

AMTDT
- amplified *Mycobacterium tuberculosis* direct test

AMV
- assisted mechanical ventilation

aMVL
- anterior mitral valve leaflet

amygdala

amyl
- a. nitrite
- A. Nitrite Aspirols

amylase
- serum a.

amyloid
- a. A protein
- a. heart disease
- a. precursor protein (APP)

amyloidoma

amyloidosis
- alveolar-septal a.
- cardiac a.
- familial a.
- mediastinal a.
- nodular pulmonary a.

NOTES

amyloidosis *(continued)*
    parenchymal a.
    pleural a.
    primary systemic a.
    pseudotumoral mediastinal a.
    pulmonary a.
    senile a.
    tracheobronchial a.
amyocardia
amyotrophic
    a. chorea
    a. lateral sclerosis (ALS)
AN
    anodal
    atrionodal
    AN region
ANA
    antinuclear antibody
anabolic steroid
Anabolin
Anacin
Anaconda
    A. device
    A. device and delivery system
anacrotic
    a. limb
    a. notch
    a. pulse
anacrotism
anadicrotic pulse
anadicrotism
anadicrotus
    pulsus a.
anaerobe
anaerobic
    a. empyema
    a. metabolism
    a. Pulsator syringe
    a. respiration
    a. threshold (AT)
anaerobiosis
Anaerobiospirillum
anaerobius
    Peptostreptococcus a.
anagrelide HCl
analgesia
    epidural a.
    extrapleural catheter a.
    intrapleural catheter a.
    intravenous a.
    patient-controlled a. (PCA)
    percutaneous extrapleural a.
analgesic
    a. nephropathy
    patient-controlled a. (PCA)
analog
    human amylin a.
    a. video acquisition station

analog-to-digital conversion
analysis, pl. **analyses**
    backscatter a.
    beat-to-beat a.
    body density a.
    centerline method of wall
     motion a.
    computerized texture a.
    Core Laboratory Ultrasound A.
     (CLOUT)
    Doppler flow a.
    Doppler spectral a.
    Doppler waveform a.
    electron microprobe a.
    fast Fourier spectral a.
    forced vital capacity a. (FVCA)
    Fourier series a.
    Fourier transform a.
    frequency-domain a.
    hemodynamic a.
    hydroxyproline a.
    image a.
    immunoprecipitin a.
    longitudinal a.
    microarray a.
    myocardial ischemia dynamic a.
     (MIDA)
    neutron activation a.
    Northern hybridization a.
    phase image a.
    point-of-care a.
    power spectral a.
    pressure-volume a.
    quantitative coronary
     angiographic a.
    respiratory gas a.
    segmental wall motion a. (SWMA)
    sensitivity a.
    Southern blot a.
    spectral a.
    sputum a.
    time-domain a.
    videodensitometric myocardial
     textural a.
    wall motion a. (WMA)
    x-ray energy microprobe a.
analyzer
    ABL 555 a.
    AVL Omni blood gas a.
    AVL Opti Critical Care A.
    AVL Opti 1 portable blood gas a.
    Beckman O_2 a.
    840 blood gas a.
    1620 blood gas a.
    BVA-100 blood volume a.
    Cat-a-Kit a.
    Cobas Fara centrifugal a.
    CO Sleuth handheld carbon
     monoxide a.

DMI a.
ERA 300 dual-chamber pacing system a.
ETCO$_2$ multigas a.
Gem Premier Plus blood gas/electrolyte a.
Handi oxygen a.
IL Synthesis a.
a. of interrated sequences (AIS)
i-STAT handheld a.
Keystone PF a.
Marquette Series 8000 Holter a.
Medigraphics 2000 a.
MiniOX IA oxygen a.
MiniOX 1000 oxygen a.
nitric oxide a. (NOA)
Omni a.
Opti 1 pH/blood gas a.
Opti 1 portable blood a.
pacing system a.
PrinterNOx nitric oxide with MKII a.
PulmoTrack respiratory sound a.
pulse-height a.
Shimadzu DAR-2400 coronary arteriographic a.
Sievers model 280 nitric oxide a.
UltraSom computerized sleep a.
Anandron
anangioplasia
anangioplastic
anaphylactic
a. antibody
a. crisis
anaphylactoid
a. purpura
a. reaction
a. syndrome of pregnancy
anaphylatoxin
chemotactic a.
anaphylaxis
eosinophil chemotactic factors of a. (ECF-A)
slow-reacting substance of a. (SRS-A)
anaplastic
a. carcinoma
a. tumor
anaplerosis
anaplerotic sequence
anapnea
anapneic

anapnotherapy
Anaprox
anaritide acetate
ANAS, anast
anastomosis
anasarca
Anastaflo shunt
anastomose
anastomosis, pl. **anastomoses** (**ANAS, anast**)
aortic a.
aorticopulmonary a.
arterial a.
arteriovenous a. (AVA)
Baffe a.
Béclard a.
bidirectional cavopulmonary a. (BCA)
bidirectional superior cavopulmonary a. (BSCA)
cavoatrial a.
cavopulmonary a.
a. clamp
cobra-head a.
Cooley intrapericardial a.
Cooley modification of Waterston a.
cruciate a.
curved end-to-end a. (CEEA)
distal a.
extracardiac cavopulmonary a.
Fontan atriopulmonary a.
Glenn a.
Hoyer a.
intermesenteric arterial a.
Kugel a.
Nakayama a.
portacaval a. (PCA)
portoportal a.
portosystemic a.
Potts a.
Potts-Smith a.
precapillary a.
a. of Riolan
Sucquet a.
Sucquet-Hoyer a.
systemic to pulmonary artery a.
total cavopulmonary a.
Waterston a.
anastomotica
arteria a.
anastomotic stricture

NOTES

anastrozole
anatomic
 a. airways
 a. assessment
 a. block
 a. dead space
 a. localization
 a. pulmonary atresia
anatomical reentry
anatomy
 coronary a.
 designed after natural a.
 native coronary a.
anatricrotic
anatricrotism
Anatuss DM
ANCA
 antineutrophil cytoplasmic antibody
ANCC, AnCC
 anodal closure contraction
Ancef
anchor
 Harpoon suture a.
ancillary measure
Ancobon
ANCOR imaging system
Ancotil
ancrod
Ancure
 A. stent-graft
 A. system
Ancylostoma
 A. braziliense
 A. caninum
 A. duodenale
Andersen
 A. syndrome
 A. triad
Anderson
 A. phasing score
 A. procedure
 A. test
Anderson-Fabry disease
Anderson-Keys method
Anderson-Wilkins (AW)
 A.-W. acuteness score
Andes virus
Andral decubitus position
Andrews-Pynchon tube
Andrews retractor
Androcur Depot
Androderm Transdermal system
Android
android obesity
Androlone
Androlone-D
Andropository Injection
Androsov vascular stapler

ANDTE, AnDTe
 anodal duration tetanus
anechoic
Anectine Chloride
Anel operation
anemia
 aplastic a.
 chronic hemolytic a.
 Cooley a.
 hemolytic a.
 Mediterranean a.
 megaloblastic a.
 microangiopathic a.
 sickle cell a.
 splenic a.
anemic
 a. anoxia
 a. hypoxia
 a. murmur
anemometer
 hot-wire a.
 mass-flow a.
anergy
 skin test a.
aneroid manometer
anesthesia
 Bier block a.
 inhalational a.
 Macintosh blade a.
anesthetic
 eutectic mixture of local a.'s
  (EMLA)
 inhalational a.
aneuploid
AneuRx
 A. fully supported modular system
 A. stent
 A. stent graft system
aneurysm
 abdominal aortic a. (AAA)
 acute dissecting a.
 ampullary a.
 anterior communicating a. (ACA)
 aortic sinus a.
 aortoiliac a.
 apical a.
 arterial a.
 arteriovenous pulmonary a.
 a. of ascending aorta (AAA)
 atherosclerotic a.
 atrial septal a. (ASA)
 a. of atrial septum (AAS)
 Berard a.
 berry a.
 bilobed a.
 brain a.
 cardiac a.
 cerebral a.
 Charcot-Bouchard a.

chronic fusiform a.
cirsoid a.
congenital aortic a.
coronary a.
Crisp a.
cylindroid a.
descending thoracic a.
dissecting aortic a.
dolichoectatic a.
ectatic a.
embolic a.
embolomycotic a.
endoluminal reconstruction of
  basilar artery fusiform a.
false aortic a.
familial intracranial a.
fusiform aortic a.
giant a.
infected a.
inferobasilar a.
inflammatory abdominal aortic a.
  (IAAA)
infrarenal abdominal aortic a.
innominate a.
interatrial septal a. (IASA)
interventricular septum a.
intracranial fusiform a.
left ventricular a. (LVA)
luetic a.
mitral valve a.
mixed a.
mouth of a.
mural a.
mycotic aortic a.
Park a.
phantom a.
popliteal a.
Pott a.
racemose a.
Rasmussen a.
Richet a.
Rodriguez a.
ruptured aortic a.
ruptured sinus of Valsalva a.
  (RSVA)
saccular a.
serpentine a.
Shekelton a.
sinus of Valsalva a.
spurious a.
stent-assisted coiling of basilar
  fusiform a.

suprasellar a.
syphilitic aortic a.
thoracic aortic a. (TAA)
thoracoabdominal aortic a.
traction a.
traumatic aortic a.
true aortic a.
ventricular a. (VA)
verminous a.
wide-necked a.
windsock a.
a. wrapping
wrapping of abdominal aortic a.
aneurysmal, aneurysmatic
  a. bone cyst
  a. bruit
  a. cough
  a. dilation
  a. hematoma
  a. murmur
  a. phthisis
  a. sac
  a. thrill
aneurysmectomy
  abdominal aortic a.
  Matas a.
aneurysmography
aneurysmoplasty
aneurysmorrhaphy
AnEX
  anodal excitation
Anexsia
ANF
  atrial natriuretic factor
ANG
  angiogenin
  angiogram
  angiography
  angiotensin
AngeCool
  A. RF catheter
  A. RF catheter ablation system
Angeflex defibrillation lead
Angeion 2000 ICD generator
**AngeLase combined mapping-laser
  probe**
Angelchik antireflux prosthesis
Angell-Shiley
  A.-S. bioprosthetic valve
  A.-S. xenograft prosthetic valve
angel's trumpet
Anger scintillation camera

NOTES

Angestat hemostasis introducer
Angetear tearaway introducer
ANG I
    angiotensin I
angialgia
angiasthenia
angiectasis, angiectasia
Ang II
    angiotensin II
ANG III
    angiotensin III
angiitis
        allergic granulomatous a.
        Churg-Strauss a.
        leukocytoclastic a.
        necrotizing a.
        nonnecrotizing a.
angina
        abdominal a.
        antecedent a.
        anxiety a.
        bandlike a.
        benign croupous a.
        Bretonneau a.
        Canadian class I–IV a.
        chronic stable a.
        classic a.
        cold-induced a.
        a. cordis
        coronary spastic a.
        crescendo a.
        a. crouposa
        a. cruris
        decubitus a.
        diet and stress management in a.
          (DSMA)
        a. dyspeptica
        a. of effort
        effort a.
        ergonovine maleate provocation a.
        esophageal a.
        exercise-induced a.
        exertional a.
        false a.
        first-effort a.
        food a.
        a. gangrenosa
        Heberden a.
        hippocratic a.
        hypercyanotic a.
        hysteric a.
        a. inversa
        ischemic rest a.
        lacunar a.
        a. laryngea
        Ludwig a.
        a. membranacea
        microvascular a.
        mixed a.

        neutropenic a.
        nocturnal a.
        nonexertional a.
        a. nosocomii
        a. notha
        office a.
        pacing-induced a.
        a. pectoris (ang pect, AP)
        a. pectoris decubitus
        a. pectoris sine dolore
        a. pectoris vasomotoria
        a. phlegmonosa
        postinfarction a.
        postprandial a.
        preinfarction a. (PIA)
        Prinzmetal variant a.
        pseudomembranous a.
        rate-dependent a.
        rebound a.
        reflex a.
        rest a.
        a. rheumatica
        a. scarlatinosa
        Schultz a.
        second-wind a.
        sexual a.
        silent a.
        a. simplex
        a. sine dolore
        smoking-induced a.
        a. spuria
        stable a. (SA)
        toilet-seat a.
        a. tonsillaris
        a. trachealis
        treadmill-induced a.
        a. ulcerosa
        unstable a. (UA)
        variable threshold a.
        variant a. (VA)
        vasomotor a.
        vasospastic a. (VSA)
        vasotonic a.
        Vincent a.
        walk-through a.
        warm-up a.
        white-coat a.
anginae
        Saccharomyces a.
angina-guided therapy
anginal
        a. equivalent
        a. pain
        a. perceptual threshold
anginiform
anginoid
anginophobia
anginosa
        syncope a.

anginose, anginous
anginosus
    status a.
    Streptococcus a.
Angio
    angiogram
    angiographic
    angiography
angioarchitecture
angioblast
angiocardiogram (ACG)
angiocardiography (ACG)
    equilibrium radionuclide a. (ERNA)
    first-pass radionuclide a.
    radionuclide a.
    transseptal a.
angiocardiokinetic
angiocardiopathy
angiocarditis
angiocatheter
    large-bore a.
Angio-Conray contrast medium
Angiocor
    A. prosthetic valve
    A. rotational thrombolizer
angiodermatitis
angiodynia
angiodynography
angiodysplasia of colon
angioedema
Angioflow high-flow catheter
angiogenesis
    myocardial a.
    therapeutic a.
angiogenic
    a. agent
    a. gene therapy agent (AGENT)
    a. squamous dysplasia
angiogenin (ANG)
Angiografin
angiogram (ANG, Angio)
    aortic root a. (ARA)
    ECG-synchronized digital
      subtraction a.
    gated nuclear a.
    pulmonary a.
    venous digital a.
    wedge a.
angiograph
angiographer
angiographic (Angio)
    a. area of lateral projection (AL)

    a. area of left anterior oblique
      projection (ALAO)
    a. area of right anterior oblique
      projection (ARAO)
    a. assessment
    a. catheter
    a. contrast
    a. instrumentation
angiographically
    a. occult abnormality
    a. occult intracranial vascular
      malformation (AOIVM)
angiography (ANG, Angio)
    a. of abdominal aorta (AAA)
    aortography a.
    balloon-occlusion pulmonary a.
    biplane orthogonal a.
    cardiac a. (CA)
    carotid a.
    cerebral a.
    color power a.
    computed tomography a. (CTA)
    contrast a.
    contrast-enhanced magnetic
      resonance a. (CEMRA)
    coronary a. (CAG)
    coronary magnetic resonance a.
    CT a.
    digital a. (DA)
    digital subtraction a. (DSA)
    directional color a. (DCA)
    3DTF magnetic resonance a.
    elective a.
    electron beam a.
    equilibrium radionuclide a. (ERNA)
    first-pass radionuclide a.
    fluorescein a.
    FluoroPlus a.
    free-breathing coronary magnetic
      resonance a.
    gated blood-pool a.
    gated radionuclide a.
    general a. (GA)
    indocyanine green a.
    internal mammary artery graft a.
    intraarterial digital subtraction a.
      (IADSA, IA-DSA)
    intraoperative digital subtraction a.
      (IDISA)
    intraoperative vascular a. (IVA)
    intravenous digital subtraction a.
      (IVDSA)

NOTES

angiography *(continued)*
    left aortic a.
    left atrial a.
    left ventricular a.
    magnetic resonance a. (MRA, MSA)
    magnetic resonance coronary a. (MRCA)
    mesenteric a.
    multigated a.
    noncardiac a.
    nonselective coronary a.
    pulmonary a. (PA, PAG)
    pulmonary wedge a.
    quantitative coronary a. (QCA)
    quantitative edge-detection a.
    radionuclide a. (RNA)
    renal a.
    renovascular a.
    rest and exercise gated nuclear a.
    rest radionuclide a.
    saphenous vein bypass graft a.
    selective a.
    subtraction a.
    surveillance a.
    synchrotron-based transvenous a.
    thermal a.
    three-dimensional time-of-flight magnetic resonance a.
    time-of-flight magnetic resonance a. (TOF MRA)
    total absence of circulation on four-vessel a.
    ultrasound a.
    ventricular a.
    wedge pulmonary a.
Angioguard catheter device
angiohypertonia
angiohypotonia
angioid
Angioject syringe
AngioJet
    A. and Merk rheolytic thrombectomy system
    A. rapid thrombectomy system
    A. saline jet/vacuum device catheter
    A. thrombectomy catheter
angiokeratoma corporis diffusum
angiokinesis
Angio-Kit catheter
angioleiomyoma
angiologia
angiology
angioma
    cavernous a.
    cherry a.
    spider a.
Angiomark contrast agent

Angiomat Illumena contrast delivery system
angiomatosis
    bacillary a.
Angiomax
Angiomedics catheter
angiomyocardiac
angionecrosis
angioneurotic edema
Angiopac
angioparalysis
angiopathic neuropathy
angiopathy
    cerebral amyloid a. (CAA)
    microvascular a. (MVA)
angiopeptin-eluting stent
angioplasia
angioplasty
    ablative laser a.
    adjunctive balloon a.
    balloon catheter a. (BCA)
    balloon coarctation a.
    balloon coronary a.
    balloon dilation a. (BDA)
    balloon laser a.
    bootstrap two-vessel a.
    brachiocephalic vessel a.
    carotid patch a.
    carotid stent-supported a. (CSSA)
    complementary balloon a.
    a. complication
    coronary artery a.
    culprit lesion a.
    culprit vessel a.
    cutting balloon a. (CBA)
    direct acute myocardial infarction a. (DAMIA)
    direct coronary a.
    directional coronary a. (DCA)
    Dotter-Judkins percutaneous transluminal a.
    excimer laser-assisted a. (ELA)
    excimer laser coronary a. (ECLA, ELCA)
    facilitated a.
    failed rescue a.
    Grüntzig balloon catheter a.
    a. guiding catheter
    high-pressure adjunctive percutaneous transluminal coronary a.
    high-risk a.
    Ho:YAG laser a.
    IVUS-guided balloon a.
    Kinsey rotation atherectomy extrusion a.
    kissing balloon a.
    laser-assisted balloon a. (LABA)
    laser balloon a. (LBA)

laser thermal a.
multilesion a.
new device a. (NDA)
one-vessel a.
Osypka rotational a.
patch a.
patch-graft a.
percutaneous balloon a.
percutaneous excimer laser
  coronary a. (PELCA)
percutaneous laser a.
percutaneous transluminal a. (PTA)
percutaneous transluminal balloon a.
  (PTBA)
percutaneous transluminal
  coronary a. (PTCA)
percutaneous transluminal renal a.
  (PTRA)
peripheral excimer laser a. (PELA)
peripheral laser a. (PLA)
plain old balloon a. (POBA)
precoronary a.
primary percutaneous transluminal
  coronary a. (pPTCA)
rescue a.
salvage a. (SA)
salvage balloon a.
smooth excimer laser coronary a.
  (SELCA)
stand-alone balloon a.
supported a.
Tactilaze a.
thulium:YAG laser a.
tibioperoneal vessel a.
transluminal a. (TAP, TLA)
transluminal coronary a.
transradial coronary a.
vibrational a.
angioplasty-related vessel occlusion
angiopneumography
angiopoietin 1, 2
AngioRad
  A. Afterloader system
  A. radiation system
angiosarcoma
angioscintigraphy
angiosclerotic gangrene
angioscope
angioscopic
  a. assessment
  a. valvulotome

angioscopy
  coronary a.
  intracoronary a.
  percutaneous intracoronary a.
  percutaneous transluminal a.
    (PTAS)
Angio-Seal
  6-French A.-S.
  A.-S. hemostatic puncture closure
    device
  A.-S. vascular closure device
Angioskop-D
Angiosol
Angiostar Plus vascular imaging
  equipment
AngioStent
angiostomy
angiotensin (ANG, AT, At)
  a. I (A1, A-I, ANG I, AT I)
  a. I-converting enzyme
  a. II (A2, A-II, Ang II, AT II)
  a. III (ANG III)
  a. II receptor blockade
  a. II receptor blocker (ARB)
  a. II type 1 (AT1)
  renin a.
  a. sensitivity test (AST)
angiotensinase
angiotensin-converting
  a.-c. enzyme (ACE)
  a.-c. enzyme antisense gene
    therapy
  a.-c. enzyme DD (ACE-DD)
  a.-c. enzyme DD, ID genotype
  a.-c. enzyme deletion/insertion
    polymorphism
  a.-c. enzyme ID (ACE-ID)
  a.-c. enzyme II (ACE-II)
  a.-c. enzyme II genotype
  a.-c. enzyme inhibitor (ACEI,
    ACEi)
angiotensinogen gene
angiotomy
Angiovist
angle
  a. between QRS and T vectors
    (QRS-T)
  blunted costophrenic a.
  cardiodiaphragmatic a.
  cardiophrenic a.
  costophrenic a.
  costovertebral a. (CVA)

NOTES

angle *(continued)*
    Ebstein a.
    flip a.
    a. of insonation
    intercept a.
    Louis a.
    Ludwig a.
    nail-to-nail bed a.
    phase a.
    Pirogoff a.
    QRS-T a.
    sternoclavicular a.
    a. tipped catheter
    tracheobronchial a.
    xiphoid a.
angled
    a. balloon catheter
    a. pigtail catheter
angor
    a. animi
    a. pectoris
Ang-O-Span
ang pect
    angina pectoris
Angstrom
    A. II ICD
    A. MD ICD
    A. MD implantable single-lead cardioverter-defibrillator
angular gyrus (AG)
angulated
    a. coarctation
    a. multipurpose catheter
angulation
    caudal plane a.
    cranial a.
    RAO a.
angusta
    aorta a.
Angus technique
anhydrase
anhydride
    a. asthma
    coumaric a.
    hexahydrophthalic a. (HHPA)
    trimellitic a.
Anhydron
anhydrous ammonia
Anichkov, Anitschkow
    A. cell
    A. myocyte
animal dander
animi
    angor a.
A-N interval
anion
    a. exchange resin
    a. gap
    superoxide a.

anisa
    Legionella a.
anisindione
anisopiesis
anisorrhythmia
anisosphygmia
anisotropic
    a. conduction
    a. reentry
anisotropy
anisoylated
    a. plasminogen streptokinase activator complex (APSAC)
    a. streptokinase-plasminogen activator complex (ASPAC)
anistreplase
anitratum
    Bacterium a.
anitratus
    Acinetobacter a.
Anitschkow *(var. of* Anichkov*)*
ankle
    a. edema
    a. exercise
ankle-arm index
ankle-brachial
    a.-b. blood pressure ratio
    a.-b. index (ABI)
    a.-b. index test
ankle-foot orthosis (AFO)
ankylosing spondylitis
anlagen
annexin V
    technetium-99m-labeled a. V.
annihilation photon
annotation
    marker a.
annular *(var. of* anular*)*
annuloaortic ectasia (AAE)
AnnuloFlex flexible annuloplasty ring
AnnuloFlo
    A. annuloplasty ring
    A. annuloplasty ring system
annuloplasty
    a. band implant
    Carpentier a.
    DeVega tricuspid valve a.
    Gerbode a.
    Kay a.
    prosthetic ring a.
    a. ring
    septal a.
    tricuspid valve a.
    Wooler-type a.
annulus *(var. of* anulus*)*
ANOC, AnOC, AOC
    anodal opening contraction

ANOCL
anodal opening clonus
anodal (AN)
a. closure contraction (ANCC, AnCC)
a. closure sound (ACS)
a. closure tetanus (ACTe)
a. duration (AD)
a. duration contraction (ADC)
a. duration tetanus (ANDTE, AnDTe)
a. excitation (AnEX)
a. opening (AO)
a. opening clonus (ANOCL, AOCI)
a. opening contraction (ANOC, AnOC, AOC)
a. opening order (AOO)
a. opening picture (AOP)
a. opening sound (AOS)
a. opening tetanus (AOT, AOTe)
anode
anomalous
a. atrioventricular
a. atrioventricular excitation
a. bronchus
a. circumflex (ACx)
a. complex
a. conduction
a. first rib thoracic syndrome
a. left coronary artery (ALCA)
a. left main coronary artery (ALMCA)
a. mitral arcade
a. movement
a. origin
a. origin of left coronary artery from pulmonary artery (ALCAPA)
a. origin of left coronary artery from pulmonary artery syndrome
a. pulmonary vein
a. pulmonary venous connection (APVC)
a. pulmonary venous drainage (APVD)
a. pulmonary venous return
a. rectification
anomaly, pl. **anomalies**
atrioventricular connection a.
coloboma, heart anomaly, choanal atresia, retardation, and genital and ear anomalies (CHARGE)
congenital conotruncal a.

conotruncal a.
coronary artery a.
DiGeorge a. (DG, DGA)
Ebstein a.
Freund a.
pulmonary valve a.
pulmonary venous connection a.
pulmonary venous return a.
Shone a.
Taussig-Bing a.
Uhl a.
ventricular inflow a.
vertebral, vascular, anal, cardiac, tracheoesophageal, renal, and limb anomalies (VACTERL)
viscerobronchial cardiovascular a.
Anopheles
anorexia nervosa
anoxemia test
anoxia
anemic a.
cerebral a.
diffusion a.
myocardial a.
stagnant a.
ANP
atrial natriuretic peptide
atrial natriuretic polypeptide
ANP-A
atrial natriuretic peptide A
ANP-B
atrial natriuretic peptide B
ANP-C
atrial natriuretic peptide C
Anrep
A. effect
A. phenomenon
ANRL
antihypertensive neutral renomedullary lipid
ANS
autonomic nervous system
ansa cervicalis
ansamycin
ANT
adenosine nucleotide translocator
antacid
antag
antagonist
antagonism
accentuated a.
antagonist (antag)

NOTES

antagonist (*continued*)
    adrenergic a.
    aldosterone a.
    beta a.
    beta-1,-2 a.
    calcium a.
    calcium channel a. (CCA)
    dihydropyridine calcium a.
    endothelin a.
    glycoprotein IIb/IIIa a.
    leukotriene a.
    mediator receptor a.
    tachykinin receptor a.
    thromboxane receptor a.
    vitamin K a.
antasthmatic
antecedent
    a. angina
    plasma thromboplastin a. (PTA)
ante cibum (AC)
antecubital
    a. approach
    a. fossa
    a. space
    a. vein
Ante-Flo
    Gelweave A.-F.
antegrade
    a. aortogram
    a. aortography
    a. approach
    a. block
    a. block cycle length
    a. collateral
    a. conduction
    a. diastolic flow
    a. double balloon/double wire
      technique
    a. internodal pathway
    a. refractory period
antegrade/retrograde cardioplegia technique
antemortem
    a. clot
    a. thrombus
antepartum monitor (APM)
anterior
    a. aortic wall (AAW)
    a. approach
    a. articular surface of dens
    a. axillary line (AAL)
    a. border of lung
    carpal arch a.
    a. cerebral artery (ACA)
    a. chamber (AC, ac)
    a. choroidal artery (AChA)
    a. circulation (AC)
    a. circumflex humeral
    a. clear space

    a. communicating aneurysm (ACA)
    a. communicating artery (ACA, ACoA, AcoA)
    a. dentis
    a. descending artery (ADA)
    a. descending coronary artery
    a. descending segmental artery of right lung
    a. fibrous trigone
    a. flail chest
    glandula lingualis a.
    a. inferior cerebellar artery (AICA)
    a. inferior communicating artery (AICA)
    a. inferior mandibular osteotomy (AIMO)
    a. internodal pathway
    a. internodal tract of Bachmann
    a. junction line
    a. lateral myocardial infarct (ALMI)
    a. leaflet (AL)
    a. leaflet of the mitral valve (ALMV)
    a. margin of pulmonary artery (APA)
    a. mitral leaflet (AML)
    a. mitral leaflet extension
    a. mitral valve leaflet (aMVL)
    a. myocardial infarction
    a. oblique (AO)
    a. oblique projection
    a. papillary muscle (APM)
    a. papillary muscle of left ventricle
    a. pulmonary leaflet (APK)
    regio cruris a.
    a. rib fracture
    a. right ventricle (ARV)
    a. sandwich patch technique
    a. surface of heart
    a. table
    a. thoracic compression
    a. thoracotomy
    a. tricuspid leaflet (ATL)
    vena circumflexa humeri a.
    a. wall (AW)
    a. wall of aortic root (AWAR)
    a. wall dyskinesis
    a. wall infarction (AWI)
    a. wall myocardial infarction (AWMI)
anteriores
    venae cardiacae a.
anteriorly directed jet
anterius
    segmentum bronchopulmonale basale a.
anteroapical dyskinesis

anterobasal wall
anterograde
    a. APERP
    a. block
    a. flow
    a. transseptal technique
anteroinferior myocardial infarction
anterolateral
    a. flail chest
    a. myocardial infarction
    a. segment
    a. wall myocardial infarct
      (ALWMI)
anteromesial hypokinesis
anteroposterior
    a. dimension
    a. paddles
    a. projection
    a. thoracic compression
    a. thoracic diameter
anteroseptal
    a. myocardial infarction (ASMI)
    a. segment
anteroventral third ventricle (Av3V)
antesystole
anthopleurin-A
anthracis
    Bacillus a.
anthraconecrosis
anthracosilicosis
anthracosis
anthracotic tuberculosis
anthracycline-induced cardiomyopathy
anthracycline toxicity
anthraquinone
anthrax
    agricultural a.
    industrial a.
    inhalational a.
    a. meningitis
    a. pneumonia
    pulmonary a.
    a. septicemia
Anthron
    A. heparinized antithrombogenic
      catheter
    A. II catheter
anthropi
    Ochrobacterium a.
anthropometric evaluation
antiadhesion
    a. antibody

    a. clone
    22-KD$_a$ pilin a.
    a. molecule
antiadrenergic
antiaggregant therapy
antialdosterone therapy
antialiasing technique
antianginal
    a. agent
    a. treatment
antiapoptosis
antiarrhythmic
    a. agent
    a. challenge
    a. drug (AAD)
    a. drug classification (Ia, Ib, Ic,
      II, III, IV)
    a. medication
    a. surgery
    a. therapy
antiarteriosclerosis polysaccharide factor
  (AAPF)
antiatherogenic effect
antiatherosclerotic
antibacterial
antibasement membrane
anti-beta 1 adrenoreceptor antibody
  (ABAb)
antibiotic (ABx, ABX, abx)
    aerosolized a.
    antipseudomonal a.
    antipseudomonas a.
    azalide class of a.'s
    inhaled a.
    macrolide a.
    nonquinolone a.
    perioperative a.
    preoperative a.
    prophylactic a.
    a. sterilized aortic valve homograft
      (ASAH)
    streptogramin a.
antibody
    agglutinating a.
    alpha Gal a.
    anaphylactic a.
    antiadhesion a.
    anti-beta 1 adrenoreceptor a.
      (ABAb)
    anti-CagA serum a.
    anticardiolipin a. (ACLA, aCLa)
    anti-CD3 a.

NOTES

antibody *(continued)*
    anti-CD11a a.
    anti-CD18 a.
    anti-CD31 a.
    anti-CD146 a.
    anticentromere a. (ACA)
    antidesmin a.
    antiDNA a.
    antidystrophin a.
    antiglomerular basement
      membrane a.
    anti-GPIb a.
    antiheart a. (AHA)
    anti-IgE a.
    anti-La a.
    antimyosin a.
    antineutrophil cytoplasmic a.
      (ANCA)
    antinuclear a. (ANA)
    antiphospholipid a. (APL)
    antireceptor a.
    anti-Ro SSA a.
    anti-Sm a.
    anti-SSA/Ro a.
    anti-SSB/La a.
    B cell a.
    beta-adrenoceptor a.
    CD18 a.
    cross-reactive a.
    digitalis-specific a.
    direct fluorescent a. (DFA)
    7E3 glycoprotein IIb/IIIa platelet a.
    7E3 monoclonal Fab a.
    fibrin-specific a.
    fluorescent antimembrane a.
      (FAMA, FAMAT)
    glycolipid a.
    huN901-DM1 a.
    IDEC-Y2B8 a.
    laminin a.
    monoclonal antifibronectin a.
    monoclonal antimyosin a.
    monoclonal a. 3G4
    a. to murine cardiac myosin
      (AMM)
    myosin-specific a.
    OKT3 a.
    panel of reactive a.'s (PRA)
    panel-reactive a. (PRA)
    perinuclear antineutrophil
      cytoplasmic a. (pANCA)
    platelet a.
    Rh a.
    sheep antidigoxin Fab a.
    streptococcal a.
    streptokinase a.
    teichoic acid a.
    thyroid a.
    tissue-specific a.
    treponemal a.
    TR-R9 antithrombin receptor
      polyclonal a.

antibradycardia
anti-CagA serum antibody
anticardiac myosin (ACM)
anticardiolipin antibody (ACLA, aCLa)
anti-CD11a antibody
anti-CD146 antibody
anti-CD18 antibody
anti-CD31 antibody
anti-CD3 antibody
anticentromere antibody (ACA)
anticholinergic
    a. agent
    a. bronchodilator
anticipated systole
anticlot therapy
anticoagulant (AC)
    circulating a. (CAC, CACh)
    lupus a.
    a. therapy (ACT)
anticoagulant-related hemorrhage
anticoagulation
    duration of a. (DURAC)
    a. regimen of aspirin
anticoagulation regimen of aspirin
antideoxyribonuclease B
antidepressant
    tricyclic a.
antidesmin antibody
antidiabetic agent
antidiuresis
    syndrome of inappropriate a.
      (SIAD)
antidiuretic hormone (ADH)
antiDNA antibody
anti-DNase B
antidromic
    a. circus movement tachycardia
    a. conduction
    a. reciprocating tachycardia
antidysrhythmic
antidystrophin antibody
antielastase
antiendotoxin therapy
antiestrogen
antifactor Xa activity
antifibrillatory
antifibrin antibody imaging
antifibrosis
antifilarial
antifoaming inhalant
antifolate
    multitargeted a.
antifungal
antigen
    Australia a.
    avian a.

a. binding
a. binding diversity
bovine serum a.
CagA a.
carcinoembryonic a. (CEA)
cephalin cholesterol a. (CCA)
circulating anodic a. (CAA)
Epstein-Barr nuclear a. (EBNA)
factor VII a. (FVIIag)
heart shock protein a.
HSP a.
human leukocyte a. (HLA)
inhalant a.
KI a.
O a.
p24 a.
PLA-I platelet a.
platelet a. (PlA)
proliferating cell nuclear a.
  (PCNA)
recall a.
serum cryptococcal a. (sCRAG)
TF a.
Thomsen-Friedenreich a.
viral capsid a. (VCA)
viral-free a. (VAF)
antigenicity
antiglomerular
a. basement membrane antibody
a. basement membrane disease
anti-GPIb antibody
antigravity suit
anti-G suit
antiheart
a. antibody (AHA)
a. antibody titer
a. muscle autoantibody (AHMA)
antihemophilic
a. factor (human)
a. factor (recombinant)
Antihist-1
antihistamine
antihypertensive
a. agent
a. diuretic therapy
a. and lipid lowering (ALL)
a. neutral renomedullary lipid
  (ANRL)
antihypotensive
anti-IgE antibody
antiinflammatory agent
antiinhibitor coagulant complex

antiischemic therapy
anti-La antibody
antileukotriene
antilymphocyte serum
antimalarial
primaquine phosphate a.
antimicrobial
a. catheter cuff
macrolide a.
a. therapy
**antimicrobial-resistant hospital-acquired
  pneumonia**
Antiminth
antimitotic
antimony
a. compound
a. pentachloride
a. pneumoconiosis
a. toxicity
a. trichloride
antimuscarinic
antimycobacterial chemotherapy
antimycotic
antimyosin
a. antibody
a. antibody imaging
a. autoantibody
a. Fab fragment
a. infarct-avid scintigraphy
a. monoclonal antibody with Fab
  fragment (AMA-Fab)
antinatriuretic
**antineutrophil cytoplasmic antibody
  (ANCA)**
antinuclear antibody (ANA)
antioncogene
antioxidant
antioxidative
antiparasitic
antiphospholipid
a. antibody (APL)
a. syndrome
antiphosphotyrosine immunoblot
antiplasmin
antiplatelet
a. agent
a. therapy
A. Trialists' Collaboration (ATC)
antipneumococcal
antipodal
antipode
antiport

NOTES

antiporter
antipressor
antiprotease
antiproteinase
antipseudomonal antibiotic
antipseudomonas antibiotic
antireceptor antibody
antireflux
    a. prosthesis
    a. therapy
antirestenotic stent
antiretroviral
anti-Rho(D) titer
anti-Ro SSA antibody
antisense oligodeoxynucleotide
antishock garment
antisialagogue
anti-Sm antibody
antisnoring
anti-SSA/Ro antibody
anti-SSB/La antibody
antistasin
antistreptokinase
antistreptolysin O (ASO)
antistreptozyme test
antitachycardia
    a. pacemaker (ATP)
    a. pacing (ATP)
antitemplate
antithrombin (AT, At)
    a. III (AT-III, AT III)
    a. III deficiency
    recombinant human a. III (rhATIII)
antithromboplastin
antithrombotic regimen
antithymocyte globulin
antitopoisomerase, antitopo
    a. I, II
    a. I, II antibody
antitoxin
    diphtheria a.
antitrypsin
    alpha-1 a. (AAT)
    a. deficiency
    M-type alpha-1 a.
    plasma alpha-1 a. (pAAT)
    recombinant alpha-1 a. (rAAT)
antituberculin
antituberculous
    a. chemotherapy
    a. drug
    a. therapy
antitubulin
antitussive
anti-VEGF
antler sign
antra (*pl. of* antrum)
antrectomy

Antrin
antrum, pl. **antra**
    cardiac a.
Anturane
Antyllus method
anular, annular
    a. abscess
    a. array transducer
    a. calcification
    a. cartilage
    a. constriction
    a. dehiscence
    a. dilation
    a. flow
    a. ligament of trachea
    a. phased array system (APAS)
    a. thrombus
anuloaortic ectasia (AAE)
anulus, annulus, pl. **anuli**
    aortic a.
    aortic valve a. (AVA)
    a. fibrosus
    a. fibrosus dexter/sinister cordis
    mitral valve a.
    a. ovalis
    tricuspid valve a.
anxiety
    a. angina
    a. attack
    a. neurosis
anxiolytic
any-plane echocardiography
AO
    abdominal aorta
    airways obstruction
    anodal opening
    anterior oblique
    aorta
    aortic opening
    atrioventricular valve opening
Ao
    aorta
AOA
    ascending aorta
AoArE
    aortic arch epinephrine
AoBP
    aortic blood pressure
AOC (*var. of* ANOC)
    anodal opening contraction
AOCI
    anodal opening clonus
AOD
    arterial occlusive disease
    arterial oxygen desaturation
    arteriosclerotic occlusive disease
AoE
    aortic epinephrine

AOIVM
 angiographically occult intracranial
  vascular malformation
AOM
 ambulatory oximetry monitoring
AOMP, AoMP
 aortic mean pressure
AOO
 anodal opening order
 atrial asynchronous
  AOO pacemaker
  AOO pacing
AOP
 anodal opening picture
 aortic pressure
AoP
 aortic pressure
AOPW, AoPW
 aortic posterior wall
aorta, pl. **aortae (AO, Ao)**
 abdominal a. (AA, AO)
 a. abdominalis
 angiography of abdominal a.
  (AAA)
 a. angusta
 arch of a.
 arcus aortae
 a. ascendens
 ascending a. (AA, AAO, ACS Ao,
  AOA, ASCAo)
 bifurcation of a.
 buckled a.
 buckling of a.
 bulb of a.
 button of a.
 a. chlorotica
 coarctation of a. (C of A, CA,
  CoA)
 cross-clamping of a.
 cystic medial necrosis of
  ascending a. (CMN-AA)
 a. descendens
 descending a. (DA, DAo, Desc Ao)
 descending thoracic a. (DTA)
 dextropositioned a.
 dissecting a.
 dissection of a.
 double-barreled a.
 dynamic a.
 Erdheim cystic medial necrosis
  of a.
 esophageal branch of thoracic a.

 kinked a.
 medionecrosis aortae
 medionecrosis of a.
 overriding a.
 porcelain a.
 primitive a.
 pseudocoarctation of a.
 a. to pulmonary artery shunt
 recoarctation of a.
 retroesophageal a.
 sacrococcygeal a.
 straddling a.
 terminal a.
 a. thoracalis
 thoracic a. (ThA)
 a. thoracica
 transposition of a. (TA)
 tuberculous mycotic aneurysm of a.
 valvula coronaria dextra valvae
  aortae
aortal
aorta-left atrium ratio
aortalgia
aortarctia
aortectasis, aortectasia
aortectomy
aortic
 a. anastomosis
 a. aneurysmal disease
 a. aneurysm clamp
 a. anulus
 a. arch (AA)
 a. arch arteriogram
 a. arch atheroma
 a. arch cannula
 a. arch epinephrine (AoArE)
 a. arch flush (AAF)
 a. arch interruption
 a. arch syndrome (AAS)
 a. arch vessel
 a. arch vessel obstruction
 a. area of auscultation
 a. arteritis syndrome
 a. assist balloon introducer
 a. atherosclerosis
 a. atresia
 a. bifurcation
 a. bioprosthetic valve
 a. blood flow (ABF)
 a. blood pressure (AoBP)
 a. body
 a. bulb

NOTES

45

aortic *(continued)*
a. catheter
a. closure (AC)
a. closure sound
a. coarctation
a. commissure
a. compliance (AC)
A. Connector system
a. counterpulsation
a. cross-clamp
a. cuff
a. cusp
a. cusp separation
a. depressor nerve (ADN)
a. dicrotic notch pressure
a. dissection (type A, B)
a. distensibility
a. ductal flow
a. dwarfism
a. ejection sound (AES)
a. embolism
a. endograft
a. end pulmonic
a. envelope
a. epinephrine (AoE)
a. facies
a. first sound (A1)
a. flow (AF)
a. flow velocity (AFV)
a. hiatus
a. homograft
a. impedance
a. incompetence (AI)
a. injury
a. intramural hematoma (AIH)
a. intramural hemorrhage (AIH)
a. isthmus
a. jet velocity
a. knob
a. knuckle
left atrial to a. (La:A)
a. and left ventricular tunnel (ALVT)
a. lumen
a. mean pressure (AOMP, AoMP)
a. nerve
a. nipple
a. notch
a. obscuration
a. opening (AO)
a. orifice
a. override
a. perfusion cannula
a. posterior wall (AOPW, AoPW)
a. pressure (AOP, AoP, AP)
a. pressure gradient
a. prosthesis
a. pullback
a. pullback pressure

a. pulse-wave velocity
a. reconstruction
a. reflex
a. regurgitation (AR)
a. regurgitation murmur
a. ring
a. root
a. root abscess
a. root angiogram (ARA)
a. root compression
a. root dimension
a. root ratio
a. root replacement (ARR)
a. rupture
a. sac
a. sclerosis
a. second sound opening snap (A2-OS)
a. second sound, pulmonary second sound (A2P2)
a. septal defect
a. sinus
a. sinus aneurysm
a. sound (AS)
a. spindle
a. stenosis
a. stenosis jet
a. stenosis murmur
a. systolic pressure (ASP)
a. thrill
a. thromboembolic disease
a. thrombosis
a. triangle
a. tube graft
a. tunica adventitious breath sounds
a. tunica intima
a. tunica media
a. valve (AOV, AoV, AV)
a. valve annulus (AVA)
a. valve area (AVA)
a. valve atresia (AVA)
a. valve closure (AVC)
a. valve disease
a. valve echocardiogram (AVE)
a. valve gradient (AVG)
a. valve leaflet
a. valve opening (AVO)
a. valve orifice (AVO)
a. valve prolapse
a. valve regurgitation
a. valve replacement (AVIR, AVR)
a. valve resistance
a. valve restenosis
a. valve rongeur
a. valve stenosis (AVS)
a. valve stroke volume (AVSV)
a. valve vegetation
a. valve velocity profile
a. valvotomy

a. valvular disease (AVD)
a. valvular insufficiency
a. valvulitis
a. valvuloplasty
a. vasa vasorum
a. window
aortic-femoral-femoral
descending thoracic a.-f.-f. (DTAF-F)
aortic-left ventricular tunnel murmur
aortic-mitral combined disease murmur
aorticopulmonary
a. anastomosis
a. septal defect (APSD)
a. shunt
a. window
aorticorenal
aorticus
hiatus a.
torus a.
aortismus abdominalis
aortitis
arthritis-associated a.
Döhle-Heller a.
giant cell a.
luetic a.
nummular a.
rheumatic a.
syphilitic a.
Takayasu a.
aortoannular ectasia
aortobifemoral (ABF)
aortobiiliac bypass
aortocarotid bypass
aortocaval
a. compression syndrome
a. fistula
aortocoronary (AC)
a. bypass (A-C, ACB)
a. bypass graft (ACBG)
a. graft (ACG)
a. saphenous vein (ACSV)
a. saphenous vein bypass graft (ACSVBG)
a. snake graft
a. venous bypass (ACVB)
aortocoronary-saphenous vein bypass
aortoenteric fistula (AEF)
aortofemoral
a. arterial runoff
a. arteriography
a. artery shunt

a. bypass (AFB)
a. bypass graft (AFBG)
aortogram
antegrade a.
digital subtraction supravalvular a.
end-on a.
flush a.
translumbar a. (TLA)
a. with distal runoff
aortography
abdominal a.
a. angiography
antegrade a.
arch a.
ascending a.
atherosclerotic a.
biplane a.
caudally angled balloon occlusion a.
digital subtraction supravalvular a.
flush a.
laid-back balloon occlusion a.
mycotic a.
retrograde a.
selective a.
single-plane a.
sinus of Valsalva a.
supravalvar a.
thoracic arch a.
transbrachial a.
translumbar a.
traumatic a.
true versus false aneurysm a.
aortoiliac
a. aneurysm
a. bypass
a. bypass graft
a. obstructive disease (AIOD)
a. occlusive disease
a. thrombosis
aortoiliofemoral
a. bypass
a. circuit
a. endarterectomy
aortolith
aortomalacia
aortomonoiliac graft
aorto-ostial lesion
aortopathy
aortoplasty
subclavian flap a. (SFA)

NOTES

aortoptosia, aortoptosis
aortopulmonary (AP)
    a. collateral
    a. collateral artery (APC)
    a. fenestration
    a. septal defect (APSD)
    a. shunt
    a. window (APW)
aortorenal bypass
aortorrhaphy
aortosclerosis
aortostenosis
aortosubclavian bypass
aortosubclavian-carotid-axilloaxillary
  bypass
aortotomy
aortovelography
    transvenous a. (TAV)
AOS
  anodal opening sound
A2-OS
  aortic second sound opening snap
AOT, AOTe
  anodal opening tetanus
AOT
  acute occlusive thrombosis
  acute occlusive thrombus
AOU
  amount of use
AOV, AoV
  aortic valve
AP
  accessory pathway
  activator protein
  active pressure
  alkaline phosphatase
  alveolar permeability
  angina pectoris
  aortic pressure
  aortopulmonary
  apical pulse
  arterial pressure
  atherosclerotic plaque
  atrial pacing
  atrioventricular pathway
A2P2
  aortic second sound, pulmonary second
  sound
A&P
  auscultation and percussion
AP-1 complex
APA
  anterior margin of pulmonary artery
APAAP
  alkaline phosphatase antialkaline
  phosphatase
APACHE
  Acute Physiology, Age, Chronic Health
  Evaluation

APACHE II, III
APACHE CV Risk Predictor
APACHE score
apallic syndrome
APAP
  self-adjusting nasal continuous positive
  airway pressure
APAS
  anular phased array system
apathetic hyperthyroidism
APB
  atrial premature beat
APBF
  accessory pulmonary blood flow
APC
  aortopulmonary collateral artery
  argon plasma coagulation
  aspirin-phenacetin-caffeine
  atrial premature contraction
    blocked APC
APCC
  aspirin-phenacetin-caffeine-codeine
APCG
  apexcardiogram
Ap4CH
  apical four-chamber plane
APD
  action potential duration
  airway pressure disconnect
  atrial premature depolarization
APE
  acute pulmonary edema
A-peak velocity
ApEn
  approximate entropy
APERP
  accessory pathway effective refractory
  period
    anterograde APERP
Apert syndrome
aperture
    laryngeal a.
    transducer a.
apex, pl. apices
    a. beat (AB)
    cardiac a.
    a. cordis
    false a.
    hypertrophied a.
    a. impulse
    left ventricular a.
    a. of lung
    a. murmur
    a. pneumonia
    a. pulmonis
    right ventricular a. (RVA)
    ventricular a.
apexcardiogram (ACG, APCG)
apexcardiography (ACG)

aphasia
    ataxic a.
    expressive a.
    global a.
    nonfluent a.
    receptive a.
    Wernicke a.
aphasic
apheresis
    low-density lipoprotein a. (LDLA)
aphonic pectoriloquy
aphrophilus
    Haemophilus a.
API
  arterial pressure index
apical (A)
    a. abscess
    a. aneurysm
    a. blunting
    a. bronchopulmonary segment
    a. bronchus
    a. diverticulum
    a. five-chamber view
      echocardiogram
    a. four-chamber
    a. four-chamber plane (Ap4CH)
    a. four-chamber view
    a. four-chamber view
      echocardiogram
    a. hematoma
    a. hypertrophy
    a. hypoperfusion on thallium scan
    a. impulse (AI)
    a. infarction
    a. interventricular septal amplitude
    a. left ventricular puncture
    a. lordotic roentgenogram
    a. mid diastolic heart murmur
    a. pleural bleb
    a. pneumonia
    a. pulse (AP)
    a. scarring
    a. shelf
    a. systolic heart murmur
    a. tailoring thoracoplasty
    a. two-chamber
    a. two-chamber view
    a. two-chamber view
      echocardiogram
apicale
    segmentum bronchopulmonale a.
apicalis

apices (*pl. of* apex)
apicolysis
    extrapleural a.
    Semb a.
apicoposterior
    a. branch of left
    a. bronchopulmonary segment
apicoposterius
    segmentum bronchopulmonale a.
apiospermum
    Scedosporium a.
APIVR
    artificial pacemaker-induced ventricular
    rhythm
APK
    anterior pulmonary leaflet
APL
    antiphospholipid antibody
aplasia
    bone marrow a.
    focal media a.
    pulmonary a.
aplastic anemia
apleuria
Aplisol
Aplitest
APM
    antepartum monitor
    anterior papillary muscle
    Nicolet VersaLab APM
APM-2000 vital signs monitor
apnea
    age-dependent a.
    age-related a.
    a. and bradycardia (A&B)
    central a.
    central sleep a. (CSA)
    deglutition a.
    end-expiratory a.
    idiopathic central sleep a.
    a. index (AI)
    initial a.
    late a.
    mixed a. (MA)
    a. monitor
    a. neonatorum
    obstructive sleep a. (OSA)
    posthyperventilation a.
    sleep a.
    traumatic a.
apnea-hypopnea index (AHI)
apneic oxygenation

NOTES

apneumatosis
apneumia
apneusis
apneustic
    a. breathing
    a. respiration
APO, Apo, apo
    apolipoprotein
ApoA, apoA
    apolipoprotein A
Apo-Amoxi
Apo-Ampi
Apo-ASA
Apo-Atenol
APOB, apoB
    apolipoprotein B
APOC, apoC
    apolipoprotein C
Apo-Capto
Apo-Cephalex
Apo-Chlorpromazine
Apo-Chlorthalidone
Apo-Clonidine
Apo-Cloxi
APOD, apoD
    apolipoprotein D
Apo-Diltiaz
Apo-Dipyridamole FC
apoE, APOE
    apolipoprotein E
      apoE test
Apo E3 isoform
Apo-Enalapril
Apo-Erythro E-C
Apo-Furosemide
Apo-Gain
Apogee CX 100 Interspec ultrasound machine
Apo-Guanethidine
Apo-Hydralazine
Apo-Hydro
Apo-Hydroxyzine
Apo-ISDN
APOJ, apoJ
    apolipoprotein J
apolipoprotein (APO, Apo, apo)
    a. A (ApoA, apoA)
    a. A1 deficiency
    a. AI
    a. AII
    a. AIV
    a. B (APOB, apoB)
    a. B48
    a. B100
    a. C (APOC, apoC)
    a. CI-CIII
    a. D (APOD, apoD)
    a. E (apoE, APOE)

    a. J (APOJ, apoJ)
    a. regulatory protein (APR)
Apollo Light Systems
Apo-Methyldopa
Apo-Metoprolol
Apo-Nadol
aponeurosis
    Sibson a.
aponeurotic
Apo-Nifed
Apo-Pen VK
Apo-Pindol
apoplectic
    a. coma
    a. cyst
apoplexy
    asthenic a.
    capillary a.
    cerebral a.
    ingravescent a.
Apo-Prazo
Apo-Prednisone
Apo-Procainamide
Apo-Propranolol
apoptosis
    cardiomyocyte a.
    ischemia/reperfusion-induced a.
apoptotic
    a. cell
    a. cell death
    a. change
    a. destruction
    a. nucleus
A-Port vascular access
Apo-Salvent
aposthematosa
    pneumonia a.
Apo-Sulfatrim
Apo-Tamox
Apo-Timol
Apo-Timop
Apo-Triazide
Apo-Verap
Apo-Zidovudine
APP
    amyloid precursor protein
apparatus
    Benedict-Roth a.
    Fell-O'Dwyer a.
    Jacquet a.
    Langendorff a.
    Nakayama anastomosis a.
    a. respiratorius
    respiratory a.
    subvalvular a.
    V-Vac suction a.
apparent
    a. diffusion coefficient (ADC)

a. diffusion coefficient imaging
a. life-threatening event (ALTE)
appearance
acromegaloid facial a. (AFA)
cluster-of-grapes a.
cottage-loaf a.
dirty-lung a.
finger-in-glove a.
ground-glass a.
hazy a.
salt and pepper a.
tree-in-winter a.
appendage
atrial a.
auricular a.
left atrial a. (LAA)
right atrial a. (RAA)
appendectomy
atrial a.
auricular a.
applanation tonometry
apple picker's disease
applesauce sign
appliance
EMA a.
mandibular advancement a. (MAA)
oral a. (OA)
OSAP a.
SNOAR a.
Snore-Ezzer oral a.
Snorex oral a.
TheraSnore oral a.
application
MCAS modular clip a.
applicator
RapidMist metered dose spray a.
apposition
mitral-septal a.
stent a.
approach
antecubital a.
antegrade a.
anterior a.
Bobath physiotherapy a.
brachial artery a.
central a.
cephalic a.
external jugular a.
femoral a.
groin a.
Lortat-Jacob a.
MIDCAB saloon door a.

open lung a.
percutaneous a.
posterior a.
radial a.
retrograde femoral a.
saloon door parasternal a.
segmented K-space a.
selective transvenous a.
stepped bur a.
tandem needle a.
transradial a.
transxiphoid a.
trap-door a.
approximate entropy (ApEn)
approximation
Friedewald a.
approximator
rib a.
APR
apolipoprotein regulatory protein
apraxia
buccolingual a.
ideational a.
ideomotor a.
limb-kinetic a.
Apresazide
Apresoline
A. injection
A. Oral
aprindine
Aprinox
Aprodine
A. Syrup
A. Tablet
A. w/C
aprotinin
APRV
airway pressure release ventilation
APSAC
anisoylated plasminogen streptokinase
activator complex
APSD
aorticopulmonary septal defect
aortopulmonary septal defect
APSP
assisted peak systolic pressure
APT
APT program
APTH
ambulatory blood pressure monitoring
and treatment of hypertension

NOTES

aptiganel
APTT, aPTT
  activated partial thromboplastin time
Apt test
APV
  average peak velocity
APVC
  anomalous pulmonary venous connection
APVD
  anomalous pulmonary venous drainage
APW
  aortopulmonary window
AQ
  acoustic quantification
    Nasacort AQ
AQLQ
  Asthma Quality of Life Questionnaire
aqua
    Rhinocort A.
Aquacare topical
aquae
aquagenic urticaria
AquaMEPHYTON injection
Aquaphyllin
aquaporin
Aqua-Seal chest drainage unit
AquaShield
Aquatensen
Aquatherm radiant heat device
Aquazide
aqueous
  a. oxygen
  a. solution for nebulization
  a. vasopressin (AVP)
AR
  acute rejection
  adrenergic receptor
  aortic regurgitation
  atrial rate
  atrial reversal
    beta-1 AR
    beta-2 AR
    AR jet height
βAR
  beta-adrenergic receptor
AR-1 catheter
ARA
  aortic root angiogram
arachidic bronchitis
arachidonate metabolism
arachidonic
  a. acid
  a. acid cascade
  a. acid metabolite
arachidonyl ethanolamide
arachnodactyly
arachnophlebectomy
  a. needle

  a. procedure
  a. surgical device
ARAD
  abnormal right axis deviation
Araki-Sako technique
Aralen Phosphate
Aramine
araneus
    nevus a.
arantii
    ductus a.
Arantius
  A. body
  body of A.
  canal of A.
  A. nodule
ARAO
  angiographic area of right anterior
  oblique projection
ARB
  angiotensin II receptor blocker
arborization block
arbovirus
arbutamine
arc
  a. of calcium
  a. welder's pneumoconiosis
arcade
  anomalous mitral a.
  arterial a.
  a. collateral
  polygonal a.
  septal a.
arcanobacterial pharyngitis
arch
  abdominothoracic a.
  a. of aorta
  aortic a. (AA)
  a. aortography
  a. arteriography
  axillary a.
  azygos a.
  carotid a.
  cervical aortic a.
  circumflex aortic a.
  congenital interrupted aortic a.
  double aortic a.
  interrupted aortic a. (IAA)
  jugular venous a.
  Langer axillary a.
  palmar a.
  pharyngeal a.
  pulmonary a.
  right aortic a.
  transverse aortic a. (TAA)
  Zimmermann a.
architecture
  lung a.
  sleep a.

arcus
   a. aortae
   corneal a.
   a. cornealis
   a. costarum
   a. lipoides
   a. senilis
ardeparin sodium
ARDS
   acute respiratory distress syndrome
   adult respiratory distress syndrome
   posttraumatic ARDS
Arduan
Ardystil syndrome
area, pl. **areae, areas**
   aortic valve a. (AVA)
   Bamberger a.
   body surface a. (BSA)
   Brodmann a. 7, 9, 24, 40
   a. of cardiac dullness (ACD)
   cross-sectional a. (CSA)
   a. diastolic pressure (ADP)
   echo-spared a.
   EEL a.
   effective balloon-dilated a. (EBDA)
   end-diastolic a. (EDA)
   endocardial surface a. (ESA)
   Erb a.
   external elastic lamina a.
   Head a.
   intrastent minimal lumen cross-
      sectional a. (ISMLCSA)
   Killian-Jamieson a.
   Krönig a.
   left atrial a. (LAA)
   left atrial appendage a.
   left ventricular end-diastolic a.
      (LVEDA)
   local organ procurement a.
   mitral annular a.
   mitral valve a. (MVA)
   mitral valve orifice a. (MVOA)
   noncontractile a. (NCA)
   plaque a.
   precoronary care a. (PCA)
   proximal isovelocity surface a.
      (PISA)
   pulmonary valve a.
   pulmonic a.
   regurgitant jet a.
   regurgitant orifice a. (ROA)
   secondary aortic a.

   sewing ring a. (SRA)
   a. of stenosis (AS)
   subxiphoid a.
   supplemental motor a. (SMA)
   a. systolic pressure (ASP)
   tricuspid valve a.
   truncoconal a.
   valve orifice a.
area-length
   a.-l. method
   a.-l. method for ejection
areflexia
   flaccid a.
Arelix
Arenaviridae virus
ARF
   acute respiratory failure
   acute rheumatic fever
ArF excimer laser
argatroban
Argesic-SA
arginine
   a. tolerance test (ATT)
   a. vasopressin (ARVP, AVP)
   a. vasotocin (AVT)
argipressin
argon
   a. beam coagulator
   a. ion laser
   a. needle
   a. plasma coagulation (APC)
   a. pumped tuneable dye laser
Argyle
   A. catheter
   A. CPAP nasal cannula
Argyle-Turkel
   A.-T. safety thoracentesis system
   A.-T. thoracentesis
Argyll Robertson pupils
ARHS
   acute right heart syndrome
ARI
   airways reactivity index
Aria
   A. coronary artery bypass graft
   A. LX CPAP system
Arimidex
A-ring
   esophageal A-r.
Aristocort
   A. Forte
   A. Forte Injection

NOTES

Aristocort *(continued)*
    A. Intralesional Injection
    A. Intralesional Suspension
    A. Oral
    A. Tablet
Aristospan
    A. Intraarticular Injection
    A. Intralesional Injection
Arixtra subcutaneous injection
ARK
    adrenergic receptor kinase
      beta ARK
ARK-1
    adrenergic receptor kinase 1
      beta ARK-1
Arkin-Z
ARL
    AIDS-related lymphoma
ARLL
    AIDS-related lymphoma of the lung
Arloing-Courmont test
arm
    blood pressure, left a. (BPLA)
    blood pressure, right a. (BPRA)
    chest and left a. (CL)
    chest and right a. (CR)
    a. cranking
    a. cycle ergometry
    a. ergometry treadmill
    a. exercise stress test
    left a. (VL)
    right a. (VR)
Arm-a-Med
    A.-a-M. endotracheal tube
    A.-a-M. Isoetharine
    A.-a-M. Metaproterenol
armamentarium
arm-ankle indices
arm-leg gradient
armored heart
armor heart
Armour Thyroid
ARMS
    access by radial artery multilink stent
Armstrong handheld pulse oximeter
arm-tongue
    a.-t. time
    a.-t. time test
aromatic
    A. Ammonia Aspirols
    a. ammonia spirit
arousal
    a. index
    respiratory effort-related a.
ARP
    absolute refractory period
ARR
    absolute risk reduction
    aortic root replacement

arr
    arrested
array
    convex linear a.
    multielement linear a.
    sock a.
    symmetrical phased a.
arrest
    a. after arrival (AAA)
    arrhythmic cardiac a. (ACA)
    asphyxial cardiac a.
    asystolic a.
    a. before arrival (ABA)
    blunt chest impact-induced
      cardiac a.
    bradyarrhythmic a.
    cardiac a. (CA)
    cardioplegic a.
    cardiopulmonary a. (CPA)
    cardiorespiratory a.
    chronic sinus a.
    circulatory a.
    cold ischemic a.
    deep hypothermia circulatory a.
      (DHCA)
    dysrhythmic cardiac a.
    heart a.
    hypothermic fibrillating a.
    intermittent sinus a.
    nonprimary cardiac a.
    out-of-hospital cardiac a. (OHCA,
      OOH/CA)
    prehospital cardiac a. (PCA)
    respiratory a.
    secondary a. (SA)
    sinoatrial a.
    sinus a. (SA)
    sudden cardiac a. (SCA)
    total circulatory a. (TCA)
    ventricular fibrillation a.
arrest-and-reversal treatment (ART)
arrested (arr)
    a. tuberculosis
Arrhigi
    point of A.
arrhythmia
    atrial a.
    atrioventricular junctional a.
    A-V nodal Wenckebach a.
    baseline a.
    burst of a.
    cardiac a. (CA)
    a. circuit
    a. circuit cryoablation
    continuous a.
    a. control device (ACD)
    cyanotic congenital heart disease a.
    exercise-induced a.
    a. focus

hypokalemia-induced a.
inducible a.
inotropic a.
juvenile a.
lethal a.
long QT a.
Lown a.
malignant a. (MA)
malignant ventricular a. (MVA)
a. mapping system
Mönckeberg a.
A. Net arrhythmia monitor
nodal a.
nonphasic sinus a.
nonsuppressible a.
paroxysmal supraventricular a.
pause-dependent a.
perpetual a.
phasic sinus a.
postperfusion a.
primary cardiac a.
reentrant ventricular a. (RVA)
reperfusion a.
respiratory a.
respiratory sinus a. (RSA)
senile a.
sinus a. (SA)
stress-related a.
suppression of a.
supraventricular a.
tachybrady a.
trigger of ventricular a. (TOVA)
vagus a.
ventricular a. (VA)
warning a.
arrhythmia-insensitive flow-sensitive alternating inversion recovery imaging
arrhythmic cardiac arrest (ACA)
arrhythmogenesis
arrhythmogenic
a. disorder
a. pulmonary vein
a. right ventricular cardiomyopathy (ARVC)
a. right ventricular disease
a. right ventricular dysplasia (ARVD)
a. site
a. substrate
a. ventricular cardiomyopathy
arrhythmogenicity
arrhythmokinesis

arrhythmology
arrival
arrest after a. (AAA)
arrest before a. (ABA)
chest pain onset to hospital a. (CPOTHA)
Arrow
A. balloon wedge catheter
A. Berman angiographic balloon
A. Flex intraaortic balloon catheter
A. Hi-flow infusion set
A. LionHeart left ventricular assist device
A. pneumothorax kit
A. Pullback atherectomy catheter
A. QuadPolar electrode catheter
A. QuadPolar pulmonary artery catheter
A. sheath
Arrow-Clarke thoracentesis device
Arrowgard
A. Blue antiseptic-coated catheter
A. Blue Line catheter
A. central venous catheter
Arrow-Howes multilumen catheter
arsenic (As)
a. poisoning
arsine gas poisoning
art, ART
arterial
artery
Artegraft natural collagen vascular graft
Artemisin
arteria, pl. **arteriae** (*See* artery)
a. anastomotica
a. anastomotica auricularis magna
a. femoris profunda (PFA)
a. genus superior lateralis
a. genus superior medialis
a. glutealis inferior
a. glutealis superior
a. laryngea
a. laryngea superior
a. lingualis
a. pericardiacophrenica
a. pharyngea
a. pulmonalis
a. pulmonalis dextra
a. pulmonalis sinistra
arterial (a, art, ART)
a. anastomosis

NOTES

arterial *(continued)*
a. aneurysm
a. arcade
a. baroreflex (ABR)
a. bleeding
a. blood (a)
a. blood flow
a. blood gas (ABG)
a. blood gas point-of-care test (ABG PCT)
a. blood pressure (ABP, aBP)
a. calcification
a. carbon dioxide pressure
a. carbon dioxide tension (PaCO$_2$)
a. cone
a. coupling
a. cutdown
a. decortication
a. desaturation
a. dicrotic notch pressure
a. dissection
a. distensibility
a. embolectomy catheter
a. embolism
a. entry site
a. filter
a. gas bubble
a. gas embolism (AGE)
a. groove
a. hyperemia
a. hypertension (AH)
a. hypotension
a. hypoxemia
a. impedance
a. insufficiency
a. line (A-line)
a. line transducer
a. mean
a. mean line
mean pulmonary a. (MPA)
a. media
a. mesocardium
a. murmur
a. needle
a. occlusion
a. occlusive disease (AOD)
a. oxygen content (CAO2)
a. oxygen desaturation (AOD)
a. oxygen partial pressure (PaO$_2$)
a. oxygen saturation (SaO$_2$)
a. oxygen tension (PaO$_2$)
a. partial pressure of CO$_2$ (PaCO$_2$)
a. pressure (AP)
a. pressure of arterial fluid (P$_A$)
a. pressure index (API)
a. pseudoaneurysm
pulmonary a. (PA, Pa)
a. pulse
a. pyemia

a. reconstruction
a. remodeling
a. runoff
a. saturation
a. sclerosis
a. sheath
a. shrinkage
a. spasm
a. spider
a. stick
a. switch operation
a. switch procedure
a. tension (TA)
a. thrill
a. thrombosis
a. vein of Soemmerring
a. wave
a. wedge
arterialization
arterialized capillary blood (ACB)
arteriectasis, arteriectasia
arteries (*pl. of* artery) **(AA, aa)**
arterioatony
arteriocapillary sclerosis
arteriogenesis
arteriogram
aortic arch a.
brachial a.
runoff a.
arteriograph
arteriographic regression
arteriography
aortofemoral a.
arch a.
biplane pelvic a.
biplane quantitative coronary a.
bronchial a.
carotid a.
catheter a.
coronary a. (CAG)
cut-film a.
digital subtraction a.
femoral a.
Judkins selective coronary a.
longitudinal a.
quantitative a.
quantitative coronary a. (QCA)
renal a.
selective a.
Sones selective coronary a.
ultrasonic a. (UA)
arteriohepatic dysplasia syndrome
arteriolar
a. hyalinosis
a. sclerosis
arteriole
afferent a.
efferent a.
ellipsoid a.

Isaacs-Ludwig a.
precapillary a.
arteriolith
arteriolitis
necrotizing a.
arteriolonecrosis
arteriolosclerosis
arteriolovenular bridge
arteriomalacia
arteriometer
arterionecrosis
hyaline a.
arteriopalmus
arteriopathy
hypertensive a.
plexogenic pulmonary a.
arterioplasty
pulmonary a.
arteriopressor
arteriopulmonary shunt
arteriorrhexis
arteriosclerosis (AS, ATS) (*See also*
atherosclerosis)
allograft a.
cerebral a.
coronary a.
decrudescent a.
generalized a. (GAS)
hyaline a.
hypertensive a.
Mönckeberg a.
nodose a.
nodular a.
nonatheromatous a.
a. obliterans
peripheral a.
senile a.
arteriosclerotic (*See also* atherosclerotic)
a. cardiovascular disease (ASCVD)
a. heart disease (AHD, ASHD)
a. occlusive disease (AOD)
a. peripheral vascular disease
(ASPVD)
a. vascular disease (ASVD)
arteriospasm
arteriosum
cor a.
ligamentum a.
arteriosus
conus a.
ductus a. (DA)
papillary muscle of conus a.

patent ductus a. (PDA)
persistent ductus a.
persistent truncus a. (PTA)
pseudotruncus a.
reversed ductus a.
truncus a. (TA)
arteriotomy
brachial a.
arteriotony
arteriovenosa
arteriovenous (A-V, AV, A/V)
a. anastomosis (AVA)
a. communication (AVC)
congenital pulmonary a.
a. crossing change
a. fistula (AVF)
a. malformation (AVM)
a. nicking
a. oxygen difference (AVD O$_2$)
a. passage time (AVP)
a. pulmonary aneurysm
a. shunt (AVS)
arteritis, pl. **arteritides**
brachiocephalic a.
coronary a.
cranial a.
a. deformans
fibrinoid a.
giant cell a.
granulomatous a.
Horton a. (HA)
a. hyperplastica
infantile a.
mesenteric a.
a. nodosa
a. obliterans
pulmonary arteritides
rheumatic a.
rheumatoid a.
syphilitic a.
Takayasu a.
temporal a.
tuberculous a.
a. umbilicalis
a. verrucosa
artery, pl. **arteries (a, art, ART)**
aberrant subclavian a.
abnormal coronary a. (ACA)
accessory obturator a.
acetabular a.
ACx coronary a.
Adamkiewicz a.

NOTES

57

artery *(continued)*
    afferent a.
    anomalous left coronary a. (ALCA)
    anomalous left main coronary a.
      (ALMCA)
    anomalous origin of left coronary
      artery from pulmonary a.
      (ALCAPA)
    anterior cerebral a. (ACA)
    anterior choroidal a. (AChA)
    anterior communicating a. (ACA,
      ACoA, AcoA)
    anterior descending a. (ADA)
    anterior descending coronary a.
    anterior inferior cerebellar a.
      (AICA)
    anterior inferior communicating a.
      (AICA)
    anterior margin of pulmonary a.
      (APA)
    aortopulmonary collateral a. (APC)
    ascending ileocolic a.
    ascending pharyngeal a.
    atrioventricular node a.
    A-V nodal a.
    axillary a.
    banding of pulmonary a.
    basal collateral a.
    basilar a. (BA)
    beading of arteries
    bilateral internal mammary a.
      (BIMA)
    bilateral internal thoracic a.
    blocked heart a.
    brachial a.
    brachiocephalic a.
    bronchial a.
    bronchopulmonary segmental a.
      (BPSA)
    callosomarginal a.
    caroticotympanic a.
    carotid a.
    celiac a.
    cephalic a.
    circumflex a.
    circumflex coronary a. (CCA,
      CFX)
    coarctation of pulmonary a.
    common carotid a.
    common femoral a.
    common hepatic a.
    common iliac a.
    common internal iliac a. (CIIA)
    complete transposition of great
      arteries (CTGA)
    congenitally corrected transposition
      of great arteries
    copper-wire a.
    corkscrew a.

    coronary a. (CA)
    cricothyroid a.
    crural a.
    CxCor a.
    deep lingual a.
    descending thoracic aorta-to-
      femoral a. (DTAFA)
    dextroposed transposition of great
      arteries
    diagonal coronary a.
    diaphragmatic a.
    direct stenting of coronary a.
      (DISCO)
    dorsal lingual branches of
      lingual a.
    Drummond marginal a.
    D-transposition of great arteries
      (D-TGA, dTGA)
    EC a.
    a. ectasia
    efferent a.
    end a.
    epicardial coronary a.
    esophageal branch of left gastric a.
    external carotid a. (ECA)
    external mammary a.
    femoral a. (FA)
    fetal-type posterior cerebral a.
    first obtuse marginal a. (OM-1)
    gastroepiploic a. (GEA)
    great a.
    hepatic a.
    Heubner recurrent a.
    ileal a.
    ileocolic a.
    iliac a.
    IM a.
    infarct a.
    infarct-related a. (IRA)
    inferior epigastric a. (IEA)
    inferior laryngeal a.
    inferior mesenteric a. (IMA)
    inferior temporal a. (ITA)
    inferior thyroid a.
    innominate a.
    intermediate circumflex a. (ICXA)
    internal carotid a. (ICA)
    internal mammary a. (IMA)
    internal maxillary a. (IMAX)
    internal thoracic a. (ITA)
    intersegmental a.
    intramural coronary a.
    jejunal a.
    Kugel anastomotic a.
    LAC a.
    LAD coronary a.
    LADD coronary a.
    LC a.
    LCC a.

LCF coronary a.
LCX coronary a.
left anterior descending a. (LADA)
left anterior descending coronary a.
  (LADCA)
left circumflex a. (LCA, LCX)
left circumflex coronary a. (LCX)
left common carotid a. (LCCA)
left coronary a. (LCA)
left internal mammary a. (LIMA)
left internal thoracic a. (LITA)
left main a. (LMA)
left main coronary a. (LMCA)
left pulmonary a. (LPA)
left subclavian a. (LSCA)
left vertebral a. (LVA)
lenticulostriate a.
LIC a.
LMC a.
LM coronary a.
LMS coronary a.
lumen of a.
lysed a.
main pulmonary a. (MPA)
mainstem coronary a.
major aortopulmonary collateral a.
  (MAPCA)
major coronary a. (MCA)
malposition of great arteries
  (MGA)
mammary a.
marginal branch of the
  circumflex a. (CFX-MARG)
marginal circumflex a.
medial basal branch of
  pulmonary a.
mesenteric a.
midcoronary a.
middle capsular a.
middle cerebral a. (MCA)
native coronary a.
Neubauer a.
nodal a.
nonatheromatous a.
normal coronary arteries (NCA)
obtuse marginal a. (OMA)
obtuse marginal coronary a.
occipital a. (OA)
OM coronary a.
parietooccipital a.
penetrator a.
perforating a.

pericardiophrenic a.
perineal a.
peripheral a.
peroneal a.
pharyngeal branch of descending
  palatine a.
pharyngeal branch of inferior
  thyroid a.
phrenic a.
PLCx coronary a.
popliteal a.
posterior cerebral a. (PCA)
posterior circumflex a. (PC)
posterior communicating a. (PCoA)
posterior descending a. (PDA)
posterior inferior cerebellar a.
  (PICA)
posterior inferior communicating a.
  (PICA)
posterior margin of pulmonary a.
  (PPA)
posterior pulmonary a. (PPA)
posterior right coronary a. (pRCA)
posterolateral segment [coronary] a.
  (PLSA)
profunda femoris a.
pulmonary a. (PA)
radial a.
ramus intermedius a.
ranine a.
renal a.
retinal a.
RIC a.
right brachial a. (RBA)
right common carotid a. (RCCA)
right coronary a. (RCA)
right gastroepiploic a. (RGEA)
right internal mammary a. (RIMA)
right internal thoracic a. (RITA)
right middle cerebral a. (R-MCA)
right pulmonary a. (RPA)
right vertebral a. (RVA)
second obtuse marginal a. (OM-2)
septal perforating a.
silver-wiring of retinal a.
single internal mammary a. (SIMA)
sinoatrial nodal a.
sinus node a.
smooth coronary a.
stenting in small arteries (SISA)
sternocleidomastoid a.
subclavian a.

NOTES

artery (continued)
    sublingual a.
    superdominant a.
    superficial external pudendal a.
    superficial femoral a. (SFA)
    superior carotid a.
    superior cerebellar a. (SCA)
    superior femoral a. (SFA)
    superior laryngeal a.
    superior mesenteric a. (SMA)
    superior thyroid a.
    terminal internal carotid a. (TICA)
    thoracodorsal a.
    tibial a.
    tortuous right coronary a.
    transposition of great arteries (TGA)
    transverse cervical a.
    umbilical a.
    unilateral absence of pulmonary a. (UAPA)
    unprotected a.
Artha-G
arthritis, pl. **arthritides**
    acute rheumatic a.
    A. Foundation Pain Reliever
    juvenile rheumatoid a.
    rheumatoid a. (RA)
arthritis-associated aortitis
Arthropan
arthropod venom
ArthroWand
Arthus-type reaction
articularis
    facies a.
articular surface of arytenoid cartilage
articulation
artifact
    aliasing a.
    bang a.
    baseline a.
    beam width a.
    blooming a.
    breast a.
    catheter impact a.
    catheter whip a.
    chemical shift a.
    coin a.
    crush a.
    cupping a.
    end-pressure a.
    flow a.
    ghosting a.
    mitral regurgitation a.
    motion a.
    muscle a.
    N/2 a.
    pacemaker stimulus a.
    phantom flow a.
    respiratory a.
    reverberation a.
    side lobe a.
    smearing a.
    susceptibility a.
    T a.
    view-aliasing a.
    wrap-around ghosting a.
    zebra a.
artifactual bradycardia
artificial
    a. blood
    a. body
    a. cardiac valve
    a. circus movement tachycardia (ACMT)
    a. heart (AH)
    a. heart energy system (AHES)
    a. larynx
    a. lung
    a. lung-expanding compound (ALEC)
    a. pacemaker
    a. pacemaker-induced ventricular rhythm (APIVR)
    a. pneumothorax
    a. respiration
    a. ventilation
Artrek
    A. automated edge-detection algorithm
    A. cineangiographic analysis system
ARV
    anterior right ventricle
ARVC
    arrhythmogenic right ventricular cardiomyopathy
ARVD
    arrhythmogenic right ventricular dysplasia
Arvidsson dimension-length method
Arvin
ARVP
    arginine vasopressin
arylesterase
arylsulfatase
arytenoidea cricoideae
arytenoid gland
Arzbaecher pill electrode
Arzco
    A. pacemaker
    A. preamplifier
    A. Tapsul pill electrode
AS
    Adams-Stokes
    aortic sound
    area of stenosis
    arteriosclerosis
    atherosclerosis

atrial septum
atrial stenosis
　AS disease
As
arsenic
ASA
acetylsalicylic acid
atrial septal aneurysm
　MSD Enteric Coated ASA
asaccharolyticus
　Peptostreptococcus a.
ASAH
antibiotic sterilized aortic valve
　homograft
asahii
　Trichosporon a.
Asaphen
Asasantine
asbestiform
asbestos
　a. bodies
　a. pleural effusion
　a. pneumoconiosis
asbestosis
　parenchymal a.
Asbron G
asc
ascending
ASCAD
atherosclerotic coronary artery disease
A-scan echography
ASCAo
ascending aorta
ascariasis
Ascaris lumbricoides
ascendens
　aorta a.
ascendentis
　plexus periarterialis arteriae
　pharyngeae a.
ascending (asc)
　a. aorta (AA, AAO, ACS Ao,
　　AOA, ASCAo)
　a. aorta to pulmonary artery shunt
　a. aorta synchronized pulsation
　　(AASP)
　a. aortic blood pressure
　a. aortic pressure (PAo)
　a. aortography
　a. ileocolic artery
　a. loop of Henle

　a. pharyngeal artery
　a. pharyngeal plexus
　a. polyneuropathy
ascent
barotrauma of a.
　A. guiding catheter
Aschner
　A. phenomenon
　A. reflex
　A. sign
Aschner-Dagnini reflex
Aschoff
　A. body
　A. cell
　A. nodule
Aschoff-Tawara node
ascites
chylous a.
a. praecox
ascorbate
　a. dilution curve
　sodium a.
ascorbic acid
Ascriptin
ASCS
acute sickle chest syndrome
ASCVD
arteriosclerotic cardiovascular disease
atherosclerotic cardiovascular disease
ASD
atrial septal defect
　ASD closure device
ASD2
secundum atrial septal defect
ASDA
American Sleep Disorders Association
ASDOS
atrial septal defect occlusion system
atrial septum defect occluder system
　ASDOS umbrella
　ASDOS umbrella occluder
ASE
American Society of Electrocardiography
asequence
ASH
asymmetric septal hypertrophy
ash
fly a.
ASHCVD
atherosclerotic hypertensive
　cardiovascular disease

NOTES

ASHD
 arteriosclerotic heart disease
 atrioseptal heart disease
Asherman chest seal
Asherson syndrome
Ashley phenomenon
Ashman
 A. beat
 A. phenomenon
Ashworth Scale
Asian influenza
a-SiC:H
 amorphous hydrogenated silicon carbide
Askin tumor
Ask-Upmark syndrome
ASM
 airways smooth muscle
Asmalix
asmaPLAN+ peak flowmeter
ASMI
 anteroseptal myocardial infarction
ASO
 antistreptolysin O
ASP
 aortic systolic pressure
 area systolic pressure
ASPAC
 anisoylated streptokinase-plasminogen
  activator complex
asparaginase
asparagine
aspartate aminotransferase (AST)
aspartic acid
aspergilloma formation
aspergillosis
 allergic bronchopulmonary a.
  (ABPA)
 bronchopulmonary a.
 chronic necrotizing a.
 invasive pulmonary a. (IPA)
 parenchymal a.
 pleural a.
 primary pleural a.
 pseudomembranous
  tracheobronchial a.
 pulmonary a.
 semiinvasive a.
 suppurative necrotizing a.
Aspergillus
 A. *avenaceus*
 A. *caesiellus*
 A. *candidus*
 A. *carneus*
 A. empyema
 A. *flavus*
 A. *fumigatus*
 A. *nidulans*
 A. *niger*
 A. *oryzae*

 A. *restrictus*
 A. *sydowi*
 A. *terreus*
 A. toxicosis
 A. tracheobronchitis
 A. *ustus*
 A. *versicolor*
asphygmia
asphyxia
 blue a.
 a. carbonica
 cyanotic a.
 a. cyanotica
 a. livida
 local a.
 a. neonatorum
 a. pallida
 secondary a.
 symmetric a.
 traumatic a.
 white a.
asphyxial cardiac arrest
asphyxiant
asphyxiate
asphyxiating thoracic dystrophy (ATD)
asphyxiation
aspirate
 bronchotracheal a.
 endotracheal a. (EA)
 needle a.
 tracheal a.
 tracheobronchial a.
aspirated and flushed
aspirating needle
aspiration
 a. biopsy
 a. biopsy cytology (ABC)
 bronchoscopic needle a. (BNA)
 diagnostic a.
 endoscopic ultrasound-guided fine-
  needle a. (EUS-FNA)
 fine-needle a. (FNA)
 fluid a.
 a. of foreign body
 foreign body a.
 gastric a.
 hydrocarbon a.
 intractable a.
 large-volume a.
 a. lung injury
 massive a.
 meconium a.
 nosocomial a.
 a. pneumonia
 a. pneumonitis
 small-volume a.
 thoracic percutaneous needle a.
  (TPNA)
 transbronchial needle a. (TBNA)

transthoracic needle a. (TTNA)
transtracheal a.

aspiration-induced respiratory disease

aspirator

Cavitron ultrasonic surgical a.
(CUSA)
Cook County a.
Schueler Model 200 A.
Ultra-Lite portable a.
Vac-Pak-II ultra-lite portable a.
Vacu-Aide home-use a.

aSpire covered stent

aspirin

anticoagulation regimen of a.
Bayer Buffered A.
buffered a.
dipyridamole and a.
enteric-coated a.
Extra Strength Bayer Enteric
500 A.
St. Joseph Adult Chewable A.
ticlopidine plus a. (T + A)
a. tolerance time (ATT)

aspirin/extended release dipyridamole

aspirin-induced asthma (AIA)

aspirin-phenacetin-caffeine (APC)

aspirin-phenacetin-caffeine-codeine
(APCC)

Aspirols

Amyl Nitrite A.
Aromatic Ammonia A.

asplenia

Asprimox

ASPVD

arteriosclerotic peripheral vascular
disease
atherosclerotic peripheral vascular disease

ASS

asthma severity score

assay

adherence a.
agar diffusion a.
Asserachrom D-DI ELISA a.
Asserachrom tPA immunologic a.
automated BNP a.
Bioclot protein S a.
BNA-100-Behring Diagnostics
immunonephelometric a.
Cardiac T rapid a.
cardiac troponin I a.
Clauss a.
CoA-set fibrin monomer a.

cTnI a.
Cushman a.
D-dimer enzyme-linked
immunosorbent a.
Enzygnost TAT ELISA a.
enzyme-linked immunosorbent a.
(ELISA)
euglobulin clot a. (ECT)
ferricytochrome a.
Hemochron high-dose thrombin
time a.
hemoSTATUS a.
Heptest clotting a.
Hybritech immunoradiometric a.
immune adherence
immunosorbent a. (IAIA)
immunoradiometric a. (IRMA)
immunoturbidimetric a.
lucigenin chemiluminescence a.
MonoClone immunoenzymetric a.
multimer a.
myoglobin a.
N High Sensitivity CRP a.
Opus cardiac troponin I a.
PCR a.
radioligand binding a.
rapid platelet function a. (RPFA)
sandwich enzyme-linked
immunosorbent a.
S-Mgb a.
Stachrom PAI chromogenic a.
thyrotoxin radioisotope a.
Tina-quant immunoturbidimetric a.
TRAP a.
TUNEL a.
Ultegra rapid platelet function a.
Velogene rapid TB a.

assembly

blood pressure a. (BPA)
Collins SurveyTach with
MicroTach a.
infant nasal cannula a. (INCA)

Asserachrom

A. D-DI ELISA assay
A. tPA immunologic assay

assessment

anatomic a.
angiographic a.
angioscopic a.
cardiovascular function a.
causality a.
Chedoke-McMaster Stroke A.

NOTES

assessment *(continued)*
    echocardiographic a.
    functional a.
    hemodynamic a.
    invasive a.
    jugular bulb catheter placement a.
    noninvasive a.
    sepsis-related organ failure a.
      (SOFA)
    sequential organ failure a. (SOFA)
    transposition a.
Assess peak flowmeter
assist
    Venturi exhalation A.
assistance
    external pressure circulatory a.
      (EPCA)
    intraaortic balloon a. (IABA)
    mechanical ventricular a. (MVA)
    ventilatory a.
assist/control
    a./c. mode ventilation
    a./c. ventilation (ACV)
assisted
    a. circulation
    a. mechanical ventilation (AMV)
    a. peak systolic pressure (APSP)
    a. respiration
    a. ventilation
Assmann
    A. focus
    A. tuberculous infiltrate
association
    American Cardiology
      Technologists A. (ACTA)
    American College of
      Cardiology/American Heart A.
      (ACC/AHA)
    American Heart A. (AHA)
    American Sleep Disorders A.
      (ASDA)
    atrioventricular a.
    CHARGE a.
    Kennedy Disease A. (KAD)
    National Home Oxygen Patients A.
AST
    angiotensin sensitivity test
    aspartate aminotransferase
    atrial overdrive stimulation rate
Astech peak flowmeter
Astelin nasal spray
astemizole
asterixis
asteroid body
asteroides
    Nocardia a.
asthenia
    neurocirculatory a.
    vasoregulatory a.

asthenic apoplexy
asthenicus
    thorax a.
asthma
    abdominal a.
    acarian a.
    adult-onset a.
    aliphatic amines a.
    allergen-induced a.
    allergic a.
    aluminum potroom a.
    alveolar a.
    anhydride a.
    aspirin-induced a. (AIA)
    atopic a.
    bacterial a.
    baker's a.
    benzalkonium chloride a.
    brittle a.
    bronchial a.
    cacoon seed a.
    cardiac a.
    a. care algorithm (ACA)
    casein a.
    castor bean a.
    cat a.
    catarrhal a.
    A. Check peak flowmeter
    Cheyne-Stokes a.
    chlorella a.
    chronic a.
    cobalt a.
    cobalt-related a.
    cockroach a.
    coffee bean a.
    cold dry air-induced a.
    cotton-dust a.
    cough variant a.
    a. crystal
    cutaneous a.
    daytime a. (DA)
    diisocyanate a.
    dust a.
    Elsner a.
    emphysematous a.
    essential a.
    exercise-induced a. (EIA)
    extrinsic a.
    factitious a.
    food a.
    Global Institute for A. (GIA)
    grinder's a.
    Heberden a.
    horse a.
    humid a.
    hyperventilation-induced a. (HIA)
    idiosyncratic a.
    infective a.
    inner city a.

intrinsic a.
irritant-induced a.
isocyanate-induced a.
kapok a.
karaya a.
Kopp a.
lycopodium a.
mall a.
meat-wrapper's a.
methylene diphenyl diisocyanate a.
Mexican bean weevil a.
Millar a.
miller's a.
miner's a.
mixed a.
nacre dust a.
nasal a.
near-fatal a. (NFA)
nervous a.
nocturnal a.
nonatopic a.
occupational a. (OA)
oil mist a.
osmotically induced a. (OIA)
pancreatin a.
a. paper
phthalic anhydride irritant-
  induced a.
pollen a.
polyether alcohol a.
poorly reversible a.
postcoital a.
potter's a.
prawn a.
A. Quality of Life Questionnaire
  (AQLQ)
red cedar a.
red soft coral a.
reflex a.
rose hips a.
Rostan a.
royal jelly-induced a.
a. severity score (ASS)
sexual a.
sheep blowfly a.
shellfish a.
soybean lecithin a.
spasmodic a.
steam-fitter's a.
steroid-dependent a.
steroid-resistant a.
stone stripper's a.

styrene a.
subclinical a.
sunflower a.
symptomatic a.
tall oil a.
tartrazine a.
thymic a.
tragacanth a.
triad a.
a. trigger
trimellitic anhydride a.
true a.
tylosin tartrate a.
Vicia sativa a.
weeping fig a.
Wichmann a.
work-aggravated a.
work-related a.
zardaverine a.
AsthmaMentor peak flowmeter
AsthmaNefrin
Asthmanex
AsthmaPACK personal asthma care kit
Asthmastik
asthmatic
brittle a.
a. bronchitis
chronic stable a.
corticosteroid-dependent a.
steroid-dependent a.
tight a.
asthmaticus
status a.
asthmatiform
asthmogen
hydrosoluble a.
occupational a.
asthmogenic
asthmoid
a. respiration
a. wheeze
Astler-Coller classification
Astra
A. profile
A. T4, T6 pacemaker
Astrand bicycle exercise stress test
Astrand-Rhyming protocol
astrocyte
astronyxis
Acanthamoeba a.
Astropulse cuff
Astro-Trace Universal adapter clip

NOTES

Astroviridae virus
Astrup blood gas value
ASV
adaptive support ventilation
autologous saphenous vein
ASVD
arteriosclerotic vascular disease
asymmetric
a. dimethylarginine (ADMA)
a. septal hypertrophy (ASH)
asymmetrical
bilateral a. (BA)
asymptomatic
a. cardiac ischemia (ACI, acute coronary insufficiency)
a. carotid bruit (ACB)
a. complex ectopy
a. coronary artery disease (ACAD)
a. left ventricular dysfunction
a. myocarditis
asynchronous
atrial a. (AOO)
a. pacing
a. pulse generator
ventricular a. (VOO)
asynchrony index
asynergy
asystole
atrial a.
Beau a.
transient a.
asystolia
asystolic arrest
AT
acute thrombosis
adenosine triphosphate
anaerobic threshold
angiotensin
antithrombin
atrial tachycardia
atropine
AT1
angiotensin II type 1
AT1 receptor C allele
At
angiotensin
antithrombin
atrial
atrium
AT I
angiotensin I
AT II
angiotensin II
ata
atmosphere absolute
Atacand
A. HCT
A. Plus tablet
atactic hemiparesis

Atakr system
Atarax Oral
AT-atropine stress echocardiography
ATA unit
ataxia
a. cordis
Friedreich a.
hereditary a.
spinocerebellar a.
ataxia-telangiectasia
ataxic
a. aphasia
a. gait
a. hemiparesis (AH)
ATB
atrial tachycardia with block
ATC
Antiplatelet Trialists' Collaboration
ATD
Amplatz thrombectomy device
asphyxiating thoracic dystrophy
ATDR
atrial tachycardia detection rate
atelectasia
atelectasis
absorption a.
acquired a.
bibasilar a.
compression a.
congenital a.
lobar a.
obstructive a.
patchy a.
platelike a.
postobstructive a.
primary a.
relaxation a.
resorption a.
rounded a.
secondary a.
segmental a.
subsegmental a.
tricuspid a.
atelectatic
a. band
a. rale
atelocardia
Aten
atenolol and chlorthalidone
ATF
activating transcription factor
At fib, Atr fib
atrial fibrillation
Atgam
atherectomy
Auth a.
a. catheter
coronary a.
coronary rotational a. (CRA)

directional a.
excimer laser coronary a.
excisional a.
extraction a.
high-speed directional coronary a.
high-speed rotational a. (HSRA)
a. index
Kinsey a.
percutaneous coronary rotational a.
 (PCRA)
percutaneous transluminal
 rotational a. (PTRA)
rotablator a. (ROTA)
rotational a. (RA)
rotational coronary a. (RCA)
transluminal extraction a. (TEA)
transluminal extraction coronary a.
atheroablation
AtheroCath
A. Bantam coronary atherectomy
 catheter
A. GTO coronary atherectomy
 catheter
Simpson peripheral A.
atheroemboli (*pl. of* atheroembolus)
atheroembolic stroke
atheroembolism
atheroembolus, pl. **atheroemboli**
atherogenesis
monoclonal theory of a.
response-to-injury hypothesis of a.
atherogenic
a. dyslipidemia
a. index (AI)
a. metabolic triad
atherogenicity index
atherolytic reperfusion guidewire
atheroma
AA a.
aortic arch a.
a. burden
complex a.
core of a.
coronary a.
intimal a.
protruding a.
atheromatous
a. cap
a. core
a. debris
a. embolism

a. gruel
a. plaque
atherosclerosis (AS, Athsc, ATS) (*See
 also* arteriosclerosis)
aortic a.
cardiac allograft a. (CAA)
coronary artery a.
de novo a.
encrustation theory of a.
lipogenic theory of a.
a. obliterans
premature a.
a. prevention and treatment
radiation-induced a.
atherosclerotic (*See also* arteriosclerosis)
a. aneurysm
a. aortic disease
a. aortography
a. cardiovascular disease (ACVD,
 ASCVD)
a. carotid artery disease
a. coronary artery disease (ACAD,
 ASCAD)
a. debris
a. heart disease (AHD)
a. hypertensive cardiovascular
 disease (ASHCVD)
a. narrowing
a. peripheral vascular disease
 (ASPVD)
a. plaque (AP)
a. plaque burden
atherosis
atherothrombosis
atherothrombotic
a. brain infarction (ABI)
a. cardiovascular disease
a. stroke
atherotome
athlete
A. guidewire
a.'s's heart
athletic heart
Athsc
atherosclerosis
AT III
antithrombin III
AT-III
antithrombin III
Ativan
Atkins-Cannard tracheal tube
Atkins diet

NOTES

ATL
anterior tricuspid leaflet
ATL UltraMark 7
echocardiographic device
ATL UltraMark IV 7.5-MHz linear
array transducer
ATL UltraMark 9 ultrasound
system
atlantis
fovea articularis inferior a.
fovea articularis superior a.
fovea dentis a.
A. SR intravascular ultrasound
imaging catheter
A. SR IVUS catheter
atlas
a. DG balloon angioplasty catheter
superior articular facet of a.
a. ULP balloon dilatation catheter
Atlee clamp
ATLS
advanced trauma life support
atm
atmosphere
atmosphere (atm)
a. absolute (ata)
ICAO standard a.
a.'s of pressure
standard a.
atmospheric pressure
atmospherization
atmotherapy
ATnativ
atomic absorption spectrometry
atomizer
atopic asthma
atopy
atorvastatin calcium
atovaquone
ATP
adenosine triphosphate
antitachycardia pacemaker
antitachycardia pacing
ATP hydrolysis
ATPase
adenosine triphosphatase
myofibrillar ATPase
SR calcium ATPase
ATP-SPECT
adenosine triphosphate single-photon
emission computed tomography
atra
Stachybotrys a.
ATRAC-II double-balloon catheter
ATRAC multipurpose balloon catheter
atracurium
Atraloc needle
Atrauclip hemostatic clip
atraumatic needle

atresia
anatomic pulmonary a.
aortic a.
aortic valve a. (AVA)
atrioventricular valve a.
bronchial a.
congenital bronchial a. (CBA)
esophageal a.
functional pulmonary a.
glottic a.
gross tracheoesophageal a.
infundibular a.
laryngeal a.
membranous pulmonary a.
mitral a.
pulmonary a. (PA)
pure pulmonary a. (PPA)
tricuspid a. (TA)
ventricular a.
atretic pulmonary valve
Atr fib (*var. of* At fib)
atria (*pl. of* atrium)
atrial (At)
a. activation mapping
a. anomalous band
a. appendage
a. appendectomy
a. arrhythmia
a. asynchronous (AOO)
a. asynchronous pacemaker
a. asystole
a. baffle operation
a. balloon septostomy
a. bigeminy
a. bolus dynamic computer
tomography
a. bradycardia
a. capture
a. capture beat
a. capture threshold
a. carotid ventricular (ACV)
a. chaotic tachycardia
a. contraction (ac)
a. cuff
a. defibrillation threshold
a. deflection
a. demand inhibited (AAI)
a. demand inhibited pacemaker
a. demand triggered (AAT)
a. demand triggered pacemaker
a. diastole
a. diastolic gallop (ADG)
a. disk
a. dissociation
a. echo
a. ectopic (AE)
a. ectopic beat
a. ectopic tachycardia (AET)
a. ectopy

a. effective refractory period (AERP)
a. ejection force
a. electrogram (AEG)
a. emptying index (AEI)
a. escape interval
a. escape rhythm
a. extrastimulus method
a. extrasystole
a. fibrillation (AF, AFib, At fib, Atr fib)
a. fibrillation cycle length (AFCL)
a. fibrillation detection
a. fibrillation-flutter (AFF)
a. fibrillation investigators
a. fibrillation threshold
a. filling fraction (AFF)
a. filling pressure
a. flutter (AF, AFL)
a. flutter response (AFR)
a. flutter response algorithm
a. fusion (AF)
a. fusion beat
a. heart rate (AHR)
a. implantable cardioverter-defibrillator (AICD, A-ICD)
a. incremental pacing
a. inhibited (AAI)
a. insufficiency (AI)
a. isthmus ablation
a. kick
a. lead impedance
a. liver pulse
a. maze procedure
a. myocardial infarction
a. myocarditis
a. myxoma
a. natriuretic factor (ANF)
a. natriuretic peptide (ANP)
a. natriuretic peptide A (ANP-A)
a. natriuretic peptide B (ANP-B)
a. natriuretic peptide C (ANP-C)
a. natriuretic polypeptide (ANP)
a. non-sensing
a. notch
a. ostium primum defect
a. overdrive pacing
a. overdrive stimulation rate (AST)
a. pacing (AP)
a. pacing stress test
a. pacing wire
a. parasystole

a. paroxysmal tachycardia
a. partition
a. premature beat (APB)
a. premature complex
a. premature contraction (APC)
a. premature depolarization (APD)
a. pressure (PA)
pulmonary venous a. (PVa)
a. pulse amplitude
a. pulse width
a. rate (AR)
a. reentry
a. refractory period
a. relaxation
a. repolarization wave
a. reversal (AR)
a. reverse remodeling
a. ring
a. sensing configuration
a. sensitivity
a. septal aneurysm (ASA)
a. septal defect (ASD)
a. septal defect occlusion system (ASDOS)
a. septal defect patch
a. septal defect umbrella
a. septal resection
a. septectomy
a. septostomy
a. septum (AS)
a. septum defect occluder system (ASDOS)
a. septum septal pacing
a. shear
a. situs inversus
a. sound
a. spike
a. standstill
a. stasis index
a. stenosis (AS)
a. stretch
a. synchronous noncompetitive pacemaker
a. synchronous pulse generator
a. synchronous ventricular inhibited (VDD)
a. synchronous ventricular inhibited pacemaker
a. synchrony
a. systole
a. tachycardia (AT)

NOTES

atrial *(continued)*

    a. tachycardia detection rate (ATDR)

    a. tachycardia with block (ATB)

    a. tachycardic response

    a. tachycardic response algorithm

    a. thrombus

    a. train pacing

    a. transport function

    a. trigeminy with aberrancy

    a. triggered

    a. triggered noncompetitive pacemaker

    a. triggered pulse generator

    a. undersensing

    a. valve

    a. vector loop

    a. venous pulse

    a. and ventricular implantable cardioverter-defibrillator (AV-ICD)

    a. ventricular nodal reentry tachycardia

    a. ventricular reciprocating tachycardia (AVRT)

    a. ventricular shunt

    a. volume constant (Vak)

    a. VOO pacemaker

atrial/aortic

    left a./a. (LA/Ao)

atrial-axis discontinuity

atrial-based pacemaker

atrial-femoral artery bypass

atrialized

    a. chamber

    a. ventricle

atrial-paced cycle length

atrial-to-pulmonary venous gradient

atrial-well technique

atriocarotid (AC)

    a. interval

atriocommissuropexy

atriocyte

atriodextrofascicular tract

atriodigital dysplasia

atriofascicular

    a. Mahaim reentrant tachycardia

    a. tract

atriography

atrio-His (A-H)

    a.-H. bypass tract

    a.-H. fiber

    a.-H. pathway

atrionodal (AN)

atrionodal bypass tract

atriopeptidase inhibitor

atriopressor reflex

atriopulmonary shunt

atrioseptal

    a. heart disease (ASHD)

    a. sign

atriosystolic murmur

atriotomy

atrioventricular (A-V, AV)

    anomalous a.

    a. association

    a. block (AVB)

    a. bundle

    a. canal (AVC)

    a. canal cushion

    a. canal defect

    a. circumflex branch (AVCx)

    complete a.

    a. conduction (AVC)

    a. conduction abnormality

    a. conduction defect

    a. conduction system (AVCS)

    a. conduction tissue

    a. connection anomaly

    a. delay (AVD)

    a. discordance

    a. dissociation (AVD)

    a. extrasystole (AVE)

    a. flow rumbling murmur

    a. furrow

    a. gradient

    a. groove

    a. interval

    a. junction (AVJ)

    a. junctional

    a. junctional ablation

    a. junctional arrhythmia

    a. junctional bigeminy

    a. junctional escape beat

    a. junctional escape complex

    a. junctional escape extrasystole

    a. junctional heart block

    a. junctional pacemaker augmentor

    a. junctional reciprocating tachycardia

    a. junctional rhythm

    a. junction motion

    a. junction rhythm (AVJR)

    a. malformation (AVM)

    a. nodal ablation

    a. nodal bigeminy

    a. nodal conduction (AVN)

    a. nodal extrasystole

    a. nodal reentrant tachycardia (AVNRT)

    a. nodal reentry (AVNR)

    a. nodal reentry tachycardia (AVNRT)

    a. nodal rhythm

    a. nodal tachycardia (AVNT)

    a. node (AVN)

    a. node artery

a. node block
a. node dysfunction (AVND)
a. node functional refractory period
   (AVNFRP)
a. node pathway
a. opening (AVO)
a. orifice
a. pathway (AP)
a. reciprocating tachycardia (AVRT)
a. reentrant tachycardia (AVRT)
a. refractory period (AVRP)
a. septal defect (AVSD)
sequential a. (SAV)
a. sequential pacemaker
a. situs concordance
a. sulcus
a. synchronous pacing
a. synchrony
a. time
a. valve (AVV)
a. valve atresia
a. valve insufficiency
a. valve opening (AO)
a. valve regurgitation
a. valve ring

atrioventricularis
crus dextrum fasciculi a.
crus sinistrum fasciculi a.
crux dextrum fasciculi a.
crux sinistrum fasciculi a.
nodus a.
truncus fascicularis a.

Atrioverter
A. implantable atrial defibrillator
A. implantable defibrillator device
Metrix A.

atrium, pl. **atria (A, At)**
accessory a.
auricles of atria
common a.
congenital single a.
a. cordis
a. cordis sinistrum
a. dextrum
electrocardiographic wave
   corresponding to a wave of
   depolarization crossing the A. (P)
Fontan right a.
a. glottidis
a. of heart
high right a.
left a. (LA)

low right a. (LRA)
low septal a.
low septal right a. (LSRA)
a. of lung
a. pulmonale
pulmonary venous a.
right a. (RA)
roof of left a.
single a.
a. sinistrum
stunned a.
systemic venous a.

Atromid-S
Atropair
atrophic
a. cardiomyopathy
a. catarrh
a. emphysema
a. laryngitis
a. papulosis
a. pharyngitis
a. thrombosis

atrophy
brown a.
cardiac a.
Erb a.
multiple system a.
olivopontocerebellar a.
optic a.
peroneal muscular a.
red a.

atropine (AT)
A.-Care
Isopto A.
a. sulfate
a. test

Atropine-Care
Atropisol
Atrostim phrenic nerve stimulator
Atrovent
A. Aerosol Inhalation
A. Inhalation Solution

ATS
arteriosclerosis
atherosclerosis
ATS Open Pivot heart valve
ATS standard aortic valve
ATS standard mitral valve

ATT
arginine tolerance test
aspirin tolerance time

NOTES

attachment
    epithelial-mucus a.
attack
    Adams-Stokes a.
    anxiety a.
    drop a.
    heart a.
    odor-triggered panic a.
    Stokes-Adams a.
    transient ischemic a. (TIA)
    vagal a.
    vasovagal a.
attenuation
    broadband ultrasound a. (BUA)
    ground-glass a. (GGA)
    heterogeneous parenchymal a.
    vascular a.
attenuator
attraction sphere
attrition murmur
ATW
    all track wire
    ATW steerable guidewire
atypical
    a. alveolar hyperplasia
    a. atrioventricular nodal reentrant
      tachycardia (AAVNRT)
    a. chest pain
    a. mycobacterial colonization
    a. pneumonia
    a. tamponade
    a. tuberculosis
    a. verrucous endocarditis
Au
    gold
audiometry
    heart rate a. (HRA)
auditory
    a. alternans
    a. fremitus
Auenbrugger sign
Auer body
Aufrecht sign
Aufricht elevator
augmentation
    flow a.
    pressure a. (PA)
    a. therapy
augmented V wave
Augmentin
augmentor
    atrioventricular junctional
      pacemaker a.
    pacemaker a.
aur, auric
    auricle
    auricular
auranofin
aureomycin sensitivity

aureus
    Staphylococcus a.
auric (*var. of* aur)
auricle (aur, auric)
    a.'s of atria
    left a. (LA)
    right a. (RA)
auricular (aur, auric)
    a. appendage
    a. appendectomy
    a. complex
    a. extrasystole
    a. fibrillation
    a. flutter
    a. premature beat
    a. standstill
    a. systole
    a. tachycardia
auricularis magna
Auriculin
auriculopressor reflex
auriculoventricular
    a. extrasystole
    a. groove
    a. interval
aurothiomalate
Aurous
    A. centimeter sizing catheter
    A. graduate sizing catheter
aus, ausc
    auscultation
auscultation (aus, ausc)
    aortic area of a.
    cardiac a.
    Korányi a.
    percussion and a. (P&A)
    a. and percussion (A&P)
auscultatory
    a. alternans
    a. gap
    a. sign
    a. sound
auscultogram
Austin
    A. Flint murmur
    A. Flint phenomenon
    A. Flint respiration
    A. Flint rumble
    A. Medical Equipment (A.M.E.)
Australia antigen
Australian Q fever
australis
    Rickettsia a.
Austrian syndrome
autacoid, autocoid
Auth atherectomy
Autima II dual-chamber pacemaker
AutoAdjust CPAP device
autoanalyzer

autoantibody
  antiheart muscle a. (AHMA)
  antimyosin a.
  cardiac a.
autobiotic
autobullectomy
  inflammatory a.
  partial a.
autocapture
  ventricular a.
AutoCapture pacing system
AutoCat intraaortic balloon pump
Autoclix
autocoid (*var. of* autacoid)
autocorrelation
  serial a. (SAC)
AutoCorr portable pulse oximeter
autocrine signaling
autodecremental
  a. mode
  a. pacing
autodigestion of connective tissue
autofluorescence bronchoscopy
autogamous
autogamy
autogenic
  a. drainage (AD)
  a. graft
autogenous vein
autograft
  pulmonary a. (PA)
Autohaler
autohypnosis
autoimmune
  a. disorder
  a. thyroid disease (AITD)
autoimmunity
  cardiac a.
Auto-Injector
  LidoPen I.M. Injection A.-I.
Autolet
autologous
  a. blood
  a. blood management system
  a. blood patch
  a. blood selective aortic arch
    perfusion (AB-SAAP)
  a. clot
  a. fat graft
  a. pericardial patch
  a. saphenous vein (ASV)

  a. transfusion
  a. vein graft-coated stent (AVGCS)
automated
  a. BNP assay
  a. border detection (ABD)
  a. boundary protection (ABP)
  a. cardiac flow measurement
    (ACM)
  a. cardiac output measurement
    (ACOM, AcomA)
  a. cervical cell screening system
  a. edge detection
automatic
  a. atrial tachycardia (AAT)
  a. beat
  a. boundary detection (ABD)
  a. capacitor formation interval
  a. cell
  a. device
  a. ectopic tachycardia
  a. exposure system
  a. external cardioverter-defibrillator
    (AECD)
  a. external defibrillator (AED)
  a. implantable cardioverter-
    defibrillator (AICD, A-ICD)
  a. implantable defibrillator (AID)
  a. internal cardioverter-defibrillator
    (AICD, A-ICD)
  a. internal defibrillator
  a. mode conversion
  a. mode conversion algorithm
  a. mode switching (AMS)
  a. mode-switching algorithm
  a. oscillometric blood pressure
    monitor
  a. pacemaker
  a. systolic blood pressure
    measurement (ABP)
  a. ventricular contraction
automaticity
  enhanced a.
  pacemaker a.
  sinus nodal a.
autonomic
  a. dysreflexia
  a. failure
  a. hyperreflexia
  a. modulation
  a. nervous system (ANS)
  a. perturbation
  pulmonary branch of a.

NOTES

autonomic *(continued)*
    a. response
    a. sensory innervation
autonomici
    rami pulmonales systematis a.
autoPEEP, intrinsic PEEP
    unintended positive end expiratory
    pressure
autoperfusion
    a. balloon
    a. balloon catheter
Autoplex
    A. Factor VIII inhibitor bypass
    product
    A. T
autoprogramming
autoradiography
    quantitative a. (QAR)
autoregulation
    cerebrovascular a.
    heterometric a.
    homeometric a.
    orthostasis a.
autosensing
AutoSet
    A. CS device
    A. Portable II
    A. Portable II CPAP system
    A. Portable II diagnosis and
    therapy device
autosomal-dominant familial aortic aneurysm disease
autosome
Autostat ligating and hemostatic clip
Auto Suture Surgiclip
auto-threshold function
autotitrating CPAP
autotitration device
autotoxic cyanosis
Autotransfuser
    Biosurge Synchronous A.
autotransfusion system
autotransplantation
Autotrans system
Autovac LF autotransfusion system
autumnal catarrh
auxocardia
A-V, AV
    arteriovenous
    atrioventricular
    A-V atrioventricular junctional
    rhythm
    A-V branch block
    A-V bundle
    A-V conduction defect
    A-V delay interval
    A-V dissociation
    A-V Gore-Tex fistula
    A-V groove

    A-V groove block
    A-V junction
    A-V junction ablation
    A-V junctional escape beat
    A-V junctional escape complex
    A-V junctional extrasystole
    A-V junctional tachycardia
    A-V nodal artery
    A-V nodal bigeminy
    A-V nodal conduction
    A-V nodal extrasystole
    A-V nodal modification
    A-V nodal reentry
    A-V nodal reentry tachycardia
    A-V nodal rhythm
    A-V nodal Wenckebach arrhythmia
    A-V node
    A-V node block
    A-V node reentrant tachycardia
    A-V node Wenckebach periodicity
    A-V reciprocating tachycardia
    A-V sequential pacemaker
    A-V synchronous pacemaker
    A-V synchrony
    A-V universal (DDD)
    A-V Wenckebach block
AV
    aortic valve
    arteriovenous
    atrioventricular
A/V
    alanine/valine
    arteriovenous
AVA
    aortic valve annulus
    aortic valve anulus
    aortic valve area
    aortic valve atresia
    arteriovenous anastomosis
    AVA 3Xi advanced venous access
    device
AVAD
    acute ventricular assist device
Avalide
Avanar
    A. intravascular ultrasound catheter
    A. IVUS catheter
Avanti introducer
Avapro HCT
avascular necrosis
AVB
    atrioventricular block
AVC
    aberrant ventricular conduction
    aortic valve closure
    arteriovenous communication
    atrioventricular canal
    atrioventricular conduction

Avco
 A. aortic balloon
 A. balloon pump
AVCS
 atrioventricular conduction system
AVCx
 atrioventricular circumflex branch
AVD
 aortic valvular disease
 atrioventricular delay
 atrioventricular dissociation
AVD O$_2$
 arteriovenous oxygen difference
AVDP
 average diastolic pressure
AVE
 aortic valve echocardiogram
 atrioventricular extrasystole
 AVE Microstent II stent
 AVE S540, S670 stent
Avelox
 A. IV
 A. tablet
avenaceus
 Aspergillus a.
average
 a. diastolic pressure (AVDP)
 a. mean pressure (AMP)
 a. peak velocity (APV)
 a. pulse magnitude
 spatial average pulse a. (I$_{sapa}$)
averaging
 digital a.
 gated a.
 signal a.
AVF
 arteriovenous fistula
aVF
 unipolar limb lead on left leg in
  electrocardiography
 aVF lead
AVG
 aortic valve gradient
AVGCS
 autologous vein graft-coated stent
AVHD
 acquired valvular heart disease
AVHS
 acquired valvular heart syndrome
avian
 a. antigen
 a. influenza A (H5N1) virus

 A. transport ventilator
 a. tuberculosis
aviator's disease
AV-ICD
 atrial and ventricular implantable
  cardioverter-defibrillator
Avicor
avidin-biotin peroxidase
AVIR
 aortic valve replacement
Avitene
avium
 Mycobacterium a.
avium-intracellulare
 Mycobacterium a.-i. (MAI)
AVJ
 atrioventricular junction
AVJR
 atrioventricular junction rhythm
AVL
 AVL Omni blood gas analyzer
 AVL Opti Critical Care Analyzer
 AVL Opti 1 portable blood gas
  analyzer
aVL
 unipolar limb lead on left leg in
  electrocardiography
 aVL lead
AVM
 arteriovenous malformation
 atrioventricular malformation
AVN
 atrioventricular nodal conduction
 atrioventricular node
AVND
 atrioventricular node dysfunction
AVNFRP
 atrioventricular node functional refractory
  period
AVNR
 atrioventricular nodal reentry
AVNRT
 atrioventricular nodal reentrant
  tachycardia
 atrioventricular nodal reentry tachycardia
AVNT
 atrioventricular nodal tachycardia
AVO
 aortic valve opening
 aortic valve orifice
 atrioventricular opening
AvoSure PT monitor

NOTES

AVOXimeter 1000E whole blood oximeter

AVP
  abnormal vasopressin
  ambulatory venous pressure
  aqueous vasopressin
  arginine vasopressin
  arteriovenous passage time

AV-Paceport thermodilution catheter

AVR
  accelerated ventricular rhythm
  aortic valve replacement

aVR
  unipolar limb lead on right arm in
    electrocardiography
      aVR lead

AVRP
  atrioventricular refractory period

AVRT
  atrial ventricular reciprocating
    tachycardia
  atrioventricular reciprocating tachycardia
  atrioventricular reentrant tachycardia

AVS
  aortic valve stenosis
  arteriovenous shunt

AVSD
  acquired ventricular septal defect
  atrioventricular septal defect

AVSV
  aortic valve stroke volume

AVT
  arginine vasotocin

avulsion

AVV
  atrioventricular valve

Av3V
  anteroventral third ventricle

AW
  Anderson-Wilkins
  anterior wall
    AW acuteness score

AWAR
  anterior wall of aortic root

A-wave spectral velocity waveform

AWI
  anterior wall infarction

AWM
  abnormal wall motion

AWMI
  anterior wall myocardial infarction

Axcis
    A. percutaneous myocardial
      revascularization system
    A. PMR system

axes (*pl. of* axis)

axial
    a. computed tomography (ACT)
    a. control
    a. interstitial disease
    a. interstitium
    a. plane

axillaris
  regio a.

axillary
    a. arch
    a. artery
    a. bifemoral bypass
    a. block
    a. lymph node
    a. nerve
    a. triangle
    a. vein

axilloaxillary bypass

axillofemoral bypass

Axiom
    A. double sump pump
    A. thoracic trocar

Axios 04 pacemaker

axis, pl. **axes**
  celiac artery a.
  clockwise rotation of electrical a.
  a. deviation
  electrical a.
  frontal a.
  horizontal long a.
  hypophyseal-pituitary-adrenal a.
  hypothalamic-pituitary-adrenal a.
    (HPAA)
  instantaneous electrical a.
  J point electrical a.
  junctional a.
  long a. (LAX)
  mean electrical a.
  mean QRS a.
  normal electrical a.
  parasternal long a.
  parasternal short a.
  P wave a.
  QRS a.
  R a.
  rightward a.
  a. shift
  short a. (SAX)
  Strong unbridling of celiac
    artery a.
  superior QRS a.
  thoracic a.
  vertical long a.
  X, Y, Z a.

Axius vacuum 2 stabilizer

Ayercillin

Ayers
    A. cardiovascular needle holder
    A. sphygmomanometer
    A. T-piece

Ayerza
> A. disease
> A. syndrome

Aygestin

Ayr
> A. saline nasal drops
> A. saline nasal gel
> A. saline nasal mist

AZ
> acquisition zoom
> AZ technology

Azactam

azalide class of antibiotics

Azan-Mallory stain

azapetine phosphate

azatadine maleate

azathioprine

azidothymidine (AZT)

azimilide
> a. dihydrochloride
> a. supraventricular arrhythmia
> program

azithromycin

azlocillin

Azmacort Oral Inhaler

azotemia
> extrarenal a.
> postrenal a.
> prerenal a.
> renal a.

AZT
> azidothymidine

AZTEC
> amplitude zone time epoch coding
> AZTEC in ECG

aztreonam

azurophil granule

azygography

azygos
> a. arch
> a. fissure
> a. lobe of right lung
> a. node
> a. vein

Azzopardi effect

NOTES

B

B bump
B bump on echocardiogram
B cell antibody
B cell lymphoma
B knuckle

b

branched

B1 cell

B₄

leukotriene B4 (LTB4, LTB₄)

B6 bronchus sign

B101 ET Tape II adhesive tape

BA

basilar artery
bilateral asymmetrical

Babbington-type nebulizer

Babcock operation

Babes-Ernst body

Babesia

B. bigemina
B. bovis
B. canis
B. divergens
B. major
B. microti
B. rodhaini

babesiosis

human b.

Babinski

downgoing B.
B. reflex
B. syndrome
upgoing B.

Babinski-Vasquez syndrome

baby

blue b.

BABYbird respirator

babygram x-ray

Babyhaler spacer device

babyPac ventilator

BAC

bronchioloalveolar carcinoma

bacampicillin hydrochloride

Baccelli sign

Bachmann

anterior internodal tract of B.
B. bundle
internodal tract of B.
B. pathway

Baci-IM injection

bacillary

b. angiomatosis
b. embolism

b. phthisis
b. pneumonia

bacille Calmette-Guérin (BCG)

bacilli (*pl. of* bacillus)

bacilliformis

Bartonella b.

Bacillus

B. alvei
B. anthracis
B. cereus
B. circulans
B. laterosporus
B. licheniformis
B. megaterium
B. pneumoniae
B. polymyxa
B. pseudodiphtheriticum
B. pumilus
B. sphaericus
B. stearothermophilus
B. subtilis
B. subtilis enzyme

bacillus, pl. bacilli

acid-fast b.
Battey b.
Bordet-Gengou b.
Calmette-Guérin b.
B. Calmette-Guérin live
B. Calmette-Guérin vaccine
enteric gram-negative b.
Friedländer b.
gram-negative b. (GNB)
gram-positive b.
influenza b.
Klebs-Loeffler b.
Koch b.
Koch-Weeks b.
Loeffler b.
Much b.
Mycobacterium intracellulare,
Battey b.
Warthin-Starry-staining bacillus
Weeks b.

bacitracin

back-bleeding

backflush

background subtraction technique

back pressure

backscatter

b. analysis
integrated b.
b. threshold
two-dimensional integrated b.

backup ventilation (BUV)

backward heart failure

Bactec
> Bactec MGIT 960 System for *Mycobacteria* testing
> BACTEC radiometry
> BACTEC system

bacteremia, bacteriemia
> streptococcal b.

bacteremic

bacteria (*pl. of* bacterium)

bacteria-free stage of bacterial endocarditis

bacterial
> b. asthma
> b. colonization
> b. endocarditis (BE, BEC)
> b. endotoxin
> b. myocarditis
> b. pericarditis
> b. pneumococcal pneumonia
> b. respiratory tract infection
> b. superinfection
> b. vegetation

bactericidal titer

bacteriemia (*var. of* bacteremia)

bacterioid

bacteriophage

bacteriostatic
> b. agent
> b. effect

bacterium, pl. bacteria
> facultative bacteria

Bacterium anitratum

Bacteroides
> B. corrodens
> B. fragilis
> B. furcosus
> B. melaninogenicus
> B. oralis
> B. pneumosintes

Bactrim DS

Bactroban Topical

BAE
> bovine aortic endothelium
> bronchial artery embolization

BAEC
> bovine aortic endothelial cell

BAEDP
> balloon aortic end-diastolic pressure

Baehr-Lohlein lesion

Baffe anastomosis

baffle
> fabric b.
> b. fenestration
> Gore-Tex b.
> intraatrial b.
> b. leak
> manual resuscitation b.
> Mustard atrial b.

> b. obstruction
> pericardial b.

baffled jet nebulizer

bag
> Ambu b.
> Douglas b.
> Hope b.
> Lifesaver disposable resuscitator b.
> manual resuscitation b.
> rebreathing b.
> SureGrip breathing b.
> Tedlar b.
> Voorhees b.

bagassosis

BagEasy disposable manual resuscitator

baggy heart

bag-mask ventilation

bagpipe sign

bag-valve-mask (BVM)
> b.-v.-m. ventilation

Bahnson aortic clamp

BAI
> breath-actuated inhaler

Bailey
> B. aortic clamp
> B. aortic valve rongeur
> B. catheter
> B. rib spreader

Bailey-Gibbon rib contractor

Bailey-Glover-O'Neill commissurotomy knife

bailout
> emergency b.
> b. situation
> b. stenting
> b. valvuloplasty

Baim pacing catheter

Bainbridge
> B. effect
> B. reflex

Bair
> B. Hugger
> B. Hugger blanket

baker's asthma

Bakes dilator

BAL
> bronchoalveolar lavage

Baladi Inverter device

balance
> micronutrient b.
> sympathovagal b.
> Wilhelmy b.

balanced coronary circulation

BALF
> bronchoalveolar lavage fluid

Balke
> B. exercise stress test
> B. treadmill protocol

B

Balke-Ware
    B.-W. test
    B.-W. treadmill protocol
Balkin Up and Over contralateral introducer with radiopaque band
ball
    carotid b.
    Esmarch b.
    fibrous b.
    fungus b.
    b. heart valve
    b. mitral commissurotomy
    NC Bandit b.
    parietal b.
    pleural fibrin b.
    b. of Reil
    sinoatrial b.
    b. valve prosthesis
    b. valve thrombus
ball-and-cage, ball-in-cage
    b.-a.-c. prosthesis
    b.-a.-c. prosthetic valve
ballerina-foot pattern
ballet
    cardiac b.
ball-in-cage (*var. of* ball-and-cage)
ballistocardiogram
ballistocardiograph (BCG)
ballistocardiography
ball-occluder valve
balloon
    Accent-DG b.
    ACS Alpha b.
    ACX b.
    b. angioplasty catheter
    b. aortic end-diastolic pressure
      (BAEDP)
    b. aortic valvotomy (BAV)
    b. aortic valvuloplasty (BAV)
    Arrow Berman angiographic b.
    b. atrial septoplasty
    b. atrial septostomy (BAS)
    autoperfusion b.
    AVCO aortic b.
    Bandit b.
    Berman angiographic b.
    Blue Max high-pressure b.
    b. catheter angioplasty (BCA)
    b. catheterization
    b. catheter sealing device
    b. coarctation angioplasty
    compliant b.

    Cook b.
    Cordis Powerflex angioplasty b.
    b. coronary angioplasty
    b. coronary occlusion (BCO)
    b. counterpulsation
    counterpulsation b.
    cutting b.
    Datascope b.
    b. dilation
    b. dilation angioplasty (BDA)
    Dispatch b.
    b. dissector
    b. distention test
    Dynasty b.
    Eliminator dilatation b.
    b. embolectomy catheter
    Express b.
    Extractor three-lumen retrieval b.
    Falcon Omniflex b.
    fixed-wire b.
    Force b.
    Hartzler Micro II b.
    Helix b.
    Hunter-Sessions b.
    b. inflation
    Inoue self-guiding b.
    Integra II b.
    intraaortic b. (IAB)
    14K b.
    Kay b.
    Kontron b.
    b. laser angioplasty
    latex b.
    Lo-Fold b.
    low-profile semi-compliant b.
    Mansfield b.
    Medtronic Evergreen b.
    Micross SL b.
    Microvasive Rigiflex TTS b.
    b. mitral commissurotomy (BMC)
    b. mitral valvuloplasty (BMV)
    Monorail Speedy b.
    Multi-Link Tristar b.
    NC b.
    noncompliant b.
    b. occlusion
    b. occlusive intravascular lysis
      enhanced recanalization
    Olbert b.
    Owens b.
    Panther b.
    PE b.

NOTES

balloon *(continued)*
    Piccolino b.
    pillow-shaped b.
    polyethylene terephthalate b.
    polyolefin copolymer b.
    polyvinyl chloride b.
    Powerflex angioplasty b.
    preperitoneal dilator b. (PDB)
    ProCross Rely b.
    b. pulmonary valvotomy
    b. pulmonary valvuloplasty (BPV)
    b. pump
    QuickFurl SL b.
    radiofrequency hot b.
    Ranger b.
    Raptor PTCA b.
    right ventricular copulsation b. (RVCB)
    b. rupture
    b. septostomy
    b. septostomy catheter
    Shadow b.
    b. shunt
    Simpson PET b.
    Simpson positron emission tomography b.
    sizing b.
    Slalom b.
    Solo b.
    Spears laser b.
    Stack autoperfusion b.
    stealth angioplasty b.
    Surpasse b.
    b. tamponade
    Target Therapeutics Stealth angioplasty b.
    b. test occlusion (BTO)
    trefoil Schneider b.
    b. tricuspid valvotomy
    Tyshak b.
    UltraFuse b.
    b. valvuloplasty (BV)
    b. valvuloplasty catheter
    b. valvuloplasty registry (BVR)
    waisting of b.
    windowed b.
    workhorse b.
balloon-expandable
    b.-e. flexible coil stent
    b.-e. intravascular stent
balloon-flotation pacing catheter
balloon-imaging catheter
ballooning
    b. mitral cusp syndrome
    b. mitral valve syndrome
    b. posterior leaflet syndrome
balloon-occlusion pulmonary angiography
Balloon-on-a-Wire dilatation system
balloon-shaped heart

balloon-tipped
    b.-t. angiographic catheter
    b.-t. flow-directed catheter
    b.-t. thermodilution catheter
Balme cough
Balminil-DM Children
Balminil Expectorant
BALT
    bronchus-associated lymphoid tissue
Baltaxe view
Baltherm catheter
Bamberger
    B. area
    B. bulbar pulse
    B. sign
Bamberger-Marie
    B.-M. disease
    B.-M. syndrome
Bamberger-Pins-Ewart sign
bambuterol
bamiphylline
Bamyl
banana-shaped left ventricle
Bancap HC
bancrofti
    Wuchereria b.
band
    A b.
    b. of adhesion
    atelectatic b.
    atrial anomalous b.
    Balkin Up and Over contralateral introducer with radiopaque b.
    contraction b.
    CPK-BB b.
    CPK-MB b.
    CPK-MM b.
    I b.
    Mach b.
    MB b.
    moderator b.
    myocardial b. (MB)
    parietal b.
    Pepper Medical tube neck b.
    pulmonary artery b.
    b. of Reil
    b. saw effect
    Vesseloops rubber b.
    Z b.
bandage
    compression b.
    Esmarch b.
    b. scissors
bandbox
    b. resonance
    b. sound
banding
    Müller b.
    PA b.

B

pulmonary artery b.
b. of pulmonary artery
Trusler rule for pulmonary
artery b.
Bandit
B. balloon
B. PTCA catheter
bandlike
b. angina
b. intrapericardial echo
bandpass filter
bandwidth
bang artifact
bangungot syndrome
bank
tissue b.
Bannister disease
Bannwarth syndrome
Banophen Oral
BAO
basilar artery occlusion
Bapadin
BAPV
basal average peak velocity
baseline average peak velocity
BAR
beta-adrenergic receptor
Baratol
barbed hook
Barbilixir
barbiturate
barbourin
Bard
B. Clamshell septal occluder
B. Clamshell septal umbrella
B. Commander PTCA guidewire
B. percutaneous cardiopulmonary
support system
B. Safety Excalibur catheter
B. sign
B. Stinger S ablation catheter
B. XT coronary stent
Bardco catheter
Bardenheurer ligation
Bard-Parker blade
bare-metal stent
barium
b. enema
b. esophagram
b. swallow
BARK
beta-adrenergic receptor kinase

barking cough
Barlow syndrome
Barnard
B. mitral valve prosthesis
B. operation
baroceptor
barograph
barometer-maker's disease
barometric pressure
baroreceptor
cardiac b.
carotid b.
perturbed carotid b.
b. reflex
b. reflex sensitivity (BRS)
b. sensitivity
b. sensitization
baroreflex
arterial b. (ABR)
biochemical b.
carotid b.
b. sensitivity (BRS)
sinoatrial b.
baroscope
barosinusitis
barospirator
barotaxis
barotrauma
b. of ascent
dental b.
b. of descent
facial b.
pulmonary b.
Barraya forceps
barrel-hooping compression
barrel-shaped
b.-s. chest
b.-s. thorax
Barrett esophagus
barrier
blood-air b.
blood-brain b. (BBB)
blood-bronchoalveolar b.
blood-bronchus b.
blood-gas b.
blood-retina b.
placental b.
Barrow classification
Barsony-Polgar syndrome
Barthel
B. ADL score
B. index

NOTES

83

Bartholin duct
Barth syndrome
Bartonella
    B. bacilliformis
    B. elizabethae
Bartter syndrome
BAS
    balloon atrial septostomy
    beta-adrenergic stimulation
basal
    b. average peak velocity (BAPV)
    b. cell carcinoma
    b. collateral artery
    b. diastolic murmur
    b. fetal heart rate (BFHR)
    b. ganglia (BG)
    b. heart rate (BHR)
    b. part of left and right inferior pulmonary
    b. segmental bronchus
    b. systolic
    b. tuberculosis
basalis communis
basaloid carcinoma
basal-septal hypertrophy
base
    b. of lung
    whole blood buffer b.
baseline
    b. arrhythmia
    b. artifact
    b. average peak velocity (BAPV)
    B. Dyspnea Index (BDI)
    b. ECG
    b. echocardiography
    b. fetal heart rate
    b. rhythm
    b. shift
    b. ST-segment abnormality
    TP b.
    b. variability
    b. variability of fetal heart rate
    wandering b.
basement membrane
baseplate
    winged b.
BASH
    body acceleration synchronous with heart rate
basic
    b. cardiac life support (BCLS)
    b. cycle length (BCL)
    b. drive cycle length
    b. fibroblast growth factor (bFGF)
    b. life support (BLS)
    b. life support ambulance
    b. life support-defibrillation (BLS-D)
Basidiomycetes

basilar
    b. artery (BA)
    b. artery occlusion (BAO)
    b. half ejection fraction
    b. rale
    b. sinus
basilaris ossis occipitalis
basilic vein
basiliximab
basipharyngeal canal
basis pulmonis
basket
    Medi-Tech multipurpose b.
    pericardial b.
basophil
basophilic vascular streaking
Bassen-Kornzweig abetalipoproteinemia
bath
    film fixer b.
    film wash b.
    fixer b.
    Haake water b.
    Nauheim b.
    wash b.
Ba theorem
bathycardia
bathypnea
Batista
    B. left ventricular reduction procedure
    B. left ventriculectomy procedure
    B. ventricular remodeling
Bato compound
batrachotoxin
Batson plexus
battery
    b. cell impedance
    b. cell voltage function
    Celsa b.
    b. elective replacement
    external pacemaker b.
    LiI b.
    lithium iodine b.
    nickel-cadmium b.
    b. status
    b. voltage
Battey
    B. bacillus
    B. disease
bat wing shadow
Bauer syndrome
baumannii
    Acinetobacter b.
Baumanometer standard mercury sphygmomanometer
Baumes symptom
bauxite
    b. pneumoconiosis
    b. pneumonoconiosis

BAV
  balloon aortic valvotomy
  balloon aortic valvuloplasty
  bicommissural aortic valve
BAVFO
  bradycardia after arteriovenous fistula
    occlusion
Baxter Health Care Continu-Flo
  infusion device
Bayer
    B. Buffered Aspirin
    B. Low Adult Strength
    B. Select Chest Cold Caplets
    B. Select Pain Relief Formula
Bayes theorem
Bayle granulation
Bayliss theory
Baylor
    B. autologous transfusion system
    B. rapid autologous transfusion
    (BRAT)
Bayou virus
Baypress
Bazett
    B. corrected QT interval
    B. correction formula
Bazin disease
BB
  bundle branch
BBB
  blood-brain barrier
  bundle branch block
BBBB
  bilateral bundle branch block
BBM
  brush border membrane
BBMV
  brush border membrane vesicle
BBR
  bundle branch reentry
B&B Trachguard antidisconnection
  device
BCA
  balloon catheter angioplasty
  bidirectional cavopulmonary anastomosis
BCD Plus cardioplegic unit
BCG
  bacille Calmette-Guérin
  ballistocardiograph
  bronchocentric granulomatosis
    BCG vaccine

BCI Capnocheck DualStream
  capnograph
BCKD
  branched chain alpha ketoacid
    dehydrogenase
BCL
  basic cycle length
Bcl-2 expression
BCLS
  basic cardiac life support
BCM
  blood-clotting mechanism
BCO
  balloon coronary occlusion
  biliary cholesterol output
B-complex
    ferrous sulfate, ascorbic acid, and
      vitamin B-c.
BCPR
  bystander cardiopulmonary resuscitation
BCS
  British Cardiac Society
B-D
    Becton-Dickinson
      B-D Potain thoracic trocar
BDA
  balloon dilation angioplasty
BDCS
  Behavioral Dyscontrol Scale
BDG
  bidirectional Glenn procedure
BDI
  Baseline Dyspnea Index
BDT
  bronchodilator
BDW
  biphasic defibrillation waveform
BE
  bacterial endocarditis
bead
    Digoxin RIA B.
beading of arteries
Beall
    B. circumflex artery scissors
    B. disk valve prosthesis
    B. mitral valve prosthesis
    B. prosthetic valve
Beall-Surgitool ball-cage prosthetic valve
beam
    b. splitter
    b. width artifact

NOTES

bean
> castor b.
> green coffee b.

beanbag shotgun round ammunition
bean-spooning task
Bear
> B. 1, 2 adult volume ventilator
> B. Cub infant ventilator
> B. 1000 ventilator

beat
> aberrantly conducted b.
> apex b. (AB)
> Ashman b.
> atrial capture b.
> atrial ectopic b.
> atrial fusion b.
> atrial premature b. (APB)
> atrioventricular junctional escape b.
> auricular premature b.
> automatic b.
> A-V junctional escape b.
> capture b.
> combination b.
> coupled premature b.
> dependent b.
> Dressler b.
> dropped b.
> echo b.
> ectopic Ashman b.
> ectopic junctional b. (EJB)
> ectopic ventricular b.
> entrained b.
> escape b.
> extrasystolic b.
> fascicular b.
> forced b.
> frequency ectopic ventricular b. (FEVB)
> fusion b.
> heart b.
> b. inclusion index (BII)
> interference b.
> interpolated b.
> isolated ectopic b.
> junctional escape b.
> junctional premature b. (JPB)
> Lown class 4a, 4b ventricular ectopic b.
> malignant b.
> missed b.
> mixed b.
> nodal b.
> nodal premature b. (NPB)
> paired b.'s
> parasystolic b.
> b.'s per minute (BPM, bpm)
> b. per second (BPS)
> postextrasystolic b.
> premature b. (PB)

> premature atrial b. (PAB)
> premature junctional b.
> premature nodal b. (PNB)
> premature ventricular b. (PVB)
> pseudofusion b.
> reciprocal b.
> retrograde b.
> salvo of b.'s
> single premature atrial b.
> skipped b.
> summation b.
> supraventricular premature b. (SVPB)
> total heart b.'s (THB)
> unifocal ventricular ectopic b. (UVEB)
> ventricular capture b.
> ventricular ectopic b. (VEB)
> ventricular escape b.
> ventricular fusion b.
> ventricular premature b. (VBP, VPB)
> VP b.

beat-by-beat
> b.-b.-b. capture
> b.-b.-b. hemodynamic monitoring

beat-to-beat
> b.-t.-b. analysis
> b.-t.-b. finger arterial pressure
> b.-t.-b. variability
> b.-t.-b. variability of fetal heart rate

Beatty-Bright friction sound
Beau
> B. asystole
> B. disease
> B. lines
> B. syndrome

Beaver
> B. blade
> B. knife

Beaver-DeBakey blade
BEB
> blind esophageal brushing

BEC
> bacterial endocarditis

Beck
> B. cardiopericardiopexy
> B. Depression Inventory
> B. epicardial poudrage
> B. I, II operation
> B. miniature aortic clamp
> B. triad

Becker disease
Becker-type tardive muscular dystrophy
Beckman
> B. ICS Nephelometer system
> B. O$_2$ analyzer

Beck-Potts aortic and pulmonic clamp

Béclard
  B. anastomosis
  B. hernia
Becloforte
beclomethasone dipropionate
Beclovent Oral Inhaler
Beconase AQ Nasal Inhaler
becquerel (Bq)
Becton-Dickinson (B-D)
  B.-D. guidewire
  B.-D. Teflon-sheathed needle
bed
  adventitial b.
  b. block
  capillary b.
  coronary b.
  cyanosis of nail b.'s
  distal b.
  myocardial b.
  nail b.
  perfusion b.
  pulmonary vascular b.
  Sanders b.
  Stress Echo b.
  time in b.
  vascular b.
  venous capacitance b.
Bedfont
  B. carbon monoxide monitor
  B. EC60 Gastrolyzer hydrogen
    monitor
bedside
  b. balloon atrial septoplasty
  b. monitor
  b. transthoracic echocardiography
beef
  b. insulin
  b. Lente Iletin II
beef-lung heparin
beer
  b. and cobalt syndrome
  b. heart
  B. law
beer-drinker's cardiomyopathy
Beer-Lambert principle
bee venom
beginning-of-life rate
behavior
  contractile b.
  type A, B b.
behavioral
  B. Dyscontrol Scale (BDCS)

  b. factor
  b. therapy
Behçet
  B. disease
  B. syndrome
Béhier-Hardy sign
beigelii
  Trichosporon b.
Belhaussen tachycardia
bell
  b. sound
  b. stethoscope
  b. tympany
Bellavar medical support stockings
belli
  Isospora b.
bell-metal resonance
bellows
  chest b.
  b. function
  b. murmur
  b. sound
Belsey
  B. esophagoplasty
  B. Mark IV fundoplication
  B. two-thirds wrap fundoplication
belt
  abdominal b.
  Alice4 RESP-EZ respiratory
    effort b.
  stroke b.
Belzer solution
Bemis air purifier
Bena-D injection
Benadryl
  B. injection
  B. Oral
  B. Topical
benafentrine
benazepril
  amlodipine and b.
  b. hydrochloride
  b. and hydrochlorothiazide
bendrofluazide
bendroflumethiazide
Benecol margarine
Benedict-Roth
  B.-R. apparatus
  B.-R. spirometer
benefit evaluation (BET)
Bengolea forceps
Benicar

NOTES

benidipine
benign
>   b. croupous angina
>   b. early repolarization (BER)
>   b. fibrous mesothelioma
>   b. intracranial hypertension

benigna
>   endocarditis b.

benignum
>   empyema b.

Benjamin
>   B. binocular laryngoscope
>   B. pediatric laryngoscope

Bennett
>   B. Cascade II Servo Controlled
>   Heated Humidifier
>   B. MA-1, PR-2 ventilator
>   Nellcor Puritan B. (NPB)
>   B. twin

Bentall
>   inclusion technique of B.
>   B. inclusion technique
>   B. operation
>   B. procedure

bent bronchus sign
Bentley
>   B. Duraflo II
>   B. transducer

Benton Lines Test
Bentson
>   B. exchange straight guidewire
>   B. floppy-tip guidewire
>   B. Plus cerebral wire guide

Bentson-Hanafee-Wilson catheter
Bentson-style guidewire
Benylin
>   B. Cough Syrup
>   B. Expectorant
>   B. Pediatric

benzalkonium chloride asthma
benzathine
>   b. benzyl penicillin
>   penicillin G b.

benzoate
>   caffeine and sodium b.

benzocaine, butyl aminobenzoate, tetracaine, and benzalkonium chloride
benzodiazepine
benzonatate
benzoporphyrin
benzothiadiazide
benzothiazepine
benzoylpas
>   calcium b.
>   b. calcium

benzthiazide
benzylpenicillin
benzylpenicilloyl polylysine (PPL)
benzyl-thiourea

bepridil hydrochloride
BER
>   benign early repolarization

beractant
beraprost sodium (BPS)
Berard aneurysm
Berg Balance Scale
Berger operation
Bergmeister papilla
Bergstrom needle biopsy technique
beriberi
>   cerebral b.
>   dry b.
>   b. heart
>   infantile b.
>   wet b.

Berkovits-Castellanos hexapolar electrode
Berlin
>   B. nosology
>   B. TAH
>   B. total artificial heart

Berman
>   B. airway
>   B. angiographic balloon
>   B. angiographic catheter

Bernheim syndrome
Berning and Steensgaard-Hansen score
Bernoulli
>   B. effect
>   B. equation
>   B. theorem

Bernstein
>   B. procedure
>   B. test

Berotec
berry aneurysm
berylliosis
beryllium-induced lung disease
Besnier-Boeck-Schaumann
>   B.-B.-S. disease
>   B.-B.-S. syndrome

BeStent
>   B. 2 coronary stent
>   B. Rival coronary stent system
>   B. Rival stent
>   B. 2 with Discrete Technology
>   coronary stent system

BESTNEB nebulizer
besylate
>   amlodipine b.
>   cisatracurium b.

BET
>   benefit evaluation

beta
>   b. adrenoceptor
>   b. adrenoceptor stimulation
>   b. agonist
>   b. antagonist
>   b. ARK

b. ARK-1
b. AR kinase1 enzyme
b. blockade
b. blocker
b. blocking agent
b. carotene
estrogen receptor b. (ER beta)
b. lactamase
b. lipoprotein
b. ray
b. receptor
b. thromboglobulin

beta-1
b.-1 AR
b.-1B adrenergic receptor (ADRA1B)
b.-1 blocker

beta-1,-2
b.-1,-2 adrenergic stimulation
b.-1,-2 antagonist
b.-1,-2 receptor

beta-2
b.-2 AR
b.-2 AR overexpression
b.-2 integrin MAC-1

beta-adrenergic
b.-a. agonist
b.-a. blockade
b.-a. blocker
b.-a. blocking agent
b.-a. receptor (βAR, BAR)
b.-a. receptor kinase (BARK)
b.-a. stimulation (BAS)

beta-adrenoceptor antibody
beta-adrenoreceptor
b.-a. agonist
b.-a. blocker
b.-a. blocking agent

beta-beta homodimer
beta-blocker therapy
Beta-Cath system
Betacel-Biotronik pacemaker
Betachron ER
beta-endorphin
17-beta-estradiol
transdermal 17-b.-e.

beta-galactosidase
11-beta-hydroxysteroid dehydrogenase
betaine diet
beta-lactam

beta-lactamase
CAZ b.-l.
b.-l. inhibitor

Betaloc Durules
betamethasone
systemic b.

betamethyliodophenyl pentadecanoic acid
beta-MHC
beta-myosin heavy chain
b.-MHC gene

beta-myosin heavy chain (beta-MHC)
Betapace
B. AF tablet
B. Oral

Betapen-VK Oral
beta-radiation
intracoronary b.-r.

Beta-Rail catheter
beta-sitosterol
BetaStent
beta-thalassemia
homozygous -t.

beta-thromboglobulin
b.-t. level
plasma b.-t.

Beta-Tim
betaxolol hydrochloride
bethanechol chloride
bethanidine
Bethea sign
Bettman-Fovash thoracotome
Beuren syndrome
bevantolol
bezafibrate
Bezalip
Bezold-Jarisch reflex
BF
blood flow
breathing frequency
BF large core bronchoscope

BFE
blood flow energy

bFGF
basic fibroblast growth factor

BFHR
basal fetal heart rate

BFR
blood flow rate

BFV
blood flow velocity

BG
basal ganglia

NOTES

BGO
    bismuth germanate
B-H
    bundle of His
        B-H interval
BH
    borderline hypertensive
BHD
    bilateral hemisphere damage
BHF
    British Heart Foundation
BHI
    breath holding index
BHIA
    brain-heart infusion agar
BHIBA
    brain-heart infusion blood agar
BHIRS
    brain-heart infusion and rabbit serum
BHR
    basal heart rate
    borderline hypertensive rat
    bronchial hyperreactivity
    bronchial hyperresponsiveness
BHT
    borderline hypertension
    butylated hydroxytoluene
BI
    brain infarct
Bianchi
    B. nodules
    B. valve
biatrial
    b. enlargement
    b. pacing
biatriatum
    cor pseudotriloculare b.
Biaxin Filmtabs
bibasally
bibasilar
    b. atelectasis
    b. coarse crackle
    b. rale
bible printer's lung
bicalutamide
BICAP
    bilateral circumactive probe
    B. unit
bicarbonate (HCO$_3$)
    sodium b.
bicarbonaturia
Bicarbon Sorin valve
bicardiogram
BiCAT
    bilateral carotid artery traction
bicaval
Bicer-Val prosthetic valve
Bichat tunic

Bicillin
    B. C-R
    B. L-A injection
bicommissural aortic valve (BAV)
Bicor catheter
bicuspid
bicuspidalis
    cuspis anterior valvae b.
bicuspidization
bicycle
    Aerodyne stationary b.
    Collins b.
    b. dynamometer
    b. echocardiography
    b. ergometer exercise stress test
    b. ergometry
    b. exercise
    MedGraphics CPE 2000 electronically braked b.
    stationary b.
    Tredex powered b.
bidimensional echocardiography
bidirectional
    b. cavopulmonary anastomosis (BCA)
    b. cavopulmonary shunt
    b. four-pole Butterworth high-pass digital filter
    b. Glenn operation
    b. Glenn procedure (BDG)
    b. isthmus conduction block
    b. shunt calculation
    b. superior cavopulmonary anastomosis (BSCA)
    b. ventricular
    b. ventricular tachycardia
Bier block anesthesia
Biermer sign
bifascicular
    b. heart block
biferious (*var. of* bisferious)
Bifidobacterium
bifid P wave
bifocal demand DVI pacemaker
bifoil balloon catheter
bifurcated
    b. aortofemoral prosthesis
    b. graft
    b. stent
    b. vein graft for vascular reconstruction
bifurcating block
bifurcatio
    b. tracheae
    b. trunci
bifurcation
    b. of aorta
    aortic b.
    carotid b.

coronary b.
b. lesion (BL)
b. lymph node
b. prosthesis
b. of pulmonary trunk
b. of trachea
tracheal b.
Y-shaped b.
bifurcational coronary lesion
bigemina
    Babesia b.
bigeminal
b. bisferious pulse
b. rhythm
bigeminus
pulsus b.
bigeminy
atrial b.
atrioventricular junctional b.
atrioventricular nodal b.
A-V nodal b.
escape-capture b.
junctional b.
nodal b.
reciprocal b.
rule of b.
ventricular b.
big endothelin
biglycan
BII
beat inclusion index
bil, bilat
bilateral
bilateral (bil, bilat)
b. adrenal hyperplasia
b. anterior flail chest
b. aortoostial coronary artery disease
b. asymmetrical (BA)
b. bundle branch block (BBBB)
b. carotid artery traction (BiCAT)
b. circumactive probe (BICAP)
b. hemisphere damage (BHD)
b. internal mammary artery (BIMA)
b. internal thoracic artery
b. lung transplant (BLT)
b. sequential single lung transplant
b. symmetrical (BS)
bile
b. acid binding resin

b. acid sequestrant
b. solubility test
bileaflet
b. prolapse
b. prosthesis
b. tilting-disk prosthetic valve
bilevel
b. positive airway pressure (BiPAP)
b. positive pressure device
Bilharzia
bilharziasis
biliary
b. cholesterol output (BCO)
b. cirrhosis
b. colic
b. disease
BiliBlanket phototherapy system
Bili mask
bilious pneumonia
bilirubinemia
bilirubin oxidative metabolite
billiard ball effect
Billingham criteria
billowing
cusp b.
b. mitral leaflet syndrome (BMLS)
mitral valve b.
b. mitral valve syndrome
bilobate
bilobectomy
bilobed aneurysm
bilobular
biloculare
cor b.
Biltricide
BIMA
bilateral internal mammary artery
bimanual precordial palpation
Bimodality Lung Oncology Team (BLOT)
binding
albumin cobalt b. (ACB)
antigen b.
fragment antigen-b. (Fab)
guanine nucleotide modulatable b.
ligand b.
table b.
Bing stylet
Bing-Taussig heart procedure
Binswanger disease
binuclear

NOTES

binucleate
bioassay
bioavailability
Biobrane adhesive
BioBypass gene-based drug delivery
　product
Biocef
Biocell RTV implant
biochanin A
biochemical baroreflex
Bioclate
Bioclot protein S assay
biocompatibility
biocompatible stent
Biocontrol Technology/Coratomic lead
Biocor
　　B. 200 high performance
　　　oxygenator
　　B. porcine valve
　　B. softshell venous reservoir
biodegradable stent
Biodex System
BioDiamond
　　B. F stent
　　B. Micro stent
　　B. S rapid exchange PTCA
　　　catheter
BiodivYsio
　　B. added support stent
　　B. AS　PC-coated stent
　　B. OC over-the-wire stent
　　B. open cell stent
　　B. PC stent
　　B. small vessel stent
　　B. SV PC-coated stent
bioelectric
　　b. current
　　b. potential
bioelectricity
bioequivalence
biofeedback
biogenesis
　　mitochondrial b.
BioGlue
　　B. protein-based surgical adhesive
　　B. surgical adhesive for aortic
　　　dissection
　　B. surgical patch
BioGold
biograft
　　Dardik B.
　　B. graft
bioimpedance
　　b. electrocardiograph
　　b. monitor
　　thoracic electrical b. (TEB)
Biolase laser adapter
biologic
　　GenStent b.

biological
　　b. aortic valve
　　b. effects of ionizing Radiation
　　b. fitness
　　b. half-life
biomarker
Biomatrix ocular implant
Bio-Medicus
　　B.-M. arterial catheter
　　B.-M. pump
Bio-Med MVP-10 pediatric ventilator
biomembrane
biondii
　　Magnolia b.
bionic baroreflex system
BioPolyMeric vascular graft
Biopore TM lead
bioprosthesis
　　Carpentier-Edwards Perimount RSR
　　　pericardial b.
　　Freestyle aortic root b.
　　freestyle stentless b.
　　Hancock II porcine b.
　　Hancock M.O. II porcine b.
　　Medtronic Intact porcine b.
　　Mosaic cardiac b.
　　pericarbon b.
　　Perimount RSR pericardial b.
　　porcine b.
　　quadricusp mitral valve b.
　　stentless porcine b.
　　Toronto SPV b.
　　X-Cell cardiac b.
bioprosthetic
　　b. endocarditis
　　b. heart valve
　　b. valve (BPV)
biopsy
　　aspiration b.
　　bite b.
　　bronchial brush b.
　　bronchoscopic lung b. (BLB)
　　bronchoscopic needle b.
　　brush b.
　　catheter-guided b.
　　controlled lung b.
　　cytological b.
　　endomyocardial b. (EMB)
　　endoscopic b.
　　excisional b.
　　fine-needle aspiration b.
　　b. forceps
　　lung b.
　　mediastinal lymph node b.
　　open lung b. (OLB)
　　percutaneous needle aspiration b.
　　percutaneous transthoracic needle b.
　　　(PTNB)

pericardial b.
pleural b.
punch b.
scalene fat pad b.
scalene lymph node b.
supraclavicular lymph node b.
surgical lung b. (SLB)
transbronchial b. (TBB, TBBX, TBBx)
transbronchial lung b. (TBLB)
transcatheter b. (TCB)
transthoracic needle b. (TNB)
transthoracic needle aspiration b.
transvenous b.
ultrasonically guided needle b. (UGNB)
ventricular b.
video-assisted thoracic surgical lung b.
wedge b.

bioptic sampling
bioptome
cardiac b.
Caves-Schultz b.
Cordis b.
Kawai b.
King b.
Konno b.
Mansfield b.
Olympus b.
Scholten endomyocardial b.
Stanford b.

Bio-Pump
biopyrrin
Biorate pacemaker
bioresorbable implant
Biosense
B. left ventricular mapping
B. NOGA catheter-based endocardial mapping system
B. revascularization approach for viable endocardium (BRAVE)

Biosense-guided laser myocardial revascularization
Biosound
B. Genesis II scanning system
B. 2000 II s.a. high-resolution ultrasound
B. 2000 II ultrasound unit
B. 3000 ultrasound unit

BioSource Cytoscreen SAA kit
Biostent

Biosurge Synchronous Autotransfuser
biosynthesis
leukotriene b.
Biot
B. breathing
B. respiration
B. sign
biotin/streptavidin system
Biotrack coagulation monitor
biotransformation
Biotronik
B. lead
B. lead connector
B. pacemaker
Bio-Vascular prosthetic valve
BI-OX III ear oximeter
BioZ
B. hemodynamic monitoring system
B. ICG Module
B. ICG Monitor
B. impedance cardiography technology
B. noninvasive cardiac function monitoring system

BioZ.com cardiac output monitor
BioZ.pc system
BioZ.sim ICG Stimulator
BioZtect sensor
BIP
bronchiolitis with interstitial pneumonitis
BiPAP
bilevel positive airway pressure
BiPAP duet system
BiPAP S/T-D 30 system
BiPAP S/T-D ventilatory support system
BiPAP unit
BiPAP Vision system
biperiden
biphasic
b. defibrillation waveform (BDW)
b. mesothelioma
b. response
b. shock
b. stridor
b. waveform
b. waveform transthoracic defibrillation
biplanar tomography
biplane
b. aortography
b. area-length method

NOTES

biplane *(continued)*
 b. fluoroscopy
 b. formula
 b. imaging
 b. orthogonal angiography
 b. pelvic arteriography
 b. quantitative coronary arteriography
 b. ventriculography

bipolar
 b. catheter
 b. circumactive probe
 b. coagulating forceps
 b. electrocardiogram (BPEC)
 b. esophageal recording
 b. generator
 b. pacemaker
 b. radiofrequency surgical ablation instrument

BiPort hemostasis introducer sheath kit
Biquin Durules
Birbeck granules
bird
 B. Ascension ventilator
 b. breeder's lung
 b. fancier's lung
 b. fever
 b.'s nest lesion
 b.'s nest vena cava filter
 b.'s nest vena cava filter
 B. sign
 B. VDR ventilator

bird's-eye catheter
birefringence
birminghamensis
 Legionella b.
birth control pill
bis-chloromethylether
bis(chloromethyl) ether
bisferiens
 pulsus b.
bisferient
bisferious, biferious
 b. pulse
bishop
 b.'s hat
 b.'s nod
 B. sphygmoscope
bishydroxycoumarin
bismesylate
 almitrine b., almitrine bimesylate
bismuth
 b. germanate (BGO)
 b. subsalicylate
Bisolvon
bisoprolol
 b. fumarate
 b. and hydrochlorothiazide
Bisping electrode

bistoury
 Jackson b.
bisulfate
 clopidogrel b.
bitartrate
 hydrocodone b.
 metaraminol b.
 norepinephrine b.
bite
 b. biopsy
 b. block
biteblock, bite block
bitolterol mesylate
Bitpad digitizer
BIVAD (*var. of* BVAD)
bivalirudin
bivalve
biventricular
 b. assist device (BVAD, BIVAD)
 b. direct cardiac compression
 b. dysfunction
 b. endomyocardial fibrosis
 b. hypertrophy (BVH)
 b. pacing
 b. pacing wire
 b. support (BVS)
Bivona
 B. Fome-Cuff tube
 B. TTS tracheostomy tube
bizarre QRS complex
Bizzari-Guiffrida laryngoscope
Björk method of Fontan procedure
Björk-Shiley (B-S)
 B.-S. aortic valve prosthesis
 B.-S. convexoconcave (BSCC)
 B.-S. convexoconcave 60-degree valve prosthesis
 B.-S. convexoconcave disk prosthetic valve
 B.-S. floating disk prosthesis
 B.-S. graft
 B.-S. heart valve holder
 B.-S. heart valve sizer
 B.-S. mitral valve
 B.-S. monostrut valve
BL
 bifurcation lesion
 buffered lidocaine
black
 b. blood magnetic resonance imaging
 B. Creek Canal virus
 b. lung
 b. lung disease
 b. phthisis
 b. pleura
 b. pleura sign
 b. tea
 b. widow spider venom

Blackfan-Diamond syndrome
blackfoot disease
Blackman window
blackout
    shallow water b.
    b. spell
black-white interface technique
blade
    Acra-Cut Spiral craniotome b.
    b. atrial septostomy
    Bard-Parker b.
    Beaver b.
    Beaver-DeBakey b.
    CLM articulating laryngoscope b.
    b. control wire holder
    DeBakey b.
    electrosurgical b.
    knife b.
    Lite B.
    Macintosh b.
    Miller b.
    RAD airway laryngeal b.
    rotating b.'s
    b. septostomy catheter
    straight b.
Blake exercise stress test
Blalock-Hanlon
    B.-H. atrial septectomy
    B.-H. operation
Blalock pulmonary stenosis clamp
Blalock-Taussig (BT)
    B.-T. operation
    B.-T. procedure
    B.-T. shunt (BTS)
blanche
    tache b.
blanch test
bland
    b. diet
    b. edema
    b. embolism
Bland-Altman method
Bland-Garland-White syndrome
blanket
    Bair Hugger b.
    bronchial mucus b.
    circulating water b.
    cooling b.
    hypothermia b.
blanking
    b. period

    postventricular atrial b. (PVAB)
    total atrial b. (TAB)
blast
    b. chest
    b. lung
    b. wave
blastoma
    pleuropulmonary b.
    pulmonary b.
Blastomyces dermatitidis
blastomycosis
    North American b.
Blazer RPM navigation and ablation catheter
BLB
    bronchoscopic lung biopsy
        BLB oxygen mask
BLE
    buffered lidocaine with epinephrine
bleb
    apical pleural b.
    emphysematous b.
    pleural b.
    sarcolemmal b.
    b. stapling
bleeding
    arterial b.
    back-b.
    cerebral b.
    b. diathesis
    extraparenchymal b.
    b. globe
    microvascular b. (MVB)
    b. time (BLT, Blx, BT)
blender
    Virtis b.
blending
    sensor b.
blennothorax
Blenoxane
bleomycin sulfate
BLES
    bovine lavage extract surfactant
blind
    b. coronary dimple
    b. cul-de-sac
    b. esophageal brushing (BEB)
    b. thoracentesis
bloater
    blue b.
bloc
    heart-lung b.

B

NOTES

95

Blocadren Oral
Bloch equation
block
    alveolar-capillary b.
    anatomic b.
    antegrade b.
    anterograde b.
    arborization b.
    atrial tachycardia with b. (ATB)
    atrioventricular b. (AVB)
    atrioventricular junctional heart b.
    atrioventricular node b.
    A-V branch b.
    A-V groove b.
    AV node b.
    A-V Wenckebach b.
    axillary b.
    bed b.
    bidirectional isthmus conduction b.
    bifascicular heart b.
    bifurcating b.
    bilateral bundle branch b. (BBBB)
    bite b.
    bundle branch b. (BBB)
    complete A-V b.
    complete heart b. (CHB)
    complete right bundle branch b.
      (CRBBB)
    conduction b.
    congenital complete heart b.
    congenital heart b. (CHB)
    congenital symptomatic A-V b.
    connector b.
    b. cycle length
    diffuse intraventricular b.
    divisional heart b.
    entrance b.
    exit b.
    familial atrioventricular b.
    fascicular heart b.
    first-degree A-V b.
    first-degree heart b.
    focal b.
    functional b.
    heart b. (HB)
    3:1 heart b.
    3:2 heart b.
    heparin b.
    His bundle heart b.
    incomplete atrioventricular b.
    incomplete bilateral bundle
      branch b. (IBBBB)
    incomplete left bundle branch b.
      (ILBBB)
    incomplete right bundle branch b.
      (IRBBB)
    infrahisian b.
    interatrial b.
    intercostal nerve b.

    intraatrial b.
    intrahisian b.
    intraventricular b. (IVB)
    left anterior bundle branch b.
      (LABBB)
    left bundle branch b.
    left bundle branch system b.
      (LBBsB)
    Luciani-Wenckebach
      atrioventricular b.
    Mobitz first-degree b.
    Mobitz second-degree b.
    Mobitz type I, II
      atrioventricular b.
    nonspecific intraventricular b.
    paraffin b.
    partial heart b.
    periinfarction b.
    Perspex b.
    protective b.
    protoplasmic b.
    pseudo-A-V b.
    rate-dependent bundle branch b.
    retrograde b.
    right bundle-branch b. (RBBB)
    right bundle branch system b.
      (RBBsB)
    second-degree A-V b.
    second-degree heart b.
    shock b.'s
    sinoatrial b. (SAB)
    sinoatrial entrance b. (SAEB)
    sinoatrial exit b.
    sinoauricular b.
    sinus exit b.
    subjunctional heart b.
    suprahisian b.
    third-degree atrioventricular b.
    third-degree A-V b.
    third-degree heart b.
    total atrioventricular b. (TAVB)
    transient heart b.
    trifascicular b.
    unidirectional b.
    unifascicular b.
    vagal b.
    ventricular b.
    voltage-dependent b.
    Wenckebach atrioventricular b.
    Wenckebach A-V b.
    Wenckebach exit b.
    Wenckebach periodicity b.
    Wilson b.
blockade
    aggressive platelet b.
    alpha-1 adrenoceptor b.
    angiotensin II receptor b.
    beta b.
    beta-adrenergic b.

left stellate ganglionic b. (LSGB)
neuromuscular b.
platelet glycoprotein IIb/IIIa b.
reuptake b.
sodium channel b.
stellate ganglion b.

blocked
b. APC
b. fascicle
b. heart artery
b. pleurisy

blocker
adrenoceptor b.
aldosterone-receptor b.
alpha-adrenergic b.
alpha-adrenoreceptor b.
angiotensin II receptor b. (ARB)
beta b.
beta-1 b.
beta-adrenergic b.
beta-adrenoreceptor b.
calcium-channel b. (CCB)
calcium entry b.
ganglionic b.
integrin b.
L-type calcium b.
platelet glycoprotein IIb/IIIa b.
renin-angiotensin b.
selectin b.
slow-channel b.
sodium-channel b.

blocking
b. vagal afferent fiber
b. vagal efferent fiber

Blom-Singer valve
blood
arterial b. (a)
arterialized capillary b. (ACB)
artificial b.
autologous b.
b. cardioplegia
b. cast
b. clot
b. column
b. count
b. dyscrasia
b. expander
b. flow (BF)
b. flow energy (BFE)
b. flow enhancement device
b. flow measurement
b. flowmeter

b. flow rate (BFR)
b. flow reserve
b. flow velocity (BFV)
Fluosol artificial b.
frank b.
b. gas
1620 b. gas analyzer
840 b. gas analyzer
b. gas sensor
mixed venous b.
b. monocyte stimulation
b. murmur
b. oxygen
b. oxygenation level-dependent
(BOLD)
b. oxygenation level-dependent
technique
b. oxygen level
oxygen saturation of hemoglobin of
arterial b.
b. patch injection
b. perfusion
b. perfusion monitor (BPM, bpm)
b. platelet thrombus
b. plate thrombus
b. pool
b. pressure (bl pr, BP, B/P)
b. pressure assembly (BPA)
b. pressure cuff (BPC)
b. pressure decrease (BPD)
b. pressure gauge (BPG)
b. pressure increase (BPI)
b. pressure index (BPI)
b. pressure, left arm (BPLA)
b. pressure and pulse (BP&P)
b. pressure recorder (BPR)
b. pressure, right arm (BPRA)
b. pump
b. replacement
b. sampling
b. sampling instrument
shear rate of b.
shunted b.
sludged b.
tonometered whole b.
b. urea nitrogen (BUN)
venous b. (VB)
b. vessel (BV)
b. vessel invasion (BVI)
b. vessel prosthesis (BVP)
b. viscosity (BlV)
b. volume (BLV, BlV)

NOTES

B

blood (*continued*)
    b. volume distribution
    b. volume expander (BVE)
    b. volume pulse (BVP)
    b. warmer
blood-air barrier
blood-borne infectious agent
blood-brain barrier (BBB)
blood-bronchoalveolar barrier
blood-bronchus barrier
blood-clot lysis time (BLT)
blood-clotting mechanism (BCM)
blood-flow probe
blood-gas barrier
bloodless phlebotomy
bloodletting
blood-pool imaging
blood-retina barrier
bloodstream infection
blood-tinged sputum
Bloodwell forceps
bloody
    b. effusion
    b. sputum
    b. tap
Bloom
    B. programmable stimulator
    B. syndrome
blooming
    b. artifact
    b. effect
BLOT
    Bimodality Lung Oncology Team
blot
    Northern b.
    slot b.
    Southern b.
    b. test
    Western b.
blow
    b. bottle
    diastolic b.
blow-by
    b.-b. oxygen
    b.-b. ventilator
blowing
    b. murmur
    b. wound
bl pr
    blood pressure
BLS
    basic life support
BLS-D
    basic life support-defibrillation
BLT
    bilateral lung transplant
    bleeding time
    blood-clot lysis time
blubbery diastolic murmur

blue
    b. asphyxia
    b. baby
    b. bloater
    code b. (CB)
    b. Cook sheath
    b. disease
    Evans b.
    b. finger syndrome
    B. FlexTip catheter
    B. Line cuffed endotracheal tube
    B. Max high-pressure balloon
    methylene b.
    b. phlebitis
    b. sclera
    Sulphan B.
    b. toe syndrome
    b. velvet syndrome
Blumenau test
Blumenthal lesion
blunt
    b. cardiac rupture
    b. chest impact-induced cardiac arrest
    b. chest injury
    b. chest trauma
    b. dissection
    b. eversion
    b. eversion carotid endarterectomy
    b. pulmonary injury
    b. thoracic trauma
    b. torso injury
blunted
    b. costophrenic angle
    b. ejection fraction
    b. exercise response
    b. systolic pulmonary venous flow
    b. systolic velocity
    b. waveform
blunting
    apical b.
    nocturnal cardiovascular b.
blush
    capillary b.
    myocardial b.
    b. phenomenon
    tumor b.
BLV
    blood volume
BlV
    blood viscosity
    blood volume
Blx
    bleeding time
BMC
    balloon mitral commissurotomy
    bone mineral content
BME
    brief maximal effort

BMI
body mass index
BMLS
billowing mitral leaflet syndrome
B-mode
B-m. echocardiography
B-m. ultrasonography
B-m. ultrasound
BMP-2
bone morphogenetic protein type 2
BMPR
bone morphogenetic protein receptor
BMR-4500SG sealed hard shell venous reservoir with Duraflo
BMST
Bruce maximum stress test
BMV
balloon mitral valvuloplasty
BNA
bronchoscopic needle aspiration
BNA-100-Behring Diagnostics immunonephelometric assay
BNP
brain natriuretic peptide
B-type natriuretic peptide
BO
bronchiolitis obliterans
boat-shaped heart
Bobath
B. exercise
B. physiotherapy approach
Bochdalek hernia
Bock ganglion
Bodai adapter
body
b. acceleration synchronous with heart rate (BASH)
aortic b.
Arantius b.
b. of Arantius
artificial b.
asbestos b.'s
Aschoff b.
aspiration of foreign b.
asteroid b.
Auer b.
Babes-Ernst b.
b. box method
Bracht-Wächter b.'s
carotid b. (CB)
central fibrous b.
creola b.

b. density analysis
Döhle inclusion b.'s
b. fat
ferruginous b.
fibrous b.
foreign b.
Gamna-Gandy b.'s
gelatin compression b.
Gordon elementary b.
Heinz b.
LCL b.'s
b. mass index (BMI)
Masson b.
Medlar b.
multilamellar b.
Negri b.
neuroepithelial b.
b. packer
paraaortic b.'s
b. of phalanx
b. plethysmograph
b. position
psammoma b.'s
psittacosis inclusion b.'s
b. surface area (BSA)
b. surface laplacian mapping (BSLM)
thoracic vertebral b.
tracheobronchial foreign b.
vagal b.
Weibel-Palade b.'s
Zuckerkandl b.'s
bodybuilder electromechanical criteria
Boeck
B. disease
B. sarcoid
Boehringer
B. Mannheim standard
B. suction regulator
Boerema hernia repair
Boerhaave
B. syndrome
B. tear
Boettcher forceps
Bogalusa criteria
boggy edema
Bogros space
Bohr
B. effect
B. equation
B. formula
B. isopleth method

B

NOTES

bois
> bruit de b.

BOLD
> blood oxygenation level-dependent
> BOLD technique

bolometer

bolster
> Teflon felt b.

Boltzmann distribution

bolus
> b. cardiac output calculation
> b. intravenous injection
> b. of medication
> b. tracking

bombesin

bond
> soldered b.

bone
> fibrous dysplasia of b.
> lingual b.
> b. marrow aplasia
> b. marrow embolism
> b. marrow injection
> b. marrow transplant
> b. mineral content (BMC)
> b. morphogenetic protein receptor (BMPR)
> b. morphogenetic protein type 2 (BMP-2)
> Paget disease of b.

Bonferroni
> B. correction
> B. method

boning
> dog b.

bony heart

Bonzel Monorail balloon catheter

bookeri
> *Alcaligenes b.*

Bookwalter retractor

booming rumble

BOOP
> bronchiolitis obliterans with organizing pneumonia

booster heart

boot
> Bunny b.
> Circulator b.
> compression b.
> Cryo/Cuff pressure b.
> gelatin compression b.
> IPC b.'s
> PNS Unna b.
> sheepskin b.

Boothby-Lovelace-Bulbulian oxygen mask

boot-shaped heart

bootstrap
> b. dilation

> b. two-vessel angioplasty
> b. two-vessel technique

border
> b. of cardiac dullness
> endocardial cardiac b.
> epicardial cardiac b.
> b. rale
> sternal b.

borderline
> b. cardiomegaly
> b. ECG
> b. hypertension (BHT)
> b. hypertensive (BH)
> b. hypertensive rat (BHR)

Bordetella pertussis

Bordet-Gengou
> B.-G. bacillus
> B.-G. test

Borg
> B. category-ratio
> B. dyspnea rating
> B. numerical scale
> B. rating of perceived exertion
> B. rating of perceived exertion scale
> B. scale (1-20)
> B. treadmill exertion scale

Born aggregometry

Bornholm disease

Borrelia burgdorferi

borreliosis
> Lyme b.

Borst side-arm introducer set

BOS
> bronchiolitis obliterans syndrome

Bosch ERG 500 ergometer

bosentan

Bostock
> B. catarrh
> B. disease

Botallo duct

both ventricles inhibited (VDI)

botryomycosis
> pulmonary b.

Böttcher space

bottle
> blow b.
> Castaneda b.
> Plasma-Plex b.
> b. sound

bottleneck stenosis

botulinum
> *Clostridium b.*

Bouchut respiration

bougie
> EndoLumina illuminated b.

bougienage
> esophageal b.

Bouillaud
    B. disease
    B. sign
    B. tinkle
bound
    creatine kinase, myocardial b.
    (CKMB)
bounding pulse
bouquet of vessels
Bourassa catheter
Bourdon gauge
Bourns-Bear ventilator
Bourns infant ventilator
Bouveret disease
Bovie electrocautery
bovine
    b. aortic endothelial cell (BAEC)
    b. aortic endothelium (BAE)
    b. heart
    b. heart valve
    b. heterograft
    b. lavage extract surfactant (BLES)
    pegademase b.
    b. pericardial valve
    b. pericardium strip
    b. serum antigen
bovinum
    cor b.
bovis
    Actinomyces b.
    Babesia b.
    Mycobacterium b.
Bowditch
    B. law
    B. phenomenon
    B. staircase effect
bowing
    leftward ventricular septal b.
    (LVSB)
    b. of mitral valve leaflet
box
    b. plot
    SunBox light b.
box-and-whisker plot
Boyce sign
Boyd
    B. perforating vein
    B. point
Boydens chamber
boydii
    Petriellidium b.
    Pseudallescheria b.

Boyle
    B. Gay-Lusac law
bozemanii
    Legionella b.
Bozzolo sign
BP
    blood pressure
    British Pharmacopoeia
    bronchopulmonary
    bypass
        BP fistula
B/P
    blood pressure
BPA
    blood pressure assembly
BPC
    blood pressure cuff
BPD
    blood pressure decrease
    bronchopulmonary dysplasia
BPEC
    bipolar electrocardiogram
BPG
    blood pressure gauge
    bypass graft
BPI
    blood pressure increase
    blood pressure index
BPLA
    blood pressure, left arm
BPM, bpm
    beats per minute
    blood perfusion monitor
BP&P
    blood pressure and pulse
BPR
    blood pressure recorder
BPRA
    blood pressure, right arm
BPS
    beat per second
    beraprost sodium
    breaths per second
    systolic blood pressure
BPSA
    bronchopulmonary segmental artery
BPV
    balloon pulmonary valvuloplasty
    bioprosthetic valve
BPXG body plethysmograph
Bq
    becquerel

B

NOTES

BR
   breathing reserve
   bronchial responsiveness
brachial
   b. arteriogram
   b. arteriotomy
   b. artery
   b. artery approach
   b. artery cutdown
   b. artery pressure (BrAP)
   b. artery thrombosis
   b. bypass
   b. catheter
   b. dance
   b. nerve
   b. plexopathy
   b. plexus
   b. plexus injury
   b. plexus tension test
   b. pulse
   b., radial, femoral (BRAFE)
   b. syndrome
   b. vein
brachial-ankle index
brachioaxillary bridge graft fistula
brachiocephalic
   b. arteritis
   b. artery
   b. ischemia
   b. system
   b. trunk
   b. vein
   b. vessel angioplasty
brachiocephalicus
   truncus b.
brachiogram
brachiosubclavian bridge graft fistula
Bracht-Wächter
   B.-W. bodies
   B.-W. lesion
brachycardia
brachytherapy
   endobronchial b.
   vascular b.
Bradbury-Eggleston syndrome
Bradshaw-O'Neill aorta clamp
Brady, brady
   bradycardia
bradyarrhythmia
bradyarrhythmic arrest
bradycardia (Brady, brady)
   b. after arteriovenous fistula
     occlusion (BAVFO)
   apnea and b. (A&B)
   artifactual b.
   atrial b.
   Branham b.
   cardiomuscular b.
   central b.

   clinostatic b.
   essential b.
   fetal b.
   idiopathic b.
   idioventricular b.
   junctional b.
   nodal b.
   b. pacing support
   postinfectious b.
   postinfective b.
   pulseless b.
   sinoatrial b.
   sinus b. (SB)
   vagal b.
   ventricular b.
bradycardia-dependent aberrancy
bradycardia-tachycardia (brady-tachy)
   b.-t. syndrome
bradycrotic
bradydactyly
bradydiastole
brady down
bradydysrhythmia (*var. of*
  bradyrhythmia)
bradykinin perfusion
bradykinin-stimulated cells
bradypnea
bradyrhythmia, bradydysrhythmia
bradysphygmia
brady-tachy
   bradycardia-tachycardia
   b.-t. syndrome (BTS)
BRAFE
   brachial, radial, femoral
   BRAFE approach for elective
     coronary stent implantation
Bragg-Paul respirator
braid-like lesion
brain
   b. aneurysm
   b. band enzyme of CPK (CPK-
     BB)
   b. death
   b. infarct (BI)
   b. murmur
   b. natriuretic peptide (BNP)
   b. stem stroke
   b. wave
brain-heart
   b.-h. infusion
   b.-h. infusion agar (BHIA)
   b.-h. infusion blood agar (BHIBA)
   b.-h. infusion and rabbit serum
     (BHIRS)
branch
   atrioventricular circumflex b.
     (AVCx)
   bundle b. (BB, BUN br)
   descending anterior b.

descending posterior b.
esophageal b.
jailed side b.
left anterior descending b. (LADB)
left bundle b. (LBB)
left coronary circumflex b. (LCXB)
b. lesion
lingual b.
marginal b. #1
obtuse marginal b. (OMB)
pharyngeal b.
posterolateral circumflex b. (PLCx)
b. pulmonary artery stenosis
b. retinal artery occlusion (BRAO)
b. retinal vein occlusion (BRVO)
right bundle b. (RBB)
b.'s of segmental bronchi
septal perforator b.
side b.
tracheal b.
b. vein occlusion (BVO)
b. vessel occlusion
b. vessel pruning
branched (b)
    b. chain alpha ketoacid
      dehydrogenase (BCKD)
branching
    airway b.
    mirror-image brachiocephalic b.
branchiogenic
branchiomere
branchiomerism
branchiomotor
Branham
    B. bradycardia
    B. sign
Branhamella catarrhalis
BRAO
    branch retinal artery occlusion
BRAP
    burst of rapid atrial pacing
BrAP
    brachial artery pressure
Brasdor method
Brasfield chest radiograph score
brash
    water b.
brasiliensis
    Nocardia b.
    Paracoccidioides b.
brassy cough

BRAT
    Baylor rapid autologous transfusion
    BRAT system
Brauer cardiolysis
Braunwald
    B. classification I–IIIB
    B. sign
BRAVE
    Biosense revascularization approach for
      viable endocardium
brawny edema
braziliense
    Ancylostoma b.
bread-and-butter
    b.-a.-b. pericardium
    b.-a.-b. textbook sign
Breas PV10 CPAP device
breast
    b. artifact
    b. pang
    thrush b.
breath
    b. excretion test
    exercise-induced shortness of b.
    b. holding
    b. holding index (BHI)
    b. holding test
    b. marker
    b. pentane test
    shortness of b. (SB, SOB)
    b. sound
    b. stacking
breath-actuated inhaler (BAI)
breather
    The Sports b.
Breathe Right nasal strip
breathhold
    b. maneuver
    b. turbo-flash tagged imaging
breathing
    apneustic b.
    b. bag sign
    Biot b.
    bronchial b.
    Cheyne-Stokes b.
    controlled b.
    controlled diaphragmatic b. (CDBR)
    b. exercise
    b. frequency (BF)
    frog b.
    glossopharyngeal b.

B

NOTES

breathing *(continued)*
    intermittent positive pressure b. (IPPB)
    Kussmaul b.
    Ondine b.
    oxygen cost of b.
    b. pacemaker
    periodic b.
    positive-negative pressure b. (PNPB)
    pursed-lip b.
    b. reserve (BR)
    resting tidal b.
    RfB System-I for controlled diaphragmatic b.
    shallow b.
    sign mechanism for ventilator b.
    sleep-disordered b. (SDB)
    b. technique
    tidal b.
    work of b. (WOB)
breath-methylated alkane contour
breaths per second (BPS)
Brechenmacher fiber
Brecher and Cronkite technique
Breeze E150 ventilation system
bregmocardiac reflex
Brehmer treatment
Bremer AirFlo Vest
brequinar sodium
Brescia-Cimino A-V fistula
Breslow-Day test for homogeneity
Brethaire Inhalation Aerosol
Brethine
    B. injection
    B. Oral
Bretonneau angina
Bretschneider-HTK cardioplegic solution
Brett syndrome
Bretylate
bretylium
    b. infusion
    b. loading
    b. therapy
    b. tosylate
Breuer-Hering
    B.-H. deflation index
    B.-H. inflation reflex
Brevibloc injection
Brevital
Bricanyl
    B. injection
    B. Turbohaler
bridge
    arteriolovenular b.
    cytoplasmic b.
    disulfide b.
    muscle b.
    myocardial b.

    Wheatstone b.
    B. X3 renal stent system
bridging
    b. collateral
    muscular b.
    myocardial b. (MB)
brief maximal effort (BME)
bright
    B. disease
    b. echo
    B. murmur
brightness modulation
Brilliant lead
Brill-Zinsser disease
B-ring
    esophageal B-r.
Brisbane method
brisk wall motion abnormality
Brite Tip catheter
British
    B. Cardiac Society (BCS)
    B. Heart Foundation (BHF)
    B. Pharmacopoeia (BP)
brittle
    b. asthma
    b. asthmatic
BRK series transseptal needle
broadband ultrasound attenuation (BUA)
Broadbent inverted sign
broad QRS complex
Brock
    B. infundibulectomy
    B. operation
    B. procedure
    B. syndrome
Brockenbrough
    B. atrial septoplasty
    B. atrial stenting
    B. curved needle
    B. effect
    B. sign
    B. technique
    B. transseptal commissurotomy
Brockenbrough-Braunwald-Morrow sign
Brockenbrough-Braunwald sign
brocresine
Broders index
Brodie abscess
Brodie-Trendelenburg tourniquet test
Brodmann
    B. area 7, 9, 24, 40
Bromanate DC
Bromanyl Cough Syrup
bromazepam
Bromfed
bromhexine hydrochloride
bromide
    ethidium b.

hydrogen b.
ipratropium b.
methyl b.
oxitropium b.
pancuronium b.
pipecuronium b.
tiotropium b.
bromocriptine
bromodiphenhydramine and codeine
Bromotuss w/Codeine Cough Syrup
brompheniramine, phenylpropanolamine, and codeine
Brompton
    B. cocktail
    B. solution
Brom repair
Bronalide
broncatar
bronchadenitis, bronchoadenitis
bronchi (*pl. of* bronchus)
bronchia (*pl. of* bronchium)
bronchial
    b. adenoma
    b. allergy
    b. arteriography
    b. artery
    b. artery embolization (BAE)
    b. asthma
    b. atresia
    b. breathing
    b. breath sounds
    b. brush biopsy
    b. brushings
    b. bud
    b. calculus
    b. carcinoma
    b. challenge test
    b. collateral
    b. collateral artery murmur
    b. crisis
    b. cyst
    b. dehiscence
    b. disruption
    b. epithelial cell
    b. fremitus
    b. gland
    b. hyperreactivity (BHR)
    b. hyperresponsiveness (BHR)
    b. inflammatory polyp
    b. lavage
    b. lumen
    b. marking

b. meniscus sign
b. microflora
b. mucous membrane
b. mucus blanket
b. mucus inhibitor
b. pneumonia
b. provocation
b. provocation test
b. rale
b. respiration
b. responsiveness (BR)
b. sarcoidosis
b. sleeve resection
b. smooth muscle
b. smooth muscle tone
b. spasm
b. stenosis
b. stump
b. stump failure
b. synechia
b. toilet
b. tree
b. tube
b. vein
b. washings
b. washings cytology
b. wheezing
bronchiales
    rami b.
    venae b.
bronchiectasia sicca
bronchiectasis
    chemical b.
    cylindrical b.
    cystic b.
    dry b.
    follicular b.
    fusiform b.
    pseudocylindrical b.
    saccular b.
    suppurative b.
    traction b.
bronchiectatic
    b. cavity
    b. rale
bronchiloquy
bronchiocele
bronchiogenic
bronchiolar
    b. adenocarcinoma
    b. carcinoma

NOTES

bronchiolar *(continued)*
   b. exocrine cell
   b. inflammatory infiltrate
bronchiole
   alveolar b.
   respiratory b.
   terminal b.
bronchiole-alveolar communication
bronchiolectasis, bronchiolectasia
   traction b.
bronchioli (*pl. of* bronchiolus)
bronchiolitis
   acute obliterating b.
   constrictive b.
   b. exudativa
   exudative b.
   b. fibrosa obliterans
   follicular b.
   infectious b.
   b. obliterans (BO)
   b. obliterans syndrome (BOS)
   b. obliterans with organizing
    pneumonia (BOOP)
   obliterative b. (OB)
   proliferative b.
   respiratory b. (RB)
   vesicular b.
   viral b.
   b. with interstitial pneumonitis
    (BIP)
bronchioloalveolar
   b. adenocarcinoma
   b. carcinoma (BAC)
bronchiolocentric
bronchiolopulmonary
bronchiolus, pl. **bronchioli**
   b. terminalis
bronchiomediastinalis
   truncus lymphaticus b.
bronchiorum
   tunica muscularis b.
bronchiostenosis
bronchitic
bronchitis
   acute bacterial exacerbation of
    chronic b. (ABECB)
   acute exacerbation of chronic b.
   acute laryngotracheal b.
   arachidic b.
   asthmatic b.
   capillary b.
   Castellani b.
   catarrhal b.
   cheesy b.
   chemical b.
   chronic asthmatic b.
   chronic obstructive b.
   croupous b.
   dry b.

   epidemic capillary b.
   ether b.
   exudative b.
   fibrinous b.
   hemorrhagic b.
   infectious asthmatic b.
   mechanic's b.
   membranous b.
   nonasthmatic eosinophilic b.
   obliterative b.
   phthinoid b.
   plastic b.
   polypoid b.
   productive b.
   pseudomembranous b.
   putrid b.
   secondary b.
   b. sicca
   simple chronic b.
   smoker's b.
   staphylococcal b.
   streptococcal b.
   suffocative b.
   vegetal b.
   verminous b.
   vesicular b.
   wheezy b.
   winter b.
Bronchitrac L flexible suction catheter
bronchium, pl. **bronchia**
bronchoadenitis (*var. of* bronchadenitis)
bronchoalveolar
   b. carcinoma
   b. lavage (BAL)
   b. lavage fluid (BALF)
   b. washings
bronchoalveolitis
bronchoaspergillosis
bronchoblastomycosis
bronchoblennorrhea
bronchocandidiasis
**Broncho-Cath double-lumen endotracheal
   tube**
bronchocavernous respiration
bronchocele
bronchocentric granulomatosis (BCG)
bronchoconstriction
   hyperpnea-induced b. (HIB)
   reflex vagal b.
bronchoconstrictive effect
bronchoconstrictor
bronchodilating agent
bronchodilation, bronchodilatation
bronchodilator (BDT)
   b. administration
   aerosolized b.
   anticholinergic b.
   b. effect
   inhaled b.

Marax b.
nebulized b.
b. response
b. therapy
bronchoedema
bronchoegophony
bronchoesophageal muscle
bronchoesophageus
musculus b.
bronchoesophagoscopy
bronchofiberscope
bronchogenic
b. adenocarcinoma
b. carcinoma
b. cyst
bronchogram
air b.
tantalum b.
bronchography
Cope method b.
inhalation b.
percutaneous transtracheal b.
broncholith
broncholithiasis
bronchomalacia
bronchomediastinal lymphatic trunk
bronchomotor
bronchophony
pectoriloquous b.
sniffling b.
whispered b.
bronchopleural fistula
bronchopleuromediastinal fistulectomy
bronchopleuropneumonia
bronchopneumonia
acute hemorrhagic b.
confluent b.
diffuse b.
focal b.
hemorrhagic b.
hypostatic b.
necrotizing b.
sequestration b.
subacute b.
tuberculous b.
virus b.
bronchopneumonic infiltrate
bronchopneumonitis
bronchoprovocation test
bronchopulmonale
segmentum b.

bronchopulmonales
nodi lymphoidei b.
bronchopulmonary (BP)
b. aspergillosis
b. carcinoid tumor
b. cyst
b. dysplasia (BPD)
b. lymph node
b. segment
b. segmental artery (BPSA)
b. spasm
b. tissue
b. tract
b. venous fistula
b. washings
bronchorrhea
Broncho Saline
bronchoscope
BF large core b.
Dumon b.
Dumon-Harrell b.
fiberoptic b.
flexible fiberoptic b.
Fujinon flexible b.
Kernan-Jackson b.
Michelson b.
Moersch b.
Negus b.
Pentax b.
Pilling b.
respiration b.
Safar b.
Storz b.
ventilation b.
Waterman b.
Yankauer b.
bronchoscopic
b. brush
b. electrocautery
b. lung biopsy (BLB)
b. needle aspiration (BNA)
b. needle biopsy
b. smear
b. ultrasound
bronchoscopist
bronchoscopy
autofluorescence b.
diagnostic b.
fiberoptic b. (FB, FOB)
flexible fiberoptic b. (FFB)
fluorescence b.
laser b.

NOTES

bronchoscopy *(continued)*
    b. quality improvement project
    rigid b.
    surveillance b.
    therapeutic b.
    ultrasound-guided b.
    virtual b. (VB)
    white light b. (WLB)
bronchospasm
    allergic b.
    exercise-induced b. (EIB)
    paradoxical b.
    reversible b.
bronchospastic
    b. component
    b. event
bronchospirography
bronchospirometer
bronchospirometry
    differential b.
bronchostenosis
bronchotracheal aspirate
bronchovascular bundle
bronchovenous fistula
bronchovesicular
    b. breath sounds
    b. marking
    b. respiration
bronchus, pl. **bronchi**
    anomalous b.
    apical b.
    basal segmental b.
    branches of segmental bronchi
    cardiac b.
    ectopic b.
    eparterial b.
    hyparterial bronchi
    intermediate b.
    b. intermedius
    left main b.
    lingular b.
    lobar b.
    bronchi lobares
    lower lobe b.
    main stem b.
    middle lobe b.
    mucosa of b.
    muscular coat of b.
    primary b.
    b. principalis dexter
    b. principalis sinister
    right main b.
    secondary b.
    segmental b.
    b. segmentalis
    stem b.
    subsegmental b.
    b. suis
    supernumerary b.

    tertiary b.
    tracheal b.
    tunica mucosa bronchi
    upper lobe b.
bronchus-associated lymphoid tissue (BALT)
bronchus-grasping forceps
Bronkodyl
Brontex Liquid
Brookfield viscometer
broth
    heart infusion b. (HIB)
    b. test
    Todd Hewitt b.
brown
    b. atrophy
    b. edema
    b. induration of lung
    b. sputum
    b. urine
Brown-Adson forceps
Brown-Dodge method
Brown-McHardy pneumatic dilator
Brozek formula
BRS
    baroreceptor reflex sensitivity
    baroreflex sensitivity
Bruce
    B. bundle
    B. exercise stress test
    B. maximum stress test (BMST)
    B. treadmill protocol
brucei
    Trypanosoma b.
Brucella melitensis
brucellosis
Brugada syndrome
Brugia
    B. malayi
    B. timori
bruit
    abdominal b.
    aneurysmal b.
    asymptomatic carotid b. (ACB)
    carotid b.
    b. d'airain
    b. de bois
    b. de canon
    b. de choc
    b. de clapotement
    b. de claquement
    b. de craquement
    b. de cuir neuf
    b. de diable
    b. de drapeau
    b. de fele
    b. de froissement
    b. de frolement
    b. de frottement

b. de galop
b. de grelot
b. de la roue de moulin
b. de Leudet
b. de lime
b. de parchemin
b. de piaulement
b. de pot fele
b. de rappel
b. de Roger
b. de scie
b. de scie ou de rape
b. de soufflet
b. de tabourka
b. de tambour
b. de triolet
epigastric b.
false b.
midepigastric b.
musical b.
Roger b.
seagull b.
systolic b.
thyroid b.
Traube b.
Verstraeten b.

Brunelli equation
**Brunnstrom-Fugl-Meyer Scale for motor
  test**
brush
Air-Lon tracheal tube b.
b. biopsy
b. border membrane (BBM)
b. border membrane vesicle
  (BBMV)
bronchoscopic b.
b. cell
Edwards-Carpentier aortic valve b.
B. electrocardiographic score
Mill-Rose protected specimen
  microbiology b.
OTW thrombolytic b.
protected specimen b. (PSB)
Brushfield spot
brushing
blind esophageal b. (BEB)
bronchial b.'s
double-sheath bronchial b.'s
microbiologic b.
protected catheter b. (PCB)
protected specimen b. (PSB)
washings and b.'s

brusque dilatation of esophagus
BRVO
branch retinal vein occlusion
Bryant ampulla
BS
bilateral symmetrical
B-S
Björk-Shiley
  B-S valve
BSA
body surface area
BSCA
bidirectional superior cavopulmonary
  anastomosis
B-scan frame
BSCC
Björk-Shiley convexoconcave
  BSCC heart valve
BSLM
body surface laplacian mapping
BT
Blalock-Taussig
bleeding time
  BT shunt
BTF-37 arterial blood filter
BTO
balloon test occlusion
BTS
Blalock-Taussig shunt
brady-tachy syndrome
B-type natriuretic peptide (BNP)
BUA
broadband ultrasound attenuation
bubble
arterial gas b.
b. contrast echocardiography
b. humidifier
b. oxygenation
b. oxygenator
bubbling rale
bubbly lung syndrome
bubonic plague
bucardia
buccal
Nitrogard B.
buccalis
  Leptotrichia b.
buccolingual apraxia
buccopharyngeal
**Buchbinder Thruflex over-the-wire
  catheter**
Buckberg cardioplegia

NOTES

buckled aorta
buckling
    b. of aorta
    chordal b.
    midsystolic b.
bud
    bronchial b.
    lung b.
Budd-Chiari syndrome
budesonide
    b. inhalation powder
    b. inhalation suspension
Buerger-Allen exercise
Buerger disease
buffer
    Krebs-Henseleit b.
buffered
    b. aspirin
    b. lidocaine (BL)
    b. lidocaine with epinephrine
    (BLE)
Bufferin
buffy coat smear
BUFUL
    bumetanide and furosemide on lipid
    BUFUL profile
Buhl desquamative pneumonia
buildup time (T_b)
bulb
    b. of aorta
    aortic b.
    carotid b.
    thrombosis of jugular b.
bulbar pulse
bulboventricular
    b. fold
    b. foramen
    b. groove
    b. loop
    b. sulcus
    b. tube
bulbus cordis
bulge
    precordial b.
    spare tire b.
bulging
    diastolic b.
    infarct b.
    systolic b.
bulla, pl. **bullae**
    emphysematous b.
    pulmonary b.
    b. resorption
Bullard intubating laryngoscope
bulldog clamp
bullectomy
    transaxillary apical b.
bullet-tip catheter
bullet wound

bullous
    b. emphysema
    b. lung disease
bull's-eye
    b.-e. plot
    b.-e. polar coordinate mapping
bumetanide and furosemide on lipid
    (BUFUL)
Bumex
bump
    B b.
    ductus b.
BUN
    blood urea nitrogen
BUN br
    bundle branch
bundle
    atrioventricular b.
    A-V b.
    Bachmann b.
    b. branch (BB, BUN br)
    b. branch block (BBB)
    b. branch fibrosis
    b. branch reentrant tachycardia
    b. branch reentry (BBR)
    bronchovascular b.
    Bruce b.
    central bronchovascular b.
    commissural b.
    Gantzer accessory b.
    b. of His (B-H)
    His b. (HB)
    image b.
    James b.
    Keith b.
    Kent b.
    Kent-His b.
    Killian b.
    left b. (LB)
    Mahaim b.
    main b.
    Marshall b.
    neurovascular b.
    right b. (RB)
    b. of Stanley Kent
    Thorel b.
    vascular b.
bundle-branch
Bunny boot
Bunyaviridae
bupivacaine
bupropion SR
bur
    diamond-coated b.
    b. hole
burden
    atheroma b.
    atherosclerotic plaque b.

ischemic b.
plaque b.
Burdick
B. ECG machine
B. electrocardiogram
Burette multiple patient delivery system
Burford-Finochietto rib spreader
burgdorferi
Borrelia b.
Burger
B. scalene triangle
B. technique for scapulothoracic
disarticulation
Bürger-Grütz
B.-G. disease
B.-G. syndrome
Burghart symptom
Burhenne steerable catheter
Burinex
Burker Avance spectrometer
Burkholderia cepacia
Burkitt lymphoma
burned out viral myocarditis
burnetii
Coxiella b.
burning pain
Burns
space of B.
Burow
B. quantitative method
B. solution
B. vein
bursa, pl. **bursae**
Calori b.
Fleischmann b.
laryngeal b.
b. subcutanea
sublingual b.
b. sublingualis
burst
b. of arrhythmia
b. atrial pacing
paroxysmal b.
b. of rapid atrial pacing (BRAP)
respiratory b.
b. shock
spider b.
b. of ventricular pacing (BVP)
b. of ventricular tachycardia
Buschke
B. disease
scleredema of B.

Buselmeier shunt
buspirone transdermal patch
Busse-Buschke disease
buster
clot b.
busulfan lung syndrome
butanedione monoxime
butorphanol
butterfly
b. catheter
b. heart valve
b. needle
b. pattern
b. shadow
Butterworth bidirectional filter
buttock claudication
button
b. of aorta
cell b.
coronary artery b.
b. electrode
Kistner tracheal b.
Moore tracheostomy b.
Panje voice b.
skin b.
b. technique
tracheal b.
tracheostomy b.
buttoned device
buttonhole
b. deformity
mitral b.
b. mitral stenosis
b. stenosis
buttress
Teflon pledget suture b.
butylated hydroxytoluene (BHT)
butyrophenone
BUV
backup ventilation
BV
balloon valvuloplasty
blood vessel
BVA-100 blood volume analyzer
BVAD, BIVAD
biventricular assist device
BVE
blood volume expander
BvgAS regulon
BvgS protein
BVH
biventricular hypertrophy

NOTES

BVI
blood vessel invasion
BVM
bag-valve-mask
BVM device
BVM ventilation
BVO
branch vein occlusion
BVP
blood vessel prosthesis
blood volume pulse
burst of ventricular pacing
BVR
balloon valvuloplasty registry
BVS
biventricular support
BVS pump
BVS-5000 biventricular support system
Bx
Bx Velocity stent with Raptor OTW delivery system
Bx Velocity with Hepacoat on Raptor stent system
ByCPR
bystander cardiac pulmonary resuscitation
bypass (BP)
aortobiiliac b.
aortocarotid b.
aortocoronary b. (A-C, ACB)
aortocoronary-saphenous vein b.
aortocoronary venous b. (ACVB)
aortofemoral b. (AFB)
aortoiliac b.
aortoiliofemoral b.
aortorenal b.
aortosubclavian b.
aortosubclavian-carotid-axilloaxillary b.
atrial-femoral artery b.
axillary bifemoral b.
axilloaxillary b.
axillofemoral b.
brachial b.
cardiopulmonary b. (CBP, CPB)
carotid-axillary b.
carotid-carotid b.
carotid-subclavian b.
b. circuit
coronary artery b. (CAB)
coronary artery b. graft (CARB)
cross femoral-femoral b.
crossover femoral-femoral b.
descending thoracic aortofemoral-femoral b.
femoral-femoral b.
femoral-popliteal b.
femoral-tibial b.
femoral-tibial-peroneal b.
femoroaxillary b.
femorofemoral crossover b.
femoropopliteal b.
femorotibial b.
gastric b. (GBP)
b. graft (BPG)
b. graft catheterization
heart-lung b.
iliopopliteal b.
infracubital b.
internal mammary artery b. (IMAB)
left heart b.
Litwak left atrial-aortic b.
low-flow cardiopulmonary b. (LFB)
b. machine
midcoronary artery b.
minimally invasive coronary artery b. (MICAB)
minimally invasive direct coronary artery b. (MIDCAB)
off-pump coronary artery b. (OPCAB)
percutaneous cardiopulmonary b. (PCPB)
percutaneous left heart b. (PLHB)
perfusion-assisted direct coronary artery b. (PADCAB)
peripheral artery b.
portacaval b. (PCB)
renal artery-reverse saphenous vein b.
reversed b.
right heart b. (RHB)
saphenous vein b. (SVB)
subclavian-carotid b.
subclavian-subclavian b.
superior mesenteric artery b.
b. surgery
b. time
total b. (TBP)
total cardiopulmonary b. (TCB)
totally endoscopic coronary artery b. (TECAB)
total revascularization off pump by coronary artery b. (TROPCAB)
b. tract
bypassable
by-product
eosinophil b.-p.
nicotine b.-p.
byssinosis
bystander
b. cardiac pulmonary resuscitation (ByCPR)
b. cardiopulmonary resuscitation (BCPR)
b. effect

C
cardiac
cardiovascular disease
chest lead in electrocardiography
cholesterol
C oxygen cylinder
C point of cardiac apex pulse
C valvular leaflet
C wave
C wave of jugular venous
3C
cranio-cerebello-cardiac syndrome
^{11}C, C-11
carbon-11
C$_4$
leukotriene C.
C1qR gene
C1r deficiency
c4b purified human complement
c7 E3 Fab
CA
cancer
carcinoma
cardiac angiography
cardiac arrest
cardiac arrhythmia
catecholamine
catecholaminergic
coarctation of aorta
coronary artery
croup-associated
CA monitor
CA virus
C of A
coarctation of aorta
CAA
cardiac allograft atherosclerosis
cerebral amyloid angiopathy
circulating anodic antigen
CAA-related hemorrhage
CAAS
Cardiovascular Angiography Analysis
System
CAB
coronary artery bypass
cabergoline
CABF
coronary artery blood flow
CABG
coronary artery bypass grafting
CABGS
coronary artery bypass graft surgery
cable
OxyLead interconnect c.
Cabot-Locke murmur

CABS
continuous ambulatory blood sampler
coronary artery bypass surgery
CAC, CACh
cardiac-accelerator center
cardiac arrest code
circulating anticoagulant
cold air challenge
cachectic endocarditis
cachecticorum
melanoderma c.
cachexia
cancer c.
cardiac c.
thyroid c.
cacoon seed asthma
CAD
computer-assisted diagnostic
coronary artery disease
coronoradiographic documentation
CADASIL
cerebral autosomal dominant arteriopathy
with subcortical infarct and
leukoencephalopathy
CADD-Plus intravenous infusion pump
**Cadence tiered therapy defibrillator
system**
Cadet
C. high voltage can implantable
cardioverter-defibrillator
C. V-115 implantable cardioverter-
defibrillator
cadherin
vascular c.
CADI
coronary artery disease index
cadmiosis
cadmium (Cd)
c. oxide
c. oxide fumes
CADR
coronary artery descriptors and restenosis
CAE
coronary artery embolism
CAEP
chronotropic exercise assessment protocol
CAESAR
computer-assisted evaluation of stenosis
and restenosis
CAESAR analysis system
caesiellus
Aspergillus c.
CAF
continuous atrial fibrillation
coronary artery fistula

113

Cafcit
> C. injection
> C. oral solution

café-au-lait spot

café coronary

Cafergot

caffeine
> c. citrate
> citrated c.
> c. citrate oral solution
> phenacetin, aspirin, and c. (PAC)
> c. and sodium benzoate

CAG
> coronary angiography
> coronary arteriography

CagA
> cytotoxin-associated gene product A
> CagA antigen

cage
> chest c.
> Faraday c.
> rib c.
> thoracic c.
> titanium c.

caged
> c. ball valve
> c. ball valve prosthesis

CAGEIN
> catheter-guided endoscopic intubation

CAH
> combined atrial hypertrophy

CAHD
> coronary arteriosclerotic heart disease

CAI
> cortical arousal index

c-a interval

Caire
> C. Sprint portable liquid oxygen device
> C. Stroller portable liquid oxygen device

caisson disease

CAL
> chronic airflow limitation

Calan SR

calcicardiogram

calcicosilicosis

calcicosis

calcific
> c. aortic stenosis (CAS)
> c. debris
> c. embolus
> c. mitral stenosis
> c. nodular aortic stenosis
> c. pericarditis

calcification
> anular c.
> arterial c.
> dystropic c.

> eggshell c.
> metastatic c.
> mitral annular c.
> mitral annulus c. (MAC)
> Mönckeberg c.
> napkin-ring c.
> pericardial c.
> pulmonary c.
> soft tissue c.
> c. of tips of the mitral valve
> valvular c.

calcified
> c. aortic valve
> c. lesion
> c. mitral leaflet
> c. nodule
> c. papillary muscle in the right ventricle
> c. pericardium
> c. plaque
> c. thrombus

Calcilean

calcineurin

calcinosis, Raynaud phenomenon, esophageal involvement, sclerodactyly, telangiectasia (CREST)

calciphylaxis

calcitonin gene-related peptide (CGRP)

calcium
> c. antagonist
> arc of c.
> atorvastatin c.
> benzoylpas c.
> c. benzoylpas
> c. channel agonist
> c. channel antagonist (CCA)
> c. channel blocking agent
> c. chloride
> coronary c.
> c. current (I_{Ca})
> c. deposit
> c. entry blocker
> fenoprofen c.
> c. gluceptate
> c. gluconate
> c. heparin (CH)
> c. ion
> c. ionophore A23187
> mitral annular c.
> myoplasmic c.
> nadroparin c.
> c. oxalate
> c. oxalate deposition
> c. paradox
> c. product
> c. rigor
> c. score
> c. sign

spotty coronary c.
c. transient
calcium-channel blocker (CCB)
Calciviridae virus
calcoaceticus
Acinetobacter c.
calcofluor stain
Calculair spirometer
calculation
bidirectional shunt c.
bolus cardiac output c.
calculator
risk c.
calculosa
pericarditis c.
calculus, pl. calculi
bronchial c.
cardiac c.
pleural c.
caldesmon
calf, pl. calves
c. aortic microsome (CAM)
c. claudication
c. cramp
c. embryonic heart cell (CEHC)
c. lung surfactant extract (CLSE)
c. pain
calfactant intratracheal suspension
Calgary Sleep Apnea Quality of Life Index
calibration
calibrator
Califf score
California disease
calipers
AccuGage vessel c.
digital c.
electronic c.
Lange c.
callosa
pericarditis c.
callosomarginal artery
Calmers
Robitussin Cough C.
Sucrets Cough C.
Calmette-Guérin
C.-G. bacillus
calmodulin
Calm-X Oral
Calmylin Expectorant
Calori bursa

calorie
ratio of ingested saturated fat and cholesterol to c.'s
calorie-restricted diet
calorimetry
myocardial indirect c.
Calot triangle
CALP
congenital absence of left pericardium
calphostin C
calsequestrin (CASQ)
Caltrac accelerometer
Caluso PEG tube
calves (*pl. of* calf)
Calypso Rely PTCA balloon angioplasty catheter
CAM
calf aortic microsome
cell adhesion molecule
child-adult-mist
circulating adhesion molecule
Cam-Ap-Es
Cambridge electrocardiograph
camera
ADAC Cirrus single-headed SPECT c.
ADAC Vertex dual-headed SPECT c.
Anger scintillation c.
DSX Sopha c.
gamma scintillation c.
multicrystal gamma c.
multiwire gamma c.
scintillation c.
Siemens Orbiter gamma c.
single-crystal gamma c.
Sopha Medical gamma c.
video c.
cameral fistula
Cameron-Haight elevator
CAMP
cyclophosphamide, doxorubicin, methotrexate, procarbazine
CAMP test
cAMP
cyclic adenosine monophosphate
Campbell De Morgan spot
camptodactyly
pericarditis, arthropathy, c. (PAC)
Camptosar
Campylobacter

C

NOTES

camsylate
> trimethaphan c.

CAN
> cardiac autonomic neuropathy
> continuous albuterol nebulization

can
> high voltage c. (HVC)
> pacemaker c.

Canadian
> C. Cardiovascular Coalition (CCC)
> C. Cardiovascular Society (CCS)
> C. Cardiovascular Society angina score (CCSAS)
> C. Cardiovascular Society classification (CCSC)
> C. Cardiovascular Society functional classification
> C. class I–IV angina
> C. Heart Classification (CHC)
> C. Registry of Atrial Fibrillation (CARAF)

canal
> c. of Arantius
> atrioventricular c. (AVC)
> basipharyngeal c.
> carotid c.
> common atrioventricular c.
> complex atrioventricular c.
> c. of Cuvier
> facial c.
> femoral c.
> hiatus of facial c.
> His c.
> Holmgren-Golgi c.
> Hunter c.
> c. of Lambert
> palatovaginal c.
> partial atrioventricular c.
> perivascular c.
> persistent common atrioventricular c.
> pharyngeal c.
> pleuroperitoneal c.
> pulmoaortic c.
> Rivinus c.'s
> van Horne c.
> ventricular c.
> Verneuil c.

canalicular period
canalization
cancer (CA)
> c. cachexia
> c. embolus
> International Staging System for Lung C. (ISSLC)
> metachronous lung c.
> nonsmall-cell lung c. (NSCLC)

> roentgenographically occult lung c. (ROLC)
> scar c.

cancerization
> field c.

Cancidas
candesartan
> c. cilexetil
> c., cilexetil and hydrochlorothiazide

Candida
> *C. albicans*
> *C. glabrata*
> *C. guilliermondii*
> *C. lusitaniae*
> *C. parapsilosis*
> *C. pneumonia*

candidemia
candidiasis
> oral c.

candidum
> *Geotrichum c.*

candidus
> *Aspergillus c.*
> *Thermoactinomyces c.*

candle flame pattern
candoxatril
candoxatrilat
candy-cane esophagus
candy wrapper edge effect
canine fossa
caninum
> *Ancylostoma c.*

canis
> *Babesia c.*
> *Toxocara c.*

cannabinoid
Cann-Ease
> C.-E. moisturizing nasal gel
> C.-E. nasal moisturizer

cannon
> C. formula
> c. sound
> C. theory
> c. wave

cannonball
> c. metastases
> c. pulse

cannula
> Abelson c.
> Aegis aortic c.
> aortic arch c.
> aortic perfusion c.
> Argyle CPAP nasal c.
> cardiovascular c.
> Cimochowski cardiac c.
> Entree thoracoscopy c.
> femoral perfusion c.
> Flexicath silicone subclavian c.
> Fluoro Tip c.

Gregg c.
Grüntzig femoral stiffening c.
Heartport endovenous drainage c.
nasal c.
O2 via nasal c.
Polystan perfusion c.
QuickDraw venous c.
RAP c.
remote access perfusion c.
Rockey ventricular c.
saphenous vein c.
Sarns aortic arch c.
Sarns soft-flow aortic c.
Sarns two-stage c.
Softip oxygen nasal c.
StraightShot arterial c.
Tibbs arterial c.
triport c.
two-stage c.
vein graft c.
vena cava c.
venous c.
Wallace Flexihub central venous
  pressure c.
washout c.
cannulate
cannulation
femoral arterial c. (FAC)
canola oil
canon
bruit de c.
canrenoate potassium
canrenone
cantering rhythm
canthomeatal slice
Cantlie line
Cantrell pentalogy
CAO
chronic airflow obstruction
coronary artery obstruction
CAO2
arterial oxygen content
CAOD
coronary artery occlusive disease
CAP
central apical part
community-acquired pneumonia
coronary artery fistula
coupled atrial pacing
cyclophosphamide, doxorubicin, cisplatin
CA4P
combretastatin A4 prodrug

cap
atheromatous c.
collagenous c.
Drixoral Cough & Congestion
  Liquid C.'s
Drixoral Cough & Sore Throat
  Liquid C.'s
fibrous c.
c. inflammation
left apical c.
mesenchymal c.
pleural c.
c. repair
Sudafed Cold & Cough Liquid C.
c. thickness
capacitance
segmental venous c. (SVC)
venous c. (VC)
c. vessel
capacitor
c. deformation
c. forming time
c. reform
capacity
aerobic c. (VO_2)
carbon monoxide diffusing c.
cerebrovascular reserve c. (CRC)
diffusing c.
diffusion c.
exercise c.
forced expiratory c. (FEC)
forced expiratory volume in 1
  second to forced vital c. ratio
  (FEV_1/FVC)
forced inspiratory c. (FIC)
forced inspiratory vital c. (FIVC)
forced vital c. (FVC)
force-generating c.
functional reserve c. (FRC)
functional residual c. (FRC)
inspiratory c. (IC)
inspiratory reserve c. (IRC)
inspiratory vital c. (IVC)
lung transfer c.
maximal breathing c.
maximal sustainable ventilatory c.
  (MSVC)
maximal vital c. (MVC)
maximum aerobic c.
maximum breathing c. (MBC)
maximum expiratory flow at 50%
  vital c. (MEF_{50})

C

NOTES

capacity *(continued)*
    membrane diffusing c. (Dm)
    metabolic vasodilatory c.
    myocardial vascular c. (MVC)
    normal vital c. (NVC)
    oxygen c.
    oxygen-binding c.
    oxygen-carrying c.
    oxygen-diffusing c.
    pulmonary diffusion c. (D_{CO})
    residual lung c.
    residual volume/total lung c.
     (RV/TLC)
    respiratory c.
    serum reserve cholesterol
     binding c. (SRCBC)
    slow vital c. (SVC)
    timed vital c.
    total lung c. (TLC)
    ventilatory c.
    vital c. (VC)
    work c.
Capastat Sulfate
capecitabine
Capelle-Durrer
    van C.-D. (VCD)
Capetown prosthetic valve
capillaritis
capillaropathy
capillary
    alveolar c.
    c. apoplexy
    c. bed
    c. blood flow (CBF)
    c. blood gas (CBG)
    c. blood sugar (CBS)
    c. blush
    c. bronchitis
    c. embolism
    extraalveolar c.
    c. filling
    c. filtration coefficient
    c. hydrostatic pressure (CHP)
    c. leak syndrome (CLS)
    peritubular c. (PTC)
    c. pressure (CP)
    c. pulse
    c. recruitment
    c. thrombi
    c. wedge pressure
Capintec nuclear VEST monitor
Capiscint
Caplan
    C. nodule
    C. syndrome
Caplets
    Advil Cold & Sinus C.
    Bayer Select Chest Cold C.
    Dimacol C.

    Dimetapp Sinus C.
    Dristan Sinus C.
capneic microorganism
Capnocheck
    C. handheld capnometer
    C. Plus NIPB monitor
    C. quantitative capnometer
***Capnocytophaga canimorsus* sepsis**
capnogram
    volumetric c.
capnograph
    BCI Capnocheck DualStream c.
    Clarity c.
    Microcap handheld c.
    Microstream c.
    Novametrix Tidal Wave
     handheld c.
    SC-300 portable c.
    SC-210 sidestream c.
    Tidal Wave handheld c.
capnography
    color c.
capnometer
    Capnocheck handheld c.
    Capnocheck quantitative c.
capnometry
    end-tidal c.
CapnoProbe sublingual CO_2 system
Capnostat CO_2 sensor
Capoten
Capozide
capped lead
capreomycin sulfate
CAPRI
    Cardiopulmonary Research Institute
caprisans
    pulsus c.
caprizant
caproate
    hydroxyprogesterone c.
capsaicin
CAPSO
    cautery-assisted palatal stiffening
    operation
capsula fibrosa glandula
capsulatum
    Histoplasma c.
capsule
    CellCept c.
    internal c.
    mycophenolate mofetil c.
    Neoral cyclosporine c.
    Ordrine AT Extended Release C.
    posterior limb of the internal c.
     (PLIC)
    Rescaps-D C.
    Tiazac extended-release c.
    Tricor c.

Tuss-Allergine Modified T.D. C.
Tussogest Extended Release C.

Capsulets

Sinumist-SR C.

CapSure

C. cardiac pacing lead
C. SP lead
C. VDD lead

CapSureFix lead

captopril

c. and hydrochlorothiazide
c. renography

capture

atrial c.
c. beat
beat-by-beat c.
c. complex
failure to c.
functional failure to c.
loss of c.
pacemaker c.
retrograde arterial c.
c. threshold
ventricular c.

caput medusae

CAQ

Childhood Asthma Questionnaire

CAR

cardiac ambulation routine
carvedilol
CAR AMP

Carabelli tube

Carabello sign

CARAF

Canadian Registry of Atrial Fibrillation

caramiphen and phenylpropanolamine

CARB

coronary artery bypass graft

carbachol

c. inhalation challenge (CIC)
c. provocation test

carbamazepine

carbapenem

carbazochrome salicylate

carbenicillin

indanyl c.

carbetapentane

chlorpheniramine, ephedrine,
phenylephrine, and c.

carbide

aluminum c.

amorphous hydrogenated silicon c.
(a-SiC:H)
cobalt in tungsten c.

carbinoxamine

c. and pseudoephedrine
c., pseudoephedrine, and
dextromethorphan

Carbocaine

carbocholine

carbocysteine

Carbodec DM

carbohydrate

c. intolerance
c. utilization test

Carbomedics

C. bileaflet prosthetic heart valve
C. cardiac valve prosthesis
C. top-hat supra-annular valve
C. valve device

carbomethoxyisopropyl isonitrile

carbon

c. dioxide (CO_2)
c. dioxide dissociation curve
c. dioxide pressure
c. dioxide production
c. dioxide tension
c. disulfide
c. monoxide (CO)
c. monoxide diffusing capacity
c. monoxide oximetry
c. monoxide sleuth
c. monoxide transfer factor (TLCO,
TLco)
pyrolytic c.

carbon-11 (^{11}C, C-11)

c.-11 acetate
c.-11 hydroxyephedrine
c.-11 labeled fatty acids
c.-11 palmitic acid radioactive
tracer

carbonate

magnesium c. ($MgCO_3$)

carbonica

asphyxia c.

carbonic anhydrase inhibitor

carboplatin, etoposide (CE)

Carbo-Seal

C.-S. ascending aortic prosthesis
C.-S. graft material

carboxyhemoglobin (COHb, $HbCO_2$)

carboxyhemoglobinemia

NOTES

carbuterol hydrochloride
carcinoembryonic antigen (CEA)
carcinogen
carcinogenesis
    field c.
carcinogenicity
carcinoid
    c. heart disease
    c. murmur
    c. plaque
    c. syndrome
    c. tumor
    c. valve disease
carcinoma, pl. **carcinomata (CA)**
    adenoid cystic c.
    adenosquamous c.
    alveolar cell c.
    anaplastic c.
    basal cell c.
    basaloid c.
    bronchial c.
    bronchiolar c.
    bronchioloalveolar c. (BAC)
    bronchoalveolar c.
    bronchogenic c.
    clear cell c.
    ductal cell c.
    epidermoid c.
    giant cell c.
    hair-matrix c.
    infiltrating lobular c.
    large cell undifferentiated c.
    lung c.
    lymphangitic c.
    lymphoepithelioma-like c.
    melanotic c.
    metastatic c.
    mucinous c.
    mucoepidermoid c.
    nasopharyngeal c.
    nonsmall-cell lung c. (NSCLC)
    oat cell c.
    papillary c.
    poorly differentiated c.
    prickle cell c.
    primary lung c.
    reserve cell c.
    scar c.
    scirrhous c.
    signet-ring cell c.
    c. simplex
    c. in situ
    small cell c.
    small cell lung c. (SCLC)
    spindle cell c.
    squamous cell bronchogenic c.
    transitional cell c.
    undifferentiated small-cell c.

    verrucous c.
    well-differentiated c.
carcinomatosa
    lymphangitis c.
carcinomatosis
    lymphangitic c. (LC)
carcinomatous
    c. neuromyopathy
    c. pericarditis
carcinosarcoma
CARD
    cardiac automatic resuscitative device
card
    cardiac
    cardiology
    TruZone asthma action plan
      wallet c.
Cardarelli sign
CARDEA data management system
Cardec DM
Cardec-S Syrup
Cardene SR
cardiac (C, card)
    C. Ablation Registry
    c. accident
    c. action potential
    c. adjustment scale (CAS)
    c. allograft
    c. allograft atherosclerosis (CAA)
    c. allograft vascular disease
      (CAVD)
    c. allograft vasculopathy (CAV)
    c. alternation
    c. ambulation routine (CAR)
    c. amyloidosis
    c. aneurysm
    c. angiography (CA)
    c. antimyosin antibody uptake
    c. antrum
    c. apex
    c. apnea monitor
    c. arrest (CA)
    c. arrest code (CAC, CACh)
    c. arrhythmia (CA)
    c. asthma
    c. atrophy
    c. auscultation
    c. autoantibody
    c. autoimmunity
    c. automatic resuscitative device
      (CARD)
    c. autonomic neuropathy (CAN)
    c. ballet
    c. baroreceptor
    c. bioptome
    c. blood-pool imaging
    c. border of dullness
    c. bronchus
    c. cachexia

c. calculus
c. care unit (CCU)
c. catheter
c. catheterization (CC)
c. catheter-microphone
c. center (CC)
c. chamber
c. cirrhosis
c. cocktail
c. compensation
c. competence
c. compression
c. conduction
c. conduction system
c. contour
c. contraction
C. Control Systems lead
c. contusion (CC)
c. cooling jacket
c. crisis
c. cushion
c. cycle (CC)
c. death
c. decompensation
c. decompression
c. decortication
c. defects, abnormal facies, thymic hypoplasia, cleft palate, hypocalcemia (CATCH-22)
c. defibrillation
c. depressant
c. depressor reflex
c. diagnostic unit (CDU)
c. diastole
c. diet
c. dilation
c. disease (CD)
c. disturbance syndrome
c. diuretic
c. dropsy
c. dullness (CD)
c. dyspnea
c. dysrhythmia (CD)
c. echodensity
c. edema
c. enlargement (CE)
c. enzyme
c. event
c. event recorder
c. examination
c. failure (CF)
c. fibrillation

FluoroPlus C.
c. function
c. gap junction protein
c. gating
c. glands of esophagus
c. glycogenosis
c. glycoside
c. hemoptysis
c. hemosiderosis
c. herniation
c. heterotaxia
c. hybrid revascularization procedure
c. hypertrophy
c. impression on lung
c. impulse
c. index (CI)
C. infarction
c. Infarction Injury Score
c. infiltration
c. insufficiency (card insuff, CI)
c. insult
c. intensive care unit (CICU)
c. interstitium
c. ischemia
c. jelly
c. laboratory panel (CLP)
c. lithomyxoma
c. liver
c. lymphatic ring
c. mapping
c. mass
c. massage
c. memory
c. metastasis
c. minute output (CMO)
c. monitoring (CM)
c. monitor strip
c. murmur (CM)
c. muscle (CM)
c. muscle wrap
c. myocyte
c. myosin
c. myxoma
c. neural crest
c. neurosis
c. notch
c. notch of left lung
c. observation unit (COU)
c. orifice
c. output (CO, $\dot{Q}$, QT, Q-T)
c. output demand

NOTES

cardiac *(continued)*
   c. output index
   c. output measurement
   c. output recorder (COR)
   c. output shock
   c. output by thermodilution
     (COTD)
   c. pacemaker
   c. pacing (CP)
   c. patch
   c. perforation
   c. performance (CP)
   c. perfusion
   c. polyp
   c. power output (CPO)
   c. preload
   c. probe
   C. Protect tomography
   c. pulmonary edema (CPE)
   c. rehabilitation (CR)
   c. rehabilitation and prevention
    program
   c. rehabilitation protocol
   c. rehabilitation unit (CRU)
   c. remodeling
   c. reserve
   c. resuscitation (CR)
   c. resuscitation team (CRT)
   c. resynchronization therapy
   c. rhythm (CR)
   c. risk factor
   c. risk index (CRI)
   c. rotation
   c. rupture
   c. sarcoidosis myocarditis
   c. sarcoma
   c. sensory nerve
   c. shadow
   c. shockwave therapy (CSWT)
   c. shock wave therapy (CSWT)
   c. shunt
   c. silhouette
   c. situs
   c. skeleton
   c. sling
   C. Society of Great Britain and
    Ireland (CSGBI)
   c. sodium channel gene
   c. souffle
   c. sound
   c. standstill
   c. status
   C. STATus CK-MB/myoglobin
    panel test
   C. STATus CK-MB test
   C. STATus rapid format troponin
    I panel test
   c. stress test (CST)
   c. stretch device

   c. stump
   c. surgery (CAS)
   c. surgery reporting system (CSRS)
   c. surgical intensive care unit
    (CSICU)
   c. sympathetic denervation
   c. sympathetic nerve (CSN)
   c. symphysis
   c. syncope
   c. systole
   c. tamponade (CT)
   c. telemetry
   c. thrombosis
   c. thrust
   c. transplant
   c. transplantation (CTx)
   C. Transplant Research Database
    (CTRD)
   C. T rapid assay
   c. troponin I (CTI, cTnI, cTn-I)
   c. troponin I assay
   c. troponin T (cTnT)
   c. tumor
   c. tumor plop
   c. ultrasound
   c. unit (CU)
   c. vagal tone
   c. valve
   c. valve prosthesis
   c. valvular incompetence
   c. variability
   c. vasculitis
   c. vein
   c. vest
   c. volume (CV)
   c. waist
   c. wall hypokinesis
   c. wall thickening
   c. work (CW)
   c. work index (CWI)
cardiaca
   adiposis c.
   steatosis c.
cardiac-accelerator center (CAC, CACh)
cardiac-specific overexpression
cardiac-thoracic unit (CTU)
cardiac troponin I (CTI, cTnI, cTn-I)
cardiac troponin T (cTnT)
cardialgia
Cardia Salt alternative
cardiataxia
cardiatelia
cardiectasia
cardiectopia
**Cardima Pathfinder mapping
  microcatheter**
cardinal
   c. symptom
   c. vein

card insuff
    cardiac insufficiency
cardioacceleration
cardioaccelerator center
cardioactive
cardioangiography
cardioarterial interval
cardioauditory syndrome
Cardiobacterium hominis
cardioballistic
CardioBeeper CB 12L cardiac monitor
Cardioblate
    C. BP, RF surgical ablation
       system
    C. RF generator
    C. surgical ablation pen
cardiocairograph
Cardiocap/5 monitor
cardiocele
cardiocentesis
cardiochalasia
CardioCoil coronary stent
Cardio-Cool myocardial protection pouch
Cardio-Cuff
cardiocyte
cardiodiaphragmatic angle
cardiodynamics
cardiodynia
cardioembolic stroke (CES)
cardioesophageal (CE)
    c. junction
    c. reflux
    c. sphincter
cardiofacial syndrome
cardiofaciocutaneous syndrome (CFC)
CardioFix
    C. pericardium patch
    C. pericardium with PhotoFix
       technology
Cardioflon suture
cardiogenesis
CardioGenesis TMR system
cardiogenic
    c. pulmonary edema
    c. sheath
    c. shock (CGS, CS)
    c. stroke
    c. syncope
Cardiografin

cardiogram
    esophageal c.
    impedance c. (IC, ICD, ICG)
cardiograph
    Minnesota Impedance C.
cardiography (CG)
    Doppler c.
    echo-Doppler c.
    impedance c. (ICG)
    ultrasonic c. (UCG, USCG)
    ultrasound c.
    variance c. (VC)
    vector c.
Cardio-Green dye
CardioGrip cardiovascular trainer
cardiohemothrombus
cardiohepatic triangle
cardiohepatomegaly
cardioinflammatory cytokine
cardioinhibitor center (CIC)
cardioinhibitory
    c. carotid sinus hypersensitivity
    c. center
    c. type
    c. vasovagal syncope
cardiokinetic
cardiokymogram
cardiokymograph
cardiokymography (CKG)
cardiol
    cardiology
CardioLab 2000 single monitor EP system
cardiolipid
cardiolipin (CL)
    c. flocculation test (CFT)
    c. microflocculation test (CMFT)
    c. natural lecithin (CNL)
    c. synthetic lecithin (CSL)
Cardiolite
    C. scan
    C. stress test
cardiolith
cardiological workspace manager (CWM)
cardiologist
    Fellow of the American College
       of C.'s (FACC)
    interventional c.
cardiology (card, cardiol)
    American College of C. (ACC)

NOTES

C

cardiology *(continued)*
    digital interchange standards for c. (DISC)
    fetal c.
    C. II stethoscope
    International Society of C. (ISC)
    International Society and Federation of C. (ISFC)
    pediatric c. (PDC, PdC)
    telecollaboration for signal analysis in c. (TECSAC)
cardiolysis
    Brauer c.
cardiomalacia
cardiomediastinal silhouette
cardiomegaly
    borderline c.
    false c.
    glycogen c.
    idiopathic c.
Cardiomemo device
cardiometry
cardiomodulorespirography (CMR)
cardiomotility
cardiomuscular bradycardia
cardiomyocyte apoptosis
cardiomyoliposis
cardiomyopathy (CM, C-M, CMP)
    African c.
    alcoholic c.
    anthracycline-induced c.
    arrhythmogenic right ventricular c. (ARVC)
    arrhythmogenic ventricular c.
    atrophic c.
    beer-drinker's c.
    cobalt c.
    concentric hypertrophic c.
    congestive c. (CCM, COCM)
    diabetic c.
    dilated c. (DCM)
    doxorubicin c.
    drug-induced c.
    false c.
    familial hypertrophic c. (FHC)
    familial hypertrophic obstructive c.
    fibroplastic c.
    genetic hypertrophic c.
    HIV c.
    hypertensive hypertrophic c.
    hypertrophic c. (HC, HCM, HCMP)
    hypertrophic obstructive c. (HOCM)
    idiopathic congestive c. (ICCM)
    idiopathic dilated c. (IDC)
    idiopathic restrictive c.
    infiltrative c.
    inflammatory c. (InfCM)
    ischemic c.

    latent c. (LCM)
    maternally inherited c.
    mildly dilated congestive c. (MDCM)
    mitochondrial c.
    nephropathic c.
    nonischemic dilated c.
    obliterative c.
    obstructive hypertrophic c. (OHC)
    pacing in c. (PIC)
    parasitic c.
    pediatric c.
    peripartal c.
    peripartum c.
    postpartum c. (PPCM)
    primary restrictive c.
    rejection c.
    restrictive c.
    right ventricular c.
    secondary c.
    spiral hypertrophic c.
    tachycardia-induced c.
    valvular c.
    viral c.
    X-linked dilated c. (XLCM)
cardiomyoplasty
    dynamic c.
cardioneural
cardioneurogenic syncope
cardioneuropathy
cardioneurosis
cardioomentopexy
cardiopaludism
CardioPass layered microporous small-bore vascular graft
cardiopath
cardiopathia nigra
cardiopathy
cardiopericardiopexy
    Beck c.
cardiopexy
    ligamentum teres c.
cardiophobia
cardiophone
cardiophony
cardiophrenia
cardiophrenic angle
cardioplegia
    adenosine-supplemented blood c.
    blood c.
    Buckberg c.
    cold blood c.
    cold crystalloid c.
    cold potassium c.
    c. cooling
    crystalloid potassium c.
    hyperkalemic c.
    c. infusion
    normothermic c.

nutrient c.
potassium chloride c.
St. Thomas Hospital c.
whole blood c.
cardioplegic
  c. arrest
  c. perfusion solution (CPS)
  c. solution
cardiopneumographic recording (CPG)
Cardiopoint needle
cardiopressor
cardioprotection
cardioprotective role
cardioptosia
cardiopulmonary (CP)
  c. arrest (CPA)
  c. blood volume (CPBV)
  c. bypass (CBP, CPB)
  c. bypass pump
  c. cerebral resuscitation (CPCR)
  c. decompression sickness (the
    chokes)
  c. exercise (CPX)
  c. exercise test (CPET)
  c. gas exchange
  c. murmur
  C. Research Institute (CAPRI)
  c. reserve (CPR)
  c. resuscitation (CPR)
  c. splanchnic nerves
  c. support (CPS)
CardioPump
  Ambu C.
cardioreparative drug agent intervention
cardiorespiratory (CR)
  c. arrest
  c. depression
  c. murmur
  c. sign
cardiorespirogram (CRG)
CardioRhythm generator
cardiorrhaphy
cardiorrhexis (CR)
cardioschisis
Cardioscint
  C. ambulatory vest detector
  C. nuclear detector
cardiosclerosis
  postinfarct c.
CardioSEAL septal occlusion system
  with QWIKLoad
cardioselectivity

Cardioserv defibrillator
cardiosphygmograph
CardioSync cardiac synchronizer
cardiosynchronous monostimulator
  (CSM)
cardiotachometer (CTM)
Cardiotec scan
CardioTek electrophysiologic tracer
  system
Cardiotest portable electrograph
cardiothoracic
  c. intensive care unit (CTICU)
  c. ratio (CT, CTR)
  c. surgery (CTS)
cardiothrombus
cardiothyrotoxicosis
cardiotocography (CTG)
cardiotomy reservoir
cardiotonic drug
cardiotoxicity
  Adriamycin c.
  doxorubicin c.
cardiotoxic myolysis
cardiotoxin
Cardiotrast
cardiotrophin-1
cardiovalvotomy
cardiovalvulitis
cardiovalvulotomy
cardiovascular (CV)
  c. accident (CVA)
  acute c. (ACV)
  C. Angiography Analysis System
    (CAAS)
  c. cannula
  c. clamp
  c. clinic (CC)
  c. collapse
  c. complication
  c. computed tomography (CVCT)
  C. Credentialing International (CCI)
  c. disability
  c. disease (C, CD, CVD)
  c. excitatory center
  c. failure (CVF)
  c. fitness
  c. function (CVFn)
  c. function assessment
  c. imaging system (CVIS)
  c. incident (CVI)
  c. inhibitory center
  c. insufficiency (CVI)

C

NOTES

cardiovascular *(continued)*
    c. intensive care unit (CVICU)
    C. and Interventional Radiological Society of Europe (CIRSE)
    c. magnetic resonance (CMR)
    c. measurement system (CMS)
    c. monitor (CVM)
    c. pressure
    c. recovery room (CVRR)
    c. reflex conditioning (CRC)
    c. reflex conditioning system (CRCS)
    c. and respiratory elements of trauma score (CVRS)
    c. self-assessment tool (CST)
    c. steady state
    c. surgery (CVS)
    c. syphilis
    c. system (CVS)
    c. technologist (CVT)
cardiovasculare
    systema c.
cardiovascular-renal (CVR)
    c.-r. disease (CVRD)
cardiovascular-respiratory (CVR)
cardioventricular pacing (CVP)
cardioversion
    chemical c.
    DC c.
    direct current c. (DCCV)
    elective c.
    electrical c.
    external c. (ECV)
    external electric c.
    internal c.
    low-energy intracardiac c.
    low-energy synchronized c.
    c. paddles
    pharmacological c.
    synchronized DC c.
    synchronized direct current c.
    c. threshold
    transthoracic direct current electrical c.
    transvenous c. (TVCV)
    transvenous internal c.
cardioverter
    Lyra 2020 implantable c.
cardioverter-defibrillator *(See also* defibrillator)
    Angstrom MD implantable single-lead c.-d.
    atrial implantable c.-d. (AICD, A-ICD)
    atrial and ventricular implantable c.-d. (AV-ICD)
    automatic external c.-d. (AECD)
    automatic implantable c.-d. (AICD, A-ICD)

automatic internal c.-d. (AICD, A-ICD)
Cadet high voltage can implantable c.-d.
Cadet V-115 implantable c.-d.
Contour LTV-135D implantable c.-d.
Contour MD implantable single-lead c.-d.
Contour V-145D implantable c.-d.
external c.-d. (ECD)
Gem III AT implantable c.-d.
Gem II VR implantable c.-d.
Guardian ATP 4210 implantable c.-d.
implantable c.-d. (ICD)
implantable automatic c.-d. (IACD)
Intermedics Res-Q implantable c.-d.
Jewel pacer-c.-d.
Lyra 2020 implantable c.-d.
Medtronic external c.-d.
Medtronic Jewel AF 7250 dual-chamber implantable c.-d.
Medtronic PCD implantable c.-d.
Micron Res-Q implantable c.-d.
MycroPhylax implantable c.-d.
nonthoracotomy lead implantable c.-d.
pacer-c.-d. (PCD)
Phylax AV dual-chamber implantable c.-d.
Phylax 06 implantable c.-d.
Powerheart automatic external c.-d.
programmable c.-d. (PCD)
PRx implantable c.-d.
Res-Q ACD implantable c.-d.
Res-Q Micron implantable c.-d.
Sentinel 2010 implantable c.-d.
subpectoral implantation of c.-d.
Telectronics ATP implantable c.-d.
tiered-therapy implantable c.-d.
tiered-therapy programmable c.-d.
transthoracic implantable c.-d.
Transvene nonthoracotomy implantable c.-d.
Ventak A-V III DR automatic implantable c.-d.
Ventak Mini II and III automatic implantable c.-d.
Ventak Prizm 2 automatic implantable c.-d.
Ventak PRx c.-d.
ventricular implantable c.-d. (V-ICD, VICD)
Ventritex Angstrom MD implantable c.-d.
Ventritex Cadence implantable c.-d.
WCD 2000 system wearable c.-d.
wearable c.-d. (WCD)

cardiovirus
CardioWest
    C. TAH
    C. total artificial heart
carditis
    coxsackievirus c.
    rheumatic c.
    streptococcal c.
    verrucous c.
Cardizem
    C. CD
    C. Injectable
    C. Lyo-Ject
    C. Monovial
    C. SR
    C. Tablet
CardoSEAL septal occlusion system
Cardura
care
    American Association for
      Respiratory C. (AARC)
    continuity of c.
    coronary c. (CC)
    emergency cardiac c. (ECC)
    end-of-life c.
    intensive coronary c. (ICC)
    kangaroo c.
    long-term c. (LTC)
    National Board for Respiratory C.
      (NBRC)
    precoronary c. (PCC)
    subacute c.
    c. vigilance (CV)
Caregiver Strain Test
**CareLink network for patient
monitoring**
carer strain
**Carey Coombs short mid-diastolic
murmur**
CARhd
    high-dose carvedilol
carina, pl. **carinae**
    c. not splayed
    c. sharp and mobile
    c. of trachea
    c. tracheae
carinal lymph node
carinatum
    pectus c.
carindacillin
Carinia domestica

carinii
    Pneumocystis c.
cariporide
Carlen double-lumen endotracheal tube
Carmalt forceps
Carmeda BioActive Surface
C-arm fluoroscopy
Carmol topical
carneae
    trabeculae c.
carneus
    Aspergillus c.
Carney
    C. complex
    C. triad
carnitine deficiency
Carnoy solution
**Carolon life support antiembolism
stockings**
carotene
    beta c.
carotenoid
caroticotympanic artery
caroticovertebral stenosis
carotid
    c. angiography
    c. angioplasty and stenting (CAS)
    c. angioplasty and stent placement
    c. arch
    c. arteriography
    c. artery
    c. artery disease
    c. artery murmur
    c. artery shunt
    c. artery stenosis (CAS)
    c. artery stenting
    c. augmentation index
    c. ball
    c. baroreceptor
    c. baroreflex
    c. bifurcation
    c. B-mode sonography
    c. body (CB)
    c. body tumor
    c. bruit
    c. bulb
    c. canal
    c. Doppler
    c. duplex scan
    c. ejection time
    c. endarterectomy (CE, CEA)
    external c. (EC)

C

NOTES

carotid (*continued*)
   c. intima-media complex
   c. occlusive disease
   c. patch angioplasty
   c. phonoangiography
   c. plaque
   c. pulse
   c. pulse amplitude (CAR AMP)
   c. pulse tracing
   c. sheath
   c. shudder
   c. sinus
   c. sinus hypersensitivity
   c. sinus hypersensitivity syndrome
   c. sinus massage
   c. sinus nerve
   c. sinus reflex
   c. sinus stimulation
   c. sinus syncope
   c. sinus test
   c. siphon
   c. steal syndrome
   c. stenosis
   c. stent
   c. stent-supported angioplasty
   (CSSA)
   c. triangle
   c. upstroke
   c. vascular disease
carotid-axillary bypass
carotid-carotid bypass
carotid-cavernous fistula (CCF)
carotid-subclavian bypass
carotodynia, carotidynia
carpal
   c. arch anterior
   c. arch dorsal
   c. arch palmar
Carpenter syndrome
Carpentier
   C. annuloplasty
   C. pericardial valve
   C. ring
   C. tricuspid valvuloplasty
Carpentier-Edwards
   C.-E. aortic valve prosthesis
   C.-E. glutaraldehyde-preserved
   porcine xenograft prosthesis
   C.-E. mitral annuloplasty valve
   C.-E. pericardial valve
   C.-E. Perimount mitral valve
   C.-E. Perimount RSR pericardial
   bioprosthesis
   C.-E. Physio annuloplasty ring
   C.-E. Physio annuloplasty ring with
   Duraflo
   C.-E. porcine prosthetic valve
   C.-E. porcine supraannular valve
carpopedal spasm

Carrel method
**Carrie coronary stent placement
  technique**
Carrington
   C. disease
   C. pneumonia
CARS
   compensatory antiinflammatory response
   syndrome
cart
   MedGraphics CPX/D metabolic c.
   metabolic c.
   resuscitation c.
   SensorMedics 2900 metabolic c.
carteolol hydrochloride
Carter equation
Cartia XT
Cartilade
cartilage
   anular c.
   articular surface of arytenoid c.
   cricoid c.
   epiglottic c.
   c.'s of larynx
   Luschka c.
   Meyer c.
   Seiler c.
   tracheal c.
   xiphoid c.
cartilagines tracheales
cartilago
   c. cricoidea
   c. sesamoidea laryngis
CARTO
   C. EP navigation system
   C. magnetic mapping system
   C. XP system
Cartrol Oral
carumonam
caruncula, pl. **carunculae**
   c. salivaris
   sublingual c.
   c. sublingualis
Carvallo sign
carvedilol (CAR)
   high-dose c. (CARhd)
Cary 118C spectrophotometer
CAS
   calcific aortic stenosis
   cardiac adjustment scale
   cardiac surgery
   carotid angioplasty and stenting
   carotid artery stenosis
   coronary artery scan
   coronary artery spasm
**CAS-8000V general angiography
  positioner**
Casale-Devereux criteria

cascade
>> AA c.
>> arachidonic acid c.
>> downstream-signaling c.
>> immune c.
>> ischemic c.
>> leukocyte-endothelial cell
>>> adhesion c.
>> c. phenomenon
>> renin-angiotensin-aldosterone c.

case
>> M6/C cylinder carrying c.

caseated tissue

caseating

caseation
>> tuberculous c.

CASE computerized exercise ECG system

casein asthma

caseous
>> c. abscess
>> c. osteitis
>> c. pneumonia
>> c. tonsillitis

CASHD
>> coronary arteriosclerotic heart disease

casing
>> Silastic electrode c.

CASL-PI MRI
>> continuous arterial spin-labeled perfusion magnetic resonance imaging

Casodex

Casoni test

caspase inhibitor

CASPER
>> computer-assisted pericardial puncture
>> computer-assisted pericardial surgery

caspofungin acetate

CASQ
>> calsequestrin

CASS
>> continuous aspiration of subglottic secretions

cast
>> blood c.

Castaneda
>> C. bottle
>> C. principle

Castellani
>> C. bronchitis
>> C. disease
>> C. point

castellanii
>> *Acanthamoeba c.*

Castellino sign

Castillo catheter

Castleman disease

castor
>> c. bean
>> c. bean asthma

Castroviejo needle holder

CAT
>> computerized axial tomography

cat
>> c. asthma
>> c. cry syndrome

catabolic illness

catabolism of rt-PA

catacrotic
>> c. pulse
>> c. wave

catacrotism

catacrotus
>> pulsus c.

catadicrotic
>> c. pulse
>> c. wave

catadicrotism

catadicrotus

Cat-a-Kit analyzer

catalase
>> superoxide c.

catamenial
>> c. hemoptysis
>> c. hemothorax
>> c. pneumothorax

cataplectic

cataplexy

Catapres Oral

Catapres-TTS Transdermal

catarrh
>> atrophic c.
>> autumnal c.
>> Bostock c.
>> hypertrophic c.
>> Laënnec c.
>> postnasal c.
>> sinus c.
>> suffocative c.

catarrhal
>> c. asthma
>> c. bronchitis
>> c. croup
>> c. laryngitis

C

NOTES

catarrhal *(continued)*
 c. pharyngitis
 c. pneumonia
catarrhalis
 Branhamella c.
 Moraxella c.
 Neisseria c.
catastrophic hemorrhage
catatricrotic pulse
catatricrotism
Catatrol
CATCH-22
 cardiac defects, abnormal facies, thymic
 hypoplasia, cleft palate, hypocalcemia
 CATCH-22 syndrome
catecholamine (CA)
 c. action
 plasma c.
 c. release
catecholaminergic (CA)
category-ratio
 Borg c.-r.
catenoid
cath
 catheter
 catheterization
 catheterize
**CATHCOR LX hemodynamic recording
system**
cathepsin G
catherization
cathespin G
8F catheter
catheter (cath)
 c. ablation
 ablation c.
 c. ablation of atrial fibrillation
 Accent balloon angioplasty c.
 ACE fixed-wire balloon c.
 Achiever balloon dilatation c.
 ACS Endura coronary dilation c.
 ACS Enhanced Torque 8/7.5-F
  Taper Tip c.
 ACS Mini c.
 ACS Monorail c.
 ACS OTW Lifestream coronary
  dilatation c.
 ACS OTW Photon coronary
  dilatation c.
 ACS OTW Photon coronary
  dilation c.
 ACS OTW Solaris coronary
  dilatation c.
 ACS OTW Solaris coronary
  dilation c.
 ACS Photon coronary dilatation c.
 ACS RX Comet angioplasty c.
 ACS RX Comet coronary
  dilatation c.

ACS RX Comet VP coronary
 dilatation c.
ACS RX Lifestream coronary
 dilation c.
ACS RX perfusion balloon c.
ACS RX Solaris coronary
 dilatation c.
ACST Tx2000 coronary
 dilatation c.
AcuNav ultrasound c.
ACX II balloon c.
c. adapter
AFocus steerable diagnostic c.
afterloading c.
Ag-AgCl$_2$ electrode bipolar c.
Ahn thrombectomy c.
Alert c.
alignment c.
AL I, II guiding c.
Amazr c.
Amcath c.
Amplatz left I, II c.
Amplatz right coronary c.
Amplatz right I, II c.
A2 multipurpose c.
AngeCool RF c.
Angioflow high-flow c.
angiographic c.
AngioJet saline jet/vacuum
 device c.
AngioJet thrombectomy c.
Angio-Kit c.
Angiomedics c.
angioplasty guiding c.
angled balloon c.
angled pigtail c.
angle tipped c.
angulated multipurpose c.
Anthron II c.
Anthron heparinized
 antithrombogenic c.
aortic c.
AR-1 c.
Argyle c.
Arrow balloon wedge c.
Arrow Flex intraaortic balloon c.
Arrowgard Blue antiseptic-coated c.
Arrowgard Blue Line c.
Arrowgard central venous c.
Arrow-Howes multilumen c.
Arrow Pullback atherectomy c.
Arrow QuadPolar electrode c.
Arrow QuadPolar pulmonary
 artery c.
arterial embolectomy c.
c. arteriography
Ascent guiding c.
atherectomy c.

AtheroCath Bantam coronary atherectomy c.
AtheroCath GTO coronary atherectomy c.
Atlantis SR intravascular ultrasound imaging c.
Atlantis SR IVUS c.
Atlas DG balloon angioplasty c.
Atlas ULP balloon dilatation c.
ATRAC-II double-balloon c.
ATRAC multipurpose balloon c.
Aurous centimeter sizing c.
Aurous graduate sizing c.
autoperfusion balloon c.
Avanar intravascular ultrasound c.
Avanar IVUS c.
AV-Paceport thermodilution c.
Bailey c.
Baim pacing c.
balloon angioplasty c.
balloon embolectomy c.
balloon-flotation pacing c.
balloon-imaging c.
balloon septostomy c.
balloon-tipped angiographic c.
balloon-tipped flow-directed c.
balloon-tipped thermodilution c.
balloon valvuloplasty c.
c. balloon valvuloplasty (CBV)
Baltherm c.
Bandit PTCA c.
Bardco c.
Bard Safety Excalibur c.
Bard Stinger S ablation c.
Bentson-Hanafee-Wilson c.
Berman angiographic c.
Beta-Rail c.
Bicor c.
bifoil balloon c.
BioDiamond S rapid exchange PTCA c.
Bio-Medicus arterial c.
bipolar c.
bird's-eye c.
blade septostomy c.
Blazer RPM navigation and ablation c.
Blue FlexTip c.
Bonzel Monorail balloon c.
Bourassa c.
brachial c.
Brite Tip c.

Bronchitrac L flexible suction c.
Buchbinder Thruflex over-the-wire c.
bullet-tip c.
Burhenne steerable c.
butterfly c.
Calypso Rely PTCA balloon angioplasty c.
cardiac c.
Castillo c.
catheter introducing forceps c.
Cath-Finder c.
Cathlon IV c.
Cathmark suction c.
CCOmbo c.
central venous c. (CV, CVC, CV cath)
cerebral ablation c.
Chilli cooled-tip ablation c.
Clark rotating cutter c.
closed end-hole c.
Closer-Closure c.
Cloverleaf c.
cobra-shaped c.
coil-tipped c.
Comet c.
conductance c.
Constellation advanced mapping c.
Cook Cardiovascular infusion c.
Cook Spectrum c.
Cook TPN c.
Cool Tip c.
Cordis BriteTip guiding c.
Cordis Ducor I, II, III c.
Cordis Predator PTCA balloon c.
Cordis Titan balloon dilatation c.
Cordis-Webster ablation c.
Cordis-Webster mapping c.
coronary angiographic c.
coronary angiography c.
coronary sinus thermodilution c.
Cournand Tip Arrow QuadPolar electrode c.
CritiCath thermodilution c.
Critikon balloon temporary pacing c.
Critikon balloon-tipped end-hole c.
Critikon balloon wedge pressure c.
CrossPoint TransAccess c.
CrossSail coronary dilatation c.
cutdown c.
Cynosar c.

C

NOTES

catheter *(continued)*

Dacron c.
Damato curve c.
c. damping
Datascope CL-II percutaneous translucent balloon c.
decapolar electrode c.
deflectable quadripolar c.
DeKock two-way bronchial c.
Desai VectorCath mapping c.
diagnostic ultrasound imaging c.
Dilaca c.
c. dilation
directional atherectomy c.
Dispatch infusion c.
Dispatch over-the-wire c.
distal balloon c. (DBC)
dog-leg c.
Doppler coronary c.
Dotter caged-balloon c.
double-balloon c.
double-chip micromanometer c.
double-J c.
double-lumen c.
double-thermistor coronary sinus c.
drill-tip c.
D114S balloon c.
dual balloon perfusion c. (DBPC)
dual-sensor micromanometric high-fidelity c.
Ducor-Cordis pigtail c.
Duett c.
duodecapolar c.
EAC c.
EchoMark angiographic c.
EDM infusion c.
Edwards c.
EID c.
eight-lumen manometry c.
Elecath electrophysiologic stimulation c.
electrode c.
El Gamal coronary bypass c.
El Gamal guiding c.
embolectomy c.
c. embolectomy
c. embolism
Encapsulon epidural c.
Endeavor nondetachable silicone balloon c.
end-hole balloon-tipped c.
end-hole 7-French c.
EndoCPB c.
EndoSonics IVUS/balloon dilation c.
Endotak C lead transvenous c.
Enhanced Torque 8F guiding c.
EnSite multielectrode array transvenous c.

Epistat double balloon c.
Eppendorf c.
e-TRAIN 110 AngioJet c.
c. exchange
expandable access c. (EAC)
Explorer 360-degree rotational diagnostic EP c.
Expo diagnostic c.
Express PTCA c.
Extra Back-up guiding c.
Extreme II peripheral excimer laser c.
8F c.
Fact coronary balloon angioplasty c.
Falcon coronary c.
Falcon Omniflex balloon c.
Falcon Omniflex PTCA c.
Falcon single-operator exchange balloon c.
Fast-Cath hemostasis introducer c.
Feldman aortic stenosis c.
7F extended-curve thermistor c.
7F fused-tip c.
fiberoptic c. delivery system
fiberoptic oximeter c.
fiberoptic pressure c.
Finesse guiding c.
Fino DVT c.
fixed-wire coronary balloon c.
Flexguard Tip c.
flexible balloon-tipped c.
Flexxicon Blue dialysis c.
flotation c.
flow-assisted short-term balloon c.
flow-directed balloon cardiovascular c.
flow-directed end-hole c.
Flow Rider flow-directed c.
fluid-filled balloon cardiovascular c.
fluid-filled balloon-tipped flow-directed c.
fluid-filled pigtail c.
7F mapping c.
2F Millar Instrument c.
focal dilatation c.
Fogarty adherent clot c.
Fogarty embolectomy c.
Fogarty graft thrombectomy c.
Foltz-Overton cardiac c.
Force balloon dilatation c.
c. fragment
Franz monophasic action potential c.
French double-lumen c.
French JR4 Schneider c.
6-French Judkins c.
6.2-French 12.5-MHz c.

7-French 20-pole deflectable
   mapping c.
French SAL c.
French shaft c.
French sizing of c.
fused-tip c.
FX miniRAIL RX PTCA c.
Ganz-Edwards coronary infusion c.
Gazelle balloon dilatation c.
Gensini coronary arteriography c.
Gensini Teflon c.
Gentle-Flo suction c.
GlideCath hydrophilic coated c.
Goeltec c.
Goodale-Lubin c.
Gorlin c.
Gould PentaCath 5-lumen
   thermodilution c.
graft-seeking c.
Grollman pulmonary artery-
   seeking c.
Groshong double-lumen c.
Grüntzig balloon c.
Grüntzig Dilaca c.
Guardian c.
c. guidewire
guiding c.
Halo XP electrophysiology c.
Hancock embolectomy c.
Hancock fiberoptic c.
Hancock hydrogen detection c.
Hancock luminal electrophysiologic
   recording c.
Hancock wedge-pressure c.
Hands-Off thermal dilution c.
Hartzler ACX II c.
Hartzler LPS dilatation c.
Hartzler Micro-600 c.
Hartzler Micro II c.
Hartzler Micro XT c.
Hartzler RX-014 balloon c.
headhunter angiography c.
Heartport endocoronary sinus c.
Heartport endovascular c.
Helix PTCA dilatation c.
HemoSplit hemodialysis c.
HemoSplit long-term dialysis c.
high-density sector basket c.
high-flow c.
high-speed rotation dynamic
   angioplasty c.
Hilal modified headhunter c.

His bundle c.
hockey-stick c.
HP SONOS 30-MHz imaging c.
c. hub
HydroCath c.
Hydrolyser hydrodynamic
   thrombectomy c.
Hydrolyser percutaneous
   thrombectomy c.
Hydromer-coated central venous c.
IAB c.
ICE c.
Imager Torque selective c.
c. impact artifact
impedance c.
implantable cardioverter-
   defibrillator c. (ICDC)
Impulse diagnostic c.
indwelling central venous c.
Infiniti c.
InfusaSleeve II c.
injection c.
Inoue balloon c.
c. instability
Integra c.
Intellicath pulmonary artery c.
intercostal c.
internal mammary artery c.
intraaortic balloon c.
intraarterial c.
intracardiac c.
intrapleural c.
intravascular ultrasound c.
intraventricular c. (IVC)
Intrepid balloon c.
Intrepid PTCA c.
c. introduction method
irrigated coiled c.
ITC balloon c.
IVUS c.
Jackman coronary sinus
   electrode c.
Jackman orthogonal c.
JL4 c.
JL5 c.
Josephson quadripolar c.
Josephson Tip Arrow QuadPolar
   electrode c.
Jostra c.
JR4 c.
JR5 c.
Judkins coronary c.

NOTES

133

catheter *(continued)*

Judkins curve LAD c.
Judkins curve LCX c.
Judkins curve STD c.
Judkins 4 diagnostic c.
Judkins guiding c.
Judkins pigtail left
  ventriculography c.
Judkins torque control c.
jugular venous c. (JVC)
Katzen long balloon dilatation c.
King guiding c.
King multipurpose c.
Konigsberg c.
Kontron balloon c.
large-bore c.
laser delivery c.
Laserprobe c.
Laserprobe-PLR Flex c.
laser transluminal angioplasty c.
  (LASTAK)
Lasso c.
left coronary c.
left heart c.
left Judkins c.
left ventricular sump c.
Lehman ventriculography c.
Levin c.
Lifestream coronary dilation c.
Livewire TC ablation c.
Livewire TC steerable
  electrophysiology c.
long ACE fixed-wire balloon c.
Long Brite Tip guiding c.
Longdwel Teflon c.
long skinny over-the-wire
  balloon c.
Lo-Profile II c.
low-profile balloon-positioning c.
low-speed rotation angioplasty c.
Lumaguide c.
LuMax Flex guiding c.
Mallinckrodt angiographic c.
c. manipulation
manometer-tipped c.
Mansfield orthogonal electrode c.
Mansfield Scientific dilatation
  balloon c.
Mansfield-Webster c.
mapping c.
c. mapping
mapping/ablation c.
Marathon guiding c.
marker c.
Maverick 2 Monorail c.
Maverick OTW c.
MaxForce balloon dilatation c.
Maxi LD PTA dilation c.

Medi-Tech balloon c.
Medi-Tech steerable c.
Medtronic Zuma guiding c.
MegaSonics PTCA c.
memory c.
Mercator atrial high-density
  array c.
Metras c.
Metricath 1000 console c.
Metricath measurement c.
Mewi-5 sidehole infusion c.
Mewissen infusion c.
MicroFerret-18 infusion c.
Micro-Guide c.
micromanometer c.
MicroMewi multiple sidehole
  infusion c.
Micross dilatation c.
Mikro-Tip micromanometer-tipped c.
Millar Doppler c.
Millar MPC-500 c.
Millenia balloon c.
Millenia PTCA c.
Miller septostomy c.
Mini-Profile c.
Mirage over-the-wire balloon c.
Molina needle c.
Monorail angioplasty c.
Monorail imaging c.
More-Flow long-term high-flow c.
MS Classique balloon dilatation c.
MTC c.
Mullins transseptal c.
multiaccess c. (MAC)
multielectrode basket c.
multielectrode impedance c.
multipolar electrode c.
Multipurpose-SM c.
multisensor c.
MVP c.
Namic c.
NarrowFlex intraaortic balloon c.
National Institutes of Health left
  ventriculography c.
National Institutes of Health
  marking c.
NavAblator c.
Naviport deflectable tip guiding c.
Navistar c.
NC Bandit c.
NC Raptor over-the-wire coaxial
  PTCA dilatation balloon c.
Neptune high-pressure PTCA
  balloon c.
NeuroVasx submicroinfusion c.
Newton c.
Nexus 2 linear ablation c.
NIH cardiomarker c.

Ninja FX series over-the-wire coaxial PTCA dilatation balloon c.
NoProfile Olbert Catheter system balloon dilatation c.
Norton flow-directed Swan-Ganz thermodilution c.
Novoste c.
Nycore pigtail c.
Nylex diagnostic c.
octapolar c.
Olbert balloon c.
Olympix II PTCA dilatation c.
Omega NV angioplasty c.
OmniCath atherectomy c.
Omni Flush c.
one-hole angiographic c.
one-hole angioplastic c.
OpenSail balloon c.
OpenSail coronary dilatation c.
Opta 5 c.
Opta Pro PTA dilatation c.
optical fiber c.
Opticath oximeter c.
Opti-Flow c.
Opti-Plast XT balloon c.
Oracle Focus imaging c.
Oracle Focus PTCA c.
Oracle Micro Plus PTCA c.
OTW HighSail coronary dilatation c.
OTW perfusion c.
over-the-needle c.
over-the-wire PTCA balloon c.
Owens balloon c.
Owens Lo-Profile dilatation c.
oximetric c.
Pace bipolar pacing c.
pacemaker c.
Paceport c.
pacing c.
ParCA c.
Parodi c.
c. patency
pediatric pigtail c.
Peel-Away banana c.
PE-MT balloon dilatation c.
Pentalumen c.
Percor Stat-DL intra-arotic balloon c.
percutaneous intraaortic balloon counterpulsation c.

percutaneous radiofrequency c.
percutaneous rotational thrombectomy c.
Performa diagnostic c.
perfusion c.
perfusion balloon c. (PBC)
Periflow balloon dilation c.
peripherally inserted c. (PIC)
Per-Q-Cath percutaneously inserted central venous c.
pervenous c.
Phantom V Plus c.
PIBC c.
Piccolino Monorail c.
pigtail rotation c.
Pinkerton .018 balloon c.
Pleurx pleural c.
plugged telescoping c.
POC Bandit c.
Polaris-DX steerable diagnostic c.
Polystan venous return c.
Positrol II c.
Powerflex Extreme PTA balloon c.
Powerflex P3 high pressure balloon c.
Predator PTCA c.
preshaped c.
Pro-Bal Protected balloon-tipped c.
probe balloon c.
probing sheath exchange c.
Procath electrophysiology c.
ProCross Rely over-the-wire balloon c.
Profile Plus balloon dilatation c.
Proflex 5 c.
pulmonary artery flotation c.
Pursuit balloon angioplasty c.
quadripolar diagnostic c.
quadripolar pacing c.
quadripolar steerable electrode c.
quadripolar steerable mapping/ablation c.
quadripolar thermocouple-equipped ablation c.
QuickFlash arterial c.
Quinton PermCath c.
Radii-T c.
radiopaque ERCP c.
Ranger over-the-wire balloon c.
Rashkind septostomy balloon c.
Rebar-18 micro c.
recessed balloon septostomy c.

NOTES

C

catheter *(continued)*

Redha-cut c.
reference c.
Ref-Star EP c.
Rentrop c.
reperfusion c.
Response electrophysiology c.
RF-generated thermal balloon c.
RF Marinr c.
rheolytic thrombectomy c.
Rhythm c.
right coronary c.
right heart c.
right Judkins c.
Rigiflex TTS balloon c.
RMI antegrade cardioplegia c.
rotational dynamic angioplasty c.
Rothbarth Uni-Flo infusion c.
Roubin infusion c.
Royal Flush Plus high-flow
  angiographic flush c.
R1 rapid exchange balloon
  dilatation c.
RX CrossSail coronary dilatation c.
RX Streak balloon c.
Sable PTCA balloon c.
Safe-Steer support c.
Sarns wire-reinforced c.
Savvy PTA dilatation c.
Schmitz-Rode c.
Scimed angioplasty c.
Scoop 1, 2 c.
self-guiding c.
self-positioning balloon c.
semirigid c.
Sensation intraaortic balloon c.
Seroma-Cath c.
serrated c.
S.E.T. thrombectomy system c.
Shadow over-the-wire balloon c.
sheath-based IVUS c.
Sherpa guiding c.
Shiley c.
SHJL4 c.
SHJR4 c.
SHJR4s c.
short monorail imaging c.
shredding embolectomy
  thrombectomy c.
sidewinder percutaneous intra-aortic
  balloon c.
Silastic c.
Simmons II, III c.
Simmons-type sidewinder c.
Simpson atherectomy c.
Simpson AtheroCath c.
Simpson-Robert c.
Slalom PTA dilatation c.
sliding rail c.

Smec balloon c.
snare c.
Softip c.
Softouch diagnostic c.
Soft-Vu Omni flush c.
Solera thrombectomy c.
Solo c.
Sones coronary c.
Sones Hi-Flow c.
Sones woven Dacron c.
Spectranetics C rapid-exchange
  laser c.
Spectranetics Extreme c.
Spring c.
Spyglass angiography c.
Stack perfusion c.
standard Lehman c.
steerable decapolar electrode c.
steerable guidewire c.
Steerocath-A ablation c.
Steerocath-Dx special procedure
  octa c.
Steerocath-T temperature ablation c.
Steri-Cath c.
Stertzer brachial c.
Stertzer guiding c.
Stinger S ablation c.
Stormer balloon c.
straight flush percutaneous c.
straight tipped c.
Sub-Microinfusion c.
Sub-4 small vessel balloon
  dilatation c.
Super Torque Plus c.
Supreme electrophysiology c.
Surpass PTCA perfusion c.
Swan-Ganz balloon flotation c.
Swan-Ganz bipolar pacing c.
Swan-Ganz flow-directed c.
Swan-Ganz Pacing TD c.
Syntel latex-free embolectomy c.
Syntel latis graft cleaning c.
systemic arterial c.
TADcath temporary transvenous
  defibrillation c.
Talon balloon dilatation c.
TEC extraction c.
TEC-guide c.
Teflon c.
Tempo diagnostic c.
Terumo SP coaxial c.
tetrapolar esophageal c.
thermodilution balloon c.
thermodilution Swan-Ganz c.
thin-walled c.
c. thrombectomy
Thrombolizer c.
through-the-needle c.
Tidal balloon c.

Titan mega XL PTCA dilatation c.
Torcon NB Advantage coronary
  angiographic c.
Torcon NB selective
  angiographic c.
torque control balloon c.
torque tube c.
Total Cross balloon c.
Tourguide guiding c.
Tracker-18 Soft Stream side-hole
  microinfusion c.
Trakstar balloon c.
transcutaneous extraction c.
transfemoral endoaortic occlusion c.
transluminal angioplasty c.
transluminal endarterectomy c.
  (TEC)
transluminal extraction c. (TEC)
Transport dilatation balloon c.
Transport drug delivery c.
transseptal c.
transtracheal oxygen c.
trefoil balloon c.
tripolar with Damato curve c.
True Sheathless intraaortic
  balloon c.
Tyshak balloon valvuloplasty c.
Uldall subclavian hemodialysis c.
ULP c.
Ultra 8 balloon c.
UltraCross profile imaging c.
UltraFuse infusion c.
Ultra ICE c.
ultra-low profile fixed-wire balloon
  dilation c.
ultrasound ablation c.
ultrasound-tipped c.
Ultra-Thin balloon c.
UMI c.
urinary c.
USCI c.
valve mapper Steerocath-Dx
  mapping c.
van Andel c.
Van Tassel c.
Vantex central venous c.
Variflex catheter c.
vascular access c.
Vaxcel c.
vector phased-array ultrasound
  tipped c.
Vector-X coronary guiding c.

Venaport coronary sinus guiding c.
ventriculoatrial shunt c.
ventriculography c.
Veripath peripheral guiding c.
vessel-sizing c.
Viggo Spectramed c.
Viking Bard c.
Viking coronary guiding c.
Visa II ST PTCA balloon c.
Vision PTCA c.
Vista Brite Tip large lumen
  guiding c.
Vitesse C c.
Vitesse Cos laser c.
Vitesse E c.
Vitesse E2 rapid-exchange c.
Vitesse PrimaFx c.
Viva Primo balloon c.
vortex effect c.
Vueport balloon-occlusion
  guiding c.
VVDL c.
waist of c.
Webster halo c.
Webster orthogonal electrode c.
wedge pressure balloon c.
c. whip
c. whip artifact
White vessel sizing c.
Wilton Webster coronary sinus
  thermodilution c.
Wilton Webster thermodilution flow
  and pacing c.
Wiseguide guide c.
WorkHorse percutaneous
  transluminal angioplasty balloon c.
WorkHorse PTCA balloon c.
woven Dacron c.
XMI thrombectomy c.
Xpeedior t120 c.
Z cardiac c.
Z-Med c.
Zuma guiding c.
Zynergy Zolution
  electrophysiology c.
catheter-based
  c.-b. revascularization
  c.-b. sensor
**catheter-directed thrombolysis and
  endovascular stent placement**
catheter-guided
  c.-g. biopsy

C

NOTES

catheter-guided *(continued)*
    c.-g. endoscopic intubation
      (CAGEIN)
catheter-guide wire
catheter-induced
    c.-i. ablation
    c.-i. coronary artery spasm
    c.-i. embolus
    c.-i. spasm (CIS)
    c.-i. thrombosis
catheterization (cath)
    balloon c.
    bypass graft c.
    cardiac c. (CC)
    combined heart c.
    coronary sinus c.
    diagnostic c. (dx cath)
    hepatic vein c.
    interventional cardiac c.
    left heart c. (LHC)
    Mullins modification of
      transseptal c.
    percutaneous transhepatic cardiac c.
    pulmonary artery c. (PAC)
    retrograde c.
    right heart c. (RHC)
    selective cardiac c.
    selective venous c. (SVC)
    subclavian approach for cardiac c.
    subclavian vein c. (SVC)
    c. technique
    transradial cardiac c.
    transseptal left heart c.
    Y wave pressure on right atrial c.
    Z point pressure on left atrial c.
    Z point pressure on right atrial c.
catheterize (cath)
catheter-microphone
    cardiac c.-m.
catheter-related
    c.-r. infection (CRI)
    c.-r. peripheral vessel spasm
catheter-snare system
catheter-tip
    c.-t. micromanometer system
    c.-t. occluder
    c.-t. spasm
Cath-Finder
    C.-F. catheter
    C.-F. catheter tracking system
Cathflo Activase
Cath-Gard
    C.-G. catheter contamination shield
    TwistLock C.-G.
CathLink 20 implanted port
Cath-Lok catheter locking device
Cathlon IV catheter
Cathmark suction catheter

cathodal
    c. closing (KC)
    c. closing contraction (KCC, KSC)
    c. closure clonus (CCCl)
    c. closure contraction (CCC)
    c. closure tetanus (CCTe)
    c. opening clonus (COCl)
    c. opening contraction (COC,
      KOC)
    c. opening tetanus (COTe)
cathode duration tetanus (CDTe)
cat-scratch disease
cattaire
    frémissement c.
cauda equina syndrome
**caudally angled balloon occlusion
  aortography**
caudal plane angulation
caudate
    c. hemorrhage
    c. hemorrhagic stroke
    c. infarct
    c. ischemic stroke
    c. nucleus
caudocephalad
caudocranial hemiaxial view
causality assessment
**cautery-assisted palatal stiffening
  operation (CAPSO)**
CAV
    cardiac allograft vasculopathy
    cyclophosphamide, doxorubicin,
      vincristine
cav
    cavity
cava, pl. **cavae**
    foramen venae cavae
    inferior vena c. (IVC)
    left inferior vena c. (LIVC)
    left superior vena c. (LSVC)
    membranous obstruction of the
      inferior vena c. (MOIVC)
    membranous obstruction of inferior
      vena c. (MOVC)
    orifice of superior vena c.
    right inferior vena c. (RIVC)
    right superior vena c. (RSVC)
    superior vena c. (SVC)
    thoracic inferior vena c. (TIVC)
    vena c. (VC)
cavae (*pl. of* cava) (*pl. of* cavum)
caval
    c. snare
    c. valve
Cavalieri method
CAVB
    complete atrioventricular block

CAVD
    cardiac allograft vascular disease
    complete atrioventricular dissociation
caveolae
    intracellular c.
Caverject injection
cavernoma
cavernous
    c. angioma
    c. hemangioma
    c. rale
    c. respiration
    c. sinus (CS)
    c. sinus thrombosis
    c. vein of penis
    c. voice
cave sickness
Caves-Schultz bioptome
CAVG
    coronary artery vein graft
CAVH
    continuous arteriovenous hemofiltration
CAVHD
    continuous arteriovenous hemodialysis
CAVHDF
    continuous arteriovenous
    hemodiafiltration
caviae
    Aeromonas c.
cavitary
    c. lesion
    c. lung disease
cavitas
    c. laryngis
    c. pharyngis
    c. pleuralis
cavitation
    pulmonary c.
cavitis
Cavitron ultrasonic surgical aspirator (CUSA)
cavity (cav)
    bronchiectatic c.
    celomic c.
    inferior laryngeal c.
    intermediate laryngeal c.
    c. of larynx
    neoplastic c.
    pharyngonasal c.
    pleural c.
    pleuroperitoneal c.

    pulmonary c.
    superior laryngeal c.
    thrombus-filled c.
    ventricular c.
CAVO
    common atrioventricular orifice
cavoatrial anastomosis
cavocaval shunt
cavography
    radionuclide superior c. (RNSC)
cavopulmonary
    c. anastomosis
    c. channel
    c. connection
    c. shunt
cavotricuspid
    c. isthmus
    c. isthmus mapping
CAVR
    continuous arteriovenous rewarming
CAVU
    continuous arteriovenous ultrafiltration
cavum, pl. **cavae**
    c. pharyngis
    c. pleurae
CAZ beta-lactamase
CB
    carotid body
    code blue
    CB lead
C4B
    human gene C4B
CBA
    congenital bronchial atresia
    cutting balloon angioplasty
CBBEST
    cutting balloon before stent
CBC
    complete blood count
CBD
    chronic beryllium disease
CBF
    capillary blood flow
    cerebral blood flow
    coronary blood flow
CBFV
    cerebral blood flow velocity
    coronary blood flow velocity
CBG
    capillary blood gas
    coronary bypass graft

C

NOTES

CBP
cardiopulmonary bypass
cyclophosphamide, bleomycin, cisplatin
CBS
capillary blood sugar
CBT
code blue team
CBV
catheter balloon valvuloplasty
central blood volume
circulating blood volume
corrected blood volume
C-C
convexoconcave
C-C heart valve
CC
cardiac catheterization
cardiac center
cardiac contusion
cardiac cycle
cardiovascular clinic
coronary care
Adalat CC
CC chemokine I-309
CCA
calcium channel antagonist
cephalin cholesterol antigen
circumflex coronary artery
CCA-IMT
common carotid artery intima-media
thickness
CCB
calcium-channel blocker
CCBV
central circulating blood volume
CCC
Canadian Cardiovascular Coalition
cathodal closure contraction
common carotid compression
cranio-cerebello-cardiac dysplasia
cranio-cerebello-cardiac syndrome
CCCl
cathodal closure clonus
CCCR
closed chest cardiac resuscitation
CCCU
comprehensive cardiac care unit
CCD
clinical cardiovascular disease
crossed cerebellar diaschisis
cumulative cardiotoxic dose
CCE
clubbing, cyanosis, and edema
CCF
carotid-cavernous fistula
cephalin-cholesterol flocculation
CCI
Cardiovascular Credentialing
International

cholesterol crystallization inhibitor
chronic coronary insufficiency
coherent contrast imaging
C-clamp
CCM
congestive cardiomyopathy
CCN
coronary care nursing
CCO
continuous cardiac output
CCOmbo catheter
CCPD
continuous cyclical peritoneal dialysis
CCPR
closed chest cardiopulmonary
resuscitation
CCS
Canadian Cardiovascular Society
CCSAS
Canadian Cardiovascular Society angina
score
CCSC
Canadian Cardiovascular Society
classification
CCTe
cathodal closure tetanus
CC-TGA
congenitally corrected transposition of
great vessels
CCTP
coronary care training program
CCU
cardiac care unit
coronary care unit
CCVD
chronic cerebrovascular disease
CCVM
congenital cardiovascular malformation
CD
cardiac disease
cardiac dullness
cardiac dysrhythmia
cardiovascular disease
conduction defect
Cardizem CD
Ceclor CD
Cd
cadmium
CD8+ T cell
CD3 cell
CD4+
CD4+ cell
CD4+ measure
CD4 cell
CD8
CD8 AIS CELLector
CD8 cell
CD18 antibody
CD20 cell

CD45 cell surface protein
CD5 cell
CD62p (p-selectin) platelet activation marker
CD63 platelet activation marker
CD68 cell
CDBR
  computerized diaphragmatic breathing retraining
  controlled diaphragmatic breathing
    CDBR respiratory muscle training
CDE
  color Doppler energy
cDGS
  complete form of DiGeorge syndrome
CDH
  congenital diaphragmatic hernia
CDI 2000 blood gas monitoring system
CDM
  change description master
cDNA
  human cloned DNA
CDP
  certified distinct part
  coronary drug project
CDTe
  cathode duration tetanus
CDU
  cardiac diagnostic unit
CE
  carboplatin, etoposide
  cardiac enlargement
  cardioesophageal
  carotid endarterectomy
CEA
  carcinoembryonic antigen
  carotid endarterectomy
  cholesterol-esterifying activity
CEAP classification
CEAT
  chronic ectopic atrial tachycardia
CECCC
  confidential enquiry into cardiac catheterization complications
Ceclor CD
cedar
    Western red c.
Cedars-Sinai classification
Cedax
Cedocard-SR
CEE
  conjugated equine estrogen

CEEA
  curved end-to-end anastomosis
    CEEA stapler
Ceelen disease
Ceelen-Gellerstedt
    C.-G. disease
    C.-G. syndrome
CeeNU Oral
cefaclor
cefadroxil monohydrate
Cefadyl
cefamandole nafate
cefazolin sodium
cefdinir
cefditoren pivoxil
cefepime HCl
cefixime
Cefizox
cefmetazole sodium
Cefobid
cefonicid sodium
cefoperazone sodium
ceforanide
Cefotan
cefotaxime sodium
cefotetan disodium
cefoxitin sodium
cefpiramide
cefpodoxime proxetil
cefprozil
ceftazidime
ceftibuten
Ceftin Oral
Ceftizox
ceftizoxime sodium
ceftriaxone sodium
cefuroxime
Cefzil
Cegka sign
CEH
    cholesterol ester hydrolase
CEHC
    calf embryonic heart cell
ceiling effect in hypertension
celecoxib
celer
    pulsus c.
Celermajer method
celerrimus
    pulsus c.
Celestin esophageal tube

NOTES

Celestone
  C. Oral
  C. Phosphate Injection
  C. Soluspan
celiac
  c. artery
  c. artery axis
  c. disease
celiacus
  truncus c.
celiprolol
cell
  c. adhesion molecule (CAM)
  adventitial c.
  air c.
  alveolar c.
  ameboid c.
  Anichkov c.
  apoptotic c.
  Aschoff c.
  automatic c.
  B1 c.
  bovine aortic endothelial c.
    (BAEC)
  bradykinin-stimulated c.
  bronchial epithelial c.
  bronchiolar exocrine c.
  brush c.
  c. button
  calf embryonic heart c. (CEHC)
  CD3 c.
  CD4 c.
  CD4+ c.
  CD5 c.
  CD8 c.
  CD20 c.
  CD68 c.
  CD8+ T c.
  chicken-wire myocardial c.
  ciliated epithelial c.
  clear c.
  c. cycle
  effector c.
  embryonal c.
  endodermal c.
  epithelial c.
  equator of c.
  foam c.
  foamy myocardial c.
  giant c.
  goblet c.
  c. granulation
  great alveolar c.
  heart failure c.
  HeLa c.
  human aortic endothelial c.
    (HAEC)
  human aortic smooth muscle c.
    (HASMC)

hyperplastic mucus-secreting
  goblet c.
IgE-sensitized c.
Kulchitsky c.
Langerhans giant c.
Langhans c.
Langhans-type giant c.
mast c.
c. membrane
c. membrane-bound adenylate
  cyclase
mesangial c.
mesenchymal intimal c.
mesothelial c.
metaplastic mucus-secreting c.
mononuclear c.
mucous c.
multinucleated giant c.
N c.
neoplastic c.
NPM c.'s
oat c.
P c.
Pelger-Huet c.
peripheral blood mononuclear c.
  (PBMC)
prolactin-producing decidual c.
pup c.
Purkinje c.
RA c.
red blood c. (RBC)
renal juxtaglomerular c.
c. respiration
Sala c.
C. Saver
C. Saver autologous blood recovery
  system
C. Saver Haemonetics
  Autotransfusion system
sensitized c.
septal c.
smooth muscle c. (SMC)
c. sorter
squamous alveolar c.
stave c.
c. strain
T c.
transitional c.
c. type
typical small c.
vacuolated c.
vascular smooth muscle c. (VSMC)
vasofactive c.
c. wall defect (CWD)
whorling of myocardial c.
CellCept
  C. capsule
  C. intravenous
  C. intravenous for injection

C. oral suspension
C. tablet
cell-coated stent
CELLector
CD8 AIS C.
cell-free extract
cell-mediated
c.-m. immune response
c.-m. immunity
cellophane rale
cell-seeded stent
Celltrifuge
cellular
c. cholesterol efflux
c. embolism
c. infiltrate
c. metaplasia
c. sheets
cellulitis
cellulose
oxidized c.
celomic cavity
celophlebitis
CELP
code excited linear prediction
CELP ECG
Celsa battery
Celsior solution
Cel-U-Jec Injection
CEMRA
contrast-enhanced magnetic resonance
angiography
Cenafed Plus Tablet
Cenflex central monitoring system
Cenolate
centenarian
center
cardiac c. (CC)
cardiac-accelerator c. (CAC, CACh)
cardioaccelerator c.
cardioinhibitor c. (CIC)
cardioinhibitory c.
cardiovascular excitatory c.
cardiovascular inhibitory c.
Chemetron HR-1 humidity c.
chest pain c. (CPC)
C.'s for Epidemiologic Studies
Depression scale (CES-D)
expiratory c.
inpatient exercise c. (IEC)
inspiratory c.
interventional cardiac c. (ICC)

Kronecker c.
musculoskeletal intervention c.
(MUSIC)
pneumotaxic c.
respiratory c.
vasoconstrictor c. (VCC)
vasodilator c. (VDC)
vasoinhibitory c. (VIC)
vasomotor c. (VMC)
Veterans Affairs Medical C.
(VAMC)
centerline method of wall motion
analysis
Centimist nebulizer
centimorgan (cM)
CentoRx
central
c. apical part (CAP)
c. apnea
c. apnea-hypopnea index
c. approach
c. baroreflex failure
c. blood volume (CBV)
c. bradycardia
c. bridging strut
c. bronchovascular bundle
c. circulating blood volume
(CCBV)
c. cyanosis
c. fibrous body
c. hypopnea
c. motor conduction time (CMCT)
c. pneumonia
c. respiration
c. retinal artery occlusion (CRAO)
c. sleep apnea (CSA)
c. sleep apnea syndrome (CSAS)
c. splanchnic venous thrombosis
(CSVT)
c. tendon of diaphragm
c. terminal electrode
c. vein
c. vein occlusion (CVO)
c. venous (CV)
c. venous catheter (CV, CVC, CV
cath)
c. venous line
c. venous oximetry
c. venous oxygen (CVO)
c. venous pressure (CVP)
c. venous temperature (CVT)
centriacinar emphysema

NOTES

centrifugal
- c. left and right ventricular assist device
- c. pump

centrilobular
- c. axial interstitial disease
- c. cyst
- c. emphysema
- c. nodule

centripetal
- c. diffusion
- c. rub (CPR)
- c. venous pulse

centroid

centronuclear myopathy

centrum tendineum diaphragmatis

Century heart-lung machine

CEP
- chronic eosinophilic pneumonia

cepacia
- *Burkholderia c.*
- *Pseudomonas c.*

Cepacia syndrome

ceph
- cephalin

cephalexin monohydrate

cephalic
- c. approach
- c. artery
- c. vasomotor response (CVR)
- c. vein

cephalin (ceph)
- c. cholesterol antigen (CCA)
- c. flocculation (CEPH FLOC)

cephalin-cholesterol flocculation (CCF)

cephalization of pulmonary flow pattern

cephalocaudad

cephalometrics

cephalometry
- lateral c.
- radiographic c.

cephalopharyngeus

cephalosporin
- fourth-generation c.
- second-generation c.
- third-generation c.

cephalothin sodium

cephapirin sodium

CEPH FLOC
- cephalin flocculation

cephradine

Ceporacin

Ceptaz

CEqual
- C. Lite cardiac rehabilitation protocol
- C. Plus cardiac rehabilitation protocol

cerebra (*pl. of* cerebrum)

cerebral
- c. ablation catheter
- c. air embolism
- c. amyloid angiopathy (CAA)
- c. aneurysm
- c. angiography
- c. anoxia
- c. apoplexy
- c. arteriosclerosis
- c. autosomal dominant arteriopathy with subcortical infarct and leukoencephalopathy (CADASIL)
- c. beriberi
- c. bleeding
- c. blood flow (CBF)
- c. blood flow velocity (CBFV)
- c. edema
- c. embolization
- c. embolus
- c. event
- c. HT
- c. hyperthermia
- c. infarct
- c. infarction
- c. ischemia
- c. lupus
- c. microangiopathy (CMA)
- c. oximetry
- c. perfusion
- c. perfusion pressure (CPP)
- c. pneumonia
- c. protective therapy
- c. rate of glucose metabolism (CMR_{gic})
- c. rate of oxygen metabolism ($CMRO_2$)
- c. red blood cell volume (CRCV)
- c. respiration
- c. thromboangiitis obliterans (CTAO)
- c. thrombosis
- c. transit time (cTT)
- c. tuberculosis
- c. vasculopathy
- c. vasospasm (CVS)
- c. venous thrombosis (CVT)

cerebritis

cerebroprotective

cerebrovascular (CV)
- c. accident (CVA)
- c. amyloid peptide (CVAP)
- c. autoregulation
- c. disease (CeVD)
- c. event
- c. ferrocalcinosis
- c. incident (CVI)
- c. infarction (CVI)
- c. insufficiency (CVI)
- c. reactivity (CVR)

c. reserve capacity (CRC)
c. resistance (CVR)
c. syncope
c. thrombosis
cerebrum, pl. **cerebrums, cerebra**
Ceredase injection
cereolysin
cereus
    Bacillus c.
Cerezyme
cerivastatin
c. sodium
c. sodium tablet
Cerose-DM
certified distinct part (CDP)
Certoparin
ceruleus
    locus c.
cervical
c. aortic arch
c. aortic knuckle
c. disk
c. heart
c. part of esophagus
c. pleura
c. plexus block for carotid
   endarterectomy surgery
c. radiculitis
c. rib syndrome
c. spine deformity
c. venous hum
c. vertebra (CV)
cervicalis
    ansa c.
cervicothoracic sympathectomy
CES
   cardioembolic stroke
CESD
   cholesterol ester storage disease
CES-D
   Centers for Epidemiologic Studies
   Depression scale
cesium chloride
cESS
   circumferential end-systolic stress
cessation
    airflow c.
    smoking c.
cestodic tuberculosis
CET
   cholesterol-ester transfer
Cetacaine

CE-TCCS
   contrast-enhanced transcranial color-
    coded real-time sonography
cetirizine
CETP
   cholesteryl ester transfer protein
CEU
   contrast-enhanced ultrasound
CeVD
   cerebrovascular disease
CF
   cardiac failure
   chest and left leg
   clotting factor
   complex fixation
   contractile force
   coronary flow
   cystic fibrosis
    Guiatuss CF
    CF lead
    CF lead in electrocardiography
    Robafen CF
    Synacol CF
CFA
   cryptogenic fibrosing alveolitis
CFC
   cardiofaciocutaneous syndrome
   chlorofluorocarbon
CFC-free
    CFC-f. delivery system
    CFC-f. product
CFQ
   Cognitive Failures Questionnaire
CFR
   coronary flow reserve
CFS
   chronic fatigue syndrome
CFT
   cardiolipin flocculation test
CFTR
   cystic fibrosis transmembrane regulator
CFVR
   coronary flow velocity reserve
CFX
   circumflex coronary artery
CFX-MARG
   marginal branch of the circumflex artery
CFZ
   clofazimine
CG
   cardiography

C

NOTES

cGMP
cyclic guanosine monophosphate
CGN
compressor-generated nebulizer
CGR biplane angiographic system
CGRP
calcitonin gene-related peptide
CGS
cardiogenic shock
CGVD
chronic graft vascular disease
CH
calcium heparin
cholesterol
chronic hypertension
continuous heparin
CH 2000 cardiac diagnostic system
CH infusion
Ch, ch
chest
Chagas heart disease
chagasic myocardiopathy
chagoma
chain
alpha-myosin heavy c. (alpha-MHC)
beta-myosin heavy c. (beta-MHC)
imaging c.
light c.
myosin heavy c.
myosin light c.
paratracheal c.
chain-compensated spirometer
challenge
antiarrhythmic c.
carbachol inhalation c. (CIC)
cold air c. (CAC, CACh)
cold dry air c.
ergonovine c.
fluid c.
histamine c.
hypercapnic c.
methacholine bronchoprovocation c.
osmotic c.
chamber
AeroChamber Plus valved
holding c.
anterior c. (AC, ac)
atrialized c.
Boydens c.
cardiac c.
c. compression
c. dilation
dual c. (DC)
EasiVent valved holding c.
false aneurysmal c.
c.'s of the heart
hyperbaric c.
monoplace c.
MR 290 humidification c.

multiplace c.
OptiChamber valved holding c.
plasma clot diffusion c. (PCDC)
rudimentary c.
c. rupture
c. stiffness
valved holding c. (VHC)
Chamberlain
C. mediastinoscopy
C. procedure
Chandler V-pacing probe
change
apoptotic c.
arteriovenous crossing c.
c. description master (CDM)
environmental c.
E-to-A c.
fibrinoid c.
fractional area c. (FAC)
Gerhardt c.
hyaline fatty c.
ischemic ECG c.
malignancy-associated c. (MAC)
myxomatous c.
nonspecific climatic c.
obstructive sleep apnea-induced
cardiovascular c.
polyneuropathy, organomegaly,
endocrinopathy, monoclonal
gammopathy and skin c.'s
(POEMS)
QRS c.
rheologic c.
serial c.
skin c.
ST segment c.'s
ST-T segment c.'s
ST-T wave c.'s
trophic c.'s
T wave c.
vascular c. (VC)
channel
cavopulmonary c.
collateral c.
common pulmonary venous c.
(CPVC)
fast c.
HERG potassium c.
ion c.
K^+ c.
lymphatic c.
marker c.
membrane c.
receptor-operated calcium c.
sarcolemmal calcium c.
slow c.
sodium c.
transmural c.
transmyocardial laser c.

transnexus c.
T-type calcium c.
voltage-dependent calcium c.
voltage-gated c.
voltage-sensitive calcium c. (VSCC)
water c.

channeling
mechanical myocardial c. (MMC)
myocardial c. (MC)
percutaneous myocardial c. (PMC)
transmyocardial mechanical c.
(TMC)

chaos theory
chaotic
c. atrial tachycardia
c. heart
c. rhythm

Chapman index
charcoal
c. heart
c. hemoperfusion

Charcot
C. sign
C. syndrome

Charcot-Bouchard
C.-B. aneurysm
C.-B. microaneurysm

Charcot-Leyden crystal
Charcot-Marie-Tooth disease
Charcot-Neumann crystal
Charcot-Robin crystal
Charcot-Weiss-Baker syndrome
Chardack-Greatbatch
C.-G. implantable cardiac pulse
generator
C.-G. pacemaker

Chardack Medtronic pacemaker
CHARGE
coloboma, heart anomaly, choanal atresia,
retardation, and genital and ear
anomalies
CHARGE association
CHARGE syndrome

charge-coupled device transducer
charge time
Charles
C. law
C. procedure

Charlson comorbidity index
Char syndrome

CHART
continuous hyperfractionated accelerated
radiotherapy

charybdotoxin
Chasers
Scot-Tussin DM Cough C.

Chassaignac axillary muscle
Chaussier tube
CHB
complete heart block
congenital heart block

CHC
Canadian Heart Classification

CHD
congenital heart disease
congestive heart disease
coronary heart disease
cyanotic heart disease

Chealamide
CHEC
community hypertension evaluation clinic

check
magnet c.

Check-Flo
C.-F. introducer
C.-F. performer introducer set for
radial artery access
C.-F. sheath obturator

checklist
Hopkins Symptom C.

Checkmate gamma brachytherapy
system
Chédiak-Higashi syndrome
Chedoke-McMaster Stroke Assessment
cheese
c. worker's lung
c. worker's lung disease

cheesy
c. bronchitis
c. pneumonia

chelate
gadolinium c.

chelator
iron c.

chelonae
Mycobacterium c.

Chemetron HR-1 humidity center
chemical
c. ablation
acaricidal c.
c. bronchiectasis
c. bronchitis

NOTES

chemical *(continued)*
    c. cardioversion
    c. exposure
    c. pleurodesis
    c. pneumonitis
    c. shift artifact
    c. shift imaging (CSI)
    c. stimulus
chemiluminescence
chemoattractant
chemoattracting
    c. agent
    c. molecule
    c. property
    c. stimuli
chemodectoma
chemokine
    CXC c.
Chemo-Port perivena catheter system device
chemoprophylaxis
    secondary c.
chemoreceptor
    peripheral c.
    c. reflex
    c. syndrome
chemoreflex
chemosensitivity
chemosis
chemotactic
    c. anaphylatoxin
    c. cytokine
    c. response
chemotaxis
    eosinophilic c.
chemotherapeutic
    c. agent
    c. index
chemotherapy (CMT)
    antimycobacterial c.
    antituberculous c.
    intraarterial c.
    molecular c.
    neoadjuvant c.
    tuberculous c.
chemotoxin
    neutrophil c.
ChemTrak AccuMeter theophylline test
Cheracol D
cherry angioma
cherry-picking procedure
chest (Ch, ch)
    alar c.
    anterior flail c.
    anterolateral flail c.
    barrel-shaped c.
    c. bellows
    bilateral anterior flail c.
    blast c.

c. cage
cobbler's c.
c. compression
c. cuirass
dirty c.
dropsy c.
emphysematous c.
empyema of c.
flail c.
foveated c.
funnel c.
c. index
keeled c.
lateral flail c.
c. lead
c. lead in electrocardiography (C)
c. and left arm (CL)
c. and left leg (CF)
noisy c.
c. pain (CP)
c. pain center (CPC)
c. pain observation unit (CPOU)
c. pain onset to hospital arrival (CPOTHA)
c. pain order sheet (CPOS)
c. pain policy (CPP)
c. pain syndrome (CPS)
c. pain of unknown etiology (CPUE)
paralytic c.
c. percussion
c. percussion and vibration
phthinoid c.
c. physical therapy (CPT)
c. physiotherapy (CPT)
pigeon c.
c. port
pressurelike sensation in c.
c. PT
pterygoid c.
quiet c.
c. radiograph (CXR, CxR)
c. and right arm (CR)
c. roentgenogram (CR)
c. roentgenography (CR)
c. shell
c. shield
tetrahedron c.
c. thump
c. tightness
c. tube (CT)
c. wall
c. wall adhesion
c. wall compliance
c. wall elastic recoil pressure (Pth)
c. wall injury
c. wall motion
c. wall patch

c. wall stimulation (CWS)
c. x-ray (CX, CXR, CxR)
chewable
E.E.S. C.
Cheyne-Stokes
C.-S. asthma
C.-S. breathing
C.-S. respiration
C.-S. sign
CHF
chronic heart failure
congestive heart failure
CHFDT
congestive heart failure data tool
Chiari
C. network
C. syndrome
Chiari-Budd syndrome
Chiba needle
chicken fat clot
chicken-wire myocardial cell
child-adult-mist (CAM)
Child classification
childhood
C. Asthma Questionnaire (CAQ)
c. nitrosopnea
c. tuberculosis
childhood-type tuberculosis
children
Balminil-DM C.
Koffex DM C.
C.'s Motrin Suspension
Chilli
C. cooled ablation system
C. cooled-tip ablation catheter
CHIME
coloboma, heart anomaly, ichthyosis, mental retardation, ear abnormality
chimeric-7E3
c.-7E3 antiplatelet therapy
c.-7E3 Fab
chimerism
hematopoietic c.
mixed hematopoietic c.
Chinese
C. licorice
C. restaurant asthma syndrome
Chlamydia
C. pecorum
C. pneumoniae
C. psittaci
C. trachomatis

Chlamydiaceae
chlamydial
Chlamydia **pneumonia**
chloral hydrate
chlorambucil
chloramine-T technique
chloramphenicol transferase
chlordiazepoxide
chlorella asthma
chloride
Adrenalin C.
ammonium c.
Anectine C.
benzocaine, butyl aminobenzoate, tetracaine, and benzalkonium c.
bethanechol c.
calcium c.
cesium c.
c. current (I_{Cl})
edrophonium c.
hydrogen c.
c. ion
methacholine c.
polyvinyl c. (PVC)
potassium c. (KCl)
c. secretion
c. shift
sodium c.
succinylcholine c.
tetraethylammonium c.
triphenyl tetrazolium c.
tubocurarine c.
vinyl c.
xenon c. (XeCl)
zinc c.
chlorine dioxide
chlormethiazole
chlorofluorocarbon (CFC)
chloroquine phosphate
chlorothiazide
c. and methyldopa
c. and reserpine
chlorotica
aorta c.
chlorotic phlebitis
chlorotrianisene
chlorpheniramine
c., ephedrine, phenylephrine, and carbetapentane
hydrocodone, phenylephrine, pyrilamine, phenindamine, c.
c. maleate

C

NOTES

chlorpheniramine *(continued)*
 c., phenylephrine, and codeine
 c., phenylephrine, and dextromethorphan
 c., phenylpropanolamine, and dextromethorphan
 c. and pseudoephedrine
 c., pseudoephedrine, and codeine
Chlorprom
Chlorpromanyl
chlorpromazine hydrochloride
chlorpropamide
chlortetracycline sensitivity
chlorthalidone
 atenolol and c.
 clonidine and c.
Chlor-Trimeton
 C.-T. injection
 C.-T. Oral
choc
 bruit de c.
Choice PT plus wire
choir
 vascular c.
chokes
CHOL, chol
 cholesterol
cholangiogram
 intravenous c. (IVC)
cholangiography
 intravenous c. (IVC, IVCH)
cholangitis
 sclerosing c.
cholecystitis
Choledyl SA
cholelithiasis
cholerae
 Vibrio c.
choleraesuis
 Salmonella c.
cholera vaccine reaction
Cholestech
 C. LDX system
 C. LDX system with TC and Glucose Panel
cholesterol (C, CH, CHOL, chol)
 c. cleft
 c. crystallization inhibitor (CCI)
 c. embolism
 c. emboli syndrome
 c. embolization
 c. ester
 c. ester hydrolase (CEH)
 c. ester storage disease (CESD)
 free c. (FC)
 low c. (lo chol)
 low fat and c. (LFC)
 c. monitoring system
 nonesterified c. (NEC)

 c. pericarditis
 c. pleurisy
 c. pneumonitis
 c. saturation index (CSI)
 serum c.
 c. stone (CS)
 c. sulfate (CS)
 c. thorax
 total c. (TC)
 total plasma c. (TPC)
cholesterol-esterifying activity (CEA)
cholesterol-ester transfer (CET)
cholesterol-lecithin (CL)
 c.-l. flocculation (CLF)
cholesterol-lowering lipid (CLL)
cholesterol-phospholipid (C/P, C/PL)
Cholesterol-Saturated Fat Index (CSFI)
cholesterol, total (CT)
cholesterol-triglyceride (C/TG)
cholesteryl
 c. ester storage disease
 c. ester transfer protein (CETP)
Cholestin
Cholestron Pro II handheld device
cholestyrame
cholestyramine resin
choline
 c. magnesium trisalicylate
 c. salicylate
 c. theophyllinate
cholinergic
 c. agent
 c. receptor
 c. response
cholinesterase inhibitor
chondral disarticulation
chondralgia
chondrocostal disarticulation
chondroitin sulfate
chondroma
chondrosarcoma
chondrosternal
chondrosternoplasty
chondroxiphoid
chorda, pl. **chordae**
 flail c.
 chordae tendineae
 chordae tendineae cordis
 chordae tendineae rupture
 c. vocalis
chordal
 c. buckling
 c. length
 c. rupture
 c. structure
 c. transfer
chordalis
 endocarditis c.
chordoplasty

chorea
>   amyotrophic c.
>   c. cordis
>   Huntington c.
>   Sydenham c.

choriocarcinoma

chorionic villus sampling

choroidopathy
>   *Pneumocystis* c.

CHP
>   capillary hydrostatic pressure

Christmas
>   C. disease
>   C. factor

chromaffin cell tumor

chromate

chromatin
>   coarse c.

chromatography
>   affinity c.
>   denaturing high performance
>   liquid c. (DHPLC)
>   gas c.
>   high-performance liquid c. (HPLC)
>   high-pressure liquid c. (HPLC)
>   Sephadex G24 c.

chromic catgut suture

chromium

chromogenic method

chromosome
>   c. 5q
>   c. 11q
>   c. 14q

chronic
>   c. airflow limitation (CAL)
>   c. airflow obstruction (CAO)
>   c. aortic stenosis
>   c. asthma
>   c. asthmatic bronchitis
>   c. atrial fibrillation
>   c. beryllium disease (CBD)
>   c. catarrhal laryngitis
>   c. catarrhal tonsillitis
>   c. cerebrovascular disease (CCVD)
>   c. constrictive pericarditis
>   c. contractile dysfunction
>   c. coronary insufficiency (CCI)
>   c. coronary occlusions
>   c. cor pulmonale
>   c. ectopic atrial tachycardia
>   (CEAT)
>   c. endocarditis

c. eosinophilic pneumonia (CEP)
c. fatigue syndrome (CFS)
c. fibrous pneumonia
c. fusiform aneurysm
c. graft vascular disease (CGVD)
c. heart failure (CHF)
c. hemolytic anemia
c. hypertension (CH)
c. hypertensive disease
c. hypertrophic emphysema
c. hyperventilation syndrome
c. idiopathic orthostatic hypotension
c. inflammatory airway disease
c. interstitial lung disease
c. lunger
c. lymphocytic thyroiditis
c. mucocutaneous moniliasis
c. myocarditis
c. necrotizing aspergillosis
c. nonvalvular atrial fibrillation
  (CNAF)
c. obstruction outflow disease
  (COOD)
c. obstructive airways disease
c. obstructive bronchitis
c. obstructive lung disease (COLD)
c. obstructive pulmonary disease
  (COPD)
c. obstructive pulmonary
  emphysema (COPE)
c. obstructive respiratory disease
  (CORD)
c. passive congestion
c. peripheral arterial disease
  (CPAD)
c. pharyngitis
c. pleurisy
c. pulmonary cystic
  lymphangiectasis
c. pulmonary edema
c. pulmonary emphysema (CPE)
c. pulmonary insufficiency of
  prematurity
c. recurrent chemical injury
c. renal failure
c. respiratory failure (CRF)
C. Respiratory Questionnaire (CRQ)
c. restrictive pulmonary disease
  (CRPD)
c. sheath
c. shock
c. sinus arrest

NOTES

C

chronic *(continued)*
    c. stable angina
    c. stable asthmatic
    c. suppurative lung disease (CSLD)
    c. tamponade
    c. thromboembolic pulmonary
      hypertension (CTEPH)
    c. thrombotic pulmonary vascular
      obstruction (CTPVO)
    c. total occlusion (CTO)
    c. upper respiratory obstruction
    c. valvular heart disease (CVHD)
    c. valvulitis
    c. venous insufficiency (CVI)
    c. ventilatory failure (CVF)
    c. volume load
chronicity
Chronicle implantable hemodynamic
  monitor
Chrono-log
    C.-l. optical aggregometer
    C.-l. platelet aggregometer
chronolog
    nebulizer c.
chronophysiology
Chronos 04 pacemaker
chronotherapeutic
chronotherapy
chronotropic
    c. effect
    c. exercise assessment protocol
      (CAEP)
    c. incompetence
    c. response
chronotropism
    negative c.
    positive c.
CHUK
    conserved helix-loop-helix ubiquitous
    kinase
Church cardiovascular scissors
Churchill-Cope reflex
Churg-Strauss
    C.-S. angiitis
    C.-S. syndrome (CSS)
    C.-S. vasculitis
Chuter endovascular device
Chvostek sign
chyliform
    c. pleural effusion
    c. pleurisy
chylomicron
    c. remnant (CMR)
    c. remnant receptor
chylomicronemia
    c. syndrome
chylopericarditis
chylopericardium
    primary isolated c.

chylopleura
chylopneumothorax
chylothorax, pl. **chylothoraces**
    traumatic c.
chylous
    c. ascites
    c. hydrothorax
    c. pericardial effusion
    c. pleural effusion
    c. pleurisy
    c. spill
chymase gene locus
CI
    cardiac index
    cardiac insufficiency
    colloidal iron
    confidence interval
    constraint-induced
    coronary insufficiency
    CI therapy
Ciaglia
    C. percutaneous tracheostomy
    introducer
    C. serial dilatation technique
Ciba-Corning 2500 CO-Oximeter
cibenzoline
CIC
    carbachol inhalation challenge
    cardioinhibitor center
cicaprost
cicatricial stenosis
cicatrization
ciclesonide
cicletanine
CICU
    cardiac intensive care unit
cidal effect
Cidecin
cidofovir
Cidomycin
cifenline succinate
cigarette
    c. cough
    c. smoke (CS)
    c. smoking
CIIA
    common internal iliac artery
cilastatin
    imipenem and c.
cilazapril
cilexetil
    candesartan c.
cilia (*pl. of* cilium)
ciliary
    c. beat frequency
    c. dysfunction
    c. efficacy
    c. impairment
    c. movement

ciliastatic
ciliated
    c. epithelial cell
    c. epithelium
ciliocytophthoria
ciliogenesis
ciliotoxicity
cilium, pl. **cilia**
cilnidipine
cilostazol
cimetidine
Cimino arteriovenous shunt
Cimino-Brescia arteriovenous fistula
Cimochowski cardiac cannula
cinchonism
cincinnatiensis
    Legionella c.
cine
    c. computed tomography
    c. CT
    c. gradient-echo MRI
    c. loop
    c. scan
    c. view
cineangiocardiography
    radionuclide c.
cineangiogram
cineangiographic system
cineangiography
    conventional c.
cinearteriography
cinebronchography
cinecamera
cinefilm
cinefluorography
cinefluoroscopy
cineless recording system
cine-MRI
cine-pulse system
cineventriculogram
cineventriculography
CineView Plus Freeland system
cinnarizine
Cinobac Pulvules
cinoxacin
Cin-Quin
CIPF
    classic interstitial pneumonitis with
    fibrosis
Cipro
    C. injection
    C. Oral

ciprofibrate
ciprofloxacin hydrochloride
ciprostene
Circadia dual-chamber rate-adaptive pacemaker
circadian
    c. blood pressure pattern
    c. disruption
    c. event recorder
    c. pacemaker
    c. periodicity
    c. rhythm
    c. variation
circannual cycle
circaseptan cycle
circle
    c. of death
    c. of Vieussens
    c. of Willis (CW)
circuit
    aortoiliofemoral c.
    arrhythmia c.
    bypass c.
    FilterLine c.
    fluidic c.
    Intertech anesthesia breathing c.
    macroreentrant c.
    output c.
    reentrant c.
    sensing c.
    shunting c.
    timing c.
circuitry
    low-prime c.
Circulaire
    C. aerosol drug delivery device
    C. aerosol drug delivery system
    C. inhaled medication delivery
     device
circulans
    Bacillus c.
circular plane
circulating
    c. adhesion molecule (CAM)
    c. anodic antigen (CAA)
    c. anticoagulant (CAC, CACh)
    c. bacterial endotoxin
    c. blood volume (CBV)
    c. endothelin
    c. interleukin-6
    c. water blanket

C

NOTES

circulation
   airway, breathing, c. (ABC)
   allantoic c.
   anterior c. (AC)
   assisted c.
   balanced coronary c.
   codominant coronary c.
   collateral c.
   compensatory c.
   coronary collateral c.
   derivative c.
   extracorporeal c. (ECC)
   fetal c.
   Fontan c.
   general c. (GC)
   left dominant coronary c.
   lesser c.
   peripheral c.
   persistent fetal c. (PFC)
   placental c.
   portal c.
   posterior c. (PC)
   pulmonary c. (PC)
   restoration of spontaneous c. (ROSC)
   return of spontaneous c. (ROSC)
   c., sensation, motion (CSM)
   systemic c.
   thebesian c.
   c. time
   transient spontaneous c. (TSC)
   c. volume
Circulator
   C. boot
   C. boot therapy
circulatory
   c. arrest
   c. collapse
   c. compromise
   compromise systemic c.
   c. congestion
   c. depression
   c. embarrassment
   c. failure
   c. hypoxemia
   c. hypoxia
   c. instability
   c. overload
   c. shock
   c. stability
   c. support system
circumaortic
   c. venous collar
   c. venous ring
circumference
   left ventricular end-diastolic c. (LVEDC)
circumferential
   c. end-systolic stress (cESS)

   c. ESS
   c. fiber shortening
   c. wall stress (CWS)
circumflex (CX)
   anomalous c. (ACx)
   c. aortic arch
   c. artery
   c. coronary (CxCor)
   c. coronary artery (CCA, CFX)
   left c. (LC, LCF, LCX)
   left atrial c. (LAC)
circumoral cyanosis
circumscribed
   c. edema
   c. pleurisy
circus
   c. movement
   c. movement tachycardia (CMT)
   c. senilis
CIRF
   cocaine-induced respiratory failure
CirKuit-Guard
   C.-G. device
   C.-G. pressure relief valve
cirrhosis
   biliary c.
   cardiac c.
   congestive c.
   Laënnec c.
   c. of liver
   stasis c.
cirrhotic
CIRSE
   Cardiovascular and Interventional Radiological Society of Europe
cirsoid
   c. aneurysm
   c. varix
CIS
   catheter-induced spasm
   coronary implant system
cisapride
cisatracurium besylate
cisplatin (DDP)
   cyclophosphamide, bleomycin, c. (CBP)
   cyclophosphamide, doxorubicin, c. (CAP)
   doxorubicin, 5-fluorouracil, c. (AFP)
   c., etoposide (PE)
   mitomycin, vinblastine, c. (MVP)
   c., vincristine, doxorubicin, etoposide (CODE)
cisterna, pl. cisternae
   cylindrical confronting c.
   perinuclear c.
   subsarcolemmal c.
   terminal c.

CIT
cold ischemic time
citicoline
citrate
caffeine c.
diethylcarbamazine c.
esprolol plus sildenafil c.
c. exchange
nesiritide c.
piperazine c.
sildenafil c.
sufentanil c.
citrated caffeine
citric acid cycle
Citrobacter
C. amalonatica
C. freundii
Citrol Smoking alternative
citrovorum rescue
CIV
continuous intravenous infusion
c-Jun
c-Jun gene
c-Jun N-terminal kinase (JNK)
CK
color kinesis
creatine kinase
CK image
CKG
cardiokymography
CKMB
creatine kinase, myocardial bound
CK-MB elevation
CL
cardiolipin
chest and left arm
cholesterol-lecithin
cycle length
CL lead
cl
clean
clear
clotting
cloudy
CLA
clarithromycin
closed loop algorithm
CLA for infusion of catecholamine
in heart stress test
Cladosporium
Claforan

Clagett
C. closure
C. procedure
clamp
Allis c.
anastomosis c.
aortic aneurysm c.
Atlee c.
Bahnson aortic c.
Bailey aortic c.
Beck miniature aortic c.
Beck-Potts aortic and pulmonic c.
Blalock pulmonary stenosis c.
Bradshaw-O'Neill aorta c.
bulldog c.
cardiovascular c.
Cooley anastomosis c.
Cooley aortic c.
Cooley-Beck vessel c.
Cooley bronchus c.
Cooley-Derra anastomosis c.
Cooley-Satinsky c.
Crafoord coarctation c.
Crile c.
Crutchfield c.
Davidson c.
DeBakey aortic aneurysm c.
DeBakey arterial c.
DeBakey-Bahnson c.
DeBakey-Bainbridge c.
DeBakey-Derra anastomosis c.
DeBakey-Harken auricle c.
DeBakey-Howard aortic
aneurysmal c.
DeBakey-Kay aortic c.
DeBakey-McQuigg-Mixter
bronchial c.
DeBakey pediatric c.
DeBakey peripheral vascular c.
DeBakey-Satinsky vena cava c.
DeBakey-Semb ligature-carrier c.
Demos tibial artery c.
Derra aortic c.
Derra vena caval c.
dreamer c.
Edwards c.
endoaortic c.
euglycemic glucose c.
Favaloro proximal anastomosis c.
Glassman c.
Grant abdominal aortic
aneurysmal c.

NOTES

clamp *(continued)*
    Grover c.
    Halsted c.
    Hartmann c.
    Heartport endoaortic c.
    Hopkins aortic c.
    Hufnagel ascending aortic c.
    Jacobson microbulldog c.
    Jacobson modified vessel c.
    Jacobson-Potts c.
    Javid carotid artery bypass c.
    Kantrowitz thoracic c.
    Kelly c.
    Kindt carotid artery c.
    Koala vascular c.
    Lambert aortic c.
    Lambert-Kay aortic c.
    Liddle aorta c.
    Mattox aorta c.
    microvascular c.
    mosquito c.
    Müller vena caval c.
    myocardial c.
    noncrushing vascular c.
    Noon A-V fistula c.
    pediatric vascular c.
    Reich-Nechtow c.
    resection c.
    Rochester Kocher c.
    Rochester Péan c.
    Ruel aorta c.
    Rumel c.
    Sarot bronchus c.
    Satinsky c.
    Schumacher aorta c.
    side biting c.
    Sideris c.
    Subramanian c.
    suprahepatic caval c.
    VascuClamp vascular c.
    vascular c.
    vessel c.
    Vorse-Webster c.
    Wylie carotid artery c.
    Wylie vascular c.
    Yasargil carotid c.
clamshell
    c. closure of atrial septal defect
    C. II device
    c. incision
    c. septal occluder
    C. septal umbrella
clandestine myocardial ischemia
clapotement
    bruit de c.
claquement
    bruit de c.
    c. d'ouverture

Clara cell secretory protein
clarithromycin (CLA)
Claritin
Claritin-D 24 Hour
Clarity
    C. capnograph
    C. multiparameter monitoring system
    C. software
Clark
    C. classification of malignant melanoma
    C. oxygen electrode
    C. rotating cutter catheter
Clarke-Hadfield syndrome
classic
    c. angina
    c. expectorant
    C. II stethoscope
    c. interstitial pneumonitis with fibrosis (CIPF)
    c. mucolytic
    c. risk factor
classification, class
    Allen and Davis c.
    Ambrose c.
    American Heart Association c.
    American Heart Association Stroke Outcome C. (AHA.SOC)
    antiarrhythmic drug c. (Ia, Ib, Ic, II, III, IV)
    Astler-Coller c.
    Barrow c.
    Braunwald c. I–IIIB
    Canadian Cardiovascular Society c. (CCSC)
    Canadian Cardiovascular Society functional c.
    Canadian Heart C. (CHC)
    CEAP c.
        clinical manifestation, etiologic factor, anatomic involvement and pathophysiologic feature
    Cedars-Sinai c.
    Child c.
    Clark c. of malignant melanoma
    Cohen-Rentrop c.
    congestive heart failure c. I-IV
    Croften c.
    DeBakey c.
    de Groot c.
    Dexter-Grossman c.
    Diamond c.
    Dukes c.
    Efron jackknife c.
    Fontaine lower limb ischemia c.
    Forrester Therapeutic C. grades I–IV

Fukunaga-Hayes unbiased
  jackknife c.
functional capacity c.
Gray-Weale plaque c.
Hannover c.
Heath-Edwards c.
Hinkle-Thaler c.
hip c.
Killip heart disease c.
Killip heart failure c.
Killip-Kimball heart failure c.
KWB hypertension c.
Levine-Harvey c.
Liebow c.
Loesche c.
Lown c.
Mallampati airway c. I-IV
Mallampati-Samsoon airway c. I-IV
Mayo c.
Minnesota ECG c.
New York Heart Association
  functional c. I–IV
Novacode serial ECG c.
NYHA functional c. I–IV
Reid c.
Rentrop c.
round-robin c.
Samsoon-Young airway c. I-IV
Samsoon-Young modification of
  Mallampati airway c.
Sellers mitral regurgitation c.
Shaher-Puddu c.
Singh-Vaughan-Williams
  arrhythmia c.
Stary histology c.
TIMI c.
Timpe and Runyon
  Mycobacteria c.
TNM c.
Vaughan-Williams antiarrhythmic
  drug c.
Walter Reed c.
Wood c.
Yacoub and Radley-Smith c.
claudicant limb
claudication
buttock c.
calf c.
intermittent c.
one-block c.
three-block c.

two-block c.
two-flights-of-stairs c.
Claudius fossa
Clauss
C. assay
C. method
clavicle
acromial articular facies of c.
acromial articular surface of c.
sternal extremity of c.
clavicular facet
clavipectoral triangle
clavulanic acid
Clavulin
clean (cl)
cleaner
VT Mercury Vac organic mercury
  vacuum c.
clear (cl)
C. Advantage Spirometry Filter
c. cell
c. cell carcinoma
c. cell tumor
Scot-Tussin Senior C.
clearance
airway c.
c. assistive device
creatinine c.
drug c.
gas c.
mucociliary c. (MCC)
peripheral zone radioaerosol c.
c. technique
tracheobronchial c.
CLeaRS cardiac lead removal system
ClearView
C. intracoronary shunt
C. intravascular arteriotomy shunt
cleavage
abnormal c. of cardiac valve
cleft
c. anterior leaflet
c. of aortic leaflet
cholesterol c.
laryngeal c.
c. limb-heart (CLH)
c. mitral valve
Schmidt-Lanterman c.
clemastine fumarate
clenched fist sign
clentiazem

NOTES

C

Cleocin
    C. HCl
    C. HCl Oral
    C. Pediatric
    C. Pediatric Oral
    C. Phosphate
    C. Phosphate Injection
clevidipine
CLF
    cholesterol-lecithin flocculation
CLH
    cleft limb-heart
    CLH syndrome
click
    ejection c. (EC)
    Hamman c.
    late systolic c. (LSC)
    metallic c.
    midsystolic c. (MSC)
    mitral c.
    mitral valve prolapse-systolic c.
      (MVP-SC)
    c. murmur
    nonejection systolic c.
    palmar c.
    pulmonary ejection c. (PEC)
    c. syndrome
    systolic c. (SC)
Clickhaler
clicking
    c. pneumothorax
    c. rale
click-murmur syndrome
clindamycin
clinic
    cardiovascular c. (CC)
    community hypertension
      evaluation c. (CHEC)
    lipid research c. (LRC)
clinical
    c. cardiovascular disease (CCD)
    c. manifestation, etiologic factor,
      anatomic involvement and
      pathophysiologic feature (CEAP
      classification)
    c. practice guidelines (CPG)
    c. pulmonary infection score
      (CPIS)
    c. research unit (CRU)
Clinitron air-fluidized therapy
clinocephaly
Clinoril
clinostatic bradycardia
clip
    Adams-DeWeese vena caval
      serrated c.
    alligator c.
    Astro-Trace Universal adapter c.
    Atrauclip hemostatic c.

    Autostat ligating and hemostatic c.
    crankshaft c.
    Elgiloy-Heifitz aneurysm c.
    Fogarty spring c.
    Horizon surgical ligating and
      marking c.
    ligation c.
    microbulldog c.
    Miles vena cava c.
    Moretz c.
    nose c.
    C. On torquer
    partial occlusion inferior vena
      cava c.
    Smith c.
    Sugar c.
    Sugita c.
    vascular c.
    vena cava c.
ClipTip reusable sensor
Clivarine
CLL
    cholesterol-lowering lipid
CLM articulating laryngoscope blade
cloacae
    Enterobacter c.
clockwise
    c. flutter
    c. loop
    c. rotation
    c. rotation of electrical axis
    c. torque
clofazimine (CFZ)
    c. palmitate
clofibrate
clofilium
clomethiazole
clone
    antiadhesion c.
clonidine
    c. and chlorthalidone
    c. hydrochloride
cloning
    DNA c.
**Cloninger Temperament and Character
  Inventory**
clonogenic technique
Clonorchis sinensis
clonus
    anodal opening c. (ANOCL,
      AOCl)
    cathodal closure c. (CCCl)
    cathodal opening c. (COCl)
clopidogrel bisulfate
clorprenaline hydrochloride
closed
    c. chest cardiac massage
    c. chest cardiac resuscitation
      (CCCR)

c. chest cardiopulmonary resuscitation (CCPR)
c. chest commissurotomy
c. chest pneumothorax
c. chest thoracostomy
c. chest water-seal drainage
c. circuit method
c. end-hole catheter
c. loop algorithm (CLA)
c. transventricular mitral commissurotomy

closed-circuit spirometer
closed-loop
c.-l. delivery
c.-l. device
c.-l. pacing
c.-l. sedative administration

closed-tube thoracostomy
Closer-Closure catheter
closing
cathodal c. (KC)
c. slope
c. snap
c. volume

clostridial myocarditis
Clostridium
C. botulinum
C. perfringens
C. septicum
C. tetani

closure
airway c.
aortic c. (AC)
aortic valve c. (AVC)
C. catheter/radiofrequency generator
Clagett c.
delayed primary c. (DPC)
double umbrella c.
early mitral valve c. (EMVC)
King ASD umbrella c.
mitral c. (Mc)
nonoperative c.
patch c.
percutaneous patent ductus arteriosus c.
premature mitral c. (PMC)
premature valve c.
primary c.
PTFE c.
pulmonic c. (PC)
saphenous vein patch c.
semilunar valve c. (SC)

threatened c.
transcatheter c. (TCC)
tricuspid c. (Tc)
umbrella c.

Clo-Sur P.A.D. dressing
clot
agonal c.
agony c.
antemortem c.
autologous c.
blood c.
c. buster
C. Buster Amplatz thrombectomy device
chicken fat c.
currant jelly c.
fibrin c.
laminated c.
c. lysis
c. lysis time (CLT)
passive c.
postmortem c.
c. retraction time
C. Stop drain

clot-bound thrombin
cloth
Dacron c.

clot-promoting factor (CPF)
clotrimazole
clotted hemothorax
clotting (cl)
c. abnormality
c. disorder
c. factor (CF)
c. time (CLT, CT)

cloud
signal-loss c.

clouded sensorium
clouding
hilar c.
mental c.

cloudy (cl)
CLOUT
Core Laboratory Ultrasound Analysis

Cloverleaf catheter
cloxacillin sodium
CLP
cardiac laboratory panel

CLS
capillary leak syndrome

CLSE
calf lung surfactant extract

NOTES

C

CLT
  clot lysis time
  clotting time
clubbing
    c., cyanosis, and edema (CCE)
    digital c.
    c. of fingers
    c. of toes
cluster
    microcalcification c. (MCC)
cluster-of-grapes appearance
C-M
  cardiomyopathy
CM
  cardiac monitoring
  cardiac murmur
  cardiac muscle
  cardiomyopathy
  congestive myocardiopathy
  continuous murmur
C/M
  counts per minute
cM
  centimorgan
CM3 cocktail
CMA
  cerebral microangiopathy
CMAD
  count median aerodynamic diameter
CMAP
  compound motor action potential
CMC
  corticomedullary contrast
CMCT
  central motor conduction time
CMD
  count median diameter
CMFT
  cardiolipin microflocculation test
CMH
  congenital malformation of the heart
CMN-AA
  cystic medial necrosis of ascending aorta
CMO
  cardiac minute output
CMP
  cardiomyopathy
CMP-NANA
  cystidine monophospho-N-
  acetylneuraminic acid
CMR
  cardiomodulorespirography
  cardiovascular magnetic resonance
  chylomicron remnant
CMR$_{gic}$
  cerebral rate of glucose metabolism
CMRO$_2$
  cerebral rate of oxygen metabolism

CMS
  cardiovascular measurement system
    CMS AccuProbe 450 system
CMSD
  congenital myocardial sympathetic
  dysinnervation
CMT
  chemotherapy
  circus movement tachycardia
CMV
  cytomegalovirus
    CMV IE-2 gene expression
    CMV IE-2 riboprobe
    CMV pneumonitis
    CMV seronegative
    CMV seropositive
CMVIG
  cytomegalovirus immune globulin
CNAF
  chronic nonvalvular atrial fibrillation
CNL
  cardiolipin natural lecithin
cNOS
  constitutive nitric oxide synthase
CNP
  C-type natriuretic peptide
CNRT
  corrected sinus node recovery time
CNT
  continuous nebulization therapy
CNTHM
  conotruncal heart malformation
CO
  carbon monoxide
  cardiac output
    CO oximeter
    CO oximetry
    CO Sleuth
    CO Sleuth carbon monoxide
    monitor
    CO Sleuth handheld carbon
    monoxide analyzer
CO$_2$
  carbon dioxide
    arterial partial pressure of CO$_2$
    (PaCO$_2$)
    CO$_2$ oximetry
    partial pressure of end-tidal CO$_2$
    (PETCO$_2$)
    pulse oximeter/end tidal CO$_2$
    (POET)
    CO$_2$ waveform
CoA
  coarctation of aorta
  coenzyme A
Coach incentive spirometer
coaching whistle

coag
> coagulation
> Rapidpoint Coag

Coag-A-Mate coagulometer

CoaguChek
> C. aPTT testing system
> C. Pro DM monitor

coagulation (coag)
> c. activity
> argon plasma c. (APC)
> diffuse intravascular c. (DIC)
> disseminated intravascular c. (DIC, DIVC)
> disseminated intravascular blood c. (DIVBC)
> c. factor
> c. forceps
> F2R blood c.
> intravascular c. (IVC)
> intravascular blood c. (IVBC)
> local intravascular c. (LIC)
> c. necrosis
> c. protein
> c. thrombosis
> c. time (CT)

coagulative myocytolysis

coagulator
> argon beam c.
> Concept bipolar c.

coagulometer
> Coag-A-Mate c.

coagulopathy
> consumption c.
> disseminated intravascular c. (DIC)
> hemorrhagic c.
> intravascular consumption c. (IVCC)

coagulum formation

coal
> c. miner's lung
> c. tar
> c. worker's pneumoconiosis (CWP)

coalescence

coalition
> Canadian Cardiovascular C. (CCC)

Coanda effect

coapt

coarct
> coarctation

coarctation (coarct)
> angulated c.
> c. of aorta (C of A, CA, CoA)

aortic c.
distorted c.
juxtaductal c.
low-plaque c.
native c.
c. of pulmonary artery
reversed c.

coarctectomy

coarse
> c. breath sounds
> c. chromatin
> c. crackle
> c. murmur
> c. rale
> c. thrill

CoA-set fibrin monomer assay

Coat-a-Count radioimmunoassay

coating
> Hydrocoat hydrophilic c.
> Pro/Pel c.
> Teflon c.

coaxial pressure

cobalt
> c. asthma
> c. cardiomyopathy
> c. exposure
> c. fumes
> c. toxicity
> c. in tungsten carbide

cobalt-induced airway disease

cobalt-related
> c.-r. asthma
> c.-r. lung disease
> c.-r. pulmonary fibrosis

Cobas Fara centrifugal analyzer

cobbler's chest

cobblestoning

Cobe-Stöckert heart-lung machine

Coblation technology

cobra-head anastomosis

cobra-shaped catheter

COC
> cathodal opening contraction

cocaine
> c. abuse
> alkaloidal c.

cocaine-induced
> c.-i. hypertension
> c.-i. myocardial infarction
> c.-i. respiratory failure (CIRF)

cocaine-related sudden death

cocci (*pl. of* coccus)

C

NOTES

coccidioidal
Coccidioides immitis
coccidioidin test
coccidioidoma
coccidioidomycosis
    disseminated c.
    meningeal c.
    miliary c.
    primary c.
    pulmonary c.
coccobacillus
coccus, pl. **cocci**
    cocci country
    gram-negative cocci
    gram-positive cocci
    cocci granuloma
Cochrane Library
cocillana
Cockayne syndrome
Cockett procedure
cockroach asthma
cocktail
    Brompton c.
    cardiac c.
    CM3 c.
    scintillation c.
COCl
    cathodal opening clonus
COCM
    congestive cardiomyopathy
coctum
    sputum c.
Codafed Expectorant
CODE
    cisplatin, vincristine, doxorubicin,
      etoposide
code
    c. blue (CB)
    c. blue team (CBT)
    cardiac arrest c. (CAC, CACh)
    c. excited linear prediction (CELP)
    ICHD pacemaker c.
    Minnesota c.
    Minnesota Q-QS c.
    pacing c.
    c. response team (CRT)
codeine
    bromodiphenhydramine and c.
    brompheniramine,
      phenylpropanolamine, and c.
    chlorpheniramine, phenylephrine,
      and c.
    chlorpheniramine, pseudoephedrine,
      and c.
    Deproist Expectorant With C.
    guaifenesin and c.
    guaifenesin, pseudoephedrine, and c.
    Guiatussin with C.
    Mallergan-VC with C.

    Phenergan With C.
    c. phosphate
    promethazine, phenylephrine, and c.
    terpin hydrate and c.
    triprolidine, pseudoephedrine, and c.
Codemaster defibrillator (Hewlett-
  Packard)
CodeMaster defibrillator (Philips)
Codiclear DH
coding
    amplitude zone time epoch c.
      (AZTEC)
codominant
    c. coronary circulation
    c. system
    c. vessel
coefficient
    apparent diffusion c. (ADC)
    capillary filtration c.
    damping c.
    c. of diffusion
    distribution c. (Kd)
    fat-absorption c.
    Hill c.
    Spearman c.
coenzyme
    c. A (CoA)
    c. Q
    c. Q10
COER-24 delivery system
coeur en sabot
Coe virus
coexistent
    c. cardiac alterations
    c. pathology
cofactor
    heparin c. (HCF)
coffee bean asthma
Cogan syndrome
Co-Gesic
Cognitive Failures Questionnaire (CFQ)
cogwheel respiration
COHb
    carboxyhemoglobin
Cohen-Rentrop classification
coherent contrast imaging (CCI)
cohesiveness
Cohn cardiac stabilizer
cohort
coil
    Cook detachable PDA c.
    detachable embolization c.
    distal shocking c.
    c. electrode
    elliptical end-capped quadrature
      radiofrequency c.
    c. embolization
    Gianturco c.
    Guglielmi detachable c.

Helmholtz head c.
Intercept vascular internal MR c.
c. obliteration
phased array receiver c.
platinum c.
prolapse c.
quadrature birdcage c.
quadrature head c.
spring c.
c. stent
c. thrombogenicity
Tornado embolization c.
coil-tipped catheter
coin
c. artifact
c. lesion
c. lesion of lung
c. percussion
c. sound
c. test
coincidence detection
coital hemoptysis
coitus-induced myocardial infarction
Colapinto compression device
colchicine
COLD
chronic obstructive lung disease
cold
c. abscess
c. agglutinin
c. agglutinin pneumonia
c. air challenge (CAC, CACh)
c. blood cardioplegia
c. crystalloid cardioplegia
c. dry air challenge
c. dry air-induced asthma
c. exposure
c. gangrene
c. hemagglutinin disease
c. ischemic arrest
c. ischemic time (CIT)
c. nodule
c. potassium cardioplegia
c. pressor test
c. pressor testing maneuver
c. spot
Sudafed Severe C.
cold-induced angina
cold-mist humidifier
Cole-Cecil murmur
colesevelam HCl
Colestid

colestipol hydrochloride
colfosceril palmitate
colic
biliary c.
colistimethate sodium
colistin
collaboration
Antiplatelet Trialists' C. (ATC)
collagen
c. deposition
endomysial c.
c. fatigue
fibrillar c.
c. plug
c. sponge
c. type I–V
c. vascular lung disease
c. vascular sealing (CVS)
collagenase
collagenolysis
collagenous
c. cap
c. pneumoconiosis
collapse
cardiovascular c.
circulatory c.
hemodynamic c.
lobar c.
massive c.
c. rale
respiratory c.
right ventricular diastolic c.
(RVDC)
c. therapy
tracheobronchial c.
collapsed lung
collapsibility
pharyngeal c.
collapsing pulse
collar
circumaortic venous c.
c. incision
c. prosthesis
c. of Stokes
collateral
adequate c.
antegrade c.
aortopulmonary c.
arcade c.
bridging c.
bronchial c.
c. channel

NOTES

collateral *(continued)*
  c. circulation
  c. filling
  c. flow
  c. hyperemia
  perfusion via c.
  reconstitution via c.
  c. respiration
  septal c.
  systemic c.
  venous c.
  c. vessel
collateralization
  compensatory c.
  pial c.
  ventilation c.
collateralizing vessel
collecting duct
collection
  expired air c.
college
  Tokyo Medical C. (TMC)
collier's
  c. lung
  c. phthisis
collimation
  x-ray scatter c.
collimator
  511-keV c.
  LEAP c.
  Picker Dyna Mo c.
  slant hole c.
Collins
  C. bicycle
  C. chain compensated gasometer
    technique
  C. respirometer
  C. solution
  C. Survey spirometer
  C. SurveyTach with MicroTach
    assembly
Collis-Nissen fundoplication
colloid
  c. oncotic pressure (COP)
  c. osmotic pressure
colloidal iron (CI)
Collostat hemostatic sponge
coloboma
  c. heart anomaly, choanal atresia,
    retardation, and genital and ear
    anomalies (CHARGE)
  c. heart anomaly, ichthyosis,
    mental retardation, ear abnormality
    (CHIME)
Colombo inverted Y technique
colon
  angiodysplasia of c.
  marginal artery of c.
colonic ischemia

colonization
  airway bacterial c.
  atypical mycobacterial c.
  bacterial c.
colony-stimulating factor (CSF)
color
  c. capnography
  c. Doppler energy (CDE)
  c. Doppler flow convergence
  c. flow Doppler
  c. flow mapping
  c. kinesis (CK)
  c. kinesis echocardiographic display
  c. kinesis image
  c. kinesis imaging
  c. M-mode Doppler
    echocardiography
  c. power angiography
  c. tissue Doppler imaging
color-coded flow mapping
colorimetric detector
colorvascular Doppler ultrasound
ColorZone
  C. Management system
  C. tape
Columbia S.K. virus
column
  blood c.
  plasma exchange c.
Coly-Mycin M Parenteral
coma
  apoplectic c.
  diabetic c.
Combicath
combination beat
combined
  c. atrial hypertrophy (CAH)
  c. heart catheterization
  c. M-mode echophonocardiography
  penicillin G benzathine and
    procaine c.
  c. ventricular hypertrophy (CVH)
Combipres
Combitube airway
Combivent inhaler
Combivir
combretastatin A4 prodrug (CA4P)
comet
  C. catheter
  c. sign
  c. tail sign
Comfeel Ulcus dressing
Comfit endotracheal tube holder
ComfortSeal mask
commissural
  c. bundle
  c. fusion
  c. mitral regurgitation
  c. splitting

commissurales
cuspides c.
commissure
aortic c.
fused c.
scalloped c.
split fused c.
valve c.
commissuroplasty
commissurotomy
ball mitral c.
balloon mitral c. (BMC)
Brockenbrough transseptal c.
closed chest c.
closed transventricular mitral c.
mitral c. (MC)
mitral balloon c.
mitral valve c.
open mitral valve c. (OMVC)
percutaneous mechanical mitral c.
percutaneous mitral c. (PMC)
percutaneous mitral balloon c.
(PMBC)
percutaneous transatrial mitral c.
percutaneous transvenous mitral c.
(PTMC)
transventricular mitral valve c.
tricuspid c.
committed mode pacemaker
common
c. atrioventricular canal
c. atrioventricular orifice (CAVO)
c. atrium
c. carotid artery
c. carotid artery intima-media
thickness (CCA-IMT)
c. carotid compression (CCC)
c. femoral artery
c. femoral vein
c. hepatic artery
c. iliac artery
c. internal iliac artery (CIIA)
c. pulmonary venous channel
(CPVC)
c. variable immunodeficiency
(CVID)
commotio cordis
communication
arteriovenous c. (AVC)
bronchiole-alveolar c.
interalveolar c.

interarterial c.
narrow c.
communis
basalis c.
truncus arteriosus c. (TAC)
community-acquired
c.-a. infection
c.-a. pneumonia (CAP)
community hypertension evaluation clinic (CHEC)
compact
c. A-V node
C. II desktop spirometer
Compactin
compages thoracis
CompAire Elite compressor nebulizer system
Companion 314 nasal CPAP
compartment
c. procedure
c. syndrome
Compazine
C. injection
C. Oral
compensated
c. congestive heart failure
c. edentulism
c. sheath
c. shock
compensating emphysema
compensation
cardiac c.
depth c.
electronic distance c.
time-gain c. (TGC)
compensatory
c. antiinflammatory response
syndrome (CARS)
c. circulation
c. collateralization
c. emphysema
c. hypertrophy
c. hypertrophy of heart
integral pulse frequency
modulation/Smith delay c.
(IPFM/SDC)
c. mechanism
c. pause
c. polycythemia
c. vessel enlargement
competence
cardiac c.

NOTES

C

165

competing risks
complement
    c. activation
    c4b purified human c.
    c. component C1r deficiency
    c. inhibitor
    c. system
complemental air
complementary
    c. air
    c. balloon angioplasty
complement-fixation test
complete
    c. atrioventricular
    c. atrioventricular block (CAVB)
    c. atrioventricular dissociation
    (CAVD)
    c. A-V block
    c. A-V dissociation
    c. blood count (CBC)
    c. form of DiGeorge syndrome
    (cDGS)
    c. heart block (CHB)
    c. pacemaker patient testing system
    (CPPTS)
    c. right bundle branch block
    (CRBBB)
    c. stent delivery platform
    Tenax-XR C.
    c. transposition of great arteries
    (CTGA)
completed myocardial infarction
completely positive deflection flutter
complex
    aberrant QRS c.
    Acinetobacter calcoaceticus-
    baumannii c.
    amphotericin B cholesteryl
    sulfate c.
    amphotericin B lipid c. (ABLC)
    anisoylated plasminogen
    streptokinase activator c. (APSAC)
    anisoylated streptokinase-plasminogen
    activator c. (ASPAC)
    anomalous c.
    antiinhibitor coagulant c.
    AP-1 c.
    c. atheroma
    atrial premature c.
    c. atrioventricular canal
    atrioventricular junctional escape c.
    auricular c.
    A-V junctional escape c.
    bizarre QRS c.
    broad QRS c.
    capture c.
    Carney c.
    carotid intima-media c.
    diphasic c.

Eisenmenger c.
electrocardiographic c. (rSr)
electrocardiographic wave c.
equiphasic c.
factor IX c. (human)
far-field QRS c.
filtered QRS c.
first positive deflection during the
    QRS c. (R)
c. fixation (CF)
frequent spontaneous premature c.
fusion c.
Ghon c.
Golgi c.
high-density lipoprotein-
    cholesterol c. (HDL-C)
HLA-DQ gene c.
HLA-DR gene c.
intermediate density lipoprotein-
    cholesterol c. (IDL-C, IDL-c)
interpolated premature c.
iron dextran c.
isodiphasic c.
junctional c.
c. lesion
LIP/PLH c.
low-density lipoprotein-cholesterol c.
    (LDL-C, LDL-c)
Lutembacher c.
MAI c.
membrane attack c. (MAC)
monophasic contour of QRS c.
monophasic negative QRS c. (QS)
multiform premature ventricular c.
Mycobacterium avium c. (MAC)
Mycobacterium avium-
    intracellulare c.
Mycobacterium fortuitum-chelonae c.
nadir of QRS c.
c. plaque
plasminogen-streptokinase c.
pleomorphic premature
    ventricular c.
polymorphic premature
    ventricular c.
polysaccharide-iron c.
premature atrial c.
premature atrioventricular
    junctional c.
premature ventricular c.
primary c.
prothrombin c. (PTC)
prothrombinase c.
QRS c.
QRS-T c.
c. of Q, R, S, waves
    corresponding to depolarization of
    ventricles (QRS)
QS c.

Ranke c.
R-on-T premature ventricular c.
RS c.
second positive deflection during
    QRS c. (R′)
Shone c.
sling ring c.
sodium ferric gluconate c.
Steidele c.
streptokinase-plasminogen c.
supraventricular premature c.
    (SVPC)
Taussig-Bing c.
thrombin-antithrombin III c.
time between the P wave and
    beginning of QRS c. (P-R)
transposition c.
VATER c.
ventricular c.
ventricular premature c. (VPC)
very low density lipoprotein-
    triglyceride c. (VLDL-TG)
compliance
aortic c. (AC)
chest wall c.
c. of heart
left ventricular chamber c.
left ventricular muscle c.
lung c.
patient c.
pulmonary c. (PC)
c., rate, oxygenation and pressure
    (CROP)
c., rate, oxygenation and pressure
    index
specific c.
static lung c.
thoracic c.
total lung c.
ventilatory c.
compliant balloon
complicated myocardial infarction
complication
angioplasty c.
cardiovascular c.
confidential enquiry into cardiac
    catheterization c.'s (CECCC)
groin c.
late angioplasty c.
noninfectious c.
c. rate
thromboembolic c. (TEC)

component
bronchospastic c.
elastic c.
harmonic c.
mitral c. (M1)
plasma thromboplastin c. (PTC,
    PTH)
thrombogenic c.
composite valve graft replacement
compound
antimony c.
artificial lung-expanding c. (ALEC)
Bato c.
c. cyst
glycyl c.
Hurler-Scheie c.
Hycomine C.
c. motor action potential (CMAP)
nitinol polymeric c.
volatile organic c. (VOC)
compPac ventilator
**comprehensive cardiac care unit
    (CCCU)**
compressed-air sickness
compressed Ivalon patch graft
compressible volume
compression
anterior thoracic c.
anteroposterior thoracic c.
aortic root c.
c. atelectasis
c. bandage
barrel-hooping c.
biventricular direct cardiac c.
c. boot
cardiac c.
chamber c.
chest c.
common carotid c. (CCC)
c. cough
direct cardiac c. (DCC)
dynamic tracheal c.
external cardiac c. (ECC)
extrinsic c.
c. gloves
high-frequency chest wall c.
    (HFCC)
intermittent pneumatic c. (IPC)
interposed abdominal c.
intrathoracic gas c.
nonuniform direct cardiac c.
sternal c.

C

NOTES

compression *(continued)*
    c. stockings
    c. thrombosis
    c. ultrasonography
compression-decompression
    active c.-d. (ACD)
compressor
    AM-50 portable air c.
    Deschamps c.
    DeVilbiss Pulmo-Aide LT c.
    Easy Air 15 c.
    Easy Neb c.
    external inflatable c.
    Freeway Lite portable aerosol c.
    Pulmo-Mist c.
    Puritan all purpose c.
compressor-generated nebulizer (CGN)
compressor-nebulizer
    Pulmo-Aide aerosol c. n.
    PulmoMate aerosol c. n.
compromise
    circulatory c.
    respiratory c.
    side branch c.
    c. systemic circulatory
    vascular c.
Compton
    C. effect
    C. scatter
Compu-Neb ultrasonic nebulizer
Compuscan Hittman computerized electrocardioscanner
computed
    c. tomographic scan
    c. tomography (CT)
    c. tomography angiographic portography (CTAP)
    c. tomography angiography (CTA)
    c. tomography in arterial portography (CTAP)
    c. tomography scanner
computer
    digital c.
computer-assisted
    c.-a. diagnostic (CAD)
    c.-a. evaluation of stenosis and restenosis (CAESAR)
    c.-a. pericardial puncture (CASPER)
    c.-a. pericardial surgery (CASPER)
computer-assisted diagnostics
computerized
    c. axial tomography (CAT)
    c. diaphragmatic breathing retraining (CDBR)
    c. sleep analysis system
    c. texture analysis
conal
    c. septal defect
    c. septum

Concato disease
concave pattern
concealed
    c. accessory conduction
    c. accessory pathway
    c. bypass tract
    c. entrainment
    c. retrograde conduction
    c. rhythm
concentration
    fractional inspired oxygen c. (FIO_2, FiO_2)
    hydrogen ion c. (pH)
    intracellular calcium c.
    lactic acid c.
    lymphocyte c.
    minimal alveolar c. (MAC)
    minimum bactericidal c.
    minimum inhibitory c. (MIC)
    plasma endothelin c.
    plasma homocysteine c.
    venous plasma norepinephrine c.
concentration-effect relation
concentrator
    NewLife Elite c.
    NewLife oxygen c.
    Puritan Bennett Aeris 590 oxygen c.
    SolAiris III, V oxygen c.
concentric
    c. hypertrophic cardiomyopathy
    c. left ventricular hypertrophy
    c. remodeling
concept
    Concept bipolar coagulator
    leading circle c.
    solid angle c.
Conchapak
concordance
    atrioventricular situs c.
    ventriculoarterial c.
concordant
    c. alternans
    c. alternation
    c. changes electrocardiogram
concretio
    c. cordis
    c. pericardii
concussion
    myocardial c.
condition
    isocapnic c.
    preexisting c.
conditioning
    cardiovascular reflex c. (CRC)
conduct
    Health On the Net code of c. (HONcode)

conductance
- c. catheter
- c. catheter method
- epicardial flow c.
- S-segment airway c.
- c. stroke volume
- upstream airway c.
- c. vessel

conducting airways

conduction
- aberrant ventricular c. (AVC)
- accelerated A-V node c.
- anisotropic c.
- anomalous c.
- antegrade c.
- antidromic c.
- atrioventricular c. (AVC)
- atrioventricular nodal c. (AVN)
- A-V nodal c.
- c. block
- cardiac c.
- concealed accessory c.
- concealed retrograde c.
- decremental c.
- c. defect (CD)
- c. delay
- delayed c.
- c. disorder
- c. disturbance
- EAVN c.
- electrotonic c.
- enhanced atrioventricular c. (EAVC)
- forward c.
- His-Purkinje c.
- c. impairment
- impulse c.
- internodal c.
- intraatrial c.
- intraventricular c.
- nondecremental retrograde ventriculoatrial c.
- orthodromic c.
- orthograde c.
- c. pathway
- Purkinje c.
- c. ratio
- retrograde atrioventricular c. (RAVC)
- retrograde VA c.
- sinoventricular c.
- c. slowing
- supernormal c.

- supranormal c.
- c. system
- c. time
- transseptal c.
- V-A c.
- c. velocity
- ventricular c.
- ventriculoatrial c. (VAC, V-AC)

conductive
- c. coupling
- c. system

conduit
- extracardiac ventriculopulmonary c.
- c. lumen
- respiratory syncytial virus c.

cone
- arterial c.
- elastic c.
- pulmonary c.

coned-down view

confidence interval (CI)

confidential enquiry into cardiac catheterization complications (CECCC)

configuration
- atrial sensing c.
- dome-and-dart c.
- doughnut c.
- horseshoe c.
- QRS complex c.
- snowman c.
- spadelike c.
- spike-and-dome c.
- ventricular sensing c.

confirmatory evaluation

confluence
- pulmonary venous c. (PVC)

confluent bronchopneumonia

congenita
- myotonia c.

congenital
- c. absence of left pericardium (CALP)
- c. adrenal hyperplasia
- c. anomaly of mitral valve
- c. aortic aneurysm
- c. aortic stenosis
- c. aspiration pneumonia
- c. atelectasis
- c. bronchial atresia (CBA)
- c. cardiovascular malformation (CCVM)
- c. central alveolar hypoventilation

NOTES

C

congenital *(continued)*
  c. central hypoventilation syndrome
  c. complete heart block
  c. conotruncal anomaly
  c. cystic adenomatoid malformation
  c. diaphragmatic hernia (CDH)
  c. heart block (CHB)
  c. heart disease (CHD, CongHD)
  c. interrupted aortic arch
  c. laryngeal stridor
  c. lobar overinflation
  c. long QT interval syndrome
  c. malformation of the heart (CMH)
  c. mitral stenosis
  c. murmur
  c. myocardial sympathetic dysinnervation (CMSD)
  c. peribronchial myofibroblastic tumor
  c. polyvalvular disease (CPVD)
  c. pseudocholinesterase deficiency
  c. pulmonary arteriovenous
  c. pulmonary arteriovenous fistula
  c. single atrium
  c. symptomatic A-V block
congenitale
  P c.
congenitally
  c. absent pericardium
  c. corrected transposition of great arteries
  c. corrected transposition of great vessels (CC-TGA)
Congestac
congestion
  active c.
  chronic passive c.
  circulatory c.
  functional c.
  hypostatic c.
  passive c.
  physiologic c.
  pulmonary c.
  pulmonary venous c. (PVC)
  venous c.
  Vicks 44D Cough & Head C.
congestive
  c. cardiomyopathy (CCM, COCM)
  c. cirrhosis
  c. edema
  c. heart disease (CHD)
  c. heart failure (CHF)
  c. heart failure classification I-IV
  c. heart failure data tool (CHFDT)
  c. myocardiopathy (CM)
  c. pulmonary disease
  c. right ventricular failure (CRVF)

CongHD
  congenital heart disease
coniofibrosis
conjoined cusp
conjugate
  polyribosylribitol phosphate-diphtheria toxoid c. (PRP-D)
conjugated equine estrogen (CEE)
connection
  accessory arteriovenous c.
  anomalous pulmonary venous c. (APVC)
  cavopulmonary c.
  Damus-Kaye-Stansel c.
  discordant atrioventricular c.
  discordant ventriculoarterial c.
  Fontan c.
  partial anomalous pulmonary venous c. (PAPVC)
  pulmonary venous c.
  systemic to pulmonary c.
  total anomalous pulmonary venous c. (TAPVC)
  total cavopulmonary c. (TCP, TCPC)
  univentricular atrioventricular c.
connective
  c. tissue
  c. tissue growth factor (CTGF)
  c. tissue lesion
connector
  Biotronik lead c.
  c. block
  Cordis c.
  Luer-Lok c.
  Medtronic c.
  unipolar c.
  Y c.
Connell airway
connexin 43
connexon distribution
connori
  Nosema c.
Conn syndrome
conotruncal
  c. abnormality
  c. anomaly
  c. heart malformation (CNTHM)
conoventricular fold and groove
Conradi-Hünermann syndrome
Conradi line
Conray contrast medium
consanguineous
consanguinity
consciousness
  loss of c.
conscious sedation
consecutive vasculitis
conservative surgery (CS)

conserved helix-loop-helix ubiquitous kinase (CHUK)
conserver, conservor
    EX-2000 DeVilbiss c.
    Hideaway oxygen c.
    high-flow oxygen c. (HFOC)
    Oxymatic electronic oxygen c.
    PulseDose EX2000D oxygen c.
    Walkabout oxygen c.
console
    Quest Medical MPS c.
consolidated lung volume
consolidation
    airspace c.
    lobular c.
    c. of lung
    patchy c.
    peribronchiolar airspace c.
    pulmonary c.
consolidative process
consonating rale
constant
    atrial volume c. (Vak)
    c. coupling
    empiric c.
    gas c. (R)
    Gorlin c.
    Hodgkin-Huxley c.
    c. tilt wave
    ventricular volume c. (vvk)
constant-flow method
constant-workload cycle exercise
Constellation advanced mapping catheter
constellatus
    Peptococcus c.
constitutive
    c. nitric oxide synthase (cNOS)
    c. secretion
constraint
    pericardial c.
constraint-induced (CI)
    c.-i. movement therapy
constriction
    anular c.
    esophageal c.
    neurohormonal arterial c.
    occult pericardial c.
    supraannular c.
constrictive
    c. bronchiolitis
    c. endocarditis
    c. heart disease
    c. pericarditis (CP)
    c. physiology
constrictor muscle of pharynx
consumption
    c. coagulopathy
    maximum oxygen c. (VO_2 max)
    myocardial oxygen c. (MVO2, MVO_2)
    oxygen c. (VO_2)
    peak exercise oxygen c. (VO_2)
    platelet c.
    volume oxygen c. (VO_2)
contact metastasis
contagiosum
    molluscum c.
Contak
    C. CD CRTD Easytrak system
    C. CD ventricular resynchronization pacemaker
    C. Renewal 3 CRTD system
    C. Renewal 3 system cardiac resynchronization therapy
content
    arterial oxygen c. (CAO2)
    bone mineral c. (BMC)
    harmonic c.
    oxygen c.
contiguous ventricular septal defect
continuity
    c. of care
    c. equation
continuous
    c. albuterol nebulization (CAN)
    c. ambulatory blood sampler (CABS)
    c. arrhythmia
    c. arterial spin-labeled perfusion magnetic resonance imaging (CASL-PI MRI)
    c. arteriovenous hemodiafiltration (CAVHDF)
    c. arteriovenous hemodialysis (CAVHD)
    c. arteriovenous hemofiltration (CAVH)
    c. arteriovenous rewarming (CAVR)
    c. arteriovenous ultrafiltration (CAVU)
    c. aspiration of subglottic secretions (CASS)
    c. atrial fibrillation (CAF)

C

NOTES

continuous *(continued)*
    c. cardiac output (CCO)
    c. cardiac output with SvO_2
    c. cyclical peritoneal dialysis (CCPD)
    c. cyclic peritoneal
    c. full-thickness linear lesion
    c. heart murmur
    c. heparin (CH)
    c. hyperfractionated accelerated radiotherapy (CHART)
    c. intravenous infusion (CIV)
    c. loop exercise echocardiogram
    c. mandatory ventilation
    c. murmur (CM)
    c. nebulization therapy (CNT)
    c. noninvasive monitoring of ventilated infants
    c. pericardial lavage
    c. positive air pressure
    c. positive airway pressure (CPAP)
    c. positive pressure ventilation
    c. progesterone
    c. ramp protocol
    c. venovenous hemofiltration (CVVH)
    c. wave Doppler echocardiogram
continuous-flow ventilation
continuous-wave
    c.-w. Doppler (CWD)
    c.-w. Doppler echocardiography
    c.-w. Doppler imaging
    c.-w. Doppler ultrasound
    c.-w. laser ablation
continuum
contour
    breath-methylated alkane c.
    cardiac c.
    c. of heart
    C. high voltage can ICD
    C. II ICD
    left-heart c.
    C. LT V-135D ICD
    c. LTV-135D implantable cardioverter-defibrillator
    C. MD implantable single-lead cardioverter-defibrillator
    Murgo pressure c.
    QRS c.
    C. V-145D ICD
    C. V-145D implantable cardioverter-defibrillator
    ventricular c.
    Ventritex C.
contracta
    vena c.
contracted heart
contractile
    c. amplitude

    c. behavior
    c. element
    c. force (CF)
    c. function
    c. protein
    c. reserve
    c. ring dysphagia
    c. work index
contractility
    increased c.
    isovolumetric c.
    left ventricular c.
    myocardial c.
    ventricular wall c.
contraction
    anodal closure c. (ANCC, AnCC)
    anodal duration c. (ADC)
    anodal opening c. (ANOC, AnOC, AOC)
    atrial c. (ac)
    atrial premature c. (APC)
    automatic ventricular c.
    c. band
    c. band necrosis
    cardiac c.
    cathodal closing c. (KCC, KSC)
    cathodal closure c. (CCC)
    cathodal opening c. (COC, KOC)
    escape ventricular c.
    Gowers c.
    high-amplitude peristaltic c. (HAPC)
    isometric c.
    isotonic c.
    junctional premature c. (JPC)
    LAA c.
    left atrial c. (LAC)
    low-amplitude c. (LAC)
    maximum voluntary c. (MVC)
    muscular c.
    nodal premature c. (NPC)
    c. pattern
    premature c.
    premature atrial c. (PAC)
    premature junctional c. (PJC)
    premature ventricular c. (PVC)
    pulse synchronized c.'s (PSC)
    rested state c. (RSC)
    R on T ventricular premature c.
    supraventricular premature c.
    synchronous atrial c.
    tertiary c.
    ventricular c. (VC)
    ventricular premature c. (VPC)
    volume c.
contractor
    Bailey-Gibbon rib c.
contracture
    premature nodal c. (PNC)

contraindication
contrast
    c. agent
    angiographic c.
    c. angiography
    corticomedullary c. (CMC)
    c. echocardiography
    half-diluted c.
    Iohexol c.
    left atrial spontaneous echo c.
    (LASEC)
    c. left ventriculography
    Levovist c.
    c. material
    c. medium
    c. medium delivery
    negative c.
    Optiray c.
    Optison c.
    c. ratio
    sonicated albumin-dextrose c.
    spontaneous echo c. (SEC)
    c. stagnation
    time-to-peak c.
    Ultravist c.
    c. venography
    c. ventriculography (CV)
contrast-enhanced
    c.-e. CT
    dynamic susceptibility c.-e. (DSC)
    c.-e. echocardiogram
    c.-e. magnetic resonance
    angiography (CEMRA)
    c.-e. transcranial color-coded real-
    time sonography (CE-TCCS)
    c.-e. ultrasound (CEU)
contrast-guided venipuncture
contrecoup injury
control
    axial c.
    CVC 123 calibration verification c.
    damping c.
    gain c.
    C. III Elite disinfectant
    pressure c. (PC)
    pressure-regulated volume c.
    (PRVC)
    QC 253 CO-oximetry c.
    quality c.
    RA 523 blood gas/CO-oximetry c.
    reject c.
    Take C.

    time-gain c. (TGC)
    time-varied gain c. (TGC, TVGC)
    torque c.
    volume c. (VC)
    c. wire
controlled
    c. breathing
    c. coughing
    c. diaphragmatic breathing (CDBR)
    c. diaphragmatic respiration
    c. lung biopsy
    c. mechanical ventilation
    c. ventricular response
controller
    flow c.
    pressure c.
    vacuum c.
    venous flow c. (VFC)
    volume c.
control-mode ventilation
ControlWire guidewire
contusion
    cardiac c. (CC)
    lung c.
    myocardial c.
    c. pneumonia
    pulmonary c.
conundrum
conus
    c. arteriosus
    c. cordis
    c. elasticus
    pulmonary c.
    tendon of c.
convalescent phase
convective
    c. cooling
    c. gas mixing
conventional
    amphotericin B (c.)
    c. cineangiography
    c. ventilation (CV)
convergence
    color Doppler flow c.
conversion
    analog-to-digital c.
    automatic mode c.
    Fontan c.
    pressure c.
converter
    scan c.
converting enzyme inhibitor

NOTES

173

convex linear array
convexoconcave (C-C)
 Björk-Shiley c.-c. (BSCC)
convulsion
ConXn
COOD
 chronic obstruction outflow disease
cooing
 c. murmur
 c. sign
Cook
 C. balloon
 C. Cardiovascular infusion catheter
 C. County aspirator
 C. detachable PDA coil
 C. flexible biopsy forceps
 C. FlexStent
 C. intracoronary stent
 C. locking stylet
 C. multiple-assessment scale
 C. pacemaker
 C. Spectrum catheter
 C. TPN catheter
cookie
 Gelfoam c.
Cook-Medley hostility scale
cool
 c. head-warm body perfusion
 c. mist
Cooley
 C. anastomosis clamp
 C. anemia
 C. aortic clamp
 C. atrial retractor
 C. bronchus clamp
 C. dilator
 C. forceps
 C. intrapericardial anastomosis
 C. modification of Waterston
  anastomosis
 C. neonatal instrument
 C. sump tube
 C. U sutures
Cooley-Beck vessel clamp
Cooley-Bloodwell-Cutter valve
Cooley-Bloodwell mitral valve prosthesis
Cooley-Cutter disk prosthetic valve
Cooley-Derra anastomosis clamp
Cooley-Satinsky clamp
cooling
 c. blanket
 cardioplegia c.
 convective c.
 core c.
 topical c.
Cool Tip catheter
cool-tip laser
Coomassie blue stain

Coombs
 C. murmur
 C. test
Coons Super Stiff long tip guidewire
Cooper ligament
Cooperman event probability
Cooper-Rand intraoral artificial larynx
coordinate
 c. reduction time encoding system
  (CORTES)
 c. system
Co-Oximeter
 Ciba-Corning 2500 Co-O.
 Co-Oximeter module
COP
 colloid oncotic pressure
 cryptogenic organizing pneumonia
 cryptogenic organizing pneumonitis
COPD
 chronic obstructive pulmonary disease
COPE
 chronic obstructive pulmonary
  emphysema
Cope
 C. method bronchography
 C. Nitinol mandril wire guide
 C. pleural biopsy needle
Copeland technique
Coping Strategies questionnaire
copious sputum
copolymer
 polyolefin c. (POC)
copper (CU)
 c. wiring
copper-62 (^{62}CU)
copper-wire
 c.-w. artery
 c.-w. effect
COR
 cardiac output recorder
cor
 coronary
 cor adiposum
 cor arteriosum
 cor biloculare
 cor bovinum
 cor hirsutum
 cor juvenum
 cor mobile
 cor pendulum
 cor pseudotriloculare biatriatum
 cor pulmonale (CP)
 cor taurinum
 cor triatriatum
 cor triatriatum dexter
 cor triatriatum dextrum
 cor triatriatum sinistrum
 cor triloculare

cor triloculare biatriatum
cor triloculare biventriculare
Coradur
CORALI
coronarography and alimentation
coral thrombus
Coratomic R wave inhibited pacemaker
Corazonix Predictor
CORD
chronic obstructive respiratory disease
cord
epidural spinal c. (ESC)
false vocal c.
Ferrein c.'s
true vocal c.
vocal c.
Cordarone
Cordis
C. Ancar pacing lead
C. bioptome
C. Bioptome sheath
C. BriteTip guiding catheter
C. connector
C. CrossFlex coronary stent
C. Ducor I, II, III catheter
C. LC Multipurpose stent system
C. Mini stent system
C. Powerflex angioplasty balloon
C. Predator PTCA balloon catheter
C. Stockert generator
C. tantalum coil stent
C. Titan balloon dilatation catheter
cordis
accretio c.
adipositas c.
angina c.
anulus fibrosus dexter/sinister c.
apex c.
ataxia c.
atrium c.
bulbus c.
chordae tendineae c.
chorea c.
commotio c.
concretio c.
conus c.
crena c.
delirium c.
diastasis c.
ectasia c.
ectopia c.
facies anterior c.

facies diaphragmatica c.
facies inferior c.
facies pulmonalis dextra/sinistra c.
facies sternocostalis c.
hypodynamia c.
ictus c.
incisura apicis c.
malum c.
myasthenia c.
myofibrosis c.
myomalacia c.
myopathia c.
palpitatio cordis
pulsus c.
steatosis c.
systema conducens c.
theca c.
trepidatio c.
tumultus c.
venae c.
vortex c.
Cordis-Webster
C.-W. ablation catheter
C.-W. mapping catheter
Cordox
cordy pulse
core
c. of atheroma
atheromatous c.
c. cooling
C. Exercise Testing Laboratory
ischemic c.
C. Laboratory Ultrasound Analysis (CLOUT)
lipid c.
c. pneumonia
c. temperature
Coreg
Core-Vent implant
Corgard
Cori disease
Corinthian stent
corkscrew artery
Corlopam
Cormed ambulatory infusion pump
corneal arcus
cornealis
arcus c.
Cornelia de Lange syndrome
Cornell
C. exercise protocol

NOTES

Cornell *(continued)*
    C. modification of the Bruce
      protocol
    C. voltage
    C. voltage-duration product criteria
corniculate tubercle
corniculum
Corometrics
    C. Doppler scanner
    C. monitor
**Corometrics-Aloka echocardiograph
  machine**
coronal
    c. cut
    c. plane
    c. slice
corona radiata
coronarism
coronaritis
coronarius
    sinus c.
**coronarography and alimentation
  (CORALI)**
coronaropathy
    dilated c.
coronary (cor)
    c. air embolism
    c. anastomotic shunt
    c. anatomy
    c. aneurysm
    c. angiographic catheter
    c. angiography (CAG)
    c. angiography catheter
    c. angioscopy
    c. arterial reserve
    c. arteriography (CAG)
    c. arteriosclerosis
    c. arteriosclerotic heart disease
      (CAHD, CASHD)
    c. arteritis
    c. artery (CA)
    c. artery angioplasty
    c. artery anomaly
    c. artery atherosclerosis
    c. artery blood flow (CABF)
    c. artery button
    c. artery bypass (CAB)
    c. artery bypass graft (CARB)
    c. artery bypass grafting (CABG)
    c. artery bypass grafting surgery
    c. artery bypass graft surgery
      (CABGS)
    c. artery bypass surgery (CABS)
    c. artery descriptors and restenosis
      (CADR)
    c. artery disease (CAD)
    c. artery disease index (CADI)
    c. artery dissection
    c. artery distensibility

c. artery dominance
c. artery ectasia
c. artery embolism (CAE)
c. artery fistula (CAF, CAP)
c. artery lesion
c. artery obstruction (CAO)
c. artery occlusion
c. artery occlusive disease (CAOD)
c. artery probe
c. artery-right ventricular fistula
c. artery risk assessment and
  treatment
c. artery scan (CAS)
c. artery spasm (CAS)
c. artery stenosis
c. artery thrombosis
c. artery vein graft (CAVG)
c. atherectomy
c. atheroma
c. bed
c. bifurcation
c. blood flow (CBF)
c. blood flow measurement
c. blood flow velocity (CBFV)
c. branch occlusion
c. bypass graft (CBG)
c. bypass graft patency
café c.
c. calcium
c. calcium scanning
c. care (CC)
c. care nursing (CCN)
c. care training program (CCTP)
c. care unit (CCU)
circumflex c. (CxCor)
c. collateral circulation
c. cushion
c. cusp
c. drug project (CDP)
c. endarterectomy
c. event
c. failure
c. flow (CF)
c. flow reserve (CFR)
c. flow reserve technique
c. flow velocity
c. flow velocity reserve (CFVR,
  CVR)
c. heart disease (CHD)
c. implant system (CIS)
c. insufficiency (CI)
c. intravascular ultrasound
c. IVUS
left circumflex c. (LCC)
left interventricular c. (LIC)
left main c. (LMC)
c. luminal stenosis
c. luminology
c. macroangiopathy

c. magnetic resonance angiography
c. microangiopathy
c. microcirculatory vasoconstriction
c. microvascular disease
c. microvessel endothelium
c. nodal rhythm
c. occlusive disease
c. ostial dimple
c. ostial stenosis
c. ostium
percutaneous transluminal c.
c. perfusate solution (CPS)
c. perfusion gradient
c. perfusion pressure (CorPP, CPP)
c. plaque regression
c. plaque rupture
c. prognosis index (CPI)
c. prognostic index
c. radiation therapy
c. recanalization
c. reflex
c. rehabilitation program (CRP)
c. remodeling
c. resistance vessel
c. revascularization
right interventricular c. (RIC)
c. ring
c. risk profile
c. roadmapping
c. rotational ablation
c. rotational atherectomy (CRA)
c. sclerosis (CS)
c. sinus (CS)
c. sinus blood flow (CSBF)
c. sinus catheterization
c. sinus electrogram
c. sinus flow
c. sinus intervention (CSI)
c. sinus lead
c. sinus occlusion pressure (CSOP)
c. sinus retroperfusion
c. sinus rhythm
c. sinus thermodilution
c. sinus thermodilution catheter
c. slow flow syndrome (CSFS)
c. spasm
c. spastic angina
c. steal
c. steal mechanism
c. steal phenomenon
c. stenting
c. sulcus

c. tendon
c. thrombolysis
c. thrombosis (CT)
c. tree
c. vascular reserve
c. vascular resistance
c. vascular turgor
c. vasculature
c. vasodilation
c. vasodilator reserve
c. vasomotion
c. vasospasm
c. vein
c. venous graft (CVG)
c. venous pressure
c. wire
coronary-pulmonary fistula (C-PF)
coronary-subclavian steal syndrome
Coronaviridae virus
coronavirus infection
coronoradiographic documentation (CAD)
corpora (*pl. of* corpus)
corporeal
CorPP
coronary perfusion pressure
corpus, pl. **corpora**
c. linguae
c. phalangis
corpuscle
Donné c.
Drysdale c.
Hassall c.
corrected
c. blood volume (CBV)
c. dextrocardia
c. ejection time (ETc)
c. pre-ejection period (PEPc)
c. Q-T
c. sinus node recovery time (CNRT)
c. time of sinoatrial node function recovery (CTSNFR)
c. TIMI frame count (CTFC)
c. transposition (CT)
c. transposition of great vessels
correction
Bonferroni c.
metabolite c.
Teichholz c.
Yates c.
corrective therapy (CT)

NOTES

Correra line
CorRestore
    C. implantable patch
    C. system
corridor procedure
Corrigan
    C. disease
    C. pneumonia
    C. pulse
    C. respiration
    C. sign
corrodens
    Bacteroides c.
    Eikenella c.
corrosive esophagitis
Cortef Oral
CORTES
    coordinate reduction time encoding
    system
    CORTES ECG
cortex, pl. **cortices**
    adrenal c.
    premotor c. (PMC)
    primary sensorimotor c. (SM1)
    sensorimotor c. (SMC)
cortical
    c. arousal index (CAI)
    c. plasticity
    c. stroke
    c. vein thrombosis
corticomedullary contrast (CMC)
corticosteroid
    inhaled c.'s (ICS)
    c. therapy
corticosteroid-dependent asthmatic
corticosteroid-treated heart
corticotropin
corticotropin-releasing factor (CRF)
cortisol
    24-hour c.
cortisone acetate
Cortone Acetate
Cortrosyn injection
Corvert injection
Corvisart
    C. disease
    C. facies
Corvita
    C. endoluminal graft
    C. endoprosthesis stent graft
Coryllos-Bethune rib shears
Coryllos-Shoemaker rib shears
Corynebacterium
    C. diphtheriae
    C. jeikeium
coryza
coryzavirus
Corzide
CoSeal resorbable synthetic sealant

Cosgrove-Edwards
    C.-E. annuloplasty system
    C.-E. annuloplasty system with
        Duraflo treatment
Cosgrove retractor
Cosmegen
CO$_2$SMO
    CO$_2$SMO capnograph/pulse oximeter
    CO$_2$SMO Plus
    CO$_2$SMO Plus continuous
      noninvasive respiratory profile
      monitor
Cosmos
    C. II DDD pacemaker
    C. II pulse generator
    C. 283 DDD pacemaker
Cosprin
cost
    oxygen c.
    Prescription Analyses and C.
      (PACT)
costal
    c. margin
    c. part of diaphragm
    c. pit of transverse process
    c. pleura
    c. pleurisy
    c. respiration
    c. surface of lung
costalis
    pleura c.
costarum
    arcus c.
costocervicalis
    truncus c.
costochondral
    c. junction
    c. syndrome
costochondrectomy
costochondritis
costoclavicular
    c. ligament
    c. maneuver
    c. rib syndrome
costodiaphragmatic
    c. recess
    c. recess of pleura
costomediastinal recess of pleura
costophrenic
    c. angle
    c. septal line
    c. sinus
    c. sulcus
costosternal syndrome
costotome
costoversion thoracoplasty
costovertebral angle (CVA)
cosyntropin

COTD
cardiac output by thermodilution
COTe
cathodal opening tetanus
cotransporter
monocarboxylate proton c.
co-trimoxazole
cottage-loaf appearance
cotton-dust asthma
cottonoid patty
cotton-wool
c.-w. exudate
c.-w. spot
Cotunnius space
COU
cardiac observation unit
couch incrementation
cough
aneurysmal c.
Balme c.
barking c.
brassy c.
cigarette c.
compression c.
c. CPR
c. CPR technique
croupy c.
decubitus c.
Diphen C.
directed c.
dog c.
dry c.
c. efficiency
extrapulmonary c.
c. fracture
habit c.
habitual c.
hacking c.
mechanical c.
minute-gun c.
Morton c.
multifactorial c.
paroxysmal c.
privet c.
productive c.
psychogenic c.
c. reflex
reflex c.
c. resonance
seal-bark c.
Silphen C.
smoker's c.

stomach c.
c. suppressant
Sydenham c.
c. syncope
tea taster's c.
c. threshold
c. transportability
trigeminal c.
c. variant asthma
wet c.
whooping c.
winter c.
coughing
controlled c.
expulsive c.
Huff c.
paroxysm of c.
quad c.
cough-specific quality of life questionnaire
cough-thrill
Coulter counter
CoumaCare
C. Coumadin management system
C. patient management system
Coumadin
coumadinization
coumaric anhydride
coumarin pulsed dye laser
Coumel tachycardia
coumestan
coumetarol
Council
National Advisory Heart C. (NAHC)
count
blood c.
complete blood c. (CBC)
corrected TIMI frame c. (CTFC)
differential blood c.
double c.
end-diastolic c. (EDC)
end-systolic c. (ESC)
first shock c.
kick c.
c. median aerodynamic diameter (CMAD)
c. median diameter (CMD)
c.'s per minute (C/M)
c. rate
relative lymphocyte c.
second through fifth shock c.

NOTES

count *(continued)*
  shock c.
  thrombolysis in myocardial
    infarction frame c.
  TIMI frame c.
  total patient shock c.
  touch shock c.
  white blood cell c.
counter
  Coulter c.
  event/episode c.
  pacing c.
  time-based c.
counterclockwise
  c. flutter
  c. rotation
counterimmunoelectrophoresis
counteroccluder
counterpressor
  Acland-Buncke c.
counter-pulsation
counterpulsation
  aortic c.
  balloon c.
  c. balloon
  enhanced external c. (EECP)
  intraaortic c. (IACP)
  intraaortic balloon c. (IABC,
    IABCP)
  intraarterial c.
  percutaneous intraaortic balloon c.
    (PIBC)
  pulmonary artery c. (PACP)
countershock
  electrical c.
counting
  double c.
count-rate linearity
country
  cocci c.
coupled
  c. atrial pacing (CAP)
  c. premature beat
  c. pulse
  c. rhythm
  c. suturing
couplet
  ventricular c.
coupling
  arterial c.
  conductive c.
  constant c.
  electromechanical c.
  excitation-contraction c.
  fixed c.
  intercellular c.
  c. interval
  neuromuscular c.
  variable c.

  vasoneuronal c.
  ventriculoarterial c.
Cournand
  C. dip
  C. needle
  C. Tip Arrow QuadPolar electrode
    catheter
Cournand-Grino angiography needle
Cournand-Potts needle
cove plane
cover
  OxiLink oximeter probe c.
Covera-HS
Cover-Strip wound closure strip
Coversyl
COX
  cyclooxygenase
  cytochrome c oxidase
Cox
  C. maze operation
  C. organism
COX-1, 2 enzyme
Coxiella
  C. burnetii
coxsackie A, B, B3, B4 virus
coxsackievirus
  c. carditis
  c. myocarditis
Cozaar
CP
  capillary pressure
  cardiac pacing
  cardiac performance
  cardiopulmonary
  chest pain
  constrictive pericarditis
  cor pulmonale
    Vancocin CP
C/P
  cholesterol-phospholipid
    C/P ratio
CPA
  cardiopulmonary arrest
CPAD
  chronic peripheral arterial disease
CPAP
  continuous positive airway pressure
    AirSep CPAP
    autotitrating CPAP
    Companion 314 nasal CPAP
    fixed-pressure CPAP
    intelligent CPAP
    nasal CPAP
    Phantom nasal mask CPAP
    Sullivan III CPAP
CPB
  cardiopulmonary bypass
CPBV
  cardiopulmonary blood volume

CPC
chest pain center
CP-Cardiosol
CPCR
cardiopulmonary cerebral resuscitation
CPE
cardiac pulmonary edema
chronic pulmonary emphysema
CPET
cardiopulmonary exercise test
C-PF
coronary-pulmonary fistula
CPF
clot-promoting factor
CPG
cardiopneumographic recording
clinical practice guidelines
CPHV OptiForm mitral valve
CPI
coronary prognosis index
CPI endocardial defibrillation/rate-sensing/pacing lead
CPI Endotak transvenous electrode
CPI Mini device
CPI/Guidant
CPI/G. lead
CPI/G. pacemaker
CPI-PRx pulse generator
CPIS
clinical pulmonary infection score
CPK
creatine phosphokinase
brain band enzyme of CPK (CPK-BB)
CPK isoenzyme
MB enzymes of CPK
muscle fraction enzyme of CPK (CPK-MM, CPK-3)
myocardial band enzymes of CPK (CPK-MB, CPK-2)
CPK-3 (*var. of* CPK-MM)
CPK-BB
brain band enzyme of CPK
CPK-BB band
CPK-MB, CPK-2
myocardial band enzymes of CPK
CPK-MB band
CPK-MB fraction
CPK-MM, CPK-3
muscle fraction enzyme of CPK
CPK-MM band

C/PL
cholesterol-phospholipid
C/PL ratio
CPO
cardiac power output
CPOS
chest pain order sheet
CPOTHA
chest pain onset to hospital arrival
CPOU
chest pain observation unit
CPP
cerebral perfusion pressure
chest pain policy
coronary perfusion pressure
CPPTS
complete pacemaker patient testing system
CPR
cardiopulmonary reserve
cardiopulmonary resuscitation
centripetal rub
cough CPR
four-phase Lifestick CPR
simultaneous compression-ventilation CPR (SCV-CPR)
CPS
cardioplegic perfusion solution
cardiopulmonary support
chest pain syndrome
coronary perfusate solution
CPS system
CPT
chest physical therapy
chest physiotherapy
CPUE
chest pain of unknown etiology
CPVC
common pulmonary venous channel
CPVD
congenital polyvalvular disease
CPX
cardiopulmonary exercise
CPX test
C-R
Bicillin C-R
CR
cardiac rehabilitation
cardiac resuscitation
cardiac rhythm
cardiorespiratory
cardiorrhexis

C

NOTES

CR (continued)
chest and right arm
chest roentgenogram
chest roentgenography
CR lead
metoprolol CR
Norpace CR
CRA
coronary rotational atherectomy
cracked-pot
c.-p. resonance
c.-p. sound
cracking
environmental stress c.
crackle
bibasilar coarse c.
coarse c.
end-inspiratory Velcro c.
pleural c.
crackling rale
cradle
foot c.
Crafoord
C. coarctation clamp
C. lobectomy scissors
Crafoord-Sellor hemostatic forceps
cramp
calf c.
cranial
c. angulation
c. arteritis
c. nerves I–XII
craniocardiac reflex
craniocaudal view
cranio-cerebello-cardiac
c.-c.-c. dysplasia (CCC)
c.-c.-c. syndrome (3C, CCC)
craniopharyngeal
c. duct
c. duct tumor
cranking
arm c.
crankshaft clip
Cranley-Grass phleborrheogram
CRAO
central retinal artery occlusion
craquement
bruit de c.
crash technique
crassamentum
Crawford graft inclusion technique
CRBBB
complete right bundle branch block
CRC
cardiovascular reflex conditioning
cerebrovascular reserve capacity
CRCS
cardiovascular reflex conditioning system

CRCV
cerebral red blood cell volume
C-reactive protein (CRP)
cream
EMLA c.
Gormel c.
Medrol Veriderm C.
crease
ear lobe c. (ELC)
creatine
c. kinase (CK)
c. kinase, myocardial bound (CKMB)
c. phosphokinase (CPK)
creatinine clearance
Creech
manner of C.
C. manner
C. technique
creep
stent c.
creeping thrombosis
Crego traction
crena cordis
crenulated tantalum wire
creola body
Creo-Terpin
crepitant rale
crepitation
crepitus
crescendo
c. angina
c. murmur
c. sleep
c. TIA
crescendo-decrescendo diamond-shaped systolic ejection murmur
crescent
sublingual c.
crescentic glomerulonephritis
CREST
calcinosis, Raynaud phenomenon, esophageal involvement, sclerodactyly, telangiectasia
CREST syndrome
crest
cardiac neural c.
supraventricular c.
vagal neural c.
CRF
chronic respiratory failure
corticotropin-releasing factor
CRG
cardiorespirogram
CRI
cardiac risk index
catheter-related infection
Cribier method
Cricket pulse oximeter

cricoesophageal tendon
cricoesophageus
 tendo c.
cricoid
 c. cartilage
 c. pressure
cricoidea
 cartilago c.
cricoideae
 arytenoidea c.
cricopharyngeal achalasia syndrome
cricothyroid
 c. artery
 c. membrane
cricothyroidotomy
cricotracheotomy
cri du chat syndrome
Crile
 C. clamp
 C. tip occluder
crimper
crimping
Crinone
crinophagy
crisis, pl. **crises**
 anaphylactic c.
 bronchial c.
 cardiac c.
 hypertensive c.
 laryngeal c.
 myasthenic c.
 pharyngeal c.
 sickle cell c.
 thoracic c.
Crisp aneurysm
crisscross
 c. atrioventricular valve
 c. fashion
 c. heart
 c. heart malposition
crista
 c. supraventricularis
 c. terminalis
criteria, sing. **criterion**
 Airlie House c.
 Akaike information c.
 Allen-Brown c.
 Billingham c.
 bodybuilder electromechanical c.
 Bogalusa c.
 Casale-Devereux c.
 Cornell voltage-duration product c.

 Dallas c.
 Duke infective endocarditis c.
 Eagle c.
 Estes ECG c.
 exclusion c.
 Framingham heart failure c.
 Gubner-Ungerleider voltage c.
 Heath-Edwards c.
 Jones c.
 12-lead voltage-duration product c.
 Penn Convention c.
 process-based c.
 pseudodisappearance criterion
 Rand appropriateness selection c.
 Rautaharju ECG c.
 Romhilt-Estes point score c.
 Saccomanno morphologic c.
 Sellers c.
 Sokolow-Lyon voltage c.
 TIMI c.
 voltage c.
 von Reyn c.
 Wilks lambda criterion
critical
 c. aortic stenosis
 c. care unit
 C. Care Ventilator
 c. coronary stenosis
 c. coupling interval
 c. flicker frequency
 c. flicker fusion
 c. rate
 c. valvular stenosis
Criticare pulse oximeter
CritiCath thermodilution catheter
Critikon
 C. automated blood pressure cuff
 C. balloon temporary pacing
  catheter
 C. balloon-tipped end-hole catheter
 C. balloon wedge pressure catheter
 C. guidewire
Crit-Scan noninvasive hematocrit
 measurement device
Crixivan
crochetage EKG pattern
Crocq disease
Croften classification
cromafiban
cromakalim
cromoglycate
 disodium c. (DSCG)

NOTES

C

cromoglycate *(continued)*
    PMS-Sodium C.
    sodium c.
cromolyn
    c. sodium
    c. sodium inhalation solution
CROP
    compliance, rate, oxygenation and
      pressure
cross
    c. femoral-femoral bypass
    yellow c.
crossbridge
    actin-myosin c.
cross-checking
    sensory c.-c.
cross-clamp
    aortic c.-c.
    c.-c. time
cross-clamping of aorta
crossed
    c. cerebellar diaschisis (CCD)
    c. embolism
CrossFlex
    C. coil stent
    C. LC-stainless steel, laser-cut
      coronary stent
Cross-Jones
    C.-J. disk prosthetic valve
    C.-J. mitral valve
cross-linkage theory
crosslinked D fragment
crossover
    femoral-femoral c.
    c. femoral-femoral bypass
CrossPoint TransAccess catheter
cross-reactive antibody
CrossSail coronary dilatation catheter
cross-sectional
    c.-s. area (CSA)
    c.-s. echocardiography (CSE, CSR)
    c.-s. two-dimensional
      echocardiogram
crosstalk pacemaker
Crosswire nitinol hydrophilic guidewire
Crotalus
croup
    catarrhal c.
    diphtheritic c.
    false c.
    membranous c.
    pseudomembranous c.
    spasmodic c.
    c. tent
croup-associated (CA)
    c.-a. virus
Croupette child tent
crouposa
    angina c.

croupous
    c. bronchitis
    c. laryngitis
    c. pharyngitis
    c. pneumonia
croupy cough
crowded oropharynx
Crow-Fukase syndrome
crowing
    c. breath sounds
    c. inspiration
Crown-Crisp index
Crown stent
CRP
    coronary rehabilitation program
    C-reactive protein
      high-sensitivity CRP
CRPD
    chronic restrictive pulmonary disease
CRQ
    Chronic Respiratory Questionnaire
CRT
    cardiac resuscitation team
    code response team
CRT-ICD
    InSync II Marquis remote
      monitoring CRT-ICD
CRU
    cardiac rehabilitation unit
    clinical research unit
cruces (*pl. of* crux)
cruciate anastomosis
crude stroke
crudum
    sputum c.
cruentum
    sputum c.
crunch
    Hamman c.
    Means-Lernan mediastinal c.
    mediastinal c.
crunching sound
crural
    c. artery
    c. diaphragm
crus, pl. **crura**
    angina c.
    c. dextrum diaphragmatic
    c. dextrum fasciculi
      atrioventricularis
    c. sinistrum diaphragmatis
    c. sinistrum fasciculi
      atrioventricularis
crush artifact
crushing chest pain
Crutchfield clamp
Cruveilhier
    C. nodes
    C. sign

Cruveilhier-Baumgarten
    C.-B. murmur
    C.-B. sign
crux, pl. **cruces**
    c. dextrum fasciculi
      atrioventricularis
    c. of heart
    c. sinistrum fasciculi
      atrioventricularis
cruzi
    Trypanosoma c.
CRVF
    congestive right ventricular failure
cryoablation
    arrhythmia circuit c.
    encircling c.
    c. lesion
cryocardioplegia
Cryocare cardiac surgical system
cryocatheter
    Freezor c.
CryoCor cryoablation system
cryocrit
Cryo/Cuff pressure boot
Cryo-Cut microtome
cryoglobulinemia
cryoprecipitate
cryopreservation
cryopreserved
    c. heart valve allograft
    c. homograft valve
    c. human aortic allograft
    c. valved allograft
    c. vein
cryoprobe
    Erbe c.
    Spembly c.
cryoprotectant
cryosurgical technique
cryotherapy
    endobronchial c.
cryptococcal
    c. myocarditis
    c. pulmonary disease
cryptococcoma
cryptococcosis
    disseminated c.
    pulmonary c.
Cryptococcus
    C. albidus
    C. histolyticus
    C. laurentii
    C. neoformans
cryptogenic
    c. fibrosing alveolitis (CFA)
    c. hemoptysis
    c. organizing pneumonia (COP)
    c. organizing pneumonitis (COP)
    c. stroke
cryptophthalmos syndrome
cryptosporidiosis
Cryptosporidium
crystal
    asthma c.
    Charcot-Leyden c.
    Charcot-Neumann c.
    Charcot-Robin c.
    Leyden c.
    piezoelectric c.
    sonomicrometer piezoelectric c.
crystalline nicotine
crystalloid
    airway, breathing, circulation,
      intravenous, c. (ABCIC)
    c. cardioplegic solution
    c. fluid
    c. potassium cardioplegia
    c. prime
    c. resuscitation
CS
    cardiogenic shock
    cavernous sinus
    cholesterol stone
    cholesterol sulfate
    cigarette smoke
    conservative surgery
    coronary sclerosis
    coronary sinus
    cycloserine
      Poly-Histine CS
CSA
    central sleep apnea
    cross-sectional area
CSAS
    central sleep apnea syndrome
CSBF
    coronary sinus blood flow
CSE
    cross-sectional echocardiography
CSF
    colony-stimulating factor
CSFI
    Cholesterol-Saturated Fat Index

C

NOTES

CSFS
coronary slow flow syndrome
CSGBI
Cardiac Society of Great Britain and
Ireland
CSI
chemical shift imaging
cholesterol saturation index
coronary sinus intervention
CSICU
cardiac surgical intensive care unit
CSL
cardiolipin synthetic lecithin
CSLD
chronic suppurative lung disease
CSM
cardiosynchronous monostimulator
circulation, sensation, motion
CSN
cardiac sympathetic nerve
CSO
ostium of coronary sinus
CSOP
coronary sinus occlusion pressure
CSR
cross-sectional echocardiography
CSRS
cardiac surgery reporting system
CSS
Churg-Strauss syndrome
CSSA
carotid stent-supported angioplasty
CST
cardiac stress test
cardiovascular self-assessment tool
CSVT
central splanchnic venous thrombosis
CSWT
cardiac shock wave therapy
cardiac shockwave therapy
CT
cardiac tamponade
cardiothoracic ratio
chest tube
cholesterol, total
clotting time
coagulation time
computed tomography
coronary thrombosis
corrected transposition
corrective therapy
CT angiography
cine CT
contrast-enhanced CT
helical CT
high-resolution CT (HRCT)
reference phantom CT
CT scan

Siemens Evolution electron beam
CT
Technicare Omega 500 CT
thin-section CT
CTA
computed tomography angiography
CTAO
cerebral thromboangiitis obliterans
isolated CTAO
CTAP
computed tomography angiographic
portography
computed tomography in arterial
portography
CTB
cytotrophoblast
CTEPH
chronic thromboembolic pulmonary
hypertension
CTFC
corrected TIMI frame count
CTG
cardiotocography
C/TG
cholesterol-triglyceride
C/TG ratio
CTGA
complete transposition of great arteries
CTGF
connective tissue growth factor
CT-guided stereotaxic technique
CTI
cardiac troponin I
CTICU
cardiothoracic intensive care unit
CTLA4Ig protein
CTM
cardiotachometer
cTnI, cTn-I
cardiac troponin I
cTnI assay
cTnT
cardiac troponin T
CTO
chronic total occlusion
C-to-E amplitude
CTPVO
chronic thrombotic pulmonary vascular
obstruction
CTR
cardiothoracic ratio
CTRD
Cardiac Transplant Research Database
CTS
cardiothoracic surgery
CTSNFR
corrected time of sinoatrial node function
recovery

cTT
cerebral transit time
CTU
cardiac-thoracic unit
CTx
cardiac transplantation
C-type natriuretic peptide (CNP)
CU
cardiac unit
copper
⁶²CU
copper-62
cubitus valgus
cuff
antimicrobial catheter c.
aortic c.
Astropulse c.
atrial c.
blood pressure c. (BPC)
Critikon automated blood
pressure c.
Dinamap blood pressure c.
endotracheal tube c.
Finapres finger c.
finger c.
c. plethysmography
pneumatic c.
c. sign
c. suctioning
c. test
tracheostomy c.
cuffed
c. endotracheal tube
c. hypertension
c. tracheostomy tube
cuffing
peribronchial c.
cuff-leak test
cuirass
chest c.
c. respirator
tabetic c.
c. ventilator
culbertsoni
Acanthamoeba c.
cul-de-sac
blind c.-d.-s.
culotte
c. coronary stenting technique
c. fashion
culprit
c. lesion

c. lesion angioplasty
c. vessel angioplasty
culture
endoscopic tissue c. (ETC)
pericardial fluid c. (PFC)
culture-negative endocarditis
cumetharol
cumethoxaethane
cumulative cardiotoxic dose (CCD)
cuneiform tubercle
Cunninghamella
cupping artifact
cuprophane membrane
cupula, pl. **cupulae**
c. of pleura
c. pleurae
pleural c.
curare
curd
soap c.
curet, curette
Curosurf intratracheal suspension
currant
c. jelly clot
c. jelly sputum
c. jelly thrombus
current
alternating c. (AC)
bioelectric c.
calcium c. (I_{Ca})
chloride c. (I_{Cl})
diastolic c.
direct c. (DC)
fast sodium c.
K c.
low energy direct c. (LEDC)
membrane c.
pacemaker c. (I_F)
pseudoalternating c.
pump c.
radiofrequency c. (RFC)
range-alternating c.
sodium c. (I_{Na})
systolic c.
toxin-insensitive c.
transient inward c.
transsarcolemmal calcium c.
Curry needle
Curschmann spiral
curse
Ondine c.

C

NOTES

curve
>actuarial survival c.
>AH c.
>ascorbate dilution c.
>carbon dioxide dissociation c.
>dissociation c.
>dose-effect curve dose-response c.
>dye-dilution c.
>flow volume c.
>Frank-Starling c.
>function c.
>green dye c.
>hemoglobin-oxygen dissociation c.
>indocyanine dilution c.
>intracardiac pressure c.
>isovolume pressure flow c. (IVPF)
>J c.
>Kaplan-Meier event-free survival c.
>left ventricular pressure-volume c.
>length-active tension c.
>length-tension c. (LT)
>mitral E velocity c.
>nitrogen c.
>oxygen dissociation c.
>oxyhemoglobin dissociation c.
>pressure-natriuresis c.
>pressure-volume c.
>pulse c.
>single-breath nitrogen c.
>Starling c.
>thermal dilution c.
>thermodilution c.
>time-activity c.
>Traube c.
>venous return c.
>venovenous dye dilution c.
>ventricular function c. (VFC)
>volume-time c.

curved
>c. end-to-end anastomosis (CEEA)
>c. tapered Tefcor movable core
>   wire guide

Curvularia lunata

CUSA
>Cavitron ultrasonic surgical aspirator

Cushing
>C. forceps
>C. pressure response
>C. reflex
>C. syndrome
>C. triad

cushingoid facies

cushion
>atrioventricular canal c.
>cardiac c.
>coronary c.
>endocardial c.
>pharyngoesophageal c.'s
>Sullivan bubble c.

Cushman assay

cusp
>accessory c.
>aortic c.
>c. billowing
>conjoined c.
>coronary c.
>c. degeneration
>c. eversion
>c. excursion
>c. fenestration
>fish-mouth c.
>left coronary c. (LCC)
>c. motion
>noncoronary c. (NCC)
>right coronary c. (RCC)

cuspides commissurales

cuspis
>c. anterior valvae bicuspidalis
>c. anterior valvae tricuspidalis

cut
>coronal c.
>DCA c.
>c. point
>sagittal c.

cutaneous
>c. asthma
>c. hyperesthesia
>c. malignancy
>c. necrotizing venulitis

cutdown
>arterial c.
>brachial artery c.
>c. catheter
>saphenous vein c. (SVC)
>c. technique
>venous c.

cut-film arteriography

Cutinova Hydro dressing

cutis
>c. laxa
>c. laxa syndrome
>c. marmorata

Cutler-Ederer method

cutpoint

cutter
>C. aortic valve prosthesis
>EZ45 thoracic linear c.
>rib c.

Cutter-Smeloff
>C.-S. aortic valve prosthesis
>C.-S. disk valve
>C.-S. mitral valve

cutting
>C. Ballon Ultra 2
>c. balloon
>c. balloon angioplasty (CBA)
>c. balloon before stent (CBBEST)

c. balloon device
c. balloon RCT
cuvette
dye c.
Cuvier
canal of C.
duct of C.
Cu/Zn superoxide dismutase
CV
cardiac volume
cardiovascular
care vigilance
central venous
central venous catheter
cerebrovascular
cervical vertebra
contrast ventriculography
conventional ventilation
CV wave of jugular venous pulse
CVA
cardiovascular accident
cerebrovascular accident
costovertebral angle
CVAP
cerebrovascular amyloid peptide
CVC
central venous catheter
CVC 123 calibration verification
control
CV cath
central venous catheter
CVCT
cardiovascular computed tomography
CVD
cardiovascular disease
C-Vest
C-V. ambulatory radionuclide
detector
C-V. radiation detector system
CVF
cardiovascular failure
chronic ventilatory failure
CVFn
cardiovascular function
CVG
coronary venous graft
CVH
combined ventricular hypertrophy
CVHD
chronic valvular heart disease
CVI
cardiovascular incident

cardiovascular insufficiency
cerebrovascular incident
cerebrovascular infarction
cerebrovascular insufficiency
chronic venous insufficiency
multiple CVIs
CVICU
cardiovascular intensive care unit
CVID
common variable immunodeficiency
partial CVID
CVIS
cardiovascular imaging system
CVIS imaging device
CVM
cardiovascular monitor
CVO
central vein occlusion
central venous oxygen
CVP
cardioventricular pacing
central venous pressure
CVP line
CVR
cardiovascular-renal
cardiovascular-respiratory
cephalic vasomotor response
cerebrovascular reactivity
cerebrovascular resistance
coronary flow velocity reserve
CVRD
cardiovascular-renal disease
CVRR
cardiovascular recovery room
CVRS
cardiovascular and respiratory elements
of trauma score
CVS
cardiovascular surgery
cardiovascular system
cerebral vasospasm
collagen vascular sealing
c-v systolic wave
CVT
cardiovascular technologist
central venous temperature
cerebral venous thrombosis
CVVH
continuous venovenous hemofiltration
CW
cardiac work
circle of Willis

NOTES

CWD
cell wall defect
continuous-wave Doppler
CWI
cardiac work index
CWM
cardiological workspace manager
CWP
coal worker's pneumoconiosis
CWS
chest wall stimulation
circumferential wall stress
CX
chest x-ray
circumflex
CXC chemokine
CxCor
circumflex coronary
CxCor artery
CXR, CxR
chest radiograph
chest x-ray
cyanide
c. antidote kit
hydrogen c. (HCN)
cyanmethemoglobin method
cyanoacrylate
n-butyl c. (n-BCA)
2-cyanoacrylate
isobutyl 2-c.
cyanochroic, cyanochrous
cyanogen bromide method
cyanosed
cyanosis
autotoxic c.
central c.
circumoral c.
edema, clubbing, and c. (ECC)
false c.
hereditary methemoglobinemic c.
late c.
c. of nail beds
peripheral c.
pulmonary c.
c. retinae
reverse differential c.
shunt c.
tardive c.
cyanotic
c. asphyxia
c. congenital heart disease
c. congenital heart disease
arrhythmia
c. heart defect
c. heart disease (CHD)
cyanotica
asphyxia c.
Cyberlith pacemaker

Cybertach
C. automatic-burst atrial pacemaker
C. 60 bipolar pacemaker
Cybex isokinetic dynamometer
cyclandelate
cyclase
adenylate c.
adenylyl c. (AC)
cell membrane-bound adenylate c.
guanylate c.
guanylyl c.
cycle
cardiac c. (CC)
cell c.
circannual c.
circaseptan c.
citric acid c.
c. ergometer
c. ergometry
forced c.
isometric period of cardiac c.
Krebs c.
c. length (CL)
c. length alternans
c. length alternation
moiety-conserved c.
ratio of expiration time and total
time of breathing c. (tE/tTOT)
ratio of inspiration time and total
time of breathing c. (tI/tTOT)
respiratory c.
restored c.
returning c.
RR c.
short-long-short c.
sound wave c.
Wenckebach c.
cycle-length window
cyclic
c. adenosine monophosphate
(cAMP)
c. guanosine monophosphate
(cGMP)
c. nucleotide adenosine
monophosphate
c. progesterone
c. respiration
cyclin A gene
cyclocumarol
cycloergometer
cycloheximide
cyclohexylamine
Cyclomen
cyclooxygenase (COX)
c. inhibitor
cyclooxygenase-1
cyclooxygenase-2
cyclopentamine hydrochloride
cyclopenthiazide

cyclopentylpropionate
    hydrocortisone c.
cyclophosphamide
    c., bleomycin, cisplatin (CBP)
    c., doxorubicin, cisplatin (CAP)
    c., doxorubicin, methotrexate,
      procarbazine (CAMP)
    c., doxorubicin, vincristine (CAV)
    vindesine, cisplatin, lomustine, c.
      (VCPC)
cyclopropane
cycloserine (CS)
cyclosporin A
cyclosporine
cyclothiazide
cyclotron-produced F-18
  fluorodeoxyglucose
CYFRA
    cytokeratin 19 fragment
    CYFRA 21-1 tumor marker
Cyklokapron
    C. injection
    C. Oral
Cylexin
cylinder
    C oxygen c.
    M6 oxygen c.
cylindrical
    c. bronchiectasis
    c. confronting cisterna
cylindroadenoma
cylindroid aneurysm
cylindroma
cylindruria
Cynosar catheter
CYP3A isoform
CYP1A2 isoform
CYP2C9 isoform
CYP2D6 isoform
CYP2C19 isoform
Cypher sirolimus-eluting coronary stent
cypionate
    hydrocortisone c.
cyproheptadine hydrochloride
cyproterone
Cyriax syndrome
cys-LT
    cysteinyl leukotriene
cyst
    aneurysmal bone c.
    apoplectic c.
    bronchial c.

    bronchogenic c.
    bronchopulmonary c.
    centrilobular c.
    compound c.
    echinococcal c.
    hemorrhagic c.
    hepatic hydatid c.
    honeycomb c.
    hydatid c.
    locular c.
    loculated c.
    mucoretention c.
    mucous retention c.
    multilocular c.
    necrotic c.
    neurenteric c.
    pericardial c.
    pleuropericardial c.
    renal c.
    retention c.
    springwater c.
    thymic c.
    Tornwaldt c.
    true c.
    unilocular c.
cystathionine synthase deficiency
cystatin C
cysteine
cysteinyl leukotriene (cys-LT)
cystic
    c. adenomatoid malformation
    c. bronchiectasis
    c. disease of lung
    c. emphysema
    c. fibrosis (CF)
    c. fibrosis transmembrane
      conductance regulator
    c. fibrosis transmembrane regulator
      (CFTR)
    c. lesion
    c. medial necrosis
    c. medial necrosis of ascending
      aorta (CMN-AA)
    c. space
cystica
    medionecrosis aortae idiopathica c.
    osteitis tuberculosa multiplex c.
cysticercosis
cystidine monophospho-*N*-
  acetylneuraminic acid (CMP-NANA)
Cytadren
cytarabine hydrochloride

NOTES

cytobrush
cytocentrifugation
cytochalasin B
cytochrome
    c. c oxidase (COX)
    c. P450 system
CytoGam
cytokeratin 19 fragment (CYFRA)
cytokine
    cardioinflammatory c.
    chemotactic c.
    c. expression
    inflammatory c.
    pleiotropic c.
    proinflammatory c.
cytokine-induced endothelial synthesis
cytological biopsy
cytology
    aspiration biopsy c. (ABC)
    bronchial washings c.
    sputum c.
cytomegalic inclusion disease
cytomegalovirus (CMV)
    c. encephalitis
    human c. (HCMV)
    c. immune globulin (CMVIG)
    c. immune globulin intravenous,
      human
    c. pneumonitis
Cytomel Oral

cytometer
cytometric indirect immunofluorescence
cytomitome
cytomorphology
cytomorphosis
cytoplasmic bridge
cytoprotective
    c. agent
    c. effect
Cytosar-U
cytosine-thymine-guanine trinucleotide
cytoskeleton
    actin c.
cytosolic protein
cytosome
cytotoxic
    c. edema
    c. gene therapy
    c. singlet oxygen
cytotoxicity
cytotoxin-associated gene product A
    (CagA)
cytotrophoblast (CTB)
Cytovene
Cytoxan
    C. injection
    C. Oral
Czaja-McCaffrey rigid stent
    introducer/endoscope

D

    diastole
    dipyridamole
    disease
    donor
        D loop
        D sleep
        D wave

2D

    two-dimensional
        2D echocardiogram
        2D echocardiography
        2D gradient-echo sequence
        2D TEE system Ultra-Neb 99

D2

    prostaglandin D2

3D

    three-dimensional
        3D IVUS
        3D segmented-FLASH imaging
        sequence
        3D SPGR image
        3D tagged magnetic resonance
        imaging
        3D time-of-flight magnetic
        resonance angiographic sequence
        3D TOF MRA

D_4

    leukotriene D_4

Do_2

    oxygen delivery

D_{CO}

    pulmonary diffusion capacity

D114S balloon catheter

D1790G mutant gene

D2L OTW balloon dilatation catheter with extended pressure range

DA

    daytime asthma
    descending aorta
    digital angiography
    ductus arteriosus

D-A

    donor-acceptor

Da

    dalton

d(A)

    primary donor

Daae disease

DAC

    Guiatuss DAC
    Guiatussin DAC
    Halotussin DAC
    Mytussin DAC

dacarbazine

daclizumab

DaCosta syndrome

Dacron

    D. catheter
    D. cloth
    D. fiber
    D. intracardiac patch
    D. onlay patch-graft
    D. tube graft

dactinomycin

DAD

    delayed afterdepolarization
    diffuse alveolar damage

dagger-shaped aortic envelope

Daggett procedure

DAH

    diffuse alveolar hemorrhage
    disordered action of heart

daidzein

Daig sheath

d'airain

    bruit d'a.

Dakin solution

Dalalone

Dale-Schwartz tube

Dale tracheostomy tube holder

dalfopristin

Dallas

    D. Classification System
    D. criteria

dalteparin

    d. sodium
    d. sodium injection

dalton (Da)

Dalton-Henry law

Dalton law

damage

    bilateral hemisphere d. (BHD)
    diffuse alveolar d. (DAD)
    enzyme-induced d.
    left brain d. (LBD)
    left hemisphere d. (LHD)
    myocardial d. (MD)
    parietal pleural d.
    regional alveolar d. (RAD)
    right brain d. (RBD)
    right hemisphere d. (RHD)
    silent ischemic brain d. (SIBD)

Damato curve catheter

D'Amato sign

DAMIA

    direct acute myocardial infarction angioplasty

Damian graft procedure

dampened waveform

D

damping
>Accudynamic adjustable d.
>catheter d.
>d. coefficient
>d. control

Damus-Kaye-Stansel (DKS)
>D.-K.-S. connection
>D.-K.-S. operation
>D.-K.-S. procedure
>D.-K.-S. procedure for single ventricle physiology

DAN
>diabetic autonomic neuropathy

danaparoid sodium

danazol

dance
>brachial d.
>hilar d.
>St. Vitus d.

dander
>animal d.

Dane particle

Danielson method

Danocrine

Danon storage disease

Dantrium

dantrolene sodium

DAo
>descending aorta

DAP
>depolarizing afterpotential
>diastolic aortic pressure

dapsone (DDS)

daptomycin for injection

Daranide

Daraprim

DAR breathing system

Dardik Biograft

darkfield microscopy

Darling disease

Darox cutaneous thoracic patch electrode

DASE
>dobutamine atropine stress echocardiography

DASH
>dietary approaches to stop hypertension

Dash single-chamber rate-adaptic pacemaker

DASI
>Duke Activity Status Index

DAT
>direct amplification test

data
>measured d.
>nonparametric d.
>pressure-volume d.

database
>Cardiac Transplant Research D. (CTRD)
>Duke Carcinoid D.
>GenBank genome sequence d.
>low-density lipoprotein receptor mutation d. (LDLR, LDL-R)

Datascope
>D. Accutor bedside monitor
>D. balloon
>D. CL-II percutaneous translucent balloon catheter
>D. pulse oximeter
>D. System 90 intraaortic balloon pump

DATI
>diastolic amplitude time index

daughter radionuclide

DaunoXome

David operation

Davidson
>D. clamp
>D. protocol exercise test
>D. scapular retractor
>D. thoracic trocar

Davies
>D. disease
>D. endomyocardial fibrosis
>D. myocardial fibrosis
>D. technique

da Vinci robotic surgical system

Davis sign

DAVM
>dural arteriovenous malformation

day
>milligram per kilogram per d.

daytime asthma (DA)

Dazamide

dazoxiben

DBC
>distal balloon catheter

DBCL
>dilute blood clot lysis
>>DBCL method

DBP
>diastolic blood pressure

DBPC
>dual balloon perfusion catheter

DC
>direct current
>dual chamber
>electric defibrillator using DC discharge
>>Bromanate DC
>>DC cardioversion
>>DC electric shock
>>Myphetane DC

DCA
>dichloroacetate
>directional color angiography

directional coronary angioplasty
    DCA cut
    DCA debulking technique
DCABG
    double coronary artery bypass graft
DCAF
    dilated cardiomyopathy and atrial
        fibrillation
DCBF
    dynamic cardiac blood flow
DCC
    direct cardiac compression
DCCV
    direct current cardioversion
DCFM
    Doppler color flow mapping
DCG
    dynamic electrocardiography
DCHS
    dysarthria-clumsy hand syndrome
DCI
    delayed cerebral ischemia
    digital cardiac imaging
**DCI-S automated coronary analysis
system**
DCLHb
    diaspirin cross-linked hemoglobin
DCM
    dilated cardiomyopathy
DCMAG-1 gene
DCOP
    distal coronary occlusion pressure
DCOR
    dopachrome oxidoreductase
DCP
    dual chamber pacemaker
DCS
    decompression sickness
    distal coronary sinus
        neurologic DCS
        pulmonary DCS
DCV
    delayed cerebral vasoconstriction
D2CV
    Doppler two-chamber view
D4CV
    Doppler four-chamber view
DDAVP, dDAVP
    DDAVP injection
    DDAVP Nasal
ddC
    dideoxycytidine

DDD
    A-V universal
    AV universal
    dual-mode, dual-pacing, dual-sensing
        DDD pacemaker
        DDD pacing
DDDR pacing
DDFP
    dodecafluoropentane
DD genotype
DDI
    DDI mode pacemaker
    DDI pacing
ddI
    didanosine
D-dimer
    D-d. enzyme-linked immunosorbent
        assay
    fibrin D-d.
    D-d. test
DDIR pacing
DDP
    cisplatin
DDR
    diastolic descent rate
DD2R
    dopamine D2 receptor
DDS
    dapsone
DE
    dobutamine echocardiography
2DE
    two-dimensional echocardiography
3DE
    three-dimensional echocardiography
De
    De Martel scissors
    De Morgan spots
de
    de Groot classification
    de la Camp sign
    de Lange syndrome
    de Musset sign (aortic aneurysm)
    de Mussy point
    de Mussy sign (pleurisy)
    de novo
    de novo atherosclerosis
    de novo coronary lesion
    de novo malignancy
    de Quervain thyroiditis
dead
    d. space

D

NOTES

dead (continued)

d. space gas volume to tidal gas volume ratio (V_{DS}/V_T)

d. space:tidal volume ratio

d. space ventilation

d. time

deadly quartet syndrome

deaired

deairing procedure

deaminase

adenosine d. (ADA)

1-deamine-4-valine-D-arginine vasopressin (dVDAVP)

dearterialization

hepatic d.

death

aborted sudden d.

apoptotic cell d.

brain d.

cardiac d.

circle of d.

cocaine-related sudden d.

ischemic sudden d.

late sudden d.

out-of-hospital sudden cardiac d. (OOH-SCD)

postresuscitative d.

pump failure d.

sudden cardiac d. (SCD)

sudden coronary d. (SCD)

sudden heart d. (SHD)

sudden unexplained d.

sudden unexplained nocturnal d. (SUND)

vascular d.

voodoo d.

DeBakey

D. aortic aneurysm clamp

D. arterial clamp

D. arterial forceps

D. Atraugrip forceps

D. ball valve prosthesis

D. blade

D. chest retractor

D. classification

D.-Derra anastomosis clamp

D.-Derra anastomosis forceps

manner of D.

D. pediatric clamp

D. peripheral vascular clamp

D. rib spreader

D. tissue forceps

D. type I, II, III, IIIa, IIIb aortic dissection

D. VAD

D. VAD continuous-axial-flow pump

D. Vasculour-II vascular prosthesis

DeBakey-Bahnson clamp

DeBakey-Bainbridge clamp

DeBakey-Colovira-Rumel thoracic forceps

DeBakey-Creech

D.-C. aneurysm repair

D.-C. manner

DeBakey-Derra

D.-D. anastomosis clamp

D.-D. anastomosis forceps

DeBakey-Diethrich coronary artery forceps

DeBakey-Harken auricle clamp

DeBakey-Howard aortic aneurysmal clamp

DeBakey-Kay aortic clamp

DeBakey-McQuigg-Mixter bronchial clamp

DeBakey-Mixter thoracic forceps

DeBakey-NASA axial-flow ventricular-assist device

DeBakey-Péan cardiovascular forceps

DeBakey-Satinsky vena cava clamp

DeBakey-Semb ligature-carrier clamp

DeBakey-Surgitool prosthetic valve

debilis

pulsus d.

debility

Debove

D. membrane

D. treatment

debris

atheromatous d.

atherosclerotic d.

calcific d.

grumous d.

pultaceous d.

valve d.

debrisoquine sulfate

debt

oxygen d.

debubbling procedure

debulking

d. device

mechanical d.

d. procedure

Decabid

Decadron

D. Injection

D. Oral

D. Phosphate

Decadron-LA

Deca-Durabolin

Decaject

Decaject-LA

decamethonium

decanoate

Hybolin D.

nandrolone d.

decapolar electrode catheter

decarboxylase
  histidine d.
decay
  isovolumic pressure d.
  pressure d.
deceleration
  early d.
  horizontal anteroposterior d.
  late d.
  d. time
  variable d.
  vertical d.
deceleration-dependent aberrancy
decerebrate posturing
DECG
  differentiated ECG
declamping
  d. shock
  d. shock syndrome
Declomycin
Decofed Syrup
Decohistine
  D. DH
  D. Expectorant
decompensate
decompensated shock
decompensation
  cardiac d.
decompression
  cardiac d.
  d. disorder
  d. illness
  microvascular d. (MVD)
  d. sickness (DCS)
  d. table
decompressive chest tube
Deconamine
  D. SR
  D. Syrup
  D. Tablet
deconditioning
Deconsal II
decontamination
decortication
  arterial d.
  cardiac d.
  d. of heart
  d. of lung
decrease
  blood pressure d. (BPD)
decreased
  d. breath sounds

  d. respiration
  d. valve excursion
decrement
decremental
  d. atrial pacing
  d. conduction
decrescendo murmur
decrudescence
decrudescent arteriosclerosis
decubitus
  d. angina
  angina pectoris d.
  d. cough
  d. ulcer
dedicated bipolar lead
Dedo-Pilling laryngoscope
deductive echocardiography
deendothelialization
deenergization
  myocyte d.
deep
  d. chest therapy
  d. Doppler velocity interrogation
  d. hypothermia circulatory arrest
    (DHCA)
  d. lingual artery
  d. lingual vein
  d. pathologic Q wave
  d. sleep
  d. venous insufficiency (DVI)
  d. venous pressure (DVP)
  d. venous thrombosis (DVT)
  d. venous thrombosis/pulmonary
    embolism (DVT/PE)
  d. white matter hyperintensity
    (DWMHI)
  d. white matter lesion (DWML)
de-epicardialization
deer-antler vascular pattern
Defares rebreathing method
defecation
  salivation, lacrimation, urination,
    and d. (SLUD)
  d. syncope
defect
  acquired ventricular septal d.
    (AVSD)
  aorticopulmonary septal d. (APSD)
  aortic septal d.
  aortopulmonary septal d. (APSD)
  atrial ostium primum d.
  atrial septal d. (ASD)

D

NOTES

defect *(continued)*
atrioventricular canal d.
atrioventricular conduction d.
atrioventricular septal d. (AVSD)
A-V conduction d.
cell wall d. (CWD)
clamshell closure of atrial septal d.
conal septal d.
conduction d. (CD)
contiguous ventricular septal d.
cyanotic heart d.
Eisenmenger reaction with septal d.
endocardial cushion d. (ECD)
extrafusion d.
factor V Leiden coagulation d.
filling d.
fixed perfusion d.
fixed-rate perfusion d.
Gerbode d.
humoral immune d.
hydrogen-detected ventricular
  septal d. (HVSD)
iatrogenic atrial septal d.
infundibular septal d.
interatrial septal d. (IASD)
interauricular septal d. (IASD)
interventricular septal d. (ISD,
  IVSD)
intimal d.
intraarterial conduction d. (IACD)
intraventricular conduction d.
  (IVCD)
isolated conduction d. (ICD)
lucent d.
match d.
muscular ventricular septal d.
  (MVSD)
myocardial long-chain fatty acid
  uptake d.
napkin-ring d.
nonsegmental perfusion d.
nonuniform rotational d. (NURD)
obstructive ventilatory d.
ostium primum d.
ostium secundum d.
panconduction d.
partial A-V canal d.
perfusion d.
periinfarction conduction d. (PICD)
perimembranous ventricular
  septal d.
primum atrial septal d.
pterygia, heart defects, autosomal
  recessive inheritance, vertebral
  defects, ear anomalies, radial d.'s
  (PHAVER)
pulmonary artery filling d. (PAFD)
pulmonary atresia with ventricular
  septal d. (PAVSD)

restrictive airways d.
restrictive ventilatory d.
reversible ischemic neurologic d.
  (RIND)
scintigraphic perfusion d.
secundum atrial septal d. (ASD2)
secundum-type atrial septal d.
septal d. (SD)
sinus venosus atrial septal d.
supracristal ventricular septal d.
Swiss cheese d.
d.'s syndrome
T cell d.
thallium uptake d.
transcatheter closure of atrial d.
transcatheter occlusion of atrial
  septal d.
ventilation/perfusion d.
ventricular septal d. (VSD)
ventricular septal heart d. (VSHD)
ventriculoseptal d. (VSD)
V̇/Q̇ d.
Defen-LA
defensiveness
emotional d. (ED)
deferoxamine mesylate
defervesce
defervescence
defibrillate
airway, breathing, circulation, d.
  (ABCD)
defibrillation (DF, DFIB)
biphasic waveform transthoracic d.
cardiac d.
Moe multiple wavelet hypothesis
  of atrial d.
d. paddles
d. patch
public access d. (PAD)
public access to d. (PAD)
d. response interval (DRI)
d. shock
d. threshold (DFT, DT)
defibrillator
Atrioverter implantable atrial d.
automatic external d. (AED)
automatic implantable d. (AID)
automatic internal d.
Cardioserv d.
Codemaster d. (Hewlett-Packard)
CodeMaster d. (Philips)
Endotak lead d.
external d.
ForeRunner d.
Gem II DR dual-chamber d.
Gem DR implantable d.
Guidant d.
Heart Aid 80 d.
HeartStart MRx d.

Hewlett-Packard d.
d. implant
implantable atrial d. (IAD)
InSync implantable cardioverter d.
Intec implantable d.
Jewel AF implantable d.
Lifepak d.
LifeVest wearable d.
manual d.
Marquette Responder 1500
multifunctional d.
Medtronic Gem automatic
implantable d.
Medtronic Micro Jewel II
implantable d.
Metrix implantable atrial d.
d. paddles
PD 2000 d.
Photon Micro DR/VR implantable
cardioverter d.
Porta Pulse 3 d.
public access d. (PAD)
semiautomatic external d. (SAED)
smart d.
transvenous implantable d.
d. unit
Ventak Prizm dual-chamber
implantable d.
Zoll PD 1200 external d.

deficiency
acetylcholinesterase d.
acid maltase d.
ADA d.
adenosine deaminase d.
alpha-1 antitrypsin d.
antithrombin III d.
antitrypsin d.
apolipoprotein A1 d.
carnitine d.
complement component C1r d.
congenital pseudocholinesterase d.
C1r d.
cystathionine synthase d.
dopamine beta-hydroxylase d.
enzymatic d.
factor III d.
familial apoA-I d.
familial HDL d.
familial high-density-lipoprotein d.
galactosidase d.
glucosidase d.
hemostatic d.

heparin cofactor II d.
hexosaminidase d.
homogentisic acid oxidase d.
HRF d.
hydroxylase d.
17-hydroxylase d.
magnesium d.
maltase d.
Owren factor V d.
protein C d.
protein-calorie d.
protein S d.
pseudocholinesterase d.
selenium d.
surfactant d.
thiamine d.
tissue plasminogen activator
release d.
vasopressor d.

deficit
neurologic d.
pulse d.
spectacular shrinking d.

Definity perflutren
deflated profile
deflation
deflazacort
deflectable quadripolar catheter
deflection
atrial d.
delta d.
His bundle d.
d. in the His bundle in
electrogram
intrinsic d.
intrinsicoid d.
QS d.
RS d.
deflector
deformans
arteritis d.
endarteritis d.
osteitis d.
deformation
capacitor d.
deformity
buttonhole d.
cervical spine d.
gooseneck outflow tract d.
hockey-stick d.
joint d.
parachute d.

NOTES

D

199

deformity *(continued)*
    pectus d.
    pigeon-breast d.
    shepherd's crook d.
degeneration
    cusp d.
    endothelial cell d.
    fibrinoid d.
    glassy d.
    Mönckeberg d.
    mucoid medial d.
    myxomatous d.
    Quain fatty d.
    spinocerebellar d.
    Wallerian d. (WD)
deglutition
    d. apnea
    d. mechanism
    d. murmur
    d. pneumonia
    d. syncope
Degos disease
degranulation
    goblet cell d.
degrees of freedom
Dehio test
dehiscence
    anular d.
    bronchial d.
    sternal d.
dehydrocholesterol (DHC)
dehydroemetine
dehydrogenase
    d. activity
    alpha-hydroxybutyrate d.
    11-beta-hydroxysteroid d.
    branched chain alpha ketoacid d.
    (BCKD)
    glucose-6-phosphate d. (G6PD)
    hydroxybutyrate d. (HBDH)
    lactate d.
    lactic d. (LDH)
    lactic acid d.
    pyruvate d. (PDH)
dehydromonocrotaline
11-dehydro-thromboxane B$_2$
Deklene II cardiovascular suture
DeKock two-way bronchial catheter
Del
    D. Mar Avionics Scanner
    D. Mar Avionics three-channel
    recorder
Delaborde tracheal dilator
Delatestryl Injection
delavirdine
delay
    atrioventricular d. (AVD)
    conduction d.
    electromechanical d.

    intramyocardial conduction d.
    intraventricular conduction d.
    ischemia-induced intramyocardial
    conduction d.
    nonspecific intraventricular
    conduction d. (NSIVCD)
delayed
    d. afterdepolarization (DAD)
    d. cerebral ischemia (DCI)
    d. cerebral vasoconstriction (DCV)
    d. conduction
    d. depolarization
    d. primary closure (DPC)
    d. pulmonary toxicity syndrome
    (DPTS)
    d. xenograft rejection (DXR)
delayed-type hypersensitivity (DTH)
Delbet sign
deletion
    allelic d.
    22q11 d.
delimitation
delineation
    endocardial border d.
DELIRIUM
    drugs, electrolytes, low temperature and
    lunacy, intoxication and intracranial
    processes, retention of urine or feces,
    infection, unfamiliar surroundings,
    myocardial infarction
delirium
    d. cordis
    D. Rating Scale
    toxic d.
delivery
    closed-loop d.
    contrast medium d.
    oxygen d. (Do_2)
    d. wire
Delmege sign
Delorme thoracoplasty
Delphian node
Delrin
    D. frame of valve prosthesis
    D. heart valve
Delsym
delta
    d. deflection
    d. wave
Delta-Cortef Oral
Deltasone Oral
deltopectoral groove
Deltran disposable transducer
Demadex
    D. injection
    D. Oral
demand
    cardiac output d.
    d. hypoxia

d. mode
myocardial oxygen d.
d. oxygen delivery system (DODS)
d. pacemaker
d. pacing
d. pulse generator
demand-triggered
ventricular d.-t. (VVD)
Demarquay sign
demeclocycline hydrochloride
dementia
multiinfarct d.
thalamic d.
vascular d.
Demerol
Demos tibial artery clamp
Demser
denatured homograft
denaturing high performance liquid chromatography (DHPLC)
dendritic lesion
Dendroaspis **natriuretic peptide (DNP)**
denervated
denervation
cardiac sympathetic d.
sinoaortic d. (SAD)
d. supersensitivity
dengue fever
Denhardt solution
denileukin diftitox
Dennis dissecting scissors
dense
d. hemiplegia
d. thrill
densitogram
ear d.
densitometry
acoustic d.
video d.
density
dependent d.
echo d.
full caloric d.
hydrogen d.
lipid core d.
power spectral d. (PSD)
proton d.
spin d.
density-exposure relationship of film
dental
d. antisnoring device
d. barotrauma

dentis
anterior d.
dentocariosa
Rothia d.
dentrificans
Alcaligenes d.
denudation
endothelial d.
Denver pleural effusion shunt
deoxycorticosterone
deoxygenated hemoglobin
2-deoxyglucose
deoxyhemoglobin
deoxyribonuclease (DNase)
human recombinant d.
deoxyribonucleic acid (DNA)
15-deoxyspergualin
dependence
nicotine d.
oxygen d.
use d.
dependency
ventilator d.
dependent
d. beat
d. density
d. edema
d. rubor
dephosphorylation
deplasmolysis
depletion
glycogen d.
volume d.
deployment
high-pressure stent d.
stent d.
depolarization
alternating failure of response, mechanical, to electrical d. (AFORMED)
atrial premature d. (APD)
delayed d.
diastolic d.
His bundle d.
intrinsic d.
myocardial d.
premature ventricular d. (PVD)
rapid d.
transient d.
ventricular ectopic d. (VED)
ventricular premature d. (VPD)
d. wave

D

NOTES

depolarization-repolarization
     VCD model of cardiac cell d.-r.
depolarizing
     d. afterpotential (DAP)
     d. drug
depolymerization
depolymerized porcine mucosal heparin
Depo-Medrol injection
Deponit Patch
Depopred injection
Depo-Provera injection
deposit
     calcium d.
     intraalveolar d.
deposition
     aerosol d.
     calcium oxalate d.
     collagen d.
     mitochondrial calcium d.
depot
     Androcur D.
     Lupron D.
Depot-Ped
     Lupron D.-P.
depreotide
     technetium d.
depressant
     cardiac d.
depressed
     d. ST segment (DEP ST SEG)
     d. ventricular function
depression
     aldosterone d.
     cardiorespiratory d.
     circulatory d.
     downhill ST segment d.
     downsloping ST segment d.
     horizontal ST segment d.
     Hospital Anxiety and D. (HAD)
     junctional d.
     myocardial d.
     postdrive d.
     P-Q segment d.
     precordial ST d.
     reciprocal ST d.
     rectilinear ST-segment d.
     respiratory d.
     spreading d. (SD)
     ST segment d. (STD)
     upsloping ST segment d.
     vascular d.
     X d.
depressor reflex
deprivation
     sleep d.
Deproist Expectorant With Codeine
DEP ST SEG
     depressed ST segment

depth
     d. compensation
     d. pressure fsw
     volumetric lung d. (Vp)
DEQ
     digital echo quantification
derivative
     d. circulation
     ergotamine d.'s
     hematoporphyrin d. (HPD)
     JTV519 1,4-benzothiazepine d.
     methanesulfonanilide d.
     purified protein d. (PPD)
     quaternary ammonium atropine d.
     thiazolidinedione d.
derived 12-lead electrocardiogram
DermaFlex Gel
Dermalon suture
dermatan sulfate
dermatitidis
     Ajellomyces d.
     Blastomyces d.
dermatitis, pl. **dermatitides**
     exfoliative d.
     livedoid d.
     stasis d.
     weeping d.
dermatomyositis
Dermatophagoides pteronyssinus
dermonecrotic
Derra
     D. aortic clamp
     D. valve dilator
     D. vena caval clamp
DES
     diethylstilbestrol
     diffuse esophageal spasm
     drug-eluting stent
Desai
     D. VectorCath mapping catheter
     D. VectorCath mapping system
desaturation
     arterial d.
     arterial oxygen d. (AOD)
     nocturnal d.
Desc Ao
     descending aorta
descendens
     aorta d.
     ramus anterior d.
     ramus posterior d.
descending
     d. anterior branch
     d. aorta (DA, DAo, Desc Ao)
     left anterior d. (LAD)
     d. necrotizing mediastinitis (DNM)
     d. phlebitis
     d. posterior branch
     d. thoracic aneurysm

d. thoracic aorta (DTA)
d. thoracic aorta-to-femoral artery (DTAFA)
d. thoracic aorta-to-femoral artery bypass graft
d. thoracic aortic-femoral-femoral (DTAF-F)
d. thoracic aortofemoral-femoral bypass

descent
barotrauma of d.
rapid Y d.
X, Y d.

Deschamps compressor
deserpidine
methyclothiazide and d.

desert fever
desethylamiodarone
desethyl amiodarone
Desferal Mesylate
desferrioxamine
desflurane
desglycinamide-9-arginine-8-vasopressin (DGAVP)
desiccation
mucous d.

designed after natural anatomy
Desilets-Hoffman
D.-H. catheter introducer
D.-H. sheath

desipramine hydrochloride
desirudin
deslanoside
desloratadine
desmethyldiazepam
desmin gene
desmoplastic
d. mesothelioma
d. small round cell tumor

desmopressin acetate
desmosine
desmosome
desoxycorticosterone
desoxyephedrine
phenacetin, aspirin, and d. (PAD)

Desoxyn
d'Espine sign
desquamation
peribronchial d.

desquamative
d. alveolitis

d. interstitial pneumonia (DIP)
d. interstitial pneumonitis (DIP)

destruction
alveolar d.
apoptotic d.
lung tissue d.
plasmatic vascular d.

desulfatohirudin
recombinant d.

desynchronized sleep
Desyrel
DET
dipyridamole echocardiography test

detachable embolization coil
detachment velocity
detection
d. algorithm
atrial fibrillation d.
automated border d. (ABD)
automated edge d.
automatic boundary d. (ABD)
coincidence d.
echocardiographic automated border d.
edge d.
d. enhancement
manual edge d.
microarousal d.
molecular coincidence d. (MCD)
shunt d.
single-photon d.

detective quantum efficiency
detector
ambulatory nuclear d.
Cardioscint ambulatory vest d.
Cardioscint nuclear d.
colorimetric d.
C-Vest ambulatory radionuclide d.
Doppler blood flow d.
multihead d.
TubeChek esophageal intubation d.
VEST ambulatory nuclear d.
VEST left ventricular function d.

detect time
Detensol
detergent worker's lung
deterioration
d. following improvement (DFI)
structural valve d. (SVD)

Determann syndrome

D

NOTES

determination
 acid-base d.
 metabolic parameter d.
detrusor-sphincter dyssynergia
Detsky
 D. modified risk index
 D. score
detumescence
Detussin liquid
deuterosome
devascularization
DeVega tricuspid valve annuloplasty
Devereux formula
Devereux-Reichek method
deviation
 abnormal left axis d. (ALAD)
 abnormal right axis d. (ARAD)
 axis d.
 left axis d. (LAD)
 right axis d. (RAD)
 ST d.
 standard d.
 ST-T d.
 tracheal d.
device
 abdominal aortic counterpulsation d. (AACD)
 abdominal left ventricular assist d. (ALVAD)
 Abiomed implantable heart-replacement d.
 ablative d.
 Ablatr temperature control d.
 acapella chest physical therapy d.
 Accutorr oscillometric d.
 Accutracker blood pressure d.
 Acorn CorCap cardiac support d.
 ACS anchor exchange d.
 acute ventricular assist d. (AVAD)
 Adams-DeWeese d.
 advanced venous access d.
 AeroChamber spacing d.
 Aerosomes drug delivery d.
 AERx drug delivery d.
 A.M.E. tongue retaining d.
 A-mode echo-tracking d.
 Amplatz thrombectomy d. (ATD)
 Amplatz ventricular septal defect d.
 Anaconda d.
 Angioguard catheter d.
 Angio-Seal hemostatic puncture closure d.
 Angio-Seal vascular closure d.
 Aquatherm radiant heat d.
 arachnophlebectomy surgical d.
 arrhythmia control d. (ACD)
 Arrow-Clarke thoracentesis d.
 Arrow LionHeart left ventricular assist d.

ASD closure d.
ATL UltraMark 7 echocardiographic d.
Atrioverter implantable defibrillator d.
AutoAdjust CPAP d.
automatic d.
AutoSet CS d.
AutoSet Portable II diagnosis and therapy d.
autotitration d.
AVA 3Xi advanced venous access d.
Babyhaler spacer d.
Baladi Inverter d.
balloon catheter sealing d.
Baxter Health Care Continu-Flo infusion d.
B&B Trachguard antidisconnection d.
bilevel positive pressure d.
biventricular assist d. (BVAD, BIVAD)
blood flow enhancement d.
Breas PV10 CPAP d.
buttoned d.
BVM d.
Caire Sprint portable liquid oxygen d.
Caire Stroller portable liquid oxygen d.
Carbomedics valve d.
cardiac automatic resuscitative d. (CARD)
cardiac stretch d.
Cardiomemo d.
Cath-Lok catheter locking d.
centrifugal left and right ventricular assist d.
Chemo-Port perivena catheter system d.
Cholestron Pro II handheld d.
Chuter endovascular d.
Circulaire aerosol drug delivery d.
Circulaire inhaled medication delivery d.
CirKuit-Guard d.
Clamshell II d.
clearance assistive d.
closed-loop d.
Clot Buster Amplatz thrombectomy d.
Colapinto compression d.
CPI Mini d.
Crit-Scan noninvasive hematocrit measurement d.
cutting balloon d.
CVIS imaging d.

DeBakey-NASA axial-flow ventricular-assist d.
debulking d.
dental antisnoring d.
Digiflator digital inflation d.
Digitrapper MkIII reflux testing d.
Dinamap automated blood pressure d.
directional atherectomy d.
displacement sensing d.
Doppler d.
double-disk ASD closure d.
double-umbrella d.
DPAP Stealth d.
Duett arterial closure d.
Duett vascular sealing d.
Durathane cardiac d.
El Gamal cardiac d.
emergency infusion d. (EID)
Enclose anastomosis assist d.
Enclose proximal anastomotic assist d.
Encore inflation d.
Endo Grasp d.
Equinox EEG acquisition d.
esophageal detection d. (EDD)
Everest disposable inflation d.
extended collection d.
extraction atherectomy d.
ExtreSafe phlebotomy d.
EZ Hold manual compression d.
FemoStop inflatable pneumatic compression d.
fiberoptic delivery d.
Finesse cardiac d.
finger photoplethysmographic d.
Flutter mucus clearance d.
ForeRunner automatic external defibrillator d.
Gianturco-Grifka vascular occlusion d.
GlideCath torque d.
Goetz cardiac d.
Goodale-Lubin cardiac d.
grip torque d.
Guidant-CPI d.
heart-assist d.
HeartMate implantable ventricular assist d.
Hemoband hemostasis d.
hemostatic occlusive leverage d. (HOLD)

hemostatic puncture closure d. (HPCD)
Horizon CPAP d.
HSRA d.
ICD-ATP d.
Imed infusion d.
ImPulse electronic oxygen conserving d.
In-Exsufflator respiratory d.
InfaMyst aerosol spray d.
Infiltrator local drug delivery d.
InspirEase d.
Inspiron d.
Insuflon d.
InSync cardiac resynchronization d.
Interceptor wire distal protection d.
interrogation d.
intraaortic balloon d.
intracaval d.
inverted buttoned d.
I-STATE bedside blood testing d.
Jewel AF implantable arrhythmia management d.
Jewel atrial fibrillation dual chamber d.
Kendall sequential compression d.
King cardiac d.
King interlocking d.
lead locking D. (LDD)
left ventricular assist d. (LVAD)
Lehman cardiac d.
LifeStick CPR d.
LifeStick resuscitation d.
Light Talker d.
Linx guidewire extension cardiac d.
Lock Clamshell d.
locking d.
D.'s, Ltd. pacemaker
mandibular advancement d. (MAD)
MDILog therapy monitoring d.
mechanical ventricular assist d. (MVAD)
Medtronic Activa tremor control therapy d.
Medtronic defibrillator implant support d.
Medtronic external tachyarrhythmia control D.
Medtronic-Hall d.
Medtronic-Hancock d.
Medtronic Hemopump cardiac assist d.

D

NOTES

device *(continued)*

Medtronic Inspire implantable d.
Medtronic Jewel AF implantable arrhythmia management d.
Medtronic Jewel 7219D and C d.
Medtronic Octopus tissue stabilizing d.
microarousal scoring d.
MicroDigitrapper-S apnea screening d.
MicroMed DeBakey ventricular assist d.
Miltner constraint compliance d.
21 Mini d.
26 Mini II d.
Monarch 25 inflation d.
motorized transducer pullback d.
mucus clearance d.
Mullins cardiac d.
Myocor Coapsys pacing assist d.
Needle-Pro needle protection d.
Nit-Occlud d.
nonthoracotomy system antitachycardia d. (NTS-AICD)
Novacor Diasys cardiac d.
Novacor left ventricular assist d.
O2 Advantage oxygen conserving d.
Octopus tissue stabilizing d.
Olcott torque d.
OxiMax pulse oximetry d.
Pavcnik Monodisk d.
Perclose vascular closure d.
percutaneous thrombolytic d. (PTD)
percutaneous ventricular assist d.
PerDUCER percutaneous pericardial access d.
personal heart d. (PHD)
PET balloon atherectomy d.
phased array ultrasonographic d.
Philips Integris 3000 biplane digital subtraction angiography d.
PhotoDerm VL d.
Pierce-Donachy Thoratec ventricular assist d.
Pleur-evac d.
PlexiPulse compression d.
pneumatic peripheral circulation improvement d. (PPCID)
POCT d.
point-of-care testing d.
portable aerosol delivery d.
portable monitoring d.
Port-A-Cath d.
PPCID sequential foot compression d.
Prima total occlusion d.
Pro/Pel coating cardiac d.

Prostar Plus percutaneous vascular surgical d.
Prostar XL hemostatic puncture closure d.
pullback atherectomy d.
pulsatile assist d. (PAD)
pulse oximetry d.
QuicKlamp hemostasis d.
radiant heat d. (RHD)
Rashkind double umbrella d.
rate-adaptive d.
Respiradyne pulmonary function d.
Res-Q arrhythmia control d.
right ventricular assist d. (RVAD)
RotaLink rotational atherectomy d.
rotary atherectomy d.
rotational atherectomy d.
Sarns ventricular assist d.
Selute Picotip steroid-eluting d.
Sentinel ICD d.
sequential compression d. (SCD)
Servo Screen 390 ventilator monitoring d.
Sideris adjustable buttoned d.
Silent Night diagnostic and screening d.
SmartFlow multiple lesion d.
snare d.
Softclix lancet d.
SomaSensor d.
Spider embolic protection d.
STARFlex d.
stent-anchoring d.
St. Jude cardiac d.
subcutaneous tunneling d.
Sub-Q-Set subcutaneous continuous infusion d.
SuperStitch d.
Surveyor recording d.
Symbion cardiac d.
Tandem cardiac d.
Taperseal hemostatic d.
TEC atherectomy d.
Techstar d.
Telectronics Guardian ATP 4210 d.
d. therapy
Thermedics cardiac d.
Thermocardiosystems left ventricular assist d.
Thoratec biventricular assist d.
Thoratec cardiac d.
Thoratec right ventricular assist d.
Threshold PEP d.
tiered-therapy antiarrhythmic d.
tongue-retaining d.
Trak Back pullback d.
Tranquility Bilevel airway patency maintenance d.

Tranquility Bilevel positive airway
 pressure therapy d.
Tranquility Quest CPAP d.
transcatheter d.
transvenous d.
Trapper catheter exchange d.
Turboaire Challenger cold-air
 bronchial provocation d.
Unilink anastomotic d.
Valleylab Force 2 electrosurgical d.
Vanguard d.
Vascugel d.
vascular hemostatic d. (VHD)
vascular sealing d.
VasoSeal vascular hemostasis d.
VasoView balloon dissection d.
venous access d. (VAD)
ventricular assist d. (VAD)
Venture demand oxygen delivery d.
Veriflex cardiac d.
Viringe vascular access flush d.
Voyager Aortic IntraClusion d.
wearable cardioverter-defibrillator d.
Wizard disposable inflation d.
Zipper antidisconnect d.

DeVilbiss
 D. nebulizer
 D. Pulmo-Aide LT compressor
devil's grip
Dew sign
Dexacort Phosphate in Respihaler
dexamethasone
 d. sodium phosphate (DSP)
 d. suppression test
 d. systemic
Dexasone L.A.
dexchlorpheniramine maleate
dexfenfluramine (dFEN)
dexiocardia (*var. of* dextrocardia)
dexmedetomidine HCl
Dexone LA
Dexon Plus suture
dexrazoxane
dexter
 bronchus principalis d.
 cor triatriatum d.
 lobus d.
 pulmo d.
Dexter-Grossman classification
dextra
 arteria pulmonalis d.
 valvula semilunaris d.

vena pulmonalis inferior d.
vena pulmonalis superior d.
dextrae
 ramus lobi medii arteriae
  pulmonalis d.
dextran
 d. 1, 70
 high molecular weight d.
 low-molecular weight d. (LMD)
 d. solution
 d. sulfate
dextri
 fissura horizontalis pulmonis d.
 foramen venarum minimarum
  atria d.
 lobus azygos pulmonis d.
 lobus medius pulmonis d.
 pars intralobaris intersegmentalis
  venae posterioris lobi superioris
  pulmonis d.
dextroamphetamine
 d. sulfate
 d. toxicity
dextrocardia, dexiocardia
 corrected d.
 false d.
 isolated d.
 mirror-image d.
 pulmonary hypoplasia, hypoplasia
  of pulmonary artery, agonadism,
  omphalocele/diaphragmatic
  defect, d. (PAGOD)
 secondary d.
 type 1-4 d.
 d. with situs inversus
dextrocardiogram
dextrogastria
dextrogram
dextro isomer
dextromethorphan (DM)
 acetaminophen and d.
 carbinoxamine, pseudoephedrine,
  and d.
 chlorpheniramine, phenylephrine,
  and d.
 chlorpheniramine,
  phenylpropanolamine, and d.
 guaifenesin and d.
 guaifenesin, phenylpropanolamine,
  and d.
 guaifenesin, pseudoephedrine,
  and d.

NOTES

D

dextromethorphan (continued)
    promethazine and d.
    pseudoephedrine and d.
dextroposed transposition of great arteries
dextropositioned aorta
dextroposition of heart
dextropropoxyphene
dextrorotation
dextrorphan
dextrose 5% in water (D5W, D-5-W, D$_5$W)
Dextrostat
Dextrostix
dextrothyroxine sodium
dextrotransposition
dextroversion of heart
dextrum
    atrium d.
    cor triatriatum d.
Dey-Dose Metaproterenol
Dey-Lute Isoetharine
DF
    defibrillation
DFA
    direct fluorescent antibody
dFEN
    dexfenfluramine
D, F, H, M gate
DFI
    deterioration following improvement
DFIB
    defibrillation
D/Flex filter
DFP
    diastolic filling period
    diastolic filling pressure
DFT
    defibrillation threshold
3DFT
    three-dimensional Fourier transform
DG
    diastolic gallop
    DiGeorge anomaly
    DiGeorge syndrome
    diglyceride
DGA
    DiGeorge anomaly
DGAVP
    desglycinamide-9-arginine-8-vasopressin
DGCR
    DiGeorge chromosome region
    DiGeorge critical region
DGS
    DiGeorge sequence
    DiGeorge syndrome
DGSCR
    DiGeorge syndrome critical region

DG/VCF
    DiGeorge/velocardiofacial
    DG/VCF syndrome
DH
    dynamic hyperinflation
    Codiclear DH
    Decohistine DH
    Dihistine DH
DHBP
    direct His bundle pacing
DHC
    dehydrocholesterol
DHCA
    deep hypothermia circulatory arrest
D.H.E. 45 injection
DHPLC
    denaturing high performance liquid chromatography
DiaBeta
diabetes
    hypertension in d. (HID)
    d. mellitus (DM)
diabetic
    d. autonomic neuropathy (DAN)
    d. cardiomyopathy
    d. coma
    d. diet
    d. gangrene
    d. nephropathy
    d. neuropathy
    d. phthisis
    d. retinopathy
    D. Tussin DM
    D. Tussin EX
    d. ulcer
diabeticorum
    necrobiosis lipoidica d.
Diabinese
diable
    bruit de d.
diacetate
    triamcinolone d.
diacylglycerate pathway
diacylglycerol lipase
diagnosis, pl. **diagnoses (Dx)**
    airway breathing, circulation, differential d.
    airway, breathing, circulation, differential d.
    preimplantation d. (PID)
diagnostic
    d. aspiration
    d. bronchoscopy
    d. catheterization (dx cath)
    computer-assisted d. (CAD)
    d. HRCT
    d. peritoneal lavage (DPL)

sleep d.
d. ultrasound imaging catheter
diagnostic-related group (DRG)
diagonal
d. coronary artery
left anterior descending d. (LADD)
diagram
Dieuaide d.
ladder d.
pressure-volume d.
Dialog pacemaker
dialysis
continuous cyclical peritoneal d.
(CCPD)
peritoneal d.
renal d.
dialyzer
Terumo d.
diameter
aerodynamic mass d. (AD)
anteroposterior thoracic d.
count median d. (CMD)
count median aerodynamic d.
(CMAD)
end-diastolic d. (EDD)
geometric mean d. (GMD)
D. Index Safety System (DISS)
internal d.
left atrial d.
left ventricular end-diastolic d.
(LVEDD)
left ventricular internal diastolic d.
(LVIDD)
luminal d.
LV end-diastolic d.
mass median aerodynamic d.
(MMAD)
mean luminal d. (MLD)
mean reference d. (MRD)
minimal luminal d. (MLD)
minimum lumen d. (MLD)
outer d. (OD)
reference vessel d. (RVD)
relative vessel d. (RVD)
right atrium d. (RAD)
right ventricular end-diastolic d.
(RVEDD)
d. stenosis (DS)
stretched d.
total end-diastolic d. (TEDD)
total end-systolic d. (TESD)

transverse cardiac d. (TCD)
transverse heart d. (THD)
diamine oxidase (DO)
diaminobenzidine tetrahydrochloride
Diamond classification
diamond-coated bur
Diamond-Forrester table
Diamond-Lite titanium instrument
diamond-shaped
d.-s. ejection murmur
d.-s. tracing
Diamox
diaphanoscopy
diaphoresis
diaphragm
central tendon of d.
costal part of d.
crural d.
dome of d.
eventrated d.
eventration of d.
left crus of d.
lumbar part of d.
d. phenomenon
right crus of d.
d. of stent
sternal part of d.
d. transducer
vertebral part of d.
diaphragma
musculus d.
diaphragmalgia
diaphragmatic
d. artery
d. dysfunction
d. excursion
d. fatigue resistance
d. flutter
d. hernia
d. myocardial infarction (DMI)
d. pacing
d. paralysis
d. pericardium
d. phenomenon
d. pleura
d. pleurisy
d. respiration
d. rupture
d. surface
d. surface of heart

D

NOTES

diaphragmatica
    facies d.
    pleura d.
diaphragmatis
    centrum tendineum d.
    crus dextrum d.
    crus sinistrum d.
    pars costalis d.
    pars lumbalis d.
Diaqua
diary
    event d.
    Holter d.
    sleep d.
DiaryCard
    MicroMedical D.
diaschisis
    crossed cerebellar d. (CCD)
Diasonics transducer
diaspirin cross-linked hemoglobin (DCLHb)
diastasis cordis
diastatic
Diastat vascular access graft
diastema
diaster
diastole (D)
    atrial d.
    cardiac d.
    electrical d.
    late d.
    ventricular d.
diastolic
    d. afterpotential
    d. amplitude time index (DATI)
    d. aortic pressure (DAP)
    d. blood pressure (DBP)
    d. blow
    d. bulging
    d. closing velocity
    d. current
    d. current of injury
    d. decrescendo murmur
    d. depolarization
    d. descent rate (DDR)
    d. doming
    d. filling
    d. filling pattern
    d. filling period (DFP)
    d. filling pressure (DFP)
    d. fluttering
    d. fluttering aortic valve
    d. function
    d. gallop (DG)
    d. gradient
    d. grunt
    d. heart disease
    d. heart failure
    d. hump

    d. hypertension
    d. motion
    d. murmur (DM, DS)
    d. overload
    d. potential (Vdia)
    d. pressure (DP, Pd)
    d. pressure-flow relationship (DPFR)
    d. pressure-time index (DPTI)
    d. pressure-volume relation
    pulmonary artery d. (PAD)
    pulsed d. (PD)
    d. relaxation
    d. reserve
    d. rumble
    d. shock
    d. slope
    d. stiffness
    d. suction
    d. thrill
    d. upstroke
    d. velocity integral (DVI)
    d. ventricular dysfunction
diastology
diathermy
diathesis, pl. **diatheses**
    allergic d.
    bleeding d.
diatrizoate
    sodium meglumine d.
diazepam
diazine
diazoxide
Dibenzyline
DIC
    diffuse intravascular coagulation
    disseminated intravascular coagulation
    disseminated intravascular coagulopathy
dichloroacetate (DCA)
    sodium d.
dichloroisoprenaline
dichloroisoproterenol
dichlorphenamide
dichotomization
dichotomy
diclofenac
dicloxacillin sodium
DICOM
    digital imaging and communications in medicine
    DICOM acquisition station
dicrotic
    d. notch (DN)
    d. pulse
    d. wave
dicrotism
dicumarol
dicumyl peroxide
didanosine (ddI)

didehydrodideoxythymidine
dideoxycytidine (ddC)
dideoxyinosine
dideoxynucleoside
dielectrography
diesel exhaust
diet
> AHA type I d.
> American Heart Association type
>   I d.
> Atkins d.
> betaine d.
> bland d.
> calorie-restricted d.
> cardiac d.
> diabetic d.
> high-fiber d.
> Karell d.
> Kempner d.
> LFC d.
> low-fat d.
> low-methionine d.
> low-salt d.
> low-sodium d.
> Mediterranean d.
> NCEP Step-One d.
> Ornish d.
> Portagen d.
> prudent d.
> renal d.
> salt-free d.
> Sauerbruch-Herrmannsdorfer-
>   Gerson d.
> South Beach d.
> Step-One D.
> Step-Two D.
> d. and stress management in
>   angina (DSMA)
> vegetarian d.
> very low-calorie d. (VLCD)

dietary
> d. approaches to stop hypertension
>   (DASH)
> d. fat
> d. fiber
> d. prevention of recurrent
>   myocardial infarction (DPR)
> d. salt
> d. sodium

Dieterle stain
diethylcarbamazine citrate

diethylenetriamine
> d. pentaacetate (DTPA)
> d. pentaacetate aerosol inhalation
>   lung scintigraphy
> d. pentaacetic acid (DPTA, DTPA)

diethylstilbestrol (DES)
Dieuaide
> D. diagram
> D. sign

difference
> alveolar-arterial PO_2 d. ($AaPO_2$)
> arterial-venous oxygen content d.
> arteriovenous oxygen d. (AVD O_2)
> nasal potential d.
> pulmonary A-V O_2 d.

differens
> pulsus d.

differential
> d. blood count
> d. blood pressure
> d. bronchospirometry
> d. pressure transducer
> d. stethoscope

differentiated ECG (DECG)
differentiation
> echocardiographic d.
> pressure pulse d.

difficulty
> rating of perceived breathing d.
>   (RPBD)

Diff-Quik stain
diffuse
> d. airways disease
> d. alveolar damage (DAD)
> d. alveolar hemorrhage (DAH)
> d. arterial ectasia
> d. bronchopneumonia
> d. cutaneous scleroderma
> d. emphysema
> d. esophageal spasm (DES)
> d. infiltrative lung disease (DILD)
> d. in-stent restenosis
> d. interstitial infiltrate
> d. interstitial lung disease (DILD)
> d. interstitial pulmonary fibrosis
> d. intimal thickening
> d. intravascular coagulation (DIC)
> d. intraventricular block
> d. lung injury
> d. malignant pleural mesothelioma
>   (DMPM)

D

NOTES

diffuse *(continued)*
    d. obstructive pulmonary syndrome (DOPS)
    d. panbronchiolitis (DPB)
    d. parenchymal disease
    d. paroxysmal slowing
    d. pleurisy
    d. pulmonary lymphangiomatosis
    d. sclerosing alveolitis
    d. vasospasm

diffusing
    d. capacity
    d. capacity of lung for carbon monoxide (DLCO)

diffusion
    d. anoxia
    d. capacity
    centripetal d.
    coefficient of d.
    d. hypoxia
    lung d.
    d. MRI
    d. respiration
    single-breath d.
    d. tensor imaging (DTI)

diffusion-weighted
    d.-w. imaging (DWI)
    d.-w. MRI

diffusometry
    NMR d.

diffusum
    angiokeratoma corporis d.

Diflucan
    D. injection
    D. Oral

diflunisal

diftitox
    denileukin d.

DIG
    Digitalis Investigation Group
    Digoxin Investigators Group

dig
    digitalis
    digoxigenin
    digoxin
    dig level

DiGeorge
    D. anomaly (DG, DGA)
    D. chromosome region (DGCR)
    D. critical region (DGCR)
    D. sequence (DGS)
    D. syndrome (DG, DGS)
    D. syndrome critical region (DGSCR)

DiGeorge/velocardiofacial (DG/VCF)
digestive system vascular disease
Digibind
    D. digoxin immune Fab fragments
    D. pneumatonometer

Digidote digoxin immune Fab fragments
Digiflator digital inflation device
digital
    d. angiography (DA)
    d. averaging
    d. calipers
    d. cardiac imaging (DCI)
    D. Cardiac Imaging system
    d. clubbing
    d. color Doppler velocity integration method
    d. color Doppler velocity profile integration
    d. computer
    d. echo quantification (DEQ)
    d. endarteropathy
    d. fluoroscopic unit
    d. imaging and communications in medicine (DICOM)
    d. interchange standards for cardiology (DISC)
    d. necrosis
    d. phase mapping (DPM)
    d. pulse plethysmography (DPP)
    d. radiography
    d. runoff
    d. smoothing
    d. subtraction
    d. subtraction angiography (DSA)
    d. subtraction arteriography
    d. subtraction echocardiography (DSE)
    d. subtraction imaging
    d. subtraction supravalvular aortogram
    d. subtraction supravalvular aortography
    d. subtraction technique
    d. vascular imaging (DVI)
    d. vascular imaging system (DVIS)
    d. vascular reactivity (DVR)
    d. videoangiography

digitalate pulse
Digitaline
Digitalis
    D. lanata
    D. purpurea
digitalis (dig)
    d. effect
    d. glycoside
    d. intoxication
    D. Investigation Group (DIG)
    d. sensitivity
    d. toxicity

digitalis-specific antibody
digitalization
digitalize
Digitek
digitization

digitized caliper method
digitizer
    Bitpad d.
digitizing pad
digitoxicity
digitoxin
Digitrapper
    D. MkIII reflux testing device
    D. MkIII sleep monitor
digit span memory test
diglyceride (DG)
digoxigenin (dig)
digoxigenin-labeled DNA probe
digoxin (dig, DO)
    d. effect
    d. immune Fab
    D. Investigators Group (DIG)
    d. level
    d. reduction product (DRP)
    D. RIA Bead
    d. toxicity
digoxin-induced hyperkalemia (DIH)
digoxin-like immunoreactive substance (DLIS)
digoxin-specific Fab
DIH
    digoxin-induced hyperkalemia
Dihistine
    D. DH
    D. Expectorant
dihydralazine
dihydrochloride
    azimilide d.
dihydrocodeine
dihydroergotamine mesylate
dihydropyridine calcium antagonist
dihydroxyphenylalanine
dihydroxypropyltheophylline
diisocyanate
    d. asthma
    methylene diphenyl d. (MDI)
    toluene d. (TDI)
Dilaca catheter
Dilacor XR
Dilantin
dilatable lesion
dilatancy
dilatation
    percutaneous transluminal d. (PTD)
    percutaneous transluminal balloon d. (PTBD)
    venous d. (VC)

dilated
    d. cardiomyopathy (DCM)
    d. cardiomyopathy and atrial fibrillation (DCAF)
    d. coronaropathy
dilation, dilatation
    aneurysmal d.
    anular d.
    balloon d.
    bootstrap d.
    cardiac d.
    catheter d.
    chamber d.
    endothelial-dependent arterial d.
    esophageal d.
    finger d.
    flow-mediated d. (FMD)
    d. of heart
    idiopathic right atrial d.
    intrapulmonary vascular d.
    left ventricular cavity d.
    lymphatic d.
    nitroglycerin-induced d.
    onion bulb d.
    oscillating d.
    portal vein d. (PVD)
    poststenosis d. (PSD)
    poststenotic d.
    reactive d.
    sequential d.
    serial d.
    d. thrombosis
    transient ischemic d. (TID)
    ventricular d.
dilator
    Achiever balloon d.
    Amplatz d.
    Bakes d.
    Brown-McHardy pneumatic d.
    Cooley d.
    Delaborde tracheal d.
    Derra valve d.
    Einhorn esophageal d.
    Garrett d.
    GlideCath d.
    Maloney mercury-filled esophageal d.
    mitral valve d.
    Mullins d.
    Nozovent nasal-valve d.
    Quantum TTC balloon d.
    Savary-Gilliard esophageal d.

D

NOTES

dilator *(continued)*
    d. and sheath technique
    Tubbs d.
    ventricular d. (VD)
    vessel d.
dilator-sheath system
Dilatrate-SR
DILD
    diffuse infiltrative lung disease
    diffuse interstitial lung disease
DILE
    drug-induced lupus erythematosus
dilevalol
Dilor
Diltia XT
diltiazem
    enalapril and d.
    d. HCl extended-release tablet
    d. hydrochloride
dilute blood clot lysis (DBCL)
dilution
    gas d.
    helium d.
    transpulmonary thermal-dye d.
    (TDD)
Dimacol Caplets
dimenhydrinate
dimension
    anteroposterior d.
    aortic root d.
    effective airspace d. (EAD)
    end-diastolic d. (EDD)
    end-systolic d. (ESD)
    left atrial d.
    left ventricular d. (LVDI)
    left ventricular end-diastolic d.
    (LVEDD)
    left ventricular end-systolic d.
    (LVESD)
    left ventricular internal d. (LVID)
    left ventricular internal diastolic d.
    (LVIDD)
    left ventricular systolic d. (LVSD)
    maximum transverse thoracic d.
    right ventricular d. (RVD)
    right ventricular internal d. (RVID)
dimensionality in imaging
3-dimensional MSPECT software
dimer
    excited d.'s
Dimetapp Sinus Caplets
dimethyl
    d. hydrazine
    d. sulfate
    d. sulfoxide
dimethylarginine
    asymmetric d. (ADMA)
    symmetric d.
1,1-dimethylbiguanide

dimethyl-L-arginine
dimorphism
dimple
    blind coronary d.
    coronary ostial d.
Dinamap
    D. Accutorr A1, A3 blood
    pressure monitor
    D. automated blood pressure device
    D. blood pressure cuff
    D. pulse oximeter
    D. system
    D. ultrasound blood pressure
    manometer
dinitrate
    isosorbide d. (ISDN)
dinitrile
    pyridazinone d.
dinucleotide
    nicotinamide adenine d. (NAD)
diode
    light-emitting d. (LED)
    Zener d.
Diomycin
Diovan HCT
dioxide
    carbon d. (CO_2)
    chlorine d.
    end-tidal carbon d. ($ETCO_2$)
    fraction of expired carbon d.
    ($FECO_2$)
    fraction of inspired carbon d.
    ($FICO_2$)
    nitrogen d. (NO_2)
    partial pressure of carbon d.
    (PCO_2)
    selenium d.
    sulfur d. (SO_2)
DIP
    desquamative interstitial pneumonia
    desquamative interstitial pneumonitis
dip
    a d.
    Cournand d.
    midsystolic d.
    d. phenomenon
    septal d.
    type I, II d.
dipalmitoyl
    d. phosphatidylcholine (DPPC)
    d. phosphatidylcholine test
dip-and-plateau pattern
diphasic
    d. complex
    d. P, T wave
Diphen Cough
Diphenhist
diphenhydramine (DPHM)
    d. hydrochloride

diphenylhydantoin
diphosphate
    adenosine d. (ADP)
    histamine d.
5′-diphosphate
2,3-diphosphoglycerate
diphosphonate
    methylene d. (MDP)
    technetium-99m methylene d.
diphtheria
    d. antitoxin
    d. and tetanus toxoid
    d., tetanus toxoids, and acellular
      pertussis vaccine
    d., tetanus toxoids, and whole-cell
      pertussis vaccine
    d., tetanus toxoids, and whole-cell
      pertussis vaccine and *Haemophilus*
      type b conjugate vaccine
diphtheriae
    Corynebacterium d.
diphtherial tonsillitis
diphtheric
    d. paralysis
    d. pharyngitis
diphtherin
diphtheritic
    d. croup
    d. laryngitis
    d. myocarditis
    d. paralysis
    d. pharyngitis
diphtheroid
diplegia
    facial d.
diplocardia
diplococci
Diplococcus pneumoniae
dipole theory
dipper pattern
Diprivan injection
dipropionate
    beclomethasone d.
Dipy
    dipyridamole
dipyridamole (D, Dipy)
    d. and aspirin
    aspirin/extended release d.
    d. echocardiography test (DET)
    d. handgrip test
    d. stress
    d. stress echocardiography

    d. thallium-201 scan
    d. thallium-201 scintigraphy
    d. thallium stress test
dipyridamole-thallium imaging (DTI)
dipyrine
direct
    d. acute myocardial infarction
      angioplasty (DAMIA)
    d. amplification test (DAT)
    d. cardiac compression (DCC)
    d. cardiac massage
    d. cardiac puncture
    d. coronary angioplasty
    d. current (DC)
    d. current cardioversion (DCCV)
    d. current electric shock
    d. embolism
    d. excitation
    d. fluorescent antibody (DFA)
    d. Fourier transformation imaging
    d. His bundle pacing (DHBP)
    d. immunofluorescent stain
    d. insertion technique
    d. laryngoscopy
    d. lead
    d. mapping sequence
    d. mechanical ventricular actuation
      (DMVA)
    d. murmur
    d. myocardial revascularization
      (DMR)
    d. percutaneous coronary
      intervention (d-PCI)
    d. respiration
    d. sinoatrial conduction time
      (DSACT, D-SACT)
    d. stenting of coronary artery
      (DISCO)
    d. stimulation
    d. thrombin inhibitor
direct-current shock ablation
directed cough
directional
    d. atherectomy
    d. atherectomy catheter
    d. atherectomy debulking technique
    d. atherectomy device
    d. color angiography (DCA)
    d. coronary angioplasty (DCA)
directly
    d. observed therapy (DOT)
    d. observed treatment (DOT)

D

NOTES

dirithromycin
Dirofilaria immitis
dirofilariasis
dirty
    d. chest
    d. film
    d. lung
    d. necrosis
dirty-lung appearance
Dirythmin
disability
    cardiovascular d.
Disalcid
disappearance slope
disarray
    myocardial d.
    myofibrillar d.
disarticulation
    Burger technique for
      scapulothoracic d.
    chondral d.
    chondrocostal d.
DISA-SPECT
    dual-isotope simultaneous acquisition
    single-photon emission computed
    tomography
DISC
    digital interchange standards for
    cardiology
disc (*var. of* disk)
discharge
    electric defibrillator using DC d.
    (DC)
    systolic d. (SD)
discission of pleura
DISCO
    direct stenting of coronary artery
discoid
disconnect
    airway pressure d. (APD)
discontinuity
    atrial-axis d.
discontinuous incremental threshold
  loading
discordance
    atrioventricular d.
    ventriculoarterial d.
discordant
    d. alternans
    d. alternation
    d. atrioventricular connection
    d. changes electrocardiogram
    d. ventriculoarterial connection
discovery
    D. DDDR pacemaker
    D. handheld spirometer
discrete
    d. coronary lesion
    d. subaortic stenosis (DSAS, DSS)

    d. subvalvular aortic stenosis
    (DSAS)
disease (D)
    Acosta d.
    acquired valvular heart d. (AVHD)
    acromegalic heart d.
    acute cardiovascular d. (ACVD)
    acute exacerbation of chronic
      obstructive pulmonary d.
    acute heart d. (AHD)
    ACV d.
    acyanotic heart d.
    Adams d.
    Adams-Stokes d.
    Addison d.
    airspace d.
    alcoholic heart muscle d.
    amyloid heart d.
    Anderson-Fabry d.
    antiglomerular basement
      membrane d.
    aortic aneurysmal d.
    aortic thromboembolic d.
    aortic valve d.
    aortic valvular d. (AVD)
    aortoiliac obstructive d. (AIOD)
    aortoiliac occlusive d.
    apple picker's d.
    arrhythmogenic right ventricular d.
    arterial occlusive d. (AOD)
    arteriosclerotic cardiovascular d.
    (ASCVD)
    arteriosclerotic heart d. (AHD,
    ASHD)
    arteriosclerotic occlusive d. (AOD)
    arteriosclerotic peripheral
      vascular d. (ASPVD)
    arteriosclerotic vascular d. (ASVD)
    AS d.
    aspiration-induced respiratory d.
    asymptomatic coronary artery d.
    (ACAD)
    atherosclerotic aortic d.
    atherosclerotic cardiovascular d.
    (ACVD, ASCVD)
    atherosclerotic carotid artery d.
    atherosclerotic coronary artery d.
    (ACAD, ASCAD)
    atherosclerotic heart d. (AHD)
    atherosclerotic hypertensive
      cardiovascular d. (ASHCVD)
    atherosclerotic peripheral vascular d.
    (ASPVD)
    atherothrombotic cardiovascular d.
    atrioseptal heart d. (ASHD)
    autoimmune thyroid d. (AITD)
    autosomal-dominant familial aortic
      aneurysm d.
    aviator's d.

axial interstitial d.
Ayerza d.
Bamberger-Marie d.
Bannister d.
barometer-maker's d.
Battey d.
Bazin d.
Beau d.
Becker d.
Behçet d.
beryllium-induced lung d.
Besnier-Boeck-Schaumann d.
bilateral aortoostial coronary
  artery d.
biliary d.
Binswanger d.
blackfoot d.
black lung d.
blue d.
Boeck d.
Bornholm d.
Bostock d.
Bouillaud d.
Bouveret d.
Bright d.
Brill-Zinsser d.
Buerger d.
bullous lung d.
Bürger-Grütz d.
Buschke d.
Busse-Buschke d.
caisson d.
California d.
carcinoid heart d.
carcinoid valve d.
cardiac d. (CD)
cardiac allograft vascular d.
  (CAVD)
cardiovascular d. (C, CD, CVD)
cardiovascular-renal d. (CVRD)
carotid artery d.
carotid occlusive d.
carotid vascular d.
Carrington d.
Castellani d.
Castleman d.
cat-scratch d.
cavitary lung d.
Ceelen d.
Ceelen-Gellerstedt d.
celiac d.
centrilobular axial interstitial d.

cerebrovascular d. (CeVD)
Chagas heart d.
Charcot-Marie-Tooth d.
cheese worker's lung d.
cholesterol ester storage d. (CESD)
cholesteryl ester storage d.
Christmas d.
chronic beryllium d. (CBD)
chronic cerebrovascular d. (CCVD)
chronic graft vascular d. (CGVD)
chronic hypertensive d.
chronic inflammatory airway d.
chronic interstitial lung d.
chronic obstruction outflow d.
  (COOD)
chronic obstructive airways d.
chronic obstructive lung d. (COLD)
chronic obstructive pulmonary d.
  (COPD)
chronic obstructive respiratory d.
  (CORD)
chronic peripheral arterial d.
  (CPAD)
chronic restrictive pulmonary d.
  (CRPD)
chronic suppurative lung d.
  (CSLD)
chronic valvular heart d. (CVHD)
clinical cardiovascular d. (CCD)
cobalt-induced airway d.
cobalt-related lung d.
cold hemagglutinin d.
collagen vascular lung d.
Concato d.
congenital heart d. (CHD,
  CongHD)
congenital polyvalvular d. (CPVD)
congestive heart d. (CHD)
congestive pulmonary d.
constrictive heart d.
Cori d.
coronary arteriosclerotic heart d.
  (CAHD, CASHD)
coronary artery d. (CAD)
coronary artery occlusive d.
  (CAOD)
coronary heart d. (CHD)
coronary microvascular d.
coronary occlusive d.
Corrigan d.
Corvisart d.
Crocq d.

D

NOTES

disease *(continued)*

cryptococcal pulmonary d.
cyanotic congenital heart d.
cyanotic heart d. (CHD)
cytomegalic inclusion d.
Daae d.
Danon storage d.
Darling d.
Davies d.
Degos d.
diastolic heart d.
diffuse airways d.
diffuse infiltrative lung d. (DILD)
diffuse interstitial lung d. (DILD)
diffuse parenchymal d.
digestive system vascular d.
Döhle d.
DRFS risk factors in coronary
  heart d.
Duke Databank for
  Cardiovascular D.
Duroziez d.
dust d.
Ebstein d.
effusive-constrictive d.
Eisenmenger d.
electrical d.
elevator d.
Emery-Dreifuss d.
endomyocardial d.
end-stage liver d. (ESLD)
end-stage renal d. (ESRD)
environmental lung d.
eosinophilic endomyocardial d.
epicardial coronary artery d.
Epstein d.
Erb-Goldflam d.
Erdheim d.
estrogen replacement for women
  with coronary artery d. (EWA)
extracranial carotid d. (ECD)
extracranial carotid arterial d.
  (ECAD)
extracranial internal carotid d.
Fabry d.
Fahr d.
family history of heart d.
fibroplastic d.
fibroproliferative d.
fish-meal worker's lung d.
flax-dresser's d.
flint d.
Fothergill d.
Friedländer d.
Friedreich d.
functional cardiovascular d.
furrier's lung d.
Gairdner d.
gallbladder d.

gannister d.
gastroesophageal reflux d. (GERD)
Gaucher d.
giant bullous d.
Gilchrist d.
global cardiac d.
glycogen storage d. (I-VIII)
Goldflam d.
Goldflam-Erb d.
gonadal d.
graft coronary d. (GCD)
graft-versus-host d. (GVHD)
grain handler's d.
granulomatous d.
Graves d.
Hamman d.
hand-foot-and-mouth d.
Hand-Schüller-Christian d.
hard metal d.
heart d. (HD)
Heller-Döhle d.
hematologic d.
hepatic d.
Hodgkin d.
Hodgson d.
Horton d.
Huchard d.
humeroperoneal neuromuscular d.
Hutinel d.
hyaline membrane d.
hypereosinophilic heart d.
hypertension secondary to renal d.
  (HSRD)
hypertensive arteriosclerotic
  cardiovascular d. (HASCVD)
hypertensive arteriosclerotic heart d.
  (HASHD)
hypertensive cardiovascular d.
  (HCVD, HTCVD)
hypertensive heart d. (HHD,
  HTHD)
hypertensive pulmonary vascular d.
  (HPVD)
hypertensive vascular d. (HTVD,
  HVD)
iatrogenic d.
idiopathic venoocclusive d.
immune-mediated d.
inflammatory airway d.
inorganic dust d.
Inter-Society Commission for
  Heart d.'s (ICHD)
interstitial lung d. (ILD)
intracranial atherosclerotic d. (IAD)
intrastent recurrent d.
intraventricular conduction d.
  (IVCD)
intrinsic d.
iron storage d.

Isambert d.
ischemic coronary d. (ICD)
ischemic heart d. (IHD)
isolated cerebral thromboangiitis
 obliterans d.
Kawasaki d.
Kennedy d.
Keshan d.
Kienbock d.
Kikuchi d.
kinky-hair d.
Krishaber d.
Kugelberg-Welander d.
Kussmaul d.
Kussmaul-Maier d.
left main d. (LMD)
left main coronary d. (LMC)
left main coronary artery d.
 (LMCAD)
left main stem coronary artery d.
 (LMS-CAD)
Legionnaire d.
Lemierre d.
Lenègre d.
Letterer-Siwe d.
leukoencephalopathy d.
Lev d.
Lewis upper limb cardiovascular d.
Libman-Sacks d.
lipid-coronary artery d. (LCAD)
Little d.
Löffler d.
lower extremity arterial d. (LEAD)
Lucas-Championnière d.
luetic d.
lupus-associated valve d.
Lutz-Splendore-Almeida d.
Lyme d.
macrovascular artery d.
maple bark d.
Marek d.
McArdle d.
metastatic d.
microvascular artery d.
Mikity-Wilson d.
mitral d. (MD)
mitral valve d. (MVD)
mixed aortic valve d. (MAVD)
mixed mitral valve d. (MMVD)
Mondor d.
Monge d.
Morgagni d.

Morquio-Brailsford d.
Moschcowitz d.
moyamoya d.
multilobar d.
multivalve d.
multivalvular d.
multivessel d. (MVD)
multivessel coronary artery d.
mushroom worker's d.
mycobacterial d.
myocardial d. (MD)
myxomatous valve d.
nail-patella d.
Naxos d.
necrotizing arterial d.
neoplastic d.
neurodegenerative d.
neuromuscular d.
Niemann-Pick d.
nonsegmental d.
nosocomial d.
obliterative vascular d.
obstructive airway d. (OAD)
obstructive lung d. (OLD)
occlusive d.
occupational lung d.
oculocraniosomatic d.
organic heart d. (OHD)
Osler-Weber-Rendu d.
Owren d.
parenchymal d.
peribronchovascular d.
pericardial d.
peripartal heart d.
peripheral arterial d. (PAD)
peripheral arterial occlusive d.
 (PAOD)
peripheral arteriosclerotic
 occlusive d. (PAOD)
peripheral atherosclerotic d.
peripheral conduction d.
peripheral interstitial d.
peripheral vascular d. (PVD)
pigeon-breeder's d.
pleural d.
Plummer d.
pneumatic hammer d.
polycystic kidney d.
polysaccharide storage d.
Pompe d.
Posadas-Wernicke d.
primary electrical d.

D

NOTES

disease *(continued)*

primary myocardial d. (PMD)
primary pleuropulmonary d.
primary pulmonary parenchymal d.
progression of coronary artery d. (PCAD)
pseudoheart d. (PsHD)
pulmonary thromboembolic d. (PTED)
pulmonary valve d.
pulmonary vascular d. (PVD)
pulmonary vascular obstructive d. (PVOD)
pulmonary venoocclusive d. (PVOD)
pulseless d.
Purkinje d.
Quincke d.
radiation-induced heart d. (RIHD)
radiation lung d.
ragpicker's d.
ragsorter's d.
Raynaud d.
reactive airways d. (RAD)
recalcitrant obstructive airways d.
Refsum d.
Reiter d.
renal artery d.
renal parenchymal d.
Rendu-Osler-Weber d.
restrictive airways d.
restrictive heart d.
restrictive lung d.
reversible obstructive airways d. (ROAD)
rheumatic heart d. (RHD)
rheumatic valvular heart d. (RVHD)
Roger d.
Rokitansky d.
Rosai-Dorfman d.
Rougnon-Heberden d.
Roussy-Lévy d.
Sandhoff d.
San Joaquin Valley d.
Schaumann d.
Shaver d.
Shoshin d.
shuttlemaker's d.
sickle cell d.
silo-filler's d.
single-vessel d. (SVD)
sinus node d.
slim d.
Sly d.
small airways d.
Spatz-Lindenberg d. (SLD)
spirochetal d.

spontaneous coronary artery d. (SCAD, sCAD)
Steinert d.
stenotic valvular heart d.
stentable d.
Still d.
Stokes-Adams d.
structural heart d. (SHD)
subacute coronary d. (SCD)
sudden death heart d. (SDHD)
sudden death ischemic heart d. (SDIHD)
Sylvest d.
synchronous endobronchial d.
Takayasu d.
Takayasu-Onishi d.
Tangier d.
target organ disease/clinical cardiovascular d. (TOD/CCD)
Taussig-Bing d.
Tay-Sachs d.
Thomsen d.
three-vessel coronary d.
thromboembolic d. (TED)
thyrocardiac d.
thyroid d.
thyrotoxic heart d.
transplant coronary artery d. (TCAD, TxCAD)
traumatic heart d.
tricuspid valve d.
TWAR d.
type I-VIII glycogen storage d.
Uhl d.
unilocular hydatid d.
unstable coronary artery d. (UCAD)
valvular heart d. (VHD)
van den Bergh d.
Vaquez d.
vascular d. (VD)
vasospastic d.
venoocclusive d. (VOD)
vertebrobasilar occlusive d.
vibration d.
von Recklinghausen d.
von Willebrand d.
warfarin-aspirin symptomatic intracranial d. (WASID)
Weber-Christian d.
Weil d.
Wenckebach d.
Werlhof d.
wheat weevil d.
Whipple d.
Wilkie d.
Wilson d.
Wilson-Kimmelstiel d.
Winiwarter-Buerger d.

winter vomiting d.
Woillez d.
Wolman d.
wood pulp worker's lung d.
woven coronary artery d.
Yamaguchi d.

disinfectant
Control III Elite d.

disintegration rate

disk, disc
atrial d.
cervical d.
intervertebral d.
Molnar d.
open atrial d.
optic d.
d. oxygenation
d. oxygenator
d. spring

disk-cage valve

Diskhaler

Diskus
Advair D.
Flovent D.
D. inhaler
Serevent D.

dislodgment, dislodgement
lead d.

dismutase
Cu/Zn superoxide d.
manganese superoxide d. (Mn-SOD)
superoxide d.

disodium
adenosine triphosphate d.
cefotetan d.
d. cromoglycate (DSCG)
edetate d.
ticarcillin d.

disopyramide phosphate

disorder
acid-base d.
arrhythmogenic d.
autoimmune d.
clotting d.
conduction d.
decompression d.
dysbaric d.
endocrine d.
Fredrickson classification of lipid d.'s
genetic d.
glycosphingolipid d.

iatrogenic d.
International Classification of Sleep D.'s (ICSD)
lipid d.
lupus anticoagulant d.
lymphocytic infiltrative d.
mendelian d.
movement d.
neurological d.
neuromuscular d.
neuromyopathic d.
panic d.
periodic limb movement d. (PLMD)
posttransplantation lymphoproliferative d. (PTLPD, PTLD)
Sheffield Screening Test for Acquired Language D.'s (STALD)
single-gene d.

disordered action of heart (DAH)

disorganization
segmental arterial d.

Disotate

dispar
Entamoeba d.

Dispatch
D. balloon
D. infusion catheter
D. over-the-wire catheter

dispenser
PlugStation earplug d.

dispersing electrode

dispersion
aerosol bolus d. (AD)
interlead QT d.
QT d. (QTd)
QT interval d.
QT/QTc d.
d. of refractoriness
Taylor d.
temporal d.

dispersive electrode

displacement
d. sensing device
d. waveform

display
color kinesis echocardiographic d.
liquid crystal d. (LCD)
PerfTrak d.
PerfTrak perfusion waveform d.

D

NOTES

**disposable percutaneous entry thinwall
  needle**
Disprin
disrupted plaque
disruption
> bronchial d.
> circadian d.
> great vessel d.
> plaque d.
> traumatic aortic d.

DISS
> Diameter Index Safety System

dissecans
> pneumonia d.

dissected tissue
dissecting
> d. aorta
> d. aortic aneurysm
> d. hematoma

dissection
> acute aortic d. (AAD)
> d. of aorta
> aortic d. (type A, B)
> arterial d.
> BioGlue surgical adhesive for
>   aortic d.
> coronary artery d.
> DeBakey type I, II, III, IIIa, IIIb
>   aortic d.
> epiphenomena of d.
> International Registry of Acute
>   Aortic D. (IRAD)
> intraluminal d.
> long d.
> spiral d.
> spontaneous cervical artery d.
>   (sCAD)
> spontaneous coronary artery d.
>   (SCAD, sCAD)
> Stanford type A,B aortic d.
> therapeutic d.
> thoracic aortic d.
> type A, B aortic d.

dissector
> balloon d.
> Holinger d.
> SAPH Finder surgical balloon d.
> SAPHtrak balloon d.
> Spacemaker balloon d.

disseminated
> d. coccidioidomycosis
> d. cryptococcosis
> d. intravascular blood coagulation
>   (DIVBC)
> d. intravascular coagulation (DIC,
>   DIVC)
> d. intravascular coagulopathy (DIC)
> d. lupus erythematosus

> d. polyarteritis
> d. tuberculosis

dissemination
> hematogenous bacterial d.
> micronodular d.

dissociation
> atrial d.
> atrioventricular d. (AVD)
> A-V d.
> complete atrioventricular d.
>   (CAVD)
> complete A-V d.
> d. curve
> electromechanical d. (EMD)
> electromyocardial d.
> incomplete atrioventricular d.
> incomplete A-V d.
> d. by interference
> interference d.
> intracavitary pressure-electrogram d.
> isorhythmic d.
> longitudinal d.

dissolution
distal
> d. akinesia
> d. anastomosis
> d. balloon catheter (DBC)
> d. bed
> d. convoluted tubule
> d. coronary occlusion pressure
>   (DCOP)
> d. coronary perfusion pressure
> d. coronary sinus (DCS)
> d. ectasia
> d. perfusion system (DPS)
> d. runoff
> d. shocking coil
> d. splenorenal shunt
> d. stenosis
> d. vascular insufficiency
> d. vessel embolization

distance
> half-power d.
> interelectrode d.
> Mahalanobis d.
> 6-minute walk d.

distant
> d. breath sounds
> d. heart sounds

distensibility
> aortic d.
> arterial d.
> coronary artery d.
> ventricular d.

distention, distension
> jugular venous d. (JVD)
> premature diastolic d.
> d. waveform

disto-occlusal (DO)

distorted coarctation
distortion
    peribronchovascular d.
    pincushion d.
distress
    respiratory d.
distribution
    blood volume d.
    Boltzmann d.
    d. coefficient (Kd)
    connexon d.
    interstitial d.
    microvascular flow d.
    nonhomogeneous pulmonary time-
      constant d.
    perilymphatic d.
    smooth pseudo-Winger-Ville d.
    (SPWVD)
    stocking-glove d.
    tracer d.
    volume of d.
distributive shock
disturbance
    conduction d.
    electrolytic d.
    d. of function occlusion syndrome
    (DOFOS)
    rhythm d.
    sleep d.
disturbed
    d. circadian blood pressure pattern
    d. flow
disulfide
    d. bridge
    carbon d.
    glutathione d.
Dittrich stenosis
Diuchlor
Diulo
Diupres
diurese
diuresis
    loop d.
diuretic
    d. agent
    cardiac d.
    high-ceiling d.
    indirect d.
    loop d.
    osmotic d.
    potassium-sparing d.
    potassium-wasting d.

    d. therapy
    thiazide d.
Diurexan
Diuril
diurnal
    d. peak flow variability
    d. rhythm
    d. sleep
    d. variation
Diutensin
divarication
DIVBC
    disseminated intravascular blood
    coagulation
DIVC
    disseminated intravascular coagulation
divergens
    Babesia d.
diversity
    antigen binding d.
diver's syncope
diverticulectomy
    Harrington esophageal d.
diverticulum, pl. **diverticula**
    apical d.
    Heister d.
    laryngotracheal d.
    tracheobronchial d.
    Zenker d.
divided respiration
diving
    d. air embolism
    d. goiter
    d. reflex
division
    vascular ring d.
divisional heart block
Dixarit
dizziness
DKS
    Damus-Kaye-Stansel
    DKS operation
DL
    double lumen
DLCO
    diffusing capacity of lung for carbon
    monoxide
DLIS
    digoxin-like immunoreactive substance
D-looping
DLP cardioplegic needle
d,l-sotalol

D

NOTES

DLT
  double lung transplant
DM
  dextromethorphan
  diabetes mellitus
  diastolic murmur
    Anatuss DM
    Carbodec DM
    Cardec DM
    Diabetic Tussin DM
    Fenesin DM
    Genatuss DM
    Hold DM
    Humibid DM
    Iobid DM
    Mytussin DM
    Pseudo-Car DM
    Robafen DM
    Silphen DM
    Siltussin DM
    Tolu-Sed DM
    Triaminic DM
    Uni-tussin DM
Dm
  membrane diffusing capacity
DM-400 Holter ECG cassette recorder
DMI
  diaphragmatic myocardial infarction
    DMI analyzer
DMPM
  diffuse malignant pleural mesothelioma
DMR
  direct myocardial revascularization
DMVA
  direct mechanical ventricular actuation
DN
  dicrotic notch
DNA
  deoxyribonucleic acid
    DNA cloning
    DNA histogram
    human cloned DNA (cDNA)
    DNA probe
    DNA sequencing
    DNA switch
DNA-coated stent
DNAR
  do not attempt resuscitation
DNase
  deoxyribonuclease
DNM
  descending necrotizing mediastinitis
DNP
  Dendroaspis natriuretic peptide
DNR
  do not resuscitate
DO
  diamine oxidase

  digoxin
  disto-occlusal
do
  do not attempt resuscitation
    (DNAR)
  do not resuscitate (DNR)
Doan's
  Extra Strength D.
  D. Original
dobutamine
  d. atropine stress echocardiography
    (DASE)
  d. echocardiography (DE)
  d. holiday
  d. hydrochloride
  d. perfusion scintigraphy
  d. stress echocardiography (DSE)
  d. stress test
dobutamine-induced ischemia
Dobutrex injection
docetaxel
Docke murmur
docking wire
dock wire
docosahexaenoic acid
documentation
  coronoradiographic d. (CAD)
  negative coronoradiographic d. (n-
    CAD)
Dodd perforating vein
dodecafluoropentane (DDFP)
dodecapeptide
Dodge area-length method
DODS
  demand oxygen delivery system
DOE
  dyspnea on exertion
dofetilide
DOFOS
  disturbance of function occlusion
  syndrome
dog
  d. boning
  d. cough
dog-leg catheter
Döhle
  D. disease
  D. inclusion bodies
Döhle-Heller aortitis
Dolacet
dolastatin
dolens
  phlegmasia alba d.
  phlegmasia cerulea d.
dolichoectatic aneurysm
dolichol
dolichostenomelia
Dolobid

dolore
    angina pectoris sine d.
    angina sine d.
DOLV
    double-outlet left ventricle
domain
    time d.
dome
    d. of diaphragm
    d. excursion
    d.-shaped
dome-and-dart configuration
domestica
    Carinia d.
dominance
    coronary artery d.
dominant positive deflection flutter
doming
    diastolic d.
    d. of leaflet
    systolic d.
    tricuspid valve d.
domino procedure
domperidone
donation
    predeposit autologous d.
Donders pressure
Donné corpuscle
donor (D)
    d. heart
    d. organ ischemic time
    primary d. (d(A))
    unrelated d. (URD)
donor-acceptor (D-A)
donor-specific transfusion
do not resuscitate (DNR)
door-to-balloon time
door-to-needle time
L-dopa
dopachrome oxidoreductase (DCOR)
Dopamet
dopamine
    d. beta-hydroxylase deficiency
    d. D2 receptor (DD2R)
    d. hydrochloride
dopaminergic
    d. agent
    d. function
Dopastat
dopexamine
Doppler
    Aloka color D.

D. auto-correlation technique
D. blood flow detector
D. cardiography
carotid D.
color flow D.
D. color flow
D. color flow mapping (DCFM)
D. color jet
D. continuity equation
continuous-wave D. (CWD)
D. coronary catheter
D. device
D. echocardiography
D. effect
D. fetal heart monitor
D. fetal stethoscope
D. flow analysis
D. flow probe
D. four-chamber view (D4CV)
FreeDop cordless D.
D. interrogation
intravascular D.
D. measurement
D. pressure
D. pressure gradient
pulsed D. echocardiography (PDE)
pulsed-wave D. (PWD)
pulsed-wave tissue D. (PWTD)
quantitative D.
D. recording
D. shift
D. signal
D. sonography (DS)
D. speckle
spectral D.
D. spectral analysis
steady D.
D. tissue imaging (DTI)
D. transducer
D. transesophageal color flow
    imaging
D. two-chamber view (D2CV)
D. ultrasonic flowmeter
D. ultrasonography
D. ultrasound
D. velocimetry
D. velocity probe
D. velocity wire
D. waveform analysis
Doppler-Cavin monitor
Doppler-derived index

D

NOTES

Doppler-guided hemorrhoidal artery ligation
Doppler peak flow velocity (Vmax)
Doppler-tipped angioplasty guidewire
Dopram injection
DOPS
  diffuse obstructive pulmonary syndrome
Doptone monitoring
d'orange
  peau d'o.
Dorendorf sign
Dorian rib stripper
Dormin Oral
dornase
  d. alfa
  pancreatic d.
Dor procedure
dorsal
  carpal arch d.
  d. lingual branches of lingual artery
  d. mesocardium
dorsalis pedis pulse
dorsi
  latissimus d.
dorsum linguae
DORV
  double-outlet right ventricle
Doryx Oral
dosage regimen
dose
  cumulative cardiotoxic d. (CCD)
  extra-fine particle d. (EFPD)
  fine particle d. (FPD)
  high heparin d. (HHD)
  maximum tolerated d. (MTD)
  MIH d.
  minimum cumulative cardiotoxic d. (MCCD)
  nonpressor d.
  priming d.
  radiation absorbed d. (rad)
  subantihypertensive d.
  threshold d.
dose-effect curve dose-response curve
Dosepak
  Medrol D.
dosimetry
dosing
  trough d.
Dos Santos needle
Dostinex
DOT
  directly observed therapy
  directly observed treatment
Dotter
  D. caged-balloon catheter
  D. effect
  D. intravascular retrieval set

D. procedure
D. technique
dottering
  d. effect
  d. of lesion
Dotter-Judkins
  D.-J. percutaneous transluminal angioplasty
  D.-J. technique
double
  d. aortic arch
  d. aortic stenosis
  d. coronary artery bypass graft (DCABG)
  d. count
  d. counting
  d. ectopic tachyarrhythmia
  d. external direct current shock
  d. flexible tipped wire guide
  d. lumen (DL)
  d. lung transplant (DLT)
  D. Play large bore double Y hemostasis valve
  d. pleurisy
  d. pneumonia
  d. product
  d. simultaneous stimulation test
  d. strength (DS)
  d. switch procedure
  d. tachycardia (DT)
  d. umbrella
  d. umbrella closure
  d. valve replacement (DVR)
  d. ventricular extrastimulus
  d. ventricular response (DVR)
  d. voice
double-balloon
  d.-b. catheter
  d.-b. (9-11) technique
  d.-b. technique
  d.-b. valvotomy
  d.-b. valvuloplasty
double-barreled aorta
double-chain rt-PA
double-chip micromanometer catheter
double-disk
  d.-d. ASD closure device
  d.-d. occluder
double-dummy technique
double-flanged valve sewing ring
double-headed stethoscope
double-inlet left ventricle
double-J
  d.-J catheter
  d.-J stent
double-lumen
  d.-l. catheter
  d.-l. endobronchial tube

d.-l. sign
venovenous d.-l. (VVDL)
double-oblique imaging
double-outlet
    d.-o. left ventricle (DOLV)
    d.-o. left ventricle malposition
    d.-o. right ventricle (DORV)
    d.-o. right ventricle malposition
double-rib fracture
double-sandwich IgM ELISA
double-sheath bronchial brushings
double-shock sound
double-syringe technique
doublet
double-thermistor coronary sinus catheter
double-umbrella device
double-wire technique
doubling time
doughnut
    d. configuration
    d. sign
Douglas
    D. bag
    D. bag collection method
    D. bag technique
d'ouverture
    claquement d'o.
dove coo musical murmur
Dow
    D. Corning tube
    D. method
Down
    D. flow generator
    D. syndrome (DS)
downgoing Babinski
downhill
    d. esophageal varix
    d. ST segment depression
down-regulation
downsloping
    d. ST segment
    d. ST segment depression
downstream
    d. sampling method
    d. segment
    d. venous pressure (DSVP)
downstream-signaling cascade
doxacurium
doxapram hydrochloride
doxazosin mesylate

doxepin hydrochloride
doxofylline
doxorubicin
    d. cardiomyopathy
    d. cardiotoxicity
    d., 5-fluorouracil, cisplatin (AFP)
    d. hydrochloride
doxorubicin-induced cardiac toxicity
Doxychel Oral
doxycycline pleurodesis
Doyen elevator
DP
    diastolic pressure
DPAP Stealth device
DPB
    diffuse panbronchiolitis
DPC
    delayed primary closure
d-PCI
    direct percutaneous coronary intervention
D-penicillamine
DPFR
    diastolic pressure-flow relationship
D-Phe-L-Pro-L-Arg-chloromethyl ketone (PPACK)
DPHM
    diphenhydramine
DPI
    dry powder inhaler
DPL
    diagnostic peritoneal lavage
DPM
    digital phase mapping
DPP
    digital pulse plethysmography
DPPC
    dipalmitoyl phosphatidylcholine
        DPPC test
DPR
    dietary prevention of recurrent myocardial infarction
DPS
    distal perfusion system
        QuickFlow DPS
DPTA
    diethylenetriamine pentaacetic acid
DPTI
    diastolic pressure-time index
DPTS
    delayed pulmonary toxicity syndrome
DR-70 tumor marker test

D

NOTES

Dräger
- D. respirometer
- D. ventilator

drag force

drain
- Clot Stop d.

drainage
- anomalous pulmonary venous d. (APVD)
- autogenic d. (AD)
- closed chest water-seal d.
- external ventricular d. (EVD)
- hemi-anomalous pulmonary venous d. (HAPVD)
- partial anomalous pulmonary venous d. (PAPVD)
- percussion and postural d. (P&PD)
- postural d. (PD)
- pulmonary venous d.
- thoracic duct d. (TDD)
- Thora-Drain III chest d.
- total anomalous pulmonary venous d. (TAPVD)
- underwater seal d.
- water-seal d.

Dramamine Oral

Drapanas mesocaval shunt

drapeau
- bruit de d.

dreamer clamp

dreaming sleep

dream pain

Drechslera hawaiiensis

dressing
- Clo-Sur P.A.D. d.
- Comfeel Ulcus d.
- Cutinova Hydro d.
- Kaltostat wound packing d.
- stent d.
- Vigilon d.
- wet-to-dry d.

Dressler
- D. beat
- D. syndrome

DRFS
- Dundee rank factor score
- DRFS risk factors in coronary heart disease

DRG
- diagnostic-related group

DRI
- defibrillation response interval

drill-tip catheter

Drinker respirator

drip
- heparin d.
- postnasal d. (PND)

Dripps-American Surgical Association score

Dristan Sinus Caplets

drive
- d. cycle length
- respiratory d.
- d. train
- ventricular d.

driveline infection

driver
- D. coronary stent
- TLC-II portable VAD d.

Drixoral
- D. Cough & Congestion Liquid Caps
- D. Cough & Sore Throat Liquid Caps
- D. Nasal

Dromos pacemaker

dromotropic effect

dronabinol

droop
- facial d.

drop
- d. attack
- Ayr saline nasal d.'s
- falling d.
- d. heart
- Rondamine-DM d.'s
- Rondec D.'s
- Tussafed d.'s

droperidol

dropout
- septal d.

dropped beat

dropsy
- cardiac d.
- d. chest
- d. of pericardium

drowned
- d. lung
- d. newborn syndrome

drowsiness
- Tylenol Cold No D.

Droxia

DRP
- digoxin reduction product

drug
- d. abuse
- antiarrhythmic d. (AAD)
- antituberculous d.
- cardiotonic d.
- d. clearance
- depolarizing d.
- d.'s, electrolytes, low temperature and lunacy, intoxication and intracranial processes, retention of urine or feces, infection, unfamiliar surroundings, myocardial infarction (DELIRIUM)
- hydrophobic d.

hypnotic d.
investigational new d. (IND)
lipophilic d.
neuroprotective d.
nondepolarizing d.
nonsteroidal antiinflammatory d.
   (NSAID)
pressor d.
sedative-hypnotic d.
sympathomimetic d.
vasoactive d.
drug-associated pericarditis
drug-eluting stent (DES)
drug-induced
d.-i. cardiomyopathy
d.-i. lupus erythematosus (DILE)
d.-i. lupus syndrome
d.-i. pericarditis
d.-i. thrombocytopenia
drug-loaded biodegradable polymer stent
drug-refractory tachycardia
Drummond
marginal artery of D.
D. marginal artery
D. sign
dry
d. beriberi
d. bronchiectasis
d. bronchitis
d. cough
d. gangrene
d. pericarditis
d. pleurisy
d. powder inhaler (DPI)
d. rale
standard temperature and
   pressure, d.
dry-powder actuator
Drysdale corpuscle
DS
diameter stenosis
diastolic murmur
Doppler sonography
double strength
Down syndrome
duration of systole
   Bactrim DS
   Septra DS
   Sulfatrim DS
%DS
percent diameter stenosis

DSA
digital subtraction angiography
DSACT, D-SACT
direct sinoatrial conduction time
DSAS
discrete subaortic stenosis
discrete subvalvular aortic stenosis
DSC
dynamic susceptibility contrast-enhanced
   DSC MRI
DSCG
disodium cromoglycate
DSE
digital subtraction echocardiography
dobutamine stress echocardiography
DSI-III screw-in lead pacemaker
DSMA
diet and stress management in angina
D-sotalol block of HERG
DSP
dexamethasone sodium phosphate
DSPA
vampire bat salivary plasminogen
   activator
DSS
discrete subaortic stenosis
DSVP
downstream venous pressure
DSX Sopha camera
DT
defibrillation threshold
double tachycardia
   defibrillation threshold (DFT, DT)
DTA
descending thoracic aorta
DTAFA
descending thoracic aorta-to-femoral
   artery
   DTAFA bypass graft
DTAF-F
descending thoracic aortic-femoral-
   femoral
2D-TCCS
two-dimensional transcranial color-coded
   sonography
3DTF
three-dimensional time-of-flight
   3DTF magnetic resonance
   angiography
   3DTF magnetic resurence
   angiography

D

NOTES

D-TGA, dTGA
D-transposition of great arteries
DTH
delayed-type hypersensitivity
DTI
diffusion tensor imaging
dipyridamole-thallium imaging
Doppler tissue imaging
DTIC-Dome
D-to-E
D-to-E amplitude
D-to-E slope
DTPA
diethylenetriamine pentaacetate
diethylenetriamine pentaacetic acid
DTPA aerosol inhalation lung
scintigraphy
D-transposition of great arteries (D-TGA, dTGA)
dual
d. atrioventricular node
d. balloon perfusion catheter
(DBPC)
d. chamber (DC)
d. chamber pacemaker (DCP)
d. echophonocardiography
d. marker
dual-chamber
d.-c. ICD
d.-c. Maximo remote monitoring
ICD
d.-c. Medtronic Kappa 400
pacemaker
d.-c. pacing
d.-c. rate-responsive
dual-coil transvenous lead
dual-demand pacemaker
dual-energy digital radiography
dual-helical slice mode
dual-isotope simultaneous acquisition single-photon emission computed tomography (DISA-SPECT)
duality
dual-lead electrocardiogram
dual-loop intraatrial reentry
dual-mode, dual-pacing, dual-sensing (DDD)
dual-sensor micromanometric high-fidelity catheter
dual-site right atrial pacing
dual-slice mode
Dubois index
Du Bois-Reymond law
Duchenne
D. muscular dystrophy
D. sign
duckbill voice prosthesis
Duckworth phenomenon
Ducor-Cordis pigtail catheter

duct
Bartholin d.
Botallo d.
collecting d.
craniopharyngeal d.
d. of Cuvier
medullary collecting d.
pharyngobranchial d.
thoracic d.
thyrolingual d.
ductal cell carcinoma
Duct-Occlud system
ductus
d. arantii
d. arteriosus (DA)
d. bump
patent d. (PD)
percutaneous occlusion of d.
d. sublinguales minores
d. sublingualis major
d. thoracicus
d. venosus
Duett
D. arterial closure device
D. catheter
D. vascular sealing device
Duffield cardiovascular scissors
Duke
D. Activity Status Index (DASI)
D. bleeding time
D. Carcinoid Database
D. Databank for Cardiovascular
disease
D. infective endocarditis criteria
D. treadmill exercise score
D. treadmill prognostic score
D. University quantitative/qualitative
evaluation system (DUQUES)
Dukes classification
dullness
absolute d. (M3)
absolute cardiac d. (ACD)
area of cardiac d. (ACD)
border of cardiac d.
cardiac d. (CD)
cardiac border of d.
left border of d. (LBD)
left border of cardiac d. (LBCD)
left lower border of cardiac d.
(LLBCD)
marked d. (M2)
percussion d.
relative cardiac d. (RCD)
right border of d. (RBD)
right border cardiac d. (RBCD)
dull pain
dumoffii
Legionella d.

Dumon
- D. bronchoscope
- D. endobronchial silicone stent
- D. tracheobronchial stent

Dumon-Harrell bronchoscope
Duncan syndrome
Dundee rank factor score (DRFS)
Dunham fan
duodecapolar catheter
duodenale
- *Ancylostoma d.*

duodenal string test
Duo-Medihaler aerosol
DuoNeb
Duostat rotating hemostatic valve
Duo-Trach Injection
DUPEL drug delivery system
duplex
- d. Doppler scan
- d. imaging
- d. pulsed-Doppler ultrasonography
- pulsus d.
- d. scanning
- d. ultrasound

DUQUES
- Duke University quantitative/qualitative evaluation system

DURAC
- duration of anticoagulation

Duracep biopsy forceps
Duraflo
- BMR-4500SG sealed hard shell venous reservoir with D.
- Carpentier-Edwards Physio annuloplasty ring with D.

Duragesic Transdermal
dural arteriovenous malformation (DAVM)
Duralyn balloon material
Duramist Plus
Duran annuloplasty ring
Durapulse pacemaker
Duraquin
Dura-Tabs
- Quinaglute D.-T.

Durathane cardiac device
duration
- action potential d. (APD)
- anodal d. (AD)
- d. of anticoagulation (DURAC)
- d. of ECG wave
- d. of exercise

- d. of expiration (T_E)
- half amplitude pulse d.
- d. of inspiration (T_I)
- monophasic action potential d. (MAPD)
- D. Nasal Solution
- P d.
- pacing d.
- pulse d. (PD)
- pulse wave d.
- d. of P wave
- P-wave d.
- QRS complex d.
- QT interval d.
- signal-averaged P-wave d. (SAPD)
- sustained rate d.
- d. of systole (DS)

Duratuss
Duratuss-G
Durham tube
Duricef
Duromedics
- D. mitral valve
- D. valve prosthesis

duropleural fistula
Duroziez
- D. disease
- D. murmur
- D. sign
- D. symptom

Durules
- Betaloc D.
- Biquin D.

durus
- pulsus d.

duskiness
dusky
dust
- d. asthma
- d. disease
- grain d.
- inorganic d.
- mushroom d.
- organic d.

duteplase
duty factor
Duval-Coryllos rib shears
Duval lung-grasping forceps
dVDAVP
- 1-deamine-4-valine-D-arginine vasopressin

D

NOTES

DVI
> deep venous insufficiency
> diastolic velocity integral
> digital vascular imaging
>> DVI pacemaker
>> DVI pacing

DVIS
> digital vascular imaging system

DVP
> deep venous pressure

DVR
> digital vascular reactivity
> double valve replacement
> double ventricular response

DVT
> deep venous thrombosis
>> residual DVT

DVT/PE
> deep venous thrombosis/pulmonary embolism

dwarfism
> aortic d.

DWI
> diffusion-weighted imaging

DWMHI
> deep white matter hyperintensity

DWML
> deep white matter lesion

Dx
> diagnosis

dx cath
> diagnostic catheterization

DX-Portable spirometry

DXR
> delayed xenograft rejection

Dyazide

dyclonine

dye
> Cardio-Green d.
> d. cuvette
> d. dilution technique
> flashlamp excited pulsed d.
> Fox green d.
> indocyanine green d.
> d. injection
> d. laser
> radiocontrast d.
> Unisperse blue d.

dye-dilution
> d.-d. curve
> d.-d. method

Dymedix sleep sensor

Dymelor

Dymer excimer delivery system

Dynabac

Dynacin Oral

DynaCirc

Dynalink biliary self-expanding stent system

dynamic
> d. aorta
> d. cardiac blood flow (DCBF)
> d. cardiomyoplasty
> d. compliance of lung
> d. CT scan
> d. electrocardiography (DCG)
> d. exercise
> d. frequency response
> d. hyperinflation (DH)
> d. intracavitary obstruction
> d. method
> d. murmur
> d. pressure
> d. range
> d. relaxation
> d. stenosis
> d. susceptibility contrast-enhanced (DSC)
> d. susceptibility contrast-enhanced MRI
> d. tracheal compression
> D. Y stent

dynamics
> fluid d.
> funnel d.
> left ventricular-left atrial crossover d.
> RR interval d.

dynamite heart

dynamometer
> bicycle d.
> Cybex isokinetic d.
> Jamar hand d.
> Jamar model 0030J4 d.

Dynapen

DynaPulse 5000A blood pressure monitor

Dynasty
> D. balloon
> D. delivery system

dynein

Dynepo

dyne seconds

dynorphin

dyphylline

Dyrenium

dysanapsis
> airway-parenchymal d.

dysanaptic growth

dysarteriotony

dysarthria
> isolated d.
> pure d. (PD)

dysarthria-clumsy hand syndrome (DCHS)

dysautonomia
> familial d.

dysbaric
>d. disorder
>d. osteonecrosis

dysbarism

dysbetalipoproteinemia
>familial d.

dyscontrol

dyscrasia
>blood d.

dysfibrinogenemia

dysfunction
>acute endothelial d.
>age-related endothelial d.
>asymptomatic left ventricular d.
>atrioventricular node d. (AVND)
>biventricular d.
>chronic contractile d.
>ciliary d.
>diaphragmatic d.
>diastolic ventricular d.
>endothelial d.
>erectile d.
>extrathoracic airway d.
>focal ventricular d.
>global ventricular d.
>intellectual d.
>irritant-associated vocal cord d.
>left ventricular d. (LVD)
>left ventricular systolic d.
>lung d.
>microvascular d.
>multiple-organ d.
>obstructive ventilatory d.
>papillary muscle d.
>postischemic d.
>restrictive ventilatory d.
>reversible left ventricular d.
>sinoatrial node d.
>sinus node d. (SND)
>valvular d.
>ventricular d.
>vocal cord d. (VCD)

dysfunctional
>d. airway immune response
>d. myocardium

dysgenesis
>gonadal d.

dysgeusia

dysinnervation
>congenital myocardial
>sympathetic d. (CMSD)

dyskinesia
>d. intermittens
>primary ciliary d. (PCD)
>d. syndrome
>tracheobronchial d.

dyskinesis
>anterior wall d.
>anteroapical d.
>left ventricular d.
>posteroinferior d.

dyskinetic segment

dyslipidemia
>atherogenic d.
>d. constellation
>Fredrickson d. type I, IIa, IIb, III, IV, V

dyslipidemic hypertension syndrome

dyslipoproteinemia

dysmetria

dysmodulation

dysmotility
>esophageal d.

dysnystaxis

dyspeptica
>angina d.

dysphagia, dysphagy
>contractile ring d.
>d. inflammatoria
>d. lusoria
>d. nervosa
>d. paralytica
>sideropenic d.
>d. spastica
>vallecular d.
>d. valsalviana

dysphasia

dysphasic

dysplasia
>angiogenic squamous d.
>arrhythmogenic right ventricular d. (ARVD)
>atriodigital d.
>bronchopulmonary d. (BPD)
>cranio-cerebello-cardiac d. (CCC)
>ectodermal d.
>fibromuscular d.
>fibrous d.
>mucoepithelial d.
>polyostotic fibrous d.
>right ventricular d.
>ventricular radial d. (VRD)
>ventriculoradial d.

D

NOTES

dysplasia *(continued)*
    vertebral defects, imperforate anus, transesophageal fistula, and radial and renal d. (VATER)
dysplasminogenemia
dysplastic
    d. mitral valvar leaflet
    d. valve
dyspnea
    American Thoracic Society classification of d.
    cardiac d.
    effort d.
    episodic d.
    exercise-induced d.
    exertional d. (ED)
    expiratory d.
    functional d.
    inspiratory d.
    Monday d.
    nocturnal d.
    nonexpansional d.
    one-flight exertional d.
    d. on exertion (DOE)
    orthostatic d.
    paroxysmal nocturnal d. (PND)
    d. of pregnancy
    progressive d.
    psychogenic d.
    pulmonary d.
    renal d.
    rest d.
    d. scale
    D. Scale questionnaire
    sighing d.
    d. target
    tracheal wall injury with intermittent stoppage of tracheostomy and episodes of d. (TWISTED)
    Traube d.
    two-flight exertional d.

dyspneic
dysreflexia
    autonomic d.
dysregulation
    thermal d.
dysrhythmia
    cardiac d. (CD)
dysrhythmic cardiac arrest
dysrhythmogenic
dyssynchronization
dyssynchronous thoracoabdominal excursion
dyssynchrony
    mechanical d.
    thoracoabdominal d.
dyssynergia
    detrusor-sphincter d.
dyssynergic
    d. myocardial segment
    d. myocardium
dyssynergy
    regional d.
    ventricular d.
dystrophin
dystrophinopathy
dystrophy
    asphyxiating thoracic d. (ATD)
    Becker-type tardive muscular d.
    Duchenne muscular d.
    Emery-Dreifuss muscular d.
    facioscapulohumeral d.
    familial asphyxiant thoracic d.
    Landouzy-Dejerine d.
    limb-girdle muscular d.
    muscular d.
    myotonic muscular d.
    reflex sympathetic d.
    Steinert myotonic d.
    thoracic asphyxiant d.
    thoracic-pelvic-phalangeal d.
dystropic calcification
dysvascular

E

E greater than A
E point on echocardiogram
E point to septal separation (EPSS)
E sign
E wave
E wave to A wave (E/A, E:A)

7E3

7E3 glycoprotein IIb/IIIa platelet antibody
7E3 monoclonal Fab antibody

44E

Vicks Pediatric Formula 44E

E$_4$

leukotriene E$_4$

E-150 Breeze ventilator

EA

endocardiographic amplifier
endotracheal aspirate

E/A, E:A

early to late diastolic filling ratio
E wave to A wave
E/A wave ratio

EABV

effective arterial blood volume

EAC

expandable access catheter
EAC catheter

EAD

early afterdepolarization
effective airspace dimension

EAE

effective arterial elastance

EAG

electroarteriography
endovascular aortic graft

Eagle

E. criteria
E. equation
E. medium
E. portable ventilation system
E. risk score index
E. spirometer

EAMI

exercise training in anterior myocardial infarction

ear

e. densitogram
e. lobe crease (ELC)
e. oximeter

earclip

early

e. afterdepolarization (EAD)
e. deceleration
e. diastolic murmur (EDM)
e. diastolic relaxation (EDR)
e. graft failure (EGF)
e. ischemic recurrence (EIR)
e. to late diastolic filling ratio (E/A, E:A)
e. lung injury
e. mitral valve closure (EMVC)
e. opening valve
e. progressing stroke (EPS)
e. pulmonary injury
e. rapid repolarization
e. recurrence of atrial fibrillation (ERAF)
e. repolarization (ER)
e. repolarization syndrome
e. return to normal activities (ERNA)
e. systolic paradox (ESP)
e. systolic wave (SE)
e. ventricular repolarization syndrome (EVRS)

early-peaking systolic murmur

EARR

extended aortic root replacement

EasiVent

E. valved holding chamber
E. valved holding chamber mask

Easprin

EAST

Emory Angioplasty versus Surgery Trial

Easy

E. Air 15 compressor
E. Dial Reg oxygen regulator
E. Neb compressor

Easy-Breathe

Easyhaler

EasyOne spirometry system

Easytrak coronary venous lead

EAT

ectopic atrial tachycardia

Eaton

E. agent
E. agent pneumonia

Eaton-Lambert syndrome

EAVC

enhanced atrioventricular conduction

EAVN

enhanced atrioventricular nodal
EAVN conduction

EBCT

electron beam computed tomography

EBDA

effective balloon-dilated area

Eberth perithelium

E

EBM
    evidence-based medicine
EBNA
    Epstein-Barr nuclear antigen
Ebola
    Reston subtype of E.
    E. virus
EBR
    embolus-to-blood ratio
Ebrantil
Ebstein
    E. angle
    E. anomaly
    E. disease
    E. malformation
    E. malformed valve
    E. sign
EBUS
    endobronchial ultrasonography
    endobronchial ultrasound
EBV
    effective blood volume
    Epstein-Barr virus
    estimated blood volume
EC
    ejection click
    external carotid
    extracorporeal
        EC artery
EC50 ToxCO breath carbon monoxide monitor
ECA
    electrocardioanalyzer
    external carotid artery
E-CABG
    endarterectomy and coronary artery bypass grafting
    endoscopic coronary artery bypass graft
ECAD
    extracranial carotid arterial disease
ecadotril
ECAT III positron tomograph
ECBV
    effective circulating blood volume
ECC
    edema, clubbing, and cyanosis
    emergency cardiac care
    external cardiac compression
    extracorporeal circulation
eccentric
    e. atrial activation
    e. hypertrophy
    e. ledge
    e. lesion
    e. narrowing
    e. stenosis
    e. stenotic jet
eccentricity index
ecchymosis, pl. **ecchymoses**

ecchymotic
    e. facies
    e. mask
Eccovision acoustic pharyngometer
ECD
    endocardial cushion defect
    external cardioverter-defibrillator
    extracranial carotid disease
    extracranial Doppler sonography
    Ventak ECD
ECF
    effective capillary flow
ECF-A
    eosinophil chemotactic factors of anaphylaxis
ECG, EKG
    electrocardiogram
    electrocardiograph
    electrocardiography (*See also* EKG)
    AZTEC in ECG
    baseline ECG
    borderline ECG
    CELP ECG
    CORTES ECG
    differentiated ECG (DECG)
    esophageal ECG
    intracardiac ECG
    ECG leads I, II, III; V1 through V6; aVF, aVL, aVR
    Micro-Tracer portable ECG
    Miniscope MS-3 pocket ECG
    Minnesota classification of ECG
    ECG monitor strip
    ECG signal-averaging technique
    ECG silence
    straight-line ECG
    ECG triggering unit
    Welch Allyn/Schiller AT-2 full-size ECG
    Welch Allyn/Schiller AT-10 hospital grade ECG
    Welch Allyn/Schiller AT-2*plus* full-size ECG
    Welch Allyn/Schiller AT-1 three channel ECG
    Welch Allyn/Schiller MS-3 pocket size ECG
ECG-synchronized digital subtraction angiogram
echinococcal cyst
echinococcosis
Echinococcus
    E. granulosus
    E. multilocularis
ECHO
    enteric cytopathogenic human orphan
    enterocytopathogenic human orphan
    ECHO virus
    ECHO virus myocarditis

Echo
    echoventriculometry
echo, pl. **echoes**
    amphoric e.
    atrial e.
    bandlike intrapericardial e.
    e. beat
    bright e.
    e. delay time (TE)
    e. density
    gradient recall e. (GRE)
    e. guidance
    high density e.
    e. intensity
    linear e.
    metallic e.
    mitral valve e. (MVE)
    motion display e.
    nodus sinuatrialis e.
    NS e.
    pericardial e.
    e. planar imaging (EPI)
    e. ranging
    e. record access (ERA)
    e. reverberation
    RT3D e.
    scattered e.
    e. score
    smokelike echoes
    specular e.
    transcutaneous e.
    transesophageal e.
    ventricular e.
    e. zone
echoaortography
echo-bright endocardium
echocardiogram
    aortic valve e. (AVE)
    apical five-chamber view e.
    apical four-chamber view e.
    apical two-chamber view e.
    B bump on e.
    continuous loop exercise e.
    continuous wave Doppler e.
    contrast-enhanced e.
    cross-sectional two-dimensional e.
    2D e.
    E point on e.
    exercise e. (EE)
    Feigenbaum e.
    long-axis parasternal view e.
    meridian e.

    M-mode e.
    Ochsner-Mahorner e.
    parasternal long-axis view e.
    parasternal short-axis view e.
    postcontrast e.
    posterior left ventricular wall
      motion on e.
    postexercise e.
    signal-averaged e.
    transthoracic e. (TTE)
    e. with saline agitation
    W wave on e.
echocardiograph
    Acuson e.
    Ultramark 9 e.
echocardiographic
    e. assessment
    e. automated border detection
    e. automated boundary detection
      system
    e. differentiation
    e. scoring system
    e. smoke
    e. strain rate imaging
    e. transducer
echocardiography (EchoCG)
    adenosine e.
    A-mode e.
    any-plane e.
    AT-atropine stress e.
    baseline e.
    bedside transthoracic e.
    bicycle e.
    bidimensional e.
    B-mode e.
    bubble contrast e.
    color M-mode Doppler e.
    continuous-wave Doppler e.
    contrast e.
    cross-sectional e. (CSE, CSR)
    2D e.
    deductive e.
    digital subtraction e. (DSE)
    dipyridamole stress e.
    dobutamine e. (DE)
    dobutamine atropine stress e.
      (DASE)
    dobutamine stress e. (DSE)
    Doppler e.
    epiaortic e.
    ergonovine e.
    esophageal e.

NOTES

E

echocardiography *(continued)*
exercise stress e. (ESE, Ex-Echo)
high-frequency epicardial e. (HFEE)
interventional e.
intracardiac e. (ICE)
intraoperative e. (IOE)
intraoperative transesophageal e.
(IOTEE)
intravenous myocardial contrast e.
(IMCE)
meridian e.
mitral valve e.
M-mode e. (MME)
multiplane transesophageal e.
myocardial contrast e. (MCE)
negative-contrast e. (NCE)
paraplane e.
pharmacologic stress e.
pulmonary valve e.
pulsed Doppler e. (PDE)
pulsed Doppler cross-sectional e.
(PD-CSE)
quantitative two-dimensional e.
real-time three-dimensional e.
sector scan e.
signal-averaged e.
SonoHeart hand-carried e.
stress e.
stress-injected sestamibi-gated
SPECT with e.
supine bicycle stress e. (SBSE)
TDI M-mode e.
three-dimensional e. (3DE)
transesophageal e. (TEE)
transesophageal contrast e.
transesophageal dobutamine stress e.
transesophageal echocardiography-
dobutamine stress e. (TEE-DSE)
transthoracic e. (TTE)
transthoracic color Doppler e.
transthoracic contrast e.
treadmill e.
two-dimensional e. (2DE)
VIDA stress e.
EchoCG
echocardiography
echodense
e. mass
e. structure
e. valve
echodensity
cardiac e.
linear e.
superimposed e.
echo-Doppler cardiography
echoendoscope
Olympus e.
echoes (*pl. of* echo)
EchoFlow blood velocity meter system

echo-free space
echogenic
e. mass
e. plaque
echogenicity
end-diastolic wall e.
EchoGen injectable emulsion
echogram
echograph
Siemens Sonoline CD e.
echography
A-scan e.
echo-guided
e.-g. pericardiocentesis
e.-g. ultrasound
echolucent plaque
EchoMark angiographic catheter
echophonocardiography
combined M-mode e.
dual e.
echophony
echoreflective
echoreflectivity
echoscanner
echoscope
echo-signal shape
echo-spared area
Echovar Doppler system
echoventriculometry (Echo)
echovirus myocarditis
Echovist
EC/IC
extracranial/intracranial
Eck fistula
ECL
euglobin clot lysis
ECLA
excimer laser coronary angioplasty
eclampsia
Eclipse
E. holmium laser
E. PTMR system
E. TMR laser
ECLS
extracorporeal life support
ECM
external cardiac massage
extracellular matrix
ECMO
extracorporeal membrane oxygenation
ECMO pump
ECMO therapy
ecNOS, eNOS
endothelial constitutive nitric oxide
synthase
ecNOS gene
ecNOS gene expression
EcoCheck oxygen monitor

ECOM
    endotracheal cardiac output monitor
    endotracheal cardiac output monitoring
economy class syndrome
Ecotrin
ECP
    effective conduction period
    endocardial potential
    eosinophil cationic protein
    exercise cardiac power
    external cardiac pressure
ECPR
    external cardiopulmonary resuscitation
ECR
    electrocardiographic response
ECS
    extracellular-like, calcium-free solution
      ECS cardioplegic solution
Ecstasy
ECT
    euglobulin clot assay
ectasia, ectasis
    alveolar e.
    annuloaortic e. (AAE)
    anuloaortic e. (AAE)
    aortoannular e.
    artery e.
    e. cordis
    coronary artery e.
    diffuse arterial e.
    distal e.
    vascular e.
ectatic
    e. aneurysm
    e. emphysema
ecto-ADPase
ectocardia
ectocardiac, ectocardial
Ectocor pacemaker
ectodermal dysplasia
ectopia
    e. cordis
    e. cordis abdominalis
    e. cordis pectoral
    e. lentis
ectopic
    e. Ashman beat
    atrial e. (AE)
    e. atrial tachycardia (EAT)
    e. bronchus
    e. impulse
    e. junctional beat (EJB)

    e. junctional tachycardia
    e. pacemaker
    e. rhythm
    e. ventricular beat
ectopy
    asymptomatic complex e.
    atrial e.
    supraventricular e.
    ventricular e.
ECV
    endocardial ventriculotomy
    external cardioversion
    extracorporeal volume
ED
    emotional defensiveness
    end-diastole
    exertional dyspnea
EDA
    end-diastolic area
EDBP
    erect diastolic blood pressure
EDC
    end-diastolic count
EDCI
    energetic dynamic cardiac insufficiency
EDCS
    end-diastolic chamber stiffness
    end-diastolic circumferential stress
EDD
    end-diastolic diameter
    end-diastolic dimension
    esophageal detection device
eddy sound
Edecrin
    E. Oral
    E. Sodium injection
edema
    acute cardiogenic pulmonary e.
     (ACPE)
    acute noncardiogenic pulmonary e.
    acute pulmonary e. (APE)
    airway e.
    alveolar e.
    angioneurotic e.
    ankle e.
    bland e.
    boggy e.
    brawny e.
    brown e.
    cardiac e.
    cardiac pulmonary e. (CPE)
    cardiogenic pulmonary e.

E

NOTES

239

edema *(continued)*
    cerebral e.
    chronic pulmonary e.
    circumscribed e.
    e., clubbing, and cyanosis (ECC)
    clubbing, cyanosis, and e. (CCE)
    congestive e.
    cytotoxic e.
    dependent e.
    fingerprint e.
    flash pulmonary e.
    florid pulmonary e.
    focal e.
    hereditary angioneurotic e. (HANE)
    high-altitude pulmonary e. (HAPE)
    high-pressure cardiogenic
      pulmonary e.
    hydrostatic e.
    idiopathic cyclic e.
    increased-permeability pulmonary e.
    interstitial pulmonary e.
    e. of lung
    lung e.
    lymphatic e.
    Milton e.
    mucosal e.
    myocardial e.
    negative pressure pulmonary e.
      (NPPE)
    neurogenic pulmonary e.
    noncardiac pulmonary e. (NCPE)
    noncardiogenic pulmonary e.
    nonpitting e.
    obstructive e.
    paroxysmal pulmonary e.
    passive e.
    pedal e.
    periodic e.
    periorbital e.
    peripheral e.
    perivascular e.
    pitting e.
    postanesthesia pulmonary e.
    postcardioversion pulmonary e.
    presacral e.
    pretibial e.
    pulmonary e. (PE)
    pulmonary interstitial e.
    Quincke e.
    reperfusion pulmonary e.
    sacral e.
    septic pulmonary e. (SPE)
    stasis e.
    subpleural e.
    tense e.
    terminal e.
    upper lobe pulmonary e. (ULPE)

    vasogenic e.
    woody e.
edema-proteinuria-hypertension (EPH)
edematous
edentulism
    compensated e.
Eder-Puestow wire
edetate disodium
edge
    e. detection
    leading e.
    shelving e.
    trailing e.
edge-detection
    e.-d. method
    e.-d. system
EDHF
    endothelium-derived hyperpolarizing
    factor
Edinburgh Handedness Inventory (EHI)
EDL
    end-diastolic length
    end-diastolic load
EDM
    early diastolic murmur
    EDM infusion catheter
Edmark
    E. mitral valve
    E. monophasic waveform
EDNF
    endogenous digitalis-like natriuretic
    factor
EDNO
    endothelium-derived nitric oxide
EDP
    end-diastolic pressure
EDPS
    esophageal-directed pressure support
EDR
    early diastolic relaxation
EDRF
    endothelium-derived relaxing factor
edrophonium chloride
EDS
    excessive daytime sleepiness
EDT
    end-diastolic thickness
EDTA
    ethylenediaminetetraacetic acid
EDV
    end-diastolic volume
EDVI
    end-diastolic volume index
Edwards
    E. catheter
    E. clamp
    E. heart valve
    E. septectomy
Edwards-Carpentier aortic valve brush

Edwards-Duromedics bileaflet heart valve
Edwards-Tapp arterial graft
EDWTH
    end-diastolic wall thickness
EE
    exercise echocardiogram
EECP
    enhanced external counterpulsation
EEE
    experimental enterococcal endocarditis
EEG
    electroencephalogram
    electroencephalograph
    electroencephalography
      Equinox digital EEG
      Neurotrac II EEG
EEL
    external elastic lamina
      EEL area
EELV
    end-expiratory lung volume
EEM
    external elastic membrane
E.E.S.
      E.E.S. Chewable
      E.E.S. Granules
      E.E.S. Oral
EET acid
EEV
    elastic equilibrium volume
EF
    ejection fraction
efaroxan
efavirenz
EFE
    endocardial fibroelastosis
Efedron
efegatran
effect
    Anrep e.
    antiatherogenic e.
    Azzopardi e.
    bacteriostatic e.
    Bainbridge e.
    band saw e.
    Bernoulli e.
    billiard ball e.
    blooming e.
    Bohr e.
    Bowditch staircase e.
    Brockenbrough e.

bronchoconstrictive e.
bronchodilator e.
bystander e.
candy wrapper edge e.
chronotropic e.
cidal e.
Coanda e.
Compton e.
copper-wire e.
cytoprotective e.
digitalis e.
digoxin e.
Doppler e.
Dotter e.
dottering e.
dromotropic e.
erectile e.
extrapyramidal side e.
Fahraeus e.
first-night e.
fish-scaling e.
founder e.
Haldane e.
Hawthorne e.
horse-race e.
implosion e.
inertial e.
inotropic e.
jet e.
late proarrhythmic e.
Mach e.
mass e.
mille feuilles e.
neurotoxic e.
nonhemodynamic e.
pendelluft e.
peripheral vasodilator e.
postantibiotic e. (PAE)
pressor e.
Prinzmetal e.
proarrhythmic e.
protooncogenic e.
Rivero-Carvallo e.
second gas e.
silver-wire e.
snare-drum e.
snowplow e.
space-occupying e.
spalling e.
squeeze e.
time-of-flight e.
tongue-rolling e.

E

NOTES

effect *(continued)*
    training e.
    vasodilator e.
    Vaughan-Williams class e.
    Venturi e.
    volume of distribution e.
    Vroman e.
    waterfall e.
    watermelon seeding e.
    Wedensky e.
    white-coat e.
    windkessel e.
    work e.
    wrecking ball e.
effective
    e. airspace dimension (EAD)
    e. arterial blood volume (EABV)
    e. arterial elastance (EAE)
    e. balloon-dilated area (EBDA)
    e. blood volume (EBV)
    e. capillary flow (ECF)
    e. circulating blood volume (ECBV)
    e. conduction period (ECP)
    e. half-life
    e. refractory period (ERP)
    e. refractory period of left ventricle (ERPLV)
    e. regurgitant orifice (ERO)
    e. renal blood flow (ERBF)
    e. systolic pressure (ESP)
effector cell
efferent
    e. arteriole
    e. artery
efficacious
efficacy
    ciliary e.
    e. of drug therapy
    therapeutic e.
    e. of treatment
efficiency
    cough e.
    detective quantum e.
    mucociliary e.
Effler-Groves mode of Allison procedure
Effler hiatal hernia repair
efflux
    cellular cholesterol e.
effort
    angina of e.
    e. angina
    brief maximal e. (BME)
    e. dyspnea
    first e.
    poor expiratory e.
    relative inspiratory e. (RIE)
    e. syndrome

effort-independent lung volume
effort-induced thrombosis
effusion
    asbestos pleural e.
    bloody e.
    chyliform pleural e.
    chylous pericardial e.
    chylous pleural e.
    eosinophilic e.
    exudative pleural e.
    hemorrhagic e.
    interlobar e.
    loculated e.
    malignant pleural e. (MPE)
    parapneumonic e.
    partially coagulated e.
    pericardial e. (PE)
    pericarditis with e.
    pleurisy with e.
    pulmonary e.
    purulent e.
    serosanguineous e.
    serous e.
    silent pericardial e.
    stranding e.
    subpulmonic e.
    transudative pleural e.
effusion-associated lymphocyte
effusive-constrictive
    e.-c. disease
    e.-c. pericarditis
Efidac/24
eflornithine
efonidipine
EFPD
    extra-fine particle dose
EFR
    extended field radiation
Efron jackknife classification
Efudex Topical
EG
    eosinophilic granuloma
EGF
    early graft failure
eGFP
    enhanced green fluorescent protein
eggcrate mattress
Eggleston method
egg-on-a-string silhouette
egg-shaped heart
eggshell
    e. calcification
    e. friability
    e. pattern
egg-yellow reaction
egg-yolk sputum
EGM
    electrogram
egobronchophony

egophony
EGT
exuberant granulation tissue
EGTA
esophagogastric tube airway
EH
enlarged heart
essential hypertension
eh
enlarged heart
EHBF
exercise hyperemia blood flow
EHC
essential hypercholesterolemia
EHI
Edinburgh Handedness Inventory
Ehlers-Danlos syndrome
EHPH
extrahepatic portal hypertension
Ehrenritter ganglion
Ehret phenomenon
ehrlichiosis
EHT
essential hypertension
EHV
electric heart vector
EI
endovascular irradiation
E:I
expiratory to inspiratory
E:I ratio
EIA
enzyme immunoassay
exercise-induced asthma
EIB
exercise-induced bronchospasm
Eichner index
Eicken method
eicosanoid excretion
eicosapentaenoic acid (EPA)
EID
emergency infusion device
EID catheter
eight-lumen manometry catheter
Eikenella corrodens
EILV
end-inspiratory lung volume
Einhorn esophageal dilator
Einthoven
E. equation
E. law
E. lead

E. string galvanometer
E. triangle
EIR
early ischemic recurrence
Eisenmenger
E. complex
E. disease
E. physiology
E. reaction
E. reaction with septal defect
E. syndrome
E. tetralogy
E. VSD
EIT
electrical impedance tomography
EJ
external jugular
EJB
ectopic junctional beat
ejected volume (EV)
ejection
area-length method for e.
e. click (EC)
e. fraction (EF)
e. fraction at rest (REF)
e. fraction during exercise (ExEF)
left ventricular e. (LVE)
e. murmur (EM)
e. period
e. phase
e. phase index
e. rate (ER)
e. shell image
e. sound (ES)
e. systolic murmur (ESM)
e. time (ET)
e. velocity
volumic e.
ejection-fraction image
Ejrup maneuver
EKG (*var. of* ECG)
electrocardiogram
electrocardiograph
EKY
electrokymogram
El
El Gamal cardiac device
El Gamal coronary bypass catheter
El Gamal guiding catheter
ELA
excimer laser-assisted angioplasty

E

NOTES

E-LAM
endothelium-leukocyte adhesion molecule
Elantan
Elastalloy Ultraflex Strecker nitinol stent
elastance
effective arterial e. (EAE)
end-systolic e.
maximum ventricular e. (Emax)
elastase
leukocyte e.
neutrophil e.
Pseudomonas e.
sputum e.
elastic
e. component
e. cone
e. equilibrium volume (EEV)
e. fibers
e. fibers in sputum
e. lamella
e. lamina
e. load
e. mandibular advancement (EMA)
e. pressure-volume (Pel-V)
e. pulse
e. recoil
e. recoil pressure
e. resistance
e. stiffness
e. stockings
e. tissue hyperplasia
elasticity
lung e.
sputum viscosity and e.
ventricular e. (VE)
elasticum
pseudoxanthoma e.
elasticus
conus e.
elastin
elastogram
intravascular e.
elastography
Elastorc catheter guidewire
Elavil
elbow flexion
ELC
ear lobe crease
ELCA
excimer laser coronary angioplasty
elderly
innocent murmur of e.
Elecath electrophysiologic stimulation catheter
Elecsys troponin T immunoassay system
elective
e. angiography

e. cardioversion
e. replacement indicator (ERI)
electric
e. cardiac pacemaker
e. defibrillator using DC discharge (DC)
General E. (GE)
e. heart vector (EHV)
e. replacement indicator (ERI)
e. storm
electrical
e. activation abnormality
e. alternans
e. alternation of heart
e. axis
e. cardioversion
e. catheter ablation
e. countershock
e. diastole
e. disease
e. failure
e. fulguration
e. heart position
e. impedance tomography (EIT)
e. injury
e. pathway
e. potential
e. systole
ElectroAcuscope
electroanatomical
e. map
e. mapping system
electroarteriography (EAG)
electrocardioanalyzer (ECA)
electrocardiogram (ECG, EKG)
ambulatory e. (AECG)
bipolar e. (BPEC)
Burdick e.
concordant changes e.
derived 12-lead e.
discordant changes e.
dual-lead e.
exercise e.
fetal e. (FECG, FEKG)
Fourier analysis of e.
His bundle e.
12-lead e.
16-lead e.
orthogonal e.
scalar e.
signal-averaged e. (SAECG)
stored e.
stress MUGA e.
thallium e.
three-channel e.
time domain signal-averaged e.
treadmill e.
unipolar e.
vector e. (VECG)

Wedensky modulated signal-averaged e.

electrocardiograph (ECG, EKG)
bioimpedance e.
Cambridge e.
MAC-VU e.
Marquette e.
Mingograf 62 6-channel e.

electrocardiographic
e. complex (rSr)
e. gated SPECT myocardial perfusion imaging
e. gating
e. lead
e. response (ECR)
e. transtelephonic monitor
e. wave
e. wave complex
e. wave corresponding to the repolarization of the ventricles (T)
e. wave corresponding to a wave of depolarization crossing the atria (P)

electrocardiography (ECG, EKG)
ambulatory e.
American Society of E. (ASE)
CF lead in e.
chest lead in e. (C)
dynamic e. (DCG)
esophageal e.
exercise e.
exercise stress e. (Ex-ECG)
fetal e.
high-resolution e. (HRE)
intracavitary e.
12-lead e.
long-term e. (LT-ECG)
myocardial e.
precordial e.
signal-averaged e. (SAECG)
stress e. (SECG)
time domain signal-averaged e.
unipolar limb lead on left leg in e. (aVF, aVL)
unipolar limb lead on right arm in e. (aVR)

electrocardiophonogram
electrocardiophonography
electrocardioscanner
Compuscan Hittman computerized e.

electrocardioversion
electrocautery
Bovie e.
bronchoscopic e.
needlepoint e.

electrochemical
e. gradient
e. polarization

electroconvulsive therapy
electrode
AE-60-I-2 implantable pronged unipolar e.
AE-85-I-2 implantable pronged unipolar e.
AE-60-KB implantable unipolar endocardial e.
AE-85-KB implantable unipolar endocardial e.
AE-60-K-10 implantable unipolar endocardial e.
AE-85-K-10 implantable unipolar endocardial e.
AE-60-KS-10 implantable unipolar endocardial e.
AE-85-KS-10 implantable unipolar endocardial e.
Arzbaecher pill e.
Arzco Tapsul pill e.
Berkovits-Castellanos hexapolar e.
Bisping e.
button e.
e. catheter
e. catheter ablation operation
central terminal e.
Clark oxygen e.
coil e.
CPI Endotak transvenous e.
Darox cutaneous thoracic patch e.
dispersing e.
dispersive e.
epicardial sock e.
esophageal pill e.
exploring e.
Fast-Patch disposable defibrillation/electrocardiographic e.
e. gel
Goetz bipolar e.
hydrogen e.'s
implantable cardioverter e.
indifferent e.
intravascular catheter e.
ion-selective e. (ISE)

E

NOTES

electrode *(continued)*
 e. jelly
 J-shaped pacemaker e.
 large-tip e.
 Laserdish e.
 Mansfield Polaris e.
 monopolar temporary e.
 multiple point e.
 multipolar catheter e.
 myocardial e.
 pacemaker e.
 e. pad
 e. paddles
 e. paste
 PE-60-I-2 implantable pronged
   unipolar e.
 PE-85-I-2 implantable pronged
   unipolar e.
 PE-60-K-10 implantable unipolar
   endocardial e.
 PE-85-K-10 implantable unipolar
   endocardial e.
 PE-60-KB implantable unipolar
   endocardial e.
 PE-85-KB implantable unipolar
   endocardial e.
 PE-85-KS-10 implantable unipolar
   endocardial e.
 platinum-iridium e.
 QuadPolar e.
 quadripolar Quad e.
 reference e.
 ring e.
 scalp e.
 screw-in epicardial e.
 screw-in sutureless myocardial e.
 Severinghaus e.
 sew-on e.
 silent e.
 silver bead e.
 silver-silver chloride e.
 stab e.
 stab-in epicardial e.
 steroid-eluting e.
 subcutaneous patch e.
 sutured plaque e.
 e. system
 temporary atrial pacemaker e.
   (TAPE)
 tined ventricular e.
 Transvene tripolar e.
 transvenous e.
 tripolar defibrillation coil e.
 unipolar defibrillation coil e.
 USCI Goetz bipolar e.
 USCI NBIH bipolar e.
 VF e.
 Vitatron catheter e.

 VL e.
 VR e.
electrodesiccation
electrode-skin interface
electrodispersive skin patch
Electrodyne pacemaker
electrodynogram
electroencephalogram (EEG)
electroencephalograph (EEG)
electroencephalography (EEG)
electrofluoroscopy
electrogenic
electrogram (EGM)
 atrial e. (AEG)
 coronary sinus e.
 deflection in the His bundle in e.
 evoked endocardial e.
 evoked ventricular e.
 far-field e.
 e. fractionation
 Furman type II e.
 high right atrium e. (HRAE)
 His bundle e. (HBE)
 intracardiac e.
 sinus node e. (SNE)
electrograph
 Cardiotest portable e.
electrokymogram (EKY)
electrokymograph
electrokymography
electrolyte
 e. imbalance
 e. and steroid cardiopathy with
   necrosis (ESCN)
electrolytic disturbance
electromagnetic
 e. interference/radiofrequency
   interference (EMI/RFI)
 e. mapping
electromanometer
electromechanical
 e. artificial heart
 e. coupling
 e. delay
 e. dissociation (EMD)
 e. interval
 e. left ventricular mapping
 e. systole
electromyocardial dissociation
electromyogram (EMG)
 kinesiological e.
electromyograph (EMG)
electromyography (EMG)
electron
 e. angiography
 e. beam computed tomography
   (EBCT)
 e. fence
 e. microprobe analysis

e. microscope
e. paramagnetic resonance
  spectroscopy
e. volt (eV)

electronic
e. calipers
e. distance compensation
e. fetal monitor
E. HouseCall system
e. pacemaker
e. pacemaker load
e. scanning

electrooculogram (EOG)
electrooculograph (EOG)
electrooculography (EOG)
electropharmacology
electrophoresis
agarose gel e.
gradient gel e.
lipoprotein e. (LEP, LPE)
polyacrylamide gel e.
protein e.
sodium dodecylsulfate
  polyacrylamide gel e. (SDS-
  PAGE)

electrophrenic respiration
electrophysiologic
e. mapping
e. test

electrophysiologist
electrophysiology (EP)
intracardiac e.
North American Society for Pacing
  and E. (NAPSE)

electrostethograph
electrosurgery
electrosurgical blade
electrotonic
e. conduction
e. transmission

electroventriculography (EVG)
electroversion
Elema
E. lead
E. pacemaker

Elema-Schonander pacemaker
element
contractile e.
length contraction compensation e.
  (LCCE)

peroxisome proliferator response e.
  (PPRE)
series elastic e.

elephantiasis
elephant-on-the-chest sensation
elevated gradient
elevation
CK-MB e.
e. of enzyme
e. MI
1-natural-log-unit e.
e. pallor of extremity
ST segment e.
transient ST segment e.
upsloping ST e.

elevator
Aufricht e.
Cameron-Haight e.
e. disease
Doyen e.
Lemmon sternal e.
Matson rib e.
Phemister e.
rib e.

ELF
epithelial lining fluid
ELF levels

elfin
e. facies
e. facies syndrome

Elgiloy-Heifitz aneurysm clip
Elgiloy stent
elimination
e. half-life
single-breath nitrogen e.

Eliminator dilatation balloon
eliprodil
ELISA
enzyme-linked immunosorbent assay
double-sandwich IgM ELISA

ELISPOT
enzyme-linked immunospot
ELISPOT test

**Elite dual-chamber rate-responsive
pacemaker**
Elixicon
Elixophyllin
elizabethae
Bartonella e.

Ellence

E

NOTES

Ellestad
    E. exercise stress test
    E. protocol
ellipse
Ellipse compact spacer
ellipsoid arteriole
elliptical
    e. end-capped quadrature
      radiofrequency coil
    e. loop
Ellis sign
Ellis-van Creveld syndrome
Eloesser flap
Elsner asthma
ELSO
    Extracorporeal Life Support Organization
Elspar
ELT
    endless loop tachycardia
Eltroxin
eluting stent
elution
    isocratic e.
    steroid e.
ELVT
    endolaser venous therapy
Elwrite pediatric lead
EM
    ejection murmur
EMA
    elastic mandibular advancement
      EMA appliance
Emax
    maximum ventricular elastance
EMB
    endomyocardial biopsy
emb
    embolism
embarrassment
    circulatory e.
    hemodynamic e.
    respiratory e.
EmboGold microsphere
embolectomy
    catheter e.
    e. catheter
    femoral e.
    pulmonary e.
    surgical e.
emboli (*pl. of* embolus)
embolic
    e. abscess
    e. aneurysm
    e. event
    e. gangrene
    e. infarct
    e. necrosis
    e. obstruction
    e. phenomenon

    e. pneumonia
    e. shower
    e. stroke
    e. thrombosis
embolism (emb)
    acute pulmonary e.
    air e. (AE)
    air pulmonary e.
    amnionic fluid e. (AFE)
    amniotic fluid e. (AFE)
    aortic e.
    arterial e.
    arterial gas e. (AGE)
    atheromatous e.
    bacillary e.
    bland e.
    bone marrow e.
    capillary e.
    catheter e.
    cellular e.
    cerebral air e.
    cholesterol e.
    coronary air e.
    coronary artery e. (CAE)
    crossed e.
    deep venous
      thrombosis/pulmonary e. (DVT/PE)
    direct e.
    diving air e.
    fat e.
    fatal pulmonary e. (FPE)
    gas e.
    hematogenous e.
    infective e.
    miliary e.
    multiple e.'s
    myxomatous pulmonary e.
    obturating e.
    oil e.
    pantaloon e.
    paradoxic e.
    paradoxical cerebral e.
    Plasmodium e.
    pulmonary e. (PE)
    pulmonary air e.
    pyemic e.
    retrograde e.
    riding e.
    saddle e.
    silent e.
    spinal e.
    straddling e.
    submassive pulmonary e.
    systemic arterial air e.
    trichinous e.
    tumor e.
    venous e.
    venous air e. (VAE)

embolization
    air e.
    bronchial artery e. (BAE)
    cerebral e.
    cholesterol e.
    coil e.
    distal vessel e.
    paradoxical e.
    plaque e.
    pulmonary e.
    septal artery e.
    septic e.
    stent e.
    subsegmental transcatheter
      arterial e. (STAE)
    e. therapy
    transcatheter e.
    transcatheter arterial e. (TAE)
embolized foreign material
embolomycotic aneurysm
embolotherapy
    transcatheter e.
embolus, pl. **emboli**
    air e.
    calcific e.
    cancer e.
    catheter-induced e.
    cerebral e.
    femoral e.
    paradoxical e.
    polyurethane foam e.
    pulmonary e.
    riding e.
    saddle e.
    threw an e.
    throw an e.
embolus-to-blood ratio (EBR)
**Embol-X arterial cannula and filter
system**
Emboshield bare wire filter
embryocardia
    jugular e.
    e. rhythm
embryologic
embryology
embryoma
embryonal cell
embryonic phenotype pattern
embryopathy
EMC
    encephalomyocarditis
    EMC virus

Emcyt
EMD
    electromechanical dissociation
Emerald diagnostic guidewire
emergency
    e. bailout
    e. bailout stent
    e. cardiac care (ECC)
    hypertensive e.
    e. infusion device (EID)
    e. medical tag (EMT)
    e. medical treatment (EMT)
    e. medical treatment and active
      labor act (EMTALA)
    e. portocaval shunt (EPCS)
    e. reperfusion
emergent thoracotomy
Emerson
    E. cuirass respirator
    E. postoperative ventilator
    E. pump
Emery-Dreifuss
    E.-D. disease
    E.-D. muscular dystrophy
emesis
    posttussive e.
emetine toxicity
EMF
    endomyocardial fibrosis
EMG
    electromyogram
    electromyograph
    electromyography
Eminase
EMI/RFI
    electromagnetic
      interference/radiofrequency interference
emission
    e. flame photometry
    single-photon e.
    stimulated acoustic e.
    vascular acoustic e.
emitter
    positron e.
EMLA
    eutectic mixture of local anesthetics
    EMLA cream
**Emory Angioplasty versus Surgery
Trial (EAST)**
emotional
    e. defensiveness (ED)
    e. stress

E

NOTES

emphysema
    alveolar duct e.
    atrophic e.
    bullous e.
    centriacinar e.
    centrilobular e.
    chronic hypertrophic e.
    chronic obstructive pulmonary e.
      (COPE)
    chronic pulmonary e. (CPE)
    compensating e.
    compensatory e.
    cystic e.
    diffuse e.
    ectatic e.
    false e.
    familial e.
    focal e.
    focal-dust e.
    gangrenous e.
    glass blower's e.
    heterogenous e.
    hypertrophic e.
    hypoplastic e.
    idiopathic unilobar e.
    infantile lobar e.
    interlobular e.
    interstitial e.
    Jenner e.
    lobar e.
    localized obstructive e.
    loculated e.
    mediastinal e.
    obstructive e.
    panacinar e.
    panlobular e.
    paracicatricial e.
    paraseptal e.
    peripheral paracicatricial e.
    predominant e.
    pulmonary e. (PE)
    pulmonary interstitial e. (PIE)
    scar e.
    senile e.
    small-lung e.
    subcutaneous e.
    surgical e.
    traumatic e.
    unilateral e.
    vesicular e.
emphysematous
    e. asthma
    e. bleb
    e. bulla
    e. chest
    e. gangrene
empiric
    e. constant
    e. therapy

Empirin
empyema
    anaerobic e.
    Aspergillus e.
    e. benignum
    e. of chest
    exudative e.
    fibrinopurulent e.
    free-flowing e.
    interlobar e.
    latent e.
    loculated e.
    metapneumonic e.
    e. necessitatis
    organizing e.
    e. of pericardium
    pleural e.
    pneumococcal e.
    postinjury e.
    postpneumonectomy tuberculous e.
    pulsating e.
    putrid e.
    sacculated e.
    streptococcal e.
    synpneumonic e.
    thoracic e.
    e. thoracis
    tuberculous e.
empyesis
    tuberculous e.
EMS
    eosinophilia-myalgia syndrome
EMT
    emergency medical tag
    emergency medical treatment
    endocardial mapping technique
EMTA
    endomethylene tetrahydrophthalic acid
EMTALA
    emergency medical treatment and active
      labor act
emulation
    pectoral e.
emulsion
    EchoGen injectable e.
    fat e.
    intravascular perfluorochemical e.
    perflenapent injectable e.
emu oil
EMVC
    early mitral valve closure
E-Mycin Oral
enalapril
    e. and diltiazem
    e. and felodipine
    e. and hydrochlorothiazide
    e. maleate
enalaprilat
enalaprilic acid

enantiomer
en bloc
> en b. bilateral lung transplant
> en b. face
> en b. face view
> en b. face view
> en b. no-touch technique

Enbrel
encainide hydrochloride
Encap
> Novo-Rythro E.

encapsulated organism
Encapsulon epidural catheter
encarditis
encased heart
encephalitis
> cytomegalovirus e.

Encephalitozoon
encephalomyelitis
encephalomyocarditis (EMC)
> e. virus

encephalopathy
> hypertensive e. (HE)
> hypoxic-ischemic e.
> metabolic e.
> subcortical vascular e. (SVE)

encircling
> e. cryoablation
> e. endocardial ventriculotomy
> e. endocardial ventriculotomy
> operation

Enclose
> E. anastomosis assist device
> E. proximal anastomotic assist
> device

encode
encoding
> respiratory ordered phase e.
> (ROPE)
> velocity e.

Encompass cardiac network
Encor
> E. lead
> E. pacemaker

Encore inflation device
encroachment
> luminal e.

encrustation theory of atherosclerosis
encysted pleurisy
end
> e. artery

Endal

endangiitis
Endantadine
endaortitis
endarterectomy
> abdominal aortic e.
> aortoiliofemoral e.
> blunt eversion carotid e.
> carotid e. (CE, CEA)
> coronary e.
> e. and coronary artery bypass
> grafting (E-CABG)
> femoral e.
> gas e.
> transient ischemic attack plus
> carotid e. (TIA + CE)
> transluminal e.
> vertebral e.

endarterial
endarteritis
> e. deformans
> Heubner specific e.
> e. obliterans
> e. proliferans
> syphilitic e.

endarteropathy
> digital e.

end-diastole (ED)
> left ventricular e.-d. (LVED)
> left ventricular dimension in e.-d.
> (LVDd)

end-diastolic
> e.-d. area (EDA)
> e.-d. chamber stiffness (EDCS)
> e.-d. circumferential stress (EDCS)
> e.-d. count (EDC)
> e.-d. diameter (EDD)
> e.-d. dimension (EDD)
> e.-d. left ventricular pressure
> e.-d. length (EDL)
> e.-d. load (EDL)
> e.-d. murmur
> e.-d. pressure (EDP)
> right ventricular e.-d. (RVED)
> e.-d. thickness (EDT)
> e.-d. velocity
> e.-d. volume (EDV)
> e.-d. volume index (EDVI)
> e.-d. wall echogenicity
> e.-d. wall enlargement
> e.-d. wall thickness (EDWTH)

Endeavor nondetachable silicone balloon catheter

E

NOTES

endemic
    e. fungal infection
    e. influenza
end-expiratory
    e.-e. apnea
    e.-e. esophageal pressure
    e.-e. film
    e.-e. lung volume (EELV)
end-flow
    right ventricular e.-f. (RVEF)
end-hole
    e.-h. balloon-tipped catheter
    e.-h. 7-French catheter
    e.-h. Tracker microcatheter
end-inspiratory
    e.-i. film
    e.-i. lung volume (EILV)
    e.-i. Velcro crackle
endless loop tachycardia (ELT)
Endo
    endocardial
    endocardium
    Endo GIA stapler
    Endo Grasp device
endoaneurysmorrhaphy
    ventricular e.
endoaortic clamp
endoaortitis
endoauscultation
endobronchial
    e. brachytherapy
    e. cryotherapy
    e. infection
    e. laser therapy
    e. obstruction
    e. tree
    e. tube
    e. tuberculosis
    e. ultrasonography (EBUS)
    e. ultrasound (EBUS)
endobronchially
endocannabinoid
endocardiac
endocardial (Endo)
    e. bipolar lead
    e. border delineation
    e. cardiac border
    e. catheter ablation
    e. cushion
    e. cushion defect (ECD)
    e. to epicardial resection operation
    e. excursion
    e. fibroelastosis (EFE)
    e. fibrosis
    e. flow
    e. mapping
    e. mapping technique (EMT)
    e. mapping of ventricular
      tachycardia

    e. motion
    e. murmur
    e. pacing
    e. potential (ECP)
    e. pressure
    e. resection
    e. sclerosis
    e. shortening
    e. stain
    e. surface area (ESA)
    e. thickening
    e. triangle
    e. tube
    e. vegetation
    e. ventriculotomy (ECV)
    e. wire
endocardial-to-endocardial resection
endocardiographic amplifier (EA)
endocardiography
endocarditic
endocarditis
    abacterial thrombotic e.
    acute bacterial e. (ABE)
    acute infective e. (AIE)
    atypical verrucous e.
    bacteria-free stage of bacterial e.
    bacterial e. (BE, BEC)
    e. benigna
    bioprosthetic e.
    cachectic e.
    e. chordalis
    chronic e.
    constrictive e.
    culture-negative e.
    enterococcal e.
    experimental enterococcal e. (EEE)
    fungal e.
    gonococcal e.
    gram-negative e.
    green strep e.
    Haemophilus e.
    infectious e.
    infective e. (IE)
    isolated parietal e.
    e. lenta
    Libman-Sacks e.
    Löffler parietal fibroplastic e.
    malignant e.
    marantic e.
    methicillin-sensitive right-sided e.
    mitral valve e.
    multivalve e.
    mural e.
    mycotic e.
    native valve e. (NVE)
    native valve fibroplastic e.
    nonbacterial thrombotic e. (NBTE)
    nonbacterial verrucous e.
    noninfective valve e.

nosocomial e.
pacemaker e.
parietal e.
e. parietalis fibroplastica (EPF)
plastic e.
polypous e.
postoperative e.
prosthetic infectious e. (PIE)
prosthetic valve e. (PVE)
pulmonic e.
rheumatic e.
rickettsial e.
right-sided e.
septic e.
staphylococcal e.
streptococcal e.
subacute bacterial e. (SBE)
subacute infective e.
syphilitic e.
terminal e.
thrombotic e.
tricuspid valve e.
tuberculous e.
ulcerative e.
valvular e.
vegetative e.
verrucous e.
endocardium (Endo)
Biosense revascularization approach
for viable e. (BRAVE)
echo-bright e.
mural e.
EndoCPB catheter
endocrine
e. disorder
e. system
endocytosis
endoderm
endodermal cell
endofibrosis
end-of-life (EOL)
e.-o.-l. care
e.-o.-l. pacemaker
e.-o.-l. rate
endogenous
e. digitalis-like natriuretic factor
(EDNF)
e. fibrinolysis
e. kinin
e. lipid
endoglin gene

endograft
aortic e.
Prograft bifurcated e.
Talent bifurcated e.
Vanguard e.
Endoknot suture
endolaryngeal
endolaser venous therapy (ELVT)
endoleak type I–IV
endolumen enlargement
EndoLumina illuminated bougie
endoluminal
e. reconstruction of basilar artery
fusiform aneurysm
e. stent graft
e. stenting
endolymphatic
e. hypertension
endolymphaticus
saccus e.
endolysosome
**endomethylene tetrahydrophthalic acid
(EMTA)**
endomyocardial
African e.
e. biopsy (EMB)
e. disease
e. fibroelastosis
e. fibrosis (EMF)
endomyocarditis
endomysial
e. collagen
e. fibrosis
endomysium
end-on aortogram
endonuclease
restriction e.
Endopath EZ45 thoracic linear stapler
endopeptidase
e. inhibitor
neutral e. (NEP)
endopericarditis
endoperimyocarditis
endoperoxide steal
endophthalmitis
endoplasmic reticulum
endopolyploidy
endoprosthesis
Wallgraft tracheobronchial e.
endorphin
Endosaph vein harvest system

E

NOTES

endoscope

    lung imaging fluorescence e. (LIFE)

    Messerklinger e.

    velopharyngeal e.

endoscopic

    e. biopsy

    e. coronary artery bypass graft (E-CABG)

    e. saphenous vein harvesting (ESVH)

    e. tissue culture (ETC)

    e. ultrasound-guided fine-needle aspiration (EUS-FNA)

    e. variceal sclerotherapy (EVS)

    e. vascular surgery (ESVS)

EndoSonics IVUS/balloon dilation catheter

Endotak

    E. C lead transvenous catheter

    E. C tripolar transvenous lead

    E. DSP lead

    E. lead defibrillator

    E. lead system

    E. pacemaker

    E. Picotip defibrillation lead

    E. Reliance lead

endotension

endothelial

    e. cell activation

    e. cell degeneration

    e. constitutive nitric oxide synthase (ecNOS, eNOS)

    e. denudation

    e. derived relaxation factor

    e. dysfunction

    e. nitric oxide synthase (eNOS)

    e. permeability

    e. purinoceptors

endothelial-dependent arterial dilation

endothelialization

endothelin (ET)

    e. A, B receptor

    e. antagonist

    big e.

    circulating e.

    myocardial e.

endothelin-1 (ET-1)

    e.-1 immunoreactivity

endothelin-2 (ET-2)

    plasma e.-2

endothelin-3 (ET-3)

endothelin-converting enzyme

endothelioma

endothelium

    bovine aortic e. (BAE)

    coronary microvessel e.

    nonfenestrated e.

endothelium-dependent

    e.-d. dilator response to substance P

    e.-d. vascular relaxation

    e.-d. vasodilation

endothelium-derived

    e.-d. hyperpolarizing factor (EDHF)

    e.-d. nitric oxide (EDNO)

    e.-d. relaxing factor (EDRF)

endothelium-independent vascular relaxation

endothelium-leukocyte adhesion molecule (E-LAM)

endothelium-mediated relaxation

endotoxemia

endotoxic sepsis

endotoxin

    bacterial e.

    circulating bacterial e.

    e. shock

endotracheal

    e. aspirate (EA)

    e. cardiac output monitor (ECOM)

    e. cardiac output monitoring (ECOM)

    e. intubation

    e. tube (ETT)

    e. tube cuff

Endotrol

    E. endotracheal tube

    E. tracheal tube

endovascular

    e. aortic graft (EAG)

    e. graft

    e. irradiation (EI)

    e. radiation therapy

    e. radiofrequency catheter ablation

    e. repair (EVR)

    e. stent grafting

endoventricular circular patch plasty

EndoWrist instrument

endpoint

    hemodynamic e.

    therapeutic e.

end-pressure artifact

endralazine

Endrate

end-stage

    e.-s. heart failure

    e.-s. liver disease (ESLD)

    e.-s. lung

    e.-s. renal disease (ESRD)

end-systole (ES)

end-systolic

    e.-s. circumferential wall stress

    e.-s. count (ESC)

    e.-s. dimension (ESD)

    e.-s. elastance

e.-s. force-length relationship (ESFL)
e.-s. force-velocity index
e.-s. left ventricular pressure
e.-s. left ventricular stress (ESS)
e.-s. length (ESL)
e.-s. murmur
e.-s. pressure (ESP)
e.-s. pressure-volume relation
e.-s. pressure-volume relationship (ESPVR)
e.-s. stress (ESS)
e.-s. stress-dimension relation
e.-s. volume (ESV)
e.-s. volume index (ESVI)
e.-s. volume ratio
e.-s. wall stress (ESWS)

end-tidal
e.-t. capnometry
e.-t. carbon dioxide ($ETCO_2$)
e.-t. sample

end-to-end
end-to-side suture
Enduron
Enduronyl Forte
enema
barium e.
Kayexalate e.
sodium polystyrene sulfonate e.

Enemol
energetic dynamic cardiac insufficiency (EDCI)
energometer
energy
blood flow e. (BFE)
color Doppler e. (CDE)
e. expenditure
internal e.
minimum defibrillation e. (MDE)
myocardial e.
e. production
radiofrequency e.
e. resolution
e. supply

Enertrax 7100 pacemaker
e-Net headpiece
enflurane
enforcer
Enforcer SDS coronary stent
engineering
tissue e.

Englert forceps

engorgement
venous e.

enhanced
e. atrioventricular conduction (EAVC)
e. atrioventricular nodal (EAVN)
e. automaticity
e. external counterpulsation (EECP)
e. external counterpulsation unit
e. green fluorescent protein (eGFP)
e. oxygenation
E. Torque 8F guiding catheter

enhancement
detection e.
leading edge e.
mean contrast e.
personalized aerobics for cardiovascular e.

enhancer
aerosol cloud e. (ACE)
universal aerosol cloud e.

enhancing lesion
enlarged heart (EH, eh)
enlargement
biatrial e.
cardiac e. (CE)
compensatory vessel e.
end-diastolic wall e.
endolumen e.
left atrial e. (LAE, LAF)
left ventricular e. (LVE)
panchamber e.
right atrial e. (RAE)
right ventricular e. (RVE)

Enlon injection
eNO, ENO
exhaled nitric oxide
expired nitric oxide

enolase
neuron-specific e. (NSE)

eNOS (*var. of* ecNOS)
endothelial nitric oxide synthase

enoxacin
enoxaparin
e. bridge therapy
e. sodium

enoximone
EnSite
E. 3000 electrophysiology workstation
E. multielectrode array transvenous catheter

E

NOTES

EnSite *(continued)*
    E. NavX intracardiac
      nonfluoroscopic navigation system
    E. 3000 system
Entamoeba
    E. dispar
    E. histolytica
entangling technique
enteral
    e. nutrition
    e. tube feeding
enteric
    e. cytopathogenic human orphan
      (ECHO)
    e. cytopathogenic human orphan
      virus
    e. fistula
    e. gram-negative bacillus
enteric-coated aspirin
enteroadherent
enteroaggregative
Enterobacter
    E. cloacae
    E. pneumonia
Enterobacteriaceae
enterococcal endocarditis
Enterococcus
    E. faecalis
    E. faecium
enterococcus, pl. **enterococci**
    vancomycin-resistant e.
enterocolitica
    Yersinia e.
enterocolitis
enterocytopathogenic human orphan
  (ECHO)
enterohemorrhagic
enteroinvasive
enteropathy
    protein-losing e. (PLE)
enterotoxin
    Escherichia coli e.
enteroviral
enterovirus
Entity pacemaker
entocyte
entoplasm
entoptic pulse
entrained beat
entrainment
    concealed e.
    epicardial e.
    high air flow with oxygen e.
      (HAFOE)
    e. mapping
    oxygen e.
    e. of tachycardia
    transient e.
    e. with concealed fusion

entrance
    e. block
    e. wound
entrapment
    lung e.
Entree
    E. thoracoscopy cannula
    E. thoracoscopy trocar
Entrophen
entropy
    approximate e. (ApEn)
entry
    air e.
    e. site
    transsarcolemmal calcium e.
Entuss-D Liquid
ENT wash
enucleation of subaortic stenosis
envelope
    aortic e.
    dagger-shaped aortic e.
    flow e.
    maximal flow-volume e. (MFVL)
    spectral e.
env gene
environment
    normobaric e.
    pharmacologic e.
environmental
    e. allergen
    e. change
    e. irritant
    e. lung disease
    e. stress cracking
    e. survey
    e. tobacco smoke (ETS)
Enzygnost
    E. F1+2 ELISA kit
    E. TAT complex kit
    E. TAT ELISA assay
enzymatic
    e. deficiency
    e. infarct size
enzyme
    allosteric modification of e.
    angiotensin-converting e. (ACE)
    angiotensin-converting e. DD (ACE-
      DD)
    angiotensin-converting e. ID (ACE-
      ID)
    angiotensin-converting e. II (ACE-
      II)
    angiotensin I-converting e.
    Bacillus subtilis e.
    beta AR kinase1 e.
    cardiac e.
    COX-1, 2 e.
    elevation of e.
    endothelin-converting e.

fibrinolytic e.
glycolytic e.
e. immunoassay (EIA)
lysosomal e.
mitochondrial e.
pancreatic e.
phosphodiesterase e.
proteolytic e.
pulmonary angiotensin I
    converting e.
sarcoplasmic reticulum-associated
    glycolytic e.'s
enzyme-induced damage
enzyme-linked
e.-l. immunosorbent assay (ELISA)
e.-l. immunospot (ELISPOT)
EOA
esophageal obturator airway
EOG
electrooculogram
electrooculograph
electrooculography
EOL
end-of-life
eosin
hematotylin and e. (H&E)
eosinophil
e. by-product
e. cationic protein (ECP)
e. chemotactic factors of
    anaphylaxis (ECF-A)
e. recruitment
eosinophilia
nonallergic rhinitis with e.
    (NARES)
peripheral blood e.
prolonged pulmonary e.
pulmonary infiltrate with e. (PIE)
pulmonary infiltration with e. (PIE)
tropical pulmonary e.
eosinophilia-myalgia syndrome (EMS)
eosinophilic
e. chemotaxis
e. effusion
e. endomyocardial disease
e. granuloma (EG)
e. granulomatosis
e. lung
e. lung syndrome
e. pneumonia
e. pneumonitis

e. pneumonopathy
e. pulmonary syndrome
EP
electrophysiology
extreme pressure
    Heartwave EP
    EP mapping
EPA
eicosapentaenoic acid
Epanutin
EPAP
expiratory positive airway pressure
eparterial bronchus
EPC
extent of pleural carcinomatosis score
EPCA
external pressure circulatory assistance
EPCS
emergency portocaval shunt
E-peak velocity
EPF
endocarditis parietalis fibroplastica
EPH
edema-proteinuria-hypertension
ephedrine
aminophylline, amobarbital, and e.
    e. sulfate
ephelis, pl. ephelides
nevi, atrial myxoma, myxoid
    neurofibromas, and ephelides
    (NAME)
ephemeral pneumonia
EPI
echo planar imaging
epiaortic echocardiography
**epibronchial right pulmonary artery
syndrome**
epicardial
e. arterial spasm
e. artery patency
e. cardiac border
e. coronary artery
e. coronary artery disease
e. defibrillator patch
e. entrainment
e. fat
e. fat pad sign
e. fat tag
e. flow
e. flow conductance
e. lead
e. pacing

E

NOTES

epicardial (*continued*)
    e. radiofrequency atrial lesion
    e. radiofrequency catheter ablation
    e. sock electrode
    e. vessel patency
epicardial-mesenchymal transformation
epicardiectomy
epicardin gene
epicardium
    left ventricular e.
Epicoccum nigrum
epidemic capillary bronchitis
epidermal growth factor
epidermidis
    Staphylococcus e.
epidermoid carcinoma
epidural
    e. analgesia
    e. spinal cord (ESC)
Epifrin
epigastric bruit
epiglottic cartilage
epiglottidis
epiglottis
epiglottitis
epiglottoplasty
epi-illuminated microscope
epilepsy
epilepticus
    status e.
epimyocarditis
epimysium
epinephrine
    aortic e. (AoE)
    aortic arch e. (AoArE)
    buffered lidocaine with e. (BLE)
    high-dose e.
    racemic e.
EpiPen
epiphenomena of dissection
epirubicin
episode
    presyncopal e.
    transient ischemic e. (TIE)
    vasovagal e.
    ventilation e.
episodic
    e. dyspnea
    e. hypertension
Epistat double balloon catheter
epistaxis
epistenocardiac pericarditis
epistenocardica
    pericarditis e.
epithelia (*pl. of* epithelium)
epithelial
    e. cell
    e. lining fluid (ELF)

    e. mucin
    e. 5′-nucleotide receptor
epithelial-mucus attachment
epithelioid
    e. hemangioendothelioma
    e. mesothelioma
epithelium, pl. **epithelia**
    ciliated e.
    human airway e.
    pulmonary e.
    sloughed bronchial e.
epitope
epituberculous infiltration
Epivir
eplerenone
Epogen
epoprostenol
    e. sodium
    e. sodium for injection
epoxyeicosatrienoic acid
epoxy resin
EPP
    equal-pressure point
    extrapleural pneumonectomy
Eppendorf catheter
eprosartan
EPS
    early progressing stroke
epsilon wave
EPSS
    E point to septal separation
Epstein-Barr
    E.-B. nuclear antigen (EBNA)
    E.-B. virus (EBV)
Epstein disease
EPT-1000 XP cardiac ablation system
eptacog alfa activated
ePTFE
    expanded polytetrafluoroethylene
    ePTFE graft
    ePTFE vascular suture
eptifibatide
Epworth sleepiness scale (ESS)
equal-pressure point (EPP)
equation
    ACSM regression e.
    alveolar-air e.
    American College of Sports
      Medicine regression e.
    Bernoulli e.
    Bloch e.
    Bohr e.
    Brunelli e.
    Carter e.
    continuity e.
    Doppler continuity e.
    Eagle e.
    Einthoven e.
    Fick e.

Ford e.
Framingham e.
Friedewald e.
Gorlin and Gorlin e.
Hagenbach extension of
  Poiseuille e.
Harris-Benedict e.
Henderson-Hasselbalch e.
Navier-Stokes e.
Nernst e.
Poiseuille e.
regression e.
Riley-Cournand e.
Rodrigo e.
Rohrer e.
Siri e.
Starling e.
Teichholz e.
Torricelli orifice e.
equator of cell
equi
  Rhodococcus e.
equilibrate
equilibration
equilibrium
  e. image
  e. multigated radionuclide
    ventriculography
  e. radionuclide angiocardiography
    (ERNA)
  e. radionuclide angiography
    (ERNA)
  voltage e.
equine rabies immunoglobulin (ERIG)
Equinox
  E. digital EEG
  E. digital EEG system
  E. EEG acquisition device
  E. occlusion balloon system
equiphasic complex
equipment
  Angiostar Plus vascular imaging e.
  Austin Medical E. (A.M.E.)
  Heart Aide Ezd noninvasive
    monitoring e.
equipotency
equipotent
equistenotic plaque
equivalency
  left main e.
equivalent
  Abell-Kendall e.

anginal e.
metabolic e.
right anterior oblique e.
ventilation e.
ventilatory e.
equol
equuli
  Actinobacillus e.
ER
  early repolarization
  ejection rate
    VoSpire ER
ERA
  echo record access
    ERA 300 dual-chamber pacing
      system analyzer
ERAF
  early recurrence of atrial fibrillation
ER alpha
  estrogen receptor alpha
Erb
  E. area
  E. atrophy
  limb-girdle dystrophy of E.
  E. point
Erbe cryoprobe
Erben reflex
ER beta
  estrogen receptor beta
ERBF
  effective renal blood flow
Erb-Goldflam disease
erbium:YAG laser
erbumine
  perindopril e.
Erdheim
  E. cystic medial necrosis
  E. cystic medial necrosis of aorta
  E. disease
  medionecrosis aortae idiopathica E.
erect diastolic blood pressure (EDBP)
erectile
  e. dysfunction
  e. effect
Ergamisol
Ergoline bicycle ergometer
ergometer
  Bosch ERG 500 e.
  cycle e.
  Ergoline bicycle e.
  Ergometrics ER 900 e.
  Gould-Godart type 18070 e.

E

NOTES

259

ergometer *(continued)*
>Lode BV Excalibur braked cycle e.
>Monark bicycle e.
>pedal-mode e.
>Siemens-Elema AG bicycle e.
>Tunturi EL400 bicycle e.

Ergometrics ER 900 ergometer
ergometry
>arm cycle e.
>bicycle e.
>cycle e.
>supine bicycle e.

ergonomic vascular access needle (EVAN)
ergonovine
>e. challenge
>e. echocardiography
>e. infusion
>e. injection
>e. maleate
>e. maleate provocation angina
>e. provocation test

ergonovine-induced
>e.-i. coronary vasospasm
>e.-i. spasm

ergoreceptor
>muscle e.

ergoreflex
ergot alkaloid
ergotamine
>e. derivative

ERI
>elective replacement indicator
>electric replacement indicator

Erie System
ERIG
>equine rabies immunoglobulin
>ERIG serum

ERK
>extracellularly responsive kinase
>extracellular-regulated kinase

Erlanger sphygmomanometer
ERNA
>early return to normal activities
>equilibrium radionuclide angiocardiography
>equilibrium radionuclide angiography
>ERNA after acute myocardial infarction

Erni sign
ERO
>effective regurgitant orifice

erosion
>intimal e.
>spark e.

erosive
>e. esophagitis
>e. reflux

ERP
>effective refractory period

ERPLV
>effective refractory period of left ventricle

ERT
>estrogen replacement therapy

ertapenem sodium
eruptive xanthoma
ERV
>expiratory reserve volume

Erwinia
Erybid
Eryc Oral
EryPed Oral
Erysipelothrix
Ery-Tab Oral
erythema
>e. marginatum
>e. migrans
>e. multiforme
>e. nodosum
>palmar e.

erythematosus
>disseminated lupus e.
>drug-induced lupus e. (DILE)
>lupus e. (LE)
>systemic lupus e. (SLE)

erythematous maculopapular rash
erythrityl tetranitrate
erythroblastosis fetalis
Erythrocin Oral
erythrocyte
>e. protoporphyrin
>e. sedimentation rate (ESR)

erythrocytosis
erythroderma
erythrogenin
erythromelalgia
erythromycin
>e. and sulfisoxazole
>systemic e.

erythropheresis
erythropoiesis
erythropoietin
>gene-activated e.
>plasma e.

Eryzole Oral
ES
>ejection sound
>end-systole
>extrasystole
>ES 300-Cardiac T ELISA troponin T immunoassay system

ESA
>endocardial surface area

ESAT-6 protein *mycobacterium tuberculosis*

ESC
    end-systolic count
    epidural spinal cord
escalator
    mucociliary e.
escape
    e. beat
    e. impulse
    e. interval
    junctional e.
    nodal e.
    e. pacemaker
    e. rhythm
    vagal e.
    ventricular e.
    e. ventricular contraction
escape-capture bigeminy
***Escherichia coli* enterotoxin**
Escherich test
ESCN
    electrolyte and steroid cardiopathy with
      necrosis
E-Scope
ESD
    end-systolic dimension
ESE
    exercise stress echocardiography
E-selectin cell adhesion molecule
ESFL
    end-systolic force-length relationship
Esimil
ESL
    end-systolic length
ESLD
    end-stage liver disease
ESM
    ejection systolic murmur
Esmarch
    E. ball
    E. bandage
    E. tourniquet
esmolol hydrochloride
esophagagram
esophagalgia
esophageae
    glandulae e.
esophageal
    e. achalasia
    e. adventitious breath sounds
    e. angina
    e. A-ring
    e. atresia

    e. bougienage
    e. branch
    e. branch of left gastric artery
    e. branch of thoracic aorta
    e. branch of vagus nerve
    e. B-ring
    e. cardiogram
    e. combination tube (ETC)
    e. constriction
    e. contraction ring
    e. detection device (EDD)
    e. dilation
    e. dysmotility
    e. ECG
    e. echocardiography
    e. electrocardiography
    e. gland
    e. hiatus
    e. lead
    e. lumen
    e. lung
    e. manometry
    e. motility
    e. mucosa
    e. nervous plexus
    e. obturator airway (EOA)
    e. opening
    e. perforation
    e. pill electrode
    e. prosthesis
    e. reflux
    e. rupture
    e. sling procedure
    e. spasm
    e. speech
    e. sphincter
    e. stricture
    e. tamponade
    e. temperature
    e. transit time
    e. varices
    e. vein
    e. web
**esophageal-directed pressure support
(EDPS)**
esophageales
    rami e.
    venae e.
esophagectomy
esophagei
    rami e.

E

NOTES

esophageus
    hiatus e.
    plexus nervosus e.
esophagi (*pl. of* esophagus)
esophagism
    hiatal e.
esophagismus
esophagitis
    corrosive e.
    e. dissecans superficialis
    erosive e.
    infectious e.
    monilial e.
    peptic e.
    reflux e.
esophagogastric
    e. junction
    e. orifice
    e. tamponade
    e. tube airway (EGTA)
    e. vestibule
esophagomyotomy
    Heller e.
esophagoplasty
    Belsey e.
    Grondahl e.
esophagoplication
esophagorespiratory fistula
esophagosalivary reflex
esophagoscope
    Foregger rigid e.
    Jesberg e.
    Lell e.
    Schindler e.
esophagoscopy
    fiberoptic e.
esophagospasm
esophagotracheal
esophagram
    barium e.
esophagus, pl. esophagi
    abdominal part of e.
    Barrett e.
    brusque dilatation of e.
    candy-cane e.
    cardiac glands of e.
    cervical part of e.
    muscular coat of e.
    nutcracker e.
    pars abdominalis esophagi
    pars cervicalis esophagi
    pars thoracica esophagi
    suspensory ligament of e.
    thoracic e.
    thoracic part of e.
    tunica mucosa esophagi
    tunica muscularis esophagi
ESP
    early systolic paradox

    effective systolic pressure
    end-systolic pressure
        ESP radiation reduction examination
        gloves
Esprit ventilator
esprolol
    e. hydrochloride
    e. plus sildenafil citrate
ESPVR
    end-systolic pressure-volume relationship
ESR
    erythrocyte sedimentation rate
ESRD
    end-stage renal disease
ESS
    end-systolic left ventricular stress
    end-systolic stress
    Epworth sleepiness scale
    European Stroke Scale
    circumferential ESS
essential
    e. asthma
    e. bradycardia
    e. brown induration of lung
    e. hemoptysis
    e. hypercholesterolemia (EHC)
    e. hypertension (EH, EHT)
    e. pulmonary hemosiderosis
    e. tachycardia
    e. thrombocytopenia
EST
    exercise stress test
    expression sequence tagged
estazolam
ester
    cholesterol e.
    N^G-nitro-L-arginine methyl e. (L-
      NAME)
Estes
    E. ECG criteria
    E. point system
    E. score
Estes-Romhilt ECG point-score system
estimated
    e. blood volume (EBV)
    e. Fick method
    e. MET
Estlander operation
estradiol
estramustine
estrogen
    conjugated equine e. (CEE)
    e. and medroxyprogesterone
    e. receptor alpha (ER alpha)
    e. receptor beta (ER beta)
    e. replacement therapy (ERT)
    e. replacement for women with
      coronary artery disease (EWA)
estrone

ESV
 end-systolic volume
ESVH
 endoscopic saphenous vein harvesting
ESVI
 end-systolic volume index
ESVS
 endoscopic vascular surgery
ESWS
 end-systolic wall stress
eszopiclone
ET
 ejection time
 endothelin
 exercise test
 exercise treadmill
ET-1
 endothelin-1
ET-2
 endothelin-2
ET-3
 endothelin-3
ETA
 ethionamide
etanercept
ETC
 endoscopic tissue culture
 esophageal combination tube
ETc
 corrected ejection time
Etch-on-a-Tube
 Photo-Mask and E.-o.-a-T.
  (PMEOAT)
ETCO$_2$
 end-tidal carbon dioxide
 ETCO$_2$ multigas analyzer
 sidestream ETCO$_2$
ETFE
 ethylene tetrafluoroethylene
ETFVL
 exercise tidal flow-volume loop
ethacrynic acid
Ethalloy needle
ethambutol hydrochloride
ethamivan
Ethamolin injection
ethane
 exhaled e.
ethanol (EtOH)
 selective septal branch injection
  of e.

ethanolamide
 arachidonyl e.
ethanolamine
 aminoethyl e.
 e. oleate
ethaverine hydrochloride
Ethavex-100
ether
 bis(chloromethyl) e.
 e. bronchitis
 e. pneumonia
 e. test
Ethibond suture
Ethicon Endopath EZ45 stapler
ethidium bromide
ethionamide (ETA)
ethmozin
Ethmozine
ethoxysclerol
ethyl alcohol
ethylene
ethylenediamine
 theophylline e.
ethylenediaminetetraacetic
 e. acid (EDTA)
 e. acid disodium salt
ethylene tetrafluoroethylene (ETFE)
ethylnorepinephrine hydrochloride
Etibi
etilefrine
etiology
 chest pain of unknown e. (CPUE)
etiopathogenesis
E-to-A change
E-to-F slope
EtOH
 ethanol
etomidate
Etopophos
etoposide
 Adriamycin, cyclophosphamide, e.
  (ACE)
 carboplatin, e. (CE)
 cisplatin, e. (PE)
 cisplatin, vincristine, doxorubicin, e.
  (CODE)
 e. phosphate
ETO Sleuth
e-TRAIN 110 AngioJet catheter
ETS
 environmental tobacco smoke

E

NOTES

ETT
- endotracheal tube
- exercise tolerance test
- exercise treadmill test

eucapneic
- e. voluntary hyperventilation

eucapnic

Eudal-SR

Euflex

euglobin clot lysis (ECL)

euglobulin
- e. clot assay (ECT)
- e. clot lysis time

euglycemia

euglycemic
- e. glucose clamp
- e. hyperinsulinemic glucose clamp test

eugonic

eukaryon

eukaryosis

eukaryote

Eulexin

eunuchoid voice

eupaverin

eupnea

Euro-Collins
- E.-C. multiorgan perfusion kit
- E.-C. solution

Europe
- Cardiovascular and Interventional Radiological Society of E. (CIRSE)

European Stroke Scale (ESS)

EUS-FNA
- endoscopic ultrasound-guided fine-needle aspiration

Eustace Smith murmur

eustachian
- e. ridge
- e. valve

eusystole

eusystolic

eutectic mixture of local anesthetics (EMLA)

euthyroid sick syndrome

euvolemic

EV
- ejected volume

eV
- electron volt

evacuation
- pleural space e.

evagination

evaluation
- Acute Physiology, Age, Chronic Health E. (APACHE)
- anthropometric e.

- benefit e. (BET)
- confirmatory e.
- medication use e. (MUE)
- noninvasive e.
- Physical Activity Scale for the Elderly E. (PASE)

EVAN
- ergonomic vascular access needle

Evans blue

EVD
- external ventricular drainage

Eve method

even-echo rephasing

event
- acute coronary e. (ACE)
- adverse e.
- apparent life-threatening e. (ALTE)
- bronchospastic e.
- cardiac e.
- cerebral e.
- cerebrovascular e.
- coronary e.
- e. diary
- embolic e.
- hard cardiac e.
- intracardiac e.
- ischemic e.
- main adverse coronary e. (MACE)
- major adverse cardiac e. (MACE)
- nonfatal cardiac e.
- e. recorder
- e. recorder monitor
- reducing e.
- respiratory e.
- serious cardiac e. (SCE)
- sleep-disordered breathing e.
- soft e.
- transient ischemic e. (TIE)
- ventricular tachycardia e. (VTE)
- wave coronary e.

event/episode counter

event-link data system

eventrated diaphragm

eventration of diaphragm

Everest disposable inflation device

EverGrip clamp insert

eversion
- blunt e.
- cusp e.

everting mattress suture

EVG
- electroventriculography

evidence-based medicine (EBM)

EVLW
- extravascular lung water

evoked
- e. endocardial electrogram
- e. ventricular electrogram

evolution
R-Test E.
E. scanner
evolutus
Peptostreptococcus e.
evolving myocardial infarction
EVR
endovascular repair
EVRS
early ventricular repolarization syndrome
EVS
endoscopic variceal sclerotherapy
EVS vascular closure system
EWA
estrogen replacement for women with
coronary artery disease
Ewald tube
Ewart sign
E-wave
E-w. spectral velocity waveform
E-w. velocity
Ewing sign
EX
Diabetic Tussin EX
Naldecon Senior EX
Ex
Touro Ex
ex
ther ex
therapeutic exercise
ex vivo
ex vivo gene transfer
EX-2000 DeVilbiss conserver
exacerbation
infective e.
recurrent infective e.
ExacTech blood glucose meter
examination
cardiac e.
funduscopic e.
limited Doppler e.
neurologic e.
parasternal e.
supraclavicular e.
suprasternal e.
EXBF
exercise hyperemia blood flow
excavatum
pectus e.
excellence
National Institute for Clinical E.
(NICE)

Excelsior 1018 microcatheter
excessive daytime sleepiness (EDS)
exchange
air e.
alanine e.
cardiopulmonary gas e.
catheter e.
citrate e.
FFA e.
gas e.
glucose e.
glutamate e.
e. guidewire
oxygen e.
perfluorocarbon-associated gas e.
(PAGE)
pulmonary gas e.
respiratory e.
sodium-potassium e.
e. technique
e. tip deflecting wire guide handle
e. transfusion
exchanger
heat/moisture e. (HME)
Na^+/H^+ e. (NHE)
ThermoVent heat and moisture e.
excimer
e. cool laser
e. gas laser
e. laser-assisted angioplasty (ELA)
e. laser coronary angioplasty
(ECLA, ELCA)
e. laser coronary atherectomy
e. sheath
e. vascular recanalization
excision
wedge e.
excisional
e. atherectomy
e. biopsy
e. cardiac surgery
excitability
supranormal e.
excitable gap
excitation
anodal e. (AnEX)
anomalous atrioventricular e.
direct e.
premature e.
reentrant e.
supranormal e.
e. wave

E

NOTES

excitation-contraction coupling
excited dimers
excitotoxic
exclusion criteria
excrescence
    Lambl e.
excretion
    absorption, distribution, metabolism, and e. (ADME)
    eicosanoid e.
    urinary equol e.
excursion
    cusp e.
    decreased valve e.
    diaphragmatic e.
    dome e.
    dyssynchronous thoracoabdominal e.
    endocardial e.
    mitral valve e. (MVE)
    phasic e.
    posterior wall e. (PWE)
    respiratory e.
Ex-ECG
    exercise stress electrocardiography
Ex-Echo
    exercise stress echocardiography
ExEF
    ejection fraction during exercise
exercise
    aerobic e. (AEX, AEx)
    ankle e.
    bicycle e.
    Bobath e.
    breathing e.
    Buerger-Allen e.
    e. capacity
    e. cardiac power (ECP)
    cardiopulmonary e. (CPX)
    constant-workload cycle e.
    duration of e.
    dynamic e.
    e. echocardiogram (EE)
    ejection fraction during e. (ExEF)
    e. electrocardiogram
    e. electrocardiography
    e. factor
    e. hyperemia blood flow (EHBF, EXBF)
    e. hyperpnea
    e. hypertension
    e. index
    e. intolerance
    isometric e.
    isotonic e.
    e. load
    low-intensity treadmill e. (LITE)
    e. LV function
    maximal resistive e. (MRE)
    mild-intensity e.

    passive vascular e. (pavex)
    peak e.
    e. prescription
    e. pressor reflex
    e. regimen
    rehabilitation e.
    So Much Improvement with a Little E. (SMILE)
    strenuous e.
    e. stress echocardiography (ESE, Ex-Echo)
    e. stress electrocardiography (Ex-ECG)
    e. stress test (EST)
    supine e.
    sustained physical e. (SPE)
    e. termination
    e. test (ET)
    e. thallium scintigraphy
    e. thallium-201 scintigraphy
    therapeutic e. (ther ex, ther ex)
    e. tidal flow-volume loop (ETFVL)
    e. tolerance
    e. tolerance test (ETT)
    e. tomographic TI-201 imaging
    e. training in anterior myocardial infarction (EAMI)
    e. treadmill (ET)
    treadmill e. (TE)
    e. treadmill test (ETT)
    unsupported arm e. (UAE)
    upright e.
exercise-induced
    e.-i. angina
    e.-i. arrhythmia
    e.-i. asthma (EIA)
    e.-i. bronchospasm (EIB)
    e.-i. dyspnea
    e.-i. fatigue
    e.-i. shortness of breath
    e.-i. silent myocardial ischemia
    e.-i. ventricular tachycardia
exerciser
exertion
    Borg rating of perceived e.
    dyspnea on e. (DOE)
    paroxysmal dyspnea on e. (PDE)
    perceived e.
    rating of perceived e. (RPE)
    shortness of breath on e. (SBE, SOBOE)
exertional
    e. angina
    e. dyspnea (ED)
    e. hypotension
    e. syncope
exfoliative dermatitis
exhalation

exhaled
    e. ethane
    e. nitric oxide (eNO, ENO)
exhaust
    diesel e.
exhaustion
    vital e.
exit
    e. block
    e. block murmur
    e. point
    e. site
    e. surgical osteosynthesis
    e. wound
exocardia
exocardial murmur
exogenous
    e. lipid
    e. lipid pneumonia
    e. obesity
    e. substrate
exon
exophthalmica
    tachycardia e.
exophthalmos
exophytic
exopneumopexy
exopolysaccharide
    mucoid e.
Exorcist technique
Exosurf Neonatal
exotoxin
    Pseudomonas e.
expandable access catheter (EAC)
expanded
    e. polytetrafluoroethylene (ePTFE)
    e. polytetrafluoroethylene vascular
      graft
expander
    blood e.
    blood volume e. (BVE)
    Hespan plasma volume e.
    hetastarch plasma e.
    plasma volume e.
    PMT AccuSpan tissue e.
    E. stent
expansion
    infarct e.
    paradoxical systolic e. (PSE)
    stent e.
    volume e.

expectorant
    Balminil E.
    Benylin E.
    Calmylin E.
    classic e.
    Codafed E.
    Decohistine E.
    Dihistine E.
    liquifying e.
    Nucofed Pediatric E.
    Phenhist E.
    Ru-Tuss E.
expectorated sputum volume
expectoration
    prune juice e.
    sputum e.
expedited recovery program
expenditure
    energy e.
    resting energy e. (REE)
experiment
    Müller e.
    Weber e.
experimental enterococcal endocarditis (EEE)
expiration
    duration of e. (T_E)
    prolongation of e.
expiratory
    e. airflow
    e. center
    e. dyspnea
    e. flow rate
    e. grunt
    e. to inspiratory (E:I)
    e. murmur
    e. positive airway pressure (EPAP)
    e. reserve volume (ERV)
    e. resistance
    e. retard
    e. rhonchi
    e. tidal flow
    e. time (T_E)
    e. trapping of air
    e. view
    e. wheezing
expired
    e. air collection
    e. gas
    e. nitric oxide (eNO, ENO)
expirograph
    Godart e.

E

NOTES

explant
explanted heart
Explorer 360-degree rotational
  diagnostic EP catheter
exploring electrode
Expo diagnostic catheter
exposure
  airway, breathing, circulation,
    disability, e. (ABCDE)
  allergen e.
  alternobaric e.
  chemical e.
  cobalt e.
  cold e.
  heptanal occupational e.
  hyperbaric e.
  hypobaric e.
  toxin e.
  workplace e.
Express
  E. balloon
  E. PTCA catheter
expression
  adenovirus-based phospholamban-
    antisense e.
  Bcl-2 e.
  CMV IE-2 gene e.
  cytokine e.
  ecNOS gene e.
  fibroblast growth factor e.
  gene e.
  P-selectin e.
  e. sequence tagged (EST)
expressive aphasia
expulsive coughing
exsanguinate
exsanguination protocol
exsanguinotransfusion
exsorption
extended
  e. aortic root replacement (EARR)
  e. collection device
  e. field radiation (EFR)
extended-release niacin/lovastatin
extender
  Taq e.
extension
  anterior mitral leaflet e.
  infarct e.
  knee e.
  Linx guidewire e.
  PSG LOC guidewire e.
  venous e. (VE)
Extentabs
  Quinidex E.
extent of pleural carcinomatosis score
  (EPC)

external
  e. branch of superior laryngeal
    nerve
  e. cardiac compression (ECC)
  e. cardiac massage (ECM)
  e. cardiac pressure (ECP)
  e. cardiopulmonary resuscitation
    (ECPR)
  e. cardioversion (ECV)
  e. cardioverter-defibrillator (ECD)
  e. carotid (EC)
  e. carotid artery (ECA)
  e. chest wall oscillation
  e. defibrillator
  e. elastic lamina (EEL)
  e. elastic lamina area
  e. elastic membrane (EEM)
  e. electric cardioversion
  e. grid
  e. high-output ramp pacing
  e. inflatable compressor
  e. intercostal
  e. jugular (EJ)
  e. jugular approach
  e. jugular vein
  e. mammary artery
  e. pacemaker
  e. pacemaker battery
  e. pressure circulatory assistance
    (EPCA)
  e. pudendal vein
  e. respiration
  e. ventricular drainage (EVD)
externum
  pericardium e.
Extra
  E. Back-up guiding catheter
  E. Sport coronary guidewire
  E. Strength Bayer Enteric 500
    Aspirin
  E. Strength Doan's
extraalveolar capillary
extracardiac
  e. cavopulmonary anastomosis
  e. murmur
  e. shunt
  e. ventriculopulmonary conduit
extracellular
  e. F-actin
  e. lipid
  e. matrix (ECM)
  e. matrix metabolism
  e. signal-regulated kinase
extracellular-like, calcium-free solution
  (ECS)
extracellularly responsive kinase (ERK)
extracellular-regulated kinase (ERK)
extracoronary
extracorporeal (EC)

e. carbon dioxide removal
e. cardiac shock wave therapy
e. circulation (ECC)
e. exchange hypothermia
e. heart
e. life support (ECLS)
E. Life Support Organization (ELSO)
e. membrane differential filtration
e. membrane oxygenation (ECMO)
e. membrane oxygenation therapy
e. membrane oxygenator
e. pump oxygenator
e. volume (ECV)

extracranial
e. carotid arterial disease (ECAD)
e. carotid disease (ECD)
e. carotid obstruction
e. Doppler sonography (ECD)
e. internal carotid disease

extracranial/intracranial (EC/IC)
e./i. bypass surgery

extract
calf lung surfactant e. (CLSE)
cell-free e.
pancreatic e.
Rauwolfia e.
shiitake mushroom e.
thyroid e.

extraction
e. atherectomy
e. atherectomy device
lactate e.
myocardial lactate e.
oxygen e.
e. reserve
transvenous catheter e.

Extractor three-lumen retrieval balloon
extraesophageal reflux
extra-fine particle dose (EFPD)
extraflexible wire
extrafusion defect
extrahepatic portal hypertension (EHPH)
extralobar
extranuclear
extraparenchymal bleeding
extrapericardial patch
extrapleural
e. air
e. apicolysis
e. catheter analgesia

e. pneumonectomy (EPP)
e. pneumothorax
e. space

extrapulmonary
e. cough
e. site
e. tuberculosis

extrapyramidal side effect
extrarenal azotemia
extrastimulation
single premature e.

extrastimulus, pl. **extrastimuli**
double ventricular e.
premature atrial e.
single e.
e. test
triple e.

extra-support guidewire
extrasystole (ES)
atrial e.
atrioventricular e. (AVE)
atrioventricular junctional escape e.
atrioventricular nodal e.
auricular e.
auriculoventricular e.
A-V junctional e.
A-V nodal e.
infranodal e.
interpolated e.
junctional e.
lower nodal e.
midnodal e.
nodal e.
premature ventricular e. (PVE)
return e.
spontaneous e.
supraventricular e. (SVC)
tip e.
upper nodal e.
ventricular e. (VE)

extrasystolic beat
extrathoracic
e. airway dysfunction
e. airway obstruction
e. neoplasm
e. rale
e. soft tissue
e. tumor

extratracheal
extravasation
plasma e.

E

NOTES

extravascular
    e. granulomatous feature
    e. lung water (EVLW)
Extreme II peripheral excimer laser catheter
extreme pressure (EP)
extremis
    in e.
extremitas anterior lienis
extremity
    elevation pallor of e.
    e. ischemia
    mottling of e.'s
ExtreSafe phlebotomy device
extrinsic
    e. allergic alveolitis
    e. asthma
    e. compression
    e. factor
    e. force
extrusion
    Kensey rotation atherectomy e.
extubation time
exuberant granulation tissue (EGT)

exudate
    cotton-wool e.
    fibrinous e.
    fluffy cotton-wool e.
exudation
    plasma protein e.
exudativa
    bronchiolitis e.
exudative
    e. bronchiolitis
    e. bronchitis
    e. empyema
    e. pleural effusion
    e. pleurisy
    e. tuberculosis
eyeball compression reflex
eyeball-heart reflex
eyeless needle
EZ45 thoracic linear cutter
ezetimibe
EZ Hold manual compression device
Ezide

F, Fr
    French
        F point of cardiac apex pulse
        F wave
6-F
        6-F Angio-Seal
        6-F Judkins catheter
7F
        7F extended-curve thermistor
          catheter
        7F fused-tip catheter
        7F mapping catheter
f
    respiratory frequency
        f wave
        f wave of jugular venous pulse
FA
    femoral artery
Fab
    fragment antigen-binding
        c7 E3 Fab
        chimeric-7E3 Fab
        digoxin immune Fab
        digoxin-specific Fab
        Fab fragment
        m7E3 Fab
FABF
    femoral artery blood flow
FABP
    fatty acid binding protein
fabric baffle
Fabry disease
FAC
    femoral arterial cannulation
    fractional area change
FACC
    Fellow of the American College of
    Cardiologists
face
        en bloc f.
        moon f.
        f. shield
        f. squeeze
        transverse artery of f.
        f. validity
facet
        clavicular f.
        inferior costal f.
        superior costal f.
        transverse costal f.
facial
        f. barotrauma
        f. canal
        f. diplegia

        f. droop
        f. vein
facies
        f. anterior cordis
        aortic f.
        f. articularis
        Corvisart f.
        f. costalis pulmonis
        cushingoid f.
        f. diaphragmatica
        f. diaphragmatica cordis
        ecchymotic f.
        elfin f.
        f. inferior cordis
        f. interlobares pulmonis
        f. medialis pulmonis
        f. mediastinalis pulmonis
        mitral f.
        f. mitralis
        mitrotricuspid f.
        f. pulmonalis dextra/sinistra cordis
        f. sternocostalis cordis
facilitated
        f. angioplasty
        f. reperfusion
facility
        long-term care f.
        LTC f.
        skilled nursing f. (SNF)
facioscapulohumeral
        f. dystrophy
        f. dystrophy of Landouzy-Dejerine
FACS
    fluorescence-activated cell sorter
FACT
        FACT coronary balloon angioplasty
          catheter
F-actin
    filamentous actin
        extracellular F-actin
factitious
        f. asthma
        f. syncope
Factive
factor
        f. I (fibrinogen)
        f. II (prothrombin)
        f. III (thromboplastin)
        f. IV (calcium ions)
        f. V (proaccelerin)
        f. VI (cannot be identified)
        f. VII (proconvertin)
        f. VIII (antihemophilic f.)
        f. VIII: (porcine)
        f. VIII:C (von Willebrand f.)

F

factor *(continued)*
    f. Xa
    f. X (Stuart f. or Stuart-Prower f.)
    f. XI (plasma thromboplastin
      antecedent f.)
    f. XII (Hageman f.)
    f. XIII (fibrin stabilizing f.)
    accelerator globin blood
      coagulation f.
    AcG blood coagulation f.
    acidic fibroblast growth f. (aFGF)
    activated f. VII (FVIIa)
    activating transcription f. (ATF)
    active-site inhibited f. VIIa
    antiarteriosclerosis polysaccharide f.
      (AAPF)
    antihemophilic f. (recombinant)
    atrial natriuretic f. (ANF)
    f. B
    basic fibroblast growth f. (bFGF)
    behavioral f.
    carbon monoxide transfer f.
      (TLCO, TLco)
    cardiac risk f.
    Christmas f.
    classic risk f.
    clot-promoting f. (CPF)
    clotting f. (CF)
    coagulation f.
    colony-stimulating f. (CSF)
    connective tissue growth f. (CTGF)
    corticotropin-releasing f. (CRF)
    f. D
    duty f.
    endogenous digitalis-like
      natriuretic f. (EDNF)
    endothelial derived relaxation f.
    endothelium-derived
      hyperpolarizing f. (EDHF)
    endothelium-derived relaxing f.
      (EDRF)
    epidermal growth f.
    exercise f.
    extrinsic f.
    fibrin-stabilizing blood
      coagulation f.
    fibroblast growth f. (FGF)
    Fletcher f.
    genetic f.
    granulocyte/macrophage colony-
      stimulating f. (GM-CSF)
    gravitation f.
    growth f.
    f. H
    Hageman f.
    heparin-binding epidermal growth f.
    histamine release inhibitory f.
      (HRIF)
    histamine-releasing f. (HRF)

    human atrial natriuretic f. (hANF)
    hypoxia-inducible f. (HIF)
    f. III deficiency
    f. II receptor (F2R)
    insulin-like growth f. (IGF)
    intravascular procoagulant f.
    f. IX complex (human)
    keratinocyte growth f. (KGF)
    lipid risk f.
    lymphocyte chemoattractant f.
      (LCF)
    monocyte chemotactic and
      activating f. (MCAF)
    Moody friction f.
    myeloid progenitor inhibitory f.
      (MPIF)
    myocardial depressant f. (MDF)
    necrosis f.
    neurohumoral f.'s
    N-terminal proatrial natriuretic f.
    f. P
    paracrine f.
    plasma thromboplastin f. (PTF)
    platelet f. 4
    platelet activating f. (PAF)
    platelet-aggregating f.
    platelet-derived growth f. (PDGF)
    platelet-derived histamine-
      releasing f. (PDHRF)
    proatherosclerotic f.
    proatrial natriuretic f. (proANF)
    proconvertin blood coagulation f.
    psychological f.
    psychosocial f.
    recombinant human vascular
      endothelial growth f. (rhVEGF)
    Rh f.
    rheumatoid f.
    risk f.
    stem cell f. (SCF)
    Stuart-Prower f.
    tissue f.
    transforming growth f. (TGF)
    transfusion f.
    tumor necrosis f. (TNF)
    vascular endothelial growth f.
      (VEGF)
    vascular permeability f. (VPF)
    f. VII antigen (FVIIag)
    f. V Leiden coagulation defect
    f. V Leiden mutation
    von Willebrand f. (vWP)
    f. XII-kallikrein-kinin system
factor-alpha
    tumor necrosis f.-a. (TNF-alpha)
factor-beta
    transforming growth f.-b.
factor-kappa-B
    nuclear f.-k.-B (NF-kappa-B)

facultative bacteria
faecalis
>   *Alcaligenes f.*
>   *Enterococcus f.*
>   *Streptococcus f.*
faecium
>   *Enterococcus f.*
faeni
>   *Micropolyspora f.*
Fagerstrom
>   F. tolerance questionnaire (FTQ)
>   F. tolerance scale
Faget sign
Fahraeus effect
Fahr disease
FAI
>   functional aerobic impairment
failed rescue angioplasty
failing lung sign
failure
>   acute congestive heart f.
>   acute heart f.
>   acute left ventricular f. (ALVF)
>   acutely decompensated congestive heart f. (AD-CHF)
>   acute renal f.
>   acute respiratory f. (ARF)
>   advanced heart f.
>   autonomic f.
>   backward heart f.
>   bronchial stump f.
>   f. to capture
>   cardiac f. (CF)
>   cardiovascular f. (CVF)
>   central baroreflex f.
>   chronic heart f. (CHF)
>   chronic renal f.
>   chronic respiratory f. (CRF)
>   chronic ventilatory f. (CVF)
>   circulatory f.
>   cocaine-induced respiratory f. (CIRF)
>   compensated congestive heart f.
>   congestive heart f. (CHF)
>   congestive right ventricular f. (CRVF)
>   coronary f.
>   diastolic heart f.
>   early graft f. (EGF)
>   electrical f.
>   end-stage heart f.
>   florid congestive heart f.
>   forward heart f.
>   heart f. (HF)
>   hepatic f.
>   high-output heart f.
>   hypercapnic respiratory f.
>   impending respiratory f.
>   insulation f.
>   left heart f. (LHF)
>   left-sided heart f.
>   left ventricular f. (LVF)
>   living with heart f. (LIhFE)
>   low-output heart f.
>   multiple-organ f.
>   multisystem organ f. (MSOF)
>   myocardial f.
>   nonhypercapnic respiratory f.
>   NYHA classification of congestive heart f.
>   organ system f.
>   pacemaker f.
>   pacing-induced heart f.
>   peripartal heart f.
>   peripartum cardiac f. (PPCF)
>   power f.
>   primary graft f. (PGF)
>   progressive pump f.
>   pulmonary f.
>   pump f.
>   refractory congestive heart f.
>   renal f.
>   respiratory f.
>   right congestive heart f. (RCHF)
>   right heart f. (RHF)
>   right-sided heart f.
>   right ventricular f. (RVF)
>   systolic heart f.
>   tachycardia-induced heart f.
>   ventilatory f.
>   ventricular f.
faint
>   f. flow
>   f. opacification
>   f. pulmonary regurgitation
fainting
>   hysterical f.
faintness
FAK
>   focal adhesion kinase
falciparum
>   *Plasmodium f.*
Falcon
>   F. coronary catheter

F

NOTES

Falcon *(continued)*
    F. Omniflex balloon
    F. Omniflex balloon catheter
    F. Omniflex PTCA catheter
    F. single-operator exchange balloon
    catheter
fallen lung sign
falling drop
falloff
    upstroke and f.
Fallot
    F. pentalogy
    pentalogy of F.
    pink tetralogy of F.
    F. tetrad
    tetralogy of F. (Tet, tet, TF, TOF,
    TOF, T of F)
    F. tetralogy (FT)
    total repair of tetralogy of F.
    F. triad
    trilogy of F.
    F. trilogy
false
    f. aneurysmal chamber
    f. angina
    f. aortic aneurysm
    f. apex
    f. bruit
    f. cardiomegaly
    f. cardiomyopathy
    f. combined hyperlipidemia
    f. croup
    f. cyanosis
    f. dextrocardia
    f. emphysema
    f. hypercholesterolemia
    f. lumen
    f. mass
    f. negative
    f. positive
    f. tendon
    f. vocal cord
FAMA, FAMAT
    fluorescence antimembrane antibody
    fluorescent antimembrane antibody
famciclovir
familial
    f. abetalipoproteinemia
    f. amyloidosis
    f. apoA-I deficiency
    f. asphyxiant thoracic dystrophy
    f. atrial myxoma
    f. atrial myxoma syndrome
    f. atrioventricular block
    f. cholestasis syndrome
    f. chylomicronemia syndrome
    f. combined hyperlipidemia (FCHL)
    f. congenital cardiac abnormality
    (FCCA)

    f. defective apolipoprotein B (FDB)
    f. dysautonomia
    f. dysbetalipoproteinemia
    f. dyslipidemic hypertension
    f. emphysema
    f. HDL deficiency
    f. high-density-lipoprotein deficiency
    f. hypercholesterolemia (FH, FHC)
    f. hyperchylomicronemia
    f. hypertension (FH)
    f. hypertriglyceridemia (FHTG)
    f. hypertrophic cardiomyopathy
    (FHC)
    f. hypertrophic obstructive
    cardiomyopathy
    f. hypobetalipoproteinemia (FHBL)
    f. hypocalciuric hypercalcemia
    f. intracranial aneurysm
    f. Mediterranean fever
    f. multifocal fibrosclerosis
    f. nephritis
    f. paroxysmal polyserositis
    f. primary pulmonary hypertension
    (FPPH)
    f. pulmonary fibrosis
    f. recurrence
    f. tachycardia
family
    f. history of heart disease
    f. history of myocardial infarction
    signal transducer and activator of
    transcription protein f.
    STAT protein f.
family-witnessed resuscitation
Famvir
fan
    Dunham f.
Fansidar
Fansimef
Faraday cage
Fareston
far-field
    f.-f. electrogram
    f.-f. QRS complex
    f.-f. R-wave sensing
    f.-f. visualization
FARI
    filtered atrial rate interval
farmer's lung
Farr test
FAS
    fetal alcohol syndrome
Fas
    F. ligand (FasL)
    F. receptor
fascia
    pectoral f.
    f. pectoralis
    Scarpa f.

fascial layer
fascicle
    blocked f.
fascicular
    f. beat
    f. heart block
    f. tachycardia
fasciculation
fasciculoventricular Mahaim fiber
fasciotomy
Fas-Fas ligand pathway
fashion
    crisscross f.
    culotte f.
    stoichiometric f.
FasL
    Fas ligand
    FasL pathway
FAST
    flow-assisted short-term
    Fourier-acquired steady-state technique
    Frenchay Aphasia Screening Test
fast
    f. channel
    f. Fourier
    f. Fourier spectral analysis
    f. Fourier transform (FFT)
    f. low-angle shot (FLASH)
    f. pathway
    f. sodium current
    f. tissue
    f. wave sleep
Fast-Cath
    F.-C. Duo introducer
    F.-C. hemostasis introducer catheter
Fast-Fit vascular stockings
fasting
    f. blood sugar
    f. plasma lipids (FPL)
    f. plasma norepinephrine
Fast-Patch disposable
defibrillation/electrocardiographic
electrode
fast-pathway radiofrequency catheter
ablation
fat
    body f.
    dietary f.
    f. embolism
    f. embolism syndrome (FES)
    f. emulsion
    epicardial f.

    high f. (HF)
    monosaturated f.
    polyunsaturated f.
    preperitoneal f.
    trans f.
    truncal distribution of body f.
fat-absorption coefficient
fatal pulmonary embolism (FPE)
fat-free mass (FFM)
fatigue
    collagen f.
    exercise-induced f.
    inspiratory muscle f.
    respiratory muscle f.
fat-laden microphages
fatty
    f. acid
    f. acid binding protein (FABP)
    f. degeneration of heart
    f. streak
faucial branches of lingual nerve
faucium
    Mycoplasma f.
Faught sphygmomanometer
Fauvel granules
FAV
    floppy aortic valve
Favaloro
    F. proximal anastomosis clamp
    F. saphenous vein bypass graft
Favaloro-Morse rib spreader
FB
    fiberoptic bronchoscopy
FBAO
    foreign body airway obstruction
FBN1 gene
FBP
    femoral blood pressure
FBPM
    forward-backward Prony method
    FBPM spectral analysis of heart
    sounds
FC
    free cholesterol
FCCA
    familial congenital cardiac abnormality
FCF
    fetal cardiac frequency
FCHL
    familial combined hyperlipidemia
FCP
    functional conduction period

F

NOTES

Fc receptor
FDB
  familial defective apolipoprotein B
FDG
  fluorodeoxyglucose
fe
  iron
    Slow fe
fear of food syndrome
feature
    alexithymic personality f.'s
    clinical manifestation, etiologic
      factor, anatomic involvement and
      pathophysiologic f. (CEAP
      classification)
    extravascular granulomatous f.
febrile
    agglutinin f.
FEC
  forced expiratory capacity
FECG
  fetal electrocardiogram
Fechtner syndrome
FECO$_2$
  fraction of expired carbon dioxide
Federici sign
feedback
    mechanoelectrical f.
    respiratory f. (RFb)
feeder vessel
feeding
    enteral tube f.
    nasogastric tube f. (NTF)
feeleii
    Legionella f.
FEES
  fiberoptic endoscopic evaluation of
    swallowing
feet of sea water (fsw)
FEF
  forced expiratory flow
FEF$_{25-75\%}$
  mean midexpiratory flow rate
FEFmax
  maximal forced expiratory flow
Feiba VH Immuno
Feigenbaum echocardiogram
FEKG
  fetal electrocardiogram
Feldman aortic stenosis catheter
fele
    bruit de f.
    bruit de pot f.
Fell-O'Dwyer apparatus
**Fellow of the American College of
  Cardiologists (FACC)**
felodipine
    enalapril and f.

Felson
    silhouette sign of F.
felt strip
female
    f. hormone
    f. pattern obesity
Femara
Femiron
femoral
    f. approach
    f. arterial cannulation (FAC)
    f. arteriography
    f. artery (FA)
    f. artery blood flow (FABF)
    f. artery occlusion
    f. artery pressure
    f. artery thrombosis
    f. blood pressure (FBP)
    brachial, radial, f. (BRAFE)
    f. canal
    f. embolectomy
    f. embolus
    f. endarterectomy
    percutaneous f.
    f. perfusion cannula
    f. pseudoaneurysm
    f. vascular injury
    f. vein
    f. vein occlusion
    f. venous sheath
    f. venous thrombosis
    f. vessel
femoral-femoral
    f.-f. bypass
    f.-f. crossover
femoral-popliteal bypass
femoral-tibial bypass
femoral-tibial-peroneal bypass
femoris
femoroaxillary bypass
femorofemoral crossover bypass
femoropopliteal
    f. bypass
    f. stenting
femorotibial bypass
FemoStop
    F. femoral compression system
    F. inflatable pneumatic compression
      device
femtoliter (fL)
fenbufen
fence
    electron beam f.
    Kirklin f.
Fenesin DM
fenestrated
    f. Fontan operation
    f. Fontan procedure
    f. tracheostomy tube

fenestration
    aortopulmonary f.
    baffle f.
    cusp f.
fenfluramine
    f. hydrochloride
    f. and phentermine (Fen-Phen)
fenofibrate
fenoldopam mesylate
fenoprofen calcium
fenoterol
Fen-Phen
    fenfluramine and phentermine
fentanyl
Feosol
Feostat
FEP-ringed Gore-Tex vascular graft
Feratab
Fergie needle
Fergon
Ferguson needle
Fergus percutaneous introducer kit
Fer-In-Sol
Fer-Iron
Fernandez reaction
Fero-Grad 500
Ferrans and Powers Quality of Life Index, cardiac version
Ferrein cords
ferricytochrome assay
ferritin
Ferrlecit
ferrocalcinosis
    cerebrovascular f.
Ferro-Sequels
ferrous
    f. fumarate
    f. gluconate
    f. salt and ascorbic acid
    f. sulfate
    f. sulfate, ascorbic acid, and vitamin B-complex
    f. sulfate, ascorbic acid, vitamin B-complex, and folic acid
ferruginous body
FES
    fat embolism syndrome
    flame emission spectroscopy
    forced expiratory spirogram
FET
    forced expiratory time

fetal
    f. alcohol syndrome (FAS)
    f. aspiration syndrome
    f. atrial wall motion
    f. bradycardia
    f. cardiac frequency (FCF)
    f. cardiology
    f. circulation
    f. electrocardiogram (FECG, FEKG)
    f. electrocardiography
    f. heart (FH, FHT)
    f. heart frequency (FHF)
    f. heart heard (FHH)
    f. heart monitor tracing
    f. heart not heard (FHNH)
    f. heart rate (FHR)
    f. heart rate nonstress test (FHRNST)
    f. heart rhythm
    f. heart sound (FHS)
    f. heart tone (FHT)
    f. magnetocardiography (FMCG)
    f. origins hypothesis
    f. oxygenation
    f. PR interval
    f. souffle
    f. tachycardia
    f. ventricular myocyte proliferative response
    f. ventricular wall motion
fetalis
    erythroblastosis f.
    hydrops f.
fetal-type
    f.-t. PCA
    f.-t. posterior cerebral artery
fetid sputum
fetocardia
FEV
    forced expiratory volume
FEV$_1$
    forced expiratory volume in 1 second
FEVB
    frequency ectopic ventricular beat
fever
    acute rheumatic f. (ARF)
    Australian Q f.
    bird f.
    dengue f.
    desert f.
    familial Mediterranean f.
    hay f.

F

NOTES

fever *(continued)*
    hemorrhagic f.
    Jaccoud dissociated f.
    Katayama f.
    Korean hemorrhagic f.
    Lassa f.
    lung f.
    Mediterranean f.
    metal fume f. (MFF)
    Monday f.
    Omsk hemorrhagic f.
    parrot f.
    pharyngoconjunctival f.
    pneumonic f.
    polymer fume f. (PFF)
    Pontiac f.
    pulmonary f.
    Q f.
    Queensland f.
    query f.
    rabbit f.
    relapsing f.
    rheumatic f. (RF)
    Rocky Mountain spotted f.
    San Joaquin Valley f.
    scarlet f.
    septic f.
    shoddy f.
    sthenic f.
    thermic f.
    threshing f.
    typhoid f.
    valley f.
    yellow f.
    zinc fume f.

FEV/FVC
    forced expiratory volume timed to forced
      vital capacity ratio

FEV$_1$/FVC
    forced expiratory volume in 1 second to
      forced vital capacity ratio

fexofenadine hydrochloride

FF
    fibrillation-flutter

FFA
    free fatty acids
      FFA exchange

FFB
    flexible fiberoptic bronchoscopy

F-18 FDG
    fluorine-18 fluorodeoxyglucose

f-f interval

FFM
    fat-free mass

FFP
    fresh frozen plasma

FFR
    fractional flow reserve

FFR$_{myo}$
    myocardial fractional flow reserve

FFT
    fast Fourier transform
    free-floating thrombus

FGF
    fibroblast growth factor

FH
    familial hypercholesterolemia
    familial hypertension
    fetal heart

FHBL
    familial hypobetalipoproteinemia

FHC
    familial hypercholesterolemia
    familial hypertrophic cardiomyopathy

FHF
    fetal heart frequency

FHH
    fetal heart heard

FHNH
    fetal heart not heard

FHR
    fetal heart rate

FHRNST
    fetal heart rate nonstress test

FHS
    fetal heart sound

FHT
    fetal heart
    fetal heart tone

FHTG
    familial hypertriglyceridemia

FI
    fundamental imaging

fib
    fibrillation

fiber
    actin f.
    afferent nerve f.'s
    atrio-His f.
    blocking vagal afferent f.'s
    blocking vagal efferent f.'s
    Brechenmacher f.
    Dacron f.
    dietary f.
    elastic f.'s
    fasciculoventricular Mahaim f.
    His-Purkinje f.'s
    James f.'s
    Kent f.'s
    laser f.
    Mahaim f.'s
    manmade vitreous f. (MMVF)
    nodoventricular f.
    parasympathetic nerve f.'s
    pseudo-Mahaim f.
    Purkinje f.'s
    f. shortening

f. shortening velocity (V_{cf})
sinospiral f.
spindle f.
terminal Purkinje f.'s
wavy f.
fiberoptic
f. bronchoscope
f. bronchoscopy (FB, FOB)
f. catheter delivery system
f. delivery device
f. endoscopic evaluation of
swallowing (FEES)
f. esophagoscopy
f. oximeter catheter
f. pressure catheter
f. rhinoscopy
fibrate
fibremia
fibric acid
fibrillar
f. collagen
f. collagen network
f. mass of Fleming
fibrillary wave
Fibrillation
fibrillation (fib)
atrial f. (AF, AFib, At fib, Atr fib)
auricular f.
Canadian Registry of Atrial F.
(CARAF)
cardiac f.
catheter ablation of atrial f.
chronic atrial f.
chronic nonvalvular atrial f.
(CNAF)
continuous atrial f. (CAF)
dilated cardiomyopathy and atrial f.
(DCAF)
early recurrence of atrial f.
(ERAF)
focal atrial f.
idiopathic ventricular f.
inducible polymorphic ventricular f.
lone atrial f.
nonprimary ventricular f.
nonvalvular atrial f. (NVAF)
paroxysmal atrial f. (PAF, PAFIB)
pharmacological intervention in
atrial f. (PIAF)
f. potential
primary ventricular f. (PVF)
prognosis in atrial f. (PIAF)

f. rhythm
spontaneous f. (SF)
spontaneous paroxysmal atrial f.
(SPAF)
f. threshold
vagal atrial f.
ventricular f. (vent fib, VF)
ventricular tachycardia/ventricular f.
(VT/VF)
fibrillation-flutter, fibrilloflutter (FF)
atrial f.-f. (AFF)
fibrillatory wave
fibrillin-1
fibrilloflutter (*var. of* fibrillation-flutter)
Fibrimage diagnostic imaging agent
fibrin
f. bodies of pleura
f. clot
f. D-dimer
f. degradation product
f. formation
f. gel
f. glue
f. monomer (FM)
f. split product
f. thrombus
fibrinogen
f. degradation product
plasma f.
radiolabeled f.
fibrinogen-fibrin
f.-f. conversion syndrome
f.-f. degradation product
fibrinogenolysis
fibrinohematic material
fibrinoid
f. arteritis
f. change
f. degeneration
f. necrosis
fibrinolysis
endogenous f.
fibrinolytic
f. abnormality
f. agent
f. enzyme
f. medium
f. reaction
f. system
f. therapy
fibrinopeptide A, B

F

NOTES

fibrinopurulent
    f. empyema
    f. phase
fibrinous
    f. acute lobar pneumonia
    f. acute pleuritis
    f. adhesion
    f. bronchitis
    f. exudate
    f. pericarditis
    f. pleurisy
fibrin-specific antibody
fibrin-stabilizing blood coagulation factor
fibroatheroma
fibroblast
    adventitial f.
    f. growth factor (FGF)
    f. growth factor expression
    human fetal lung f. (HFL)
fibrobronchoscope
fibrobullous
fibrocalcification
fibrocalcific lesion
fibrocystic
    f. lung
    f. sarcoidosis
fibroelastoma
    papillary f. (PES)
fibroelastosis
    endocardial f. (EFE)
    endomyocardial f.
    primary endocardial f.
fibrofatty plaque
fibrogenesis
fibroid
    f. heart
    f. lung
    f. phthisis
fibroma
fibromuscular dysplasia
fibromusculoelastic lesion
fibronectin
fibroplastic
    f. cardiomyopathy
    f. disease
fibroplastica
    endocarditis parietalis f. (EPF)
fibroproliferative disease
fibrosa
    intervalvular f.
fibrosarcoma
fibrosclerosis
    familial multifocal f.
fibrosing
    f. alveolitis
    f. mediastinitis
fibrosis
    adeno-associated virus for cystic f.

    African endomyocardial f.
    amiodarone pulmonary f.
    biventricular endomyocardial f.
    bundle branch f.
    classic interstitial pneumonitis with f. (CIPF)
    cobalt-related pulmonary f.
    cystic f. (CF)
    Davies endomyocardial f.
    Davies myocardial f.
    diffuse interstitial pulmonary f.
    endocardial f.
    endomyocardial f. (EMF)
    endomysial f.
    familial pulmonary f.
    focal f.
    hard metal-related lung f.
    idiopathic alveolar f. (IAF)
    idiopathic interstitial f.
    idiopathic pulmonary f. (IPF)
    interstitial f.
    interstitial pulmonary f. (IPF)
    Löffler endocardial f.
    lung f.
    mediastinal f.
    myocardial f. (MF)
    nonspecific idiopathic pulmonary f.
    nonspecific lung f.
    parahilar f.
    parenchymal f.
    partial intermixed f.
    periarteriolar f.
    peribronchial f.
    perielectrode f.
    perimyocytic f.
    perivascular f.
    progressive interstitial pulmonary f.
    progressive massive f. (PMF)
    pulmonary f.
    radiation f.
    rejection-associated pulmonary f.
    subendocardial f.
    tropical endomyocardial f.
fibrosum
    pericardium f.
fibrosus
    anulus a.
fibrothorax
fibrotic
    f. mass
    f. scar
fibrous
    f. ball
    f. body
    f. cap
    f. cap lesion
    f. capsule of thyroid gland
    f. dysplasia
    f. dysplasia of bone

f. infiltrate
f. mediastinitis
f. pericarditis
f. pericardium
f. plaque
f. pneumonia
f. ring
f. skeleton
f. subaortic stenosis

FIC
forced inspiratory capacity

Fick
F. cardiac output
F. equation
F. oxygen method
F. principle
F. relationship
F. technique

FICO$_2$
fraction of inspired carbon dioxide

Fiedler myocarditis

field
f. cancerization
f. carcinogenesis
f. flow velocity
near f.
stippling of lung f.
f. of view (FOV)

FIF
forced inspiratory flow

fifth Korotkoff sound (K5)

fight-or-flight
f.-o.-f. reaction
f.-o.-f. response

figure-of-eight
f.-o.-e. abnormality
f.-o.-e. heart
f.-o.-e. intraatrial reentry
f.-o.-e. suture

filamentous actin (F-actin)

filariasis

Filcard vena cava filter

filiform
f. pulse
f. stenosis

filiformis
pulsus f.

filling
capillary f.
collateral f.
f. defect
diastolic f.

f. fraction
f. gallop
LAA f.
parameterized diastolic f. (PDF)
period of ventricular f.
f. pressure (FP)
rapid f.
retrograde f.
f. rumble
ventricular f.

film
absorbable gelatin f.
density-exposure relationship of f.
dirty f.
end-expiratory f.
end-inspiratory f.
f. fixer bath
f. oxygenation
f. processing
Repel-CV bioresorbable adhesion-
barrier f.
scout f.
serial cut f.'s
f. wash bath

Filmtabs
Biaxin F.'s
Rondec F.

Filoviridae virus

filter
arterial f.
bandpass f.
bidirectional four-pole Butterworth
high-pass digital f.
bird's nest vena cava f.
BTF-37 arterial blood f.
Butterworth bidirectional f.
Clear Advantage Spirometry F.
D/Flex f.
Emboshield bare wire f.
Filcard vena cava f.
Gianturco-Roehm bird's nest vena
cava f.
Greenfield IVC f.
Greenfield vena cava f.
Gunther Tulip vena cava MrEye f.
heparin arterial f.
Interface arterial blood f.
Jostra arterial blood f.
Kim-Ray Greenfield caval f.
KoKo Moe pulmonary function f.
LeukoNet F.
low-pass f.

F

NOTES

filter *(continued)*
    mediastinal sump f.
    Millipore f.
    Mobin-Uddin vena cava f.
    MultiSPIRO Clear Advantage
      pulmonary function f.
    nitinol f.
    Re/Flex f.
    Simon nitinol inferior vena cava f.
    Simon nitinol IVC f.
    temporary f.
    third-order Butterworth f.
    TrapEase permanent vena cava f.
    triple-bandpass f.
    umbrella f.
    vena cava f.
    Vena Tech LGM f.
    Vitalograph Bacterial/Viral F.
    Wiener f.
    William Harvey arterial blood f.
filtered
    f. atrial rate interval (FARI)
    f. QRS complex
filtering
    four-pole Butterworth f.
FilterLine
    F. circuit
    F. sampling technology
FilterWatch sensor
**FilterWire EX embolic protection
system**
filtragometry
filtration
    extracorporeal membrane
      differential f.
    gel f.
    tangential flow f. (TFF)
    x-ray beam f.
FIM
    functional independence measure
final
    f. common pathway
    f. rapid repolarization
Finapres
    F. blood pressure monitor
    F. finger cuff
    F. technique
finder
    lumen f.
fine-needle
    f.-n. aspiration (FNA)
    f.-n. aspiration biopsy
fine particle dose (FPD)
Finesse
    F. cardiac device
    F. guiding catheter
finger
    clubbing of f.'s

    f. cuff
    f. dilation
    f. oximetry
    F. Phantom pulse oximeter testing
      system
    f. photoplethysmographic device
    f. systolic blood pressure (FSBP)
finger-in-glove appearance
fingernail
    watch-crystal f.
fingerprint
    f. edema
FingerPrint handheld pulse oximeter
finned pacemaker lead
Finochietto
    F. forceps
    F. retractor
    F. rib spreader
Finochietto-Geissendorfer rib retractor
Fino DVT catheter
FIO_2, FiO_2
    fractional inspired oxygen concentration
    fraction of inspired oxygen
firing
    laser f.
    repetitive atrial f. (RAF)
first
    f. effort
    f. heart sound (S_1)
    f. obtuse marginal artery (OM-1)
    f. pass view
    f. positive deflection during the
      QRS complex (R)
    F. Response manual resuscitator
    f. shock count
first-degree
    f.-d. A-V block
    f.-d. heart block
first-effort angina
first-line therapy
first-night effect
first-order kinetics
first-pass
    f.-p. radionuclide angiocardiography
    f.-p. radionuclide angiography
    f.-p. technique
first-phase tilt
first-third filling fraction
Fischer
    F. pneumothoracic needle
    F. sign
    F. symptom
Fischl index
FISH
    fluorescent in situ hybridization
fish
    f. meal lung
    f. oil

Fisher
>   F. Micro-capillary Tube Reader
>   F. murmur

fishhook lead
fish-meal worker's lung disease
fish-mouth
>   f.-m. cusp
>   f.-m. incision
>   f.-m. mitral stenosis

fishnet pattern
fish-scaling effect
F$_2$-isoprostane
fissura
>   f. horizontalis pulmonis dextri
>   f. obliqua pulmonis

fissure
>   azygos f.
>   horizontal f.
>   inferior accessory f.
>   f. of lung
>   major f.
>   minor f.
>   oblique f.
>   plaque f.
>   f. sign
>   sphenoidal f.
>   Sylvian f.
>   tissue f.

fissuring
>   plaque f.

fist percussion
fistula, pl. **fistulae, fistulas**
>   aortocaval f.
>   aortoenteric f. (AEF)
>   arteriovenous f. (AVF)
>   A-V Gore-Tex f.
>   BP f.
>   brachioaxillary bridge graft f.
>   brachiosubclavian bridge graft f.
>   Brescia-Cimino A-V f.
>   bronchopleural f.
>   bronchopulmonary venous f.
>   bronchovenous f.
>   cameral f.
>   carotid-cavernous f. (CCF)
>   Cimino-Brescia arteriovenous f.
>   congenital pulmonary
>   arteriovenous f.
>   coronary artery f. (CAF, CAP)
>   coronary artery-right ventricular f.
>   coronary-pulmonary f. (C-PF)
>   duropleural f.

>   Eck f.
>   enteric f.
>   esophagorespiratory f.
>   Gore-Tex AF f.
>   gross tracheoesophageal f.
>   H-type tracheoesophageal f.
>   pancreaticopleural f.
>   pancreatopleural f.
>   pleuroesophageal f.
>   pulmonary arteriovenous f. (PAF,
>   PAVF)
>   renal f.
>   silent coronary artery f.
>   solitary pulmonary arteriovenous f.
>   spontaneous closure of f.
>   subclavian arteriovenous f.
>   systemic pulmonary f. (SPF)
>   TE f.
>   tracheoesophageal f. (TEF)
>   traumatic f.

fistulectomy
>   bronchopleuromediastinal f.

fistulous opening
FITC
>   fluorescein isothiocyanate

Fitch obturator
fitness
>   biological f.
>   cardiovascular f.

Fitzgerald forceps
FIVC
>   forced inspiratory vital capacity

five-chamber view
fixation
>   complex f. (CF)
>   f. mechanism

fixative
>   Saccomanno f.

fixed
>   f. airflow obstruction
>   f. coupling
>   f. orifice resistor
>   f. perfusion defect

fixed-pressure CPAP
fixed-rate
>   f.-r. mode
>   f.-r. pacemaker
>   f.-r. perfusion defect
>   f.-r. pulse generator

fixed-wire
>   f.-w. balloon

F

NOTES

fixed-wire *(continued)*
    f.-w. balloon dilatation system
    f.-w. coronary balloon catheter
fixer bath
FL
    flow limitation
fL
    femtoliter
flabby airways
flaccid areflexia
Flack node
flagellar
flagellum, pl. **flagella**
Flagyl Oral
flail
    f. chest
    f. chorda
    f. leaflet
    f. mitral leaflet (FML)
    f. mitral valve
    f. segment
FLAIR
    fluid-attenuated inversion recovery
    FLAIR image
flame emission spectroscopy (FES)
flame-shaped hemorrhage
flap
    Abbe f.
    Eloesser f.
    intimal f.
    intraluminal f.
    Linton f.
    liver f.
    microvascular free f.
    pericardial f.
    subclavian f.
    f. tracheostomy
flapping
    f. sound
    f. tremor
    f. valve syndrome
flare
    wheal and f.
flaring
    alar f.
    nasal f.
FLASH
    fast low-angle shot
    F. MRI
    F. sequence
flash
    F. portable spirometer
    f. pulmonary edema
flashing checkerboard test
flashlamp excited pulsed dye
flashlamp-pulsed Nd:YAG laser
flask-shaped heart
flat
    f. diastolic slope

    f. tube pressure sensor
    f. wire coil stent
flatfile
flattening
    T wave f.
flavonoid
flavus
    Aspergillus f.
flax-dresser's disease
flea-bitten kidney
flecainide
fleeting infiltrate
Fleet Phospho-Soda
Fleischmann bursa
Fleischner
    F. lines
    F. syndrome
Fleisch pneumotachograph
Fleming
    fibrillar mass of F.
Fletcher factor
Flex
    F. DIC tracheostomy tube
    F. stent
    F. Tip guidewire
Flexguard Tip catheter
Flexguide intubation guide
flexibility
flexible
    f. balloon-tipped catheter
    f. coil stent
    f. fiberoptic bronchoscope
    f. fiberoptic bronchoscopy (FFB)
    f. guidewire
    f. myocardial biopsy forceps
Flexicath silicone subclavian cannula
flexion
    elbow f.
    hip f.
    shoulder horizontal f.
    trunk forward f.
Flexor
    F. Check-Flo introducer set
    F. introducer
FlexStent
    Cook F.
Flextend
    F. pacing lead
    F. steroid-eluting, transvenous
        pace/sense lead
Flexxicon Blue dialysis catheter
flicker fusion threshold
flight
    time of f. (TOF)
Flimm-Fighter
flint disease
Flint murmur

flip
- f. angle
- LDH f.

flipped T wave

flitter

floating lead

flocculation
- cephalin f. (CEPH FLOC)
- cephalin-cholesterol f. (CCF)
- cholesterol-lecithin f. (CLF)

flock worker's lung

Flolan injection

FloMap
- F. guidewire
- F. velocimeter

Flonase

flooding
- alveolar f.

floppy
- f. aortic valve (FAV)
- f. guidewire
- f. mitral valve (FMV)
- f. valve syndrome

floppy-tipped guidewire

flora
- mixed f.
- oral f.
- respiratory f.
- tracheobronchial f.

Flo-Rester vascular occluder

Florex medical compression stockings

florid
- f. congestive heart failure
- f. pulmonary edema

Florinef Acetate

FloSeal Matrix hemostatic sealant

flosequinan

flotation
- f. catheter
- f. catheter technique

Flo-Thru shunt

Flovent
- F. aerosol
- F. Diskus
- F. HFA metered-dose inhaler
- F. Rotadisk

flow
- f. acceleration
- accessory pulmonary blood f. (APBF)
- f. across orifice
- adequate blood f.

- aliasing f.
- antegrade diastolic f.
- anterograde f.
- anular f.
- aortic f. (AF)
- aortic blood f. (ABF)
- aortic ductal f.
- arterial blood f.
- f. artifact
- f. augmentation
- blood f. (BF)
- blunted systolic pulmonary venous f.
- capillary blood f. (CBF)
- cerebral blood f. (CBF)
- collateral f.
- f. controller
- f. convergence method
- coronary f. (CF)
- coronary artery blood f. (CABF)
- coronary blood f. (CBF)
- coronary sinus f.
- coronary sinus blood f. (CSBF)
- disturbed f.
- Doppler color f.
- dynamic cardiac blood f. (DCBF)
- effective capillary f. (ECF)
- effective renal blood f. (ERBF)
- endocardial f.
- f. envelope
- epicardial f.
- exercise hyperemia blood f. (EHBF, EXBF)
- expiratory tidal f.
- faint f.
- femoral artery blood f. (FABF)
- forced expiratory f. (FEF)
- forced inspiratory f. (FIF)
- forced midexpiratory f. (FMF)
- forearm blood f.
- great cardiac vein f. (GCVF)
- hepatofugal f.
- hepatopetal f.
- high f. (HF)
- holodiastolic f.
- infradiaphragmatic venous f.
- f. injector
- isovolume f.
- laminar blood f.
- left ventricular minute f. (LVMF)
- limb blood f.

F

NOTES

flow *(continued)*
    f. limitation (FL)
    f. mapping
    f. mapping technique
    maximal forced expiratory f. (FEFmax)
    maximal midexpiratory f. (MMEF, MMF)
    mean forced midexpiratory f.
    mean inspiratory f. (MIF)
    mitral regurgitant f. (MRF)
    mitral valve f. (MVF)
    myocardial blood f. (MBF)
    pansystolic f.
    peak f. (PF)
    peak cough f. (PCF)
    peak expiratory f. (PEF)
    peak inspiratory f. (PIF)
    peak tidal expiratory f. (PTEF)
    peak tidal inspiratory f. (PTIF)
    percent predicted peak expiratory f. (%PEF)
    perigraft f.
    peripheral blood f. (PBF)
    petal-fugal f.
    portal venous f. (PVF)
    pressure-compensated f.
    f. profile
    pulmonary blood f. (PBF, Qp)
    pulmonary capillary blood f. (Qc, Qpc)
    pulmonary venous f. (PVF)
    pulsatile f.
    f. rate
    f. ratio
    ratio of tidal expiratory flow at 25% of tidal volume and peak tidal expiratory f. (TEF$_{25}$/PTEF)
    regional cerebral blood f. (rCBF)
    regional myocardial blood f. (RMBF)
    renal cortical blood f. (RCBF)
    renal plasma f. (RPF)
    f. reserve
    F. Rider flow-directed catheter
    shunt f. (SF)
    shunted blood to total blood f. (QSQT)
    splanchnic blood f.
    systemic blood f. (Qs, SBF)
    thrombolysis in myocardial infarction f.
    tidal f.
    time to peak expiratory f. (tPTEF)
    time to peak inspiratory f. (tPTIF)
    TIMI f.
    total coronary f. (TCF)
    total pulmonary blood f. (TPBF)
    transvalvular f.

    tricuspid valve f.
    f. velocity
    f. volume curve
    f. volume loop
    vortex f.
    f. wire
    Wright peak f.
flow-assisted
    f.-a. short-term (FAST)
    f.-a. short-term balloon catheter
flow-delivery waveform
flow-directed
    f.-d. balloon cardiovascular catheter
    f.-d. end-hole catheter
FloWire
    F. Doppler guidewire
flow-limiting stenosis
flow-mediated
    f.-m. dilation (FMD)
    f.-m. vasodilation
flowmeter *(See also* meter)
    AirZone peak f.
    asmaPLAN+ peak f.
    Assess peak f.
    Astech peak f.
    Asthma Check peak f.
    AsthmaMentor peak f.
    blood f.
    Doppler ultrasonic f.
    FM color-coded f.
    Gould electromagnetic f.
    laser Doppler f.
    Narcomatic f.
    Parks 800 bidirectional Doppler f.
    peak f. (PFM)
    Periflux PF 1 D blood-f.
    Personal Best peak f.
    PocketPeak peak f.
    SensorMedics mass flow sensor heated wire f.
    Spir-O-Flow peak f.
    Thorpe f.
    Transonic f.
    TruZone peak f.
    Youlten nasal inspiratory peak f.
flowmetry
    laser-Doppler f.
    magnetic resonance f. (MRF)
    pulsed Doppler f.
flow-responsive remodeling
flow-sensing
    f.-s. pneumotachograph
    f.-s. spirometer
flow-time registration
Flowtron
    F. DVT pump
    F. DVT pump system
flow-volume
    tidal breathing f.-v. (TBFV)

Floxin
>F. injection
>F. Oral

floxuridine

FLU
>flunisolide

flucloxacillin

fluconazole

fluctuations
>heart rate f. (HRF)

flucytosine

Fludara

fludrocortisone acetate

fluens
>pulsus f.

fluffy
>f. alveolar infiltrate
>f. cotton-wool exudate

fluffy-cuffed tube

fluid
>arterial pressure of arterial f. (P_A)
>f. aspiration
>bronchoalveolar lavage f. (BALF)
>f. challenge
>crystalloid f.
>f. dynamics
>epithelial lining f. (ELF)
>interstitial f.
>intravascular f. (IVF)
>intravenous f. (IVF)
>isotonic f.
>f. mechanics
>partial pressure of arterial f. (PA)
>pericardial f. (PF)
>periciliary f.
>pleural f.
>pulmonary edema f. (PEF)
>respiratory tract lining f. (RTLF)
>retained lung f. (RLF)
>f. shift
>standard perfusion f. (SPF)
>f. therapy
>ventricular f. (VF)
>vesicular f.
>viscoelastic f.

fluid-attenuated
>f.-a. inversion recovery (FLAIR)
>f.-a. inversion recovery image

fluid-filled
>f.-f. balloon cardiovascular catheter
>f.-f. balloon-tipped flow-directed
>catheter

>f.-f. pigtail catheter
>f.-f. pressure monitoring guidewire

fluidic circuit

fluindione

fluke
>lung f.

Flumadine Oral

flumazenil

FluMist

flunarizine

flunisolide (FLU)
>f. HFA

flunitrazepam

Fluogen

fluorescein
>f. angiography
>f. isothiocyanate (FITC)

fluorescence
>f. antimembrane antibody (FAMA, FAMAT)
>f. bronchoscopy
>laser-induced arterial f. (LIAF)
>f. polarization
>f. spectroscopy

fluorescence-activated cell sorter (FACS)

fluorescence-guided smart laser

fluorescent
>f. antimembrane antibody (FAMA, FAMAT)
>f. in situ hybridization (FISH)
>f. treponemal antibody absorption (FTA-ABS)
>f. treponemal antibody absorption test

fluoride
>hydrogen f.
>f. toxicity

fluorine-18 fluorodeoxyglucose (F-18 FDG)

fluorocarbon poisoning

5-fluorocytosine

fluorodeoxyglucose (FDG)
>cyclotron-produced F-18 f.
>fluorine-18 f. (F-18 FDG)

2-fluoro-2-deoxyglucose

fluorodeoxyuridine (FUDR)

fluorodopamine positron emission tomographic scanning

fluorogenic

fluorography
>spot-film f.

fluorohydrocortisone

F

NOTES

fluorometry
Fluoropassiv thin-wall carotid patch
Fluoroplex Topical
FluoroPlus
> F. angiography
> F. Cardiac

fluoroquinolone
fluoroscopic
> f. guidance
> f. isthmus ablation
> f. visualization

fluoroscopy
> biplane f.
> C-arm f.
> kV f.

Fluoro Tip cannula
5-fluorouracil (5-FU)
Fluosol artificial blood
Fluotec vaporizer
fluoxetine hydrochloride
fluoxymesterone
flurazepam
flush
> aortic arch f. (AAF)
> f. aortogram
> f. aortography
> f. and bathe technique
> heparin f.
> mahogany f.
> malar f.
> warm heparinized saline f.

flushed
> aspirated and f.

flushing
> f. time
> vasomotor f. (VMF)

flutamide
fluticasone
> f. propionate (FP)
> f. propionate and salmeterol
> inhalation powder

flutter
> atrial f. (AF, AFL)
> auricular f.
> clockwise f.
> completely positive deflection f.
> counterclockwise f.
> f. cycle length
> diaphragmatic f.
> dominant positive deflection f.
> impure f.
> inferior-axis f.
> isthmus-dependent atrial f.
> mediastinal f.
> F. mucus clearance device
> pure f.
> f. R interval
> ventricular f. (VF)
> f. wave

flutter-fibrillation waves
Fluviral
flux
> soldering f.
> transmembrane calcium f.

fluxionary hyperemia
Fluzone
fly ash
flying W sign
FM
> fibrin monomer
> FM color-coded flowmeter

FMCG
> fetal magnetocardiography

FMD
> flow-mediated dilation

FMF
> forced midexpiratory flow

FMIV
> forced mandatory intermittent ventilation

FML
> flail mitral leaflet

FMLP
> formyl methionyl leucyl phenylalanine
> FMLP receptor

fMRI
> functional magnetic resonance imaging

FMV
> floppy mitral valve

FNA
> fine-needle aspiration

FO
> foramen ovale
> forced oscillation

foam
> f. cell
> polyurethane f.
> f. stability test

foamy
> f. macrophage
> f. myocardial cell

FOB
> fiberoptic bronchoscopy

focal
> f. adhesion kinase (FAK)
> f. atrial fibrillation
> f. block
> f. bronchopneumonia
> f. dilatation catheter
> f. eccentric stenosis
> f. edema
> f. emphysema
> f. fibrosis
> f. media aplasia
> f. motion abnormality
> f. myocytosis of heart
> f. vasospasm
> f. ventricular dysfunction

focal-dust emphysema

FocalSeal-L surgical sealant
focus, pl. **foci**
F. Angioplasty Catheter Technology
arrhythmia f.
Assmann f.
Ghon f.
Kampmeier foci
Simon foci
Foerster forceps
Fogarty
F. adherent clot catheter
F. embolectomy catheter
F. forceps
F. graft thrombectomy catheter
F. spring clip
Foix-Cavany-Marie syndrome
fold
bulboventricular f.
Marshall f.
pleuroperitoneal f.
Rindfleisch f.
vestibular f.
vestigial f.
folded-lung syndrome
Folgard RX
folic acid
follicular
f. bronchiectasis
f. bronchiolitis
f. pharyngitis
follow-up
Foltz-Overton cardiac catheter
Fome-Cuf tracheostomy tube
fomivirsen
fondaparinux sodium
**Fontaine lower limb ischemia
  classification**
Fontan
F. atriopulmonary anastomosis
F. circulation
F. connection
F. conversion
F. modification of Norwood
  procedure
F. operation
F. repair
F. right atrium
Fontan-Baudet procedure
Fontan-Kreutzer procedure
food
f. angina
f. asthma

F. Guide Pyramid
sodium content of f.
whole-grain f.
foot
f. cradle
superficial medial artery of f.
trash f.
f. ulcer
footprint of transducer
Foradil Aerolizer
foramen, pl. **foramina**
bulboventricular f.
f. diaphragmatis sellae
Galen f.
interventricular f. (IVF)
jugular f. (JF)
Lannelongue f.
f. of Luschka
f. of Monro
f. of Morgagni
oval f.
f. ovale (FO)
f. quadratum
f. rotundum
round f.
f. secundum
thebesian foramina
f. of veins of heart
vena caval f.
f. venae cavae
f. venarum minimarum atria dextri
force
atrial ejection f.
F. balloon
F. balloon dilatation catheter
contractile f. (CF)
drag f.
extrinsic f.
left ventricular f.
life f.
myocardial contraction f. (MCF)
peak twitch f.
potentiated twitch f.
P terminal f.
f. and rhythm (F and R)
shear f.
Starling f.
twitch f.
unpotentiated twitch f.
Venturi f.
forced
f. beat

F

NOTES

289

forced *(continued)*
- f. cycle
- f. expiratory capacity (FEC)
- f. expiratory flow (FEF)
- f. expiratory maneuver
- f. expiratory spirogram (FES)
- f. expiratory technique
- f. expiratory time (FET)
- f. expiratory volume (FEV)
- f. expiratory volume in 1 second (FEV$_1$)
- f. expiratory volume in 1 second to forced vital capacity ratio (FEV$_1$/FVC)
- f. expiratory volume timed to forced vital capacity ratio (FEV/FVC)
- f. inspiratory capacity (FIC)
- f. inspiratory flow (FIF)
- f. inspiratory vital capacity (FIVC)
- f. ischemia-reperfusion transition
- f. mandatory intermittent ventilation (FMIV)
- f. midexpiratory flow (FMF)
- f. oscillation (FO)
- f. oscillation technique (FOT)
- f. respiration
- f. vital capacity (FVC)
- f. vital capacity analysis (FVCA)

force-frequency relation
force-generating capacity
force-length relation
forceps
- Barraya f.
- Bengolea f.
- biopsy f.
- bipolar coagulating f.
- Bloodwell f.
- Boettcher f.
- bronchus-grasping f.
- Brown-Adson f.
- Carmalt f.
- coagulation f.
- Cook flexible biopsy f.
- Cooley f.
- Craafoord-Sellor hemostatic f.
- Cushing f.
- DeBakey arterial f.
- DeBakey Atraugrip f.
- DeBakey-Colovira-Rumel thoracic f.
- DeBakey-Derra anastomosis f.
- DeBakey-Diethrich coronary artery f.
- DeBakey-Mixter thoracic f.
- DeBakey-Péan cardiovascular f.
- DeBakey tissue f.
- Duracep biopsy f.
- Duval lung-grasping f.
- Englert f.

- Finochietto f.
- Fitzgerald f.
- flexible myocardial biopsy f.
- Foerster f.
- Fogarty f.
- Fraenkel f.
- Gerald f.
- Gerbode f.
- Harken f.
- Hopkins f.
- Jawz disposable biopsy f.
- Julian thoracic f.
- Kahler bronchial biopsy f.
- Magill f.
- McGill f.
- Mount-Mayfield f.
- National Institutes of Health mitral valve-grasping f.
- NIH mitral valve-grasping f.
- Pilling Weck Y-stent f.
- Potts bronchial f.
- renal artery f.
- Samuels f.
- Scholten biopsy f.
- Tuttle thoracic f.
- Varco thoracic f.

force-velocity-length relation
force-velocity relation
force-velocity-volume relation
Ford equation
forearm blood flow
Foregger
- F. laryngoscope
- F. rigid esophagoscope

foregut
foreign
- f. body
- f. body airway obstruction (FBAO)
- f. body aspiration

ForeRunner
- F. automatic external defibrillator device
- F. defibrillator

foreshortening
fork
- f. stent
- f. stenting technique

Forlanini treatment
form
- M pattern on right atrial wave f.
- myocardial infarction in dumbbell f.
- pentamidine in aerosol f.
- wave f.

formaldehyde
format
- quad screen f.
- scanning f.

formation
  aspergilloma f.
  coagulum f.
  fibrin f.
  hyaline membrane f.
  impulse f.
  rouleau f.
  sinus node f. (SNF)
forme fruste
formicans
  pulsus f.
formicant pulse
formononetin
formoterol
  f. fumarate
  f. fumarate powder for inhalation
formula, pl. **formulas, formulae**
  Bayer Select Pain Relief F.
  Bazett correction f.
  biplane f.
  Bohr f.
  Brozek f.
  Cannon f.
  Devereux f.
  Framingham f.
  Fridericia f.
  Friedewald f.
  Ganz f.
  geometric cube f.
  Gorlin hydraulic f.
  Hakki f.
  Hamilton-Stewart f.
  heart rate correction f.
  Impact specialized feeding f.
  Janz f.
  f. of Mirsky
  Penn f.
  Poiseuille resistance f.
  Sramek f.
  Teichholz f.
  Triaminic AM Decongestant F.
  Vicks Formula 44 Pediatric F.
  Yeager f.
formulation
  Sicilian Gambit f.
formyl methionyl leucyl phenylalanine (FMLP)
Forney syndrome
Forrester
  F. syndrome
  F. Therapeutic Classification grades I–IV

forskolin
  adenylate cyclase stimulator f.
Fortaz
Forte
  Aristocort F.
  Enduronyl F.
  Robinul F.
fortis
  pulsus f.
Fortovase
fortuitum
  Mycobacterium f.
forward
  f. conduction
  f. flow of velocity
  f. heart failure
  f. pressure waveform
  f. stroke volume (FSV)
  f. triangle method
  f. triangle technique
forward-backward Prony method (FBPM)
foscarnet
Foscavir injection
fos **gene**
fosinopril
fosinoprilat
fosinoprilic acid
fosinopril sodium
FOSQ
  Functional Outcomes of Sleep Questionnaire
fossa, pl. **fossae**
  antecubital f.
  canine f.
  Claudius f.
  Gerdy hyoid f.
  f. glandulae lacrimalis
  Malgaigne f.
  f. ovalis
  supraclavicular f.
FOT
  forced oscillation technique
Fothergill disease
foundation
  British Heart f. (BHF)
  Heart Disease Research f. (HDRF)
  HON F.
  National Heart f. (NHF)
founder effect
four-beam laser Doppler probe

NOTES

four-chamber
    apical f.-c.
    f.-c. view
four-day syndrome
four-hour scan
Fourier
    F. analysis of electrocardiogram
    F. series analysis
    F. transform
    F. transform analysis
    F. two-dimensional imaging
Fourier-acquired steady-state technique (FAST)
four-legged cage valve
Fourmentin thoracic index
Fournier gangrene
four-phase Lifestick CPR
four-pole Butterworth filtering
fourth
    f. heart sound (S_4)
    f. Korotkoff sound (K4)
fourth-generation cephalosporin
FOV
    field of view
fovea
    f. articularis inferior atlantis
    f. articularis superior atlantis
    f. costalis inferior
    f. costalis processus transversi
    f. costalis superior
    f. dentis atlantis
foveated chest
Fowler
    F. single-breath test
    F. solution
    F. thoracoplasty
Fox green dye
FP
    filling pressure
    fluticasone propionate
FPD
    fine particle dose
FPE
    fatal pulmonary embolism
FPL
    fasting plasma lipids
FPPH
    familial primary pulmonary hypertension
F and R
    force and rhythm
F2R
    factor II receptor
        F2R blood coagulation
Fr (*var. of* F)
    French
fractal
fraction
    atrial filling f. (AFF)
    basilar half ejection f.

blunted ejection f.
CPK-MB f.
ejection f. (EF)
f. of expired carbon dioxide ($FECO_2$)
filling f.
first-third filling f.
global ejection f.
global left ventricular ejection f.
heparin-precipitable f. (HPF)
f. of inspired carbon dioxide ($FICO_2$)
f. of inspired oxygen (FIO_2, FiO_2)
intrapulmonary shunt f. (Q_s/Q_t)
left atrial active emptying f.
left ventricular ejection f. (LVEF)
light pen-determined ejection f.
lipoprotein-deficient f. (LPDF)
MB f.
oxygen extraction f. (OEF)
physiologic dead space f.
physiologic shunt f.
regurgitant f.
residual volume f. (RVF)
rest ejection f.
right ventricular ejection f. (REF, RVEF)
shortening f.
Teichholz ejection f.
ventricular ejection f. (VEF)
ventriculogram-derived ejection f.
ventriculographic ejection f.
fractional
    f. area change (FAC)
    f. flow reserve (FFR)
    f. inspired oxygen concentration (FIO_2, FiO_2)
    f. myocardial shortening
    f. velocity reserve (FVR)
fractionation
    electrogram f.
fracture
    anterior rib f.
    cough f.
    double-rib f.
    J retention wire f.
    lead f.
    outlet strut f. (OSF)
    pacemaker lead f.
    plaque f.
    posterior rib f.
    rib f.
    sternal f.
Fraenkel
    F. forceps
    F. node
    F. pneumococcus
fragile X-mental retardation (FRAX-MR)

fragilis
    Bacteroides f.
fragilitas sanguinis
fragility
    hereditary capillary f. (HCF)
fragment
    f. antigen-binding (Fab)
    antimyosin Fab f.
    antimyosin monoclonal antibody
      with Fab f. (AMA-Fab)
    catheter f.
    crosslinked D f.
    cytokeratin 19 f. (CYFRA)
    Digibind digoxin immune Fab f.'s
    Digidote digoxin immune Fab f.'s
    Fab f.
fragmentation
    maximum atrial f. (MAF)
    f. myocarditis
    f. of myocardium
    sleep f.
    ventricular diastolic f. (VDF)
Fragmin injection
frame
    B-scan f.
Framingham
    F. equation
    F. formula
    F. heart failure criteria
    F. risk index
Francisco
    Nipponese in Honolulu and San F.
      (Ni-Hon-San)
Francisella tularensis
frank
    f. blood
    F. ECG lead placement system
    F. XYZ orthogonal lead
    F. XYZ orthogonal lead system
Frankel treatment
Frank-Starling
    F.-S. curve
    F.-S. law
    F.-S. mechanism
    F.-S. reserve
Frank-Straub-Wiggers-Starling principle
Fräntzel murmur
Franzen needle guide
Franz monophasic action potential catheter
frappage
Fraser Harlake respirometer

Fraunhofer zone
Fraxiparin
FRAX-MR
    fragile X-mental retardation
    FRAX-MR syndrome
FRC
    functional reserve capacity
    functional residual capacity
Fredrickson
    F. classification of lipid disorders
    F. dyslipidemia type I, IIa, IIb,
      III, IV, V
free
    f. cholesterol (FC)
    f. fatty acids (FFA)
    f. protoporphyrin
    f. radical
    f. root
    f. thyrotoxin index
    f. wall
free-beam laser
free-breathing coronary magnetic resonance angiography
Freedom
    Accu-Chek II F.
    degrees of F.
FreeDop
    F. cordless Doppler
    F. portable Doppler unit
free-floating
    f.-f. thrombus (FFT)
    f.-f. vena caval thrombus
free-flowing empyema
freeing up of adhesion
free-radical scavenger
Freestyle
    F. aortic root bioprosthesis
    F. bioprosthetic heart valve
    F. stentless aortic heart valve
    F. stentless bioprosthesis
free-wall accessory pathway
Freeway Lite portable aerosol compressor
Freezor
    F. CryoAblation system
    F. cryocatheter
Freitag stent
frémissement cattaire
fremitus
    auditory f.
    bronchial f.
    friction f.

F

NOTES

fremitus *(continued)*
    hydatid f.
    pectoral f.
    pericardial f.
    pleural f.
    rhonchal f.
    subjective f.
    tactile f.
    tussive f.
    vocal f.
French (F, Fr)
    F. catheter size 3-34
    F. double-lumen catheter
    F. JR4 Schneider catheter
    F. paradox
    F. SAL catheter
    F. scale
    F. shaft catheter
    F. sheath
    F. sizing of catheter
Frenchay
    F. Activities Index
    F. Aphasia Screening Test (FAST)
6.2-French 12.5-MHz catheter
frequency
    breathing f. (BF)
    ciliary beat f.
    critical flicker f.
    f. domain imaging
    dynamic f. response
    f. ectopic ventricular beat (FEVB)
    fetal cardiac f. (FCF)
    fetal heart f. (FHF)
    fundamental f.
    heart f. (Hfr)
    high pulse repetition f. (HiPRF)
    Larmor f.
    natural f.
    pulse repetition f. (PRF)
    resonant f.
    respiratory f. (f)
    f. response
    f. shifter
    f. to tidal volume (f/V_t)
    f. tracer
frequency-domain analysis
frequens
    pulsus f.
frequent spontaneous premature complex
fresh frozen plasma (FFP)
Fresnel zone
Freund
    F. anomaly
    F. operation
freundii
    Citrobacter f.
Frey-Sauerbruch rib shears

friability
    eggshell f.
friable wall
friction
    f. fremitus
    f. murmur
    f. rub
    f. sound
Fridericia formula
Friedewald
    F. approximation
    F. equation
    F. formula
Friedländer
    F. bacillus
    F. bacillus pneumonia
    F. disease
    F. pneumobacillus
Friedreich
    F. ataxia
    F. disease
    F. sign
frog breathing
froissement
    bruit de f.
frolement
    bruit de f.
frond
    papillary f.
    sea f.
frontal axis
frosted heart
frosting heart
frothy sputum
frottement
    bruit de f.
frozen thorax
FRP
    functional refractory period
fructosamine
Frumil
frusemide
fruste
    forme f.
frustrate systole
FS-069 contrast agent
FSBP
    finger systolic blood pressure
FSV
    forward stroke volume
fsw
    feet of sea water
        depth pressure fsw
FT
    Fallot tetralogy
FTA-ABS
    fluorescent treponemal antibody absorption
        FTA-ABS test

fTCD
    functional transcranial Doppler
      sonography
FTQ
    Fagerstrom tolerance questionnaire
5-FU
    5-fluorouracil
fucose residue
fucosidosis
FUDR
    fluorodeoxyuridine
fugax
    amaurosis partialis f.
Fugl-Meyer
    F.-M. motor test scale
    F.-M. motor test score
Fujinon flexible bronchoscope
**Fukunaga-Hayes unbiased jackknife
classification**
fulguration
    electrical f.
full
    f. caloric density
    f. compensatory pause
    f. PSG
fuller's earth pneumoconiosis
full-thickness linear lesion
fully automatic pacemaker
fulminans
    purpura f.
fulminant myocarditis
fumagillin
fumarate
    bisoprolol f.
    clemastine f.
    ferrous f.
    formoterol f.
    ibutilide f.
fumes
    cadmium oxide f.
    cobalt f.
    metallic oxide f.
    soldering f.
fumigatus
    Aspergillus f.
function
    atrial transport f.
    auto-threshold f.
    battery cell voltage f.
    bellows f.
    cardiac f.
    cardiovascular f. (CVFn)

    contractile f.
    f. curve
    depressed ventricular f.
    diastolic f.
    dopaminergic f.
    exercise LV f.
    global left ventricular f.
    hepatic f.
    intramyocardial f.
    left atrial appendage f.
    left ventricular f. (LVF)
    left ventricular systolic/diastolic f.
    lung f.
    mechanical contractile f.
    mitochondrial f.
    myocardial f.
    neurohormonal f.
    parasympathetic f.
    perturbed autonomic nervous
      system f.
    phagocytic f.
    preserved left ventricular systolic f.
    probability density f. (PDF)
    pulmonary f. (PF)
    pump f.
    renal f.
    respiratory f.
    resting systolic f.
    right ventricular f.
    sigh f.
    sinus node f.
    stress perfusion and rest f.
    systolic f.
    valvular f.
    ventilatory f.
    ventricular f. (VF)
functional
    f. aerobic impairment (FAI)
    f. assessment
    f. block
    f. capacity classification
    f. cardiovascular disease
    f. conduction period (FCP)
    f. congestion
    f. dyspnea
    f. failure to capture
    f. image
    f. imaging
    f. independence measure (FIM)
    f. magnetic resonance imaging
      (fMRI)
    f. magnetic stimulation

F

NOTES

functional *(continued)*
    f. mitral regurgitation
    f. MRI
    f. murmur
    F. Outcomes of Sleep Questionnaire (FOSQ)
    f. pacing abnormality
    f. pain
    f. pulmonary atresia
    f. recovery
    f. refractory period (FRP)
    f. reserve capacity (FRC)
    f. residual air
    f. residual capacity (FRC)
    f. status
    f. subtraction
    f. transcranial Doppler sonography (fTCD)
    f. undersensing
functionalism
fundamental
    f. frequency
    f. imaging (FI)
fundoplication
    Belsey Mark IV f.
    Belsey two-thirds wrap f.
    Collis-Nissen f.
    Nissen f. (NF)
    Nissen 360-degree wrap f.
    Rossetti modification of Nissen f.
fundus, pl. **fundi**
funduscopic examination
fungal
    f. endocarditis
    f. infection
fungating mass
fungi (*pl. of* fungus)
Fungizone Intravenous
fungoides
    mycosis f.
fungus, pl. **fungi**
    f. ball
funic
    f. pulse
    f. souffle
funnel
    f. chest
    f. dynamics

    mitral f.
    vascular f.
Furadantin
furcosus
    Bacteroides f.
furifosmin
Furman type II electrogram
furoate
    mometasone f.
furosemide
Furoside
furrier's
    f. lung
    f. lung disease
furrow
    atrioventricular f.
    Schmorl f.
Fusarium solani
fused commissure
fused-tip catheter
fusidic acid
fusiform
    f. aortic aneurysm
    f. bronchiectasis
fusion
    atrial f. (AF)
    f. beat
    commissural f.
    f. complex
    critical flicker f.
    entrainment with concealed f.
    f. QRS
Fusobacterium
    F. necrophorum
    F. nucleatum
f/V$_t$
    frequency to tidal volume
FVC
    forced vital capacity
FVCA
    forced vital capacity analysis
FVIIa
    activated factor VII
FVIIag
    factor VII antigen
FVR
    fractional velocity reserve
FX miniRAIL RX PTCA catheter

G
gallop
G protein
3G4
G5
G5 massage and percussion machine
G5 Neocussor percussor
G₂

G_2
prostaglandin G_2
GA
general angiography
Ga
gallium
⁶⁸Ga

^{68}Ga
gallium-68
GABA
gamma-aminobutyric acid
Gabbay-Frater valve suture
Gad hypothesis
gadodiamide
gadolinium chelate
gadolinium-diethylenetriamine pentaacetic acid (Gd-DTPA)
gadoteridol injection
Gaertner (*var. of* Gärtner)
Gaffky scale
gag
g. gene
g. reflex
gain
g. control
time-compensated g.
time compensation g. (TCG)
time-varied g. (TVG)
Gairdner disease
Gaisböck syndrome
gait
ataxic g.
gaiter perforator
galactophlebitis
galactose
galactosidase deficiency
Galanti-Giusti colorimetric method
Galaxy IVUS imaging system
Galen foramen
Galileo
G. intravascular radiotherapy system
G. ventilator
gallamine triethiodide
Gallavardin
G. murmur
G. phenomenon
gallbladder disease

gallinatum
pectus g.
gallium (Ga)
g. imaging
radiolabeled g.
g. scan
gallium-67
g.-67 imaging
g.-67 scan
g.-67 scintigraphy
gallium-68 (⁶⁸Ga)

^{68}Ga
gallop (G)
atrial diastolic g. (ADG)
diastolic g. (DG)
filling g.
presystolic g. (PSG)
protodiastolic g.
g. rhythm
S_3 g.
S_4 g.
S_7 g.
g. sound
summation g. (S_7)
systolic g.
ventricular g. (VG)
gallopamil
gallop, murmur, rub (GMR)
galop
bruit de g.
GALT
gut-associated lymphoid tissue
galvanometer
Einthoven string g.
gambiense
Trypanosoma g.
Gambro
G. Lundia Minor hemodialyzer
G. oxygenator
Gamimune N
gamma
g. globulin
g. hydroxybutyrate (GHB)
g. knife
g. radiation
g. radiation therapy system
g. ray
g. scintillation camera
gamma-aminobutyric acid (GABA)
gamma-1b
interferon g-1b
Gammagard S/D
Gammar-P IV
gammopathy
polyclonal g.

G

297

Gamna-Gandy bodies
ganciclovir (GCV)
ganglion, pl. **ganglia, ganglions**
  basal ganglia (BG)
  Bock g.
  Ehrenritter g.
  g. inferius nervi
  g. inferius nervi vagi
  left stellate g.
  petrosal g.
  pharyngeal branch of
    pterygopalatine g.
  pterygopalatine g.
  stellate g.
  g. superius nervi
  Wrisberg g.
ganglionectomy
ganglionic blocker
ganglions (*pl. of* ganglion)
ganglioside
gangliosidosis
gangrene
  angiosclerotic g.
  cold g.
  diabetic g.
  dry g.
  embolic g.
  emphysematous g.
  Fournier g.
  gas g.
  hot g.
  intracardiac gas g.
  Raynaud g.
gangrenosa
  angina g.
gangrenous
  g. emphysema
  g. pharyngitis
  g. pneumonia
gannister disease
gantry
Gantzer accessory bundle
Ganz-Edwards coronary infusion
  catheter
Ganz formula
gap
  anion g.
  auscultatory g.
  g. conduction phenomenon
  excitable g.
  g. junction
  silent g.
Garamycin injection
Garatec
Garfield-Holinger laryngoscope
gargoylism
garlic
  Kwai G.

garment
  antishock g.
  Jobst pressure g.
  pneumatic antishock g. (PASG)
garnet
  yttrium-aluminum-g. (YAG)
Garrett dilator
Gärtner, Gaertner
  G. method
  G. tonometer
  G. vein phenomenon
GAS
  generalized arteriosclerosis
gas, pl. **gases**
  alveolar g.
  arterial blood g. (ABG)
  blood g.
  capillary blood g. (CBG)
  g. chromatography
  g. chromatography-mass
    spectrometry (GC-MS)
  g. clearance
  g. clearance measurement
  g. clearance method
  g. constant (R)
  g. dilution
  g. embolism
  g. endarterectomy
  g. exchange
  expired g.
  g. gangrene
  ideal alveolar g.
  inspired g.
  intrathoracic g.
  mixed expired g.
  serial blood g.
  suffocating g.
  thoracic g.
  g. trapping
gaseous
  g. microemboli
  g. pulse
Gas-Lyte ABG syringe
gasometer
gasometric
gasometry
gasp reflex
gastri
  Mycobacterium g.
gastric
  g. aspiration
  g. bypass (GBP)
  g. inhibitory polypeptide (GIP)
  g. insufflation
  g. lung
gastric-intrapleural pressure (Pg-Ppl)
gastrocardiac syndrome
Gastrocrom
gastroepiploic artery (GEA)

gastroesophageal
- g. reflux (GER)
- g. reflux disease (GERD)
- g. scintigraphy
- g. sphincter
- g. vestibule

gastropneumonic

gastropulmonary

gate
- acquisition g.
- D, F, H, M g.

gated
- g. averaging
- g. blood-pool angiography
- g. blood-pool imaging
- g. blood-pool scanning
- g. blood-pool scintigraphy
- g. cardiac scan
- g. computed tomography
- g. equilibrium ventriculography, frame-mode acquisition
- g. equilibrium ventriculography, list-mode acquisition
- g. list mode
- g. nuclear angiogram
- g. radionuclide angiography
- g. SPECT
- g. sweep magnetic resonance imaging
- g. system
- g. technique
- g. view

gatifloxacin

gating
- cardiac g.
- electrocardiographic g.
- in-memory g.
- g. mechanism
- prospective g.
- respiratory g.
- R wave g.
- g. signal

Gaucher disease

gauge
- blood pressure g. (BPG)
- Bourdon g.
- mercury-in-Silastic strain g.
- pounds per square inch g. (psig)
- Silastic strain g.

gaussian

gauze
- Surgicel g.
- Xeroform g.

Gazelle balloon dilatation catheter

GBP
- gastric bypass
- GBP scintigraphy

GC
- general circulation

GCD
- graft coronary disease

GCI
- global cerebral ischemia

GC-MS
- gas chromatography-mass spectrometry

Gc protein

GCS
- Glasgow Coma Scale
- graduated compression stockings

GCV
- ganciclovir
- great cardiac vein

GCVF
- great cardiac vein flow

Gd-DTPA
- gadolinium-diethylenetriamine pentaacetic acid

Gd-DTPA-enhanced MRI

GDP
- guanosine 5′-diphosphate

GE
- General Electric
  - GE CT Advantage high-speed CT system
  - GE 9800 CT scanner
  - GE Electric Advantx system
  - GE Lightspeed CT scanner
  - GE Signa Horizon SR 120 whole-body scanner
  - GE Signa 1.5-T MRI
  - GE Signa 1.5-T MRI system

GEA
- gastroepiploic artery
- GEA graft

gel
- agarose g.
- aluminum hydroxide g.
- Ayr saline nasal g.
- Cann-Ease moisturizing nasal g.
- DermaFlex G.
- electrode g.
- fibrin g.

G

NOTES

gel *(continued)*
    g. filtration
    H.P. Acthar G.
    mucous g.
    Nasal Moist G.
    SDS-polyacrylamide g.
gelatin
    absorbable g.
    g. compression body
    g. compression boot
    g. sponge
    g. sponge slurry
    zinc g.
gelatinase
    92-kDa g.
gelatinous
    g. acute pneumonia
    g. infiltration
    g. sputum
gel-filtered platelet (GFP)
Gelfoam
    G. cookie
    G. sponge
    thrombin-soaked G.
    G. Topical
Gelpi retractor
gelsolin
Gelweave
    G. Ante-Flo
    G. 3 branch Plexus
    G. graft
    G. Valsalva
Gem
    G. II DR dual-chamber defibrillator
    G. II VR implantable cardioverter-
      defibrillator
    G. DR implantable defibrillator
    G. III AT implantable cardioverter-
      defibrillator
    G. Premier Plus blood
      gas/electrolyte analyzer
    G. SensiCath blood gas monitoring
      system
gemcitabine
Gemcor
gemfibrozil
gemifloxacin mesylate
Gemzar
Genac Tablet
Genahist Oral
Genatuss DM
genavense
    Mycobacterium g.
GenBank
    G. genome sequence database
    G. information system
gene
    actin g.
    angiotensinogen g.

    beta-MHC g.
    cardiac sodium channel g.
    c-Jun g.
    C1qR g.
    cyclin A g.
    DCMAG-1 g.
    desmin g.
    D1790G mutant g.
    ecNOS g.
    endoglin g.
    env g.
    epicardin g.
    g. expression
    FBN1 g.
    fos g.
    gag g.
    HER2/neu g.
    human ether-a-go-go-related g.
      (HERG)
    human preproendothelin-1 g.
    IL-4 g.
    Jumonji g.
    Jun g.
    kallikrein g.
    methylenetetrahydrofolate
      reductase g.
    MTHFR g.
    MTP g.
    MyBP-C g.
    myosin-binding protein C g.
    g. polymorphism
    g. secretor
    sodium channel g.
    g. therapy
    g. therapy product
    g. transcription
    g. transfection
    g. transfer injection site
    TT form of MTP g.
    tuple-1 g.
    zinc finger g.
gene-activated erythropoietin
general
    g. angiography (GA)
    g. circulation (GC)
    G. Electric (GE)
    g. ward
    G. Well-Being Index
generalized
    g. arteriosclerosis (GAS)
    g. tuberculosis
generation
    neointimal g.
    thrombin g.
generator
    Angeion 2000 ICD g.
    asynchronous pulse g.
    atrial synchronous pulse g.
    atrial triggered pulse g.

bipolar g.
Cardioblate RF g.
CardioRhythm g.
Chardack-Greatbatch implantable
  cardiac pulse g.
Closure catheter/radiofrequency g.
Cordis Stockert g.
Cosmos II pulse g.
CPI-PRx pulse g.
demand pulse g.
Down flow g.
fixed-rate pulse g.
implantable pulse g.
Intec AID cardioverter-
  defibrillator g.
magnet application over pulse g.
Maxilith pacemaker pulse g.
Medtronic pulse g.
Microlith pacemaker pulse g.
Microny II SR+ pulse g.
Minilith pacemaker pulse g.
multiprogrammable pulse g.
PCD ICD g.
g. pocket
pulse g.
quadripolar Itrel 2 pulse g.
Radionics radiofrequency g.
radionuclide g.
rate-responsive pulse g.
Regency SR, SR+ pulse g.
SensorMedics g.
single-chamber pulse g.
small-particle aerosol g. (SPAG)
standby pulse g.
subpectoral implantation of pulse g.
Synchrony II, III DDDR pulse g.
tantalum-178 g.
Trilogy DC, DR, SR pulse g.
ventricular inhibited pulse g.
ventricular synchronous pulse g.
ventricular triggered pulse g.
VNUS Closure
  catheter/radiofrequency g.
VPAP II ST-A bilevel flow g.
x-ray g.
GenESA
  G. closed-loop delivery system
  G. system for radionuclide imaging
    stress test
genetic
  g. disorder
  g. factor

g. heterogeneity
g. hypertension (GH)
g. hypertrophic cardiomyopathy
g. locus
g. transmission
Genic coronary stent delivery system
geniculate
genioglossal
  g. advancement
  g. advancement procedure
genioglossus
genistein
Gen-Minoxidil
Gen-Nifedipine
genomic
genotype
  ACE-II g.
  ACE-DD g.
  ACE-ID g.
  angiotensin-converting enzyme II g.
  angiotensin-converting enzyme DD,
    ID g.
  DD g.
  methylenetetrahydrofolate
    reductase g.
  mitochondrial g.
  MTHFR g.
  QQ, QR, TT g.
Gen-Pindolol
Genpril
Gensini
  G. coronary arteriography catheter
  G. index
  G. score
  G. Teflon catheter
GenStent biologic
gentamicin sulfate
Gen-Timolol
Gentle-Flo suction catheter
Gentran
Genus stent
Geocillin
geometric
  g. cube formula
  g. mean diameter (GMD)
geometry
  left ventricular g.
  normal g.
  g. of stenosis
  ventricular g.
Geopen
George-Lewis technique

G

NOTES

George Washington strut
geotrichosis
Geotrichum candidum
GER
  gastroesophageal reflux
Gerald forceps
Gerbode
    G. annuloplasty
    G. defect
    G. forceps
GERD
  gastroesophageal reflux disease
Gerdy
    G. hyoid fossa
    G. intraauricular loop
Gerhardt
    G. change
    G. syndrome
    G. triangle
Geriatric Depression Scale
geriatrician
Gerlach tonsil
germanate
    bismuth g. (BGO)
germanium-68 external source
germanium sesquioxide
germ cell tumor
gerontology
gestational hypertension
GEWS
  Gianturco expandable wire stent
Gey fixative solution
GFP
  gel-filtered platelet
GFR
  glomerular filtration rate
GFT
  gradient field transform
GFX
  grepafloxacin
    GFX 2 coronary stent system
    GFX Micro stent III
    GFX over-the-wire coronary stent
GGA
  ground-glass attenuation
GG/DM
    Kolephrin GG/DM
GH
  genetic hypertension
GHB
  gamma hydroxybutyrate
Ghon
    G. complex
    G. focus
    G. primary lesion
    G. tubercle
ghosting artifact
ghost vessel

GIA
  Global Institute for Asthma
giant
    g. aneurysm
    g. bullous disease
    g. cell
    g. cell aortitis
    g. cell arteritis
    g. cell carcinoma
    g. cell interstitial pneumonitis
    (GIP)
    g. cell myocarditis
    g. cell pneumonia
    g. TU fusion wave
    g. T wave
    g. v wave
    g. a wave
Gianturco
    G. coil
    G. expandable wire stent (GEWS)
    G. Z stent
Gianturco-Grifka vascular occlusion device
Gianturco-Roehm bird's nest vena cava filter
Gianturco-Roubin
    G.-R. Flex II stent
    G.-R. Flex-Stent coronary stent
Gibbon-Landis test
Gibson
    G. circularity index
    G. murmur
    G. rule
Giemsa stain
Giertz-Shoemaker rib shears
GIK
  glucose, insulin, and potassium
Gilchrist disease
Gill-Jonas modification of Norwood procedure
gingivalis
    Porphyromonas g.
Ginneken
    Wilders-Jongsma-van G. (WJG)
GIP
  gastric inhibitory polypeptide
  giant cell interstitial pneumonitis
  glucose insulin, potassium
G$_i$ protein
girdle-like action
gitalin
giving-in/giving-up response
GKI
  glucose potassium insulin
glabrata
    Candida g.
    Torulopsis g.
gland
    adrenal g.

arytenoid g.
bronchial g.
esophageal g.
fibrous capsule of thyroid g.
Knoll g.
laryngeal g.
levator muscle of thyroid g.
Nuhn g.
pharyngeal g.
Philip g.
Rivinus g.
sublingual g.
submucosal g.
thyroid g.
tracheal g.

glandula, pl. **glandulae**
capsula fibrosa g.
glandulae esophageae
glandulae laryngeae
g. lingualis anterior
glandulae pharyngeales
g. sublingualis
glandulae tracheales

glandular pharyngitis
Glanzmann thrombasthenia
glare
veiling g.
Glasgow
G. Coma Scale (GCS)
G. sign
glass blower's emphysema
Glassman clamp
glassy degeneration
Glattelast compression pantyhose
Glaxo Wellcome Diskhaler inhaler
glebae
Acanthamoeba g.
Glenn
G. anastomosis
G. anastomosis procedure
G. operation
G. shunt
glibenclamide
GlideCath
G. dilator
G. entry needle
G. guide wire
G. hydrophilic coated catheter
G. sheath
G. syringe
G. torque device

Glidewire
G. Gold surgical guidewire
long taper/stiff shaft G.
Microvasive G.
Radifocus G.
Terumo Radifocus G.
glipizide
glissonitis
glistening yellow coronary plaque
global
g. amnesia
g. aphasia
g. cardiac disease
g. cerebral ischemia (GCI)
g. ejection fraction
g. hypokinesis
G. Institute for Asthma (GIA)
g. left ventricular ejection fraction
g. left ventricular function
G. Therapeutics V-Flex stent
g. tissue hypoxia
g. ventricular dysfunction
globe
bleeding g.
globin
accelerator g. (AcG)
globoid heart
globular
g. heart
g. sputum
g. thrombus
globulin
antithymocyte g.
cytomegalovirus immune g. (CMVIG)
gamma g.
intravenous gamma g. (IVGG)
intravenous immune g.
lymphocyte immune g.
Minnesota antilymphocyte g. (MAG)
rabbit antithymocyte g.
respiratory syncytial virus IV immune g.
Rho(D) immune g.
globus
g. hystericus
g. pharyngis
glomangiosis
pulmonary g.
glomeriform

NOTES

G

glomerular
> g. filtration rate (GFR)
> g. hyperfiltration

glomerulonephritis
> acute g. (AGN)
> crescentic g.
> mesangial proliferative g.
> pauciimmune g.

glomerulosa

glomerulosclerosis

glomus
> g. pulmonale
> g. tumor

glossectomy

glossopharyngeal
> g. breathing
> g. nerve
> g. neuralgia

glossopharyngeo
> ramus communicans cum nervo g.

glossopharyngeus, pl. **glossopharyngei**

glottic atresia

glottidis
> atrium g.

glottis respiratoria

glove
> compression g.'s
> ESP radiation reduction
>   examination g.'s

gloved
> g. finger sign
> g. fist technique

glucagon

glucarate
> technetium g.

gluceptate
> calcium g.

Gluck rib shears

glucocorticoid-induced hypertension

glucocorticoid resistance

glucocorticosteroid

glucometer

gluconate
> calcium g.
> ferrous g.
> potassium g.
> quinidine g.

Glucophage

glucoronate
> trimetrexate g.

glucose
> g. exchange
> g., insulin, and potassium (GIK)
> g. insulin, potassium (GIP)
> g. intolerance
> g. metabolism (rMRGlu)
> g. potassium insulin (GKI)
> sarcolemmal g.

> g. transporter 4
> g. uptake

glucose-6-phosphate dehydrogenase (G6PD)

glucose-6-phosphatase

glucosidase deficiency

Glucotrol

GlucoWatch

glucuronate

glue
> fibrin g.

Glu-plasminogen

glutamate exchange

glutamer-250
> hemoglobin g.-250

glutamic-oxaloacetic transaminase (GOT)

glutaraldehyde

glutaraldehyde-tanned
> g.-t. bovine collagen tube
> g.-t. bovine heart valve
> g.-t. porcine heart valve

glutathione (GSH)
> g. disulfide

gluteal
> left ventrolateral g. (LVLG)

glutethimide

Glutose

glyburide

glyceraldehyde 3-phosphate

glycerin

glyceroltrinitrate, glyceryl trinitrate (GTN)

glyceryl
> g. guaiacolate

glycinate
> theophylline sodium g.

glycine site

glycocalicin
> g. index
> plasma g.

glycocalix, glycocalyx

glycoconjugate
> respiratory g. (RGC)

glycogen
> g. cardiomegaly
> g. depletion
> g. loading
> g. phosphorylase
> g. storage disease (I-VIII)
> g. synthase

glycogenosis
> cardiac g.
> g. type III

glycol
> polyethylene g. (PEG)
> recombinant polyethylene g. (r-PEG)

glycolated

glycolipid antibody

glycolysis
glycolytic enzyme
glycometabolic state
glycopeptide teicoplanin
glycoprotein (GP)
> histidine-rich g.
> g. IIb/IIIa antagonist
> g. IIb/IIIa inhibitor
> g. IIb/IIIa receptor
> multikringle g.
> platelet membrane g.
> platelet receptor g.

glycopyrrolate
glycoside
> cardiac g.
> digitalis g.

glycosphingolipid disorder
glycosylated hemoglobin
glycosylation of intracellular proteins
glycoxidation
glycyl compound
glycyrrhizinic acid
Glydeine
Glynase PresTab
Glyrol
Glytuss
GM-CSF
> granulocyte/macrophage colony-
> stimulating factor

GMD
> geometric mean diameter

GMP
> guanosine monophosphate

GMR
> gallop, murmur, rub

GMS
> Grocott methenamine silver
> GMS stain

GNB
> gram-negative bacillus

goblet
> g. cell
> g. cell degranulation
> g. cell hypertrophy
> g. cell metaplasia

Godart expirograph
Godwin tumor
Goeltec catheter
Goethlin test
Goetz
> G. bipolar electrode
> G. cardiac device

goiter
> diving g.
> plunging g.
> suffocative g.
> wandering g.

Golaski knitted Dacron graft
Golaski-UMI vascular prosthesis
gold (Au)
> g. marker
> g. salt

gold-195m radionuclide
Goldberg-MPC mediastinoscope
Goldblatt
> G. kidney
> G. phenomenon
> two-kidney G.

gold-coated Inflow coronary stent
Golden
> G. sign of S
> G. S sign

Goldenhar syndrome
Goldflam disease
Goldflam-Erb disease
Goldman
> G. cardiac risk index score
> G. index of risk
> G. risk-factor index

Goldner trichrome stain
Goldscheider percussion
GoldSeal nasal mask
Goldsmith operation
Goldstein hemoptysis
Golgi
> G. complex
> G. tendon organ

Gomco thoracic drainage pump
gomenol
Gomori methenamine silver stain
gonadal
> g. disease
> g. dysgenesis

gondii
> *Toxoplasma* g.

gonion to pogonion (GO-POG)
gonococcal endocarditis
gonorrhoeae
> *Neisseria* g.

Goodale-Lubin
> G.-L. cardiac device
> G.-L. catheter

GoodKnight 418A, 418G, 418P CPAP system

G

NOTES

goodness-of-fit test
Goodpasture syndrome
goose-honk murmur
gooseneck, goose neck
    g. outflow tract deformity
    g. snare
Goosen vascular punch
GO-POG
    gonion to pogonion
gordonae
    Mycobacterium g.
Gordon elementary body
Gore-Tex
    G.-T. AF fistula
    G.-T. baffle
    G.-T. bifurcated vascular graft
    G.-T. cardiovascular patch
    G.-T. jump graft
    G.-T. shunt
    G.-T. soft tissue patch
    G.-T. surgical membrane
    G.-T. tube
Goris background subtraction technique
Gorlin
    G. catheter
    G. constant
    G. and Gorlin equation
    G. hydraulic formula
    G. syndrome
gormanii
    Legionella g.
Gormel Cream
goserelin
GOT
    glutamic-oxaloacetic transaminase
Gott
    G. butterfly heart valve
    G. shunt
Gott-Daggett heart valve prosthesis
Gould
    G. electromagnetic flowmeter
    G. Instrument Systems spirometer
    G. PentaCath 5-lumen
        thermodilution catheter
    G. Statham pressure transducer
Gould-Godart type 18070 ergometer
gout
gouty phlebitis
Gowers
    G. contraction
    G. sign
    G. syndrome
GP
    glycoprotein
gp91^{phox} protein
G6PD
    glucose-6-phosphate dehydrogenase
grabbing technique

gracile habitus
gradational step exercise stress test
grade
    g. 1-6 murmur
    Sellers g.
    thrombus g.
    TIMI flow g. 0–3
    TIMI myocardial perfusion g.
graded exercise test (GXT)
gradient
    A-a g.
    alveolar arterial g. (AAG)
    alveolar-arterial oxygen g. (A-a 02)
    alveolocapillary partial pressure g.
    aortic pressure g.
    aortic valve g. (AVG)
    arm-leg g.
    atrial-to-pulmonary venous g.
    atrioventricular g.
    coronary perfusion g.
    diastolic g.
    Doppler pressure g.
    g. echo-cine MRI
    electrochemical g.
    elevated g.
    g. field transform (GFT)
    g. gel electrophoresis
    hemodynamic g.
    interatrial pressure g. (IAPG)
    intracavitary pressure g.
    intraventricular g.
    mean diastolic g. (MDG)
    mitral g.
    mitral valve g. (MVG)
    peak instantaneous Doppler g.
    peak systolic g. (PSG)
    peak transaortic valve g.
    portal pressure g. (PPG)
    pressure g.
    pulmonary bed g.
    pulmonary valve g. (PVG)
    g. recall echo (GRE)
    g. recalled acquisition in a steady
      state (GRASS)
    g. reduction
    residual g.
    g. reversal image
    systolic g.
    transaortic valve g.
    transcardiac g.
    transmitral g.
    transprosthetic g.
    transpulmonary g. (TPG)
    transstenotic pressure g.
    transvalvular aortic g.
    transvalvular pressure g. (TPG)
    ventricular g.
gradient-echo imaging

grading
> Stary histology g.

graduated compression stockings (GCS)
Graduate measuring wire guide
graft
> activated g.
> albumin-coated vascular g.
> aldehyde-tanned bovine carotid
> artery g.
> aortic tube g.
> aortocoronary g. (ACG)
> aortocoronary bypass g. (ACBG)
> aortocoronary saphenous vein
> bypass g. (ACSVBG)
> aortocoronary snake g.
> aortofemoral bypass g. (AFBG)
> aortoiliac bypass g.
> aortomonoiliac g.
> Aria coronary artery bypass g.
> Artegraft natural collagen
> vascular g.
> autogenic g.
> autologous fat g.
> bifurcated g.
> Biograft g.
> BioPolyMeric vascular g.
> Björk-Shiley g.
> bypass g. (BPG)
> CardioPass layered microporous
> small-bore vascular g.
> compressed Ivalon patch g.
> coronary artery bypass g. (CARB)
> coronary artery vein g. (CAVG)
> coronary bypass g. (CBG)
> g. coronary disease (GCD)
> coronary venous g. (CVG)
> Corvita endoluminal g.
> Corvita endoprosthesis stent g.
> Dacron tube g.
> descending thoracic aorta-to-femoral
> artery bypass g.
> Diastat vascular access g.
> double coronary artery bypass g.
> (DCABG)
> DTAFA bypass g.
> Edwards-Tapp arterial g.
> endoluminal stent g.
> endoscopic coronary artery
> bypass g. (E-CABG)
> endovascular g.
> endovascular aortic g. (EAG)
> ePTFE g.

> expanded polytetrafluoroethylene
> vascular g.
> Favaloro saphenous vein bypass g.
> FEP-ringed Gore-Tex vascular g.
> GEA g.
> Gelweave g.
> Golaski knitted Dacron g.
> Gore-Tex bifurcated vascular g.
> Gore-Tex jump g.
> Hancock pericardial valve g.
> Hancock vascular g.
> Hemashield Gold 1, 4 branch
> AAA g.
> Hemashield Gold Microvel knitted
> double velour g.
> Hemashield Vantage vascular g.
> Hemobahn endovascular prosthesis
> stent-g.
> HUV bypass g.
> IEA g.
> IMA g.
> Impra Distaflo bypass g.
> inferior epigastric artery g.
> Inoue triple-branched stent g.
> InterGard vascular g.
> internal mammary artery g.
> internal thoracic artery g.
> Ionescu-Shiley vascular g.
> ITA g.
> Jostent coronary stent g.
> jump g.
> Kimura cartilage g.
> knitted polyester crimped g.
> left internal mammary artery g.
> left internal thoracic artery g.
> LIMA g.
> LITA g.
> lower extremity bypass g.
> mammary artery g.
> mandrel g.
> Meadox g.
> Medtronic AneuRx stent g.
> mesenteric bypass g.
> Microknit arterial g.
> Microknit patch g.
> Microvel double velour g.
> minimally invasive direct coronary
> artery bypass g. (MIDCABG)
> modified human graft umbilical
> vein g.
> nonvalved g.
> Passager stent g.

G

NOTES

graft *(continued)*

pedicle g.
Perma-Flow coronary bypass g.
polytetrafluoroethylene stent g.
portacaval H g.
post g. (PG)
predilated polytetrafluoroethylene g.
PTFE stent g.
radial artery g.
g. rejection
renal artery bypass g.
reversed saphenous vein g.
right internal mammary artery g.
right internal thoracic artery g.
RIMA g.
RITA g.
saphenous vein g. (SVG)
single coronary artery bypass g.
  (SCABG)
skip g.
snake g.
stent g. (SG)
straight tube g.
subclavian artery bypass g.
T g.
Talent g.
Teflon g.
thoracic stent g.
transluminally placed endovascular
  branched stent g.
triple coronary artery g. (TCAG)
triple coronary artery bypass g.
  (TCABG)
two-piece bifurcated intraluminal g.
Ultramax woven velour vascular g.
Vanguard III endovascular aortic g.
Varivas R denatured homologous
  vein g.
VascuLink vascular access g.
g. vasculopathy
Vascutek Gelseal vascular g.
Vascutek knitted vascular g.
Vascutek woven vascular g.
vein g.
velour collar g.
venous bypass g. (VBG)
vertebral artery bypass g.
Vitagraft vascular g.
Weavenit patch g.
woven Dacron fabric g.
woven Dacron tube g.
Y g.
Y-shaped g.

GraftAssist vein-graft holder

grafting

coronary artery bypass g. (CABG)
endarterectomy and coronary artery
  bypass g. (E-CABG)
endovascular stent g.

minimally invasive coronary
  bypass g. (MICABG)
Port-Access coronary artery
  bypass g.
saphenous vein bypass g. (SVBG)

graft-seeking catheter
graft-versus-host disease (GVHD)
Graham

G. law
G. Steell murmur

grain

g. dust
g. handler's disease
refined g.

gram-negative

g.-n. bacillus (GNB)
g.-n. cocci
g.-n. endocarditis
g.-n. organism
g.-n. pericarditis

gram-positive

g.-p. bacillus
g.-p. cocci
g.-p. organism

Gram stain
granarius

Sitophilus g.

Grancher

G. sign
G. triad

granoplasm
**Grant abdominal aortic aneurysmal
  clamp**
granular

g. cell tumor
g. pharyngitis
g. respiration

granulation

Bayle g.
cell g.
g. stenosis
g. tissue

granule

aleuronoid g.
azurophil g.
Birbeck g.'s
E.E.S. G.'s
Fauvel g.'s
Much g.'s

Granulex
granulocyte activation
**granulocyte/macrophage colony-
  stimulating factor (GM-CSF)**
granulocytopenia
granulocytopenic host
granuloma

cocci g.
eosinophilic g. (EG)
hyalinizing g.

interstitial g.
necrotizing g.
noncaseating g.
pulmonary hyalinizing g.
sarcoid g.
granulomatosis
allergic angiitis and g.
bronchocentric g. (BCG)
eosinophilic g.
Langerhans cell g.
lymphomatoid g. (LYG)
talc g.
Wegener g. (WG)
granulomatous
g. arteritis
g. disease
g. hepatitis
g. inflammation
g. mediastinitis
g. pneumonitis
granulosus
Echinococcus g.
**graphite furnace atomic absorption
spectroscopy**
GRASS
gradient recalled acquisition in a steady
state
GRASS MRI
Grass S88 muscle stimulator
gratus
Strophanthus g.
Gräupner method
Graves disease
gravis
myalgia g.
myasthenia g.
gravitation factor
gray (Gy)
g. hepatization
g. induration
g. infiltration
g. scale
grayout spell
gray-scale ultrasound
Gray-Weale plaque classification
GRE
gradient recall echo
great
g. alveolar cell
g. artery
g. cardiac vein (GCV)
g. cardiac vein flow (GCVF)

G. Ormond Street tracheostomy
g. vessel
g. vessel disruption
g. vessel tear
green
g. coffee bean
g. dye curve
g. sputum
g. strep endocarditis
Greene sign
Greenfield
G. IVC filter
G. vena cava filter
Gregg
G. cannula
G. phenomenon
grelot
bruit de g.
grepafloxacin (GFX)
grid
external g.
Griesinger sign
Griess test
Griggs tracheostomy
grinder's
g. asthma
g. phthisis
grip
devil's g.
NEO-fit endotracheal tube g.
G. Technology stent crimping
process
g. torque device
gripping heart
griseofulvin
groaning murmur
Grocco sign
Grocott
G. methenamine silver (GMS)
G. stain
groin
g. approach
g. complication
**Grollman pulmonary artery-seeking
catheter**
Grönblad-Strandberg syndrome
Grondahl esophagoplasty
Grondahl-Finney operation
Groningen voice prosthesis
groove
arterial g.
atrioventricular g.

G

NOTES

groove *(continued)*
  auriculoventricular g.
  A-V g.
  bulboventricular g.
  conoventricular fold and g.
  deltopectoral g.
  Harrison g.
  laryngotracheal g.
  nasopharyngeal g.
  pharyngotympanic g.
  terminal g.
  vascular g.
  venous g.
  Waterston g.
Groshong double-lumen catheter
gross
  g. tracheoesophageal atresia
  g. tracheoesophageal fistula
Grossman
  G. scale
  G. sign
ground-glass
  g.-g. appearance
  g.-g. attenuation (GGA)
  g.-g. opacification
  g.-g. opacity
  g.-g. pattern
group
  diagnostic-related g. (DRG)
  Digitalis Investigation G. (DIG)
  Digoxin Investigators G. (DIG)
  NICE g.
Grover clamp
growth
  dysanaptic g.
  g. factor
  g. hormone
gruberi
  Naegleria g.
gruel
  atheromatous g.
grumous debris
grunt
  diastolic g.
  expiratory g.
Grüntzig
  G. balloon catheter
  G. balloon catheter angioplasty
  G. Dilaca catheter
  G. femoral stiffening cannula
  G. technique
GSH
  glutathione
GS Modular pulmonary testing system
GSNO
  S-nitrosoglutathione
G-strophanthin
G-suit

GTN
  glyceroltrinitrate
GTP
  guanosine triphosphate
  guanosine 5′-triphosphate
guaiacolate
  glyceryl g.
Guaifed
guaifenesin
  g. and codeine
  g. and dextromethorphan
  hydrocodone and g.
  hydrocodone, pseudoephedrine,
   and g.
  g. and phenylpropanolamine
  g., phenylpropanolamine, and
   dextromethorphan
  g., phenylpropanolamine, and
   phenylephrine
  g. and pseudoephedrine
  g., pseudoephedrine, and codeine
  g., pseudoephedrine, and
   dextromethorphan
  theophylline and g.
Guaifenex
  G. LA
  G. PSE
Guaimax-D
Guai-Vent/PSE
guanabenz acetate
guanadrel sulfate
guanethidine
  g. monosulfate
  g. sulfate
guanfacine
  g. acetate
  g. hydrochloride
Guangzhou GD-1 prosthetic valve
guanine nucleotide modulatable binding
guanosine
  g. 5′-diphosphate (GDP)
  g. monophosphate (GMP)
  g. triphosphate (GTP)
  g. 5′-triphosphate (GTP)
guanylate cyclase
guanylyl cyclase
Guardian
  G. AICD
  G. ATP 4210 implantable
   cardioverter-defibrillator
  G. catheter
  G. ICD
  G. pacemaker
Guardwire
  G. angioplasty system
  G. emboli containment system
GuardWire
  PercuSurge G.
  G. Plus system

guar gum
Gubner-Ungerleider
    G.-U. voltage
    G.-U. voltage criteria
Guéneau de Mussy point
guggulipid
Guglielmi detachable coil
Guiatex
Guiatuss
    G. AC
    G. CF
    G. DAC
Guiatuss-DM
Guiatussin
    G. DAC
    G. with Codeine
guidance
    echo g.
    fluoroscopic g.
Guidant
    G. CRM pacemaker
    G. defibrillator
    G. Heart Rhythm Technologies
    Linear Ablation system
    G. Multi-Link Tetra coronary stent
    system
    G. stent
    G. TRIAD three-electrode energy
    defibrillation system
Guidant-CPI device
guide
    ACS LIMA g.
    Amplatz tapered extra stiff wire g.
    Amplatz tube g.
    Amplatz ultra stiff wire g.
    Bentson Plus cerebral wire g.
    Cope Nitinol mandril wire g.
    curved tapered Tefcor movable
    core wire g.
    double flexible tipped wire g.
    Flexguide intubation g.
    Franzen needle g.
    Graduate measuring wire g.
    Lunderquist extra stiff wire g.
    McNamara renal exchange wire g.
    movable core straight safety
    wire g.
    Müller catheter g.
    New York catheter exchange
    wire g.
    Reuter tip deflecting wire g.
    Roadrunner extra-support wire g.

    tapered movable core curved
    wire g.
    Tefcor movable core straight
    wire g.
    Torq-Flex wire g.
    variable stiffness wire g.
    Vista Brite Tip IG introducer g.
    wire g.
guided imagery
guidelines
    ACC/AHA pacemaker
    implantation g.
    American College of
    Cardiology/American Heart
    Association Task Force on
    Practice g.
    American Heart Association g.
    clinical practice g. (CPG)
    implantation g.
    McGoon g.
    National Cholesterol Education
    Panel g.
    NCEP g.
    NCEP-II g.
guider
GuideRight guidewire
guidewire, guide wire (gw)
    ACS Amplatz g.
    ACS exchange g.
    ACS extra-support g.
    ACS Hi-Torque Balance
    middleweight g.
    ACS LIMA g.
    Amplatz Super Stiff g.
    Amplex g.
    atherolytic reperfusion g.
    Athlete g.
    ATW steerable g.
    Bard Commander PTCA g.
    Becton-Dickinson g.
    Bentson exchange straight g.
    Bentson floppy-tip g.
    Bentson-style g.
    catheter g.
    ControlWire g.
    Coons Super Stiff long tip g.
    Critikon g.
    Crosswire nitinol hydrophilic g.
    Doppler-tipped angioplasty g.
    Elastorc catheter g.
    Emerald diagnostic g.
    exchange g.

NOTES

G

guidewire *(continued)*

Extra Sport coronary g.
extra-support g.
flexible g.
Flex Tip g.
FloMap g.
floppy g.
floppy-tipped g.
FloWire Doppler g.
fluid-filled pressure monitoring g.
Glidewire Gold surgical g.
GuideRight g.
Hi-Torque Floppy exchange g.
Hi-Torque Floppy II g.
Hi-Torque Floppy intermediate g.
Hi-Torque Standard g.
hydrophilic coated g.
HydroSteer hydrophilic g.
intravascular Doppler-tipped g.
J g.
J-tip g.
Kayak hydrophilic g.
Linx exchange g.
Linx extension g.
g. loop
Magic Torque g.
Magnum g.
Micropuncture g.
Microvasive stiff piano wire g.
Mirage hydrophilic g.
Monorail g.
Newton g.
g. perforation
Phantom g.
Platinum Plus g.
PressureWire g.
Prima laser g.
Radifocus catheter g.
g. reflection
Reflex steerable g.
Safe-Steer g.
safety g.
Schwarten LP g.
Seeker g.
Shinobi steerable g.
silk g.
Silver Speed hydrophilic g.
Sniper hydrophilic Nitinol g.
SOS g.
Spectranetics Prima laser g.
Stabilizer balanced performance g.
Stabilizer marker wire steerable g.
Stabilizer Plus steerable g.
Stabilizer XS steerable g.
stainless steel g.
steerable angioplastic g.
Tapered Torque g.

g. technique
Teflon-coated g.
Terumo Crosswire PTCA g.
Tomcat PTCA g.
g. traversal test
Ultra-Select nitinol PTCA g.
Wholey Hi-Torque Floppy g.
Wholey Hi-Torque modified J g.
Wholey Hi-Torque standard g.
Wizdom ST steerable g.

guiding catheter
Guillain-Barré syndrome
guilliermondii

Candida g.

guillotine

rib g.

Guiraudon corridor operation
gulae

plexus g.

Gulf War syndrome
gum

g. acacia
g. elastic bougie introducer
guar g.
Nicorette G.
nicotine g.
polacrilex chewing g.

Gunn crossing sign
gunshot wound
Gunther Tulip vena cava MrEye filter
gurgling rale
Gurvich biphasic waveform
gut-associated lymphoid tissue (GALT)
guttural

g. pulse
g. rale

GVHD

graft-versus-host disease

gw

guidewire

GXT

graded exercise test

Gy

gray

gynoid obesity
gyri (*pl. of* gyrus)
Gyrocaps

Slo-Phyllin G.

Gyroscan HP Philips 15S whole-body system
gyrus, pl. gyri

angular g. (AG)
inferior frontal g. (IFG)
middle frontal g. (MFG)
superior temporal g. (STG)
supramarginal g. (SMG)

H
heart
heparin
H space
H spike
H wave
H zone

h
h peak
h plateau
h wave

H1 receptor

H₂
prostaglandin H_2

HA
Hispanic American
Horton arteritis

Haake water bath

HAART
highly active antiretroviral therapy

Haber-Weiss reaction

habit
alimentary h.'s
h. cough

Habitrol Patch

habitual cough

habitus
gracile h.

HACEK
Haemophilus aphrophilus, Actinobacillus actinomycetemcomitans, Cardiobacterium hominis, Eikenella corrodens, and *Kingella kingae*

hacking cough

HAD
Hospital Anxiety and Depression

HADS
Hospital Anxiety and Depression Scale

HAEC
human aortic endothelial cell

H-Ae interval

haematobium
Schistosoma h.

Haemolite autologous blood recovery system

haemolyticus
Haemophilus h.

Haemonetics
H. Cell Saver
H. Cell Saver system

haemophilum
Mycobacterium h.

Haemophilus
H. aphrophilus

H. aphrophilus, Actinobacillus actinomycetemcomitans, Cardiobacterium hominis, Eikenella corrodens, and *Kingella kingae* (HACEK)
H. endocarditis
H. haemolyticus
H. influenzae
H. parahaemolyticus
H. parainfluenzae (HPI)
H. pertussis
H. type b conjugate vaccine

Hafnia

HAFOE
high air flow with oxygen entrainment

Hageman factor

Hagenbach extension of Poiseuille equation

hair-matrix carcinoma

hairspray thesaurosis

hairy heart

Hakki formula

Halbrecht syndrome

Haldane
H. effect
H. transformation

Haldane-Priestley
H.-P. sample
H.-P. tube

Hales piesimeter

half amplitude pulse duration

half-diluted contrast

half-life
biological h.-l.
effective h.-l.
elimination h.-l.

half-normal saline

half-power distance

Halfprin

half-time
h.-t. method
pressure h.-t. (PHT)

half-value layer

Hall
H. prosthetic heart valve
H. sign
H. valvulotome

Haller plexus

Hallion test

Hall-Kaster prosthetic valve

hallucination
hypnagogic h.

halo
h. sheathing

H

313

halo *(continued)*
    h. sign
    H. XP electrophysiology catheter
halofantrine
halogenated
    h. hydrocarbon
    h. hydrocarbon propellant
haloperidol
Haloscale respirometer
Halotestin
halothane
Halotussin DAC
Halsted clamp
Haltran
hamartoma
    myocardial h.
    pulmonary h.
Hamburger test
Hamilton-Stewart formula
Hamilton ventilator
Hamman
    H. click
    H. crunch
    H. disease
    Hamman-Rich syndrome (HRS)
    H. murmur
    H. sign
    H. syndrome
Hamman-Rich syndrome (HRS)
Hammersmith mitral prosthesis
hammocking of posterior mitral leaflet
Hampton hump
Ham test
Hancock
    H. bipolar balloon pacemaker
    H. embolectomy catheter
    H. fiberoptic catheter
    H. hydrogen detection catheter
    H. II porcine bioprosthesis
    H. II tissue valve
    H. luminal electrophysiologic
        recording catheter
    H. mitral valve prosthesis
    H. modified orifice valve
    H. M.O. II bioprosthesis porcine
        valve
    H. M.O. II porcine bioprosthesis
    H. pericardial valve graft
    H. porcine heterograft
    H. temporary cardiac pacing wire
    H. vascular graft
    H. wedge-pressure catheter
hand
    h. agitated solution
    h. injection
hand-foot-and-mouth disease
handgrip
    h. apexcardiographic test (HAT)

    isometric h.
    h. stress
handheld
    h. nebulizer
    8500 h. pulse oximeter
Handi
    H. oxygen analyzer
    H. oxygen sensor
handle
    exchange tip deflecting wire
        guide h.
Hand-Schüller-Christian disease
Hands-Off
    H.-O. infusion port heparin-coated
        thermodilution catheter with
        TwistLock
    H.-O. thermal dilution catheter
HANE
    hereditary angioneurotic edema
hANF
    human atrial natriuretic factor
hanging heart
hangout interval
Hank's balanced salt solution
Hanley-McNeil method
Hanning window
Hannover classification
hANP
    human atrial natriuretic peptide
Hans Rudolph nonbreathing valve
Hantaan virus
hantavirus pulmonary syndrome
HAP
    high-altitude peristalsis
    hospital-acquired pneumonia
HAPC
    high-amplitude peristaltic contraction
HAPE
    high-altitude pulmonary edema
HAPE-r
    high-altitude pulmonary edema resistant
HAPE-s
    high-altitude pulmonary edema
        susceptible
haploinsufficiency
haplotype
    HLA-DQA1 gene h.
    HLA-DQB1 gene h.
happy tachypnea
HAPVC
    hemi-anomalous pulmonary venous
        connection
    hemi-anomalous pulmonary venous
        connection (HAPVC)
HAPVD
    hemi-anomalous pulmonary venous
        drainage

HAPVR
    hemi-anomalous pulmonary venous
        return
hard
    h. cardiac event
    h. metal disease
    h. metal pneumoconiosis
    h. metal-related lung fibrosis
    h. pulse
hardening
    x-ray beam h.
HAREM
    heparin assay rapid easy method
Hare syndrome
Harken
    H. ball valve
    H. forceps
    H. rib spreader
HARM
    heparin assay rapid method
harmonic
    h. component
    h. content
    h. gray-scale imaging
    h. imaging (HI)
    h. imaging mode
    h. imaging ultrasound technique
    h. phase (HARP)
    h. phase image
    h. power Doppler imaging
harness
    Heart Hugger sternum support h.
HARP
    harmonic phase
    Hospital Admission Risk Profile
    HARP image
Harpoon suture anchor
Harrington esophageal diverticulectomy
Harris adapter
Harris-Benedict equation
Harrison groove
harsh
    h. murmur
    h. respiration
Hartmann
    H. clamp
    H. solution
HARTS
    heat-activated recoverable temporary
        stent
Hartzler
    H. ACX II catheter

    H. LPS dilatation catheter
    H. Micro-600 catheter
    H. Micro II balloon
    H. Micro II catheter
    H. Micro XT catheter
    H. RX-014 balloon catheter
Harvard pump
harvester's lung
harvesting
    endoscopic saphenous vein h.
        (ESVH)
    saphenous vein h. (SVH)
Harvey Elite stethoscope
HASCVD
    hypertensive arteriosclerotic
        cardiovascular disease
HASHD
    hypertensive arteriosclerotic heart disease
Hashimoto thyroiditis
HASMC
    human aortic smooth muscle
    human aortic smooth muscle cell
Hassall corpuscle
HAST
    high-altitude simulation test
HAT
    handgrip apexcardiographic test
    heparin-associated thrombocytopenia
hat
    bishop's h.
Hatafuku fundus onlay patch
    esophageal repair
hatchetti
    Acanthamoeba h.
Hatle method
HATT
    heparin-associated thrombocytopenia and
        thrombosis
hawaiiensis
    Drechslera h.
Hawksley random zero mercury
    sphygmomanometer
hawthorn
Hawthorne effect
Hayek oscillator
Hayfebrol Liquid
hay fever
Haynes 25 material
haze
    hilar h.
    perihilar h.

NOTES

H

hazy
    h. appearance
    h. infiltrate
    h. lesion
HB
  heart block
  His bundle
Hb
  hemoglobin
    Hb oximetry
HbCO$_2$
  carboxyhemoglobin
HBDH
  hydroxybutyrate dehydrogenase
HBE
  His bundle electrogram
HBO
  hyperbaric oxygen
    HBO therapy
HbO$_2$
  oxyhemoglobin
    HbO$_2$ oximetry
HbOC vaccine
HBOT
  hyperbaric oxygen therapy
HBP
  heartbeat period
  high blood pressure
HBT Sleuth portable hydrogen monitor
HC
  hypercholesterolemia
  hypertrophic cardiomyopathy
HCF
  heparin cofactor
  hereditary capillary fragility
HCl
  hydrochloride
    anagrelide HCl
    cefepime HCl
    colesevelam HCl
    dexmedetomidine HCl
    levalbuterol HCl
    moxifloxacin HCl
    sotalol HCl
    verapamil HCl
HCM, HCMP
  hypertrophic cardiomyopathy
HCMV
  human cytomegalovirus
HCN
  hydrogen cyanide
HCO$_3$
  bicarbonate
HCT, HCTZ
  hydrochlorothiazide
    Atacand HCT
    Avapro HCT
    Diovan HCT
    Lotensin HCT

HCTS
  high cholesterol and tocopherol
    supplement
HCVD
  hypertensive cardiovascular disease
HD
  heart disease
HDH
  heart disease history
HDL
  high-density lipoprotein
    isolated low HDL
    nascent HDL
    pre-beta 1 HDL
HDLBP
  high-density lipoprotein binding protein
HDL-C
  high-density lipoprotein-cholesterol
    complex
HDL-c
  high-density lipoprotein-cell surface
HDLP
  high-density lipoprotein
HDM
  house dust mite
    HDM allergen
HDRF
  Heart Disease Research Foundation
HDU
  high-dependency unit
HE
  hypertensive encephalopathy
H&E
  hematotylin and eosin
    H&E stain
He
  heart
Head
    H. area
    H. lines
    H. paradoxical reflex
    H. zone
headache
    migraine h.
    syncopal migraine h.
head-down tilt test
headgear
    Velstretch/Velcro h.
headhunter angiography catheter
head-out water immersion
headpiece
    e-Net h.
head-tilt
    h.-t. chin-lift maneuver
    h.-t. method
head-up
    h.-u. tilt (HUT)
    h.-u. tilt-induced syncope

h.-u. tilt-table test (HUTTT)
h.-u. tilt test

Heaf test
healed
    h. myocardial infarct (HMI)
    h. tuberculosis
healing
    per primam h.
    per secundum h.
health
    H. behavior model
    H. level seven (HL7)
    H. Locus of Control Scale
    National Institutes of H. (NIH)
    H. On the Net (HON)
    H. On the Net code of conduct
    (HONcode)
healthcare
health-related quality of life (HRQL, HRQOL)
heard
    fetal heart h. (FHH)
    fetal heart not h. (FHNH)
heart (H, He, HT, ht)
    abdominal h.
    h. action of heart (DAH)
    acute margin of h.
    H. Aid 80 defibrillator
    H. Aide Ezd noninvasive
    monitoring equipment
    air-driven artificial h.
    Akutsu III total artificial h.
    ALVAD artificial h.
    anterior surface of h.
    armor h.
    armored h.
    h. arrest
    artificial h. (AH)
    athlete's h.
    athletic h.
    atrium of h.
    h. attack
    baggy h.
    balloon-shaped h.
    h. beat
    beer h.
    beriberi h.
    Berlin total artificial h.
    h. block (HB)
    boat-shaped h.
    bony h.
    booster h.

boot-shaped h.
bovine h.
CardioWest total artificial h.
cervical h.
h. chamber remodeling
chambers of the h.
chaotic h.
charcoal h.
compensatory hypertrophy of h.
compliance of h.
congenital malformation of the h.
  (CMH)
contour of h.
contracted h.
corticosteroid-treated h.
crisscross h.
crux of h.
decortication of h.
dextroposition of h.
dextroversion of h.
diaphragmatic surface of h.
dilation of h.
h. disease (HD)
h. disease history (HDH)
H. Disease Research Foundation
  (HDRF)
donor h.
drop h.
dynamite h.
egg-shaped h.
electrical alternation of h.
electromechanical artificial h.
encased h.
enlarged h. (EH, eh)
explanted h.
extracorporeal h.
h. failure (HF)
h. failure cell
H. Failure Knowledge Test
H. Failure Society of America
  (HFSA)
fatty degeneration of h.
fetal h. (FH, FHT)
fibroid h.
figure-of-eight h.
flask-shaped h.
focal myocytosis of h.
foramen of veins of h.
h. frequency (Hfr)
frosted h.
frosting h.
globoid h.

NOTES

H

heart *(continued)*

globular h.
gripping h.
hairy h.
h. and hand syndrome
hanging h.
3:2 h. block
3:1 h. block
height of h. (Ht)
Hershey total artificial h.
holiday h.
Holmes h.
horizontal h.
H. Hugger sternum support harness
hyperthyroid h.
hypoplastic h.
hypoplastic left h. (HPLH)
icing h.
implantable artificial h. (IAH)
h. infusion (HI)
h. infusion broth (HIB)
intermediate h.
intracorporeal h.
irritable h.
Jarvik 7, 8 artificial h.
Jarvik 7-70 artificial h.
Jarvik 2000 artificial h.
H. Laser
h. laser revascularization
H. Laser system
H. Laser for TMR
law of the h.
left h. (LH)
left auricle of h.
left margin of h.
Liotta total artificial h.
h., liver and kidneys (H-L-K)
h. loop
h. and lung (H&L)
h. massage
mechanical h.
mechanical alternation of h.
h. minute output (HMO)
movable h.
moyamoya of h.
h. murmur (HM)
myocytolysis of h.
myxedema h.
H. nebulizer
Norwood operation for hypoplastic left-sided h.
obtuse margin of h.
one-ventricle h.
orthotopic univentricular artificial h.
ox h.
h. palpitations
paracorporeal h.
parchment h.
pear-shaped h.

pectoral h.
pendulous h.
h. position
postischemic h.
pulmonary h.
h. pump
Quain fatty h.
h. rate (HR, HRT)
h. rate audiometry (HRA)
h. rate correction formula
h. rate fluctuations (HRF)
H. Rate 1-2-3 monitor
h. rate-pressure product
h. rate range (HRR)
h. rate recovery (HRR)
h. rate reserve (HRR)
h. rate retardation index (HRRI)
h. rate-systolic blood pressure product (RPP)
h. rate turbulence
h. rate variability (HRV)
h. rate variability test
recipient h.
h. reflex
reinnervation in transplanted h.
rheumatism of h.
right h. (RH)
right auricle of h.
right margin of h.
round h.
sabot h.
semihorizontal h.
semivertical h.
senescent h.
septation of h.
h. shock protein antigen
skeleton of h.
skin h.
snowman h.
soldier's h.
h. sounds (HS)
h. sounds S_1, S_2, S_3, S_4
stiff h.
stone h.
h. stroke
superoinferior h.
suspended h.
swinging h.
Symbion Jarvik-7 artificial h.
Symbion J-7 70-mL ventricle total artificial h.
h. synchronized evoked potential (HSEP)
systemic h.
tabby cat h.
h. tamponade
Taussig-Bing h.
teardrop h.
three-chambered h.

thrush breast h.
tiger h.
tiger lily h.
tobacco h.
h. tones (ht)
total artificial h. (TAH)
total implantation of artificial h. (TIAH)
h. transplant (HT)
h. transplantation (HT)
transverse section of h.
Traube h.
triatrial h.
trilocular h.
univentricular h.
upstairs-downstairs h.
Utah total artificial h.
h. valve
h. valve prosthesis
valvular disease of h. (VDH)
venous h.
vertical h.
Vienna total artificial h.
h. volume (HV)
waist of h.
wandering h.
water-bottle h.
h. weight (HW)
wooden-shoe h.
heart-assist device
heartbeat
AE h.
h. period (HBP)
HeartCard
H. monitor
H. 3X cardiac event recorder
heart-hand syndrome
heart-lung
h.-l. bloc
h.-l. bypass
h.-l. machine
h.-l. resuscitation (HLR)
h.-l. transplant (HLT, HLTx)
h.-l. transplantation (HLT)
HeartMate
H. implantable pneumatic left ventricular assist system
H. implantable ventricular assist device
H. LVAD
H. pump

H. vented electric left ventricular assist system
Heartport
H. catheter system
H. endoaortic clamp
H. endocoronary sinus catheter
H. endopulmonary vent
H. endovascular catheter
H. endovenous drainage cannula
H. Port-Access system
H. technique
HeartSaver VAD
Heartscan heart attack prediction test
HeartStart MRx defibrillator
Heartstream FR2 AED with attenuated defibrillation pad
Heartwave EP
Heartwire lead
heat
h. load
h. shock protein (HSP, Hsp, hsp)
h. shock protein 47 (HSP47)
h. stroke
heat-activated recoverable temporary stent (HARTS)
Heath-Edwards
H.-E. classification
H.-E. criteria
heating
ohmic h.
resistive h.
volume h.
heat/moisture exchanger (HME)
heat-treated
Profilnine H.-T.
heave
parasternal h.
precordial h.
right ventricular h.
heavy
h. chain cardiac myosin (MYHC)
h. chain cardiac myosin alpha (MYHCA)
h. metal
Heberden
H. angina
H. asthma
H. node
Hecht pneumonia
HED
hydroxyephedrine
heel strike

NOTES

H

319

Hegglin syndrome
HEHR
    highest equivalent heart rate
height
    AR jet h.
    h. of heart (Ht)
    left ventricle outflow h. (LVOH)
    right hemidiaphragm h.
    Z score weight-Z score h.
Heim-Kreysig sign
Heimlich
    H. chest drainage valve
    H. heart valve
    H. maneuver
    H. sign
Heinecke method
Heiner syndrome
Heinz body
Heister diverticulum
HeLa cell
helical
    h. coil stent
    h. CT
    h. CT scanning
    h. CT venography
helices (*pl. of* helix)
Helicobacter pylori
Helionetics/Acculase excimer laser
  transmyocardial revascularization
heliox
    helium-oxygen mixture
    H. nebulizer
Helistat
Helistent
helium
    h. dilution
    h. dilution method
    h. washout
helium-oxygen mixture (heliox)
helix, pl. **helices**
    amphipathic h.
    H. balloon
    H. PTCA dilatation catheter
Helixate
Heller-Belsey operation
Heller-Döhle disease
Heller esophagomyotomy
Heller-Nissen operation
HELLP
    hemolysis, elevated liver enzymes, and
    low platelets
        HELLP syndrome
Helmholtz head coil
helminth
helminthic myocarditis
Helminthosporium
HELP
    heparin-induced extracorporeal low-
    density lipoprotein precipitation

hemadostenosis
Hemaflex
    H. PTCA sheath with obturator
    H. sheath
hemagglutinin
Hema Metrics
hemangioendothelioma
    epithelioid h.
hemangioma
    cavernous h.
    lobular capillary h.
    sclerosing h.
hemangioma-thrombocytopenia syndrome
hemangiomatosis
hemangiosarcoma
Hemaquet
    H. introducer
    H. PTCA sheath with obturator
    H. sheath
hemarthrosis
Hemashield
    H. Gold 1, 4 branch AAA graft
    H. Gold Microvel knitted double
    velour graft
    H. Vantage vascular graft
hemathorax
hematin
hematocrit
hematogenous
    h. bacterial dissemination
    h. embolism
    h. metastasis
    h. nodule
    h. tuberculosis
hematologic disease
hematoma
    aneurysmal h.
    aortic intramural h. (AIH)
    apical h.
    dissecting h.
    intramural h. (IH)
    intraparenchymal h.
    irregular h.
    lobular h.
    parenchymal h. (PH)
    periaortic h.
    pouch h.
    pulmonary h.
    retroperitoneal h.
    round h.
    subdural h. (SDH)
hematopoiesis
hematopoietic
    h. chimerism
    h. system
hematoporphyrin derivative (HPD)
hematosis
hematotylin
    h. and eosin (H&E)

hematotylin-eosin stain
hematuria
hemi-anomalous
> h.-a. pulmonary venous connection (HAPVC)
> h.-a. pulmonary venous drainage (HAPVD)
> h.-a. pulmonary venous return (HAPVR)

hemianopia
hemiaxial view
hemiazygos vein
hemiblock
> left anterior h. (LAH)
> left anterior superior h. (LASH)
> left middle h.
> left posterior h.
> left posterior inferior h. (LPIH)
> left septal h.

hemic
> h. hypoxia
> h. murmur
> h. systole

hemicardia
hemidesmosome
hemidiaphragm
> h. paralysis
> tenting of h.

hemi-Fontan
> h.-F. operation
> h.-F. procedure

hemifundoplication
> Toupet h.

hemin
hemineglect
> motor-exploratory h.

hemiosteoporosis
hemiparesis
> atactic h.
> ataxic h. (AH)
> pure motor h. (PMH)

hemiplegia
> dense h.

hemisphere
> left h. (LH)

hemisystole
hemithorax
hemitruncus
hemizygosity
hemizygous
Hemobahn endovascular prosthesis stent-graft

Hemoband hemostasis device
hemochromatosis
Hemochron
> H. high-dose thrombin time assay
> H. monitor

hemoclastic reaction
hemoclip
> Samuels h.

hemoconcentrator
HemoCue photometer
hemocyanin
> keyhole-limpet h.

Hemocyte
hemocytometer
hemodiafiltration
> continuous arteriovenous h. (CAVHDF)

hemodialysis
> continuous arteriovenous h. (CAVHD)

hemodialyzer
> Gambro Lundia Minor h.

hemodilution
> isovolemic h.
> normovolemic h.

hemodynamic
> h. abnormality
> h. analysis
> h. assessment
> h. collapse
> h. embarrassment
> h. endpoint
> h. gradient
> h. instability
> intraoperative h.'s
> h. maneuver
> h. measurement
> h. mental stress response
> h. monitoring (HM)
> h. principle
> h. profile
> pulmonary h.'s
> h. stability
> systemic h.'s
> h. tolerance
> transvalvular h.'s
> h. vise

hemodynamically
> h. significant stenosis
> h. weighted MRI (HW)

Hemofil M

NOTES

H

hemofiltration
>   continuous arteriovenous h. (CAVH)
>   continuous venovenous h. (CVVH)

hemoglobin (Hb)
>   deoxygenated h.
>   diaspirin cross-linked h. (DCLHb)
>   h. glutamer-250
>   glycosylated h.
>   oxygenated h.
>   pyridoxalated stroma-free h. (SFHb)

hemoglobin-based therapeutic system
hemoglobinemia
hemoglobin-oxygen dissociation curve
hemoglobinuria
>   paroxysmal nocturnal h. (PNH)

Hemolink investigational hemoglobin product or blood substitute
hemolysis
>   h., elevated liver enzymes, and low platelets (HELLP)
>   h., elevated liver function tests and low platelets syndrome

hemolytic anemia
HemoMatic blood collection monitor
hemomediastinum
hemoperfusion
>   charcoal h.
>   pump-assisted coronary h.

hemopericardium
>   traumatic h.

hemophagocytic histiocyte
hemopneumopericardium
hemopneumothorax
hemopoietic
hemoptysis
>   cardiac h.
>   catamenial h.
>   coital h.
>   cryptogenic h.
>   essential h.
>   Goldstein h.
>   oriental h.

Hemopump
>   H. cardiac assist system
>   Johnson & Johnson H.
>   Medtronic H.
>   Nimbus H.

hemorheology
hemorrhage
>   anticoagulant-related h.
>   aortic intramural h. (AIH)
>   CAA-related h.
>   catastrophic h.
>   caudate h.
>   diffuse alveolar h. (DAH)
>   flame-shaped h.'s
>   hypertensive intracerebral h. (HIH)
>   intracavitary h.

>   intracerebral h. (ICH)
>   intracranial h. (ICH)
>   intramural h. (IMH)
>   intraparenchymal h.
>   intrapericardial h.
>   intraventricular h. (IVH)
>   multiple lobar h. (MLH)
>   parenchymal h. (PH)
>   peribronchovascular h.
>   petechial h.
>   postoperative h. (POH)
>   primary intracerebral h. (PICH)
>   pulmonary alveolar h.
>   recurrent lobar h. (RLH)
>   reperfusion-induced h.
>   splinter h.
>   spontaneous intracerebral h. (SICH)
>   subarachnoid h. (SAH)
>   supratentorial intracerebral h.
>   symptomatic h. (SHT)
>   thrombolysis-related intracranial h. (TICH)
>   traumatic h.

hemorrhagic
>   h. bronchitis
>   h. bronchopneumonia
>   h. coagulopathy
>   h. cyst
>   h. effusion
>   h. fever
>   h. hereditary telangiectasia
>   h. hypotension
>   h. infarction (HI)
>   h. pericarditis
>   h. pleurisy
>   h. sputum
>   h. stroke
>   h. transformation (HT)

hemosiderin-laden macrophage
hemosiderosis
>   cardiac h.
>   essential pulmonary h.
>   idiopathic pulmonary h. (IPH)
>   pulmonary h.
>   transfusional h.

HemoSplit
>   H. hemodialysis catheter
>   H. long-term dialysis catheter

hemostasis valve
hemostat
>   Kelly h.
>   Mayo h.
>   microfibrillar collagen h.
>   mosquito h.
>   straight h.

hemostatic
>   h. deficiency
>   h. occlusive leverage device (HOLD)

h. puncture closure device (HPCD)
h. sheath
hemoSTATUS assay
HemoTec activated clotting time monitor
Hemotene
hemothorax, pl. **hemothoraces (HTX)**
catamenial h.
clotted h.
Hemovac
hen-cluck stertor
Henderson-Hasselbalch equation
Henke space
Henle
ascending loop of H.
H. elastic membrane
H. fenestrated membrane
H. loop
Henle-Coenen test
Henoch-Schönlein
H.-S. purpura
H.-S. syndrome
H.-S. vasculitis
Henry-Gauer response
Henry law
hep
hepatitis
HEPA
high-efficiency particulate air
Hepacoat stent
heparin (H, HP)
h. arterial filter
h. assay rapid easy method (HAREM)
h. assay rapid method (HARM)
beef-lung h.
h. block
calcium h. (CH)
h. cofactor (HCF)
h. cofactor II deficiency
continuous h. (CH)
depolymerized porcine mucosal h.
h. drip
h. and early patency
h. flush
immobilized h.
h. infusion
h. injection
h. lock (HL)
low-dose h. (LDH)
low-dose unfractionated h. (LDUH)
low-molecular weight h. (LMWH)

low-molecular weight h. (LMWH)
minimal intermittent h. (MIH)
h. neutralizing activity (HNA)
standard h. (SH)
unfractionated h. (UFH)
heparin-associated
h.-a. thrombocytopenia (HAT)
h.-a. thrombocytopenia and thrombosis (HATT)
heparin-binding epidermal growth factor
heparin-dihydroergotamine
heparin-induced
h.-i. extracorporeal low-density lipoprotein precipitation (HELP)
h.-i. platelet activation (HIPA)
h.-i. thrombocytopenia (HIT)
h.-i. thrombocytopenia and thrombosis (HITT)
h.-i. thrombosis-thrombocytopenia syndrome (HITTS)
heparinization
intermittent h. (IH)
heparinized saline
heparin-precipitable fraction (HPF)
HEPAtech air purification system
hepatic
h. artery
h. dearterialization
h. disease
h. failure
h. function
h. hydatid cyst
h. hydrothorax
h. lipase
h. lipoprotein lipase
h. sphincter
h. vein
h. vein catheterization
hepaticopulmonary
hepatis
porta h.
hepatitis (hep)
h. A, B, C, D, E
granulomatous h.
viral h.
hepatization
gray h.
red h.
yellow h.
hepatocyte
hepatoesophageum
ligamentum h.

NOTES

H

323

hepatofugal flow
hepatojugular
    h. reflex
    h. reflux (HJR)
    h. reflux test
hepatoma
hepatomegaly
hepatopetal flow
hepatopneumonic
hepatopulmonary syndrome (HPS)
hepatosplenomegaly
hepatotoxicity
HEPES
    hydroxyethyl piperazine-ethanesulfonic
    acid
hep-lock injection
heptahelical protein G
heptahydrate
    magnesium sulfate h.
heptanal occupational exposure
heptapeptide
Heptest clotting assay
HER2/neu gene
Herceptin
hereditary
    h. angioneurotic edema (HANE)
    h. ataxia
    h. capillary fragility (HCF)
    h. hemorrhagic telangiectasia (HHT)
    h. methemoglobinemic cyanosis
heredopathia atactica polyneuritiformis
HERG
    human ether-a-go-go-related gene
    HERG potassium channel
Hering
    nerve of H.
    H. phenomenon
Hering-Breuer reflex
Hermansky-Pudlak syndrome
Herner syndrome
hernia
    Béclard h.
    Bochdalek h.
    congenital diaphragmatic h. (CDH)
    diaphragmatic h.
    hiatal h.
    Larrey h.
    Morgagni h.
    paraesophageal h.
    rolling h.
    Serafini h.
    sliding hiatal h.
    Velpeau h.
herniation
    cardiac h.
heroics
heroic snoring
heroin
herpangina pharyngitis

herpes
    h. simplex
    h. simplex pneumonia
    h. simplex pneumonitis
    h. simplex virus (HSV)
    h. zoster
Herpesviridae
herpetic
Hershey total artificial heart
herzstoss
Herzyme
Hespan plasma volume expander
Hess capillary test
hetastarch plasma expander
20-HETE
    20-hydroxyeicosatetraenoic acid
heterochronicus
    pulsus h.
heterogeneity
    genetic h.
heterogeneous
    h. parenchymal attenuation
    h. plaque
heterogenous emphysema
heterograft
    bovine h.
    Hancock porcine h.
    porcine h.
heterologous
    h. cardiac transplant
    h. surfactant
heterometric autoregulation
heterophony
    phase h.
heterophyiasis
heteroscedastic
heterotaxia
    cardiac h.
heterotaxy
    h. syndrome
    visceral h.
heterotopic
    h. cardiac transplant
    h. heart transplant (HHT)
    h. stimulus
heterotrimeric protein G
heterotropic heart transplantation (HHT)
heterotypic adhesion
heterozygosity
heterozygote
heterozygous familial hypercholesterolemia (hFH)
Heubner
    H. recurrent artery
    H. specific endarteritis
Hewlett-Packard (HP)
    H.-P. 77020 A phased-array sector
    scanner

H.-P. 78720 A SDN monitor
H.-P. biplane 5-MHz probe
H.-P. defibrillator
H.-P. ear oximeter
H.-P. 500, 1000 Echo-Doppler machine
H.-P. 5 MHz phased-array TEE system
H.-P. omniplane 5-MHz probe
H.-P. 2500 SONOS ultrasound
H.-P. SONOS 1000, 1500, 2500 ultrasound system
Hexabrix contrast material
Hexadrol Phosphate
hexafluoride
sulfur h. (SF_6)
hexahydrophthalic anhydride (HHPA)
Hexalen
hexamethonium
hexamethylmelamine
hexaxial reference system
hexokinase reaction
Hexonate
hexosaminidase deficiency
HF
heart failure
high fat
high flow
HF infrared laser
HFA
hydrofluoroalkane
flunisolide HFA
Proventil HFA
Ventolin HFA
HFCC
high-frequency chest wall compression
HFCWO
high-frequency chest wall oscillation
HFCWO ventricular resynchronizer
HFEE
high-frequency epicardial echocardiography
HFH
homozygous familial hypercholesterolemia
hFH
heterozygous familial hypercholesterolemia
HFJV
high-frequency jet ventilation
HFL
human fetal lung fibroblast

HFO
high-frequency oscillation
HFOC
high-flow oxygen conserver
H-form myocardial infarction
HFPPV
high-frequency positive pressure ventilation
Hfr
heart frequency
HFSA
Heart Failure Society of America
HFV
high-frequency ventilation
Hg
mercury
^{195m}Hg
mercury-195m
HHCS
high-altitude hypertrophic cardiomyopathy syndrome
HHD
high heparin dose
hypertensive heart disease
H_1-H_2 interval
HHPA
hexahydrophthalic anhydride
HHS
hyperkinetic heart syndrome
HHT
hereditary hemorrhagic telangiectasia
heterotopic heart transplant
heterotropic heart transplantation
hypertensive hypervolemic therapy
HI
harmonic imaging
heart infusion
hemorrhagic infarction
HIA
hyperventilation-induced asthma
hiatal
h. esophagism
h. hernia
hiatus
aortic h.
h. aorticus
esophageal h.
h. esophageus
h. of facial canal
HIB
heart infusion broth
hyperpnea-induced bronchoconstriction

NOTES

H

hibernating myocardium
hibernation
    myocardial h.
HibTITER
Hib-VAX
Hi-Care closed suction and pulmonary
  hygiene system
HIC-CPR
  high-impulse compression
  cardiopulmonary resuscitation
hiccup, hiccough
HICOR system
HI-CPR
  high-impulse cardiopulmonary
  resuscitation
HID
  hypertension in diabetes
Hideaway oxygen conserver
HIF
  hypoxia-inducible factor
Hi-Flex lead
high
    h. air flow with oxygen
    entrainment (HAFOE)
    h. arched palate
    h. blood pressure (HBP)
    h. cholesterol and tocopherol
    supplement (HCTS)
    h. density echo
    h. fat (HF)
    h. flow (HF)
    h. heparin dose (HHD)
    h. lung volume
    h. molecular weight dextran
    h. pressure connecting tube
    h. pulse repetition frequency
    (HiPRF)
    h. regional wall motion velocity
    (Vhigh)
    h. right atrium
    h. right atrium electrogram
    (HRAE)
    h. spatial resolution
    h. vacuum (HV)
    h. voltage can (HVC)
high-altitude
    h.-a. hypertrophic cardiomyopathy
    syndrome (HHCS)
    h.-a. peristalsis (HAP)
    h.-a. pulmonary edema (HAPE)
    h.-a. pulmonary edema resistant
    (HAPE-r)
    h.-a. pulmonary edema susceptible
    (HAPE-s)
    h.-a. simulation test (HAST)
high-amplitude peristaltic contraction
  (HAPC)
high-ceiling diuretic

high-density
    h.-d. electroanatomical and
    entrainment mapping
    h.-d. lipoprotein (HDL, HDLP)
    h.-d. lipoprotein binding protein
    (HDLBP)
    h.-d. lipoprotein-cell surface (HDL-
    c)
    h.-d. lipoprotein-cholesterol complex
    (HDL-C)
    h.-d. sector basket catheter
high-dependency unit (HDU)
high-dose
    h.-d. carvedilol (CARhd)
    h.-d. epinephrine
    h.-d. steroid
high-efficiency particulate air (HEPA)
high-energy
    h.-e. laser
    h.-e. transthoracic shock
high-esophageal pH probe
highest equivalent heart rate (HEHR)
high-fat meal
high-fiber diet
high-flow
    h.-f. catheter
    h.-f. oxygen conserver (HFOC)
high-frequency
    h.-f. burst pacing
    h.-f. chest wall compression
    (HFCC)
    h.-f. chest wall oscillation
    (HFCWO)
    h.-f. chest wall oscillation
    ventricular resynchronizer
    h.-f. epicardial echocardiography
    (HFEE)
    h.-f. jet ventilation (HFJV)
    h.-f. jet ventilator
    h.-f. murmur
    h.-f. oscillation (HFO)
    h.-f. oscillation ventilator
    h.-f. oscillatory ventilation
    h.-f. percussive ventilation
    h.-f. positive pressure ventilation
    (HFPPV)
    h.-f. ventilation (HFV)
3100B high-frequency oscillatory
  ventilator
high-grade stenosis
high-impulse
    h.-i. cardiopulmonary resuscitation
    (HI-CPR)
    h.-i. compression cardiopulmonary
    resuscitation (HIC-CPR)
high-intensity transient signal (HITS)
highly active antiretroviral therapy
  (HAART)

high-output
    h.-o. extended aerosol respiratory therapy
    h.-o. heart failure
high-performance liquid chromatography (HPLC)
high-pitched murmur
high-pressure
    h.-p. adjunctive percutaneous transluminal coronary angioplasty
    h.-p. balloon stenting
    h.-p. cardiogenic pulmonary edema
    h.-p. inflation technique
    h.-p. liquid chromatography (HPLC)
    h.-p. neurologic syndrome (HPNS)
    h.-p. stent deployment
high-ramp protocol
high-renin essential hypertension (HREH)
high-resolution
    h.-r. B-mode ultrasonography
    h.-r. computed tomography (HRCT)
    h.-r. CT (HRCT)
    h.-r. deep penetration 2D intracardiac ultrasound
    h.-r. electrocardiography (HRE)
    h.-r. thin section computed tomographic
high-risk
    h.-r. angioplasty
    h.-r. phenotype
    h.-r. repolarization abnormality
high-sensitivity
    h.-s. C-reactive protein
    h.-s. CRP
high-speed
    h.-s. directional coronary atherectomy
    h.-s. rotational atherectomy (HSRA)
    h.-s. rotation dynamic angioplasty catheter
    h.-s. volumetric imaging
HIH
    hypertensive intracerebral hemorrhage
Hilal
    H. embolization microcoil
    H. modified headhunter catheter
hilar
    h. adenopathy
    h. clouding
    h. dance
    h. haze

    h. lymphadenopathy
    h. lymph node
Hill
    H. coefficient
    H. phenomenon
    H. sign
Hillis-Müller maneuver
hills-and-valley morphology
Hi-Lo
    H.-L. Evac endotracheal tube
    H.-L. Jet tracheal tube
Hilton sac
hilum
    h. convergence sign
    h. of lung
    h. of lymph node
    h. nodi lymphatici
    h. overlay sign
    pulmonary h.
    h. pulmonis
hilus tuberculosis
Hines-Brown test
hinge point
Hinkle-Thaler classification
hip
    h. classification
    h. flexion
HIPA
    heparin-induced platelet activation
hippocratic
    h. angina
    h. sound
    h. succussion
HiPRF
    high pulse repetition frequency
hirsutum
    cor h.
hirudin
    recombinant h. (r-hirudin)
Hirudo medicinalis
His
    bundle of H. (B-H)
    H. bundle (HB)
    H. bundle ablation
    H. bundle catheter
    H. bundle deflection
    H. bundle depolarization
    H. bundle electrocardiogram
    H. bundle electrogram (HBE)
    H. bundle heart block
    H. bundle potential
    H. canal

NOTES

H

His (*continued*)
    H. perivascular space
    H. spindle
His-Hass procedure
Hispanic American (HA)
His-Purkinje
    H.-P. conduction
    H.-P. fiber
    H.-P. system
    H.-P. tissue
Histalet Syrup
histaminase
histamine
    h. acid phosphate
    h. challenge
    h. diphosphate
    h. provocation
    h. release inhibitory factor (HRIF)
histamine-releasing factor (HRF)
His-Tawara node
histidine decarboxylase
histidine-rich glycoprotein
histiocyte
    hemophagocytic h.
    palisading h.
histiocytoma
    malignant fibrous h. (MFH)
histiocytosis
    Langerhans cell h.
    primary pulmonary h. X
    pulmonary Langerhans cell h.
histocompatibility agent B27
Histocryl Blue tissue adhesive
histogram
    DNA h.
    h. mode
histologic
histolytica
    Entamoeba h.
    Torula h.
histolyticus
    Cryptococcus h.
histomorphometry
histopathology
Histoplasma
    H. capsulatum
    H. myocarditis
histoplasmic pericarditis
histoplasmosis
    African h.
    progressive disseminated h. (PDH)
history
    heart disease h. (HDH)
    natural h.
    pack-year smoking h.
    smoking h.
histotoxic hypoxia
Histussin D Liquid
His-ventricle (HV, H-V)

    H.-v. conduction time
    His-ventricle interval
HIT
    heparin-induced thrombocytopenia
Hitachi
    H. PCT-3600W PET system
    H. U-2000 spectrophotometer
Hi-Torque
    H.-T. balance middleweight
    universal guide wire
    H.-T. Floppy exchange guidewire
    H.-T. Floppy II guidewire
    H.-T. Floppy intermediate guidewire
    H.-T. Standard guidewire
HITS
    high-intensity transient signal
HITT
    heparin-induced thrombocytopenia and
    thrombosis
HITTS
    heparin-induced thrombosis-
    thrombocytopenia syndrome
Hitzenberg test
HIV
    human immunodeficiency virus
    HIV cardiomyopathy
HIV-1 riboprobe
HIVAGEN test
Hivid
HJR
    hepatojugular reflux
HL
    heparin lock
    hyperlipidemia
HL7
    health level seven
H&L
    heart and lung
HLA
    human leukocyte antigen
    HLA-6
    HLA-129
    HLA-A11
HLA-DQA1 gene haplotype
HLA-DQB1 gene haplotype
HLA-DQ gene complex
HLA-DR gene complex
HLHS
    hypoplastic left heart syndrome
H-L-K
    heart, liver and kidneys
HLR
    heart-lung resuscitation
HLT
    heart-lung transplant
    heart-lung transplantation
    human lipotropin
HLTx
    heart-lung transplant

HLV
    hypoplastic left ventricle
HLVS
    hypoplastic left ventricle syndrome
HM
    heart murmur
    hemodynamic monitoring
    Holter monitoring
HMCAS
    hyperdense middle cerebral artery sign
HME
    heat/moisture exchanger
        Tracheolife HME
HMG-CoA
    hydroxymethylglutaryl coenzyme A
    3-hydroxy-3-methylglutaryl coenzyme A
HMG CoA-reductase inhibitor
HMI
    healed myocardial infarct
HMO
    heart minute output
HMSAS
    hypertrophic muscular subaortic stenosis
HNA
    heparin neutralizing activity
HO
    Holt-Oram
        HO syndrome
hoarseness
hockey-stick
        h.-s. catheter
        h.-s. deformity
        h.-s. tricuspid valve
HOCM
    hypertrophic obstructive cardiomyopathy
Hodgkin disease
Hodgkin-Huxley
        H.-H. constant
        H.-H. model
Hodgkin-Key murmur
Hodgson disease
Hoffman reflex
hoist
HOLD
    hemostatic occlusive leverage device
Hold DM
holder
        Ayers cardiovascular needle h.
        Björk-Shiley heart valve h.
        blade control wire h.
        Castroviejo needle h.

        Comfit endotracheal tube h.
        Dale tracheostomy tube h.
        GraftAssist vein-graft h.
        Lewy chest h.
        LifePort endotracheal tube h.
        Marsupial Pouch postsurgical
            drain h.
        needle h.
        NEO-fit neonatal endotracheal
            tube h.
        Thomas LT endotracheal tube h.
        Thomas Quick Block endotracheal
            tube h.
        Vital-Ryder microvascular needle h.
        Watson heart valve h.
        wire h.
holding
        breath h.
hole
        bur h.
holiday
        dobutamine h.
        h. heart
        h. heart syndrome
Holinger
        H. anterior commissure
            laryngoscope
        H. dissector
holism
Hollenberg treadmill exercise score
Hollenhorst plaque
hollow viscus
Holmes heart
Holmes-Rahe scale
Holmgren-Golgi canal
holmium laser
**holmium:yttrium-aluminum-garnet
(Ho:YAG)**
holodiastolic
        h. decrescendo murmur
        h. flow
        h. flow reversal
holography
        ultrasound h.
holosystolic murmur (HSM)
Holter
        H. diary
        Marquette three-channel laser H.
        H. monitor
        H. monitoring (HM)
        H. tube

NOTES

H

Holter-guided antiarrhythmic drug therapy
Holt-Oram (HO)
    H.-O. syndrome (HOS)
Holzknecht space
Homans sign
homatropine
    hydrocodone and h.
home-based cardiac rehabilitation
homeometric autoregulation
homeostasis
home unattended polysomnography
hominis
    Actinobacillus h.
    Cardiobacterium h.
    Mycoplasma h.
    Pentatrichomonas h.
HomMed
    H. monitor
    H. monitoring system
homocysteine
    plasma h.
    total h. (tHcy)
homocystine
homocystinuria syndrome
homodimer
    alpha-alpha h.
    beta-beta h.
homogeneity
    Breslow-Day test for h.
    tracer h.
homogeneous plaque
homogentisic acid oxidase deficiency
homograft
    antibiotic sterilized aortic valve h. (ASAH)
    aortic h.
    denatured h.
    homovital h.
    h. insertion for pulmonary regurgitation
    mitral valve h.
    pulmonary artery h.
homologous cardiac transplant
homoscedastic
homotypic adhesion
homovital homograft
homozygosity
homozygote
homozygous
    h. beta-thalassemia
    h. familial hypercholesterolemia (HFH)
HON
   Health On the Net
    HON Foundation
HONcode
   Health On the Net code of conduct

honeycomb
    h. cyst
    h. lesion
    h. lung
    h. pattern
honeycombing
    h. of lung
    subpleural h.
Hong Kong influenza
honk
    precordial h.
    systolic h.
honking murmur
hood O$_2$
Hood stoma stent
hook
    Adson h.
    barbed h.
    Pitie-Salpetriere saphenous vein h.
hook-and-loop fastener strap
Hooke law
Hoover sign
Hope
    H. bag
    H. continuous & Heliox nebulizer
    H. resuscitator
    H. sign
Hopkins
    H. aortic clamp
    H. forceps
    H. Symptom Checklist
Horder spots
horehound lozenge
Horizon
    H. AutoAdjust CPAP system
    H. CPAP device
    H. LT CPAP system
    H. nasal CPAP system
    H. PFT spirometer
    H. surgical ligating and marking clip
horizontal
    h. anteroposterior deceleration
    h. fissure
    h. heart
    h. long axis
    h. long-axis tomogram
    h. long-axis view
    h. ST segment
    h. ST segment depression
    h. VAS
hormone
    adrenocorticotropic h. (ACTH)
    antidiuretic h. (ADH)
    female h.
    growth h.
    mineralocorticoid h.
    natriuretic h.
    parathyroid h.

h. replacement therapy (HRT)
syndrome of inappropriate
    antidiuretic h. (SIADH)
thyroid-stimulating h. (TSH)

Horner
  H. sign
  H. syndrome
horripilation
horse asthma
horse-race effect
horseshoe
  h. configuration
  h. lung
Horton
  H. arteritis (HA)
  H. disease
HOS
  Holt-Oram syndrome
hose
  Juzo h.
  TED h.
Hosmer-Lemeshow Goodness-of-Fit test
hospital
  H. Admission Risk Profile (HARP)
  H. Anxiety and Depression (HAD)
  H. Anxiety and Depression Scale
    (HADS)
hospital-acquired
  h.-a. infection
  h.-a. pneumonia (HAP)
host
  granulocytopenic h.
  humoral h.
  immunocompetent h.
  nonimmunocompromised h.
host-generated neutrophils recruitment
hot
  h. gangrene
  h. nose sign
  h. potato voice
  h. spot
Hotelling T2 test
hot-tip laser probe
hot-wire
  h.-w. anemometer
  h.-w. pneumotachometer
Hounsfield unit (HU)
hour
  Claritin-D 24 h.

24-hour
  24-h. ambulatory
    electrocardiographic recorder
  24-h. cortisol
12-hour antiplatelet therapy
hourglass
  h. murmur
  h. pattern
  h. stenosis
house
  h. dust mite (HDM)
  h. dust mite allergen
Housecall transtelephonic monitoring
  system
Howard method
Howel-Evans syndrome
Howell test
Ho:YAG
  holmium:yttrium-aluminum-garnet
    Ho:YAG laser
    Ho:YAG laser angioplasty
Hoyer anastomosis
HP
  heparin
  Hewlett-Packard
  hypersensitivity pneumonitis
    HP SONOS 30-MHz imaging
      catheter
    HP SONOS 2500 transducer
HPA
  hypothalamic-pituitary-adrenal
HPAA
  hypothalamic-pituitary-adrenal axis
H.P. Acthar Gel
HPCD
  hemostatic puncture closure device
HPD
  hematoporphyrin derivative
5-HPETE acid
HPF
  heparin-precipitable fraction
HPI
  Haemophilus parainfluenzae
H'P interval
HPLC
  high-performance liquid chromatography
  high-pressure liquid chromatography
HPLH
  hypoplastic left heart
HPN
  hypertension

NOTES

H

hpn
hypertension
HPNS
high-pressure neurologic syndrome
H-proline
HPS
hepatopulmonary syndrome
HPV
human papillomavirus
hypoxic pulmonary vasoconstriction
HPVD
hypertensive pulmonary vascular disease
H-Q interval
H-QRS interval
HR, HRT
heart rate
HRA
heart rate audiometry
HRAE
high right atrium electrogram
H-R conduction time
HRCT
high-resolution computed tomography
high-resolution CT
diagnostic HRCT
HRCT scan
HRE
high-resolution electrocardiography
HREH
high-renin essential hypertension
HRF
heart rate fluctuations
histamine-releasing factor
HRF deficiency
HRIF
histamine release inhibitory factor
Hrmax
maximal heart rate
HRQL, HRQOL
health-related quality of life
HRR
heart rate range
heart rate recovery
heart rate reserve
HRRI
heart rate retardation index
HRS
Hamman-Rich syndrome
HRSUB
submaximal heart rate
HRT (*var. of* HR)
heart rate
hormone replacement therapy
hyperfractionated radiation
HRV
heart rate variability
power spectrum of HRV
HRV test

HS
heart sounds
HSAS
hypertrophic subaortic stenosis
HSEP
heart synchronized evoked potential
HSM
holosystolic murmur
HSP, Hsp, hsp
heat shock protein
HSP antigen
HSP47
heat shock protein 47
HSRA
high-speed rotational atherectomy
HSRA device
HSRD
hypertension secondary to renal disease
HSS
hypertrophic subaortic stenosis
HSV
herpes simplex virus
HSV meningitis
HSV pneumonia
HT
heart
heart transplant
heart transplantation
hemorrhagic transformation
hypertension
hypertensive
cerebral HT
5HT
5-hydroxytryptamine
Ht
height of heart
ht
heart
heart tones
HTCVD
hypertensive cardiovascular disease
HTG
hypertriglyceridemia
HTHD
hypertensive heart disease
HTLV
human T-cell lymphotropic virus
HTLV-I, II
HTN
hypertension
hypertensive nephropathy
HTVD
hypertensive vascular disease
HTX
hemothorax
hypertension
H-type tracheoesophageal fistula
HU
Hounsfield unit

hub
  catheter h.
  h. and spoke referral system
Huchard
  H. disease
  H. sign
Hudson
  H. Lifesaver resuscitator
  H. Multi-Vent
Huff coughing
Hufnagel
  H. ascending aortic clamp
  H. prosthetic valve
Hugger
  Bair H.
Hughes-Stovin syndrome
Hull triad
hum
  cervical venous h.
  venous h.
human
  h. airway epithelium
  h. amylin analog
  h. analog amylin AC137
  antihemophilic factor (h.)
  h. aortic endothelial cell (HAEC)
  h. aortic smooth muscle (HASMC)
  h. aortic smooth muscle cell
    (HASMC)
  h. atrial natriuretic factor (hANF)
  h. atrial natriuretic peptide (hANP)
  h. babesiosis
  h. cloned DNA (cDNA)
  h. cosmid library
  h. cytomegalovirus (HCMV)
  cytomegalovirus immune globulin
    intravenous, h.
  h. ether-a-go-go-related gene
    (HERG)
  h. fetal lung fibroblast (HFL)
  h. gene C4B
  h. immunodeficiency virus (HIV)
  h. leukocyte antigen (HLA)
  h. lipotropin (HLT)
  h. lymphocyte antigen typing
  h. menopausal gonadotropin
    coenzyme A reductase inhibitor
  h. neuropeptide
  h. papillomavirus (HPV)
  h. pooled AAT
  h. preproendothelin-1 gene
  h. recombinant deoxyribonuclease

  h. T-cell lymphotropic virus
    (HTLV)
  h. umbilical vein (HUV)
  Velosulin H.
Humate-P
Humatin
humeral
  anterior circumflex h.
humeroperoneal neuromuscular disease
Humibid
  H. DM
  H. L.A.
  H. Sprinkle
humid asthma
humidification
humidified oxygen
humidifier
  Bennett Cascade II Servo
    Controlled Heated H.
  bubble h.
  cold-mist h.
  jet h.
  h. lung
  Mistogen passover h.
  passover h.
  Respironics Oasis h.
  Sullivan HumidAire heated h.
  ThermoFlo h.
  Whisper Mist h.
humidity
  absolute h.
  relative h.
humming murmur
humming-top murmur
humoral
  h. host
  h. immune defect
hump
  Hampton h.
Humulin L, N, R, U insulin
huN901-DM1 antibody
hunger
  air h.
Hunt
  H. angiographic trocar
  H. and Hess grades I through V
    aneurysm grading system
Hunter
  H. canal
  H. detachable balloon occluder
  H. operation
  H. syndrome

NOTES

H

Hunter-Hurler syndrome
Hunter-Sessions balloon
hunting reaction
Huntington chorea
Hurler-Scheie compound
Hurler syndrome
Hurricaine spray
Hürthle
    H. cell tumor
    H. manometer
Hustead needle
HUT
    head-up tilt
Hutinel disease
HUTTT
    head-up tilt-table test
HUV
    human umbilical vein
        HUV bypass graft
Huygens principle
H-V
    His-ventricle
        H.-V. conduction time
        H.-V. interval
HV
    heart volume
    high vacuum
    His-ventricle
    hypervolemic
HVC
    high voltage can
HVD
    hypertensive vascular disease
HVR
    hypoxic ventilatory response
HVS
    hyperventilation syndrome
HVSD
    hydrogen-detected ventricular septal
    defect
HW
    heart weight
    hemodynamically weighted MRI
hyaline
    h. arterionecrosis
    h. arteriosclerosis
    h. fatty change
    h. membrane disease
    h. membrane formation
    h. thrombus
hyalinizing granuloma
hyalinosis
    arteriolar h.
hyaloserositis
    progressive multiple h.
hyaluronan
hyaluronic
    h. acid
    h. acid polymer

hyaluronidase
Hyate:C
Hybolin Decanoate
Hybond ECL nitrocellulose membrane
hybrid
    h. revascularization
    h. unit
hybridization
    fluorescent in situ h. (FISH)
    in situ h.
Hybritech immunoradiometric assay
Hycamtin
HycoClear Tuss
Hycodan
Hycomine Compound
Hycotuss Expectorant Liquid
HYD
    hydrocortisone
hydantoin
hydatid
    h. cyst
    h. fremitus
hydralazine
    h. hydrochloride
    h. and hydrochlorothiazide
hydralazine, hydrochlorothiazide, and
    reserpine
Hydrap-ES
hydrate
    chloral h.
    terpin h.
hydration
    systemic h.
hydraulic
    h. resistance
    h. vein stripper
hydrazine
    dimethyl h.
Hydrea
hydride
    lithium h.
hydrobromic acid
hydrobromide
    hydroxyamphetamine h.
hydrocarbon
    h. aspiration
    halogenated h.
    polycyclic aromatic h. (PAH)
    h. toxicity
HydroCath catheter
Hydrocet
hydrochloric acid
hydrochloride (HCl)
    acebutolol h.
    acecainide h.
    alfentanil h.
    amantadine h.
    amiloride h.
    amiodarone h.

amprolium h.
bacampicillin h.
benazepril h.
bepridil h.
betaxolol h.
bromhexine h.
carbuterol h.
carteolol h.
chlorpromazine h.
ciprofloxacin h.
clonidine h.
clorprenaline h.
colestipol h.
cyclopentamine h.
cyproheptadine h.
cytarabine h.
demeclocycline h.
desipramine h.
diltiazem h.
diphenhydramine h.
dobutamine h.
dopamine h.
doxapram h.
doxepin h.
doxorubicin h.
encainide h.
esmolol h.
esprolol h.
ethambutol h.
ethaverine h.
ethylnorepinephrine h.
fenfluramine h.
fexofenadine h.
fluoxetine h.
guanfacine h.
hydralazine h.
idarubicin h.
isoprenaline h.
isoprophenamine h.
isopropylarterenol h.
isoproterenol h.
isoxsuprine h.
labetalol h.
levamisole h.
lidocaine h.
lincomycin h.
lomefloxacin h.
mecamylamine h.
mechlorethamine h.
mefloquine h.
meperidine h.
mepivacaine h.

methamphetamine h.
methoxamine h.
methoxyphenamine h.
metoclopramide h.
mexiletine h.
minocycline h.
mitoxantrone h.
moexipril h.
Mustargen H.
nalmefene h.
naloxone h.
nicardipine h.
nortriptyline h.
oxytetracycline h.
papaverine h.
phenoxybenzamine h.
phentolamine h.
phenylephrine h.
phenylpropanolamine h.
prazosin h.
prenalterol h.
procainamide h.
procaine h.
promethazine h.
propafenone h.
propranolol h.
protokylol h.
protriptyline h.
pyridoxine h.
quinapril h.
rimantadine h.
sematilide h.
sertraline h.
sotalol h.
spirapril h.
terazosin h.
tetracaine h.
thioridazine h.
ticlopidine h.
tiprenolol h.
tizanidine h.
tocainide h.
tolazoline h.
trazodone h.
vancomycin h.
verapamil h.
yohimbine h.
hydrochlorothiazide (HCT, HCTZ)
amiloride and h.
benazepril and h.
bisoprolol and h.
candesartan, cilexetil and h.

NOTES

H

hydrochlorothiazide *(continued)*
    captopril and h.
    enalapril and h.
    hydralazine and h.
    irbesartan and h.
    h. and lisinopril
    lisinopril and h.
    losartan and h.
    losartan potassium/h.
    methyldopa and h.
    moexipril and h.
    propranolol and h.
    quinapril and h.
    h. and reserpine
    h. and spironolactone
    h. and triamterene
    valsartan and h.
Hydrocoat hydrophilic coating
hydrocodone
    h. and acetaminophen
    h. bitartrate
    h. and guaifenesin
    h. and homatropine
      , h. phenylephrine,
    pyrilamine, phenindamine,
    chlorpheniramine
    h. and phenylpropanolamine
    h. and pseudoephedrine
    h., pseudoephedrine, and
    guaifenesin
Hydrocort
hydrocortisone (HYD)
    h. cyclopentylpropionate
    h. cypionate
    h. hydrogen succinate
    h. sodium phosphate
    h. sodium succinate
    systemic h.
Hydrocortone
    H. Acetate
    H. Acetate Injection
    H. Phosphate
    H. Phosphate Injection
hydrocyanic acid
HydroDIURIL
HydroDot neuromonitoring system
hydroflumethiazide and reserpine
hydrofluoric acid
hydrofluoroalkane (HFA)
hydrogen
    h. appearance time
    h. bromide
    h. chloride
    h. cyanide (HCN)
    h. density
    h. electrodes
    h. fluoride
    h. inhalation technique
    h. ion concentration (pH)

    h. peroxide
    h. sulfide
hydrogen-3 mazindol
hydrogen-detected ventricular septal defect (HVSD)
Hydrogesic
hydrolase
    cholesterol ester h. (CEH)
    lysosomal h.
Hydrolyser
    H. hydrodynamic thrombectomy catheter
    H. percutaneous thrombectomy catheter
hydrolysis
    ATP h.
    h. of surfactant
hydromediastinum
Hydromer-coated central venous catheter
Hydromet
hydromorphone
hydronephrosis
Hydropane
Hydro Par
hydropericarditis
hydropericardium
Hydrophen
hydrophilic
    h. agent
    h. coated guidewire
hydrophobic
    h. drug
hydropneumatosis
hydropneumopericardium
hydropneumothorax
hydrops
    h. fetalis
    h. pericardii
hydroquinidine
Hydro-Serp
Hydroserpine
hydrosoluble asthmogen
hydrosphere
hydrosphygmograph
hydrostatic
    h. edema
    h. suction
HydroSteer hydrophilic guidewire
Hydro-T
hydrothorax
    chylous h.
    hepatic h.
Hydrotropine
hydroxide
    potassium h. (KOH)
hydroxocobalamin
hydroxyamphetamine hydrobromide
hydroxyapatite

hydroxybutyrate
  h. dehydrogenase (HBDH)
  gamma h. (GHB)
hydroxychloroquine sulfate
18-hydroxycorticosterone
20-hydroxyeicosatetraenoic acid (20-HETE)
hydroxyephedrine (HED)
  carbon-11 h.
hydroxyethyl
  h. piperazine-ethanesulfonic acid (HEPES)
  h. piperazine-ethenesulfonic acid
  h. starch
17-hydroxylase deficiency
hydroxylase deficiency
hydroxyl radical
hydroxymethylglutaryl
  h. coenzyme A (HMG-CoA)
  h. coenzyme A reductase inhibitor
3-hydroxy-3-methylglutaryl
  3-h.3-m. coenzyme A (HMG-CoA)
  3-h.3-m. coenzyme A reductase
  3-h.3-m. coenzyme A reductase inhibitor
hydroxyprogesterone caproate
hydroxyproline analysis
5-hydroxypropafenone
hydroxytoluene
  butylated h. (BHT)
5-hydroxytryptamine (5HT)
hydroxyurea
hydroxyzine
  theophylline, ephedrine, and h. (TEH)
Hylorel
Hylutin injection
Hynes pharyngoplasty
hyoid
  mandibular plane to h. (MP-H)
  h. myotomy
  h. suspension
hyopharyngeus
Hypaque
hyparterial bronchi
hyperabduction syndrome
hyperacute
  h. rejection
  h. T wave
hyperadrenergic activity
hyperaldosteronism

hyperalgesia
hyperalimentation
  intravenous h. (IVH)
hyperalphalipoproteinemia
hyperammonemia
hyperapobetalipoproteinemia
hyperapolipoprotein B syndrome
hyperbaric
  h. chamber
  h. exposure
  h. oxygen (HBO)
  h. oxygenation
  h. oxygen therapy (HBOT)
  h. pressure
hyperbradykinism
hypercalcemia
  familial hypocalciuric h.
  h. syndrome
hypercalciuria
hypercapnia
  oxygen-induced h.
  permissive h. (PHC)
hypercapnic
  h. acidosis
  h. challenge
  h. respiratory failure
  h. stimulus
  h. ventilatory response
hypercarbia
  oxygen-induced h.
hypercardia
hyperchloremic acidosis
hypercholesterolemia (HC)
  essential h. (EHC)
  false h.
  familial h. (FH, FHC)
  heterozygous familial h. (hFH)
  homozygous familial h. (HFH)
  polygenic h.
  h. (types IIa, IIb)
hypercholesterolemic
hyperchylomicronemia
  familial h.
hypercirculation
hypercoagulability
hypercoagulable state
hypercontractile
hypercontractility
hypercortisolemia
hypercortisolism

NOTES

H

337

hypercyanotic
  h. angina
  h. spell
hyperdense middle cerebral artery sign (HMCAS)
hyperdiastole
hyperdicrotic
hyperdicrotism
hyperdynamic
  h. septic shock
  h. state
hyperemia
  active h.
  adenosine-induced h.
  arterial h.
  collateral h.
  fluxionary h.
  passive h.
  peristatic h.
  postocclusion h.
  reactive h.
  venous h.
hyperemic velocity
hypereosinophilia syndrome
hypereosinophilic
  h. heart disease
  h. syndrome
hyperesthesia
  cutaneous h.
hyperestrogenemia
hyperfibrinogenemia
hyperfiltration
  glomerular h.
Hyperflex tracheostomy tube
hyperfractionated radiation (HRT)
hypergammaglobulinemia
HyperGEN
  hypertension genetic epidemiology network
hyperglobulinemia
hyperglycemia
hyperhomocystinemia
hyperinfection
hyperinflated
hyperinflation
  dynamic h. (DH)
hyperinsulinemia
hyperinsulinemic euglycemic clamp metabolic state
hyperinsulinism
hyperintense heterogeneous signal
hyperintensity
  deep white matter h. (DWMHI)
  patchy h.
  periventricular h. (PVH, PVHI)
  pontine h. (PHI)
  punctate h.
  white matter h. (WMHI)
hyperirritability

hyperkalemia
  digoxin-induced h. (DIH)
hyperkalemic cardioplegia
hyperkinemia
hyperkinesia
hyperkinesis
hyperkinetic
  h. heart syndrome (HHS)
  h. pulse
  h. state
hyperlactatemia
hyperleukocytosis
hyperlipidemia (HL)
  false combined h.
  familial combined h. (FCHL)
  multiple lipoprotein-type h.
  polygenic h.
  WHO/Fredrickson classification of primary h.
hyperlipoproteinemia type I, IIa, IIb, III, IV, V
hyperlucency
hyperlucent
  h. lung
  h. lung syndrome
hypermagnesemia
hypermetabolism
hypernatremia
hypernitrosopnea
hyperoxaluria
hyperoxia
hyperparathyroidism
hyperperfusion syndrome
hyperphosphatemia
hyperpiesis, hyperpiesia
hyperpietic
hyperpigmentation
hyperplasa
  lymphoid interstial pneumonia/pulmonary lymphoid h. (LIP/PLH)
hyperplasia
  adrenal h.
  atypical alveolar h.
  bilateral adrenal h.
  congenital adrenal h.
  elastic tissue h.
  intimal h. (IH)
  intravascular papillary endothelial h. (IPEH)
  lymphoid h.
  mucous gland h.
  multifocal micronodular pneumocyte h.
  neointimal h.
  nodular lymphoid h.
  reactive mesothelial h.
  type II cell h.

hyperplastic
  h. mucus-secreting goblet cell
  h. osteoarthritis
hyperplastica
  arteritis h.
hyperpnea
  exercise h.
  h.-induced bronchoconstriction (HIB)
  isocapnic h.
hyperpnea-induced bronchoconstriction (HIB)
hyperpolarization
  afterspike h. (AHP)
hyperreactivity
  airways h. (AHR)
  bronchial h. (BHR)
  nonspecific bronchial h.
  work-related bronchial h.
hyperreflexia
  autonomic h.
hyperreninemia
hyperresonance
hyperresonant
hyperresponsive airways
hyperresponsiveness
  airways h. (AHR)
  bronchial h. (BHR)
hypersecretion
  airway h.
  mucus h.
hypersecretory
hypersensitive carotid sinus syndrome
hypersensitivity
  aminosalicylic acid h.
  cardioinhibitory carotid sinus h.
  carotid sinus h.
  delayed-type h. (DTH)
  h. myocarditis
  h. pneumonia
  h. pneumonitis (HP)
  h. vasculitis
hyperserotonemia
  vasculocardiac syndrome of h.
hypersignal
hypersomnia
  idiopathic h.
hypersomnolence
hypersphyxia
Hyperstat IV
hypersystole
hypersystolic

hypertelorism
hypertension (HPN, hpn, HT, HTN, HTX, hypn)
  accelerated h.
  acquired pulmonary h.
  adrenal h.
  alveolar h.
  ambulatory blood pressure
    monitoring and treatment of h.
    (APTH)
  arterial h. (AH)
  benign intracranial h.
  borderline h. (BHT)
  ceiling effect in h.
  chronic h. (CH)
  chronic thromboembolic
    pulmonary h. (CTEPH)
  cocaine-induced h.
  cuffed h.
  h. in diabetes (HID)
  diastolic h.
  dietary approaches to stop h.
    (DASH)
  endolymphatic h.
  episodic h.
  essential h. (EH, EHT)
  exercise h.
  extrahepatic portal h. (EHPH)
  familial h. (FH)
  familial dyslipidemic h.
  familial primary pulmonary h.
    (FPPH)
  genetic h. (GH)
  h. genetic epidemiology network
    (HyperGEN)
  gestational h.
  glucocorticoid-induced h.
  high-renin essential h. (HREH)
  hypoxic pulmonary h.
  idiopathic h.
  idiopathic portal h. (IPH)
  idiopathic pulmonary h. (IPH)
  induced h.
  International Society of H. (ISH)
  intracranial h. (ICH)
  intrathoracic h.
  isolated systolic h.
  labile h.
  left atrial h.
  low renin essential h. (LREH)
  malignant h. (MH)
  masked h.

NOTES

H

339

hypertension *(continued)*
  mineralocorticoid-induced h.
  neuromuscular h.
  nonprimary pulmonary h.
  obesity h.
  obliterative pulmonary h. (OPH)
  office h.
  oral contraceptive-induced h.
  orthostatic h.
  Page episodic h.
  pale h.
  paroxysmal h.
  pediatric h.
  portal h. (PHT)
  portopulmonary h.
  postcapillary h.
  postpartum h.
  precapillary pulmonary h.
  pregnancy-induced h. (PIH)
  primary h.
  primary pulmonary h. (PPH)
  pulmonary h. (PH, PHT)
  pulmonary artery h. (PAH)
  pulmonary venous h. (PVH, PVHI)
  recalcitrant h.
  red h.
  renal h.
  renoprival h.
  renovascular h. (RVH)
  resistant h.
  resting h.
  retrograde h.
  sal and water dependent h.
  secondary pulmonary h.
  h. secondary to renal disease
    (HSRD)
  splenoportal h.
  h. standard
  stress-related h.
  superimposed pregnancy-induced h.
    (SPIH)
  systemic vascular h.
  systemic venous h.
  systolic h.
  thromboembolic pulmonary h.
  venous h.
  white-coat h.
hypertensive (HT)
  h. agent
  h. arteriopathy
  h. arteriosclerosis
  h. arteriosclerotic cardiovascular
    disease (HASCVD)
  h. arteriosclerotic heart disease
    (HASHD)
  borderline h. (BH)
  h. cardiovascular disease (HCVD,
    HTCVD)
  h. crisis

  h. emergency
  h. encephalopathy (HE)
  h. heart disease (HHD, HTHD)
  h. hypertrophic cardiomyopathy
  h. hypervolemic therapy (HHT)
  h. intracerebral hemorrhage (HIH)
  h. nephropathy (HTN)
  h. pulmonary polyarteritis
  h. pulmonary vascular disease
    (HPVD)
  h. retinopathy
  spontaneously h. (SH)
  h. urgency
  h. vascular disease (HTVD, HVD)
  h. vasculopathy
hyperthermia
  cerebral h.
  whole-body h.
hyperthyroid heart
hyperthyroidism
  amiodarone-induced h.
  apathetic h.
hypertonic
  h. saline
  h. saline inhalation
hypertonica
  polycythemia h.
hypertriglyceridemia (HTG)
  familial h. (FHTG)
hypertriglyceridemic waist
hypertrophic
  h. adenoid
  h. cardiomyopathy (HC, HCM,
    HCMP)
  h. catarrh
  h. emphysema
  h. muscular subaortic stenosis
    (HMSAS)
  h. obstructive cardiomyopathy
    (HOCM)
  h. pulmonary osteoarthropathy
  h. smooth muscle layer
  h. subaortic stenosis (HSAS, HSS)
hypertrophied
  h. apex
  h. myocardium
hypertrophy
  adenotonsillar h.
  apical h.
  asymmetric septal h. (ASH)
  basal-septal h.
  biventricular h. (BVH)
  cardiac h.
  combined atrial h. (CAH)
  combined ventricular h. (CVH)
  compensatory h.
  concentric left ventricular h.
  eccentric h.
  goblet cell h.

idiopathic myocardial h. (IMH)
isolated septal h. (ISH)
left atrial h. (LAH)
left ventricular h. (LVH)
lipomatous h.
mucous gland h.
myocardial cell h.
myocyte h.
pressure-overload h.
right atrial h. (RAH)
right ventricular h. (RVH)
secondary septal h.
septal h.
stretch-induced cardiomyocyte h.
submucosal gland h.
trabecular h.
transcoronary ablation of septal h.
 (TASH)
ventricular h. (VH)
volume load h.
hyperuricemia
hyperuricemic nephropathy
hyperventilation
alveolar h.
eucapneic voluntary h.
isocapnic h.
h. maneuver
h. syndrome (HVS)
hyperventilation-induced asthma (HIA)
hyperviscosity syndrome
hypervitaminosis
hypervolemia
hypervolemic (HV)
hypha, pl. **hyphae**
hyphemia
hypn
hypertension
hypnagogic hallucination
hypnagogue
hypnalgia
hypnic
hypnology
Hypnomidate
hypnopompic
hypnosis
hypnotic drug
hypoadrenalism
hypoaeration
hypoalbuminemia
hypoaldosteronism
hyporeninemic h.
hypoalphalipoproteinemia

hypobaric
h. exposure
h. hypoxia
hypobetalipoproteinemia
familial h. (FHBL)
hypocalcemia
cardiac defects, abnormal facies,
 thymic hypoplasia, cleft palate, h.
 (CATCH-22)
hypocapnia
hypocapnic
hypocarbia
hypochloremia
hypochloremic metabolic alkalosis
hypochlorite
hypocholesterolemia
hypochondrial reflex
hypochondriasis
hypodynamia cordis
hypoechoic
hypofunction
hypogammaglobulinemia
hypoglossal nerve
hypoglycemia
hypoglycemic
h. agent
h. syncope
hypokalemia-induced arrhythmia
hypokalemic periodic paralysis
hypokinemia
hypokinesis, hypokinesia
anteromesial h.
cardiac wall h.
global h.
inferobasilar h.
hypokinetic pulse
hypomagnesemia
hyponatremia
hyponatremic-hypertensive syndrome
hypoparathyroidism
hypoperfused myocardium
hypoperfusion
myocardial h.
tissue h.
hypopharyngeal obstruction
hypophosphatemia
hypophyseal-pituitary-adrenal axis
hypophyseos
pars pharyngea h.
hypopiesis
orthostatic h.

NOTES

H

341

hypoplasia
> isthmic h.
> mitral valve h.
> h. of right ventricle
> right ventricular h.

hypoplasminogenemia

hypoplastic
> h. emphysema
> h. heart
> h. left heart (HPLH)
> h. left heart syndrome (HLHS)
> h. left ventricle (HLV)
> h. left ventricle syndrome (HLVS)

hypopnea
> central h.
> obstructive h.

hypopneic

hyporeninemia

hyporeninemic hypoaldosteronism

hyposphygmia

hypostasis
> pulmonary h.

hypostatic
> h. bronchopneumonia
> h. congestion
> h. pneumonia

hyposystole

hypotension
> acute severe h.
> arterial h.
> chronic idiopathic orthostatic h.
> exertional h.
> hemorrhagic h.
> idiopathic orthostatic h. (IOH)
> intractable h.
> orthostatic h.
> postprandial h.
> postural h.
> pulmonary artery h. (PAH)
> sympathetic orthostatic h. (SOH)
> vasodilatory h.
> vasovagal h.

hypotensive agent

hypothalamic-pituitary-adrenal (HPA)
> h.-p.-a. axis (HPAA)

hypothermia
> h. blanket
> extracorporeal exchange h.
> h. mattress
> moderate h.
> topical h.

hypothermic fibrillating arrest

hypothesis, pl. hypotheses
> fetal origins h.
> Gad h.
> leading circle h.
> lipid h.
> Lyon h.
> Moe multiple wavelet h.

> monoclonal h.
> multiple wavelet h.
> null h.
> premature ventricular complex-trigger h.
> response-to-injury h.
> sulfhydryl depletion h.
> Wu-Hoak h.

hypothrombogenic

hypothyroidism
> subclinical h.

hypotonia

hypotonicity

hypotonus, hypotony

Hypovase

hypoventilation
> alveolar h.
> congenital central alveolar h.
> nocturnal h.
> pulmonary alveolar h. (PAH)

hypovolemia

hypovolemic shock

hypoxanthine

hypoxemia
> arterial h.
> circulatory h.
> intraoperative h.
> refractory h.
> REM sleep-related h.
> rest h.
> h. test

hypoxia
> altitude h.
> alveolar h.
> anemic h.
> circulatory h.
> demand h.
> diffusion h.
> global tissue h.
> hemic h.
> histotoxic h.
> hypobaric h.
> hypoxic h.
> ischemic h.
> myocyte h.
> sleep h.
> stagnant h.
> h. warning system

hypoxia-inducible factor (HIF)

hypoxic
> h. hypoxia
> h. lap swimming
> h. pulmonary hypertension
> h. pulmonary vasoconstriction (HPV)
> h. spell
> h. syncope
> h. vasoconstriction
> h. ventilatory response (HVR)

hypoxic-ischemic encephalopathy
hypoxidosis
hysteresis
    airway h.
    pacemaker h.
    pacing h.
    rate h.
hysterical
    h. fainting
    h. syncope
hysteric angina

hystericus
    globus h.
hysterosystole
Hy-Tape waterproof adhesive tape
Hytinic
Hytrin
Hytuss
Hytuss-2X
Hyzaar
Hyzine-50 Injection

NOTES

H

I-123, ^{123}**I**
    iodine-123
        I-123 BMIPP imaging
        I-123 metaiodobenzylguanidine
        I-123 MIBG
        I-123 MIBG uptake
I-125, ^{125}**I**
    iodine-125
        I.-125 metaiodobenzylguanidine
        I.-125 MIBG
I-131, ^{131}**I**
    iodine-131
I-309
    CC chemokine I-309
^{123}**I**
    ^{123}I-MIBG-SPECT
^{125}**I** (*var. of* I-125)
I_{Cl}
    chloride current
I_{Na}
    sodium current
I_{tp}
    temporal peak intensity
        Itp pulse
I_F
    pacemaker current
I_{Ca}
    calcium current
I_{sata}
    spatial average, temporal average
     intensity
        Isata pulse
I_{sapt}
    spatial peak, temporal average intensity
        Isapt pulse
I_{sapa}
    spatial average pulse average
I_{ta}
    temporal average intensity
        Ita pulse
I_{sp}
    spatial peak intensity
        Isp pulse
I_{sppa}
    spatial peak pulse average intensity
I_{sa}
    spatial average intensity
        Isa pulse
IA
    intraaortic
    intraarterial
    intraatrial
    intraauricular

IAA
    interrupted aortic arch
IAAA
    inflammatory abdominal aortic aneurysm
IAB
    intraaortic balloon
        IAB catheter
IABA
    intraaortic balloon assistance
IABC, IABCP
    intraaortic balloon counterpulsation
IABP
    intraaortic balloon pulsation
    intraaortic balloon pump
    intraaortic balloon pumping
IAC CPR
    interposed abdominal compression
     cardiopulmonary resuscitation
IACD
    implantable automatic cardioverter-
     defibrillator
    intraarterial conduction defect
IACI
    idiopathic arterial calcification of infancy
IACP
    intraaortic counterpulsation
IAD
    implantable atrial defibrillator
    intracranial atherosclerotic disease
        Metrix IAD
IADL
    impairment of activities of daily living
    instrumental activities of daily living
        Lawton IADL
IADSA, IA-DSA
    intraarterial digital subtraction
     angiography
IAF
    idiopathic alveolar fibrosis
IAH
    implantable artificial heart
IAIA
    immune adherence immunosorbent assay
iANP
    immunoreactive atrial natriuretic peptide
IAO
    intermittent aortic occlusion
IAPG
    interatrial pressure gradient
IAQ
    indoor air quality
IART
    intraatrial reentry tachycardia

IAS
  interatrial septum
  interatrial shunting
IASA
  interatrial septal aneurysm
IASD
  interatrial septal defect
  interauricular septal defect
iatrogenic
    i. atrial septal defect
    i. disease
    i. disorder
    i. pneumothorax
IAV
  intraarterial vasopressin
I band
IBBBB
  incomplete bilateral bundle branch block
Iberet-Folic-500
iberiotoxin
IBI
  internal borderzone infarct
ibopamine
IBP
  intraaortic balloon pumping
IBPMS
  indirect blood pressure measuring system
ibuprofen
    pseudoephedrine and i.
Ibuprohm
Ibu-Tab
ibutilide fumarate
IC
  impedance cardiogram
  inspiratory capacity
  intracardiac
ICA
  internal carotid artery
ICAM
  intercellular adhesion molecule
ICAM-1
  intercellular adhesion molecule-1
ICAO
  International Civil Aviation Organization
    ICAO standard atmosphere
ICAT
  intracoronary aspiration thrombectomy
icatibant pretreatment
ICC
  immunocytochemistry
  intensive coronary care
  interventional cardiac center
ICCM
  idiopathic congestive cardiomyopathy
ICCU
  intensive coronary care unit
ICD
  impedance cardiogram
  implantable cardioverter-defibrillator

  ischemic coronary disease
  isolated conduction defect
    Angstrom II ICD
    Angstrom MD ICD
    Contour high voltage can ICD
    Contour II ICD
    Contour LT V-135D ICD
    Contour V-145D ICD
    dual-chamber ICD
    dual-chamber Maximo remote
      monitoring ICD
    Guardian ICD
    internet monitoring of ICD
    ICD lead
    Photon DR dual-chamber ICD
    remotely monitored ICD
    Res-Q Micron ICD
    single-chamber Maximo remote
      monitoring ICD
    Telectronics Guardian ATP II ICD
    transthoracically implanted ICD
    Ventritex Cadence ICD
    Vitatron Diamond ICD
ICD-9
  International Classification of Diseases,
    Ninth Revision
ICD-ATP
  implantable cardioverter-
    defibrillator/atrial tachycardia pacing
    ICD-ATP device
ICDC
  implantable cardioverter-defibrillator
    catheter
ICE
  intracardiac echocardiography
    ICE catheter
iced
    i. saline
    i. saline lavage
ice mapping
ice-pick view
ICEUS
  intracaval endovascular ultrasonography
ICG
  impedance cardiogram
  impedance cardiography
ICG-PDR
  indocyanine green plasma disappearance
    rate
ICH
  intracerebral hemorrhage
  intracranial hemorrhage
  intracranial hypertension
    infratentorial ICH
    supratentorial ICH
ICHD
  Inter-Society Commission for Heart
    Diseases
    ICHD pacemaker code

ichorous pleurisy
ICI
  intracardiac infection
icing heart
ICM
  intelligent cardiovascular monitor
  isolated cardiovascular malformation
ICO
  impedance cardiac output
  intracellular organism
ICP
  intracranial pressure
ICR
  intracardiac catheter recording
ICRT
  intracoronary radiation therapy
ICS
  inhaled corticosteroids
  intracellular-like, calcium-bearing
    crystalloid solution
    ICS cardioplegic solution
ICSD
  International Classification of Sleep
    Disorders
ICSK
  intracoronary streptokinase
ICSO
  intermittent coronary sinus occlusion
ICT
  intracardiac thrombus
icteric sputum
ictometer
ICTP
  type I collagen telopeptide
ictus
    i. cordis
    i. sanguinis
ICUS
  intracoronary ultrasound
ICV
  internal cerebral vein
ICVP
  inferior vena cava pressure
ICXA
  intermediate circumflex artery
ID
  immunodiffusion
Idamycin PFS
idarubicin hydrochloride
IDC
  idiopathic dilated cardiomyopathy

IDDM
  insulin-dependent diabetes mellitus
ideal alveolar gas
ideational apraxia
IDEC-Y2B8 antibody
ideomotor apraxia
idiojunctional rhythm
idionodal rhythm
idiopathic
    i. acute eosinophilic pneumonia
    i. alveolar fibrosis (IAF)
    i. arterial calcification of infancy
      (IACI)
    i. arteritis of Takayasu
    i. bradycardia
    i. brown induration
    i. cardiomegaly
    i. central sleep apnea
    i. congestive cardiomyopathy
      (ICCM)
    i. cyclic edema
    i. dilated cardiomyopathy (IDC)
    i. disease of myocardium (IDM)
    i. hypereosinophilic syndrome
      (IHES)
    i. hyperkinetic heart syndrome
      (IHHS)
    i. hypersomnia
    i. hypertension
    i. hypertrophic subaortic stenosis
      (IHSS)
    i. interstitial fibrosis
    i. interstitial pneumonia
    i. long Q-T interval syndrome
    i. mitral valve prolapse (IMVP)
    i. myocardial hypertrophy (IMH)
    i. myocarditis
    i. orthostatic hypotension (IOH)
    i. pericarditis
    i. portal hypertension (IPH)
    i. pulmonary fibrosis (IPF)
    i. pulmonary hemosiderosis (IPH)
    i. pulmonary hypertension (IPH)
    i. restrictive cardiomyopathy
    i. right atrial dilation
    i. thrombocytopenia
    i. thrombocytopenic purpura (ITP)
    i. unilobar emphysema
    i. venoocclusive disease
    i. ventricular fibrillation
    i. ventricular tachycardia (IVT)
idiosyncratic asthma

NOTES

idioventricular
    i. bradycardia
    i. kick
    i. rhythm (IVR)
    i. tachycardia
IDIS
    intraoperative digital subtraction
IDISA
    intraoperative digital subtraction
      angiography
IDL
    intermediate-density lipoprotein
IDL-C, IDL-c
    intermediate density lipoprotein-
      cholesterol complex
IDM
    idiopathic disease of myocardium
idoxuridine
IDV
    intermittent demand ventilation
IE
    infective endocarditis
I:E
    inspiratory to expiratory ratio
      I:E ratio
IE-2 riboprobe
IEA
    inferior epigastric artery
      IEA graft
IEC
    inpatient exercise center
IEL
    internal elastic lamina
IEM
    internal elastic membrane
      IEM rupture
IETT
    immediate exercise treadmill testing
Ifex
IFG
    inferior frontal gyrus
IFL
    inferior frontal lobe
IFN
    interferon
ifosfamide
IFP
    intimal fibrous proliferation
Ig
    immunoglobulin
Igaki-Tamai stent
IgE
    immunoglobulin E
      serum IgE
IgE-sensitized cell
IGF
    insulin-like growth factor
IGF-1 overexpression

IgG
    immunoglobulin G
      ACLA IgG
      IgG avidity test
IgG1–4
IgM
    immunoglobulin M
      ACLA IgM
IGT
    impaired glucose tolerance
IH
    intermittent heparinization
    intimal hyperplasia
    intramural hematoma
IHD
    ischemic heart disease
      IHD QUERI
IHDI
    ischemic heart disease index
IHES
    idiopathic hypereosinophilic syndrome
IHHS
    idiopathic hyperkinetic heart syndrome
IHR
    intrinsic heart rate
IHSS
    idiopathic hypertrophic subaortic stenosis
IIFT
    intraoperative intraarterial fibrinolytic
      therapy
IJ
    internal jugular
Ikorel
IL
    interleukin
      IL Synthesis analyzer
IL-10
      IL-10 production
      recombinant human IL-10 (rhuIL-
      10)
IL-4 gene
ILBBB
    incomplete left bundle branch block
ILCOR
    International Liaison Committee on
      Resuscitation
ILD
    interstitial lung disease
ileal artery
ileocolic artery
Iletin
    beef Lente I. II
ileus
    meconium i.
ILHDL
    isolated low high-density lipoprotein
iliac
    i. artery
    i. artery occlusion

I

i. steal
i. vein
i. vein thrombosis
iliofemoral venous system
iliopopliteal bypass
Illinois Test of Psycholinguistic Abilities (ITPA)
illness
catabolic i.
decompression i.
illusion
Iloprost
Ilosone
Ilotycin
ILUS
intraluminal ultrasound
IM
innocent murmur
internal mammary
intramuscular
IM artery
Rocephin IM
IMA
inferior mesenteric artery
internal mammary artery
IMA graft
IMA retractor
IMAB
internal mammary artery bypass
image
i. aliasing
amplitude i.
i. analysis
i. bundle
CK i.
color kinesis i.
3D SPGR i.
ejection-fraction i.
ejection shell i.
equilibrium i.
FLAIR i.
fluid-attenuated inversion
recovery i.
functional i.
gradient reversal i.
harmonic phase i.
HARP i.
i. intensifier
paradox i.
parametric i.
phase i.
phase-encoded velocity i.

postpump i.
prepump i.
regional ejection fraction i. (REFI)
respiratory-gated 2 D segmented-
FLASH MRCA i.
SE i.
short-axis i.
stress washout myocardial
perfusion i.
supine rest gated equilibrium i.
three-dimensional spoiled gradient-
recalled acquisition i.
T1-weighted i.
VMap dynamic flow-based i.
Image-Measure morphometry software
Imagent contrast agent
imager
SONOS 2000, 5500 ultrasound i.
Imager Torque selective catheter
imagery
guided i.
ImageView system
ImageVue software
imaging
acoustic i.
ADC i.
adenosine nuclear perfusion i.
adenosine radionuclide perfusion i.
i. agent
Aloka color Doppler system for
blood flow i.
antifibrin antibody i.
antimyosin antibody i.
apparent diffusion coefficient i.
arrhythmia-insensitive flow-sensitive
alternating inversion recovery i.
biplane i.
black blood magnetic resonance i.
blood-pool i.
breathhold turbo-flash tagged i.
cardiac blood-pool i.
i. chain
chemical shift i. (CSI)
coherent contrast i. (CCI)
color kinesis i.
color tissue Doppler i.
continuous arterial spin-labeled
perfusion magnetic resonance i.
(CASL-PI MRI)
continuous-wave Doppler i.
diffusion tensor i. (DTI)
diffusion-weighted i. (DWI)

NOTES

imaging *(continued)*
digital cardiac i. (DCI)
digital subtraction i.
digital vascular i. (DVI)
dimensionality in i.
dipyridamole-thallium i. (DTI)
direct Fourier transformation i.
Doppler tissue i. (DTI)
Doppler transesophageal color
flow i.
double-oblique i.
3D tagged magnetic resonance i.
duplex i.
echocardiographic strain rate i.
echo planar i. (EPI)
electrocardiographic gated SPECT
myocardial perfusion i.
exercise tomographic TI-201 i.
Fourier two-dimensional i.
frequency domain i.
functional i.
functional magnetic resonance i.
(fMRI)
fundamental i. (FI)
gallium i.
gallium-67 i.
gated blood-pool i.
gated sweep magnetic resonance i.
gradient-echo i.
harmonic i. (HI)
harmonic gray-scale i.
harmonic power Doppler i.
high-speed volumetric i.
I-123 BMIPP i.
indium-111-labeled lymphocyte i.
infarct-avid i.
Integris cardiovascular i.
krypton-81m ventilation i.
long-echo-train-length fast-spin-
echo i., long-ETL FSE i. (long-
ETL FSE imaging)
magnetic resonance i. (MRI)
magnetic source i. (MSI)
mask-mode cardiac i.
MCD i.
myocardial perfusion i. (MPI)
native tissue harmonic i.
nuclear magnetic resonance i.
(NMRI)
nuclear perfusion i.
parametric i.
perfusion-weighted i.
pharmacologic stress perfusion i.
phase i.
planar myocardial i.
planar thallium i.
platelet i.
power motion i.
pulsed Doppler tissue i.

pulse inversion harmonic i.
PYP i.
pyrophosphate i.
radionuclide i.
radiopharmaceutical i.
real-time perfusion i.
redistribution i.
rest-redistribution thallium-201 i.
rubidium-82 i.
second harmonic i. (SHI)
sestamibi perfusion i.
single-photon emission computed
tomographic i.
single-photon emission
tomography i.
SPECT i.
SPET i.
spin-echo i.
stress-redistribution-reinjection
thallium-201 i.
stress SPECT perfusion i.
stress thallium-201 myocardial
perfusion i.
tagged magnetic resonance i.
^{99m}Tc-sestamibi i.
^{99m}Tc-tetrofosmin i.
teboroxime i.
technetium-99m MIBI i.
technetium-99m-tetrofosmin i.
technetium (Tc)-99m sestamibi
tomographic i.
thallium perfusion i.
thallium SPECT i.
three-dimensional tagged magnetic
resonance i.
tissue Doppler i. (TDI)
tomographic radionuclide i.
transient response i. (TRI)
transmission i.
triggered harmonic power
Doppler i.
ultrasonic integrated backscatter i.
velocity-encoded cine-magnetic
resonance i. (VE-cMRI)
ventilation/perfusion i.
video i.
i. window
xenon lung ventilation i.
IMAI
internal mammary artery implant
Imatron CT scanner
IMAX
internal maxillary artery
imazodan
imbalance
acid-base i.
electrolyte i.
protease-antiprotease i.
sympathovagal i.

IMCE
  intravenous myocardial contrast echocardiography
imciromab pentetate
Imdur
Imed
  I. Gemini PCI-IV pump
  I. infusion device
  I. infusion pump
I-Methasone
imglucerase
IMGU
  insulin-mediated glucose uptake
IMH
  idiopathic myocardial hypertrophy
  intramural hemorrhage
IMI
  impending myocardial infarction
  inferior myocardial infarction
I-123-MIBG
  iodine-123 metaiodobenzylguanidine
imidazoline
  i. receptor (I-receptor)
  i. receptor agonist
imipenem and cilastatin
imipramine
immediate
  i. exercise treadmill testing (IETT)
  i. silhouette
immersion
  head-out water i.
immitis
  Coccidioides i.
  Dirofilaria i.
immobilized heparin
immotile cilia syndrome
ImmuCyst
immune
  i. adherence immunosorbent assay (IAIA)
  i. cascade
  i. thrombocytopenia
immune-mediated
  i.-m. disease
  i.-m. membranous nephritis
  i.-m. vasculitis
immunity
  cell-mediated i.
Immuno
  Feiba VH I.
immunoassay
  AfeCTA i.

enzyme i. (EIA)
  nifedipine enzyme i.
  NT-proBNP ELISA enzyme i.
  Thrombus Precursor Protein i.
immunoblot
  antiphosphotyrosine i.
immunoblotting
immunochemical abnormality
immunocompetent host
immunocompromised
immunocytochemistry (ICC)
immunodeficiency
  common variable i. (CVID)
immunodetected
immunodiffusion (ID)
immunofluorescence
  cytometric indirect i.
immunofluorescent technique
immunoglobulin (Ig)
  i. E (IgE)
  equine rabies i. (ERIG)
  i. G (IgG)
  i. M (IgM)
  respiratory syncytial virus i. (RSV-IG)
  varicella-zoster i. (VZIG)
immunological theory
immunometric sandwich method
immunonephelometry
  rate i.
immunoperoxidase stain
immunoprecipitation
immunoprecipitin analysis
immunoprophylaxis
immunoradiometric assay (IRMA)
immunoreactive
  i. arginine-vasopressin (IR-AVP)
  i. atrial natriuretic peptide (iANP, IrANP)
immunoreactivity
  endothelin-1 i.
immunoregulator
  IMREG-1 i.
immunoseparation
immunosorbent
immunospot
  enzyme-linked i. (ELISPOT)
immunostaining technique
immunosuppressant
immunosuppression
  postinjury i.
  i. therapy

NOTES

immunosuppressive
immunotherapy
immunoturbidimetric assay
Imovax vaccine
impact
    I. portable aspirator model 326
    I. specialized feeding formula
impaction
    mucoid i.
Impact specialized feeding formula
impaired
    i. glucose tolerance (IGT)
    i. relaxation mitral flow pattern
impairment
    i. of activities of daily living
      (IADL)
    ciliary i.
    conduction i.
    functional aerobic i. (FAI)
    memory i.
    restrictive functional i.
    ventricular systolic i.
impedance
    acoustic i.
    i. aggregometry
    aortic i.
    arterial i.
    atrial lead i.
    battery cell i.
    i. cardiac output (ICO)
    i. cardiogram (IC, ICD, ICG)
    i. cardiography (ICG)
    i. catheter
    lead i.
    i. modulus
    pacemaker i.
    pacing lead i.
    i. plethysmography (IPG)
    thoracic i.
    i. threshold valve (ITV)
    transthoracic i.
    i. variables
    vascular i.
    ventricular i.
impeller pump
impending
    i. myocardial infarction (IMI)
    i. respiratory failure
imperfecta
    osteogenesis i.
implant
    adrenal medullary i.
    annuloplasty band i.
    Biocell RTV i.
    Biomatrix ocular i.
    bioresorbable i.
    Core-Vent i.
    defibrillator i.
    internal mammary artery i. (IMAI)

    polytf i.
    SynerGraft i.
    Zoladex I.
implantable
    i. artificial heart (IAH)
    i. atrial defibrillator (IAD)
    i. automatic cardioverter-defibrillator
      (IACD)
    i. cardioverter-defibrillator (ICD)
    i. cardioverter-defibrillator/atrial
      tachycardia pacing (ICD-ATP)
    i. cardioverter-defibrillator catheter
      (ICDC)
    i. cardioverter-defibrillator lead
    i. cardioverter electrode
    i. left ventricular assist system
      (IPLVAS)
    i. loop recorder
    i. pulse generator
implantation
    BRAFE approach for elective
      coronary stent i.
    i. guidelines
    i. metastasis
    prophylactic implantable
      cardioverter-defibrillator i.
    rescue stent i.
    i. response
    stent i.
    i. test (IT)
    transcatheter valve i.
implosion effect
Import vascular access port
impotence
    vasculogenic i.
Impra Distaflo bypass graft
impressio cardiaca pulmonis
ImPressure ultrasound pressure sensor
improvement
    deterioration following i. (DFI)
impulse
    afferent i.
    apex i.
    apical i. (AI)
    cardiac i.
    i. conduction
    I. diagnostic catheter
    ectopic i.
    escape i.
    i. formation
    overlapping biphasic i. (OLBI)
    pacing i. (PI)
    paradoxic rocking i.
    point of maximal i. (PMI)
    point of maximum i. (PMI)
    i. propagation
    right parasternal i.
    i. summation
    systolic apical i.

ImPulse electronic oxygen conserving device
impure flutter
IMREG-1 immunoregulator
IMT
  intimal-medial thickness
Imulyse tPA ELISA kit
IMV
  intermittent mandatory ventilation
  intermittent mechanical ventilation
IMVP
  idiopathic mitral valve prolapse
¹¹¹In
  indium-111
in
  in extremis
  in situ hybridization
  in situ thrombosis
  in vitro
  in vitro allergy test
  in vitro pharmacology
  in vivo
  in vivo gene transfer
inactivated poliovirus vaccine
inactivation
  recovery from i.
  tumor suppressor gene i.
inactive tuberculosis
inactivity
  physical i.
inaequalis
  pulsus i.
inamrinone
inappropriate sinus tachycardia (IST)
INCA
  infant nasal cannula assembly
  INCA system
Incardia valve system
incentive
  i. spirometer
  i. spirometry
incessant
  i. atrial tachycardia
  i. ventricular tachycardia
inch
  pounds per square i. (psi)
incidence
  peak i.
incident
  cardiovascular i. (CVI)
  cerebrovascular i. (CVI)

  i. pressure waveform
  vascular i.
incidental murmur
incision
  clamshell i.
  collar i.
  fish-mouth i.
  ladder i.
  longitudinal midline i.
  median sternotomy i.
  pleuropericardial i.
  racquet i.
  stab i.
  sternal-splitting i.
  stocking-seam i.
  thoracotomy i.
  transverse i.
incisura
  i. apicis cordis
  i. cardiaca pulmonis sinistri
  i. pulse
incline
  treadmill i.
inclusion
  Rocha-Lima i.
  i. technique of Bentall
incognitus
  Mycoplasma i.
incompetence, incompetency
  aortic i. (AI)
  cardiac valvular i.
  chronotropic i.
  mitral i. (MI)
  muscular i.
  pulmonary i.
  pulmonic i.
  pyloric i.
  relative i.
  tricuspid i. (TI)
  valvular i.
incomplete
  i. atrioventricular block
  i. atrioventricular dissociation
  i. A-V dissociation
  i. bilateral bundle branch block (IBBBB)
  i. left bundle branch block (ILBBB)
  i. right bundle branch block (IRBBB)
  i. thrombosis

NOTES

incongruens
>pulsus i.

incontinentia pigmenti syndrome

increase
>blood pressure i. (BPI)

increased
>i. afterload
>i. contractility

increased-permeability pulmonary edema

increment
>work rate i.

incremental
>i. atrial pacing
>i. shuttle walking test (ISWT)
>i. threshold loading
>i. ventricular pacing

incrementation
>couch i.

incrementing response

IND
>investigational new drug
>IND status

Indacrinone

indanyl carbenicillin

indapamide

indecainide

Indeflator Plus 20

Inderal LA

Inderide

indeterminate single ventricle

index, pl. **indices, indexes**
>airways reactivity i. (ARI)
>ankle-arm i.
>ankle-brachial i. (ABI)
>apnea i. (AI)
>apnea-hypopnea i. (AHI)
>arm-ankle indices
>arousal i.
>arterial pressure i. (API)
>asynchrony i.
>atherectomy i.
>atherogenic i. (AI)
>atherogenicity i.
>atrial emptying i. (AEI)
>atrial stasis i.
>Barthel i.
>Baseline Dyspnea I. (BDI)
>beat inclusion i. (BII)
>blood pressure i. (BPI)
>body mass i. (BMI)
>brachial-ankle i.
>breath holding i. (BHI)
>Breuer-Hering deflation i.
>Broders i.
>Calgary Sleep Apnea Quality of Life I.
>cardiac i. (CI)
>cardiac output i.
>cardiac risk i. (CRI)

cardiac work i. (CWI)
carotid augmentation i.
central apnea-hypopnea i.
Chapman i.
Charlson comorbidity i.
chemotherapeutic i.
chest i.
Cholesterol-Saturated Fat I. (CSFI)
cholesterol saturation i. (CSI)
compliance, rate, oxygenation and pressure i.
contractile work i.
coronary artery disease i. (CADI)
coronary prognosis i. (CPI)
coronary prognostic i.
cortical arousal i. (CAI)
Crown-Crisp i.
Detsky modified risk i.
diastolic amplitude time i. (DATI)
diastolic pressure-time i. (DPTI)
Doppler-derived i.
Dubois i.
Duke Activity Status I. (DASI)
Eagle risk score i.
eccentricity i.
Eichner i.
ejection phase i.
end-diastolic volume i. (EDVI)
end-systolic force-velocity i.
end-systolic volume i. (ESVI)
exercise i.
Fischl i.
Fourmentin thoracic i.
Framingham risk i.
free thyrotoxin i.
Frenchay Activities I.
General Well-Being I.
Gensini i.
Gibson circularity i.
glycocalicin i.
Goldman risk-factor i.
heart rate retardation i. (HRRI)
infarct size i. (ISI)
ischemic heart disease i. (IHDI)
isovolumetric phase i.
isovolumic i.
ITPA i.
late potential parameter i.
laterality i. (LI)
left atrial emptying i. (LAEI)
left cardiac work i. (LCWI)
left ventricular diastolic phase i.
left ventricular ejection time i. (LVETI)
left ventricular mass i.
left ventricular stroke volume i. (LVSVI)
left ventricular stroke work i. (LVSWI)

left ventricular systolic i. (LVSI)
left ventricular work i. (LVWI)
i. lesion
Lewis i.
lipid-laden macrophage i.
MB i.
mean cardiac i. (MCI)
mean rate ejection i. (MREI)
Miller i.
mitral valve closure i.
movement arousal i. (MAI)
multifactorial cardiac risk i.
  (MCRI)
myocardial band i.
myocardial jeopardy i.
oxygen consumption i.
oxygen desaturation i. (ODI)
oxyhemodynamic i.
palliative prognostic i.
penetrating cardiac trauma i.
  (PCTI)
penile-brachial pressure i.
performance i. (PI)
Pneumonia Severity I. (PSI)
polysomnographic i.
ponderal i.
Positive Symptom Distress I.
  (PSDI)
Pourcelot i.
preejection period i. (PEPI)
pulmonary vascular resistance i.
  (PVRI)
pulsatility i. (PI)
QTI:QT i.
Quality of Well-Being I.
Quetelet i.
rapid shallow breathing i. (RSBI)
regional wall motion i.
Reid i.
relaxation time i.
respiratory disturbance i. (RDI)
right ankle i.
right atrial inversion time i.
  (RAITI)
right cardiac work i. (RWCI)
right ventricular end-diastolic
  volume i. (RVEDVI)
right ventricular end-systolic
  volume i. (RVESVI)
right ventricular stroke work i.
  (RVSWI)
risk i.

Ritchie Articular I.
Robinson i.
Röhrer body mass i. (RI)
saturation i.
Schneider i.
segmental pressure i.
semiquantitative i.
shock i.
Sleep Apnea Quality of Life I.
  (SAQLI)
smoothness i.
sphericity i.
ST/HR i.
stiffness i.
stroke i. (SI)
stroke volume i. (SVI)
stroke work i. (SWI)
i. of suspicion
systemic vascular resistance i.
  (SVRI)
systolic pressure time i. (SPTI)
tension-time i.
TIMI frame count i.
total apexcardiographic relaxation
  time i. (TARTI)
total peripheral resistance i. (TPRI)
i. value
vascular resistance i.
venous disability i. (VDI)
venous filling i. (VFI)
ventricular perfusion i. (VQI)
ventricular stroke work i.
viability i.
volume thickness i. (VTI)
wall motion i. (WMI)
wall motion score i. (WMSI)
warfarin dose i. (WDI)
weaning i. (WI)
Wood units i.
Youden i.

indicator
  i. dilution method
  i. dilution technique
  elective replacement i. (ERI)
  electric replacement i. (ERI)
  operative hypertension i. (OHI)
  quality-of-care i.
  SPI-Lite sleep position i.
  xylol pulse i.
indifferent electrode
indinavir

NOTES

indirect
　　i. blood pressure measuring system (IBPMS)
　　i. diuretic
　　i. lead
　　i. murmur
indium-111 (^{111}In)
　　i.-111 scintigraphy
indium-111-labeled lymphocyte imaging
Indocin
　　I. I.V. injection
　　I. Oral
indocyanine
　　i. dilution curve
　　i. green
　　i. green angiography
　　i. green dye
　　i. green indicator dilution technique
　　i. green method
　　i. green plasma disappearance rate (ICG-PDR)
indomethacin
indoor air quality (IAQ)
indoramin
induced
　　i. hypertension
　　i. pneumothorax
inducibility
inducible
　　i. arrhythmia
　　i. nitric oxide synthase (iNOS)
　　i. nitric oxide synthetase (iNOS)
　　i. polymorphic ventricular fibrillation
　　i. polymorphic ventricular tachycardia
induction
　　rapid sequence i. (RSI)
　　sputum i.
induration
　　gray i.
　　idiopathic brown i.
　　red i.
indurative
　　i. myocarditis
　　i. pleurisy
　　i. pneumonia
industrial anthrax
indux
　　rale i.
indwelling
　　i. central venous catheter
　　i. line
inelastic load
inert gas narcosis
inertia
inertial effect
In-Exsufflator respiratory device
InfaMyst aerosol spray device

infancy
　　idiopathic arterial calcification of i. (IACI)
infant
　　i. airflow and effort sensor
　　i. Ambu resuscitator
　　continuous noninvasive monitoring of ventilated i.'s
　　I. Flow noninvasive nasal CPAP system
　　i. nasal cannula assembly (INCA)
　　i. respiratory distress syndrome (IRDS)
　　I. Resuscitation system
　　I. Star 100, 200 ventilator
　　I. Star Ventilator 500/950
infantile
　　i. arteritis
　　i. beriberi
　　i. lobar emphysema
infarct (*See also* infarction)
　　acute multiple brain i.'s (AMBI)
　　anterior lateral myocardial i. (ALMI)
　　anterolateral wall myocardial i. (ALWMI)
　　i. artery
　　i. artery patency
　　brain i. (BI)
　　i. bulging
　　caudate i.
　　cerebral i.
　　embolic i.
　　i. expansion
　　i. extension
　　healed myocardial i. (HMI)
　　insular i.
　　internal borderzone i. (IBI)
　　internal capsule i.'s
　　lacunar i.
　　partial anterior circulation i. (PACI)
　　perforating artery i. (PAI)
　　pontine i. (PI)
　　posterior circulation i. (POCI)
　　posterior wall i. (PWI)
　　pulmonary i.
　　red i.
　　i. scar
　　silent cerebral i. (SCI)
　　i. size index (ISI)
　　subcortical junctional i.
　　i. thinning
　　total anterior circulation i. (TACI)
　　watershed i.
　　i. zone wall motion
infarct-avid
　　i.-a. hot-spot scintigraphy

i.-a. imaging
i.-a. myocardial scintigraphy
infarction (*See also* infarct)
acute coronary i. (ACI)
acute diaphragmatic myocardial i.
age-undetermined myocardial i.
anterior myocardial i.
anterior wall i. (AWI)
anterior wall myocardial i.
  (AWMI)
anteroinferior myocardial i.
anterolateral myocardial i.
anteroseptal myocardial i. (ASMI)
apical i.
atherothrombotic brain i. (ABI)
atrial myocardial i.
cardiac i.
cerebral i.
cerebrovascular i. (CVI)
coitus-induced myocardial i.
completed myocardial i.
complicated myocardial i.
diaphragmatic myocardial i. (DMI)
dietary prevention of recurrent
  myocardial i. (DPR)
drugs, electrolytes, low temperature
  and lunacy, intoxication and
  intracranial processes, retention of
  urine or feces, infection,
  unfamiliar surroundings,
  myocardial i. (DELIRIUM)
ERNA after acute myocardial i.
evolving myocardial i.
exercise training in anterior
  myocardial i. (EAMI)
family history of myocardial i.
hemorrhagic i. (HI)
H-form myocardial i.
impending myocardial i. (IMI)
inferior myocardial i. (IMI)
inferior wall i. (IWI)
inferior wall myocardial i. (IWMI)
inferolateral myocardial i.
inferoposterior myocardial i.
ischemic cerebral i.
juvenile myocardial i.
lacunar i. (LI)
large-vessel i. (LVI)
lateral medullary i. (LMI)
lateral myocardial i. (LMI)
malignant middle cerebral artery i.
  (mMCAI)

medial medullary i. (MMI)
myocardial i. (MI)
National Registry of Myocardial I.
  (NRMI)
non-Q-wave myocardial i. (NQMI,
  NQWMI)
non-ST segment elevation
  myocardial i. (NSTEMI)
non-ST segment myocardial i.
  (non-STEMI)
nontransmural myocardial i. (NTMI)
old myocardial i. (OMI)
perioperative myocardial i. (PMI)
posterior myocardial i.
postmyocardial i.
predictive index for myocardial i.
  (PIMI)
primary i. (PI)
pulmonary i. (PI)
Q-wave myocardial i. (QMI)
recent myocardial i. (RMI)
recurrent myocardial i.
right ventricle i. (RVI)
right ventricular i.
Roesler-Bressler i.
ruled out for myocardial i.
  (romied)
rule out myocardial i. (ROMI)
silent brain i. (SBI)
silent cerebral i. (SCI)
silent myocardial i. (SMI)
small-vessel i. (SVI)
ST-elevation acute myocardial i.
  (STEAMI)
striatocapsular i.
ST-segment elevation myocardial i.
  (STEMI)
stuttering myocardial i.
subacute myocardial i.
subendocardial i. (SEI)
subendocardial myocardial i.
  (SEMI)
threatened myocardial i. (TMI)
thrombotic brain i. (TBI)
through-and-through myocardial i.
transmural anterior myocardial i.
  (TAMI)
transmural inferior myocardial i.
  (TIMI)
transmural myocardial i. (TMI)
unstable angina/non-Q-wave
  myocardial i. (UA/NQMI)

NOTES

infarction *(continued)*
    watershed i.
    i. with shock
infarctlet
infarct-related
    i.-r. artery (IRA)
    i.-r. vessel
Infasurf
InfCM
    inflammatory cardiomyopathy
infected
    i. aneurysm
    i. myxoma
    i. secretion
infection
    acute lower respiratory tract i.
      (ALRI)
    adenoviral type 40/41 i.
    bacterial respiratory tract i.
    bloodstream i.
    catheter-related i. (CRI)
    community-acquired i.
    coronavirus i.
    driveline i.
    endemic fungal i.
    endobronchial i.
    fungal i.
    hospital-acquired i.
    intracardiac i. (ICI)
    laryngeal i.
    laryngotracheal i.
    latent tuberculosis i. (LTBI)
    MAC i.
    MAI i.
    miliary i.
    Mycobacterium avium complex i.
    Mycobacterium avium-
      intracellulare i.
    mycotic i.
    nosocomial i.
    opportunistic i.
    pleuropulmonary i.
    primary i.
    pyogenic i.
    recurrent respiratory i. (RRI)
    respiratory tract i.
    rhinocerebral i.
    secondary i.
    spirochetal i.
    staphylococcal i.
    streptococcal i.
    Streptococcus pyogenes i.
    surgical site i. (SSI)
    systemic i.
    upper respiratory i. (URI)
    varicella-zoster i.
    viral respiratory i.
infectious
    i. asthmatic bronchitis

    i. bronchiolitis
    i. endocarditis
    i. esophagitis
    i. mononucleosis
infective
    i. asthma
    i. embolism
    i. endocarditis (IE)
    i. exacerbation
    i. pericarditis
    i. thrombosis
    i. thrombus
INFeD injection
inferior
    i. accessory fissure
    arteria glutealis i.
    i. border of lung
    i. constrictor muscle of pharynx
    i. costal facet
    i. costal pit
    i. epigastric artery (IEA)
    i. epigastric artery graft
    i. esophageal sphincter
    fovea costalis i.
    i. frontal gyrus (IFG)
    i. frontal lobe (IFL)
    i. ganglion of glossopharyngeal
      nerve
    i. laryngeal artery
    i. laryngeal cavity
    i. laryngeal vein
    i. lingular bronchopulmonary
      segment
    i. lobe of left/right lung
    macular arteriole i.
    i. mesenteric artery (IMA)
    i. mesenteric artery retractor
    i. mesenteric vascular occlusion
    i. myocardial infarction (IMI)
    i. parietal/superior temporal lobe
      (IPSTL)
    i. phrenic lymph node
    i. temporal artery (ITA)
    i. thyroid artery
    i. thyroid vein
    i. tracheobronchial lymph node
    i. triangle sign
    i. vena cava (IVC)
    i. vena cava occlusion
    i. vena cava pressure (ICVP)
    i. vena cava reconstruction (IVCR)
    i. vena cava thrombosis (IVCT)
    i. venacavography (IVCV)
    vena laryngea i.
    i. wall infarction (IWI)
    i. wall myocardial infarction
      (IWMI)
inferior-axis flutter

inferiores
> nodi lymphoidei phrenici i.
> nodi lymphoidei
> tracheobronchiales i.

inferioris
> rami esophageales arteriae
> thyroideae i.

inferius
> tuberculum thyroideum i.

inferoapical
inferobasal wall
inferobasilar
> i. akinesis
> i. aneurysm
> i. hypokinesis

inferolateral
> i. myocardial infarction
> i. segment

inferoposterior myocardial infarction
inferoseptal segment
infestans
> *Triatoma i.*

infestation
> parasitic i.

infiltrate
> alveolar i.
> Assmann tuberculous i.
> bronchiolar inflammatory i.
> bronchopneumonic i.
> cellular i.
> diffuse interstitial i.
> fibrous i.
> fleeting i.
> fluffy alveolar i.
> hazy i.
> inflammatory cellular i.
> infraclavicular i.
> interstitial i.
> linear i.
> lobar i.
> migratory pulmonary i.
> nodular i.
> patchy i.
> peribronchiolar inflammatory i.
> perivascular eosinophilic i.
> perivascular lymphocytic i.
> reticulonodular i.
> strandy i.
> streaky i.
> Wasserman-positive pulmonary i.

infiltrating lobular carcinoma

infiltration
> cardiac i.
> epituberculous i.
> gelatinous i.
> gray i.
> inflammatory cell i.
> patchy i.
> perivascular i. (PVI)
> subepicardial fatty i.

infiltrative cardiomyopathy
Infiltrator local drug delivery device
Infiniti
> I. catheter
> I. catheter introducer system

Infinix
> I. DP-i vascular x-ray
> I. NB-i vascular x-ray
> I. VC-i vascular x-ray

inflammation
> adhesive i.
> cap i.
> granulomatous i.
> lymphoplasmacytic i.
> neutrophil-induced pulmonary i.
> peribronchiolar granulomatous i.

inflammatoria
> dysphagia i.

inflammatory
> i. abdominal aortic aneurysm
> (IAAA)
> i. adhesion
> i. airway disease
> i. autobullectomy
> i. cardiomyopathy (InfCM)
> i. cell infiltration
> i. cellular infiltrate
> i. cytokine
> i. marker
> i. mediator
> i. myofibroblastic tumor
> i. pericarditis
> i. pseudotumor (IPT)
> i. reaction

inflation
> balloon i.
> oscillating balloon i.
> i. pressure
> i. reflex

inflow
> i. tract
> turbulent diastolic mitral i.

influenza, pl. **influenzae**

NOTES

influenza *(continued)*
  i. A, B, C virus
  Asian i.
  i. bacillus
  endemic i.
  Hong Kong i.
  Port Charles i.
  Russian i.
  Texas i.
  i. tracheobronchitis
  Victoria i.
  i. virus pneumonia
  i. virus vaccine
influenzae
  Haemophilus i.
  nontypeable *Haemophilus* i. (NTHI)
influenzal pneumonia
Influenzavirus **A, B, C**
influx
  transsarcolemmal calcium i.
infraclavicular
  i. infiltrate
  i. triangle
infracristal
infracubital bypass
infradiaphragmatic
  i. portion
  i. venous flow
infrahisian
  i. block
  i. conduction system
infranodal extrasystole
infrared
  near i.
  i. thermography
  i. thermometer
infrared-pulsed laser
infrarenal abdominal aortic aneurysm
infrasegmental vein
infratentorial ICH
infrequens
  pulsus i.
infundibula (*pl. of* infundibulum)
infundibular
  i. atresia
  i. obstruction
  i. pulmonary stenosis (IPS)
  i. septal defect
  i. stenosis
  i. wedge resection
infundibulectomy
  Brock i.
infundibulum, pl. **infundibula**
  i. of lung
  tendo infundibuli
  tendon of i.
Infusaid infusion pump
InfusaSleeve
  I. II catheter

  Kaplan-Simpson I.
  LocalMed I.
Infuse-A-Port pump
infuser
infusion
  Adenoscan i.
  adrenomedullin i.
  brain-heart i.
  bretylium i.
  cardioplegia i.
  CH i.
  continuous intravenous i. (CIV)
  ergonovine i.
  heart i. (HI)
  heparin i.
  intracoronary acetylcholine i.
  IO i.
  isoproterenol i.
  nitroprusside i.
  volume i.
ingravescent apoplexy
inguinalis
  regio i.
INH
  isoniazid
inhalant
  antifoaming i.
  i. antigen
inhalation
  i. agent
  Atrovent Aerosol I.
  i. bronchography
  i. challenge test
  formoterol fumarate powder for i.
  hypertonic saline i.
  isoproterenol sulfate i.
  NebuPent I.
  oxygen i.
  i. pneumonia
  i. therapy
  tobramycin solution for i.
  toxic fume i.
  i. tuberculosis
inhalational
  i. anesthesia
  i. anesthetic
  i. anthrax
inhaled
  i. antibiotic
  i. bronchodilator
  i. corticosteroids (ICS)
  i. radioaerosol technique
Inhale deep lung delivery system
inhaler
  AeroBid Oral Aerosol I.
  Aerodose insulin i.
  AERx i.
  Albuterol spiros i.
  Azmacort Oral I.

Beclovent Oral I.
Beconase AQ Nasal I.
breath-actuated i. (BAI)
Combivent i.
Diskus i.
dry powder i. (DPI)
Flovent HFA metered-dose i.
Glaxo Wellcome Diskhaler i.
Intal Oral I.
ipratropium i.
metered-dose i. (MDI)
metered-solution i. (MSI)
nicotine i.
Nicotrol I.
pressurized metered-dose i. (pMDI)
Tape Based i.
Vancenase AQ I.
Vanceril Oral I.

Inhibace

inhibited
atrial i. (AAI)
atrial demand i. (AAI)
atrial synchronous ventricular i.
  (VDD)
both ventricles i. (VDI)
i. pacing
ventricular i. (VVI)

inhibition
leukotriene i.
magnet i.
neutral endopeptidase i. (NEP-I,
  NEPi)
phosphodiesterase III i. (PDE3I)
potassium i.

inhibitor
ACE i.
acyl-CoA:cholesterol
  acyltransferase i.
alpha-2-plasmin i.
alpha-1 proteinase i.
angiotensin-converting enzyme i.
  (ACEI, ACEi)
atriopeptidase i.
beta-lactamase i.
bronchial mucus i.
carbonic anhydrase i.
caspase i.
cholesterol crystallization i. (CCI)
cholinesterase i.
complement i.
converting enzyme i.
cyclooxygenase i.

direct thrombin i.
endopeptidase i.
glycoprotein IIb/IIIa i.
HMG CoA-reductase i.
human menopausal gonadotropin
  coenzyme A reductase i.
hydroxymethylglutaryl coenzyme A
  reductase i.
3-hydroxy-3-methylglutaryl coenzyme
  A reductase i.
Kuntiz-type i.
leukotriene i.
lipoprotein-associated coagulation i.
MAO i.
mast cell i.
matrix metalloproteinase i. (MMPI)
metalloproteinase i.
monoamine oxidase i. (MAOI)
mucus i.
Na^+/H^+ exchange i. (NHEI)
neutral endopeptidase i.
oxysterol i.
PDE isoenzyme i.
phosphodiesterase i. (PDE, PDE-I)
phosphodiesterase isoenzyme i.
plasminogen activator i. (PAI)
platelet aggregation i.
platelet glycoprotein IIb/IIIa i.
platelet IIb/IIIa i.
protease i. (PI)
proton pump i.
reductase i.
renin i.
secretory leukocyte protease i.
  (SLPI)
secretory leukoprotease i. (SLPI)
secretory leukoproteinase i. (SLPI)
thromboxane synthetase i.
tissue factor pathway i. (TFPI)
tissue plasminogen activator i.
  (tPAI)
vasopeptidase i. (VPI)

inhibitor-1
plasminogen activator i.-1 (PAI-1)

inhomogeneity

initial apnea

initiative
ischemic heart disease quality
  enhancement research I. (IHD
  QUERI)
NIH *Xenopus* I.

NOTES

initiative *(continued)*
  quality enhancement research I.
    (QUERI)
  Women's Health I. (WHI)
injectable
  Cardizem I.
injection
  Abbokinase i.
  Activase i.
  Adenocard i.
  Adrucil i.
  A-hydroCort i.
  A-methaPred i.
  Amikin i.
  Andropository i.
  Apresoline i.
  AquaMEPHYTON i.
  Aristocort Forte i.
  Aristocort Intralesional i.
  Aristospan Intraarticular i.
  Aristospan Intralesional i.
  Arixtra subcutaneous i.
  Baci-IM i.
  Bena-D i.
  Benadryl i.
  Bicillin L-A i.
  blood patch i.
  bolus intravenous i.
  bone marrow i.
  Brethine i.
  Brevibloc i.
  Bricanyl i.
  Cafcit i.
  i. catheter
  Caverject i.
  Celestone Phosphate i.
  CellCept intravenous for i.
  Cel-U-Jec i.
  Ceredase i.
  Chlor-Trimeton i.
  Cipro i.
  Cleocin Phosphate i.
  Compazine i.
  Cortrosyn i.
  Corvert i.
  Cyklokapron i.
  Cytoxan i.
  dalteparin sodium i.
  daptomycin for i.
  DDAVP i.
  Decadron i.
  Delatestryl i.
  Demadex i.
  Depo-Medrol i.
  Depopred i.
  Depo-Provera i.
  D.H.E. 45 i.
  Diflucan i.
  Diprivan i.

  Dobutrex i.
  Dopram i.
  Duo-Trach i.
  dye i.
  Edecrin Sodium i.
  Enlon i.
  epoprostenol sodium for i.
  ergonovine i.
  Ethamolin i.
  Flolan i.
  Floxin i.
  Foscavir i.
  Fragmin i.
  gadoteridol i.
  Garamycin i.
  hand i.
  heparin i.
  hep-lock i.
  Hydrocortone Acetate i.
  Hydrocortone Phosphate i.
  Hylutin i.
  Hyzine-50 i.
  Indocin I.V. i.
  INFeD i.
  Intropin i.
  iopromide i.
  isosorbide dinitrate i.
  Kefurox i.
  Kenalog i.
  Key-Pred i.
  Key-Pred-SP i.
  Lasix i.
  lepirudin rDNA i.
  Levophed i.
  Lincocin i.
  Lincorex i.
  Lovenox i.
  meropenem for i.
  Minocin I.V. i.
  mycophenolate mofetil intravenous
    for i.
  Narcan i.
  Nebcin i.
  negative-contrast i.
  Neosar i.
  Neutrexin i.
  Normodyne i.
  Nydrazid i.
  Oncovin i.
  Osmitrol i.
  Pentam-300 i.
  Permapen i.
  Phenergan i.
  Pitressin i.
  Prednisol TBA i.
  Priscoline i.
  Prodrox i.
  Prostin VR Pediatric i.
  Refludan i.

Retrovir i.
Reversol i.
Rifadin i.
root i.
Solu-Cortef i.
Solu-Medrol i.
Sotradecol i.
Sublimaze i.
Tac-3 i.
Tensilon i.
Terramycin I.M. i.
tinzaparin sodium i.
Toposar i.
Trandate i.
Triam-A i.
Triam Forte i.
Triamonide i.
Tridil i.
Tri-Kort i.
Trilog i.
Trilone i.
Triostat i.
Ultravist i.
Ureaphil i.
Vancocin i.
Vancoled i.
VePesid i.
Vibramycin i.
Vistaril i.
Vumon i.
Wycillin i.
Zinacef i.

injector

flow i.
Medrad Mark IV angiographic i.
Mill-Rose esophageal i.
modified Mark IV R-wave-triggered power i.
power i.
pressure i.
Viamonte-Hobbs dye i.

injury

acute chemical i.
acute lung i. (ALI)
aortic i.
aspiration lung i.
blunt chest i.
blunt pulmonary i.
blunt torso i.
brachial plexus i.
chest wall i.
chronic recurrent chemical i.

contrecoup i.
diastolic current of i.
diffuse lung i.
early lung i.
early pulmonary i.
electrical i.
femoral vascular i.
intrathoracic i.
ischemic-reperfusion i.
late lung i.
late pulmonary i.
lipid-induced lung i.
lung i.
median nerve i.
mesangial immune i.
myocardial i.
penetrating chest i.
phrenic nerve crush i.
pulmonary parenchymal i.
radionecrosis i.
reperfusion i.
I. Severity Score (ISS)
systolic current of i.
thermal i.
thoracic crush i.
vascular i.
ventilator-associated lung i. (VALI)
ventilator-induced lung i. (VILI)

inlet

thoracic i.
ventricular i.

in-memory gating

inner

i. city asthma
i. wall (IW)

Innervasc expandable vascular access system

innervation

autonomic sensory i.

innocent

i. heart murmur
i. murmur (IM)
i. murmur of elderly

Innohep

innominate

i. aneurysm
i. artery
i. vein

Innovace

Innovar

inoculation

inogatran

NOTES

INOmax
inorganic
>   i. acid
>   i. acid vapor
>   i. dust
>   i. dust disease
>   i. murmur

iNOS
>   inducible nitric oxide synthase
>   inducible nitric oxide synthetase

inosine
inositol triphosphate
inotrope
>   negative i.

inotropic
>   i. agent
>   i. arrhythmia
>   i. effect
>   i. support

inotropy
Inoue
>   I. balloon catheter
>   I. balloon mitral valvotomy
>   I. balloon technique
>   I. endovascular stent-graft
>   I. self-guiding balloon
>   I. single-balloon technique
>   I. triple-branched stent graft

INOvent delivery system
inpatient exercise center (IEC)
INR
>   international normalized ratio
>   target INR

insert
>   AirSep Ultimate nasal seal gel i.
>   EverGrip clamp i.
>   Koala vascular i.

insertion
>   percutaneous catheter i.
>   retrograde catheter i.
>   route of i.
>   wire i.

insipidus
>   nephrogenic diabetes i.

insomnia
insomniac
insonation
>   angle of i.

insonified
Inspector large bore in-line hemostasis valve
InSpectra tissue spectrometer
inspiration
>   crowing i.
>   duration of i. (T_I)
>   sustained maximal i. (SMI)

inspirator
inspiratory
>   i. airflow

i. capacity (IC)
i. center
i. dyspnea
expiratory to i. (E:I)
i. to expiratory ratio (I:E)
i. flow rate
i. limb
i. loading
i. murmur
i. muscle fatigue
i. occlusion pressure
i. positive airway pressure (IPAP)
i. rale
i. reserve capacity (IRC)
i. reserve volume (IRV)
i. resistance and positive expiratory pressure (IR-PEP)
i. stridor
i. threshold load (ITL)
i. time (T_I)
i. view
i. vital capacity (IVC)

InspirEase device
inspired gas
inspirometer
Inspiron
>   I. device
>   I. incentive spirometer

inspissated
instability
>   catheter i.
>   circulatory i.
>   hemodynamic i.
>   microsatellite i.

instantaneous
>   i. electrical axis
>   i. spectral peak velocity
>   i. vector

Insta-Pulse heart rate monitor
in-stent
>   i.-s. neointimal proliferation
>   i.-s. restenosis (ISR)
>   i.-s. thrombosis

InStent VascuCoil stent
instillation
>   intracavitary i.
>   lavage i.

institute
>   Cardiopulmonary Research I. (CAPRI)
>   National Heart I. (NHI)
>   National Heart, Lung, Blood I. (NHLBI)
>   Texas Heart I. (THI)

instrument
>   activating adjusting i. (AAI)
>   bipolar radiofrequency surgical ablation i.
>   blood sampling i.

Cooley neonatal i.'s
Diamond-Lite titanium i.'s
EndoWrist i.
KinetiX i.'s
K x-ray fluorescence i.
Matsuda titanium surgical i.'s
Micrins microclamp i.
Multi-Dop X/TCD transcranial
  Doppler i.
Pneumo-Needle reusable i.
thrombolytic predictive i. (TPI)
Yesavage depression i.
instrumental activities of daily living
  (IADL)
instrumentation
angiographic i.
insudate
insufficiency
acute coronary i. (ACI)
  asymptomatic cardiac ischemia
aortic valvular i.
arterial i.
atrial i. (AI)
atrioventricular valve i.
cardiac i. (card insuff, CI)
cardiovascular i. (CVI)
cerebrovascular i. (CVI)
chronic coronary i. (CCI)
chronic venous i. (CVI)
coronary i. (CI)
deep venous i. (DVI)
distal vascular i.
energetic dynamic cardiac i.
  (EDCI)
left ventricular i. (LVI)
mitral i. (MI)
mitral valve i. (MVI)
multivalve i.
myocardial i.
periprosthetic valve aortic i.
pulmonary i.
pulmonic i.
renal i.
respiratory i.
rheumatic mitral i.
Sternberg myocardial i.
tricuspid i. (TI)
valvular i.
velopharyngeal i.
venous valvular i.
insufflation
gastric i.

thoracoscopic talc i.
tracheal gas i. (TGI)
insufflator
Insuflon device
insula, pl. **insulae**
insular infarct
insulation
i. failure
lead i.
insulin
beef i.
glucose potassium i. (GKI)
Lente Iletin I, II i.
NPH Iletin i.
pork i.
i. preparation
regular purified pork i.
i. resistance
i. resistance syndrome
I. Riabead II radioimmunoassay
i. shock
insulin-dependent diabetes mellitus
  (IDDM)
insulin-like growth factor (IGF)
insulin-mediated glucose uptake (IMGU)
insult
cardiac i.
vascular i.
InSync
I. cardiac resynchronization device
I. II Marquis remote monitoring
  CRT-ICD
I. implantable cardioverter
  defibrillator
I. multisite cardiac stimulator
intact valve
Intal
I. Nebulizer Solution
I. Oral Inhaler
Intec
I. AID cardioverter-defibrillator
  generator
I. implantable defibrillator
Integra
I. catheter
I. II balloon
integral
diastolic velocity i. (DVI)
paced depolarization i.
i. pulse frequency modulation
  (IPFM)

NOTES

integral *(continued)*
    i. pulse frequency modulation/Smith delay compensatory (IPFM/SDC)
    systolic velocity i. (SVI)
    velocity time i.
integrated
    i. backscatter
    i. bipolar sensing
    i. lead system
integration
    digital color Doppler velocity profile i.
    vertical i.
integrator
    Medical Graphics pneumotachograph with volume i.
Integrilin
integrin
    i. blocker
    i. signaling
integrin-dependent pathway
Integris
    I. cardiac imaging system
    I. cardiovascular imaging
    I. 3D RA
    I. H5000 digital x-ray imaging system
Integrity
    I. AFx AutoCapture pacing system
    I. AFx DR model 5346 pacemaker
intellectual dysfunction
Intellicath pulmonary artery catheter
intelligence quotient (IQ)
intelligent
    i. cardiovascular monitor (ICM)
    i. CPAP
intensifier
    image i.
intensity
    echo i.
    intravascular signal i.
    peak myocardial video i. (PMVI)
    pulse average i. (Ipa)
    reduced signal i.
    spatial average i. (I_{sa})
    spatial average, temporal average i. (I_{sata})
    spatial peak i. (I_{sp})
    spatial peak pulse average i. (I_{sppa})
    spatial peak, temporal average i. (I_{sapt})
    temporal average i. (I_{ta})
    temporal peak i. (I_{tp})
    waxing and waning in i.
intensive
    i. coronary care (ICC)
    i. coronary care unit (ICCU)
intensivist

intentionem
    per primam i.
    per secundum i.
intention to treat (ITT)
interaction
    adhesin-receptor i.
    leukocyte-endothelial cell i.
    lung-liver i.
interalveolar
    i. communication
    i. septa
interarterial
    i. communication
    i. shunt
interarytenoid notch
interatrial
    i. block
    i. conduction time
    i. pressure gradient (IAPG)
    i. septal aneurysm (IASA)
    i. septal defect (IASD)
    i. septum (IAS)
    i. shunting (IAS)
interauricular septal defect (IASD)
intercadence
intercadent
intercalary
intercellular
    i. adhesion molecule (ICAM)
    i. adhesion molecule-1 (ICAM-1)
    i. coupling
intercept
    i. angle
    I. vascular internal MR coil
Interceptor wire distal protection device
intercidens
    pulsus i.
intercostal
    i. catheter
    external i.
    internal i.
    i. mammary vessel
    i. nerve block
    i. retraction
    i. space
intercostale
    spatium i.
intercurrens
    pulsus i.
interdependence
    ventricular i.
interectopic interval
interelectrode
    i. distance
    i. space
interest
    region of i. (ROI)
interface
    I. arterial blood filter

electrode-skin i.
lung-wall i.
Monarch Mini Mask nasal i.
sputum-epithelium i.
Ultimate Seal gel i.
interfascicular fibrous tissue
interference
i. beat
i. dissociation
dissociation by i.
electromagnetic
interference/radiofrequency i.
(EMI/RFI)
interferon (IFN)
i. alfa-2a,-2b
i. alfa-2b and ribavirin combination
pack
i. alpha
alpha-i.
i. gamma-1b
interferon alfa-2a,-2b
InterGard vascular graft
interlaced scanning
interlead
i. QT dispersion
i. QT variability
interleukin (IL)
IL-1-11
circulating IL-6
PEG IL-2
interlobar
i. effusion
i. empyema
i. pleurisy
i. surface of lung
interlobular
i. emphysema
i. pleurisy
interlobularis
pneumonia i.
intermediary vesicle
intermediate
i. bronchus
i. circumflex artery (ICXA)
i. coronary syndrome
i. density lipoprotein-cholesterol
complex (IDL-C, IDL-c)
i. heart
i. laryngeal cavity
i. probability
intermediate-density lipoprotein (IDL)

Intermedics
I. atrial antitachycardia pacemaker
I. lead
I. Marathon dual-chamber rate-
responsive pacemaker
I. Marathon VVI single-chamber
pacemaker
I. Res-Q implantable cardioverter-
defibrillator
I. Stride pacemaker
intermedius
bronchus i.
ramus i.
intermesenteric arterial anastomosis
intermittence, intermittency
intermittens
dyskinesia i.
intermittent
i. aortic occlusion (IAO)
i. claudication
i. coronary sinus occlusion (ICSO)
i. demand ventilation (IDV)
i. heparinization (IH)
i. mandatory ventilation (IMV)
i. mechanical ventilation (IMV)
i. percussive ventilation (IPV)
i. pneumatic compression (IPC)
i. positive pressure (IPP)
i. positive pressure breathing
(IPPB)
i. positive pressure ventilation
(IPPV)
i. pulse
i. sinus arrest
interna
lamina elastica i.
internal
i. adhesive pericarditis
i. borderzone infarct (IBI)
i. branch of superior laryngeal
nerve
i. capsule
i. capsule infarcts
i. cardioversion
i. carotid artery (ICA)
i. cerebral vein (ICV)
i. diameter
i. elastic lamina (IEL)
i. elastic membrane (IEM)
i. elastic membrane rupture
i. energy
i. intercostal

NOTES

internal *(continued)*
    i. jugular (IJ)
    i. jugular vein
    i. mammary (IM)
    i. mammary artery (IMA)
    i. mammary artery bypass (IMAB)
    i. mammary artery catheter
    i. mammary artery graft
    i. mammary artery graft
      angiography
    i. mammary artery implant (IMAI)
    i. mammary vessel
    i. maxillary artery (IMAX)
    i. pneumatic stabilization
    i. pudendal vein
    i. reed switch
    i. respiration
    i. thoracic artery (ITA)
    i. thoracic artery graft
    i. thoracic vein
    i. workrate

international
    Cardiovascular Credentialing I.
      (CCI)
    I. Civil Aviation Organization
      (ICAO)
    I. Classification of Diseases, Ninth
      Revision (ICD-9)
    I. Classification of Sleep Disorders
      (ICSD)
    I. Cooperative Pulmonary Embolism
      Registry
    I. Liaison Committee on
      Resuscitation (ILCOR)
    i. normalized ratio (INR)
    I. Registry of Acute Aortic
      Dissection (IRAD)
    I. Society of Cardiology (ISC)
    I. Society and Federation of
      Cardiology (ISFC)
    I. Society for Heart and Lung
      Transplantation (ISHLT)
    I. Society for Heart Transplantation
      (ISHT)
    I. Society of Hypertension (ISH)
    I. Staging System for Lung Cancer
      (ISSLC)
    I. Standards Organization (ISO)

internet monitoring of ICD

internodal
    i. conduction
    i. pathway
    i. tract of Bachmann

internum
    pericardium i.

interpleural space

interpolated
    i. beat

    i. extrasystole
    i. premature complex

interposed
    i. abdominal compression
    i. abdominal compression
      cardiopulmonary resuscitation (IAC
      CPR)

interposition of Dacron tube

interpulmonary septum

interpulse
    i. interval (IPI)
    i. potential (Ipp)

interquartile range

interrogation
    deep Doppler velocity i.
    i. device
    Doppler i.
    stereoscopic i.

interrupted
    i. aortic arch (IAA)
    i. pledgeted suture
    i. respiration

interruption
    aortic arch i.

intersegmental
    i. artery
    i. part of pulmonary vein

intersegmentales
    partes i.

Intersept cardiotomy reservoir

**Inter-Society Commission for Heart
  Diseases (ICHD)**

interstitial
    i. distribution
    i. emphysema
    i. fibrosis
    i. fluid
    i. granuloma
    i. infiltrate
    i. lung disease (ILD)
    i. marking
    i. nodule
    i. pattern
    i. and perivascular collagen
      network
    i. plasma cell pneumonia
    i. pneumonitis
    i. pulmonary edema
    i. pulmonary fibrosis (IPF)
    i. space

interstitium
    axial i.
    cardiac i.
    lung i.
    peripheral i.

intersystole

intersystolic period

Intertach II pacemaker

Intertech anesthesia breathing circuit

InterTherapy intravascular ultrasound interval
    A-A i.
    A_1-A_2 i.
    A-C i.
    AH i.
    A_2 incisural i.
    A-N i.
    A_2 to opening snap i.
    atrial escape i.
    atriocarotid i.
    atrioventricular i.
    auriculoventricular i.
    automatic capacitor formation i.
    A-V delay i.
    Bazett corrected QT i.
    B-H i.
    c-a i.
    cardioarterial i.
    confidence i. (CI)
    coupling i.
    critical coupling i.
    defibrillation response i. (DRI)
    electromechanical i.
    escape i.
    fetal PR i.
    f-f i.
    filtered atrial rate i. (FARI)
    flutter R i.
    H-Ae i.
    hangout i.
    H_1-H_2 i.
    His-ventricle i.
    H'P i.
    H-Q i.
    H-QRS i.
    H-V i.
    interectopic i.
    interpulse i. (IPI)
    isoelectric i.
    isometric i.
    isovolumic i.
    JT i.
    long PP i.
    long QT i.
    magnet pacing i.
    NN i.
    pacemaker escape i.
    passive i.
    P-H i.
    P-J i.

    postsphygmic i.
    P-P i.
    P-Q i.
    P-R i.
    presphygmic i.
    prolongation of P-R i.
    Q-H i.
    Q-M i.
    QR i.
    QRB i.
    QRS i.
    QRS-T i.
    Q-S_2 i.
    QT i.
    QTc i.
    QU i.
    right ventricular systolic time i.
    R-P i.
    R-R i.
    R-R' i.
    RS-T i.
    short coupling i.
    shortening of P-R i.
    sphygmic i.
    S-QRS i.
    S_1-S_2 i.
    ST i.
    stimulus-T i.
    symptom-free i.
    systolic time i. (STI)
    TP i.
    V-A i.
    V-H i.
interval-dependent potentiation
interval-strength relation
intervalvular fibrosa
intervention
    cardioreparative drug agent i.
    coronary sinus i. (CSI)
    direct percutaneous coronary i. (d-PCI)
    myocardial infarction triage and i. (MITI)
    percutaneous coronary i. (PCI)
    Society for Cardiac Angiography and I.'s (SCAI)
    vagomimetic i.
interventional
    i. cardiac catheterization
    i. cardiac center (ICC)
    i. cardiologist

NOTES

interventional *(continued)*
    i. echocardiography
    i. radiology
interventricular (I.V.)
    i. foramen (IVF)
    i. septal defect (ISD, IVSD)
    i. septal motion
    i. septal rupture
    i. septal thickness (IVS)
    i. septum (IVS)
    i. septum aneurysm
    i. sulcus
    i. vein
intervertebral disk
interview
    Alexithymia Provoked Response I.
    structured I.
intestinal
    i. ischemia
    i. lipodystrophy
intima
    aortic tunica i.
intimal
    i. atheroma
    i. defect
    i. erosion
    i. fibrous proliferation (IFP)
    i. fláp
    i. hyperplasia (IH)
    i. proliferation
    i. tear
    i. thickening
intimal-medial
    i.-m. thickening
    i.-m. thickness (IMT)
intolerance
    carbohydrate i.
    exercise i.
    glucose i.
intoxication
    alcohol i.
    digitalis i.
intraalveolar
    i. deposit
    i. pressure
intraaortic (IA)
    i. balloon (IAB)
    i. balloon assistance (IABA)
    i. balloon catheter
    i. balloon counterpulsation (IABC, IABCP)
    i. balloon device
    i. balloon pulsation (IABP)
    i. balloon pump (IABP)
    i. balloon pumping (IABP, IBP)
    i. counterpulsation (IACP)
intraarterial (IA)
    i. catheter
    i. chemotherapy

    i. conduction defect (IACD)
    i. counterpulsation
    i. digital subtraction angiography (IADSA, IA-DSA)
    i. gene transfer
    i. thrombosis
    i. vasopressin (IAV)
intraatrial (IA)
    i. activation sequence
    i. baffle
    i. block
    i. conduction
    i. conduction time
    i. reentrant tachycardia
    i. reentry tachycardia (IART)
    i. shunting
intraauricular (IA)
intrabronchial
intracardiac (IC)
    i. accelerometer
    i. amobarbital sodium procedure
    i. atrial activation sequence
    i. catheter
    i. catheter recording (ICR)
    i. ECG
    i. echocardiography (ICE)
    i. electrogram
    i. electrophysiology
    i. event
    i. gas gangrene
    i. infection (ICI)
    i. lead
    i. mapping
    i. mass
    i. navigation
    i. pacing
    i. pressure
    i. pressure curve
    i. shunt
    i. sucker
    i. thrombus (ICT)
    i. tumor
intracaval
    i. device
    i. endovascular ultrasonography (ICEUS)
intracavitary
    i. air meniscus
    i. electrocardiography
    i. hemorrhage
    i. instillation
    i. pressure-electrogram dissociation
    i. pressure gradient
intracavity mass
intracellular
    i. calcium concentration
    i. caveolae
    i. lipid
    i. magnesium

i. organism (ICO)
i. tyrosine protein kinase
intracellulare
   Mycobacterium i.
intracellular-like, calcium-bearing
   crystalloid solution (ICS)
intracerebral hemorrhage (ICH)
IntraCoil self expanding nitinol stent
intracoronary
   i. acetylcholine infusion
   i. angioscopy
   i. artery radiation
   i. aspiration thrombectomy (ICAT)
   i. beta-radiation
   i. Doppler flow wire
   i. radiation therapy (ICRT, IRT)
   i. sonicated meglumine
   i. stenting
   i. stenting of de novo narrowing
   i. stent placement
   i. streptokinase (ICSK)
   i. thrombolysis balloon
      valvuloplasty
   i. ultrasonography
   i. ultrasound (ICUS)
   i. vascular ultrasound (IVUS)
intracorporeal heart
intracranial
   i. atherosclerotic disease (IAD)
   i. fusiform aneurysm
   i. hemorrhage (ICH)
   i. hypertension (ICH)
   i. microembolic signal
   i. pressure (ICP)
intractable
   i. aspiration
   i. hypotension
intragraft thrombus
intrahisian block
intralesion restenosis
Intralipid
intralobar
intralobular line
intraluminal
   i. dissection
   i. flap
   i. plaque
   i. thrombus
   i. ultrasound (ILUS)
IntraLuminal Safe-Steer system
intramucosal pH

intramural
   i. coronary artery
   i. hematoma (IH)
   i. hemorrhage (IMH)
   i. thrombosis
   i. thrombus
intramuscular (IM)
intramyocardial
   i. conduction delay
   i. function
   i. pressure
   i. sinusoid
   i. vessel
intraoperative
   i. cell salvage
   i. digital subtraction (IDIS)
   i. digital subtraction angiography
      (IDISA)
   i. echocardiography (IOE)
   i. hemodynamics
   i. hypoxemia
   i. intraarterial fibrinolytic therapy
      (IIFT)
   i. mapping
   i. transesophageal echocardiography
      (IOTEE)
   i. vascular angiography (IVA)
intraosseous (IO)
intraparenchymal
   i. hematoma
   i. hemorrhage
intraparietal sulcus (IPS)
intrapericardial
   i. hemorrhage
   i. pressure (IPP)
   i. sign
intraperitoneal rupture
intraplaque LDL oxidation
intrapleural
   i. catheter
   i. catheter analgesia
   i. oncotic pressure
   i. rupture
   i. sealed drainage unit
   i. space
intrapulmonary
   i. percussive ventilation (IPV)
   i. rheumatoid nodule
   i. shunt
   i. shunt fraction (Q_s/Q_t)
   i. shunting

NOTES

intrapulmonary *(continued)*
    i. vascular dilation
    i. vein (IPV)
intrapulmonic
intrarectal
intrastent
    i. minimal lumen cross-sectional area (ISMLCSA)
    i. recurrent disease
    i. restenosis (IR)
intrathoracic
    i. gas
    i. gas compression
    i. hypertension
    i. injury
    i. pressure
    i. PTLPD
    i. thyroid
intratracheal tube
intrauterine
    i. pneumonia
    i. respiration
intravariability
intravasation
    venous i.
intravascular (I.V., i.v.)
    i. aggregate
    i. blood coagulation (IVBC)
    i. bronchoalveolar tumor
    i. catheter electrode
    i. coagulation (IVC)
    i. consumption coagulopathy (IVCC)
    i. Doppler
    i. Doppler-tipped guidewire
    i. elastogram
    i. fetal air sign
    i. fluid (IVF)
    i. foreign body retrieval
    i. gene transfer
    i. mass (IVM)
    i. MRI
    i. oxygenator (IVOX)
    i. papillary endothelial hyperplasia (IPEH)
    i. perfluorochemical emulsion
    i. pressure (IVP)
    i. procoagulant factor
    i. red light therapy (IRLT)
    i. signal intensity
    i. stent
    i. thrombus
    i. ultrasound (IVUS)
    i. ultrasound catheter
    i. volume
intravenous (I.V., i.v.)
    i. analgesia
    CellCept i.
    i. cholangiogram (IVC)

    i. cholangiography (IVC, IVCH)
    i. digital subtraction angiography (IVDSA)
    i. fluid (IVF)
    Fungizone I.
    i. gamma globulin (IVGG)
    i. glucose tolerance test (IVGTT)
    i. hyperalimentation (IVH)
    i. immune globulin
    i. immunoglobulin therapy
    i. myocardial contrast echocardiography (IMCE)
    Saventrine I.
    i. vasopressin (IVV)
intravenously enhanced computed tomography (IVCT)
intraventricular (I.V., IVT)
    i. aberration
    i. block (IVB)
    i. catheter (IVC)
    i. conduction
    i. conduction defect (IVCD)
    i. conduction delay
    i. conduction disease (IVCD)
    i. conduction pattern
    i. gradient
    i. hemorrhage (IVH)
intravital capillary video microscopy
Intrepid
    I. balloon catheter
    I. PTCA catheter
intrinsic
    i. asthma
    i. deflection
    i. depolarization
    i. disease
    i. heart rate (IHR)
    i. positive end-expiratory pressure (PEEPi)
    i. sympathomimetic activity
intrinsicoid deflection
intrinsic PEEP *(var. of* autoPEEP)
introduced
    percutaneously i.
introducer
    Angestat hemostasis i.
    Angetear tearaway i.
    aortic assist balloon i.
    Avanti i.
    Check-Flo i.
    Ciaglia percutaneous tracheostomy i.
    Desilets-Hoffman catheter i.
    Fast-Cath Duo i.
    Flexor i.
    gum elastic bougie i.
    Hemaquet i.
    I. II sheath
    LPS Peel-Away i.

Maximum hemostasis i.
Micropuncture Peel-Away i.
Mullins catheter i.
Nottingham i.
PD Access with Peel-Away
  needle i.
split-sheath i.
TFX Medical safety needle with i.
Tuohy-Borst i.
Ultimum hemostasis i.
UMI transseptal Cath-Seal
  catheter i.
USCI i.

introducer/endoscope
Czaja-McCaffrey rigid stent i./e.

intron
i. 16
i. A

Intropin injection
intubated patient
intubation
catheter-guided endoscopic i.
  (CAGEIN)
endotracheal i.
lighted stylet i.
mainstem i.
nasotracheal i.
O'Dwyer i.
orotracheal i.
rapid-sequence i.
retrograde translaryngeal i.
RSI orotracheal i.
i. time
tracheal i.

intubator
intussusception
Invacare
I. nasal prongs
I. Venture HomeFill complete
  home oxygen system

Invanz
invasion
blood vessel i. (BVI)

invasive
i. assessment
i. management
i. monitoring
i. pressure measurement
i. pulmonary aspergillosis (IPA)

inventory
Beck Depression i.

Cloninger Temperament and
  Character i.
Edinburgh Handedness i. (EHI)
State-Trait Anxiety i. (STAI)

inversa
angina i.

inverse-ratio ventilation (IRV)
Inversine
inversion
right atrial i. (RAI)
shallow T wave i.
i. spin-echo pulse sequence (ISE)
T wave i.
U wave i.
ventricular i.

inversus
atrial situs i.
dextrocardia with situs i.
levocardia with situs i.
situs i.
visceroatrial situs i.

inverted
i. buttoned device
i. T wave
i. V technique

investigational
i. new drug (IND)
i. new drug status

investigator
atrial fibrillation i.

Invirase
INVM
isolated noncompaction of ventricular
  myocardium

involvement
right atrial i. (RAI)

inward-going rectification
INX stent
IO
intraosseous
IO infusion

Iobid DM
iodide
metocurine i.
potassium i.
saturated solution of potassium i.
  (SSKI)

iodine
lithium i. (LiI)
radiolabeled i.

iodine-123 (I-123)

NOTES

373

iodine-123 *(continued)*
    i.-123 heptadecanoic acid radioactive tracer
    i.-123 metaiodobenzylguanidine (I-123-MIBG)
    i.-123 metaiodobenzylguanidine uptake
iodine-125 (I-125, ^{125}I)
    i.-125 isotope
iodine-131 (I-131, ^{131}I)
    i.-131 MIBG scintigraphy
iodophenylpentadecanoic acid
iodoquinol
IOE
    intraoperative echocardiography
IOH
    idiopathic orthostatic hypotension
Iohexol contrast
Iomeron
ion
    calcium i.
    i. channel
    chloride i.
    potassium i.
    i. pump
    sodium i.
Ionescu
    I. method
    I. trileaflet valve
Ionescu-Shiley
    I.-S. pericardial patch
    I.-S. pericardial valve
    I.-S. pericardial xenograft
    I.-S. valve prosthesis
    I.-S. vascular graft
ionic mechanism
ionizing radiation (IR)
ionophore
    calcium i. A23187
ion-selective electrode (ISE)
iopamidol
Iopamiro
iopromide injection
I-orthoiodohippurate
IOTEE
    intraoperative transesophageal echocardiography
iothalamate meglumine contrast medium
ioversol
ioxaglate
    i. meglumine
    i. meglumine contrast medium
    i. sodium
    sodium meglumine i.
IPA
    invasive pulmonary aspergillosis
Ipa
    pulse average intensity

IPAP
    inspiratory positive airway pressure
IPC
    intermittent pneumatic compression
    ischemic preconditioning
    IPC boots
IPEH
    intravascular papillary endothelial hyperplasia
IPF
    idiopathic pulmonary fibrosis
    interstitial pulmonary fibrosis
IPFM
    integral pulse frequency modulation
IPFM/SDC
    integral pulse frequency modulation/Smith delay compensatory
IPG
    impedance plethysmography
IPH
    idiopathic portal hypertension
    idiopathic pulmonary hemosiderosis
    idiopathic pulmonary hypertension
IPI
    interpulse interval
IPLVAS
    implantable left ventricular assist system
IPP
    intermittent positive pressure
    intrapericardial pressure
Ipp
    interpulse potential
IPPB
    intermittent positive pressure breathing
IPPV
    intermittent positive pressure ventilation
ipratropium
    i. and albuterol
    i. bromide
    i. inhaler
IPS
    infundibular pulmonary stenosis
    intraparietal sulcus
ipsilateral stroke
IPSTL
    inferior parietal/superior temporal lobe
IPT
    inflammatory pseudotumor
IPV
    intermittent percussive ventilation
    intrapulmonary percussive ventilation
    intrapulmonary vein
IQ
    intelligence quotient
    I. nasal mask
IR
    intrastent restenosis
    ionizing radiation
    ischemia-reperfusion

I/R
   ischemia/reperfusion
IRA
   infarct-related artery
IRAD
   International Registry of Acute Aortic
   Dissection
IrANP
   immunoreactive atrial natriuretic peptide
IR-AVP
   immunoreactive arginine-vasopressin
IRBBB
   incomplete right bundle branch block
irbesartan and hydrochlorothiazide
IRC
   inspiratory reserve capacity
IRDS
   infant respiratory distress syndrome
I-receptor
   imidazoline receptor
Ireland
      Cardiac Society of Great Britain
      and I. (CSGBI)
Irex Exemplar ultrasound
iridium strand
iridodonesis
irinotecan
irinotecan
Iris
      I. coronary stent
      I. II stent
IRLT
   intravascular red light therapy
IRMA
   immunoradiometric assay
      IRMA blood gas analysis system
      IRMA SL blood glucose strip
      tester
iron (fe)
   i. chelator
   colloidal i. (CI)
   i. dextran complex
   i. lung
   serum i.
   i. storage disease
IR-PEP
   inspiratory resistance and positive
   expiratory pressure
irradiation
      endovascular i. (EI)
      prophylactic brain i. (PCI)
      total axial node i. (TANI)

   total body i. (TBI)
   total lymphoid i. (TLI)
irregular
   i. discrete lesion
   i. hematoma
   i. rhythm
irregularis
   pulsus i.
irregularly
   i. irregular cardiac rhythm
   i. irregular pulse
irrespirable
irreversible
   i. airway obstruction
   i. shock
Irri-Cath suction system
irrigated
   i. catheter ablation
   i. coiled catheter
irrigation
irritable heart
irritant
   environmental i.
   nonspecific i.
   i. receptor
   respiratory i.
   i. rhinitis
   i. sinusitis
irritant-associated vocal cord
   dysfunction
irritant-induced asthma
IRT
   intracoronary radiation therapy
IRV
   inspiratory reserve volume
   inverse-ratio ventilation
Isaacs-Ludwig arteriole
Isambert disease
ISC
   International Society of Cardiology
ischemia
   acute cardiac i. (ACI)
   asymptomatic cardiac i. (ACI,
      acute coronary insufficiency)
   brachiocephalic i.
   cardiac i.
   cerebral i.
   clandestine myocardial i.
   colonic i.
   delayed cerebral i. (DCI)
   dobutamine-induced i.
   exercise-induced silent myocardial i.

NOTES

ischemia *(continued)*
    extremity i.
    global cerebral i. (GCI)
    intestinal i.
    left ventricular i. (LVI)
    left ventricular subendocardial
      myocardial i. (LVSEMI)
    limb i.
    low-flow i.
    manifest i.
    mental stress-induced i.
    mesenteric i.
    mucosal i.
    myocardial i. (MI)
    nonocclusive mesenteric i.
    psychophysiological interventions in
      myocardial i. (PIMI)
    recurrent mesenteric i.
    regional i.
    silent myocardial i.
    subendocardial i.
    transient mesenteric i.
    vertebrobasilar territory i. (VBI)
ischemia-driven revascularization
ischemia-guided medical therapy
ischemia-induced
    i.-i. intracellular acidosis
    i.-i. intramyocardial conduction
      delay
ischemia-reperfusion (IR)
ischemia/reperfusion (I/R)
ischemia/reperfusion-induced apoptosis
ischemic
    i. burden
    i. cardiomyopathy
    i. cascade
    i. cerebral infarction
    i. contracture of left ventricle
    i. core
    i. coronary disease (ICD)
    i. ECG change
    i. event
    i. heart disease (IHD)
    i. heart disease index (IHDI)
    i. heart disease life stress
      monitoring program
    i. heart disease quality
      enhancement research initiative
      (IHD QUERI)
    i. hypoxia
    i. leukoaraiosis
    i. mitral regurgitation
    i. myocardium
    i. necrosis
    i. paralysis
    i. penumbra
    i. pericarditis
    i. preconditioning (IPC)
    i. rest angina

    i. stroke
    i. sudden death
    i. threshold
    i. zone
ischemic-reperfusion injury
ischemic-type preconditioning stimulus
ISD
    interventricular septal defect
ISDN
    isosorbide dinitrate
ISE
    inversion spin-echo pulse sequence
    ion-selective electrode
iseganan HCl oral solution
isethionate
    aerosolized pentamidine i.
    pentamidine i.
    piritrexim i.
ISFC
    International Society and Federation of
      Cardiology
ISH
    International Society of Hypertension
    isolated septal hypertrophy
ISHLT
    International Society for Heart and Lung
      Transplantation
ISHT
    International Society for Heart
      Transplantation
ISI
    infarct size index
Ismelin
ISMLCSA
    intrastent minimal lumen cross-sectional
      area
IS-5-MN
    isosorbide-5-mononitrate
Ismo
ISO
    International Standards Organization
isoactin switch
isobutyl 2-cyanoacrylate
isocapnia
isocapnic, isocapneic
    i. condition
    i. hyperpnea
    i. hyperventilation
isocenter system
isochoric
isocratic elution
isocyanate
    methyl i.
isocyanate-induced asthma
isodiphasic complex
isoechoic
isoelectric
    i. interval
    i. line

i. period
i. point
i. ST segment
isoenzyme
CPK i.
i. of lactate dehydrogenase found in the heart, erythrocytes, and kidneys (LD1)
myocardial muscle creatine kinase i.
isoetharine
Arm-a-Med I.
Dey-Lute I.
I. Inhalation Solution USP 1%
isoflavone
isoflurane
isoform
Apo E3 i.
CYP1A2 i.
CYP3A i.
CYP2C9 i.
CYP2C19 i.
CYP2D6 i.
isoglycemia
isointense heterogeneous signal
isolated
i. cardiovascular malformation (ICM)
i. cerebral thromboangiitis obliterans disease
i. conduction defect (ICD)
i. CTAO
i. dextrocardia
i. dysarthria
i. ectopic beat
i. heat perfusion
i. low HDL
i. low high-density lipoprotein (ILHDL)
i. noncompaction of left ventricular myocardium
i. noncompaction of ventricular myocardium (INVM)
i. parietal endocarditis
i. septal hypertrophy (ISH)
i. systolic hypertension
i. T wave
i. volume responder (IVR)
isomer
dextro i.
isomerism

isometric
i. contraction
i. contraction period
i. exercise
i. handgrip
i. handgrip test
i. interval
i. period of cardiac cycle
i. relaxation period
i. sports
i. systolic tension (IST)
isometrically contracting myocardial preparation
isomyosin switch
isoniazid (INH)
rifampin and i.
isonitrile
carbomethoxyisopropyl i.
methoxyisobutyl i. (MIBI)
technetium-99m hexakis 2-methoxyisobutyl i.
technetium-99m methoxyisobutyl i.
Isopaque
isoprenaline
i. hydrochloride
i. sulfate
isoprophenamine hydrochloride
isopropylarterenol hydrochloride
8-iso-prostaglandin F$_{2alpha}$
isoproterenol
i. hydrochloride
i. infusion
i. and phenylephrine
i. stress test
i. sulfate
i. sulfate inhalation
i. tilt-table test
isoproterenol-induced vasovagal syncope
Isoptin SR
Isopto Atropine
Isordil
isorhythmic dissociation
isosorbide
i. dinitrate (ISDN)
i. dinitrate injection
i. mononitrate
isosorbide-5-mononitrate (IS-5-MN)
Isospora belli
Isostent stent
isothiocyanate
fluorescein i. (FITC)

NOTES

isotonic
- i. contraction
- i. exercise
- i. fluid

isotope
- iodine-125 i.

isotypic
Isovex
isovolemic hemodilution
isovolume
- i. flow
- i. pressure flow curve (IVPF)
- i. shifting

isovolumetric
- i. contractility
- i. phase index
- i. relaxation
- i. relaxation period (IVRP)
- i. time (IVT)

isovolumic
- i. index
- i. interval
- i. pressure decay
- i. relaxation
- i. relaxation period
- i. relaxation time (IVRT)
- i. systole

Isovue contrast medium
isoxsuprine hydrochloride
ISR
- in-stent restenosis

isradipine
israelii
- *Actinomyces i.*

ISS
- Injury Severity Score

ISSLC
- International Staging System for Lung Cancer

IST
- inappropriate sinus tachycardia
- isometric systolic tension

I-STATE bedside blood testing device
i-STAT handheld analyzer
isthmectomy
isthmic hypoplasia
isthmus, pl. **isthmi**
- aortic i.
- cavotricuspid i.
- Krönig i.
- i. line
- posterior i.
- septal i.
- subeustachian i.
- thyroid i.
- tricuspid-inferior vena cava i.

isthmus-dependent atrial flutter
Isuprel Mistometer

ISWT
- incremental shuttle walking test

IT
- implantation test

ITA
- inferior temporal artery
- internal thoracic artery
  - ITA graft

ITC balloon catheter
iterative presyncope
ITL
- inspiratory threshold load

ITP
- idiopathic thrombocytopenic purpura

ITPA
- Illinois Test of Psycholinguistic Abilities
  - ITPA index

itraconazole
ITT
- intention to treat

ITV
- impedance threshold valve

I.V.
- interventricular
- intravascular
- intravenous
- intraventricular
  - Avelox IV
  - Gammar-P IV
  - Hyperstat IV
  - Merrem IV
  - moxifloxacin HCl I.V.
  - Vasotec IV

i.v.
- intravascular
- intravenous

IVA
- intraoperative vascular angiography

Ivalon
- I. plug
- I. sponge

IVB
- intraventricular block

IVBC
- intravascular blood coagulation

IVC
- inferior vena cava
- inspiratory vital capacity
- intravascular coagulation
- intravenous cholangiogram
- intravenous cholangiography
- intraventricular catheter
  - IVC thrombosis

IVCC
- intravascular consumption coagulopathy

IVCD
- intraventricular conduction defect
- intraventricular conduction disease

IVCH
intravenous cholangiography
IVCR
inferior vena cava reconstruction
IVCT
inferior vena cava thrombosis
intravenously enhanced computed
tomography
IVCV
inferior venacavography
IVDSA
intravenous digital subtraction
angiography
Ivemark syndrome
ivermectin
IVF
interventricular foramen
intravascular fluid
intravenous fluid
IVGG
intravenous gamma globulin
IVGTT
intravenous glucose tolerance test
IVH
intravenous hyperalimentation
intraventricular hemorrhage
IV-Heart nebulizer
IVM
intravascular mass
IVOX
intravascular oxygenator
IVP
intravascular pressure
IVPF
isovolume pressure flow curve

IVR
idioventricular rhythm
isolated volume responder
IVRP
isovolumetric relaxation period
IVRT
isovolumic relaxation time
IVS
interventricular septal thickness
interventricular septum
IVSD
interventricular septal defect
IVT
idiopathic ventricular tachycardia
intraventricular
isovolumetric time
IVUS
intracoronary vascular ultrasound
intravascular ultrasound
IVUS catheter
coronary IVUS
3D IVUS
IVUS-guided balloon angioplasty
IVV
intravenous vasopressin
Ivy bleeding time
IW
inner wall
IWI
inferior wall infarction
IWMI
inferior wall myocardial infarction

NOTES

J

joule
J curve
J exchange wire
J guidewire
J & J stent
J junction
J point electrical axis
J retention wire
J retention wire fracture
J wave

J5 lipopolysaccharidase

JA

juxtaarticular
JA lesion

Jaa Amp

Jaa-Prednisone

Jabaley-Stille Super Cut Scissors

Jaccoud

J. dissociated fever
J. sign

jacket

cardiac cooling j.
Medtronic cardiac cooling j.

Jackman

J. coronary sinus electrode catheter
J. orthogonal catheter

Jackson

J. bistoury
J. safety triangle
J. sign
J. syndrome

Jacobaeus procedure

Jacobson

J. microbulldog clamp
J. modified vessel clamp

Jacobson-Potts clamp

Jacquet apparatus

Jaeger body test

Jaffe method

jail

stent j.

jailed side branch

Jak

Janus kinase

Jako laryngoscope

Jak/STAT pathway

Jamar

J. hand dynamometer
J. model 0030J4 dynamometer

James

J. accessory tracts
J. bundle
J. exercise protocol
J. fiber

Jamshidi needle

Janeway

J. lesion
J. sphygmomanometer

Janus

J. kinase (Jak)
J. kinase/signal transducer and activator of transcription
J. syndrome

Janz formula

japonicum

Schistosoma j.

Jarvik

J. 7, 8 artificial heart
J. 7-70 artificial heart
J. 2000 artificial heart

Jatene

J. arterial switch procedure
J. technique

Javid

J. carotid artery bypass clamp
J. shunt

jaw reflex (JR)

jaw-thrust/head-tilt maneuver

Jawz disposable biopsy forceps

Jebsen Hand Function Test

jeikeium

Corynebacterium j.

jejunal artery

jejunostomy

percutaneous endoscopic j. (PEJ)

jelly

cardiac j.
electrode j.

Jenkins Activity Survey

Jenner emphysema

jeopardized myocardium

jeopardy

myocardial j.
j. score

JER

junctional escape rhythm

jerk

myoclonic j.

jerky

j. pulse
j. respiration

Jervell and Lange-Nielsen syndrome

Jesberg esophagoscope

JET

junctional ectopic tachycardia

jet

anteriorly directed j.
aortic stenosis j.
Doppler color j.

J

jet *(continued)*
        eccentric stenotic j.
        j. effect
        j. humidifier
        j. lesion
        mitral regurgitant j.
        mosaic j.
        j. nebulizer
        patent ductus arteriosus flow j.
        regurgitant j.
        residual j.
        saline j.
        signal-void j.
        stenotic j.
        tricuspid regurgitant j.
        turbulent j.
        j. velocity
        j. ventilation
Jeune syndrome
Jewel
        J. AF implantable arrhythmia
        management device
        J. AF implantable defibrillator
        J. atrial fibrillation dual chamber
        device
        J. pacer-cardioverter-defibrillator
        J. PCD
JF
    jugular foramen
jimsonweed
Jinotti closed suctioning system
JL4
    Judkins left 4
        JL4 catheter
JL5
    Judkins left 5
        JL5 catheter
J-loop technique
JNK
    c-Jun N-terminal kinase
Jobst
        J. extremity pump
        J. pressure garment
        J. Vairox gradient compression
        vascular stockings
Job syndrome
Johnson
        J. & Johnson coronary stent
        J. & Johnson hemopump
        J. & Johnson Interventional
        Systems
        J. and Johnson Interventional
        Systems stent
    joint
        j. deformity
        Joint National Committee on
        Prevention, Detection, Evaluation,

        and Treatment of High Blood
        Pressure
        tuberculosis of bones and j.'s
Joklik medium
Jomed stent
**Jonas modification of Norwood
    procedure**
Jones criteria
Jonnson maneuver
jordanis
        Legionella j.
Jorgenson thoracic scissors
josamycin
Josephson
        J. quadripolar catheter
        J. Tip Arrow QuadPolar electrode
        catheter
Jostent
        J. coronary stent
        J. coronary stent graft
Jostra
        J. arterial blood filter
        J. cardiotomy reservoir
        J. catheter
joule (J)
JPB
    junctional premature beat
JPC
    junctional premature contraction
JR
    jaw reflex
    junctional rhythm
JR4
    Judkins right 4
        JR4 catheter
JR5
    Judkins right 5
        JR5 catheter
JRT
    junctional recovery time
JS
    junctional slowing
J-shaped
        J-s. pacemaker electrode
        J-s. tube
JT
    junctional tachycardia
        JT interval
J-tip guidewire
JTV519 1,4-benzothiazepine derivative
Judkins
        J. coronary catheter
        J. curve LAD catheter
        J. curve LCX catheter
        J. curve STD catheter
        J. 4 diagnostic catheter
        J. guiding catheter
        J. left 4 (JL4)
        J. left 5 (JL5)

J. pigtail left ventriculography catheter
J. right 4 (JR4)
J. right 5 (JR5)
J. selective coronary arteriography
J. technique
J. torque control catheter

Judkins-Sones technique

jugular

j. bulb catheter placement assessment
j. embryocardia
external j. (EJ)
j. foramen (JF)
internal j. (IJ)
j. vein (JV)
j. vein pulse (JVP)
j. venous arch
j. venous catechol spillover
j. venous catheter (JVC)
j. venous distention (JVD)
j. venous pressure (JVP)
j. venous pulsations (JVP)
j. venous pulse
j. venous pulse tracing (JVPT)

jugulodigastric lymph node

juice

Minute Maid Premium Heart Wise orange j.
purple grape j.

Julian thoracic forceps

Jumonji gene

jump graft

jumping thrombosis

junction

adherens j.
atrioventricular j. (AVJ)
A-V j.
cardioesophageal j.
costochondral j.
esophagogastric j.
gap j.
J j.
loose j.
QRS-ST j.
saphenofemoral j.
sinotubular j.
ST j.
sternochondral j.
tight j.
tracheoesophageal j.

triadic j.
venoatrial j.

junctional

atrioventricular j.
j. axis
j. bigeminy
j. bradycardia
j. complex
j. depression
j. ectopic tachycardia (JET)
j. escape
j. escape beat
j. escape rhythm (JER)
j. extrasystole
j. parasystole
j. premature beat (JPB)
j. premature contraction (JPC)
j. reciprocating tachycardia
j. recovery time (JRT)
j. rhythm (JR)
j. slowing (JS)
j. tachycardia (JT)

***Jun* gene**

Junod procedure

Juquitiba virus

jute worker's lung

juvenile

j. arrhythmia
j. myocardial infarction
j. pattern
j. rheumatoid arthritis

juvenum

cor j.

juxtaarticular (JA)

j. lesion

juxtacapillary receptor

juxtacardiac pleural pressure

juxtaductal coarctation

juxtaesophageal lymph node

juxtapulmonary-capillary receptor

Juzo

J. hose
J. shrinker
J. stockings

JV

jugular vein

JVC

jugular venous catheter

JVD

jugular venous distention

JVP

jugular vein pulse

NOTES

JVP *(continued)*
    jugular venous pressure
    jugular venous pulsations

JVPT
    jugular venous pulse tracing
J-wire lead

K

potassium
    K current
    K 54 lead
    K stylet
    K x-ray fluorescence instrument

K4

fourth Korotkoff sound

K5

fifth Korotkoff sound

KAAT II Plus intraaortic balloon pump

KabiVitrum

KAD

Kennedy Disease Association

Kahler bronchial biopsy forceps

Kairos pacemaker

Kales scoring method

kaliuresis

kallidinogenase inactivator unit

kallikrein

    k. 1 (KLK1)
    k. gene
    k. inactivating unit (KIU)

kallikrein-bradykinin system

kallikrein-kinin (KK)

Kallmann syndrome

Kaltostat

    K. wound packing dressing
    K. wound packing material

Kamen-Wilkinson endotracheal tube

Kampmeier foci

Kampo medicine

kanamycin

kangaroo

    k. care
    K. pump

kansasii

    Mycobacterium k.

Kantor-Berci video laryngoscope

Kantrowitz

    K. pacemaker
    K. thoracic clamp

kaolin

    k. partial thromboplastin time (KPTT)
    k. pneumoconiosis

kaolin-cephalin clotting time (KCCT)

kaolinosis

Kaon

Kaopectate

Kaplan-Meier

    K.-M. event-free survival curve
    K.-M. method

Kaplan-Simpson InfusaSleeve

kapok asthma

Kaposi sarcoma (KS)

Kappa 400 Series pacemaker

karaya asthma

Karell

    K. diet
    K. treatment

Karhunen-Loeve procedure

Karhunen-Loéve transform (KLT)

Karl Storz D-LIGHT AF autofluorescence system

Karmen units

Karmody venous scissors

Karnofsky rating scale

Karolinska quality of life questionnaire

Karplus sign

Kartagener

    K. syndrome
    K. triad

Kasabach-Merritt syndrome

Kasser-Kennedy method

Katayama fever

Kattus

    K. exercise stress test
    K. treadmill protocol

Katz activities of daily living score

Katzen

    K. infusion wire
    K. long balloon dilatation catheter

Katz-Wachtel phenomenon

Kaufman pneumonia

Kawai bioptome

Kawasaki

    K. disease
    K. syndrome

Kawashima intraventricular tunnel

Kay

    K. annuloplasty
    K. balloon

Kayak hydrophilic guidewire

Kayexalate enema

Kay-Shiley caged-disk valve

KC

cathodal closing

KCC

cathodal closing contraction

KCCT

kaolin-cephalin clotting time

KCG

kinetocardiogram

K⁺ channels

KCl

potassium chloride

Kd

distribution coefficient

K

kDa, kd
kilodalton
92-kDa gelatinase
Kearns-Sayre syndrome
keel
McNaught k.
keeled chest
Keflex
Keftab
Kefurox injection
Kefzol
Keith
K. bundle
K. node
Keith-Flack node
Keith-Wagener-Barker (KWB)
Kellner questionnaire
Kellock sign
Kelly
K. clamp
K. hemostat
keloidal
Kempner diet
Kenalog injection
Kendall
K. nasal prongs
K. sequential compression device
Kennedy
K. area-length method
K. disease
K. Disease Association (KAD)
Kensey rotation atherectomy extrusion
Kent
K. bundle
K. bundle ablation
bundle of Stanley K.
K. fiber
K. pathway
K. potential
Kent-His bundle
Kentrox RV 65 cm lead
keratinocyte growth factor (KGF)
keratin pearls
Kerley A, B, C lines
Kerlone Oral
Kernan-Jackson bronchoscope
Kern technique
kerosene pneumonitis
Keshan disease
ketamine
ketanserin
Ketek
ketoacidosis
ketoconazole
ketone
D-Phe-L-Pro-L-Arg-chloromethyl k. (PPACK)
ketoprofen
ketorolac

ketotifen
Kety-Schmidt method
keV
kiloelectron volt
key
K. pulse rate (KPR)
ResCue K.
keyhole-limpet hemocyanin
keyhole surgery
Key-Pred Injection
Key-Pred-SP injection
Keystone PF analyzer
kg
kilogram
KGF
keratinocyte growth factor
kg/m²
kilogram per meter squared
KI antigen
kick
atrial k.
k. count
idioventricular k.
kidney
flea-bitten k.
Goldblatt k.
heart, liver and k.'s (H-L-K)
isoenzyme of lactate dehydrogenase found in the heart, erythrocytes, and k.'s (LD1)
polycystic k.
Kiel classification of lymphoma
Kienbock
K. disease
K. phenomenon
Kifa catheter material
Kikuchi disease
killer
natural k. (NK)
Killian bundle
Killian-Jamieson area
Killian-Lynch laryngoscope
Killip
K. heart disease classification
K. heart failure classification
Killip-Kimball heart failure classification
kilodalton (kDa, kd)
45-kilodalton protein
kiloelectron volt (keV)
kilogram (kg)
milliliter per k. (mL/kg)
k. per meter squared (kg/m²)
kilohm (kOhm)
kilojoule (kJ)
kilopascal (kPa)
kilopond (kp)
kilopond-meter (kpm)
kilovolt (kV)
kilowatt (kW)

Kimmelstiel-Wilson syndrome
Kim-Ray
    K.-R. Greenfield caval filter
    K.-R. thermodilution
Kimura cartilage graft
kinase
    adrenergic receptor k. (ARK)
    adrenergic receptor k. 1 (ARK-1)
    beta-adrenergic receptor k. (BARK)
    c-Jun N-terminal k. (JNK)
    conserved helix-loop-helix
      ubiquitous k. (CHUK)
    creatine k. (CK)
    extracellularly responsive k. (ERK)
    extracellular-regulated k. (ERK)
    extracellular signal-regulated k.
    focal adhesion k. (FAK)
    intracellular tyrosine protein k.
    Janus k. (Jak)
    mitogen-activated protein k.
      (MAPK)
    phosphorylase k.
    protein k. (PKase)
    protein k. A (PKA)
    protein k. C (PKC)
    protooncogenic protein k.
    Ras mitogen-activated protein k.
    serine k.
    serum creatine k.
    Src k.
    threonine protein k.
Kindt carotid artery clamp
kinesiological electromyogram
kinesis
    color k. (CK)
kinetic
    first-order k.'s
    k. therapy
    zero-order k.'s
KinetiX
    K. instrument
    K. ventilation monitor
kinetocardiogram (KCG)
kinetocardiograph
King
    K. ASD umbrella closure
    K. biopsy method
    K. bioptome
    K. cardiac device
    K. double umbrella closure system
    K. guiding catheter

    K. of Hearts Express 3X cardiac
      event recorder
    K. of Hearts Holter monitor
    K. interlocking device
    K. multipurpose catheter
kingae
    Haemophilus aphrophilus,
      Actinobacillus
      actinomycetemcomitans,
      Cardiobacterium hominis,
      Eikenella corrodens, and
      Kingella k. (HACEK)
kinin
    endogenous k.
kininogen
kinked aorta
kinky-hair disease
Kinsey
    K. atherectomy
    K. rotation atherectomy extrusion
      angioplasty
Kinyoun stain
Kirklin fence
Kirkorian-Touboul method
Kirstein method
Kisch reflex
kissing
    k. balloon angioplasty
    k. balloon technique
    k. stenting
    k. stents
    k. tonsils
Kistner tracheal button
kit
    ACE k.
    AeroGear asthma action k.
    Alatest Latex-specific IgE allergen
      test k.
    Arrow pneumothorax k.
    AsthmaPACK personal asthma
      care k.
    BioSource Cytoscreen SAA k.
    BiPort hemostasis introducer
      sheath k.
    cyanide antidote k.
    Enzygnost F1+2 ELISA k.
    Enzygnost TAT complex k.
    Euro-Collins multiorgan
      perfusion k.
    Fergus percutaneous introducer k.
    Imulyse tPA ELISA k.
    MDI k.

K

NOTES

kit (*continued*)

    No Pour Pak suction catheter k.
    Oncor ApopTaq k.
    percutaneous access k. (PAK)
    percutaneous catheter introducer k.
    Per-fit percutaneous tracheostomy k.
    Pleurx pleural catheter/home
      drainage k.
    Portex Per-fit tracheostomy k.
    Pro-Vent arterial blood gas k.
    Pro-Vent arterial blood sampling k.
    Pulsator dry heparin arterial blood
      gas k.
    TintElize PAI-1 ELISA k.
    TriPort hemostasis introducer
      sheath k.
    Vari-Lase endovenous laser
      procedure k.
    Virgo anticardiolipin screening
      ELISA test k.
    Yamasa assay k.

KIU

    kallikrein inactivating unit

kJ

    kilojoule

KK

    kallikrein-kinin
    KK system

KL-6

    serum KL-6

Klebsiella

    K. oxytoca
    K. pneumoniae
    K. pneumoniae subsp. *ozaenae*
    K. rhinoscleromatis

Klebsiella **pneumonia**
Klebs-Loeffler bacillus
Kleihauer-Betke test
Kleihauer test
Klein transseptal introducer sheath
Klein-Waardenburg syndrome
Klinefelter syndrome
Klippel-Feil syndrome
Klippel-Trenaunay-Weber syndrome
KLK1

    kallikrein 1

KLT

    Karhunen-Loéve transform

knee

    k. extension
    medial inferior artery of k.
    medial superior artery of k.

knife, pl. **knives**

    A-K diamond k.
    Bailey-Glover-O'Neill
      commissurotomy k.
    Beaver k.
    k. blade
    gamma k.

    Lebsche sternal k.
    roentgen k.
    UltraCision ultrasonic k.
    valvotomy k.
    k. wound

KnightStar 335 respiratory-support system
knitted

    k. polyester crimped graft
    k. sewing ring
    k. vascular prosthesis

knives (*pl. of* knife)
knob

    aortic k.

knock

    pericardial k. (PK)

Knoll gland
knuckle

    aortic k.
    B k.
    cervical aortic k.
    k. sign

Ko-Airan bleeding control procedure
Koala

    K. vascular clamp
    K. vascular insert

Koate-HP
KOC

    cathodal opening contraction

Koch

    K. bacillus
    K. node
    K. old tuberculin
    K. phenomenon
    triangle of K.
    K. triangle

Kocher-Cushing reflex
Koch-Weeks bacillus
Koelner Vitaport accelerometer
Koffex

    K. DM
    K. DM Children

Kogenate
KOH

    potassium hydroxide

Kohlrausch vein
kOhm

    kilohm

Kohn pore
KoKo Moe pulmonary function filter
Kolephrin GG/DM
Kolmogorov-Smirnov procedure
Kondoleon-Sistrunk elephantiasis procedure
Konica KFDR-S laser film scanner
Konigsberg catheter
Konno

    K. biopsy method
    K. bioptome

K. operation
K. procedure
Kontron
K. balloon
K. balloon catheter
K. intraaortic balloon pump
Konyne 80
Koplik spot
Kopp asthma
Korányi
K. auscultation
K. sign
Korean hemorrhagic fever
Korotkoff phase I–V
Kostmann syndrome
Kotonkan virus
Kozak sequence
kp
kilopond
kPa
kilopascal
kpm
kilopond-meter
KPR
key pulse rate
KPTT
kaolin partial thromboplastin time
^{81m}Kr
krypton-81m
Krebs
K. cycle
K. solution
Krebs-Henseleit
K.-H. buffer
K.-H. solution
Kreiselman unit
Kreysig sign
kringle
Krishaber disease
Krogh apparatus spirometer
Kronecker center
Krönig
K. area
K. isthmus
Krukenberg vein
krypton-81m (**^{81m}Kr**)
k. ventilation imaging
KS
Kaposi sarcoma

KSC
cathodal closing contraction
k-space segmentation
K-Sponge
Kugel
K. anastomosis
K. anastomotic artery
Kugelberg-Welander
K.-W. disease
K.-W. syndrome
Kuhn
K. mask
K. tube
Kuhnt postcentral vein
Kulchitsky cell
Kuntiz-type inhibitor
Kuntz
nerve of K.
Kurten vein stripper
Kussmaul
K. breathing
K. disease
K. paradoxical pulse
K. respiration
K. sign
K. symptom
K. syndrome
Kussmaul-Kien respiration
Kussmaul-Maier disease
kV
kilovolt
kV fluoroscopy
Kveim
K. antigen skin test
K. reaction
Kveim-Siltzbach test
kW
kilowatt
Kwai garlic
kwashiorkor-like malnutrition
KWB
Keith-Wagener-Barker
KWB hypertension classification
Kwelcof
kymogram
kymograph
kymography
kymoscope
kyphoscoliosis

K

NOTES

L

L 67 lead
L loop

LA

left atrium
left auricle
long acting
Dexone LA
Guaifenex LA
Inderal LA

L.A.

long acting
Dexasone L.A.
Humibid L.A.
Solurex L.A.

LAA

left atrial appendage
left atrial area
LAA contraction
LAA filling
LAA thrombi

La:A

left atrial to aortic
La:A ratio

LA/Ao

left atrial/aortic
LA/Ao ratio

LABA

laser-assisted balloon angioplasty

LABBB

left anterior bundle branch block

Labbe neurocirculatory syndrome

label

open l. (OL)

labeled

l. FFA scintigraphy
open l. (OL)

labeling

TdT-mediated dUTP nick-end l.
(TUNEL)

labetalol hydrochloride

labile

l. blood pressure
l. hypertension
l. pulse

lability

transient pulmonary vascular l.
(TPLV)

laboratory

Core Exercise Testing L.
Venereal Disease Research L.
(VDRL)

Laborde method

labored respiration

Labrador lung

Labtron stethoscope

LABV

left atrial ball valve

LAC

left atrial circumflex
left atrial contraction
low-amplitude contraction
LAC artery

laceration

parenchymal l.

lacidipine

lacrimalis

fossa glandulae l.

lacrymans

Serpula l.

LACS

lacunar syndrome

lactamase

beta l.

lactate

amrinone l.
l. dehydrogenase
l. extraction
milrinone l.
Ringer l.
sodium l.
l. threshold

lactea

macula l.

lactic

l. acid
l. acid concentration
l. acid dehydrogenase
l. acidosis
l. acid transport
l. dehydrogenase (LDH)

LactiCare-HC

Lactobacillus

lacuna, pl. **lacunae**

l. pharyngis

lacunar

l. angina
l. infarct
l. infarction (LI)
l. stroke
l. syndrome (LACS)

LAD

left anterior descending
left axis deviation
LAD coronary artery

LADA

left anterior descending artery

LADB

left anterior descending branch

L

LADCA
>left anterior descending coronary artery

LADD
>left anterior descending diagonal
>>LADD coronary artery

ladder
>>l. diagram
>>l. incision
>>L. of Life score

LADP
>left anterior descending arterial pressure

LAE
>left atrial enlargement

LAEDV
>left atrial end diastolic volume

LAEI
>left atrial emptying index

Laënnec
>>L. catarrh
>>L. cirrhosis
>>L. pearl
>>L. sign

Laerdal resuscitator

LAESV
>left atrial end systolic volume

laevis
>>*Xenopus l.*

LAF
>left atrial enlargement

LAFS
>long-axis fractional shortening

Laguna Negra virus

LAH
>left anterior hemiblock
>left atrial hypertrophy

laid-back
>>l.-b. balloon occlusion aortography
>>l.-b. view

laidlawii
>>*Acholeplasma l.*

LAIS laser

laiteuse
>>tache l.

lakes
>>venous l.

LAM
>left atrial myxoma
>lymphangioleiomyomatosis

LAMA
>laser-assisted microanastomosis

LAMB
>lentigines, atrial myxoma, mucocutaneous myxomas, and blue nevi
>>LAMB syndrome

Lambert
>>L. aortic clamp
>>canal of L.

Lambert-Beer law

Lambert-Eaton myasthenic syndrome

Lambert-Kay aortic clamp

lambertosis

Lambl excrescence

lamella
>>elastic l.

lamifiban

lamina, pl. **laminae**
>>elastic l.
>>l. elastica interna
>>external elastic l. (EEL)
>>internal elastic l. (IEL)

laminar blood flow

laminated
>>l. clot
>>l. connective tissue
>>l. thrombus

laminin antibody

laminography

lamivudine (3TC)
>>zidovudine and l.

lamp
>>Wood l.

Lamprene

Lam procedure

LAN
>local area network

Lanaphilic topical

lanata
>>*Digitalis l.*

lanatoside C

Lancisi sign

Landolfi sign

Landouzy-Dejerine
>>L.-D. dystrophy
>>facioscapulohumeral dystrophy of L.-D.
>>L.-D. syndrome

Landry-Guillain-Barré syndrome

LANE
>lidocaine, atropine, naloxone, epinephrine [drugs that may be administered via endotracheal tube]

lanetoplase

Lange calipers

Langendorff
>>L. apparatus
>>L. heart preparation

Langer axillary arch

Langerhans
>>L. cell granulomatosis
>>L. cell histiocytosis
>>L. giant cell

Langevin updating procedure

Langhans cell

Langhans-type giant cell

Lannelongue foramen

lanoteplase

Lanoxicaps

Lanoxin

lanreotide
lansingensis
    Legionella l.
lanuginosum
LANV
    left atrial neovascularization
Lanz low-pressure cuff endotracheal tube
LAO
    left anterior oblique
    left atrial overload
        LAO position
LAP
    laser-assisted palatoplasty
    left atrial pressure
laparotomy sponge
Laplace
    L. law
    L. mechanism
    L. principle
    L. relationship
Laplacian mapping
lapping murmur
Lap Sac
LAPW
    left atrial posterior wall
LAR
    Sandostatin LAR
Largactil
large
    l. bore Tuohy-Borst side-arm adapter
    l. cell carcinoma with rhabdoid phenotype
    l. cell undifferentiated carcinoma
    l. vessel
large-bore
    l.-b. angiocatheter
    l.-b. catheter
    l.-b. chest tube
    l.-b. slotted aspirating needle
    l.-b. trocar
large-caliber chest tube
large-tip electrode
large-vessel infarction (LVI)
large-volume aspiration
L-arginine
Lariam
Larmor frequency
Laron syndrome (LS)

Larrey
    L. hernia
    L. space
larva migrans
laryngalgia
laryngea
    angina l.
    arteria l.
    prominentia l.
    protuberantia l.
laryngeae
    glandulae l.
laryngeal
    l. aperture
    l. atresia
    l. bursa
    l. cleft
    l. cough reflex test (LCR)
    l. crisis
    l. gland
    l. infection
    l. mask airway (LMA)
    l. nerve
    l. part of pharynx
    l. pouch
    l. prominence
    l. rale
    l. reflex
    l. stridor
    l. syncope
    l. tonsil
    l. vein
    l. ventricle
    l. vertigo
    l. web
laryngectomee
larynges (*pl. of* larynx)
laryngeus
    Syngamus l.
laryngis (*gen. of* larynx)
    cartilago sesamoidea l.
    cavitas l.
    membrana fibroelastica l.
    musculi l.
    sacculus l.
    tunica mucosa l.
    ventriculus l.
    vestibulum l.
laryngismus
    l. paralyticus
    l. stridulus

NOTES

393

laryngitis
- atrophic l.
- catarrhal l.
- chronic catarrhal l.
- croupous l.
- diphtheritic l.
- membranous l.
- phlegmonous l.
- l. sicca
- l. stridulosa
- subglottic l.
- syphilitic l.
- tuberculous l.
- vestibular l.

Laryngoflex reinforced endotracheal tube

laryngomalacia

laryngopharynx

laryngoscope
- Benjamin binocular l.
- Benjamin pediatric l.
- Bizzari-Guiffrida l.
- Bullard intubating l.
- Dedo-Pilling l.
- Foregger l.
- Garfield-Holinger l.
- Holinger anterior commissure l.
- Jako l.
- Kantor-Berci video l.
- Killian-Lynch l.
- Lindholm operating l.
- Machida fiberoptic l.
- Macintosh l.
- Magill l.
- Ossoff-Karlan l.
- shadow-free l.
- Shapshay-Healy l.
- Storz-Hopkins l.

laryngoscopy
- direct l.
- mirror-image l.
- suspension l.

laryngospasm

laryngotracheal
- l. diverticulum
- l. groove
- l. infection

laryngotracheitis

laryngotracheobronchitis

larynx, gen. **laryngis**, pl. **larynges**
- artificial l.
- cartilages of l.
- cavity of l.
- Cooper-Rand intraoral artificial l.
- Nu-Vois artificial l.
- saccule of l.
- tuberculosis of l.
- ventricular band of l.
- vestibule of l.

LASEC
- left atrial spontaneous echo contrast

laser
- l. ablation
- alexandrite l.
- ArF excimer l.
- argon ion l.
- argon pumped tuneable dye l.
- l. balloon angioplasty (LBA)
- l. bronchoscopy
- l. capture microdissection (LCM)
- cool-tip l.
- coumarin pulsed dye l.
- l. delivery catheter
- l. Doppler flowmeter
- dye l.
- Eclipse holmium l.
- Eclipse TMR l.
- erbium:YAG l.
- excimer cool l.
- excimer gas l.
- l. fiber
- l. firing
- flashlamp-pulsed Nd:YAG l.
- fluorescence-guided smart l.
- free-beam l.
- Heart L.
- HF infrared l.
- high-energy l.
- holmium l.
- Ho:YAG l.
- infrared-pulsed l.
- LAIS l.
- low-energy l.
- Lumonics YAG l.
- l. maze operation
- microsecond pulsed flashlamp pumped dye l.
- mid-infrared pulsed l.
- Nd:YAG l.
- neodymium:yttrium-aluminum-garnet l.
- PhotoGenica V-Star l.
- pulsed dye l.
- Q-switched Nd:YAG l.
- l. revascularization
- ruby l.
- Spectranetics l.
- spectroscopy-directed l.
- Surgilase 150 l.
- THC:YAG l.
- l. thermal angioplasty
- thulium-holmium-chromium:yttrium-aluminum-garnet l.
- thulium-holmium:YAG l.
- l. transluminal angioplasty catheter (LASTAK)
- l. tube
- tunable pulsed dye l.

ultraviolet l.
XeCl excimer l.
xenon chloride excimer l.
YAG l.

laser-assisted
l.-a. balloon angioplasty (LABA)
l.-a. microanastomosis (LAMA)
l.-a. palatoplasty (LAP)
l.-a. uvulopalatopharyngoplasty (LAUPPP)
l.-a. uvulopalatoplasty (LAUP)

Laserdish
L. electrode
L. pacing lead

laser-Doppler flowmetry
laser-induced
l.-i. arterial fluorescence (LIAF)
l.-i. thrombosis

Laserpor pacing lead
Laserprobe catheter
Laserprobe-PLR Flex catheter
LASH
left anterior superior hemiblock

Lasix
L. injection
L. Oral
L. Special

Lassa
L. fever
L. virus

Lasso catheter
LASTAK
laser transluminal angioplasty catheter

LAT
left atrial thrombus

late
l. afterdepolarization
l. angioplasty complication
l. apical systolic murmur
l. apnea
l. arterial switch
l. cyanosis
l. deceleration
l. diastole
l. diastolic murmur
l. diastolic potential (LDP)
l. lung injury
l. potential parameter
l. potential parameter index
l. proarrhythmic effect
l. progressing stroke (LPS)
l. pulmonary injury

l. reperfusion
l. silhouette
l. sudden death
l. systole
l. systolic click (LSC)
l. systolic murmur (LSM)

latent
l. cardiomyopathy (LCM)
l. empyema
l. pleurisy
systolic wave, l. (SL)
l. tuberculosis infection (LTBI)

late-peaking systolic murmur
lateral
l. basal bronchopulmonary segment
l. basal segmental artery of right lung
l. cephalometry
l. flail chest
l. jugular lymph node
l. medullary infarction (LMI)
l. mesocardium
l. myocardial infarction (LMI)
l. pharyngeal space
l. sac
l. thrombus
l. ventricular nerve (LVN)
l. view
l. wall (LW)

laterale
segmentum bronchopulmonale basale l.
spatium pharyngeum l.

laterales
venae circumflexae femoris l.

lateralis
arteria genus superior l.
ramus anterior l.

laterality index (LI)
lateropharyngeum
spatium l.

laterosporus
Bacillus l.

latex balloon
lathyrogen
Lathyrus odoratus
Latino
latissimus
l. dorsi
l. dorsi muscle
l. dorsi procedure

L

NOTES

LATP
: left atrial transmural pressure

LATPT
: left atrial transesophageal pacing test

Latrodectus Mactans

Laubry-Soulle syndrome

laudanosine

LAUP
: laser-assisted uvulopalatoplasty

LAUPPP
: laser-assisted uvulopalatopharyngoplasty

Laurell
: L. method
: rocket immunoelectrophoretic method of L.

Laurence-Moon-Bardet-Biedl syndrome

Laurence-Moon-Biedl syndrome

laurentii
: *Cryptococcus l.*

lavage
: bronchial l.
: bronchoalveolar l. (BAL)
: continuous pericardial l.
: diagnostic peritoneal l. (DPL)
: iced saline l.
: l. instillation
: pericardial l.
: pleural l.
: tracheobronchial l.

LAW
: left atrial wall

law
: all or none l.
: Beer L.
: Bowditch l.
: Boyle Gay-Lusac l.
: Charles l.
: Dalton l.
: Dalton-Henry l.
: Du Bois-Reymond l.
: Einthoven l.
: Frank-Starling l.
: Graham l.
: l. of the heart
: Henry l.
: Hooke l.
: Lambert-Beer L.
: Laplace l.
: Louis l.
: Marey l.
: Ohm l.
: Poiseuille l.
: Starling l.
: Sutton l.
: Torricelli l.

Lawton
: L. IADL
: L. Instrumental Activities of Daily Living scale

LAX
: long axis

laxa
: cutis l.

LAX-DSS
: long axis-discrete subaortic stenosis

layer
: adventitial l.
: fascial l.
: half-value l.
: hypertrophic smooth muscle l.
: M cell l.
: mucous l.
: peribronchiolar l.
: subendocardial l.

lazaroid

LB
: left bundle

LBA
: laser balloon angioplasty

LBB
: left bundle branch

LBBsB
: left bundle branch system block

LBCD
: left border of cardiac dullness

LBD
: left border of dullness
: left brain damage

LBNP
: lower body negative pressure

LBP
: low blood pressure

LBT
: loaded breathing test

LBV
: lung blood volume

LC
: left circumflex
: lymphangitic carcinomatosis
: LC artery
: LC Plus reusable nebulizer
: LC STAR reusable nebulizer

LCA
: left circumflex artery
: left coronary artery

LCAD
: lipid-coronary artery disease

LCAT
: lecithin cholesterol acetyltransferase
: lecithin cholesterol acyltransferase

LCATA
: lecithin cholesterol acetyltransferase alpha

LCC
: left circumflex coronary
: left coronary cusp
: LCC artery

LCCA
  left common carotid artery
LCCE
  length contraction compensation element
LCD
  liquid crystal display
LCF
  left circumflex
  lymphocyte chemoattractant factor
    LCF coronary artery
LCL
  Levinthal-Coles-Lillie
    LCL bodies
LCM
  laser capture microdissection
  latent cardiomyopathy
LCO
  left coronary ostium
  low cardiac output
LCOS
  low cardiac output syndrome
LCR
  laryngeal cough reflex test
  ligase chain reaction
LCS
  left coronary sinus
LCVA
  left hemisphere stroke
LCWI
  left cardiac work index
LCX
  left circumflex
  left circumflex artery
  left circumflex coronary artery
    LCX coronary artery
LCXB
  left coronary circumflex branch
LD1
  isoenzyme of lactate dehydrogenase
    found in the heart, erythrocytes, and
    kidneys
LDD
  lead locking device
LDH
  lactic dehydrogenase
  low-dose heparin
    LDH flip
LDL
  low-density lipoprotein
    LDL direct blood test
    native LDL (n-LDL)

  oxidative modification of LDL
    (oxLDL, ox-LDL)
  oxidized LDL
  LDL pattern B
LDLA
  low-density lipoprotein apheresis
LDL-C, LDL-c
  low-density lipoprotein-cholesterol
    complex
LDL/HDL
  low-density lipoprotein/high density
    lipoprotein
    LDL/HDL radio
LDLP
  low-density lipoprotein
LDLR, LDL-R
  low-density lipoprotein receptor
  low-density lipoprotein receptor mutation
    database
LDP
  late diastolic potential
LDUH
  low-dose unfractionated heparin
LE
  lupus erythematosus
LEAD
  lower extremity arterial disease
3.3 lead
lead
      3.3 l.
      A 67 l.
      ABC l.
      Accufix II DEC pacing l.
      Accufix pacemaker l.
      active fixation pacemaker l.
      Aescula left ventricular l.
      Aescula LV l.
      American Pacemaker Corporation l.
      Angeflex defibrillation l.
      aVF l.
      aVL l.
      aVR l.
      Biocontrol Technology/Coratomic l.
      Biopore TM l.
      Biotronik l.
      Brilliant l.
      capped l.
      CapSure cardiac pacing l.
      CapSureFix l.
      CapSure SP l.
      CapSure VDD l.
      Cardiac Control Systems l.

NOTES

L

lead *(continued)*
  CB l.
  CF l.
  chest l.
  CL l.
  Cordis Ancar pacing l.
  coronary sinus l.
  CPI endocardial defibrillation/rate-
    sensing/pacing l.
  CPI/Guidant l.
  CR l.
  dedicated bipolar l.
  direct l.
  l. dislodgment
  dual-coil transvenous l.
  Easytrak coronary venous l.
  Einthoven l.
  electrocardiographic l.'s
  Elema l.'s
  Elwrite pediatric l.
  Encor l.
  endocardial bipolar l.
  Endotak C tripolar transvenous l.
  Endotak DSP l.
  Endotak Picotip defibrillation l.
  Endotak Reliance l.
  epicardial l.
  esophageal l.
  l. extraction system
  finned pacemaker l.
  fishhook l.
  Flextend pacing l.
  Flextend steroid-eluting, transvenous
    pace/sense l.
  floating l.
  l. fracture
  Frank XYZ orthogonal l.
  Heartwire l.
  Hi-Flex l.
  ICD l.
  l. impedance
  implantable cardioverter-
    defibrillator l.
  indirect l.
  l. insulation
  Intermedics l.
  intracardiac l.
  J-wire l.
  K 54 l.
  Kentrox RV 65 cm l.
  L 67 l.
  Laserdish pacing l.
  Laserpor pacing l.
  left ventricular transvenous l.
  Lewis l.
  Lifeline l.
  limb l.
  l. locking device (LDD)
  Low-Flex l.

Mason-Likar placement of ECG l.
Medtronic l.'s
Microtip l.
modified chest l. (MCL)
monitor l.'s
MR l.
myocardial l.
Myopore l.
nonintegrated transvenous
  defibrillation l.
Oscor pacing l.
Osypka atrial l.
over-the-wire pacing l.
pacemaker l.'s
Pacesetter/St. Jude l.
Pacesetter Tendril DX steroid-
  eluting active-fixation pacing l.
pediatric l.
permanent cardiac pacing l.
Pisces l.
l. placement
l. poisoning
Polyflex l.
PolySafe A-track l.
Precept l.
precordial l.
l. reversal
reversed arm l.'s
scalar l.'s
screw-in l.
screw-on l.
segmented ring tripolar l.
semidirect l.
silicone l.
single-pass l.
Sorin l.
Sprint Model 6942, 6943
  tachyarrhythmia l.
SRT l.
standard limb l.
steroid-eluting pacemaker l.
Stop at Ring l.
Stop at Tip l.
SVC l.
Sweet Tip bipolar l.
Synox fractal pacemaker l.
Target Tip l.
Telectronics Accufix pacing l.
temporary pervenous l.
Tendril DX implantable pacing l.
Tendril DX steroid-eluting active-
  fixation pacing l.
Tendril SDX model 1688 active-
  fixation pacing l.
Terox RV l.
ThinLine EZ bipolar pacemaker l.
ThinLine EZ pacing l.
three-turn epicardial l.
l. threshold

TIJ l.
transcutaneous l.
Transvene l.
transvenous defibrillator l.
tripolar l.
two-turn epicardial l.
unipolar limb l.'s
unipolar precordial l.
Uni-Silicone l.
V l.
ventral lead 1, 2, 3, 4, 5, 6 (V1-V6)
ventricular l.
Vitatron l.
V-Pace transluminal pacing l.
V1-V6 EKG l.'s
Wilson l.

12-lead
12-l. electrocardiogram
12-l. electrocardiography
12-l. voltage-duration product criteria
16-lead electrocardiogram
leading
l. circle concept
l. circle hypothesis
l. edge
l. edge enhancement
lead-letter marker
lead/zirconium/titanium (LZT)
leaflet
adherent l.
anterior l. (AL)
anterior mitral l. (AML)
anterior mitral valve l. (aMVL)
anterior pulmonary l. (APK)
anterior tricuspid l. (ATL)
aortic valve l.
bowing of mitral valve l.
calcified mitral l.
cleft anterior l.
cleft of aortic l.
C valvular l.
doming of l.
dysplastic mitral valvar l.
flail l.
flail mitral l. (FML)
hammocking of posterior mitral l.
mitral l.
mitral valve l. (MVL)
l. motion
posterior l.

posterior mitral l. (PML)
posterior mitral valve l. (PMVL, pMVL)
posterior pulmonary l. (PPL)
posterior tricuspid l. (PTL)
prolapsed middle scallop of posterior l.
prolapsing mitral l. (PML)
prolapsing mitral valvar l.
tethered l.
l. thickening
tricuspid valvular l.
valvular l.
l. vegetation
leak
alveolar l.
baffle l.
paraprosthetic l.
perivalvular l.
shunt l.
silent trace l.
leakage
perivalvular l. (PVL)
spectral l.
LEAP
low energy all-purpose
LEAP collimator
Lebsche sternal knife
lecithin
cardiolipin natural l. (CNL)
cardiolipin synthetic l. (CSL)
l. cholesterol acetyltransferase (LCAT)
l. cholesterol acetyltransferase alpha (LCATA)
lecithin/sphingomyelin (L/S)
Lecompte maneuver
LED
light-emitting diode
LEDC
low energy direct current
ledge
eccentric l.
limbic l.
Lee-White method
left
l. anterior bundle branch block (LABBB)
l. anterior descending (LAD)
l. anterior descending arterial pressure (LADP)

L

NOTES

left (*continued*)

l. anterior descending artery (LADA)
l. anterior descending branch (LADB)
l. anterior descending coronary artery (LADCA)
l. anterior descending diagonal (LADD)
l. anterior hemiblock (LAH)
l. anterior oblique (LAO)
l. anterior oblique position
l. anterior oblique projection
l. anterior superior hemiblock (LASH)
l. aortic angiography
l. apical cap
apicoposterior branch of l.
l. arm (VL)
l. atrial abnormality
l. atrial active emptying fraction
l. atrial active emptying volume
l. atrial angiography
l. atrial to aortic (La:A)
l. atrial/aortic (LA/Ao)
l. atrial appendage (LAA)
l. atrial appendage area
l. atrial appendage flow velocity
l. atrial appendage function
l. atrial appendage stunning
l. atrial area (LAA)
l. atrial ball valve (LABV)
l. atrial circumflex (LAC)
l. atrial contraction (LAC)
l. atrial diameter
l. atrial dimension
l. atrial emptying index (LAEI)
l. atrial end diastolic volume (LAEDV)
l. atrial end systolic volume (LAESV)
l. atrial enlargement (LAE, LAF)
l. atrial hypertension
l. atrial hypertrophy (LAH)
l. atrial isolation procedure
l. atrial maximal volume
l. atrial minimal volume
l. atrial myxoma (LAM)
l. atrial neovascularization (LANV)
l. atrial overload (LAO)
l. atrial partitioning
l. atrial posterior wall (LAPW)
l. atrial pressure (LAP, PLa, Pla)
l. atrial spontaneous echo contrast (LASEC)
l. atrial thrombus (LAT)
l. atrial transesophageal pacing test (LATPT)
l. atrial transmural pressure (LATP)

l. atrial wall (LAW)
l. atrium (LA)
l. auricle (LA)
l. auricle of heart
l. axis deviation (LAD)
l. border of cardiac dullness (LBCD)
l. border of dullness (LBD)
l. brain damage (LBD)
l. bundle (LB)
l. bundle branch (LBB)
l. bundle branch block
l. bundle branch system block (LBBsB)
l. cardiac work index (LCWI)
l. circumflex (LC, LCF, LCX)
l. circumflex artery (LCA, LCX)
l. circumflex coronary (LCC)
l. circumflex coronary artery (LCX)
l. common carotid artery (LCCA)
l. coronary artery (LCA)
l. coronary artery of stomach
l. coronary catheter
l. coronary circumflex branch (LCXB)
l. coronary cusp (LCC)
l. coronary ostium (LCO)
l. coronary sinus (LCS)
l. crus of diaphragm
l. dominant coronary circulation
l. foot electrode in vectorcardiography
l. heart (LH)
l. heart blood volume (LHBV)
l. heart bypass
l. heart catheter
l. heart catheterization (LHC)
l. heart failure (LHF)
l. heart strain (LHS)
l. hemisphere (LH)
l. hemisphere damage (LHD)
l. hemisphere stroke (LCVA)
l. inferior pulmonary vein
l. inferior vena cava (LIVC)
l. internal jugular vein
l. internal mammary artery (LIMA)
l. internal mammary artery graft
l. internal thoracic artery (LITA)
l. internal thoracic artery graft
l. interventricular coronary (LIC)
l. Judkins catheter
l. lateral projection
l. lateral ventricular preexcitation (LLVP)
l. leg (VF)
l. lower border of cardiac dullness (LLBCD)
l. lower lobe (LLL)

l. lower pulmonary vein (LLPV)
l. main (LM)
l. main artery (LMA)
l. main bronchus
l. main coronary (LMC)
l. main coronary artery (LMCA)
l. main coronary artery disease (LMCAD)
l. main coronary disease (LMC)
l. main coronary occlusion
l. main coronary stenosis
l. main disease (LMD)
l. main equivalency
l. main stem (LMS)
l. main stem coronary artery disease (LMS-CAD)
l. marginal (LM)
l. marginal coronary artery occlusion (LMCAO)
l. margin of heart
l. median (LM)
l. median vein
l. middle hemiblock
l. portal view (LPV)
l. posterior hemiblock
l. posterior inferior hemiblock (LPIH)
l. posterior ventricular preexcitation (LPVP)
l. pulmonary artery (LPA)
l. pulmonary veins (LPV)
l. recurrent laryngeal nerve
l. septal hemiblock
l. septum (LS)
l. stellate ganglion
l. stellate ganglionic blockade (LSGB)
l. subclavian artery (LSCA)
l. superior pulmonary vein
l. superior vena cava (LSVC)
l. upper lobe (LUL)
l. upper pulmonary vein (LUPV)
l. ventricle (LV)
l. ventricle outflow (LVO)
l. ventricle outflow height (LVOH)
l. ventricular (LV)
l. ventricular aneurysm (LVA)
l. ventricular angiography
l. ventricular apex
l. ventricular assist device (LVAD)
l. ventricular assist system (LVAS)

l. ventricular assist system implantable pump
l. ventricular bypass pump (LVBP)
l. ventricular cavity dilation
l. ventricular cavity obstruction ring
l. ventricular chamber compliance
l. ventricular contractility
l. ventricular developed pressure (LVDP)
l. ventricular diastolic phase index
l. ventricular diastolic pressure (LVDP)
l. ventricular diastolic relaxation
l. ventricular diastolic volume (LVDV)
l. ventricular dimension (LVDI)
l. ventricular dimension in end-diastole (LVDd)
l. ventricular dysfunction (LVD)
l. ventricular dyskinesis
l. ventricular ejection (LVE)
l. ventricular ejection fraction (LVEF)
l. ventricular ejection time (LVEJT, LVET)
l. ventricular ejection time index (LVETI)
l. ventricular end-diastole (LVED)
l. ventricular end-diastolic area (LVEDA)
l. ventricular end-diastolic circumference (LVEDC)
l. ventricular end-diastolic diameter (LVEDD)
l. ventricular end-diastolic dimension (LVEDD)
l. ventricular end-diastolic pressure (LVEDP, LVEP)
l. ventricular end-diastolic volume (LVEDV)
l. ventricular end-systolic dimension (LVESD)
l. ventricular end-systolic stress
l. ventricular end-systolic volume (LVESV)
l. ventricular enlargement (LVE)
l. ventricular epicardium
l. ventricular failure (LVF)
l. ventricular filling pressure (LVFP)
l. ventricular force

L

NOTES

left *(continued)*

l. ventricular function (LVF)
l. ventricular geometry
l. ventricular hypertrophy (LVH)
l. ventricular infarct volume (LVIV)
l. ventricular inflow tract obstruction
l. ventricular insufficiency (LVI)
l. ventricular internal diastolic diameter (LVIDD)
l. ventricular internal diastolic dimension (LVIDD)
l. ventricular internal dimension (LVID)
l. ventricular ischemia (LVI)
l. ventricular-left atrial crossover dynamics
l. ventricular mass (LVM)
l. ventricular mass index
l. ventricular minute flow (LVMF)
l. ventricular muscle compliance
l. ventricular myxoma
l. ventricular outflow tract (LVOT)
l. ventricular outflow tract obstruction (LVOTO)
l. ventricular outflow tract velocity
l. ventricular output
l. ventricular peak filling rate (LVPFR)
l. ventricular posterior wall (LVPW)
l. ventricular power
l. ventricular pressure (LVP, PLV)
l. ventricular pressure-volume curve
l. ventricular puncture
l. ventricular reduction (LVR)
l. ventricular relaxation
l. ventricular-right atrial communication murmur
l. ventricular strain (LVS)
l. ventricular stroke volume (LVSV)
l. ventricular stroke volume index (LVSVI)
l. ventricular stroke work (LVSW)
l. ventricular stroke work index (LVSWI)
l. ventricular subendocardial myocardial ischemia (LVSEMI)
l. ventricular sump catheter
l. ventricular systolic/diastolic function
l. ventricular systolic dimension (LVSD)
l. ventricular systolic dysfunction
l. ventricular systolic index (LVSI)
l. ventricular systolic output (LVSO)
l. ventricular systolic performance
l. ventricular systolic pressure (LVSP)
l. ventricular tension (LVT)
l. ventricular transvenous lead
l. ventricular unloading
l. ventricular volume (LVV)
l. ventricular wall (LVW)
l. ventricular wall motion (LVWM)
l. ventricular wall motion abnormality
l. ventricular wall stress
l. ventricular wall thickness (LVWT)
l. ventricular work (LVW)
l. ventricular work index (LVWI)
l. ventriculography
l. ventrolateral gluteal (LVLG)
l. vertebral artery (LVA)

left-heart contour
left-sided

l.-s. heart failure
l.-s. innominate trunk

left-to-right shunt
leftward ventricular septal bowing (LVSB)
leg

chest and left l. (CF)
left l. (VF)
peripheral pulses palpable both l.'s (PPPBL)

Legionella

L. anisa
L. birminghamensis
L. bozemanii
L. cincinnatiensis
L. dumoffii
L. feeleii
L. gormanii
L. jordanis
L. lansingensis
L. longbeachae
L. micdadei
L. oakridgensis
L. pneumonia
L. pneumoniae
L. pneumophila
L. wadsworthii

legionellosis
Legionnaire

L. disease
L. pneumonia

Legroux remission
Lehman

L. cardiac device
L. ventriculography catheter

leiomyoma, pl. **leiomyomata**
leiomyosarcoma
Leishmania

leishmaniasis
leisure time physical activity (LTPA)
Leitner syndrome
Lell esophagoscope
lemakalim
Lemierre
    L. disease
    L. syndrome
Lemmon sternal elevator
LemonPrep electrode lotion
Lenègre
    L. disease
    L. syndrome
length
    antegrade block cycle l.
    atrial fibrillation cycle l. (AFCL)
    atrial-paced cycle l.
    basic cycle l. (BCL)
    basic drive cycle l.
    block cycle l.
    chordal l.
    l. contraction compensation element (LCCE)
    cycle l. (CL)
    drive cycle l.
    end-diastolic l. (EDL)
    end-systolic l. (ESL)
    flutter cycle l.
    lesion l. (LL)
    paced cycle l.
    pacing cycle l. (PCL)
    sinus cycle l. (SCL)
    sinus node cycle l. (SNCL)
    l. of stay (LOS)
    tachycardia cycle l.
    ventricular tachycardia cycle l. (VTCL)
    Wenckebach cycle l.
length-active tension curve
length-dependent activation
length-resting tension relation
length-tension
    l.-t. curve (LT)
    l.-t. relation
LENI
    lower extremity noninvasive
Lennert lymphoma
lenta
    endocarditis l.
Lente Iletin I, II insulin
lenticulostriate artery

lentiginosis
lentigo, pl. **lentigines**
    lentigines, atrial myxoma, mucocutaneous myxomas, and blue nevi (LAMB)
    lentigines, electrocardiographic abnormalities, ocular hypertelorism, pulmonary stenosis, abnormalities of genitalia, retardation of growth, and deafness (LEOPARD)
lentis
    ectopia l.
Lenz syndrome
Leocor hemoperfusion system
LEOPARD
    lentigines, electrocardiographic abnormalities, ocular hypertelorism, pulmonary stenosis, abnormalities of genitalia, retardation of growth, and deafness
    LEOPARD syndrome
LEP
    lipoprotein electrophoresis
lepirudin
    l. rDNA
    l. rDNA injection
leprae
    Mycobacterium l.
lepromin test
leptin
leptospiral pneumonia
leptospirosis
Leptotrichia buccalis
lercanidipine
Leredde syndrome
Leriche syndrome
Lerman-Means scratch
lesion
    aorto-ostial l.
    Baehr-Lohlein l.
    bifurcation l. (BL)
    bifurcational coronary l.
    bird's nest l.
    Blumenthal l.
    Bracht-Wächter l.
    braid-like l.
    branch l.
    calcified l.
    cavitary l.
    coin l.
    complex l.
    connective tissue l.

L

NOTES

lesion *(continued)*
    continuous full-thickness linear l.
    coronary artery l.
    cryoablation l.
    culprit l.
    cystic l.
    deep white matter l. (DWML)
    dendritic l.
    de novo coronary l.
    dilatable l.
    discrete coronary l.
    dottering of l.
    eccentric l.
    enhancing l.
    epicardial radiofrequency atrial l.
    fibrocalcific l.
    fibromusculoelastic l.
    fibrous cap l.
    full-thickness linear l.
    Ghon primary l.
    hazy l.
    honeycomb l.
    index l.
    irregular discrete l.
    JA l.
    Janeway l.
    jet l.
    juxtaarticular l.
    l. length (LL)
    Libman-Sacks l.
    linear l.
    Lohlein-Baehr l.
    long l.
    macrovascular coronary l.
    monotypic l.
    mucocutaneous l.
    multifocal l.
    nonbacterial thrombotic
      endocardial l.
    nonstentable l.
    onion scale l.
    ostial l.
    parenchymal l.
    plexiform l.
    polypoidal l.
    pulmonary coin l.
    punctate mucosal l.
    restenosis l.
    satellite l.
    shunt-dependent l.
    smooth l.
    space-occupying l.
    spot l.
    stenotic l.
    stentable l.
    synchronous airway l.'s
    tandem l.
    target l.
    type Va, Vb, Vc l.

    ulcerated l.
    vegetative l.
    wear-and-tear l.
    wire-loop l.
lesser
    l. circulation
    l. resection
LET
    lidocaine, epinephrine and tetracaine
    lidocaine epinephrine and tetracaine
    LET solution
lethal arrhythmia
letrozole
Letterer-Siwe disease
leucine
leucovorin
Leudet
    bruit de L.
leukemia
    acute lymphocytic l. (ALL)
    acute myelocytic l. (AML)
leukemic cell lysis pneumopathy
Leukeran
leukoaraiosis
    ischemic l.
leukocidin
leukocyte
    l. elastase
    polymorphonuclear l. (PMN)
leukocyte-endothelial
    l.-e. cell adhesion cascade
    l.-e. cell adhesion molecule
    l.-e. cell interaction
leukocytoblastic vasculitis
leukocytoclastic angiitis
leukocytosis
    transient l.
leukoencephalopathy
    cerebral autosomal dominant
      arteriopathy with subcortical
      infarct and l. (CADASIL)
    l. disease
    progressive multifocal l. (PML)
LeukoNet Filter
leukostasis
    pulmonary l.
Leukotrap red cell storage system
leukotriene
    l. A_4
    l. antagonist
    l. B_4 (LTB4, LTB_4)
    l. biosynthesis
    l. C_4
    cysteinyl l. (cys-LT)
    l. D_4
    l. E
    l. E_4
    l. inhibition
    l. inhibitor

l. modifier
l. synthesis
leumedin
leuprolide acetate
Leutrol
Lev
L. disease
L. syndrome
levalbuterol
l. HCl
l. HCl inhalation solution
levamisole hydrochloride
Levaquin
Levatol
levator muscle of thyroid gland
LeVeen
L. peritoneovenous shunt
L. plaque-cracker
L. valve (LVV)
level
air-fluid l.
beta-thromboglobulin l.
blood oxygen l.
dig l.
digoxin l.
ELF l.'s
malondialdehyde l.
multiple shunt l.'s
myofibrillar calcium l.
peak and trough l.'s
plasma nicotine l.
plasma thyroxine l. (PTL)
predose l.
reflecting l.
renin l.
sarcolemmal l.
serum renin l.
total homocysteine l. (tHcy)
triglyceride l.
trough and peak l.'s
level-dependent
blood oxygenation l.-d. (BOLD)
Levenberg-Marquardt algorithm
Levin catheter
Levine
L. grade 1–6 cardiac murmur
L. sign
Levine-Harvey classification
Levinson-Durbin recursion
Levinthal-Coles-Lillie (LCL)
levoatriocardinal vein

levocardia
l. malposition
mixed l.
l. with situs inversus
levocardiogram
levodopa
Levo-Dromoran
levofloxacin
levogram
levoisomerism
Levophed injection
levorphanol
levosimendan
Levo-T
Levothroid
levothyroxine
levotransposition
levoversion
Levovist
L. contrast
L. echocontrast agent
Levoxyl
Levy Chimeric Faces Test
Lewis
L. index
L. lead
L. lines
P substance of L.
L. thoracotomy
L. upper limb cardiovascular
disease
Lewis-Pickering test
Lewis-Tanner procedure
Lewy chest holder
Lewy-Rubin needle
Lexxel
Leyden crystal
LFB
low-flow cardiopulmonary bypass
LFC
low fat and cholesterol
LFC diet
LFCT
lung-to-finger circulation time
LFT
liver function test
LGV
lymphogranuloma venereum
LH
left heart
left hemisphere

L

NOTES

L/H
     lung-to-heart
     L/H ratio
LHBV
     left heart blood volume
LHC
     left heart catheterization
LHD
     left hemisphere damage
LHF
     left heart failure
LHMT
     low-range heparin management test
LHS
     left heart strain
LI
     lacunar infarction
     laterality index
LIAF
     laser-induced arterial fluorescence
Liberator locking stylet
Libman-Sacks
     L.-S. disease
     L.-S. endocarditis
     L.-S. lesion
     L.-S. syndrome
library
     Cochrane L.
     human cosmid l.
LIC
     left interventricular coronary
     local intravascular coagulation
     LIC artery
licheniformis
     Bacillus l.
lichenoides
     tuberculosis l.
licorice
     Chinese l.
Liddle
     L. aorta clamp
     L. syndrome
lidocaine
     l., atropine, naloxone, epinephrine
        [drugs that may be administered
        via endotracheal tube] (LANE)
     buffered l. (BL)
     l. epinephrine and tetracaine (LET)
     l. hydrochloride
Lidodan
lidoflazine
LidoPen I.M. Injection Auto-Injector
Liebermann-Burchard test
Liebermeister
     L. rule
     L. sign
Liebow
     L. classification
     usual interstitial pneumonia of L.

lienis
     extremitas anterior l.
     porta l.
lifarizine
LIFE
     lifestyle intervention, food and exercise
        program
     lung imaging fluorescence endoscope
life
     L. Care Pump
     l. change unit
     l. force
     health-related quality of l. (HRQL,
        HRQOL)
     Mini Asthma Quality of L.
        (MAQOL)
     quality of l.
     stroke-specific quality of l. (SS-
        QOL)
     L. Suit
     l. support
Lifecare PLV-100 ventilator
lifeguard lung
Lifeline lead
LIFE-Lung System
Lifepak
     L. defibrillator
     L. 5, 7 monitor/defibrillator
Lifepath
     L. AAA endovascular graft system
     L. stent-graft
LifePort endotracheal tube holder
Lifesaver disposable resuscitator bag
Lifescan
LifeShirt monitor
LifeStick
     L. CPR device
     L. resuscitation device
Lifestream coronary dilation catheter
lifestyle
     l. intervention, food and exercise
        program (LIFE)
     sedentary l.
LifeVest wearable defibrillator
life-years
     quality-adjusted l.-y. (QALY)
LIFT
lift
     parasternal systolic l.
     tongue-jaw l.
ligament
     Cooper l.
     costoclavicular l.
     Marshall l.
     pericardiosternal l.
     pulmonary l.
     Teutleben l.

ventricular l.
vestibular l.

ligamentum, pl. **ligamenta**
ligamenta anularia trachealia
l. arteriosum
l. hepatoesophageum
l. latum pulmonis
l. phrenicocolicum
l. pulmonale
l. teres cardiopexy

ligand
l. binding
Fas l. (FasL)
macromolecular l.
l. plus 1, 2, 3

ligase chain reaction (LCR)

ligation
Bardenheurer l.
l. clip
Doppler-guided hemorrhoidal
 artery l.
Linton radical vein l.
thoracic duct l.
variceal l.
varicose vein stripping and l.

ligature
Stannius l.

light
L. chain
L.-emitting diode (LED)
L. microscopy
L. pen
L. pen-determined ejection fraction
Questran L.
L. reflexion rheography
L. stroke
L. Talker device
L. wand

Lightcriteria

lighted
l. stylet
l. stylet intubation

light-emitting diode (LED)

lightwire

lignan

Lignieres test

lignocaine
M l.

LIhFE
living with heart failure
LIHFE questionnaire

LiI
lithium iodine
LiI battery

Likert
L. 5-point scale
L. scale (LS)

Lilienthal-Sauerbruch
L.-S. retractor
L.-S. rib spreader

Lillehei-Kaster
L.-K. cardiac valve prosthesis
L.-K. mitral valve prosthesis
L.-K. pivoting-disk prosthetic valve

Lillehei-Nakib toroidal valve

Lillehei pacemaker

Lillehi-Nakib toroidal valve

Lilliput oxygenator

LIMA
left internal mammary artery
LIMA graft

LIMA-Lift tool

LIMA-Loop tool

limb
anacrotic l.
l. blood flow
claudicant l.
inspiratory l.
l. ischemia
l. lead
l. salvage
thoracic l.

limb-girdle
l.-g. dystrophy of Erb
l.-g. muscular dystrophy

limb-heart
cleft l.-h. (CLH)

limbic ledge

limb-kinetic apraxia

lime
bruit de l.

limit
Nyquist l.

limitation
airflow l.
chronic airflow l. (CAL)
flow l. (FL)

limited
l. Doppler examination
l. treadmill test (LTT)
l. ventricular reserve

limonite pneumoconiosis

L

NOTES

Lincocin
> L. injection
> L. Oral

lincomycin hydrochloride
Lincorex injection
lincosamide
Linctus With Codeine phosphate
Lindbergh pump
Lindesmith operation
Linde Walker Oxygen Program
Lindholm
> L. operating laryngoscope
> L. tracheal tube

line
> anterior axillary l. (AAL)
> anterior junction l.
> arterial l. (A-line)
> arterial mean l.
> Beau l.'s
> Cantlie l.
> central venous l.
> Conradi l.
> Correra l.
> costophrenic septal l.
> CVP l.
> Fleischner l.
> Head l.'s
> indwelling l.
> intralobular l.
> isoelectric l.
> isthmus l.
> Kerley A, B, C l.'s
> Lewis l.'s
> Linton l.
> M l.'s
> midaxillary l.
> midclavicular l. (MCL)
> paraspinal l.
> pleural l.
> pleuroesophageal l.
> posterior junction l.
> l. sepsis
> septal l.
> tram l.
> Z l.
> Zahn l.'s
> zero velocity l.

linear
> l. ablation
> l. echo
> l. echodensity
> l. infiltrate
> L. KGT tonometer
> l. lesion
> l. local shortening map
> l. phonocardiograph
> l. stenosis

linearity
> amplitude l.
> count-rate l.

linear-phased radiofrequency catheter ablation
linezolid
Lingraphica
> L. aphasic treatment
> L. system treatment technology

linguae
> corpus l.
> dorsum l.
> radix l.
> raphe l.
> septum l.
> tunica mucosa l.
> venae dorsales l.
> vena profunda l.
> vinculum l.

lingual
> l. bone
> l. branch
> l. branch of facial nerve
> l. plexus
> l. quinsy
> l. thyroid
> l. tonsil
> l. vein

lingualis
> arteria l.
> plexus periarterialis arteriae l.
> rami isthmi faucium nervi l.
> tonsilla l.

lingualplasty
lingula, pl. **lingulae**
> l. of left lung
> l. pulmonis sinistri

lingular
> l. bronchus
> l. pneumonia

lingularis
> vena l.

linguofacialis
> truncus l.

linoleic acid
linsidomine
Linton
> L. flap
> L. line
> L. radical vein ligation
> L. vein stripper

Linx
> L. exchange guidewire
> L. extension guidewire
> L. extension wire
> L. guidewire extension
> L. guidewire extension cardiac device

liothyronine

liotrix
Liotta-BioImplant low profile
  bioprosthesis prosthetic valve
Liotta total artificial heart
LIP
  lymphocytic interstitial pneumonitis
  lymphoid interstitial pneumonia
  lymphoid interstitial pneumonitis
lipase
  diacylglycerol l.
  hepatic l.
  hepatic lipoprotein l.
  lipoprotein l. (LL, LPL)
lipedema
lipemia
  postprandial l. (PPL)
lipid
  l.-A
  l. accumulation
  antihypertensive neutral
    renomedullary l. (ANRL)
  bumetanide and furosemide on l.
    (BUFUL)
  cholesterol-lowering l. (CLL)
  l. core
  l. core density
  l. disorder
  endogenous l.
  exogenous l.
  extracellular l.
  fasting plasma l. (FPL)
  l. hypothesis
  intracellular l.
  neutral l. (NL)
  l. panel
  l. peroxidation product
  l. peroxide
  l. pneumonia
  renomedullary l.
  l. research clinic (LRC)
  l. risk factor
  sarcolemma l.
  l. solubility
  l. triad
  vasodepressor l. (VDL)
lipid-coronary artery disease (LCAD)
Lipidil
  L. Micro
  L. Supra
lipid-induced lung injury
lipid-laden
  l.-l. macrophage

  l.-l. macrophage index
  l.-l. plaque
lipid-lowering
  l.-l. agent
  l.-l. therapy
lipidosis, pl. **lipidoses**
lipid-rich plaque
Lipitor
lipoarabinomannan
lipocardiac
lipodystrophy
  intestinal l.
lipofuscinosis
  neuronal ceroid l.
lipogenic theory of atherosclerosis
lipohyalinosis
lipoides
  arcus l.
lipoid pneumonia
lipolysis
lipoma, pl. **lipomata**
lipomatous hypertrophy
lipoparticle
lipoperoxide
lipophilic drug
lipophilicity
  properties of l.
lipopolysaccharidase
  J5 l.
lipopolysaccharide (LPS)
  l. vaccine
lipopolysaccharide-induced
  thrombocytopenia
lipoprotein (LP, Lp)
  l. A (LPA, Lp(a))
  alpha l.
  l. B (LPB, Lp(b))
  beta l.
  l. electrophoresis (LEP, LPE)
  high-density l. (HDL, HDLP)
  intermediate-density l. (IDL)
  isolated low high-density l.
    (ILHDL)
  l. lipase (LL, LPL)
  l. lipase activity (LPLA)
  low-density l. (LDL, LDLP)
  low-density lipoprotein/high
    density l. (LDL/HDL)
  malondialdehyde modified low-
    density l. (MDA-LDL)
  microsomal l. (MLP)
  native low-density l.

L

NOTES

lipoprotein *(continued)*
>non-high density l. (NHDL)
>normal low-density l. (NLDL)
>oxidized low-density l. (OxLDL)
>pre-beta l.
>l. receptor-related protein (LRP)
>remnant l. (RLP)
>remnant-like particle l.
>RLP l.
>small low-density l.
>total cholesterol/high-density l.'s (TC/HDL)
>triglyceride rich l. (TRL, TRLP)
>very high density l. (VHDL)
>very low density l. (VLDL)
>l. X (LPX, Lp-X)

lipoprotein-associated coagulation inhibitor
lipoprotein-deficient fraction (LPDF)
lipoproteinemia
liposarcoma
liposomal
>amphotericin B (liposomal)

Liposorber LA-15 system
Liposyn
lipothymia
lipotropin
>human l. (HLT)

Lipovnik virus
lipoxygenase
>5-l.
>l. pathway

LIP/PLH
>lymphoid interstial pneumonia/pulmonary lymphoid hyperplasa
>LIP/PLH complex

lip pursing
Liprostin
Liquaemin
liquefaciens
>*Serratia* l.

liquefaction necrosis
Liquibid
liquid
>Brontex L.
>l. crystal display (LCD)
>Detussin l.
>Entuss-D l.
>Hayfebrol l.
>Histussin D l.
>Hycotuss Expectorant L.
>oxygen-carrying perfluorochemical l.
>Rhinosyn l.
>Rhinosyn-PD l.
>Ryna l.
>l. scintillation spectrophotometer

liquifying expectorant

Liqui-Gels
>Alka-Seltzer Plus Flu & Body Aches Non-Drowsy L.-G.
>Robitussin Severe Congestion L.-G.

LiquiVent
LIS
>lung injury score

lisinopril
>hydrochlorothiazide and l.
>l. and hydrochlorothiazide

Lissajou loop
Listeria monocytogenes
list mode
LITA
>left internal thoracic artery
>LITA graft

LITE
>low-intensity treadmill exercise
>LITE protocol

Lite Blade
liter
>millimoles per l. (mmol/L)
>l. per minute (Lpm)
>l. per minute per meter squared (Lpm/m^2)

lithium
>l. hydride
>l. iodine (LiI)
>l. iodine battery

lithium-powered pacemaker
lithomyxoma
>cardiac l.

Litten
>L. diaphragm sign
>L. phenomenon

Little disease
Littman
>L. class II pediatric stethoscope
>L. defibrillation pad

Litwak left atrial-aortic bypass
LIVC
>left inferior vena cava

live
>Bacillus Calmette-Guérin l.

livedo
>l. reticularis
>l. vasculitis

livedoid dermatitis
liver
>cardiac l.
>cirrhosis of l.
>l. flap
>l. function test (LFT)
>l. palm
>right triangular ligament of l.

Livewire
>L. TC ablation catheter
>L. TC steerable electrophysiology catheter

livida
>   asphyxia l.

Livierato
>   L. reflex
>   L. sign
>   L. test

living
>   activities of daily l. (ADL)
>   impairment of activities of daily l. (IADL)
>   instrumental activities of daily l. (IADL)
>   l. related transplant (LRT)
>   l. with heart failure (LIhFE)

LL
>   lesion length
>   lipoprotein lipase

LLBCD
>   left lower border of cardiac dullness

LLL
>   left lower lobe

L-looping of the ventricle

LLPV
>   left lower pulmonary vein

LLVP
>   left lateral ventricular preexcitation

LM
>   left main
>   left marginal
>   left median
>   LM coronary artery

LMA
>   laryngeal mask airway
>   left main artery

LMA-Unique laryngeal mask

LMC
>   left main coronary
>   left main coronary disease
>   LMC artery

LMCA
>   left main coronary artery

LMCAD
>   left main coronary artery disease

LMCAO
>   left marginal coronary artery occlusion

LMD
>   left main disease
>   low-molecular weight dextran

LMI
>   lateral medullary infarction
>   lateral myocardial infarction

LMS
>   left main stem
>   LMS coronary artery

LMS-CAD
>   left main stem coronary artery disease

LMWH
>   low-molecular weight heparin

L-NAME
> N^G-nitro-L-arginine methyl ester

L-NMMA
> N^G-monomethyl-L-arginine

load
>   chronic volume l.
>   elastic l.
>   electronic pacemaker l.
>   end-diastolic l. (EDL)
>   exercise l.
>   heat l.
>   inelastic l.
>   inspiratory threshold l. (ITL)
>   whole-body amyloid l.

loaded breathing test (LBT)

loading
>   bretylium l.
>   discontinuous incremental threshold l.
>   glycogen l.
>   incremental threshold l.
>   inspiratory l.
>   methionine l.
>   rapid fluid l.
>   relaxation l.
>   saline l.
>   volume l.

lobar
>   l. atelectasis
>   l. bronchus
>   l. collapse
>   l. emphysema
>   l. infiltrate
>   l. pneumonia

lobares
>   bronchi l.

lobe
>   inferior frontal l. (IFL)
>   inferior parietal/superior temporal l. (IPSTL)
>   left lower l. (LLL)
>   left upper l. (LUL)
>   nonprimary l.
>   right lower l. (RLL)
>   right middle l. (RML)

L

NOTES

lobe (*continued*)
  right upper l. (RUL)
  side l.
lobectomize
lobectomy
  sleeve l.
  video-assisted thoracic surgical non-rib-spreading l. (VNSSL)
lobeline sulfate
lobular
  l. capillary hemangioma
  l. consolidation
  l. hematoma
  l. pneumonia
lobule
  pulmonary l.
  secondary pulmonary l.
  superior parietal l. (SPL)
lobus
  l. azygos pulmonis dextri
  l. dexter
  l. medius pulmonis dextri
local
  l. area network (LAN)
  l. asphyxia
  l. intravascular coagulation (LIC)
  l. organ procurement area
  l. reaction
  l. syncope
  l. thrombotic response
LocaLisa technique
localization
  anatomic l.
localized
  l. obstructive emphysema
  l. pericarditis
  l. sacculation
LocalMed
  L. catheter infusion sleeve
  L. InfusaSleeve
Lochol
lo chol
  low cholesterol
LoCholest
loci (*pl. of* locus)
lock
  heparin l. (HL)
  l. pericardiocentesis set and tray
Lock-A-Card
Lock Clamshell device
locking
  l. device
  l. stylet
LOCM
  low osmolality contrast material
  low osmolality contrast media
locular cyst
loculated
  l. cyst

l. effusion
l. emphysema
l. empyema
loculation
locus, pl. **loci**
  l. ceruleus
  chymase gene l.
  genetic l.
  quantitative trait l. (QTL)
lodaxamide
Lode BV Excalibur braked cycle ergometer
Loeffler bacillus
Loesche classification
lofexidine
Löffler
  L. disease
  L. endocardial fibrosis
  L. parietal fibroplastic endocarditis
  L. pneumonia
  L. syndrome
Löfgren syndrome
Lo-Fold balloon
logarithmic
  l. dynamic range
  l. phonocardiograph
Lohlein-Baehr lesion
Lombardi sign
lomefloxacin hydrochloride
lomustine
London
  L. School of Hygiene Cardiovascular Rose Questionnaire
  L. School of Hygiene and Tropical medicine sphygmomanometer
lone atrial fibrillation
long
  l. ACE fixed-wire balloon catheter
  l. axial oblique view
  l. axis (LAX)
  l. axis-discrete subaortic stenosis (LAX-DSS)
  L. Bare Stent Registry
  L. Brite Tip guiding catheter
  l. dissection
  l. iliac artery occlusion
  l. lesion
  l. PP interval
  l. pulse
  l. QT (LQT)
  l. QT1 (LQT1)
  l. QT2 (LQT2)
  l. QT arrhythmia
  l. QT interval
  l. QT syndrome (LQTS)
  l. QTU syndrome
  l. skinny over-the-wire balloon catheter
  l. taper/stiff shaft Glidewire

long-acting
    l.-a. nitrate
    Sinex l.-a.
long acting (LA, L.A.)
long-axis
    l.-a. fractional shortening (LAFS)
    l.-a. parasternal view
      echocardiogram
    l.-a. shortening velocity
    l.-a. view
longbeachae
    Legionella l.
Longdwel Teflon catheter
long-echo-train-length fast-spin-echo imaging (long-ETL FSE imaging)
long-ETL FSE imaging
    long-echo-train-length fast-spin-echo
      imaging
longitudinal
    l. analysis
    l. arteriography
    l. dissociation
    l. midline incision
    l. narrowing
    l. relaxation time
long-leg venography technique
Longmire valvotomy
long-term
    l.-t. care (LTC)
    l.-t. care facility
    l.-t. electrocardiography (LT-ECG)
    l.-t. oxygen therapy (LTOT)
long-time recording
Loniten Oral
loop
    atrial vector l.
    bulboventricular l.
    cine l.
    clockwise l.
    D l.
    l. diuresis
    l. diuretic
    elliptical l.
    exercise tidal flow-volume l.
      (ETFVL)
    flow volume l.
    Gerdy intraauricular l.
    guidewire l.
    heart l.
    Henle l.
    L l.
    Lissajou l.

    maximum flow-volume l. (MFVL)
    maxi-vessel l.'s
    memory l.
    l. monitor
    P l.
    pressure-volume l.
    QRS l.
    reentrant l.
    rigid monopolar l.
    sewing ring l.
    T l.
    tidal l.
    tidal flow-volume l. (TFVL)
    U l.
    Uresil radiopaque silicone band
      vessel l.'s
    U-shaped catheter l.
    vector l.
    ventricular pressure-volume l.
    video l.
loose junction
Lopid
Lopressor
Lo-Profile II catheter
Lo-Pro tracheal tube
Lorabid
loracarbef
loratadine
lorazepam
lorcainide
Lorcet Plus
Lore-Lawrence trachea tube
Lortat-Jacob approach
LOS
    length of stay
    low cardiac output syndrome
losartan
    l. and hydrochlorothiazide
    l. potassium
    l. potassium/hydrochlorothiazide
loss
    age-related bone l.
    l. of capture
    l. of consciousness
    signal l.
    volume l.
lossy algorithm
Lotensin HCT
lotion
    LemonPrep electrode l.
lotrafiban
Lotrel

L

NOTES

Louis
> L. angle
> L. law

Louisiana pneumonia
lovastatin
Lovenox injection
Loven reflex
low
> l. blood pressure (LBP)
> l. cardiac output (LCO)
> l. cardiac output syndrome (LCOS, LOS)
> l. cholesterol (lo chol)
> l. energy all-purpose (LEAP)
> l. energy direct current (LEDC)
> l. fat and cholesterol (LFC)
> l. flow rate
> l. osmolality contrast material (LOCM)
> l. osmolality contrast media (LOCM)
> L. Profile Port vascular access
> l. renin essential hypertension (LREH)
> l. right atrium (LRA)
> l. septal atrium
> l. septal right atrium (LSRA)

low-amplitude contraction (LAC)
low-chloride St. Thomas solution
low-density
> l.-d. lipoprotein (LDL, LDLP)
> l.-d. lipoprotein apheresis (LDLA)
> l.-d. lipoprotein-cholesterol complex (LDL-C, LDL-c)
> l.-d. lipoprotein/high density lipoprotein (LDL/HDL)
> l.-d. lipoprotein receptor (LDLR, LDL-R)
> l.-d. lipoprotein receptor mutation database (LDLR, LDL-R)

low-dose
> l.-d. bile-acid sequestrant
> l.-d. dobutamine cine MRI
> l.-d. heparin (LDH)
> l.-d. unfractionated heparin (LDUH)

Lowell pleural needle
Löwenberg cuff sign
low-energy
> l.-e. intracardiac cardioversion
> l.-e. laser
> l.-e. synchronized cardioversion

Lowenstein medium
lower
> l. airways
> l. body negative pressure (LBNP)
> l. extremity arterial disease (LEAD)
> l. extremity bypass graft
> l. extremity noninvasive (LENI)

> l. infection point
> l. lobe bronchus
> l. lobe of lung
> l. nodal extrasystole
> l. nodal rhythm
> l. respiratory tract
> l. respiratory tract smear
> l. ribs
> L. rings

lowering
> antihypertensive and lipid l. (ALL)

Lower-Shumway cardiac transplant
low-esophageal pH probe
low-fat diet
Low-Flex lead
low-flow
> l.-f. cardiopulmonary bypass (LFB)
> l.-f. ischemia

low-frequency murmur
low-intensity treadmill exercise (LITE)
low-methionine diet
low-molecular
> l.-m. weight dextran (LMD)
> l.-m. weight heparin (LMWH)
> l.-m. weight heparin (LMWH)

Lown
> L. arrhythmia
> L. class 4a, 4b ventricular ectopic beat
> L. classification
> L. grading system
> L. technique
> L. and Woolf method

Lown-Edmark waveform
Lown-Ganong-Levine syndrome
low-output heart failure
low-pass filter
low-pitched murmur
low-plaque coarctation
low-pressure tamponade
low-prime circuitry
low-profile
> l.-p. balloon-positioning catheter
> l.-p. semi-compliant balloon

low-ramp protocol
low-range heparin management test (LHMT)
low-reflow phenomenon
low-risk chest pain (LRCP)
low-salt
> l.-s. diet
> l.-s. syndrome

low-sodium
> l.-s. diet
> l.-s. syndrome

low-speed rotation angioplasty catheter
low-viscosity mucus
lozenge
> horehound l.

Lozide
Lozol
LP, Lp
 lipoprotein
 lung perfusion
  LP stent
LPA
 left pulmonary artery
 lipoprotein A
Lp(a)
 lipoprotein A
LPB, Lp(b)
 lipoprotein B
LPDF
 lipoprotein-deficient fraction
LPE
 lipoprotein electrophoresis
L-phenylalanine mustard
LPIH
 left posterior inferior hemiblock
LPL
 lipoprotein lipase
LPLA
 lipoprotein lipase activity
Lpm
 liter per minute
Lpm/m^2
 liter per minute per meter squared
LPS
 late progressing stroke
 lipopolysaccharide
  LPS Peel-Away introducer
LPV
 left portal view
 left pulmonary veins
LPVP
 left posterior ventricular preexcitation
LPX, Lp-X
 lipoprotein X
LQT
 long QT
  LQT syndrome
LQT1
 long QT1
LQT2
 long QT2
LQTS
 long QT syndrome
LRA
 low right atrium
LRC
 lipid research clinic

LRCP
 low-risk chest pain
LREH
 low renin essential hypertension
LRP
 lipoprotein receptor-related protein
LRT
 living related transplant
LS
 Laron syndrome
 left septum
 Likert scale
L/S
 lecithin/sphingomyelin
  L/S ratio
LSC
 late systolic click
LSCA
 left subclavian artery
L-selectin
LSGB
 left stellate ganglionic blockade
LSM
 late systolic murmur
LSRA
 low septal right atrium
LSVC
 left superior vena cava
LT
 length-tension curve
 lung transplant
LTB4, LTB$_4$
 leukotriene B4
 leukotriene B$_4$
LTBI
 latent tuberculosis infection
LTC
 long-term care
  LTC facility
LT-ECG
 long-term electrocardiography
LTOT
 long-term oxygen therapy
LTPA
 leisure time physical activity
LTT
 limited treadmill test
LTx
 lung transplant
L-type calcium blocker
lubeluzole

L

NOTES

lubricant
RotaGlide l.
lubricity
Lucas-Championnière disease
lucency
lucent defect
Luciani-Wenckebach atrioventricular block
luciferase reporter phages
lucigenin
l. chemiluminescence assay
Ludiomil
Ludwig
L. angina
L. angle
Luer-Lok
L.-L. connector
L.-L. needle
L.-L. needle tip
L.-L. port
Luer tracheal tube
lues
luetic
l. aneurysm
l. aortitis
l. disease
Lufyllin
Lugol solution
Lukens thymus retractor
Luke procedure
LUL
left upper lobe
Lumaguide catheter
LuMax Flex guiding catheter
lumbar
l. part of diaphragm
l. sympathectomy
lumbricoides
Ascaris l.
lumen, pl. **lumina**
airway l.
aortic l.
l. of artery
bronchial l.
conduit l.
double l. (DL)
esophageal l.
false l.
l. finder
pharyngeal tracheal l. (PTL)
plaque l.
single l.
vessel l.
luminal
l. diameter
l. encroachment
l. narrowing
l. recoil
l. widening

Luminal Sodium
luminescence
luminogram
luminology
coronary l.
Lumonics YAG laser
lunata
Curvularia l.
Lunderquist
L. exchange wire
L. extra stiff wire guide
lung
l. abscess
l. acinus
aerated l.
AIDS-related lymphoma of the l. (ARLL)
air-conditioner l.
aluminum l.
anterior border of l.
anterior descending segmental artery of right l.
apex of l.
l. architecture
artificial l.
atrium of l.
azygos lobe of right l.
base of l.
bible printer's l.
l. biopsy
bird breeder's l.
bird fancier's l.
black l.
blast l.
l. blood volume (LBV)
brown induration of l.
l. bud
l. carcinoma
cardiac impression on l.
cardiac notch of left l.
cheese worker's l.
coal miner's l.
coin lesion of l.
collapsed l.
collier's l.
l. compliance
consolidation of l.
l. contusion
costal surface of l.
cystic disease of l.
decortication of l.
detergent worker's l.
l. diffusion
dirty l.
drowned l.
dynamic compliance of l.
l. dysfunction
edema of l.
l. edema

l. elasticity
l. elastic recoil
l. elastic recoil pressure (Pel)
end-stage l.
l. entrapment
eosinophilic l.
esophageal l.
essential brown induration of l.
farmer's l.
l. fever
fibrocystic l.
fibroid l.
l. fibrosis
fish meal l.
fissure of l.
flock worker's l.
l. fluke
l. function
furrier's l.
gastric l.
harvester's l.
heart and l. (H&L)
hilum of l.
honeycomb l.
honeycombing of l.
horseshoe l.
humidifier l.
hyperlucent l.
l. imaging fluorescence endoscope
  (LIFE)
inferior border of l.
inferior lobe of left/right l.
infundibulum of l.
l. injury
l. injury score (LIS)
interlobar surface of l.
l. interstitium
iron l.
jute worker's l.
Labrador l.
lateral basal segmental artery of
  right l.
lifeguard l.
lingula of left l.
lower lobe of l.
malt worker's l.
l. marking
mason's l.
l. mass
l. mechanics
medial surface of l.
mediastinal part of l.

mesentery of l.
middle lobe of right l.
miller's l.
miner's l.
mold worker's l.
l. morphometry
mushroom worker's l.
l. nodule
oblique fissure of l.
l. perfusion (LP, Lp)
pigeon breeder's l.
pigeon fancier's l.
pigment induration of l.
pizza l.
polycystic l.
posterior basal segmental artery of
  right l.
postperfusion l.
pump l.
l. reexpansion
respirator l.
l. retractor
rheumatoid l.
root of l.
l. scan
l. scanning
scleroderma l.
shock l.
silo-filler's l.
silver polisher's l.
l. sliding
stiff l.
l. stone
superior lobe of right/left l.
thresher's l.
l. tissue destruction
l. transfer capacity
l. transplant (LT, LTx)
transverse fissure of right l.
trapped l.
trench l.
tuberculosis of l.'s
unilateral hyperlucency of l.
unilateral hyperlucent l.
unilateral nonfunctioning l.
l. unit
upper lobe of l.
l. uptake
uremic l.
vanishing l.
vernal edema of l.

NOTES

lung *(continued)*

    vertebral part of the costal surface of l.
    l. volume
    l. volume reduction surgery (LVRS)
    l. washings
    welder's l.
    wet l.
    white l.
    wood pulp worker's l.

lunger

    chronic l.

lung-liver interaction
Lungmotor
lung-to-finger circulation time (LFCT)
lung-to-heart (L/H)
lung-wall interface
lungworm
lunula, pl. **lunulae**
lupoid
Lupron

    L. Depot
    L. Depot-Ped

lupus

    l. anticoagulant
    l. anticoagulant disorder
    cerebral l.
    l. erythematosus (LE)
    l. pernio
    l. pleuritis

lupus-associated valve disease
LUPV

    left upper pulmonary vein

Lurselle
Luschka

    L. cartilage
    foramen of L.
    L. tonsil

lusitaniae

    Candida l.

lusitropic abnormality
lusitropy
lusoria

    dysphagia l.

Lutembacher

    L. complex
    L. syndrome

lutetium

    motexafin l.
    l. texaphyrin

Lutz-Splendore-Almeida disease
Luxtec fiberoptic system
LV

    left ventricle
    left ventricular
        LV end-diastolic diameter

LVA

    left ventricular aneurysm
    left vertebral artery

LVAD

    left ventricular assist device
        HeartMate LVAD
        Novacor LVAD
        vented-electric HeartMate LVAD

LVAS

    left ventricular assist system

LVBP

    left ventricular bypass pump

LVD

    left ventricular dysfunction

LVDd

    left ventricular dimension in end-diastole

LVDI

    left ventricular dimension

LVDP

    left ventricular developed pressure
    left ventricular diastolic pressure

LVDV

    left ventricular diastolic volume

LVE

    left ventricular ejection
    left ventricular enlargement

LVED

    left ventricular end-diastole

LVEDA

    left ventricular end-diastolic area

LVEDC

    left ventricular end-diastolic circumference

LVEDD

    left ventricular end-diastolic diameter
    left ventricular end-diastolic dimension

LVEDP

    left ventricular end-diastolic pressure

LVEDV

    left ventricular end-diastolic volume

LVEF

    left ventricular ejection fraction

LVEJT

    left ventricular ejection time

LVEP

    left ventricular end-diastolic pressure

LVESD

    left ventricular end-systolic dimension

LVESV

    left ventricular end-systolic volume

LVET

    left ventricular ejection time

LVETI

    left ventricular ejection time index

LVF

    left ventricular failure
    left ventricular function

LVFP

    left ventricular filling pressure

LVH
  left ventricular hypertrophy
LVI
  large-vessel infarction
  left ventricular insufficiency
  left ventricular ischemia
LVID
  left ventricular internal dimension
LVIDD
  left ventricular internal diastolic diameter
  left ventricular internal diastolic
    dimension
LVIV
  left ventricular infarct volume
LVLG
  left ventrolateral gluteal
LVM
  left ventricular mass
LVMF
  left ventricular minute flow
LVN
  lateral ventricular nerve
LVO
  left ventricle outflow
LVOH
  left ventricle outflow height
LVOT
  left ventricular outflow tract
LVOTO
  left ventricular outflow tract obstruction
LVP
  left ventricular pressure
LVPFR
  left ventricular peak filling rate
LVPmax
  maximum left ventricular pressure
LVPmin
  minimum left ventricular pressure
LVPW
  left ventricular posterior wall
LVR
  left ventricular reduction
LVRS
  lung volume reduction surgery
LVS
  left ventricular strain
LVSB
  leftward ventricular septal bowing
LVSD
  left ventricular systolic dimension

LVSEMI
  left ventricular subendocardial
    myocardial ischemia
LVSI
  left ventricular systolic index
LVSO
  left ventricular systolic output
LVSP
  left ventricular systolic pressure
LVSV
  left ventricular stroke volume
LVSVI
  left ventricular stroke volume index
LVSW
  left ventricular stroke work
LVSWI
  left ventricular stroke work index
LVT
  left ventricular tension
LVV
  left ventricular volume
  LeVeen valve
LVW
  left ventricular wall
  left ventricular work
LVWI
  left ventricular work index
LVWM
  left ventricular wall motion
LVWT
  left ventricular wall thickness
LW
  lateral wall
lwoffi
  Acinetobacter l.
lycopene
Lycoperdon
lycoperdonosis
lycopodium **asthma**
LYG
  lymphomatoid granulomatosis
Lyme
  L. borreliosis
  L. disease
  L. titer
lymphadenitis
  tuberculous l.
lymphadenopathy
  hilar l.
lymphangiectasis
  chronic pulmonary cystic l.

L

NOTES

lymphangioendothelioma
lymphangioleiomyomatosis (LAM)
    pulmonary l.
lymphangioma
lymphangiomatosis
    diffuse pulmonary l.
lymphangiomyomatosis
    pulmonary l.
lymphangitic
    l. carcinoma
    l. carcinomatosis (LC)
    l. spread
lymphangitis carcinomatosa
Lymphapress compression therapy
lymphatic
    l. channel
    l. dilation
    l. edema
    obtuse marginal l.
    subclavian l.
lymphatici
    hilum nodi l.
lymphedema praecox
lymph node
lymphocyte
    l. chemoattractant factor (LCF)
    l. concentration
    effusion-associated l.
    l. immune globulin
    T l.
    l. transformation test
lymphocytic
    l. infiltrative disorder
    l. interstitial pneumonitis (LIP)
lymphoepithelioma-like carcinoma
lymphogranuloma venereum (LGV)
lymphohematogenous drainage system
lymphoid
    l. alveolitis
    l. hyperplasia
    l. interstial pneumonia/pulmonary
      lymphoid hyperplasa (LIP/PLH)
    l. interstitial pneumonia (LIP)
    l. interstitial pneumonitis (LIP)
lymphokine
lymphoma
    African Burkitt l.
    AIDS-related l. (ARL)
    B cell l.
    Burkitt l.
    Kiel classification of l.
    Lennert l.
    nodular sclerosing Hodgkin l.

    noncleaved cell l.
    non-Hodgkin l.
    primary effusion l.
    primary pulmonary non-Hodgkin l.
      (PPL)
    pulmonary l.
    pyothorax-associated l.
lymphomatoid granulomatosis (LYG)
lymphoplasma
lymphoplasmacytic inflammation
lymphoreticular granulomatous vasculitis
lymphosarcoma
lymphotoxin
Lyo-Ject
    Cardizem L.-J.
    L.-J. syringe
Lyon-Horgan procedure
Lyon hypothesis
lyophilize
lyophilized powder
Lyra
    L. 2020 implantable cardioverter
    L. 2020 implantable cardioverter-
      defibrillator
    L. laser system
lysate
lyse
lysed artery
lysine
    l. acetylsalicylate
lysine-binding site
lysis
    clot l.
    dilute blood clot l. (DBCL)
    euglobin clot l. (ECL)
    myofibrillar l.
    spontaneous l.
    l. time
Lysodren
lysophosphatidic acid
lysophosphatidylcholine scavenger
lysophospholipase
lysosomal
    l. enzyme
    l. hydrolase
lysosome
lysozyme
lys-plasminogen
    recombinant l.-p.
Lyssavirus
lysylbradykinin
LZT
    lead/zirconium/titanium

M
  murmur
    M cell layer
    M lignocaine
    M lines
    M pattern on right atrial wave
      form
    M protein
M1
  mitral component
M2
  marked dullness
M3
  absolute dullness
M$_1$
  mitral first sound
M$_2$
  mitral second sound
M6/C cylinder carrying case
M6 oxygen cylinder
m7E3 Fab
MA
  malignant arrhythmia
  mixed apnea
mA
  milliampere
MAA
  macroaggregated albumin
  mandibular advancement appliance
    MAA perfusion lung scintigraphy
MABP
  mean arterial blood pressure
MAC
  malignancy-associated change
  membrane attack complex
  minimal alveolar concentration
  mitral annulus calcification
  multiaccess catheter
  Mycobacterium avium complex
    MAC infection
MAC-1
  beta-2 integrin MAC-1
MacCallum patch
MACE
  main adverse coronary event
  major adverse cardiac event
Macewen sign
Mach
  M. band
  M. effect
Machado-Guerreiro test
Machida fiberoptic laryngoscope
machine
  Apogee CX 100 Interspec
    ultrasound m.

  Burdick ECG m.
  bypass m.
  Century heart-lung m.
  Cobe-Stöckert heart-lung m.
  Corometrics-Aloka
    echocardiograph m.
  G5 massage and percussion m.
  heart-lung m.
  Hewlett-Packard 500, 1000 Echo-
    Doppler m.
  May-Gibbon heart-lung m.
  Respironics CPAP m.
  Respitrace m.
  Sullivan V Elite Real Time Clock
    CPAP m.
  Toshiba electrocardiography m.
machinery murmur
Macintosh
  M. blade
  M. blade anesthesia
  M. laryngoscope
Mackenzie polygraph
Mackler tube
Macleod syndrome
MacNamara protocol
macroaggregated
  m. albumin (MAA)
  m. albumin perfusion lung
    scintigraphy
macroangiopathy
  coronary m.
Macrobid
macrocardia
Macrodantin
Macrodex
macroembolus
macroglobulin
  alpha-2 m.
macroglobulinemia
  Waldenström m.
macroglossia
macrolide
  m. antibiotic
  m. antimicrobial
  m. antimicrobial agent
macromolecular ligand
macromolecule
macrophage
  alveolar m.
  foamy m.
  hemosiderin-laden m.
  m. inflammatory protein (MPI)
  m. inflammatory protein-1 (MIP-1)
  lipid-laden m.
  tissue-infiltrating m. (TIM)

M

macroreentrant
- m. atrial tachycardia
- m. circuit

macrosteatosis

macrovascular
- m. artery disease
- m. coronary lesion

MACS
- maximum aortic cusp separation

Mac stent

macula, pl. **maculae**
- m. albida
- m. lactea
- m. tendinea

macular arteriole inferior

maculopapular rash

MAC-VU electrocardiograph

MAD
- mandibular advancement device

MadCAM-1
- mucosal addresin cell adhesion molecule-1

MADRS
- Montgomery-Asberg Depression Rating Scale

Maestro implantable cardiac pacemaker

MAF
- maximum atrial fragmentation

MAG
- Minnesota antilymphocyte globulin

Magellan monitor

Magic
- M. Torque guidewire
- M. Wallstent
- M. Wallstent stent

Magill
- M. forceps
- M. laryngoscope
- M. Safety Clear Plus endotracheal tube

magna
- arteria anastomotica auricularis m.
- auricularis m.

Magnascanner
- Picker M.

magnesium
- m. carbonate ($MgCO_3$)
- m. deficiency
- intracellular m.
- m. oxide
- m. salicylate
- serum m.
- m. sulfate
- m. sulfate heptahydrate
- m. supplementation

magnet
- m. application over pulse generator
- m. check
- m. inhibition

- m. pacing interval
- m. rate
- m. wire

magnetic
- m. heart vector (MHV)
- m. moment
- m. relaxation time
- m. resonance angiography (MRA, MSA)
- m. resonance coronary angiography (MRCA)
- m. resonance flowmetry (MRF)
- m. resonance imaging (MRI)
- m. resonance signal
- m. resonance spectography
- m. resonance spectroscopy (MRS)
- m. resonance venography (MRV)
- m. source imaging (MSI)
- m. valve resistor

magnetite pneumoconiosis

magnetization
- spatial modulation of m. (SPAMM)

magnetocardiogram (MCG)
- vector m. (VMCG)

magnetocardiograph (MC)

magnetocardiography (MC)
- fetal m. (FMCG)

Magnevist

magnification

magnitude
- average pulse m.
- peak m.

Magnolia biondii

Magnum guidewire

magnus
- pulsus m.

Magovern-Cromie ball-cage prosthetic valve

Mag-Ox 400

Mahaim
- M. bundle
- M. fiber

Mahaim-type tachycardia

Mahalanobis distance

Maharishi Vedic medicine

Mahler
- M. Baseline Dyspnea Index questionnaire
- M. sign

mahogany flush

MAI
- movement arousal index
- *Mycobacterium avium-intracellulare*
- MAI complex
- MAI infection

Maillard reaction

main
- m. adverse coronary event (MACE)
- m. bundle

left m. (LM)
m. portal vein (MPV)
m. pulmonary artery (MPA)
m. renal vein
m. stem bronchus
unprotected left m. (ULM)

mainstem
m. coronary artery
m. intubation

maintained
adequate hemostasis m.

major
m. adverse cardiac event (MACE)
m. aortopulmonary collateral artery
(MAPCA)
Babesia m.
m. coronary artery (MCA)
ductus sublingualis m.
m. fissure
pectoralis m.

malabsorption
maladie de Roger
malaise
malar flush
malaria
malariae
Plasmodium m.
malarial pneumonitis
malayi
Brugia m.
maleate
azatadine m.
chlorpheniramine m.
dexchlorpheniramine m.
enalapril m.
ergonovine m.
methysergide m.
nomifensine m.
timolol m.
trimipramine m.
male pattern obesity
malformation
angiographically occult intracranial
vascular m. (AOIVM)
arteriovenous m. (AVM)
atrioventricular m. (AVM)
congenital cardiovascular m.
(CCVM)
congenital cystic adenomatoid m.
conotruncal heart m. (CNTHM)
cystic adenomatoid m.
dural arteriovenous m. (DAVM)

Ebstein m.
isolated cardiovascular m. (ICM)
Mondini pulmonary
arteriovenous m.
neural crest m.
pulmonary arteriovenous m.
(PAVM)
Taussig-Bing m.
Uhl m.

malfunction
pacemaker m.

Malgaigne fossa
malignancy
cutaneous m.
de novo m.
mesenchymal m.
posttransplantation m.
primary cardiac m.

malignancy-associated
m.-a. change (MAC)
m.-a. phlebitis

malignant
m. arrhythmia (MA)
m. beat
m. carcinoid syndrome
m. endocarditis
m. fibrous histiocytoma (MFH)
m. hypertension (MH)
m. middle cerebral artery infarction
(mMCAI)
m. pleural effusion (MPE)
m. pleural mesothelioma (MPM)
m. superior vena caval syndrome
m. SVC syndrome
m. thrombocytopenia
m. vasovagal syndrome
m. ventricular arrhythmia (MVA)
m. ventricular tachyarrhythmia
m. ventricular tachycardia

malinger
malingerer
Mallampati
M. airway classification I-IV
M. score

Mallampati-Samsoon airway classification
I-IV
mall asthma
malleable retractor
Mallergan-VC with Codeine
Mallinckrodt
M. angiographic catheter

M

NOTES

Mallinckrodt (*continued*)
    M. cuffed endotracheal tube
    M. Hi-Care Pulmonary Hygiene
      system
    M. radioimmunoassay
Mallory stain
Mallory-Weiss
    M.-W. syndrome
    M.-W. tear
malmoense
    Mycobacterium m.
malnutrition
    alcoholic m.
    kwashiorkor-like m.
    myocardial m.
    protein-calorie m.
malondialdehyde (MDA)
    m. level
    m. modified low-density lipoprotein
      (MDA-LDL)
Maloney mercury-filled esophageal
  dilator
malonylcoenzyme A, malonyl-CoA
malperfused segment
malperfusion phenomenon
malpighian vesicle
malposition
    crisscross heart m.
    double-outlet left ventricle m.
    double-outlet right ventricle m.
    m. of great arteries (MGA)
    levocardia m.
    mesocardia m.
    single ventricle m.
maltase deficiency
Malteno valve
maltophilia
    Pseudallescheria m.
    Pseudomonas m.
    Stenotrophomonas m.
    Xanthomonas m.
malt worker's lung
malum cordis
mammary
    m. artery
    m. artery graft
    internal m. (IM)
    m. souffle
    m. souffle murmur
    m. souffle sound
man
    radiation equivalent in m. (rem)
management
    invasive m.
    postprocedural m.
    real-time position m. (RPM)
    ventilator m.
manager
    cardiological workspace m. (CWM)

mandatory
    m. minute volume (MMV)
    synchronized intermittent m.
mandibular
    m. advancement appliance (MAA)
    m. advancement device (MAD)
    m. plane to hyoid (MP-H)
mandibulopharyngeal
Mandol
mandrel, mandril
    m. graft
mandrin
maneuver
    Addison m.
    Adson m.
    breathhold m.
    cold pressor testing m.
    costoclavicular m.
    Ejrup m.
    forced expiratory m.
    head-tilt chin-lift m.
    Heimlich m.
    hemodynamic m.
    Hillis-Müller m.
    hyperventilation m.
    jaw-thrust/head-tilt m.
    Jonnson m.
    Lecompte m.
    Mattox m.
    Miller m.
    modified Miller m. (MM)
    Müller m.
    nonpanting m.
    panting m.
    peak expiratory m.
    Sellick m.
    submaximal m.
    Valsalva m. (VS)
maneuverability
manganese superoxide dismutase (Mn-
  SOD)
manidipine
manifest
    m. ischemia
    Morse m.
    m. vector
manifold
manipulation
    catheter m.
manmade vitreous fiber (MMVF)
mannequin
manner
    Creech m.
    m. of Creech
    m. of DeBakey
    DeBakey-Creech m.
Mannkopf sign
manofluorography (MFG)

manometer
> aneroid m.
> Dinamap ultrasound blood
> > pressure m.
>
> Hürthle m.
> Mercury medical airway
> > pressure m.
>
> Posey Cufflator tracheal cuff
> > inflator and m.
>
> single-patient use m.
> m.-tipped catheter

manometer-tipped catheter
manometry
> esophageal m.

Mansfield
> M. balloon
> M. bioptome
> M. orthogonal electrode catheter
> M. Polaris electrode
> M. Scientific dilatation balloon
> > catheter
>
> M. Valvuloplasty Registry

Mansfield-Webster catheter
mansoni
> *Schistosoma m.*

Mantoux test
manual
> M. defibrillator
> M. edge detection
> M. resuscitation baffle
> M. resuscitation bag
> M. ventilation

manubrium
MAO
> monoamine oxidase
> MAO inhibitor

MAOI
> monoamine oxidase inhibitor

MAP
> mean airway pressure
> mean aortic pressure
> mean arterial pressure
> minimum audible pressure
> mitogen-activated protein
> monophasic action potential

map
> electroanatomical m.
> linear local shortening m.
> maximum voltage m.
> polar coordinate m.

MAPCA
> major aortopulmonary collateral artery

MAPD
> monophasic action potential duration

MAPK
> mitogen-activated protein kinase
> MAPK pathway

maple bark disease
mapping
> activation sequence m.
> advanced cardiac m.
> atrial activation m.
> Biosense left ventricular m.
> body surface laplacian m. (BSLM)
> bull's-eye polar coordinate m.
> cardiac m.
> catheter m.
> m. catheter
> cavotricuspid isthmus m.
> color-coded flow m.
> color flow m.
> digital phase m. (DPM)
> Doppler color flow m. (DCFM)
> electromagnetic m.
> electromechanical left ventricular m.
> electrophysiologic m.
> endocardial m.
> entrainment m.
> EP m.
> flow m.
> high-density electroanatomical and
> > entrainment m.
>
> ice m.
> intracardiac m.
> intraoperative m.
> Laplacian m.
> MRI velocity m.
> multisite m.
> noncontact endocardial m.
> pulsed-wave Doppler m.
> retrograde atrial activation m.
> Revelation microcatheter for EP m.
> simultaneous catheter m.
> spectral temporal m.
> spectral turbulence m.
> tachycardia pathway m.
> ventricular m.

mapping/ablation catheter
maprotiline
MAQOL
> Mini Asthma Quality of Life
> MAQOL questionnaire

MAR algorithm

M

NOTES

marantic
    m. endocarditis
    m. thrombosis
    m. thrombus
marasmic
    m. thrombosis
    m. thrombus
marasmus
Marathon guiding catheter
Marax bronchodilator
Marbach-Weil technique
Marburg virus
marcescens
    Serratia m.
Marcillin
Marek disease
Marey law
Marfan syndrome
margarine
    Benecol m.
    sitostanol ester m.
Margesic H
margin
    costal m.
    rib m.
    right costal m. (RCM)
marginal
    m. artery of colon
    m. artery of Drummond
    m. branch #1
    m. branch of the circumflex artery
      (CFX-MARG)
    m. circumflex artery
    left m. (LM)
    obtuse m. (OM)
    m. rale
marginatum
    erythema m.
margo
    m. anterior pulmonis
    m. inferior pulmonis
Marie-Bamberger syndrome
Marie syndrome
marine oil
Marinol
marinum
    Mycobacterium m.
Marion-Clatworthy side-to-end vena caval shunt
mark
    alignment m.
    M. IV respiratory pacemaker
    M. VII cooling vest
    M. V ProVis injection system
marked dullness (M2)
marker
    m. annotation
    breath m.
    m. catheter

    CD63 platelet activation m.
    CD62p (p-selectin) platelet
      activation m.
    m. channel
    CYFRA 21-1 tumor m.
    dual m.
    gold m.
    inflammatory m.
    lead-letter m.
    plaque m.
    predictive survival m.
    radiopaque end m.
    Recath bypass graft m.
    serum m.
    tumor m.
    vein graft ring m.
marking
    bronchial m.
    bronchovesicular m.
    interstitial m.
    lung m.
    perihilar m.
    pulmonary vascular m.
    vascular m.
Markov process
Marlex mesh
marmorata
    cutis m.
marneffei
    Penicillium m.
Maroteaux-Lamy syndrome
Marpres
Marquest Respirgard II nebulizer
Marquette
    M. Case-12 electrocardiographic
      system
    M. Case-12 exercise system
    M. electrocardiograph
    M. 8000 Holter monitor
    M. Holter recorder
    M. Responder 1500 multifunctional
      defibrillator
    M. Series 8000 Holter analyzer
    M. three-channel laser Holter
    M. treadmill
Marriott method
Marshall
    M. bundle
    M. fold
    M. ligament
    M. oblique vein
marsupialization
Marsupial Pouch postsurgical drain holder
Martorell syndrome
Mary Allen Engle ventricle
MAS
    meconium aspiration syndrome

mesoatrial shunt
Motor Assessment Scale
Masimo Set
mask
 Accurox m.
 ACE detachable m.
 AeroChamber m.
 AirMed m.
 Bili m.
 BLB oxygen m.
 Boothby-Lovelace-Bulbulian
  oxygen m.
 ComfortSeal m.
 EasiVent valved holding
  chamber m.
 ecchymotic m.
 GoldSeal nasal m.
 IQ nasal m.
 Kuhn m.
 LMA-Unique laryngeal m.
 meter m.
 MiniMe nasal m.
 Mirage nasal m.
 Nasal-Aire ventilator nasal
  insert m.
 Nic the Dragon aerosol m.
 nonrebreather m.
 nonrebreathing m.
 oxygen m.
 partial rebreathing m.
 PEP m.
 Phantom nasal m.
 RBS face m.
 rebreathing m.
 Rendell-Baker face m.
 Rudolph Full Face m.
 SCRAM face m.
 Series 7900 mouth breathing
  face m.
 Series 8900 nasal and mouth
  breathing face m.
 Sullivan Mirage nasal m.
 thermoplastic head m.
 Ultimate nasal m.
 Venti m.
 ventilation m.
 Venturi m.
 Vickers Ventimask Mark 2 m.
masked hypertension
mask-mode
 m.-m. cardiac imaging
 m.-m. subtraction

Mason-Likar
 M.-L. 12-lead ECG system
 M.-L. limb lead modification
 M.-L. placement of ECG lead
mason's lung
mass
 achromatic m.
 cardiac m.
 echodense m.
 echogenic m.
 m. effect
 false m.
 fat-free m. (FFM)
 fibrotic m.
 fungating m.
 intracardiac m.
 intracavity m.
 intravascular m. (IVM)
 left ventricular m. (LVM)
 lung m.
 m. median aerodynamic diameter
  (MMAD)
 myocardial m.
 pleural m.
 ventricular m.
 volumic m.
massage
 cardiac m.
 carotid sinus m.
 closed chest cardiac m.
 direct cardiac m.
 external cardiac m. (ECM)
 heart m.
 open chest cardiac m.
 vapor m.
mass-flow anemometer
Massier solution
massive
 m. aspiration
 m. collapse
 m. pneumonia
 m. thrombus
Masson
 M. body
 M. trichrome stain
MAST
 military antishock trousers
mast
 m. cell
 m. cell inhibitor
 m. cell protease
Mastadenovirus

NOTES

master
    change description m. (CDM)
    M. exercise stress test
    M. Flow Pumpette pump
    M. two-step exercise test
MasterLab Pro pneumotachograph spirometer
MasterScreen BabyBody plethysmograph
mastocytosis syndrome
MAT
    multifocal atrial tachycardia
Matas
    M. aneurysmectomy
    M. test
match defect
matching
    afterload m.
    ventilation/perfusion m.
material
    Carbo-Seal graft m.
    contrast m.
    Duralyn balloon m.
    embolized foreign m.
    fibrinohematic m.
    Haynes 25 m.
    Hexabrix contrast m.
    Kaltostat wound packing m.
    Kifa catheter m.
    low osmolality contrast m. (LOCM)
    MycroMesh graft m.
    Myoview contrast m.
    nonionic contrast m.
    Soludrast contrast m.
    vasodepressor m. (VDEM, VDM)
    vasoexcitor m. (VEM)
    Zenotech graft m.
maternal heart rate (MHR)
maternally inherited cardiomyopathy
matrix, pl. **matrices**
    extracellular m. (ECM)
    m. metalloproteinase (MMP)
    m. metalloproteinase inhibitor (MMPI)
    m. mode
    myocardial collagen m.
    subendothelial m.
    m. synthesis
    vascular m.
matrix-degrading
    m.-d. neutral metalloproteinase
    m.-d. neutral MMP
Matson-Alexander rib stripper
Matson rib elevator
Matsuda titanium surgical instrument
matter
    white m. (WM)

Mattox
    M. aorta clamp
    M. maneuver
mattress
    eggcrate m.
    hypothermia m.
    Roho m.
    m. suture
    TheraKair m.
maturation
    affinity m.
Maugeri syndrome
MAVD
    mixed aortic valve disease
Maverick
    M. 2 Monorail M.
    M. OTW catheter
Mavik
MAVIS
    mobile artery and vein imaging system
MAVR
    mitral and aortic valve replacement
max
    maximum
        VO_2 max
            maximum oxygen consumption
Maxair Inhalation Aerosol
Maxaquin Oral
MaxEPA
MaxForce balloon dilatation catheter
Maxi LD PTA dilation catheter
Maxilith pacemaker pulse generator
maxillomandibular
    m. advancement (MMA)
    m. advancement procedure
    m. osteotomy (MMO)
maximal
    m. breathing capacity
    m. exercise systolic pressure (MESP)
    m. exercise test (MET)
    m. expiratory flow rate (MEFR)
    m. expiratory flow volume (MEFV)
    m. expiratory mouth pressure (P_{Emax})
    m. expiratory pressure (MEP)
    m. flow-volume envelope (MFVL)
    m. forced expiratory flow (FEFmax)
    m. heart rate (Hrmax, MHR)
    m. inspiratory flow rate (MIFR)
    m. inspiratory mouth pressure (P_{Imax})
    m. inspiratory pressure (MIP)
    m. midexpiratory flow (MMEF, MMF)
    m. midexpiratory flow rate (MMEFR)

m. resistive exercise (MRE)
m. response plateau (MRP)
m. sniff-induced esophageal pressure
m. sniff-induced gastric pressure
m. sniff-induced transdiaphragmatic pressure
m. sustainable ventilatory capacity (MSVC)
m. treadmill stress test (MTST)
m. treadmill test
m. treadmill testing (MTT)
m. velocity (V_{MAX}, Vmax)
m. ventilation (MV)
m. ventilation rate (MVR)
m. vital capacity (MVC)

Maxima Plus plasma resistant fiber oxygenator

maximum (max)
m. aerobic capacity
m. aortic cusp separation (MACS)
m. atrial fragmentation (MAF)
m. breathing capacity (MBC)
m. closure pressure (MCP)
m. contraction pattern (MCP)
m. determined heart rate (MDHR)
m. diastolic potential (MDP)
m. digital pulse (MDP)
m. exercise tolerance test (METT)
m. expiratory airflow-static lung elastic recoil pressure (MFSR)
m. expiratory flow at 50% vital capacity (MEF_{50})
m. expiratory pressure (MEP)
m. flow rate
m. flow-volume loop (MFVL)
M. hemostasis introducer
m. inspiratory pressure (MIP)
m. left ventricular pressure (LVPmax)
m. medical therapy
m. midexpiratory flow rate (MMEF, MMF)
m. negative potential
m. oxygen consumption (VO_2 max)
m. oxygen uptake
m. predicted heart rate (MPHR)
m. pulse rate (MPR)
m. sensory rate
m. tolerated dose (MTD)
m. transverse thoracic dimension
m. velocity (V_{MAX}, Vmax)

m. venous outflow (MVO)
m. ventricular elastance (Emax)
m. voltage map
m. voluntary contraction (MVC)
m. voluntary ventilation (MVV)
m. walking time

Maxi-Myst vaporizer
Maxipime
maxi-vessel loops
Maxzide
Mayaro virus
Mayer wave
May-Gibbon heart-lung machine
May-Grünwald-Giemsa stain
Mayo
M. classification
M. exercise treadmill protocol
M. hemostat

maze
m. ablation
m. III surgery
m. procedure

Mazicon
mazindol
hydrogen-3 m.

MB
microbubble
myocardial band
myocardial bridging
MB band
MB enzymes of CPK
MB fraction
MB index

MBA hemostasis valve
MBAR
myocardial beta adrenergic receptor
MBC
maximum breathing capacity
MBF
myocardial blood flow
MBIP
model-based image processing
MBP
mean arterial blood pressure
mean blood pressure
MBPM
modified backward Prony method
MBq
megabecquerel
MBTS
modified Blalock-Taussig shunt

M

NOTES

MBV
  mitral balloon valvotomy
MC
  magnetocardiograph
  magnetocardiography
  microcirculation
  mitral commissurotomy
  myocardial channeling
  myocarditis
Mc
  mitral closure
MCA
  major coronary artery
  middle cerebral artery
MCAF
  monocyte chemotactic and activating
   factor
MCAO
  middle cerebral artery occlusion
McArdle
    M. disease
    M. syndrome
MCAS modular clip application
MCC
  microcalcification cluster
  mucociliary clearance
MCCD
  minimum cumulative cardiotoxic dose
McCort sign
MCCU
  mobile coronary care unit
MCD
  molecular coincidence detection
    MCD imaging
McDowall reflex
MCE
  myocardial contrast echocardiography
MCES
  multiple cholesterol emboli syndrome
MCF
  myocardial contraction force
MCFSR
  mean circumferential fiber-shortening
   rate
MCG
  magnetocardiogram
McGill
    M. forceps
    M. Pain Questionnaire
McGill-Melzack Pain Questionnaire
McGinn-White sign
McGoon
    M. guidelines
    M. technique
McHenry protocol
MCI
  mean cardiac index
mCi
  millicurie

MCICU
  medical coronary intensive care unit
MCL
  midclavicular line
  modified chest lead
McNamara
    M. protocol
    M. renal exchange wire guide
McNaught keel
MCP
  maximum closure pressure
  maximum contraction pattern
  monocyte chemoattractant protein
  mucin clot prevention
MCP-1
  monocyte chemoattractant protein-1
  monocyte chemotactic protein-1
McPheeters treatment
MC4-R
  melanocortin-4 receptor
MCRI
  multifactorial cardiac risk index
MCT
  methylcholine challenge testing
    MCT Oil
MCV
  mean corpuscular volume
MD
  mitral disease
  myocardial damage
  myocardial disease
MDA
  malondialdehyde
MDA-LDL
  malondialdehyde modified low-density
   lipoprotein
MDBP
  mean resting diastolic blood pressure
MDCM
  mildly dilated congestive cardiomyopathy
MDCT
  multidetector computed tomography
M/D 4 defibrillator system
MDE
  minimum defibrillation energy
MDEBP
  mean daily erect blood pressure
MDF
  myocardial depressant factor
MDG
  mean diastolic gradient
MDHR
  maximum determined heart rate
MDI
  metered-dose inhaler
  methylene diphenyl diisocyanate
    MDI kit
    MDI spacer

MDILog
  M. microelectronic monitor
  M. therapy monitoring device
MDM
  middiastolic murmur
MDP
  maximum diastolic potential
  maximum digital pulse
  methylene diphosphonate
MDR
  multidrug-resistant
MDRSP
MDR-TB
  multidrug-resistant tuberculosis
MDS
  minimum data set
  myocardial depressant substance
  MDS system
MDSBP
  mean daily supine blood pressure
MDUO
  myocardial disease of unknown origin
MDV
  myocardial Doppler velocity
MDW
  monophasic defibrillation waveform
mEAD
  monophasic action potential early
  afterdepolarization
Meadows syndrome
Meadox
  M. graft
  M. graft sizer
  M. Teflon felt pledget
  M. woven velour prosthesis
meal
  high-fat m.
mean
  m. airway pressure (MAP)
  m. aortic pressure (MAP)
  arterial m.
  m. arterial blood pressure (MABP, MBP)
  m. arterial pressure (MAP)
  m. atrial rate
  m. atrial rate algorithm
  m. blood pressure (MBP)
  m. cardiac index (MCI)
  m. circumferential fiber-shortening rate (MCFSR)
  m. contrast enhancement
  m. corpuscular volume (MCV)

m. daily erect blood pressure (MDEBP)
m. daily supine blood pressure (MDSBP)
m. diastolic gradient (MDG)
m. diastolic left ventricular pressure
m. electrical axis
m. forced midexpiratory flow
m. inspiratory flow (MIF)
m. intravascular pressure (MIP)
m. left atrial pressure (MLAP)
m. luminal diameter (MLD)
m. manifest vector
m. maternal arterial blood pressure (MMAP)
m. midexpiratory flow rate ($FEF_{25-75\%}$)
m. nocturnal saturation
m. normalized systolic ejection rate
m. pressure (PM)
m. pulmonary arterial (MPA)
m. pulmonary artery pressure (MPAP, PAPm)
m. pulmonary artery wedge pressure (MPAWP)
m. pulmonary venous pressure (MPVP)
m. QRS axis
m. rate ejection index (MREI)
m. reference diameter (MRD)
m. resting diastolic blood pressure (MDBP)
m. right atrial pressure (MRAP)
right ventricular m. (RVM)
m. right ventricular pressure (MRVP)
m. systemic arterial pressure (MSAP)
m. systolic ejection rate (MSER)
m. systolic left ventricular pressure
MEANS
  modular electrocardiogram analysis system
Means-Lernan mediastinal crunch
measles pneumonia
measure
  adjunctive m.
  ancillary m.
  CD4+ m.
  functional independence m. (FIM)

M

NOTES

measured
    m. data
    m. output
measurement
    automated cardiac flow m. (ACM)
    automated cardiac output m.
      (ACOM, AcomA)
    automatic systolic blood
      pressure m. (ABP)
    blood flow m.
    cardiac output m.
    coronary blood flow m.
    Doppler m.
    gas clearance m.
    hemodynamic m.
    invasive pressure m.
    M-mode m.
    morphometric m.
    nonpanting m.
    physiologic m.
    PR-AC m.
    pressure m.
    quantitative coronary angiography
      caliper m.
    Reid index m.
    spectral Doppler velocity m.
    splenic perfusion m.
    TDCO m.
    thermodilution m.
    transstenotic pressure gradient m.
    venous flow m.
measuring
    sinus node recovery time,
      direct m. (SNRTd)
    sinus node recovery time,
      indirect m. (SNRTi)
meat, eggs, dairy, invisible fat,
  condiments, snacks (MEDICS)
meat-wrapper's asthma
mebendazole
mecamylamine hydrochloride
mechanical
    m. alternation
    m. alternation of heart
    m. cardiopulmonary resuscitation
    m. contractile function
    m. cough
    m. debulking
    m. dyssynchrony
    m. heart
    m. myocardial channeling (MMC)
    m. obstruction
    m. pleurodesis
    m. prosthesis
    m. thrombectomy
    m. trauma
    m. valve
    m. VAS
    m. ventilation (MV)

    m. ventilatory support
    m. ventricular assistance (MVA)
    m. ventricular assist device
      (MVAD)
    m. visual analogue scale
mechanics
    fluid m.
    lung m.
mechanic's bronchitis
mechanism
    m. of action
    blood-clotting m. (BCM)
    compensatory m.
    coronary steal m.
    deglutition m.
    fixation m.
    Frank-Starling m.
    gating m.
    ionic m.
    Laplace m.
    peeling-back m.
    pinchcock m.
    postsynaptic cholinergic m.
    reentrant m.
    sinus m.
    Starling m.
    steal m.
    triggering m.
    vertical deceleration m.
    wave-speed m.
mechanocardiography
mechanoelectrical feedback
mechanoreceptor
mechanoreflex
mechanosensor
mechanotransduction
mechlorethamine hydrochloride
meclofenamate sodium
meconium
    m. aspiration
    m. aspiration syndrome (MAS)
    m. ileus
Medex
    M. coronary C1 stent
    M. transducer
MedGraphics
    M. Breeze PF software
    M. Cardio O2 system
    M. CPE 2000 electronically braked
      bicycle
    M. CPX/D metabolic cart
    M. model 1085 body
      plethysmograph
media (*pl. of* medium)
medial
    m. basal branch of pulmonary
      artery
    m. inferior artery of knee
    m. medullary infarction (MMI)

m. necrosis
m. superior artery of knee
m. surface of lung
m. tear

mediale

segmentum bronchopulmonale
basale m.

medialis

arteria genus superior m.

median

left m. (LM)
m. nerve injury
m. sternotomy
m. sternotomy incision
m. survival time (MST)

medianus

ramus m.

mediastinal

m. adenopathy
m. amyloidosis
m. crunch
m. emphysema
m. fibrosis
m. flutter
m. lymph node
m. lymph node biopsy
m. part of lung
m. pleura
m. pleurisy
m. shadow
m. shift
m. space
m. sump filter
m. thickening
m. wedge
m. widened
m. widening

mediastinale

septum m.

mediastinalis

pleura m.

mediastinitis

acute m.
descending necrotizing m. (DNM)
fibrosing m.
fibrous m.
granulomatous m.

mediastinoscope

Goldberg-MPC m.

mediastinoscopy

Chamberlain m.

mediastinotomy

mediastinum

superior vascular m.

mediator

inflammatory m.
pyrogenic m.
m. receptor antagonist
vasoactive m.

MedicAIR

M. Plus spirometer
M. Plus spirometry station

medical

m. coronary intensive care unit
(MCICU)
M. Graphics Cardiopulmonary
Exercise System 2001
M. Graphics pneumotachograph
with volume integrator
m. intensive care unit (MICU)
Quest M.
M. Research Council questionnaire

medicamentosa

rhinitis m.

medication

antiarrhythmic m.
bolus of m.
m. monitoring event system
(MEMS)
mucoactive m.
presyncopal m.
m. use evaluation (MUE)

medicinalis

Hirudo m.

medicine

American College of Sports M.
(ACSM)
digital imaging and communications
in m. (DICOM)
evidence-based m. (EBM)
Kampo m.
Maharishi Vedic m.
Society of Nuclear M. (SNM)

Medicon rib spreader
Medicopaste bandage
MEDICS

meat, eggs, dairy, invisible fat,
condiments, snacks

Medi-Facts system
Medigraphics 2000 analyzer
**Medilog 4000 ambulatory ECG
recorder**
Medinol NIR stent
mediolysis

M

NOTES

medionecrosis
> m. of aorta
> m. aortae
> m. aortae idiopathica cystica

MediPort
Medi-Strumpf stockings
meditation
Medi-Tech
> M.-T. balloon catheter
> M.-T. catheter system
> M.-T. multipurpose basket
> M.-T. steerable catheter
> M.-T. wire

Mediterranean
> M. anemia
> M. diet
> M. Diet Pyramid
> M. fever

medium, pl. **media**
> Adenoscan contrast m.
> Amipaque contrast m.
> Angio-Conray contrast m.
> aortic tunica media
> arterial media
> m. chain triglycerides
> Conray contrast m.
> contrast m.
> Eagle m.
> fibrinolytic m.
> iothalamate meglumine contrast m.
> ioxaglate meglumine contrast m.
> Isovue contrast m.
> Joklik m.
> Lowenstein m.
> low osmolality contrast media (LOCM)
> metrizamide contrast m.
> nonionic contrast m.
> Optiray contrast m.
> SHU-454 contrast m.
> SonoVue ultrasound contrast media
> media thickness
> Urografin-76 contrast m.

Medivent
> M. self-expanding coronary stent
> M. vascular stent

Medlar body
MedNova NeuroShield cerebral protection system
Medos mechanical circulatory support system
medoxomil
> olmesartan m.

Medrad Mark IV angiographic injector
Medrol
> M. Dosepak
> M. Oral
> M. Vederm Cream

medroxyprogesterone
> m. acetate (MPA)
> estrogen and m.
> estrogen, m.

Medtronic
> M. Activa tremor control therapy device
> M. Activitrax rate-responsive unipolar ventricular pacemaker
> M. AneuRx stent graft
> M. AVE S660 coronary stent
> M. BeStent stent
> M. bipolar pacemaker
> M. cardiac cooling jacket
> M. Cardiorhythm Atakr II RF ablation system
> M. connector
> M. defibrillator implant support device
> M. Elite DDDR pacemaker
> M. Elite II pacemaker
> M. Evergreen balloon
> M. external cardioverter-defibrillator
> M. external tachyarrhythmia control device
> M. Gem automatic implantable defibrillator
> M. Hancock II tissue valve
> M. Hemopump
> M. Hemopump cardiac assist device
> M. Hemopump system
> M. Inspire implantable device
> M. Intact bioprosthetic valve
> M. Intact porcine bioprosthesis
> M. Interactive Tachycardia Terminating system
> M. interventional vascular stent
> M. Jewel AF 7250 dual-chamber implantable cardioverter-defibrillator
> M. Jewel AF implantable arrhythmia management device
> M. Jewel 7219D and C device
> M. Kappa 400 pacemaker
> M. lead
> M. Micro Jewel II implantable defibrillator
> M. Mosaic bioprosthetic valve
> M. Octopus tissue stabilizing device
> M. Octopus 2+ tissue stabilizing system
> M. PCD implantable cardioverter-defibrillator
> M. pulse generator
> M. Pulsor Intrasound pain reliever
> M. radiofrequency receiver
> M. SynchroMed pump
> M. temporary pacemaker

M. Thera DR pacemaker
M. Thera i-series cardiac
  pacemaker
M. tip
M. Zuma guiding catheter
Medtronic-Hall
  M.-H. device
  M.-H. heart valve prosthesis
  M.-H. monocuspid tilting-disk valve
  M.-H. prosthetic heart valve
  M.-H. tilting-disk valve prosthesis
Medtronic-Hancock device
medulla, pl. **medullae**
  adrenal m.
  m. oblongata
  rostral ventrolateral m. (RVLM)
  rostral ventromedial m. (RVMM)
  ventrolateral m. (VLM)
medullary collecting duct
medusae
  caput m.
Med-Xcor stent
MEF$_{50}$
  maximum expiratory flow at 50% vital
  capacity
mefenamic acid
mefloquine hydrochloride
Mefoxin
MEFR
  maximal expiratory flow rate
MEFV
  maximal expiratory flow volume
megabecquerel (MBq)
megacardia
Megace
megaelectron volt (MeV)
megaesophagus
megahertz (MHz)
megaloblastic anemia
megalocardia
MegaSonics PTCA catheter
megaterium
  Bacillus m.
megaunit (MU)
megestrol acetate
meglumine
  intracoronary sonicated m.
  ioxaglate m.
Meier-Magnum system
Meigs syndrome
meizothrombin

melaninogenica
  Prevotella m.
melaninogenicus
  Bacteroides m.
melanocortin-4 receptor (MC4-R)
melanoderma cachecticorum
melanoma
  Clark classification of malignant m.
  m. inhibitory activity (MIA)
  m. inhibitory activity protein
melanotic carcinoma
melena
melenic stool
melioidosis
melitensis
  Brucella m.
Mellaril
mellitus
  diabetes m. (DM)
  insulin-dependent diabetes m.
    (IDDM)
  noninsulin-dependent diabetes m.
    (NIDDM)
melphalan
Melrose solution
Meltzer
  M. method
  M. sign
Melzack-Wall gate theory
membranacea
  angina m.
  pars m.
membranaceous
membrana fibroelastica laryngis
membrane
  adventitious m.
  alveolar-capillary m.
  alveolar hyaline m.
  alveolocapillary m.
  antibasement m.
  m. attack complex (MAC)
  basement m.
  bronchial mucous m.
  brush border m. (BBM)
  cell m.
  m. channel
  cricothyroid m.
  cuprophane m.
  m. current
  Debove m.
  m. diffusing capacity (Dm)
  external elastic m. (EEM)

M

NOTES

membrane *(continued)*
    Gore-Tex surgical m.
    Henle elastic m.
    Henle fenestrated m.
    Hybond ECL nitrocellulose m.
    internal elastic m. (IEM)
    polyacrylonitrile m.
    m. potential
    Preclude pericardial m.
    m. rupture
    sarcolemmal m.
    schneiderian respiratory m.
    serous m.
    m. stabilization
    suprapleural m.
    syncytiovascular m. (SVM)
membrane-bound membrane-type metalloproteinase (MT-MMP)
membrane-stabilizing activity
membranotomy
    transatrial m. (TM)
membranous
    m. bronchitis
    m. croup
    m. laryngitis
    m. obstruction of inferior vena cava (MOVC)
    m. obstruction of the inferior vena cava (MOIVC)
    m. pharyngitis
    m. pulmonary atresia
    m. septum
    m. wall of trachea
memory
    cardiac m.
    m. catheter
    m. impairment
    m. loop
Memotherm stent
MEMS
    medication monitoring event system
Menadol
mendelian disorder
Mendelson syndrome
Menghini needle
Ménière syndrome
meningeal coccidioidomycosis
meningitic respiration
meningitidis
    Neisseria m.
meningitis, pl. **meningitides**
    anthrax m.
    HSV m.
    Mollaret m.
meningococcal
    m. pericarditis
    m. vaccine
meningococcemia
meningococcus

meningoencephalitis
meningotheloid nodule
meniscus, pl. **menisci**
    intracavitary air m.
menopause
mental
    m. clouding
    m. status
    m. stress
    m. stress-induced ischemia
MEP
    maximal expiratory pressure
    maximum expiratory pressure
    motor provoked potential
meperidine hydrochloride
mephentermine
Mephyton Oral
mepivacaine hydrochloride
Mepron
mEq
    milliequivalent
MER
    murmur/energy ratio
meralluride
mercaptomerin sodium
6-mercaptopurine
Mercator atrial high-density array catheter
Mercuhydrin
mercury (Hg)
    M. medical airway pressure manometer
    millimeter of m. (mmHg)
    m. poisoning
    m. vapor
mercury-in-rubber strain gauge plethysmograph
mercury-in-Silastic strain gauge
mercury-195m (^{195m}Hg)
Merendino technique
Meridia
meridian
    m. echocardiogram
    m. echocardiography
    M. pacemaker
meridional wall stress
merodiastolic
meromyosin
meropenem for injection
merosystolic
Merrem IV
Mersilene braided nonabsorbable suture
MES
    microembolic signal
mesangial
    m. cell
    m. immune injury
    m. proliferative glomerulonephritis
mesangium

mesaortitis
mesarteritis
    Mönckeberg m.
mesenchymal
    m. cap
    m. intimal cell
    m. malignancy
mesenchymal-derived tumor
mesenchyme
mesenteric
    m. angiography
    m. arteritis
    m. artery
    m. artery occlusion
    m. bypass graft
    m. ischemia
    m. vascular occlusion
mesentery of lung
mesh
    m. stent
    tantalum m.
mesna
mesoatrial shunt (MAS)
mesocardia malposition
mesocardium
    arterial m.
    dorsal m.
    lateral m.
mesocaval shunt
mesoderm
    precardiac m.
mesodermal tumor
mesodiastolic
mesophlebitis
mesopneumonium
mesopulmonum
mesosystolic
mesothelial
    m. cell
    m. tumor
mesothelioma
    benign fibrous m.
    biphasic m.
    desmoplastic m.
    diffuse malignant pleural m.
     (DMPM)
    epithelioid m.
    malignant pleural m. (MPM)
    pleural m.
    sarcomatoid m.
MESP
    maximal exercise systolic pressure

messenger
    m. ribonucleic acid (mRNA)
    second m.
Messerklinger endoscope
Mestinon
mesylate
    bitolterol m.
    deferoxamine m.
    Desferal M.
    dihydroergotamine m.
    doxazosin m.
    gemifloxacin m.
    phentolamine m.
    saquinavir m.
    tirilazad m.
MET
    maximal exercise test
    metabolic equivalent of task
    multistage exercise test
     estimated MET
Meta
    M. DDDR pacemaker
    M. II pacemaker
    M. MV pacemaker
    M. rate-responsive pacemaker
metaanalysis
metabolator
metabolic
    m. acidosis
    m. alkalosis
    m. cart
    m. encephalopathy
    m. equivalent
    m. equivalent of task (MET)
    m. parameter determination
    m. rate meter
    m. syncope
    m. syndrome
    m. vasodilatory capacity
metabolism
    aerobic m.
    anaerobic m.
    arachidonate m.
    cerebral rate of glucose m.
     (CMR_{glc})
    cerebral rate of oxygen m.
     ($CMRO_2$)
    extracellular matrix m.
    glucose m. (rMRGlu)
    myocardial m.
    oxidative m.

M

NOTES

metabolism *(continued)*
    respiratory m.
    substrate m.
metabolite
    arachidonic acid m.
    bilirubin oxidative m.
    m. correction
    prostacyclin m.
metaboreceptor
metaboreflex
    muscle m.
    m. response
metachronous lung cancer
metadata
metaiodobenzylguanidine (MIBG)
    I-123 m.
    I-125 m.
metal
    m. fume fever (MFF)
    heavy m.
    m. sewing ring
    trace m.
metallic
    m. breath sounds
    m. click
    m. echo
    m. oxide fumes
    m. rale
    m. tinkle
metalloproteinase
    m. inhibitor
    matrix m. (MMP)
    matrix-degrading neutral m.
    membrane-bound membrane-type m.
      (MT-MMP)
    tissue inhibitor of m. (TIMP)
    tissue inhibitor of m.-3 (TIMP-3)
metamorphosing respiration
metam sodium
metamyelocyte
MetaPhor agarose
metaplasia
    cellular m.
    goblet cell m.
    peribronchiolar m.
metaplastic mucus-secreting cell
metapneumonic
    m. empyema
    m. pleurisy
metaproterenol
    Arm-a-Med M.
    Dey-Dose M.
    m. sulfate
metaraminol bitartrate
metarteriole
metastasectomy
    pulmonary m.
metastasis, pl. **metastases**
    cannonball metastases

    cardiac m.
    contact m.
    hematogenous m.
    implantation m.
    tumor, node, m. (TNM)
metastatic
    m. calcification
    m. carcinoid syndrome
    m. carcinoma
    m. disease
    m. nodule
    m. phenotype
    m. pneumonia
    m. sarcoma
metazoal myocarditis
Metenix
metenkephalin
meter
    ExacTech blood glucose m.
    m. mask
    metabolic rate m.
    MicroRint portable airway
      resistance m.
    MultiSPIRO The Peak peak
      flow m.
    OxySAT oxygen saturation m.
    m. per second (m/s, m/sec)
    m. per second squared (m/s^2)
    pH M.
    ventilation m.
metered-dose
    m.-d. inhaler (MDI)
    m.-d. spray
metered-solution inhaler (MSI)
metformin
methacholine
    m. bronchoprovocation challenge
    m. challenge test
    m. chloride
    m. reaction
    m. reactivity
    m. response
    reversal speed of
      bronchoconstriction in response
      to m. (r-Sm)
    speed of bronchoconstriction in
      response to m. (Sm)
methamphetamine hydrochloride
methanesulfonanilide derivative
methanesulfonate
    phentolamine m.
methemoglobin
methemoglobinemia
methicillin-sensitive right-sided
  endocarditis
methicillin sodium
methimazole
methionine loading

method

Alfieri m.
Allain m.
Anderson-Keys m.
Antyllus m.
area-length m.
Arvidsson dimension-length m.
atrial extrastimulus m.
biplane area-length m.
Bland-Altman m.
body box m.
Bohr isopleth m.
Bonferroni m.
Brasdor m.
Brisbane m.
Brown-Dodge m.
Burow quantitative m.
Carrel m.
catheter introduction m.
Cavalieri m.
Celermajer m.
chromogenic m.
Clauss m.
closed circuit m.
conductance catheter m.
constant-flow m.
Cribier m.
Cutler-Ederer m.
cyanmethemoglobin m.
cyanogen bromide m.
Danielson m.
DBCL m.
Defares rebreathing m.
Devereux-Reichek m.
digital color Doppler velocity
  integration m.
digitized caliper m.
Dodge area-length m.
Douglas bag collection m.
Dow m.
downstream sampling m.
dye-dilution m.
dynamic m.
edge-detection m.
Eggleston m.
Eicken m.
estimated Fick m.
Eve m.
Fick oxygen m.
flow convergence m.
forward-backward Prony m.
  (FBPM)

forward triangle m.
Galanti-Giusti colorimetric m.
Gärtner m.
gas clearance m.
Gräupner m.
half-time m.
Hanley-McNeil m.
Hatle m.
head-tilt m.
Heinecke m.
helium dilution m.
heparin assay rapid m. (HARM)
heparin assay rapid easy m.
  (HAREM)
Howard m.
immunometric sandwich m.
indicator dilution m.
indocyanine green m.
Ionescu m.
Jaffe m.
Kales scoring m.
Kaplan-Meier m.
Kasser-Kennedy m.
Kennedy area-length m.
Kety-Schmidt m.
King biopsy m.
Kirkorian-Touboul m.
Kirstein m.
Konno biopsy m.
Laborde m.
Laurell m.
Lee-White m.
Lown and Woolf m.
Marriott m.
Meltzer m.
modified backward Prony m.
  (MBPM)
Monte Carlo multiway sensitivity
  analysis m.
Murphy m.
Narula m.
Ogata m.
Oliver-Rosalki m.
open circuit m.
Orsi-Grocco m.
oxygen step-up m.
Pachon m.
Penaz volume-clamp m.
Penn m.
phenylephrine ramp m.
planimetry m.
polarographic m.

M

NOTES

method *(continued)*
    prick-test m.
    prism m.
    Prony m. (PM)
    proximal flow convergence m.
    pulse m.
    Purmann m.
    pyramid m.
    m. of Quinones
    Rackley m.
    Raff-Glantz derivative m.
    rebreathing m.
    Rechtschaffen scoring m.
    Roche-Microwell plate
      hybridization m.
    root inclusion m.
    Sandler-Dodge area-length m.
    Satterthwaite m.
    Scarpa m.
    Schiller m.
    Schüller m.
    Shimazaki area-length m.
    Sigma m.
    Silvester m.
    sliding scale m.
    Stanford biopsy m.
    steady-state m.
    Stegemann-Stalder m.
    Strauss m.
    Theden m.
    thermodilution m.
    Thom flap laryngeal
      reconstruction m.
    Thompson-Hatina m.
    Thrombo-Wellcotest m.
    triphenyl tetrazolium staining m.
    TUNEL m.
    Van Slyke m.
    von Claus chronometric m.
    V-slope m.
    Wardrop m.
    Weir m.
    Weiss logarithmic m.
    Welcker m.
    Westergren m.
    Willett-Stampfer m.
    Wilson-White m.
methohexital
methotrexate
methoxamine
    m. hydrochloride
methoxsalen
methoxyisobutyl
    m. isonitrile (MIBI)
    m. isonitrile single-photon emission
      computed tomography (MIBI-
      SPECT)
2-methoxyisobutyl isonitrile
    technetium hexakis 2-m. i.

methoxyphenamine hydrochloride
8-methoxypsoralen
methyclothiazide
    m. and cryptenamine tannates
    m. and deserpidine
    m. and pargyline
methyl
    m. bromide
    m. isocyanate
    m. prednisolone
methylcholine challenge testing (MCT)
methyldichloroarsine
methyldopa
    chlorothiazide and m.
    m. and hydrochlorothiazide
methylene
    m. blue
    m. diphenyl diisocyanate (MDI)
    m. diphenyl diisocyanate asthma
    m. diphosphonate (MDP)
methylenetetrahydrofolate
    m. reductase (MTHFR)
    m. reductase gene
    m. reductase genotype
methylisocyanate
methylphenidate
methylprednisolone (MTP)
    m. acetate
    sodium m.
    m. succinate
methyltestosterone
methylxanthine
methysergide maleate
Meticorten Oral
metoclopramide hydrochloride
metocurine iodide
metolazone
metoprolol
    m. CR
    m. succinate
    m. tartrate
Metras catheter
Metricath
    M. 1000 console catheter
    M. measurement catheter
Metrics
    Hema M.
Metrix
    M. atrial defibrillation system
    M. Atrioverter
    M. IAD
    M. implantable atrial defibrillator
metrizamide contrast medium
metrocyte
metronidazole
METT
    maximum exercise tolerance test
metyrosine
Metzenbaum scissors

MeV
   megaelectron volt
Mevacor lovastatin tablet
mevalonate acid
mevinolin
Mewi-5 sidehole infusion catheter
Mewissen infusion catheter
Mexican bean weevil asthma
mexiletine hydrochloride
Mexitil
Meyer cartilage
Meyerding retractor
Mezlin
mezlocillin sodium
MF
   myocardial fibrosis
MFAT
   multifocal atrial tachycardia
MFF
   metal fume fever
MFG
   manofluorography
   middle frontal gyrus
MFH
   malignant fibrous histiocytoma
MFSR
   maximum expiratory airflow-static lung
    elastic recoil pressure
MFT
   multifocal atrial tachycardia
MFVL
   maximal flow-volume envelope
   maximum flow-volume loop
mg
   milligram
MGA
   malposition of great arteries
Mgb
   myoglobulin
MgCO₃
   magnesium carbonate
MH
   malignant hypertension
MHA-TP test
MHHP
   Minnesota Heart Health Program
MHR
   maternal heart rate
   maximal heart rate
MHV
   magnetic heart vector

MHz
   megahertz
MI
   mitral incompetence
   mitral insufficiency
   myocardial infarction
   myocardial ischemia
    elevation MI
MIA
   melanoma inhibitory activity
    MIA protein
mibefradil
MIBG
   metaiodobenzylguanidine
    I-123 MIBG
    I-125 MIBG
MIBI
   methoxyisobutyl isonitrile
    MIBI SPECT
    MIBI stress test
    technetium-99m MIBI
MIBI-SPECT
   methoxyisobutyl isonitrile single-photon
    emission computed tomography
    ^{99M}Tc MIBI-SPECT
MIC
   minimum inhibitory concentration
MICAB
   minimally invasive coronary artery
   bypass
    MICAB surgery
MICABG
   minimally invasive coronary bypass
   grafting
mica pneumoconiosis
Micardis
micdadei
    Legionella m.
    Tatlockia m.
Michelson bronchoscope
miconazole
MICRhoGAM
Micrins
    M. microclamp insrument
    M. microsurgical suture
Micro
    M. Delta/Max Delta system
    M. DiaryCard spirometer
    M. II stent
    Lipidil M.
    M. Minix pacemaker

M

NOTES

Micro *(continued)*
  M. Mist nebulizer
  M. Plus spirometer
microaerosol
MicroAir
  M. handheld nebulizer
  M. ultrasonic nebulizer system
microalbuminuria
microanastomosis
  laser-assisted m. (LAMA)
microaneurysm
  Charcot-Bouchard m.
microangiopathic anemia
microangiopathy
  cerebral m. (CMA)
  coronary m.
  thrombotic m. (TMA)
microarousal
  m. detection
  m. scoring
  m. scoring device
microarray
  m. analysis
  oligonucleotide m.
microaspiration
microatelectasis
microatheroma
microatheromatosis
microballoon
microbiologic brushing
microbleed
microbrushing
microbubble (MB)
  m. persistence
microbulldog clip
microcalcification
  m. cluster (MCC)
Microcap handheld capnograph
microcardia
microcatheter
  Cardima Pathfinder mapping m.
  end-hole Tracker m.
  Excelsior 1018 m.
  Pathfinder mini m.
  Revelation endocardial m.
  Terumo SP hydrophilic-polymer-
    coated m.
  Tracker m.
microcavitation
microcentrum
MicroChamber
microcirculation (MC)
microcirculatory
  m. adaptation
  m. vasoconstriction
MicroCO carbon monoxide monitor
Micrococcus
microcoil
  Hilal embolization m.

microcontaminant
microcrystal
microdialysis
**MicroDigitrapper-S apnea screening
  device**
microdissection
  laser capture m. (LCM)
microelectrode
  tungsten m.
microemboli
  gaseous m.
microembolic signal (MES)
microembolism
microembolization
MicroFerret-18 infusion catheter
microfibril
microfibrillar collagen hemostat
microfilaria
microfilter
  OmniFilter percutaneous
    guidewire m.
microflora
  bronchial m.
MicroGard, MicroGARD, Microgard
**MicroGas 7650 transcutaneous
  monitoring system**
micrognathia
Micro-Guide catheter
microhemagglutination *Treponema
  pallidum*
microinfarct
microinvasive
microjoule
Micro-K
Microknit
  M. arterial graft
  M. patch graft
  M. vascular graft prosthesis
**MicroLab ML3500 desktop diagnostic
  spirometer**
microlaryngoscope
microlaryngoscopy
  Thornell m.
Microlith
  M. pacemaker pulse generator
  M. P pacemaker
microlithiasis
  pulmonary alveolar m. (PAM)
MicroLoop
  M. II handheld spirometer
  M. ML3535
  M. pocket spirometer
MicroLysus system
micromanometer
  m. catheter
  m. catheter system
  catheter-tip m. system
micromanometry

MicroMed DeBakey ventricular assist device
MicroMedical DiaryCard
MicroMewi multiple sidehole infusion catheter
Micromonospora
micron
    m. needle
    M. Res-Q implantable cardioverter-defibrillator
Micronase
micronebulizer
microneurography
microneutralization test
micronized progesterone
micronodular dissemination
micronutrient balance
Microny
    M. II SR+ pacemaker
    M. II SR+ pulse generator
    M. K SR pacemaker
microorganism
    capneic m.
microparticle
microphage
    fat-laden m.
Micropolyspora faeni
Micropuncture
    M. guidewire
    M. introducer needle
    M. introducer set
    M. Peel-Away introducer
microreentry
MicroRint portable airway resistance meter
microsatellite instability
microscope
    acoustic m.
    electron m.
    epi-illuminated m.
    scanning electron m. (SEM)
microscopic polyangiitis (MPA)
microscopy
    darkfield m.
    intravital capillary video m.
    light m.
microsecond pulsed flashlamp pumped dye laser
microsnare
    Amplatz gooseneck m.
microsomal
    m. lipoprotein (MLP)

    m. triglyceride transfer protein (MTP)
microsome
    calf aortic m. (CAM)
MicroSpacer, Microspacer
microsphere
    EmboGold m.
    perflexane lipid m.
    perflutren lipid m.'s
    m. perfusion scintigraphy
    polystyrene latex m.
    radiolabeled m.
    Ultrasound Contrast M.
microspheres
microsphygmy
microsphyxia
Micross
    M. dilatation catheter
    M. SL balloon
microsteatosis
Microstream capnograph
Microsulfon
MicroTach pneumotach
microthromboembolism
    pulmonary m.
microthrombosis
microthrombus
microti
    Babesia m.
    Mycobacterium m.
Microtip lead
microtome
    Cryo-Cut m.
    Stadie-Riggs m.
Micro-Tracer portable ECG
microvascular
    m. angina
    m. angiopathy (MVA)
    m. artery disease
    m. bleeding (MVB)
    m. clamp
    m. decompression (MVD)
    m. dysfunction
    m. flow distribution
    m. free flap
    m. permeability
Microvasive
    M. Glidewire
    M. Rigiflex TTS balloon
    M. stiff piano wire guidewire
Microvel double velour graft
Microvena goose neck snare

M

NOTES

MicroVent ventilator
microvessel
microvolt T-wave alternans
microwave cardiac ablation system
Microzide
micturition syncope
MICU
  medical intensive care unit
mid
MIDA
  myocardial ischemia dynamic analysis
Midamor
midaxillary line
midazolam
MIDCAB
  minimally invasive direct coronary artery
  bypass
    MIDCAB procedure
    MIDCAB saloon door approach
    MIDCAB surgery
    MIDCAB system
MIDCABG
  minimally invasive direct coronary artery
  bypass graft
midclavicular line (MCL)
midcoronary
  m. artery
  m. artery bypass
  m. segment
middiastolic
  m. murmur (MDM)
  m. rumble
middle
  m. capsular artery
  m. cerebral artery (MCA)
  m. cerebral artery occlusion
    (MCAO)
  m. constrictor muscle of pharynx
  m. frontal gyrus (MFG)
  m. lobe bronchus
  m. lobe of right lung
  m. lobe syndrome
  m. ribs
midepigastric bruit
midexpiratory phase
mid-infrared pulsed laser
midinspiratory
midline shift
midlung zone
midnodal
  m. extrasystole
  m. rhythm
midodrine
midriff
midsagittal plane
midsystolic
  m. buckling
  m. buckling of mitral valve
  m. click (MSC)

  m. click syndrome
  m. closure of aortic valve
  m. dip
  m. murmur (MSM)
  m. notching
midventricle
midventricular (MV)
midwall shortening
MIF
  mean inspiratory flow
MIFR
  maximal inspiratory flow rate
migraine
  m. headache
  m. stroke
  syncopal m.
  m. syncope
migrans
  erythema m.
  larva m.
  thrombophlebitis m. (TPM)
  visceral larva m.
migrated tumor
migrating
  m. pacemaker
  m. phlebitis
migration
  neural crest m.
  stent m.
migratory
  m. pneumonia
  m. pulmonary infiltrate
  m. thrombus
MIH
  minimal intermittent heparin
    MIH dose
Mikity-Wilson disease
Mikro-Tip
  M.-T. micromanometer-tipped
    catheter
  M.-T. transducer
mild-intensity exercise
mildly dilated congestive
  cardiomyopathy (MDCM)
Miles vena cava clip
miliary
  m. coccidioidomycosis
  m. embolism
  m. infection
  m. pattern
  m. tuberculosis
milieu
military
  m. antishock trousers (MAST)
  m. pattern
milk
  m. scan
  m. scintigraphy
  m. spots

milk-alkali syndrome
mill
>   m. house murmur
>   m. wheel murmur

Millar
>   M. asthma
>   M. Doppler catheter
>   M. Mikro-Tip catheter pressure transducer
>   M. MPC-500 catheter
>   M. TCB-500 transducer

mille feuilles effect
Millenia
>   M. balloon catheter
>   M. portable vital sign monitor
>   M. PTCA catheter

Miller
>   M. blade
>   M. elastic stain
>   M. Fisher variant of Guillain-Barré syndrome
>   M. index
>   M. maneuver
>   M. septostomy catheter

milleri
>   *Streptococcus m.*

miller's
>   m. asthma
>   m. lung

milliamperage
milliampere (mA)
millicurie (mCi)
milliequivalent (mEq)
milligram (mg)
>   m. per kilogram per day

millijoule (mJ)
Milliknit
>   M. Dacron prosthesis
>   M. vascular graft prosthesis

milliliter (mL)
>   nanograms per m.
>   m. per kilogram (mL/kg)

millimeter of mercury (mmHg)
millimole (mmol)
>   m. per liter (mmol/L)

million
>   m. international unit (MIU)
>   part per m. (ppm)

milliosmole (mOsm)

Millipore filter
millisecond (ms, msec)
milliunit (mU)
millivolt (mV)
Mill-Rose
>   M.-R. esophageal injector
>   M.-R. protected specimen microbiology brush

millwheel
milrinone lactate
Miltex rib spreader
Miltner constraint compliance device
Milton edema
Mima-Herellea
mimetic
mineralocorticoid hormone
mineralocorticoid-induced hypertension
miner's
>   m. asthma
>   m. lung
>   m. phthisis

Mingograf
>   M. 62 6-channel electrocardiograph
>   M. 82 recorder

Mingograph
Mini
>   M. Asthma Quality of Life (MAQOL)
>   21 M. device
>   26 M. II device

mini
>   m. arousal
>   m. stroke

miniballoon
minicoil
MINI Crown stent
minidefibrillator
Mini-Gamulin Rh
MiniHEART low-flow nebulizer
Minilith pacemaker pulse generator
minimae
>   venae cardiacae m.
>   venae cordis m.

minimal
>   m. alveolar concentration (MAC)
>   m. intermittent heparin (MIH)
>   m. leak technique
>   m. luminal diameter (MLD)
>   m. vascular resistance (MVR)

minimally
>   m. invasive coronary artery bypass (MICAB)

M

NOTES

minimally *(continued)*

    m. invasive coronary bypass grafting (MICABG)
    m. invasive direct coronary artery bypass (MIDCAB)
    m. invasive direct coronary artery bypass graft (MIDCABG)
    m. invasive direct coronary artery bypass procedure
    m. invasive direct coronary bypass
    m. invasive procedure (MIP)
    m. invasive valve repair (MIVR)
    m. invasive valve replacement (MIVR)

MiniMe nasal mask

Mini-Motionlogger Actigraph

minimum

    m. audible pressure (MAP)
    m. bactericidal concentration
    m. cumulative cardiotoxic dose (MCCD)
    m. data set (MDS)
    m. data set system
    m. defibrillation energy (MDE)
    m. inhibitory concentration (MIC)
    m. left ventricular pressure (LVPmin)
    m. lumen diameter (MLD)

MiniOX

    M. IA oxygen analyzer
    M. 1000 oxygen analyzer
    M. 3000 oxygen monitor

Minipress

Mini-Profile catheter

Miniscope MS-3 pocket ECG

ministernotomy

Mini-Torr Plus NIPB monitor

Minitran Patch

Minizide

Minnesota

    M. antilymphocyte globulin (MAG)
    M. classification of ECG
    M. code
    M. criteria for high R wave
    M. ECG classification
    M. Heart Health Program (MHHP)
    M. Impedance Cardiograph
    M. Leisure Time Physical Activity Questionnaire
    M. Living with Heart Failure questionnaire
    M. Q-QS code

Minocin

    M. I.V. injection
    M. Oral

minocycline hydrochloride

minor

    m. fissure
    pectoralis m.

minores

    ductus sublinguales m.

minoxidil

Minoxigaine

Mintezol

minute

    alveolar ventilation per m. (V_A)
    beats per m. (BPM, bpm)
    counts per m. (C/M)
    liter per m. (Lpm)
    M. Maid Premium Heart Wise orange juice
    m. output
    oxygen consumption per m. (VO_2)
    physiological dead space ventilation per m. (V_D)
    pulses per m. (ppm)
    m. ventilation (V_E)
    m. volume

6-minute

    6-m. corridor walk test
    6-m. walk distance
    6-m. walking test (6MWT, 6-MWT)

minute-gun cough

10-minute supine/30-minute tilt test

Miochol-E

miosis

miosphygmia

MIP

    maximal inspiratory pressure
    maximum inspiratory pressure
    mean intravascular pressure
    minimally invasive procedure

MIP-1

    macrophage inflammatory protein-1

mirabilis

    Proteus m.

Mirage

    M. hydrophilic guidewire
    M. nasal mask
    M. over-the-wire balloon catheter

Mirostipen

MIRP

    myocardial infarction rehabilitation program

mirror

    m. movement
    van Helmont m.

mirror-image

    m.-i. brachiocephalic branching
    m.-i. dextrocardia
    m.-i. laryngoscopy
    m.-i. lung syndrome

Mirsky

    formula of M.
    M. thick wall model

MIRU

    myocardial infarction research unit

misery perfusion
mismatch
    ventilation/perfusion m.
    V̇/Q̇ m.
mismatching
    afterload m.
missed
    m. beat
    m. ostium sequence (MOS)
missense mutation
miss rate
mist
    Ayr saline nasal m.
    cool m.
    Primatene M.
    m. tent
Mistogen
    M. nebulizer
    M. passover humidifier
Mistometer
    Isuprel M.
mit
    mitral
mite
    house dust m. (HDM)
MITI
    myocardial infarction triage and
    intervention
mitis
    Streptococcus m.
mitochondrial
    m. biogenesis
    m. calcium deposition
    m. cardiomyopathy
    m. enzyme
    m. function
    m. genotype
    m. oxidative phosphorylation
    m. respiration
mitochondrion, pl. **mitochondria**
mitogen-activated
    m.-a. kinase pathway
    m.-a. protein (MAP)
    m.-a. protein kinase (MAPK)
mitogenic radiation
mitomycin, vinblastine, cisplatin (MVP)
mitotane
mitoxantrone hydrochloride
mitral (mit)
    m. annular area
    m. annular calcification
    m. annular calcium

m. annulus calcification (MAC)
m. annulus motion
m. and aortic valve replacement
    (MAVR)
m. atresia
m. balloon commissurotomy
m. balloon valvotomy (MBV)
m. buttonhole
m. click
m. closure (Mc)
m. commissurotomy (MC)
m. component (M1)
m. disease (MD)
m. E-to-F slope
m. E velocity curve
m. E-wave transmission
m. facies
m. first sound (M_1)
m. funnel
m. gradient
m. incompetence (MI)
m. insufficiency (MI)
m. leaflet
m. leaflet tip
m. opening (Mo)
m. opening snap (MOS)
m. orifice (MO)
posterior m. (PM)
m. prolapse murmur
m. prosthesis
m. reflux (MR)
m. regurgitant flow (MRF)
m. regurgitant jet
m. regurgitation (MR)
m. regurgitation artifact
m. regurgitation murmur
m. restenosis
m. second sound (M_2)
m. sounds (MS)
m. stenosis (MS)
m. stenosis murmur
m. tap
m. valve aneurysm
m. valve anulus
m. valve area (MVA)
m. valve billowing
m. valve closure index
m. valve commissurotomy
m. valve dilator
m. valve disease (MVD)
m. valve echo (MVE)
m. valve echocardiography

M

NOTES

mitral *(continued)*
    m. valve endocarditis
    m. valve excursion (MVE)
    m. valve flow (MVF)
    m. valve gradient (MVG)
    m. valve homograft
    m. valve hypoplasia
    m. valve insufficiency (MVI)
    m. valve leaflet (MVL)
    m. valve opening (MVO)
    m. valve orifice (MVO)
    m. valve orifice area (MVOA)
    m. valve prolapse (MPV, MVP)
    m. valve prolapse syndrome
    (MVPS)
    m. valve prolapse-systolic click
    (MVP-SC)
    m. valve regurgitation
    m. valve replacement (MVR)
    m. valve valvotomy
    m. valvotomy
    m. valvulitis
    m. valvuloplasty
mitrale
    P m.
mitralis
    facies m.
mitralism
mitralization
mitral-septal apposition
Mitroflow Synergy PC stented
  pericardial valve
mitrotricuspid facies
MIU
    million international unit
Mivacron
mivacurium
mivazerol
MIVR
    minimally invasive valve repair
    minimally invasive valve replacement
mix
    oncology m.
mixed
    m. alveolar-interstitial pneumonitis
    m. aneurysm
    m. angina
    m. aortic valve disease (MAVD)
    m. apnea (MA)
    m. asthma
    m. beat
    m. expired gas
    m. flora
    m. hematopoietic chimerism
    m. levocardia
    m. mitral valve disease (MMVD)
    m. neurally mediated syncope
    m. thrombus
    m. venous blood

    m. venous oxygen saturation
    (SvO_2)
mixed-dust pneumoconiosis
mixing
    convective gas m.
mixture
    helium-oxygen m. (heliox)
mizoribine
mJ
    millijoule
mL
    milliliter
MLAP
    mean left atrial pressure
MLD
    mean luminal diameter
    minimal luminal diameter
    minimum lumen diameter
MLH
    multiple lobar hemorrhage
M-line protein
mL/kg
    milliliter per kilogram
MLP
    microsomal lipoprotein
MLR
    myocardial laser revascularization
      MLR procedure
MM
    modified Miller maneuver
MMA
    maxillomandibular advancement
MMAD
    mass median aerodynamic diameter
MMAP
    mean maternal arterial blood pressure
MMC
    mechanical myocardial channeling
mMCAI
    malignant middle cerebral artery
    infarction
MME
    M-mode echocardiography
MMEF, MMF
    maximal midexpiratory flow
    maximum midexpiratory flow rate
MMEFR
    maximal midexpiratory flow rate
MMF
    mycophenolate mofetil
mmHg
    millimeter of mercury
MMI
    medial medullary infarction
MMO
    maxillomandibular osteotomy
M-mode
    motion mode
      M-mode echocardiogram

M-mode echocardiography (MME)
M-mode measurement
omnidirectional M-mode
M-mode strip chart recording
M-mode transducer

mmol
millimole

mmol/L
millimoles per liter

MMP
matrix metalloproteinase
matrix-degrading neutral MMP

MMPI
matrix metalloproteinase inhibitor

MMR
myocardial metabolic rate

MMV
mandatory minute volume

MMVD
mixed mitral valve disease

MMVF
manmade vitreous fiber

Mn-SOD
manganese superoxide dismutase

MO
mitral orifice

MO$_2$
myocardial oxygen
MO$_2$ utilization

Mo
mitral opening

Mobidin

mobile
m. artery and vein imaging system (MAVIS)
carina sharp and m.
cor m.
m. coronary care unit (MCCU)
m. myxoma
m. vegetation

mobilization
secretion m.

Mobin-Uddin
M.-U. filter system
M.-U. sieve
M.-U. vena cava filter

Mobitz
M. first-degree block
M. second-degree block
M. type I, II atrioventricular block

modafinil

modality
pacing m.
therapeutic m.

mode
A m.
AAI rate-responsive m.
AAT m.
autodecremental m.
demand m.
dual-helical slice m.
dual-slice m.
fixed-rate m.
gated list m.
harmonic imaging m.
histogram m.
list m.
mask m.
matrix m.
motion m. (M-mode)
noise-reversion m.
OOO m.
overdrive m.
pacing m.
passive m.
patient activator m.
rate-drop response m.
RDR m.
m. switch
m. switching
triggered m.
VDD m.
VDI pacing m.
VVD m.
VVT m.

model
health behavior m.
Hodgkin-Huxley m.
Mirsky thick wall m.
Torricelli m.
Tracheostomy T.O.M.
anatomical m.
windkessel m.
WJG pacemaker m.

model-based image processing (MBIP)

moderate hypothermia

moderate-ramp protocol

moderator band

modification
A-V nodal m.
Mason-Likar limb lead m.
Mullins m.

M

NOTES

modified

   m. backward Prony method (MBPM)

   m. Blalock-Taussig shunt (MBTS)

   m. brachial technique

   m. Bruce protocol

   m. chest lead (MCL)

   m. Ellestad protocol

   m. Fontan procedure

   m. human graft umbilical vein graft

   m. Mark IV R-wave-triggered power injector

   m. Miller maneuver (MM)

   m. multifactorial index of cardiac risk

   m. Rashkind PDA occluder

   m. Seldinger technique

   m. shuttle test

   m. treadmill exercise test (MTET)

modifier

   leukotriene m.

MODS

   multiple-organ dysfunction syndrome

modular electrocardiogram analysis system (MEANS)

modulated

   pulse position m. (PPM)

modulation

   autonomic m.

   brightness m.

   integral pulse frequency m. (IPFM)

   pulse amplitude m. (PAM)

   pulse time m. (PTM)

   pulse with m. (PWM)

   rate m.

modulator

   selective estrogen receptor m. (SERM)

module

   BioZ ICG M.

   Co-Oximeter m.

   OmniCell catheter m.

   Research Pneumotach System instrumentation m.

modulus

   impedance m.

   Peterson elastic m.

   Young m.

Moduretic

Moe

   multiple reentrant wavelet hypothesis of M.

   M. multiple wavelet hypothesis

   M. multiple wavelet hypothesis of atrial defibrillation

Moersch bronchoscope

moexipril

   m. hydrochloride

   m. and hydrochlorothiazide

mofetil

   mycophenolate m. (MMF)

moiety-conserved cycle

moist

   Nasal M.

   m. rale

moisturizer

   Cann-Ease nasal m.

   RoEzIt skin m.

MOIVC

   membranous obstruction of the inferior vena cava

mold worker's lung

molecular

   m. chemotherapy

   m. coincidence detection (MCD)

molecule

   antiadhesion m.

   cell adhesion m. (CAM)

   chemoattracting m.

   circulating adhesion m. (CAM)

   endothelium-leukocyte adhesion m. (E-LAM)

   E-selectin cell adhesion m.

   intercellular adhesion m. (ICAM)

   leukocyte-endothelial cell adhesion m.

   proatherothrombogenic m.

   P-selectin cell adhesion m.

   soluble adhesion m.

   soluble intracellular adhesion m. (sICAM)

molecule-1

   intercellular adhesion m.-1 (ICAM-1)

   mucosal addresin cell adhesion m.-1 (MadCAM-1)

   vascular cell adhesion m.-1 (VCAM-1)

Molina needle catheter

Mol-Iron

Mollaret meningitis

mollis

   pulsus m.

molluscum contagiosum

Molnar disk

Moloney murine leukemia virus

molsidomine

molybdenum

moment

   magnetic m.

Momentum DR pacemaker

mometasone furoate

Monaghan

   M. respirator

   M. 300 ventilator

Monaldi drainage system
Monarch
    M. 25 inflation device
    M. Mini Mask nasal interface
Monark bicycle ergometer
Mönckeberg
    M. arrhythmia
    M. arteriosclerosis
    M. calcification
    M. degeneration
    M. mesarteritis
    M. sclerosis
    M. syndrome
Monday
    M. dyspnea
    M. fever
Mondini pulmonary arteriovenous
  malformation
Mondor
    M. disease
    M. syndrome
Monge disease
Monilia albicans
monilial esophagitis
moniliasis
    chronic mucocutaneous m.
moniliformis
    Streptobacillus m.
Monitan
monitor
    Accucap CO_2/O_2 m.
    Accucom cardiac output m.
    Accutorr multiparameter m.
    Accutracker II ambulatory blood
      pressure m.
    Acuson V5M transesophageal
      echocardiographic m.
    aerosol inhalation m. (AIM)
    AID-Check m.
    ambulatory Holter m.
    AMI infant apnea m.
    antepartum m. (APM)
    APM-2000 vital signs m.
    apnea m.
    Arrhythmia Net arrhythmia m.
    automatic oscillometric blood
      pressure m.
    AvoSure PT m.
    Bedfont carbon monoxide m.
    Bedfont EC60 Gastrolyzer
      hydrogen m.
    bedside m.

    bioimpedance m.
    Biotrack coagulation m.
    BioZ.com cardiac output m.
    BioZ ICG M.
    blood perfusion m. (BPM, bpm)
    CA m.
    Capintec nuclear VEST m.
    Capnocheck Plus NIPB m.
    cardiac apnea m.
    CardioBeeper CB 12L cardiac m.
    Cardiocap/5 m.
    cardiovascular m. (CVM)
    Chronicle implantable
      hemodynamic m.
    CoaguChek Pro DM m.
    Corometrics m.
    CO Sleuth carbon monoxide m.
    CO_2SMO Plus continuous
      noninvasive respiratory profile m.
    Datascope Accutor bedside m.
    Digitrapper MkIII sleep m.
    Dinamap Accutorr A1, A3 blood
      pressure m.
    Doppler-Cavin m.
    Doppler fetal heart m.
    DynaPulse 5000A blood
      pressure m.
    EcoCheck oxygen m.
    EC50 ToxCO breath carbon
      monoxide m.
    electrocardiographic
      transtelephonic m.
    electronic fetal m.
    endotracheal cardiac output m.
      (ECOM)
    event recorder m.
    Finapres blood pressure m.
    HBT Sleuth portable hydrogen m.
    HeartCard m.
    Heart Rate 1-2-3 m.
    Hemochron m.
    HemoMatic blood collection m.
    HemoTec activated clotting
      time m.
    Hewlett-Packard 78720 A SDN m.
    Holter m.
    HomMed m.
    Insta-Pulse heart rate m.
    intelligent cardiovascular m. (ICM)
    KinetiX ventilation m.
    King of Hearts Holter m.
    m. leads

M

NOTES

monitor *(continued)*
LifeShirt m.
loop m.
Magellan m.
Marquette 8000 Holter m.
MDILog microelectronic m.
MicroCO carbon monoxide m.
Millenia portable vital sign m.
MiniOX 3000 oxygen m.
Mini-Torr Plus NIPB m.
MRM-2 oxygen consumption m.
Nellcor Symphony blood
  pressure m.
Neotrend multiparameter blood
  gas m.
$NICO_2$ noninvasive cardiac
  output m.
noninvasive m.
NOxBOX m.
Ohmeda 6200, 6300 CO_2 m.
One Touch blood glucose m.
OSD m.
OxyData Plus oxygen m.
PAM2, PAM3 m.
Paratrend 7 continuous blood
  gas m.
Paratrend 7+ multiparameter blood
  gas m.
patient m.
Physios CTM 01 cardiac
  transplant m.
Pick and Go m.
Polar Vantage XL heart rate m.
Porta-Resp m.
Pressurometer blood pressure m.
PrinterNOx nitric oxide/nitrogen
  dioxide m.
Propaq Encore vital signs m.
Pulse Pro heart rate m.
Puritan Bennett 7250 metabolic m.
Q-TRAK IAQ m.
RIP portable sleep m.
SpaceLabs Holter m.
TCM30 transcutaneous oxygen m.
Tensys T-line blood pressure m.
three-channel Holter m.
transcutaneous oxygen m. (TCOM)
transtelephonic exercise m. (TEM)
VentCheck handheld respiratory m.
VenTrak respiratory mechanics m.
ventricular arrhythmia m. (VAM)
VEST ambulatory ventricular
  function m.
video m.
V.I.P. Bird volume m.
VitalCare 506DX m.
Vitalograph BreathCO M.
Vitalograph pulmonary m.

monitor/defibrillator
Lifepak 5, 7 m./d.
monitoring
ambulatory m.
ambulatory blood pressure m.
  (ABPM)
ambulatory electrocardiographic m.
  (AEM)
ambulatory Holter m. (AHM)
ambulatory oximetry m. (AOM)
beat-by-beat hemodynamic m.
cardiac m. (CM)
CareLink network for patient m.
Doptone m.
endotracheal cardiac output m.
  (ECOM)
hemodynamic m. (HM)
Holter m. (HM)
invasive m.
NIBP m.
physiologic m.
physiological m.
pleural space m.
precordial electrocardiographic m.
  (PEM)
pulse oximetry m. (POM)
transtelephonic ambulatory m.
  (TAM)
transtelephonic arrhythmia m.
  (TTM)
transtelephonic cardiac event m.
transthoracic intracardiac m. (TIM)
Monneret pulse
monoamine
m. oxidase (MAO)
m. oxidase inhibitor (MAOI)
monobactam
monocarboxylate
m. proton cotransporter
m. transporter
monocardiogram
Mono-Cedocard
Monoclate-P
monoclonal
m. antibody 3G4
m. antifibronectin antibody
m. antimyosin antibody
m. hypothesis
m. theory of atherogenesis
MonoClone immunoenzymetric assay
monocrotaline
monocrotic pulse
monocrotism
monocrotus
pulsus m.
monocyte
m. chemoattractant protein (MCP)
m. chemoattractant protein-1 (MCP-
  1)

m. chemotactic and activating
factor (MCAF)
m. chemotactic protein-1 (MCP-1)
surface adherent m. (SAM)
transcardiac m.
monocytic leukemoid reaction
monocytogenes
Listeria m.
monodisperse
Monodox Oral
monofilament
m. absorbable suture
m. polypropylene suture
Semmes-Weinstein m.
monoform tachycardia
Mono-Gesic
monohydrate
cefadroxil m.
cephalexin m.
Monojector
Monoket
Monolyth oxygenator
monomer
actin m.
fibrin m. (FM)
monometer-tipped catheter
N^G**-monomethyl-L-arginine (L-NMMA)**
monomorphic ventricular tachycardia
(MVT)
mononeuritis multiplex
Mononine
mononitrate
isosorbide m.
mononuclear cell
mononucleosis
infectious m.
monophasic
m. action potential (MAP)
m. action potential duration
(MAPD)
m. action potential early
afterdepolarization (mEAD)
m. contour of QRS complex
m. defibrillation waveform (MDW)
m. negative QRS complex (QS)
m. pulse
m. shock therapy
m. waveform
monophonic wheeze
monophosphate
adenosine m. (AMP)
cyclic adenosine m. (cAMP)

cyclic guanosine m. (cGMP)
cyclic nucleotide adenosine m.
guanosine m. (GMP)
monoplace chamber
monopolar temporary electrode
Monopril
Monorail
M. angioplasty catheter
M. guidewire
M. imaging catheter
M. Speedy balloon
monoresistance
monosaturated
m. fat
m. fatty acid
monostimulator
cardiosynchronous m. (CSM)
Monostrut cardiac valve prosthesis
monosulfate
guanethidine m.
monotest
R-lactate enzyme m.
monotherapy
monotypic lesion
monounsaturated fatty acid (MUFA)
Mono-Vacc
Monovial
Cardizem M.
M. drug delivery system
monoxide
carbon m. (CO)
diffusing capacity of lung for
carbon m. (DLCO)
partial pressure of carbon m.
(PCO)
monoxide-oximetry
monoxime
butanedione m.
Monro
foramen of M.
Monte Carlo multiway sensitivity
analysis method
montelukast sodium
Montgomery
M. Safe-T-Tube
M. speaking valve
M. tracheostomy
Montgomery-Asberg Depression Rating
Scale (MADRS)
Moody friction factor
moon face

M

NOTES

Moore
  M. procedure
  M. tracheostomy button
Moraxella
  M. catarrhalis
  M. nonliquefaciens
morbidity
morbid obesity
Morbillivirus
morcellation
Morch respirator
More-Flow long-term high-flow catheter
Morestin syndrome
Moretz clip
Morgagni
  M. disease
  foramen of M.
  M. hernia
  M. nodule
Morgagni-Adams-Stokes
  M.-A.-S. syncope
  M.-A.-S. syndrome
Morganella morganii
morganii
  Morganella m.
moribund
moricizine
moriens
  ultimum m.
morphine
morphogenesis
morphologic
morphology
  hills-and-valley m.
  QRS m.
  valvular m.
  windsock m.
morphometric measurement
morphometry
  aerosol-derived airway m. (ADAM)
  airway m.
  lung m.
Morquio-Brailsford disease
Morquio syndrome
morrhuate sodium
Morrow procedure
Morse manifest
mortality rate (MR)
mortis
  myocardial rigor m.
Morton cough
MOS
  missed ostium sequence
  mitral opening snap
mosaic
  M. cardiac bioprosthesis
  m. jet
  m. jet signals
  m. pattern

  m. perfusion
  M. porcine bioprosthetic heart
    valve
Moschcowitz
  M. disease
  M. sign
  M. test
Moses sign
Mosher life-saving tracheal tube
mOsm
  milliosmole
mosquito
  m. clamp
  m. hemostat
moss-agate sputum
Mosso sphygmomanometer
motexafin lutetium
motility
  esophageal m.
  receptor for hyaluronan-mediated m.
    (RHAMM)
motion
  abnormal wall m. (AWM)
  m. artifact
  atrioventricular junction m.
  chest wall m.
  circulation, sensation, m. (CSM)
  cusp m.
  diastolic m.
  m. display echo
  endocardial m.
  fetal atrial wall m.
  fetal ventricular wall m.
  infarct zone wall m.
  interventricular septal m.
  leaflet m.
  left ventricular wall m. (LVWM)
  mitral annulus m.
  m. mode (M-mode)
  paradoxic wall m.
  plaque m.
  precordial m.
  regional wall m. (RWM)
  right ventricular wall m.
  segmental wall m. (SWM)
  septal wall m.
  systolic m. (SM)
  systolic anterior m. (SAM)
  tricuspid annular m. (TAM)
  ventricular wall m. (VWM)
  wall m. (WM)
  whorl m.
motoneuron
motor
  M. Assessment Scale (MAS)
  M. Club Assessment test of motor
    activity
  m. neglect
  m. provoked potential (MEP)

motor-exploratory hemineglect
motoricity
motorized transducer pullback device
MOTT
    mycobacteria other than tuberculosis
mottled
mottling
    m. of extremities
    quantum m.
Moulaert
    muscle of M.
moulin
    bruit de la roue de m.
Mounier-Kuhn syndrome
mountain sickness
Mount-Mayfield forceps
mouse
    pleural m.
mousetail pulse
mouth of aneurysm
mouthguard
    Snorex m.
mouthpiece
    Pneumotach disposable m.
    SafeTway pediatric m.
mouth-to-face shield ventilation
mouth-to-mask ventilation
mouth-to-mouth
    m.-t.-m. respiration
    m.-t.-m. resuscitation
    m.-t.-m. ventilation
mouth-to-nose ventilation
mouth-to-stoma ventilation
movable
    m. core straight safety wire guide
    m. heart
    m. pulse
Movat
    M. pentachrome
    M. stain
MOVC
    membranous obstruction of inferior vena cava
movement
    air m.
    ameboid m.
    anomalous m.
    m. arousal index (MAI)
    ciliary m.
    circus m.
    m. disorder

    mirror m.
    movement science physiotherapy
    nonrapid eye m. (NREM)
    periodic leg m. (PLM)
    precordial m.
    quality of m. (QOM)
    rapid eye m. (REM)
    m.-related cortical potential (MRCP)
    sustained outward m. (SOM)
    vessel wall m.
movement-related cortical potential (MRCP)
moxalactam
moxibustion
moxifloxacin
    m. HCl
    m. HCl I.V.
    m. HCl tablet
moxonidine
moyamoya
    m. disease
    m. of heart
Moynahan syndrome
MPA
    main pulmonary artery
    mean pulmonary arterial
    medroxyprogesterone acetate
    microscopic polyangiitis
    MPA pressure
MPAP
    mean pulmonary artery pressure
MPAWP
    mean pulmonary artery wedge pressure
MPE
    malignant pleural effusion
MP-H
    mandibular plane to hyoid
MPHR
    maximum predicted heart rate
MPI
    macrophage inflammatory protein
    myocardial perfusion imaging
MPIF
    myeloid progenitor inhibitory factor
MPM
    malignant pleural mesothelioma
MPO
    myeloperoxidase
MPR
    maximum pulse rate
M-protein serotype

M

NOTES

MPS
    myocardial perfusion scintigraphy
    myocardial protection system
MPT
    multiple-parameter telemetry
MPV
    main portal vein
    mitral valve prolapse
MPVP
    mean pulmonary venous pressure
MR
    mitral reflux
    mitral regurgitation
    mortality rate
    myocardial revascularization
        MR 290 humidification chamber
        MR lead
MRA
    magnetic resonance angiography
        3D TOF MRA
        TOF MRA
MRAP
    mean right atrial pressure
MRCA
    magnetic resonance coronary
     angiography
        respiratory gated MRCA
MRCP
    movement-related cortical potential
MRD
    mean reference diameter
MRE
    maximal resistive exercise
MREI
    mean rate ejection index
MRF
    magnetic resonance flowmetry
    mitral regurgitant flow
MRI
    magnetic resonance imaging
        CASL-PI MRI
        cine gradient-echo MRI
        diffusion MRI
        diffusion-weighted MRI
        DSC MRI
        dynamic susceptibility contrast-
         enhanced MRI
        FLASH MRI
        functional MRI
        Gd-DTPA-enhanced MRI
        GE Signa 1.5-T MRI
        gradient echo-cine MRI
        GRASS MRI
        hemodynamically weighted MRI
         (HW)
        intravascular MRI
        low-dose dobutamine cine MRI
        perfusion imaging MRI
        perfusion-weighted MRI (PWI)

        Philips ACS NT 1.5 Gyroscan
         MRI
        Siemens Magnetom 1.5-T MRI
        spin-echo MRI
        Toshiba MRT 200 MRI
        T2-weighted MRI
        MRI velocity mapping
MRI-identified stroke
MRM-2 oxygen consumption monitor
mRNA
    messenger ribonucleic acid
        osteopontin mRNA
        skeletal alpha-actin mRNA
MRP
    maximal response plateau
MRS
    magnetic resonance spectroscopy
MRV
    magnetic resonance venography
MRVP
    mean right ventricular pressure
MS
    mitral sounds
    mitral stenosis
        MS Classique balloon dilatation
         catheter
Ms
    murmurs
m/s
    meter per second
m/s²
    meter per second squared
ms, msec
    millisecond
MSA
    magnetic resonance angiography
MSAP
    mean systemic arterial pressure
MSC
    midsystolic click
MS-CIS SV stent
MSCT
    multislice spiral computed tomography
MSD Enteric Coated ASA
m/sec
    meter per second
msec (*var. of* ms)
    millisecond
MSER
    mean systolic ejection rate
MSI
    magnetic source imaging
    metered-solution inhaler
MSLT
    multiple sleep latency test
MSM
    midsystolic murmur
MSNA
    muscle sympathetic nerve activity

MSOF
multisystem organ failure
MSPECT
myocardial single photon emission
tomography
MSPS
myocardial stress perfusion scintigraphy
MSS
muscular subaortic stenosis
MST
median survival time
MSU
myocardial substrate uptake
MSVC
maximal sustainable ventilatory capacity
MT
mural thrombosis
mural thrombus
MTB
Mycobacterium tuberculosis
MTC catheter
MTD
maximum tolerated dose
MTD test
MT-100 ECG Holter system
MTET
modified treadmill exercise test
MTHFR
methylenetetrahydrofolate reductase
MTHFR gene
MTHFR genotype
MT-MMP
membrane-bound membrane-type
metalloproteinase
MTP
methylprednisolone
microsomal triglyceride transfer protein
MTP gene
MTST
maximal treadmill stress test
MTT
maximal treadmill testing
M-type alpha-1 antitrypsin
MU
megaunit
mU
milliunit
Much
M. bacillus
M. granules
mucicarmine stain

mucin
m. clot prevention (MCP)
epithelial m.
mucinous
m. adenocarcinoma
m. carcinoma
mucoactive
m. medication
m. therapy
mucociliary
m. clearance (MCC)
m. efficiency
m. escalator
m. system
m. transport
mucocutaneous
m. lesion
m. lymph node syndrome
mucoepidermoid carcinoma
mucoepithelial dysplasia
Muco-Fen DM, LA
mucogenicum
Mycobacterium m.
mucoid
m. exopolysaccharide
m. impaction
m. medial degeneration
m. sputum
mucokinetic
mucolipidosis, pl. **mucolipidoses**
mucolytic
classic m.
peptide m.
mucomembranous
Mucomyst
mucopolysaccharide
acid m. (AMP)
mucopolysaccharidosis,
pl. **mucopolysaccharidoses**
mucopurulent sputum
mucopus
Mucor
Mucoraceae
mucoregulatory agent
mucoretention cyst
mucormycosis
pulmonary m.
mucosa
airway m.
m. of bronchus
esophageal m.
region of respiratory m.

M

NOTES

mucosa *(continued)*
    respiratory m.
    tracheal m.
mucosal
    m. addresin cell adhesion
      molecule-1 (MadCAM-1)
    m. edema
    m. ischemia
mucoserous
Mucosil
mucous
    m. cell
    m. desiccation
    m. gel
    m. gland hyperplasia
    m. gland hypertrophy
    m. layer
    m. plugging
    m. rale
    m. retention cyst
    m. sheets
    m. thread
mucoviscidosis
mucus
    m. clearance device
    m. hypersecretion
    m. inhibitor
    low-viscosity m.
    oyster mass of m.
    m. plug
    m. production
    m. retention
    m. secretion
    tenacious m.
    thick and sticky m.
    m. transport
    viscid m.
    m. viscosity
MUE
    medication use evaluation
Muerto Canyon virus
MUFA
    monounsaturated fatty acid
muffled heart sounds
MUGA
    multiple gated acquisition
    MUGA cardiac blood pool scan
    MUGA exercise stress test
    MUGA scanning
Müller
    M. banding
    M. catheter guide
    M. experiment
    M. maneuver
    M. sign
    M. test
    M. vena caval clamp
Mullins
    M. blade and balloon septostomy

    M. blade technique
    M. cardiac device
    M. catheter introducer
    M. dilator
    M. modification
    M. modification of transseptal
      catheterization
    M. sheath/dilator
    M. sheath system
    M. transseptal catheter
    M. transseptal catheterization sheath
multiaccess catheter (MAC)
multiaxis accelerometer
multibreath nitrogen washout technique
multicellular stent
Multicor II cardiac pacemaker
multicrystal gamma camera
multidetector computed tomography
   (MDCT)
multidisciplinary pulmonary
   rehabilitation program
Multi-Dop X/TCD transcranial Doppler
   instrument
multidrug resistance
multidrug-resistant (MDR)
    m.-r. tuberculosis (MDR-TB)
multielectrode
    m. basket catheter
    m. impedance catheter
    m. probe
multielement linear array
multifactorial
    m. cardiac risk index (MCRI)
    m. cough
MULTIFIT computer-based chronic
   illness management system
multifocal
    m. atrial tachycardia (MAT,
      MFAT, MFT)
    m. lesion
    m. micronodular pneumocyte
      hyperplasia
    m. supraventricular tachyarrhythmia
multiform
    m. premature ventricular complex
    m. tachycardia
multiforme
    erythema m.
    recurrent glioblastoma m. (RGM)
multigated angiography
Multigon 500M non-contrast-enhanced
   TCD
multihead detector
multiinfarct dementia
multikringle glycoprotein
multilamellar body
multilesion angioplasty
Multi-Link
    M.-L. Ascent stent

M.-L. coronary stent system
M.-L. Duet stent
M.-L. Frontier coronary stent
system
M.-L. Penta coronary stent system
M.-L. Pixel stent system
M.-L. Solo stent
M.-L. Tetra coronary stent system
M.-L. Tristar balloon
M.-L. Tristar stent system
M.-L. Zeta coronary stent system
multilobar disease
multilocular cyst
multilocularis
Echinococcus m.
multimer assay
multinucleated giant cell
multiplace chambers
multiplanar reconstruction technique
**multiplane transesophageal
echocardiography**
multiple
m. cholesterol emboli syndrome
(MCES)
m. CVIs
m. embolisms
m. gated acquisition (MUGA)
m. gated acquisition cardiac blood
pool scan
m. lentigines syndrome
m. lipoprotein-type hyperlipidemia
m. lobar hemorrhage (MLH)
m. point electrode
m. reentrant wavelet hypothesis of
Moe
m. sclerosis
m. shunt levels
m. sleep latency test (MSLT)
m. system atrophy
m. wavelet hypothesis
multiple-balloon valvuloplasty
multiple-organ
m.-o. dysfunction
m.-o. dysfunction syndrome
(MODS)
m.-o. failure
multiple-parameter telemetry (MPT)
multiple-trauma patient
multiplex
mononeuritis m.
m. neuropathy

multipolar
m. catheter electrode
m. electrode catheter
multiprogrammable pulse generator
Multipurpose-SM catheter
multisensor catheter
multi-sideport catheter infusion set
multisite
m. biventricular pacing
m. mapping
multislice spiral computed tomography
(MSCT)
MultiSPIRO
M. Clear Advantage pulmonary
function filter
M. computerized spirometry
M. DX-Portable Plus spirometry
M. The Peak peak flow meter
multistage
m. exercise test (MET)
m. maximal effort exercise stress
test
multisystem organ failure (MSOF)
multitargeted antifolate
Multitest cell-mediated immunity system
multivalve
m. disease
m. endocarditis
m. insufficiency
m. operation
m. pathology
multivalvular
m. disease
m. disease murmur
Multi-Vent
Hudson M.-V.
multivessel (MV)
m. coronary artery disease
m. coronary artery obstruction
m. disease (MVD)
multiwire gamma camera
multocida
Pasteurella m.
MUO
myocardiopathy of unknown origin
mupirocin
muqueux
mural
m. aneurysm
m. endocarditis
m. endocardium
m. thrombi

M

NOTES

459

mural *(continued)*
    m. thrombosis (MT)
    m. thrombus (MT)
Murat sign
Murgo pressure contour
mu rhythm
murmur (M)
    accidental m.
    amphoric m.
    anemic m.
    aneurysmal m.
    aortic-left ventricular tunnel m.
    aortic-mitral combined disease m.
    aortic regurgitation m.
    aortic stenosis m.
    apex m.
    apical mid diastolic heart m.
    apical systolic heart m.
    arterial m.
    atriosystolic m.
    atrioventricular flow rumbling m.
    attrition m.
    Austin Flint m.
    basal diastolic m.'s
    bellows m.
    blood m.
    blowing m.
    blubbery diastolic m.
    brain m.
    Bright m.
    bronchial collateral artery m.
    Cabot-Locke m.
    carcinoid m.
    cardiac m. (CM)
    cardiopulmonary m.
    cardiorespiratory m.
    Carey Coombs short mid-
      diastolic m.
    carotid artery m.
    click m.
    coarse m.
    Cole-Cecil m.
    congenital m.
    continuous m. (CM)
    continuous heart m.
    cooing m.
    Coombs m.
    crescendo m.
    crescendo-decrescendo diamond-
      shaped systolic ejection m.
    Cruveilhier-Baumgarten m.
    decrescendo m.
    deglutition m.
    diamond ejection m.
    diamond-shaped ejection m.
    diastolic m. (DM, DS)
    diastolic decrescendo m.
    direct m.
    Docke m.

dove coo musical m.
Duroziez m.
dynamic m.
early diastolic m. (EDM)
early-peaking systolic m.
ejection m. (EM)
ejection systolic m. (ESM)
end-diastolic m.
endocardial m.
end-systolic m.
Eustace Smith m.
exit block m.
exocardial m.
expiratory m.
extracardiac m.
Fisher m.
Flint m.
Fräntzel m.
friction m.
functional m.
Gallavardin m.
Gibson m.
goose-honk m.
grade 1-6 m.
Graham Steell m.
groaning m.
Hamman m.
harsh m.
heart m. (HM)
hemic m.
high-frequency m.
high-pitched m.
Hodgkin-Key m.
holodiastolic decrescendo m.
holosystolic m. (HSM)
honking m.
hourglass m.
humming m.
humming-top m.
incidental m.
indirect m.
innocent m. (IM)
innocent heart m.
inorganic m.
inspiratory m.
lapping m.
late apical systolic m.
late diastolic m.
late-peaking systolic m.
late systolic m. (LSM)
left ventricular-right atrial
  communication m.
Levine grade 1–6 cardiac m.
low-frequency m.
low-pitched m.
machinery m.
mammary souffle m.
middiastolic m. (MDM)

midsystolic m. (MSM)
mill house m.
mill wheel m.
mitral prolapse m.
mitral regurgitation m.
mitral stenosis m.
multivalvular disease m.
muscular m.
musical m.
noninvasive m.
nun's venous hum m.
obstructive m.
organic m.
outflow m.
pansystolic m.
Parrot m.
patent ductus arteriosus m.
pathologic m.
pericardial m.
physiologic m.
pleuropericardial m.
prediastolic m.
presystolic m. (PM, PSM)
primary pulmonary hypertension m.
protodiastolic m.
pulmonary m., pulmonic m.
rasping m.
reduplication m.
regurgitant m.
respiratory m.
Roger m.
rumbling diastolic m.
scratchy m.
seagull m.
seesaw m.
Steell m.
stenosal m.
Still m.
subclavian m.
subclavicular m.
systolic m. (SM)
systolic apical m.
systolic ejection m. (SEM)
systolic regurgitant m.
to-and-fro m.
transmitted m.
Traube m.
tricuspid m.
vascular m.
venous m.
ventricular septal defect m.
vesicular m.

water wheel m.
whooping m.
murmur/energy ratio (MER)
murmurs (Ms)
Murphy
    M. method
    M. percussion
Murray score
muscarinic
    m. agonist
    m. receptor
    m. stimulation
muscle
    accessory inspiratory m.
    airways smooth m. (ASM)
    anterior papillary m. (APM)
    m. artifact
    m. bridge
    bronchial smooth m.
    bronchoesophageal m.
    cardiac m. (CM)
    Chassaignac axillary m.
    m. ergoreceptor
    m. fraction enzyme of CPK (CPK-MM, CPK-3)
    human aortic smooth m. (HASMC)
    latissimus dorsi m.
    m. metaboreflex
    m. of Moulaert
    Oehl m.
    papillary m. (PM)
    pectinate m.
    pleuroesophageal m.
    posterior cricoarytenoid m.
    posterior papillary m. (PPM)
    rectus abdominis m.
    Reisseisen m.
    m. relaxant
    ribbon m.'s
    serratus anterior m.
    short-axis plane, papillary m. (SAX-PM)
    skeletal m.
    m. stiffness
    strap m.
    m. sympathetic nerve activity (MSNA)
    m. of thorax
    m. trabeculation
    trachealis m.
    transversus nuchae m.
    venous smooth m.

M

NOTES

muscular
- m. bridging
- m. coat of bronchus
- m. coat of esophagus
- m. coat of trachea
- m. contraction
- m. dystrophy
- m. incompetence
- m. murmur
- m. subaortic stenosis (MSS)
- m. venous pump
- m. ventricular septal defect (MVSD)

musculi (*pl. of* musculus)
musculi laryngis
musculoskeletal
- m. intervention center (MUSIC)
- m. pain

musculus, pl. **musculi**
- m. bronchoesophageus
- m. diaphragma
- m. levator glandulae thyroideae
- m. pleuroesophageus

mushroom
- m. dust
- m. worker's disease
- m. worker's lung

MUSIC
- musculoskeletal intervention center

musical
- m. bruit
- m. murmur
- m. rale

Musset sign
mustard
- M. atrial baffle
- M. atrial repair
- M. atrial switch operation
- L-phenylalanine m.
- nitrogen m.
- M. procedure

Mustard-Senning procedure
Mustargen Hydrochloride
Mutamycin
mutant allele
mutation
- factor V Leiden m.
- missense m.
- nonsense m.
- SCN5A m.
- thrombophilic factor V Leiden m.

mute
- m. reflex
- m. toe sign

muzolimine
MV
- maximal ventilation
- mechanical ventilation

midventricular
multivessel

mV
- millivolt

MVA
- malignant ventricular arrhythmia
- mechanical ventricular assistance
- microvascular angiopathy
- mitral valve area

MVAD
- mechanical ventricular assist device

MVB
- microvascular bleeding

MVC
- maximal vital capacity
- maximum voluntary contraction
- myocardial vascular capacity

MVD
- microvascular decompression
- mitral valve disease
- multivessel disease
- myocardial vasodilation

MVE
- mitral valve echo
- mitral valve excursion

MVF
- mitral valve flow

MVG
- mitral valve gradient

MVI
- mitral valve insufficiency

MVL
- mitral valve leaflet

MVO
- maximum venous outflow
- mitral valve opening
- mitral valve orifice

MVO2, MVO$_2$
- myocardial oxygen consumption

MVOA
- mitral valve orifice area

MVP
- mitomycin, vinblastine, cisplatin
- mitral valve prolapse
  - MVP catheter

MVPS
- mitral valve prolapse syndrome

MVP-SC
- mitral valve prolapse-systolic click

MVR
- maximal ventilation rate
- minimal vascular resistance
- mitral valve replacement

MVSD
- muscular ventricular septal defect

MVT
- monomorphic ventricular tachycardia

MVV
- maximum voluntary ventilation

MWT
    myocardial wall thickness
6MWT, 6-MWT
    6-minute walking test
    six-minute walk test
myalgia gravis
Myambutol
myasthenia
    m. cordis
    m. gravis
    m. gravis pseudoparalytica
myasthenic crisis
MyBP-C
    myosin-binding protein C
    MyBP-C gene
mycetoma
MycoAKT latex bead agglutination test
mycobacteria
    nontuberculous m. (NTM)
    m. other than tuberculosis (MOTT)
mycobacterial disease
Mycobacterium
    M. abscessus
    M. africanum
    M. avium
    M. avium complex (MAC)
    M. avium complex infection
    M. avium-intracellulare (MAI)
    M. avium-intracellulare complex
    M. avium-intracellulare infection
    M. bovis
    M. chelonae
    M. fortuitum
    M. fortuitum-chelonae complex
    M. gastri
    M. genavense
    M. gordonae
    M. haemophilum
    M. intracellulare
    M. intracellulare, Battey bacillus
    M. kansasii
    M. leprae
    M. malmoense
    M. marinum
    M. microti
    M. mucogenicum
    M. peregrinum
    M. phlei
    M. scrofulaceum
    M. simiae
    M. smegmatis
    M. szulgai

    M. terrae
    M. thermoresistible
    M. tuberculosis (MTB)
    M. ulcerans
    M. vaccae
    M. xenopi
Mycobutin Oral
mycology
mycophenolate
    m. mofetil (MMF)
    m. mofetil capsule
    m. mofetil intravenous for injection
    m. mofetil oral suspension
    m. mofetil tablet
Mycoplasma
    M. faucium
    M. hominis
    M. incognitus
    M. pneumoniae
    M. xenopi
mycoplasmal pneumonia
mycoplasmosis
mycosis, pl. **mycoses**
    m. fungoides
    Posadas m.
    pulmonary m.
Mycostatin Topical
mycotic
    m. aortic aneurysm
    m. aortography
    m. endocarditis
    m. infection
MycroMesh graft material
MycroPhylax implantable cardioverter-defibrillator
mydriatic
myectomy
    septal m.
myeloid progenitor inhibitory factor (MPIF)
myeloma
myelonecrosis
myeloperoxidase (MPO)
myelosuppression
Myers Solution
MYHC
    heavy chain cardiac myosin
MYHCA
    heavy chain cardiac myosin alpha
Mykrox
Myleran
myocardia (*pl. of* myocardium)

M

NOTES

myocardial
m. abscess
m. adrenergic signaling
m. angiogenesis
m. anoxia
m. band (MB)
m. band enzymes of CPK (CPK-MB, CPK-2)
m. band index
m. bed
m. beta adrenergic receptor (MBAR)
m. blood flow (MBF)
m. blush
m. bridge
m. bridging (MB)
m. cell hypertrophy
m. channeling (MC)
m. clamp
m. cold-spot perfusion scintigraphy
m. collagen matrix
m. concussion
m. contractility
m. contraction force (MCF)
m. contraction state
m. contrast echocardiography (MCE)
m. contusion
m. creatine phosphate
m. damage (MD)
m. depolarization
m. depressant factor (MDF)
m. depressant substance (MDS)
m. depression
m. disarray
m. disease (MD)
m. disease of unknown origin (MDUO)
m. Doppler velocity (MDV)
m. echodensity
m. edema
m. electrode
m. endothelin
m. energy
m. failure
m. fiber shortening
m. fibrosis (MF)
m. fibrous scar
m. fractional flow reserve (FFR$_{myo}$)
m. free wall rupture
m. function
m. hamartoma
m. hibernation
m. hypoperfusion
m. indirect calorimetry
m. infarction (MI)
M. Infarction Data Acquisition System
m. infarction in dumbbell form
m. infarction rehabilitation program (MIRP)
m. infarction research unit (MIRU)
m. infarction triage and intervention (MITI)
m. infiltrative process
m. infundibular stenosis
m. injury
m. insufficiency
m. ischemia (MI)
m. ischemia dynamic analysis (MIDA)
m. ischemic syndrome
m. jeopardy
m. jeopardy index
m. lactate extraction
m. laser revascularization (MLR)
m. laser revascularization procedure
m. lead
m. long-chain fatty acid uptake defect
m. malnutrition
m. mass
m. metabolic rate (MMR)
m. metabolism
m. muscle creatine kinase isoenzyme
m. necrosis
m. oxygen (MO$_2$)
m. oxygen consumption (MVO2, MVO$_2$)
m. oxygen demand
m. oxygen supply
m. oxygen uptake
m. perforation
m. perfusion
m. perfusion imaging (MPI)
m. perfusion scintigraphy (MPS)
m. protection
m. protection system (MPS)
m. remodeling
m. repolarization
m. reserve
m. revascularization (MR)
m. rigor mortis
m. salvage
m. scar tissue
m. single photon emission tomography (MSPECT)
m. sinusoid
m. sparing
m. stiffness
m. stress perfusion scintigraphy (MSPS)
m. stunning
m. substrate uptake (MSU)
m. tension
m. tissue
m. vascular capacity (MVC)

m. vasodilation (MVD)
m. viability
m. viability scintigraphy
m. VIDA
m. wall thickness (MWT)
myocardiograph
myocardiopathy
    alcoholic m.
    chagasic m.
    congestive m. (CM)
    m. of unknown origin (MUO)
myocardiorrhaphy
myocarditic
myocarditis (MC)
    acute isolated m.
    asymptomatic m.
    atrial m.
    bacterial m.
    burned out viral m.
    cardiac sarcoidosis m.
    chronic m.
    clostridial m.
    coxsackievirus m.
    cryptococcal m.
    diphtheritic m.
    ECHO virus m.
    echovirus m.
    Fiedler m.
    fragmentation m.
    fulminant m.
    giant cell m.
    helminthic m.
    Histoplasma m.
    hypersensitivity m.
    idiopathic m.
    indurative m.
    metazoal m.
    parenchymatous m.
    peripartum m.
    protozoal m.
    rheumatic m.
    rickettsial m.
    spirochetal m.
    syphilitic m.
    toxic m.
    tuberculoid m.
    viral m. (VM)
myocardium, pl. **myocardia**
    dysfunctional m.
    dyssynergic m.
    fragmentation of m.
    hibernating m.

hypertrophied m.
hypoperfused m.
idiopathic disease of m. (IDM)
ischemic m.
isolated noncompaction of left
    ventricular m.
jeopardized m.
postischemic m.
reperfused m.
senescent m.
spongy m.
stunned m.
underperfused m.
viable m.
vulnerable m.
myocardosis
    Reisman m.
myoclonic jerk
Myocor Coapsys pacing assist device
myocyte
    amplifying m.
    Anichkov m.
    cardiac m.
    m. deenergization
    m. hypertrophy
    m. hypoxia
    m. magnesium stores
    m. metabolic activity
    m. necrosis
myocytolysis
    coagulative m.
    m. of heart
myoendocarditis
myofascial
myofibril
myofibrillar
    m. ATPase
    m. calcium level
    m. disarray
    m. lysis
myofibroblast
myofibrosis cordis
myofilament
    m. calcium responsiveness
    m. contractile activation
myogenic theory
myoglobin assay
myoglobinuria
myoglobulin (Mgb)
    m. cardiac diagnostic test
myoglobulinuria
myointimal plaque

M

NOTES

myolysis
    cardiotoxic m.
myomalacia cordis
myopathia cordis
myopathy
    centronuclear m.
    myotubular m.
    nemaline m.
    tachycardia-induced m.
myopericarditis
myoplasmic calcium
myoplasty
myopleuropericarditis
Myopore lead
myopotential oversensing
Myoscint
MyoSIGHT dedicated nuclear cardiology camera system
myosin
    antibody to murine cardiac m. (AMM)
    anticardiac m. (ACM)
    cardiac m.
    m. heavy chain
    heavy chain cardiac m. (MYHC)
    m. light chain
myosin-binding
    m.-b. protein C (MyBP-C)
    m.-b. protein C gene
myosin-specific antibody
myositis
Myosplint procedure
MYOtherm XP cardioplegia delivery system
myotomy
    hyoid m.
    septal m.
myotomy-myectomy-septal resection
myotonia congenita
myotonic muscular dystrophy

myotubular myopathy
Myoview contrast material
MyoVive
Myphetane DC
myringoplasty
    venous graft m. (VGM)
myrtillus
    Vaccinium m.
Mytussin
    M. AC
    M. DAC
    M. DM
myurous pulse
myurus
    pulsus m.
myxedema
    m. heart
    pretibial m.
myxedematous
myxoma, pl. **myxomata**
    atrial m.
    cardiac m.
    familial atrial m.
    infected m.
    left atrial m. (LAM)
    left ventricular m.
    mobile m.
    petrified cardiac m.
    right atrial m.
    right ventricular m.
    stone like m.
    m. tumor
    ventricular m.
myxomatous
    m. change
    m. degeneration
    m. proliferation
    m. pulmonary embolism
    m. valve disease

N

N cell
N High Sensitivity CRP assay
N region

N-13

nitrogen-13
N-13 ammonia
N-13 ammonia positron emission tomography
N-13 ammonia uptake

N$_2$

nitrogen-13
N$_2$ oximetry

N-20 terminal peptide
N/2 artifact
n-3 fatty acid
n-6 fatty acid
N95-Companion accessory
_N_-acetylneuraminic acid
_N_-acetyl procainamide (NAPA)
Nachlas tube
NACPTAR

North American Cerebral Transluminal Angioplasty Registration

nacre dust asthma
NACT

National Alliance of Cardiovascular Technologists

NAD

nicotinamide adenine dinucleotide

nadir of QRS complex
nadolol
Nadopen-V
NADPH

nicotinamide adenine dinucleotide phosphate

nadroparin calcium
Naegleria gruberi
NAEP

National Asthma Education Program

NAEPP

National Asthma Education and Prevention Program

nafamostat
nafate

cefamandole n.

nafazatrom
nafcillin sodium
naftidrofuryl
Nagle exercise stress test
Na$^+$/H$^+$

Na$^+$/H$^+$ exchange inhibitor (NHEI)
Na$^+$/H$^+$ exchanger (NHE)

NAHC

National Advisory Heart Council

nail

n. bed
cyanosis of n. beds
n. pulse

nail-fold skin
nail-patella disease
nail-to-nail bed angle
NaK-ATPase

sodium-potassium adenotriphosphatase
sodium-potassium pump

Nakayama

N. anastomosis
N. anastomosis apparatus

nalbuphine hydrochloride
Naldecon Senior EX
Nalfon
nalidixic acid
nalmefene hydrochloride
naloxone hydrochloride
naltrexone
NAME

nevi, atrial myxoma, myxoid neurofibromas, and ephelides
NAME syndrome

Namic

N. angiographic syringe
N. catheter

nandrolone decanoate
NANIPER

nonallergic noninfectious perennial rhinitis

nanograms per milliliter
nanomole (nmol)
nanoporous
Nanos 01 pacemaker
NAPA

N-acetyl procainamide

nape

transverse muscle of n.

napkin-ring

n.-r. calcification
n.-r. defect
n.-r. stenosis

Naprosyn
naproxen
NAPSE

North American Society for Pacing and Electrophysiology

Naqua
Narcan injection
Narco

N. Biosystems recorder
N. Physiograph-6B recorder

narcolepsy
Narcomatic flowmeter

N

narcosis
> inert gas n.
> nitrogen n.

narcotic

NARES
> nonallergic rhinitis with eosinophilia

narrow communication

narrow-complex tachycardia

narrowed pulse pressure

NarrowFlex intraaortic balloon catheter

narrowing
> atherosclerotic n.
> eccentric n.
> intracoronary stenting of de
> novo n.
> longitudinal n.
> luminal n.
> nonatheromatous arterial n.
> ostial n.
> restenotic n.
> systolic coronary artery n. (SCAN)

Narula method

NAS
> no added salt

Nasabid

Nasacort AQ

Nasal

nasal
> n. airways
> n. asthma
> n. cannula
> n. continuous positive airway
> pressure (NCPAP, nCPAP)
> n. CPAP
> n. CPAP system
> DDAVP N.
> Drixoral N.
> n. flaring
> N. Moist
> N. Moist Gel
> n. nicotine spray (NNS)
> n. nocturnal ventilation (NNV)
> n. part of pharynx
> n. polyposis
> n. pool technique
> n. positive pressure ventilation
> (NPPV)
> n. potential difference
> n. prongs
> n. steroid (NS)
> triamcinolone inhalation, n.

Nasal-Aire ventilator nasal insert mask

Nasalcrom Nasal Solution

Nasalide Nasal Aerosol

nasalis
> regio n.

Nasarel

nascent HDL

nasi
> ala n.
> regio respiratoria tunicae
> mucosae n.

nasobronchial reflex

nasogastric
> n. tube
> n. tube feeding (NTF)

nasopharyngeal (NP)
> n. carcinoma
> n. groove
> n. reflux
> n. secretion
> n. wash

nasopharyngitis

nasopharyngoscopy

nasopharynx

nasotracheal
> n. intubation
> n. suction
> n. tube

Nathan test

national
> N. Advisory Heart Council
> (NAHC)
> N. Alliance of Cardiovascular
> Technologists (NACT)
> N. Asthma Education and
> Prevention Program (NAEPP)
> N. Asthma Education Program
> (NAEP)
> N. Board for Respiratory Care
> (NBRC)
> N. Cardiovascular Network (NCN)
> N. Cholesterol Education Panel
> guidelines
> N. Cholesterol Education Program
> (NCEP)
> N. Health and Nutrition
> Examination Survey I
> N. Health Service (NHS)
> N. Heart Foundation (NHF)
> N. Heart Institute (NHI)
> N. Heart, Lung, Blood Institute
> (NHLBI)
> N. Heart, Lung, Blood
> Institute/National Asthma
> Education Prevention Program
> (NHLBI/NAEPP)
> N. High Blood Pressure Education
> Program (NHBPEP)
> N. Home Oxygen Patients
> Association
> N. Hospital Network
> N. Institute for Clinical Excellence
> (NICE)
> N. Institutes of Health (NIH)
> N. Institutes of Health left
> ventriculography catheter

N. Institutes of Health marking catheter

N. Institutes of Health mitral valve-grasping forceps

N. Institutes of Health Stroke Scale (NIHSS)

N. Institutes of Neurological Disorders and Stroke (NINDS)

N. Lung Health Education Program (NLHEP)

N. Nosocomial Infection Surveillance

N. Registry of Myocardial Infarction (NRMI)

N. Society of Cardiovascular Technologists (NSCT)

native

n. coarctation

n. coronary anatomy

n. coronary artery

n. LDL (n-LDL)

n. low-density lipoprotein

n. tissue harmonic imaging

n. valve

n. valve endocarditis (NVE)

n. valve fibroplastic endocarditis

n. vessel

Natrecor

Natrilix

natriuresis

natriuretic

n. hormone

n. peptide

natural

n. frequency

n. history

n. killer (NK)

n. resistance macrophage-associated protein (Nramp)

1-natural-log-unit elevation

Naturetin

Naughton

N. cardiac exercise treadmill test

N. graded exercise stress test

N. treadmill protocol

Nauheim

N. bath

N. treatment

NavAblator catheter

Navelbine

Navidrex

Navier-Stokes equation

navigation

intracardiac n.

navigator echo signal

Naviport deflectable tip guiding catheter

Navistar catheter

Naxos disease

n-BCA

n-butyl cyanoacrylate

NBRC

National Board for Respiratory Care

NBTE

nonbacterial thrombotic endocarditis

n-butyl cyanoacrylate (n-BCA)

NC

noncardiac

NC balloon

NC Bandit ball

NC Bandit catheter

NC Raptor over-the-wire coaxial PTCA dilatation balloon catheter

NCA

noncontractile area

normal coronary arteries

n-CAD

negative coronoradiographic documentation

NCC

noncoronary cusp

NCE

negative-contrast echocardiography

NCEP

National Cholesterol Education Program

NCEP guidelines

NCEP Step-One Diet

NCEP-II guidelines

NCN

National Cardiovascular Network

NCPAP, nCPAP

nasal continuous positive airway pressure

Aladdin[II] NCPAP

NCPAP therapy

NCPE

noncardiac pulmonary edema

NCV

nerve conduction velocity

NDA

new device angioplasty

Nd:YAG

neodymium:yttrium-aluminum-garnet

Nd:YAG laser

N

NOTES

NE
    norepinephrine
near
    n. field
    n. infrared
    n. patient test (NPT)
    n. syncope
near-fainting
near-fatal asthma (NFA)
near-field visualization
near-gain
near-infrared
    n.-i. cerebral oximetry
    n.-i. spectroscopy (NIRS, NIS)
near-syncope
nebacumab
Nebcin injection
nebivolol
NebuChamber
Nebuhaler
Nebules
    Ventolin N.
nebulization
    aqueous solution for n.
    continuous albuterol n. (CAN)
    wet n.
nebulized
    n. bronchodilator
    n. Ig therapy
    n. tobramycin
nebulizer
    Acorn II n.
    AeroEclipse breath actuated n.
    aerosol n.
    AeroSonic personal ultrasonic n.
    AeroTech II n.
    air-powered n.
    Babbington-type n.
    baffled jet n.
    BESTNEB n.
    Centimist n.
    n. chronolog
    compressor-generated n. (CGN)
    Compu-Neb ultrasonic n.
    DeVilbiss n.
    handheld n.
    Heart n.
    Heliox n.
    Hope continuous & Heliox n.
    IV-Heart n.
    jet n.
    LC Plus reusable n.
    LC STAR reusable n.
    Marquest Respirgard II n.
    MicroAir electronic n.
    MicroAir handheld n.
    Micro Mist n.
    MiniHEART low-flow n.
    Mistogen n.

    Pari LC Plus reusable n.
    Pari LC Star reusable n.
    Pari Proneb Ultra n.
    PermaNeb reusable n.
    Proneb Ultra n.
    Pulmo-Aide n.
    Respirgard II n.
    Schuco n.
    Sidestream high-efficiency n.
    small-volume n. (SNV, SVN)
    Sonix 2000 ultrasonic n.
    Twin Jet n.
    ultrasonic n. (USN)
    UniHeart IV universal n.
    Updraft handheld n.
    VixOne small-volume n.
NebuPent Inhalation
NEC
    nonesterified cholesterol
Necator americanus
necessitatis
    empyema n.
neck
    transverse artery of n.
necrobacillosis
necrobiosis lipoidica diabeticorum
necrobiotic nodule
necrolysis
    toxic epidermal n.
necrophorum
    Fusobacterium n.
necrophorus
    Sphaerophorus n.
necropsy
necrosis, pl. **necroses**
    avascular n.
    coagulation n.
    contraction band n.
    cystic medial n.
    digital n.
    dirty n.
    electrolyte and steroid cardiopathy
      with n. (ESCN)
    embolic n.
    Erdheim cystic medial n.
    n. factor
    fibrinoid n.
    ischemic n.
    liquefaction n.
    medial n.
    myocardial n.
    myocyte n.
    pressure n.
    renal cortical n.
    tissue n.
    tubular n.
necrotic cyst
necrotisans
    phlebitis nodularis n.

necrotizing
- n. angiitis
- n. arterial disease
- n. arteriolitis
- n. bronchopneumonia
- n. granuloma
- n. granulomatous vasculitis
- n. pneumonia

nedocromil sodium

needle
- Abrams n.
- Adson aneurysm n.
- Aldrete n.
- arachnophlebectomy n.
- argon n.
- arterial n.
- n. aspirate
- aspirating n.
- Atraloc n.
- atraumatic n.
- Becton-Dickinson Teflon-sheathed n.
- BRK series transseptal n.
- Brockenbrough curved n.
- butterfly n.
- Cardiopoint n.
- Chiba n.
- Cope pleural biopsy n.
- Cournand n.
- Cournand-Grino angiography n.
- Cournand-Potts n.
- Curry n.
- disposable percutaneous entry thinwall n.
- DLP cardioplegic n.
- Dos Santos n.
- ergonomic vascular access n. (EVAN)
- Ethalloy n.
- eyeless n.
- N.'s Eye snare
- Fergie n.
- Ferguson n.
- Fischer pneumothoracic n.
- 27G n.
- GlideCath entry n.
- n. holder
- Hustead n.
- Jamshidi n.
- large-bore slotted aspirating n.
- Lewy-Rubin n.
- Lowell pleural n.
- Luer-Lok n.
- Menghini n.
- micron n.
- Micropuncture introducer n.
- O'Brien airway n.
- olive-tipped n.
- PercuCut biopsy n.
- percutaneous cutting n.
- pilot n.
- polytef-sheathed n.
- Potts n.
- Potts-Cournand n.
- Ranfac n.
- Riley n.
- Rochester n.
- Ross n.
- Rotex n.
- Safe Step blood-collection n.
- scalp vein n.
- Securcut aspiration biopsy n.
- Seldinger n.
- slotted n.
- standard n.
- steel-winged butterfly n.
- Stifcore aspiration n.
- Stifcore biopsy injection n.
- THI n.
- thin-walled n.
- thoracentesis n.
- n. thoracostomy
- TMC n.
- transseptal n.
- Tru-Cut biopsy n.
- Venflon n.
- Vim-Silverman n.
- Wang transbronchial n.
- Wasserman n.
- Zavala lung biopsy n.

needlepoint electrocautery

Needle-Pro needle protection device

NEEP
- negative end-expiratory pressure

nefazodone

Neff percutaneous access set

negative
- n. chronotropism
- n. contrast
- n. coronoradiographic documentation (n-CAD)
- n. deflection that follows an R wave (S)

NOTES

N

negative *(continued)*
    n. end-expiratory pressure (NEEP)
    n. expiratory pressure (NEP)
    false n.
    n. inotrope
    n. intrapleural pressure
    n. predictive value (NPV)
    n. pressure pulmonary edema (NPPE)
    n. pressure ventilation (NPV)
    n. remodeling
    n. treppe
    n. T, U wave
negative-contrast
    n.-c. echocardiography (NCE)
    n.-c. injection
    n.-c. intravascular ultrasound
NegGram
neglect
    motor n.
    perceptual-sensory n.
    unilateral spatial n. (USN)
    visuospatial n.
Negri body
Negus bronchoscope
Neisseria
    N. catarrhalis
    N. gonorrhoeae
    N. meningitidis
neisserial
nelfinavir
Nellcor
    N. N200 pulse oximeter
    N. Puritan Bennett (NPB)
    N. Symphony blood pressure monitor
    N. Symphony pulse oximeter
nemaline myopathy
Nembutal
neoadjuvant chemotherapy
neoangiogenesis
neocapillarization
Neo-Codema
neodymium:yttrium-aluminum-garnet (Nd:YAG)
    n.-a.-g. laser
neoendothelium
NEO-fit
    NEO-f. endotracheal tube grip
    NEO-f. neonatal endotracheal tube holder
neoformans
    Cryptococcus n.
neoglottis
neointima
neointimal
    n. generation
    n. hyperplasia
    n. hyperplastic response

    n. proliferation
    n. ridge
    n. tear
    n. thickening
    n. tissue
neolumen
neomycin sulfate
neonatal
    Exosurf N.
    N. Y TrachCare
neonate respiratory distress syndrome (NRDS)
neonatorum
    apnea n.
    asphyxia n.
neoplasia
neoplasm
    extrathoracic n.
neoplastic
    n. cavity
    n. cell
    n. disease
    n. pericarditis
neopterin
    serum n.
Neoral cyclosporine capsule
Neosar injection
Neo-Sert umbilical vessel catheter insertion set
Neo-Synephrine 12 Hour Nasal Solution
NeoTect
Neo-Therm neonatal skin temperature probe
Neothylline
Neotrend
    N. multiparameter blood gas monitor
    N. system
neovascularity
    plaque n.
neovascularization
    left atrial n. (LANV)
NeoVO2R infant volume control resuscitator
NEP
    negative expiratory pressure
    neutral endopeptidase
nephritis, pl. **nephritides**
    familial n.
    immune-mediated membranous n.
    tuberculous n.
Nephro-Fer
nephrogenesis
nephrogenic diabetes insipidus
nephrogram
nephron
nephropathic cardiomyopathy
nephropathy
    analgesic n.

diabetic n.
hypertensive n. (HTN)
hyperuricemic n.
nephrosclerosis
nephrostolithotomy
nephrotic syndrome
nephrotoxicity
NEP-I, NEPi
    neutral endopeptidase inhibition
neprilysin
Neptune high-pressure PTCA balloon catheter
Nernst equation
nerve
    accelerator n.
    accompanying artery of ischiadic n.
    accompanying artery of median n.
    n. action potential
    aortic n.
    aortic depressor n. (ADN)
    axillary n.
    brachial n.
    cardiac sensory n.
    cardiac sympathetic n. (CSN)
    cardiopulmonary splanchnic n.'s
    carotid sinus n.
    n. conduction velocity (NCV)
    cranial n.'s I–XII
    esophageal branch of vagus n.
    external branch of superior laryngeal n.
    faucial branches of lingual n.
    glossopharyngeal n.
    n. of Hering
    hypoglossal n.
    inferior ganglion of glossopharyngeal n.
    internal branch of superior laryngeal n.
    n. of Kuntz
    laryngeal n.
    lateral ventricular n. (LVN)
    left recurrent laryngeal n.
    lingual branch of facial n.
    pharyngeal branch of glossopharyngeal n.
    pharyngeal branch of vagus n.
    phrenic n.
    right recurrent laryngeal n.
    sensory n.
    sympathetic n.
    thoracic n.

    trigeminal n.
    ulnar n.
    vagus n.
nervi
    ganglion inferius n.
    ganglion superius n.
nervorum
    vasa n.
nervosa
    anorexia n.
    dysphagia n.
nervous
    n. asthma
    n. respiration
    n. system
    n. tachypnea
nesiritide citrate
nest of veins
net
    n. absorption
    Health On the N. (HON)
Netherton syndrome
netilmicin sulfate
network
    advanced heart failure shared clinical experience n. (AHF SCENE)
    Chiari n.
    Encompass cardiac n.
    fibrillar collagen n.
    hypertension genetic epidemiology n. (HyperGEN)
    interstitial and perivascular collagen n.
    local area n. (LAN)
    National Cardiovascular N. (NCN)
    National Hospital N.
    Organ Procurement and Transplantation N. (OPTN)
    Purkinje n.
Neubauer artery
neuf
    bruit de cuir n.
Neupogen
neural
    n. crest malformation
    n. crest migration
neuralgia
    glossopharyngeal n.
neurally
    n. mediated syncopal syndrome
    n. mediated syncope (NMS)

N

NOTES

neurally (*continued*)
  n. mediated vasovagal syncope (NMVS)
neurapraxia
neurenteric cyst
neuritis
  optic n.
neuroblastoma
neurocardiac syncope
neurocardial syncope
neurocardiogenic syncope
neurocirculatory asthenia
neurodegenerative disease
neurodiagnostics
neuroendocrine
  n. theory
  n. tumor
neuroepithelial body
neurofibroma
neurofibromatosis
neurogenic
  n. abnormality
  n. pulmonary edema
  n. theory
  n. tumor
neurohormonal
  n. arterial constriction
  n. function
neurohormone
neurohumoral
  n. factors
  n. stimulus
neurokinin A (NKA)
neuroleptic
neurologic
  n. DCS
  n. deficit
  n. examination
  n. status
  n. syncope
neurological disorder
neuromediated syncope
neuromuscular
  n. blockade
  n. blocking agent (NMBA)
  n. coupling
  n. disease
  n. disorder
  n. hypertension
neuromyopathic disorder
neuromyopathy
  carcinomatous n.
neuronal ceroid lipofuscinosis
neuron-specific enolase (NSE)
neuropathy
  angiopathic n.
  cardiac autonomic n. (CAN)
  diabetic n.
  diabetic autonomic n. (DAN)

  multiplex n.
  peripheral n.
  vasculitic n.
neuropeptide
  human n.
  n. Y
Neuroperfusion pump
neuroprotection
neuroprotective
  n. agent
  n. drug
neurosis, pl. **neuroses**
  anxiety n.
  cardiac n.
Neurostar angiography system
neurosyphilis
neuroticism
neurotoxic effect
Neurotrac
  N. II EEG
  N. II neurologic monitoring system
neurotransmission
  sympathetic n.
neurotransmitter substance
neurovascular bundle
NeuroVasx submicroinfusion catheter
neutral
  n. endopeptidase (NEP)
  n. endopeptidase inhibition (NEP-I, NEPi)
  n. endopeptidase inhibitor
  n. lipid (NL)
Neutrexin injection
neutron activation analysis
neutropenia
neutropenic angina
neutrophil
  n. chemotoxin
  n. elastase
  polymorphonuclear n. (PMN)
  segmented n.'s
neutrophilia
  pleural fluid n.
neutrophil-induced pulmonary inflammation
NEV
  noninvasive extrathoracic ventilator
nevi (*pl. of* nevus)
nevi, atrial myxoma, myxoid neurofibromas, and ephelides (NAME)
Neville
  N. stent
  N. tracheal prosthesis
nevirapine (NVP)
nevus, pl. **nevi**
  n. araneus
  nevi, atrial myxoma, myxoid neurofibromas, and ephelides (NAME)

lentigines, atrial myxoma,
mucocutaneous myxomas, and
blue nevi (LAMB)

new

N. device angioplasty (NDA)
N. York catheter exchange wire
guide
N. York Heart Association
functional classification I–IV

newborn

persistent pulmonary hypertension
of n. (PPHN)
respiratory distress syndrome of
the n.
transient tachypnea of n. (TTNB)

NewLife

N. Elite concentrator
N. oxygen concentrator

Newport

N. E100M ventilator
N. Wave V200 ventilator

Newton

N. catheter
N. guidewire

NexStent carotid stent

Nexus

N. coronary stent
N. 2 linear ablation catheter

NF

Nissen fundoplication

NFA

near-fatal asthma

NF-ATc protein

NF-kappa-B

nuclear factor-kappa-B

**N-geneous automated HDL cholesterol
test**

NH

nodal-His
nodohisian
NH region
NH region of A-V node

NHBPEP

National High Blood Pressure Education
Program

NHDL

non-high density lipoprotein

NHE

Na^+/H^+ exchanger

NHEI

Na^+/H^+ exchange inhibitor

NHF

National Heart Foundation

NHI

National Heart Institute

NHLBI

National Heart, Lung, Blood Institute

NHLBI/NAEPP

National Heart, Lung, Blood
Institute/National Asthma Education
Prevention Program

NHS

National Health Service

niacin

niacinamide

niacin/lovastatin

extended-release n.

Niaspan

NIBP

noninvasive blood pressure
NIBP monitoring

NiCad

nickel-cadmium

nicardipine hydrochloride

Nic the Dragon aerosol mask

NICE

National Institute for Clinical Excellence
NICE group

nickel

salt of n.

nickel-cadmium (NiCad)

n.-c. battery

Nickerson-Kveim test

nicking

arteriovenous n.

Nicks procedure

Nicoderm Patch

nicofuranose

Nicoladoni-Branham sign

Nicoladoni sign

Nicolet VersaLab APM

**$NICO_2$ noninvasive cardiac output
monitor**

nicorandil

Nicorette

N. Gum
N. Plus

Nicostatin

nicotinamide

n. adenine dinucleotide (NAD)
n. adenine dinucleotide phosphate
(NADPH)

2-nicotinamidoethyl nitrate

N

NOTES

nicotine
    n. by-product
    crystalline n.
    n. dependence
    n. gum
    n. inhaler
    n. nasal spray
    n. transdermal patch
Nicotinex
nicotinic acid
Nicotrol
    N. Inhaler
    N. NS nasal spray
    N. Patch
nicoumalone
NIDDM
    noninsulin-dependent diabetes mellitus
nidulans
    Aspergillus n.
nidus
Niemann-Pick disease
nifedipine enzyme immunoassay
Niferex
niger
    Aspergillus n.
night
    N. Owl pocket polygraph
    n. terrors
nightsweat
nigra
    cardiopathia n.
nigrum
    Epicoccum n.
NIH
    National Institutes of Health
    NIH cardiomarker catheter
    NIH mitral valve-grasping forceps
    NIH *Xenopus* Initiative
Nihon
    N. Kohden polygraph system
    N. Kohden polysomnogram
Ni-Hon-San
    Nipponese in Honolulu and San
    Francisco
NIHSS
    National Institutes of Health Stroke Scale
Nikaidoh-Bex technique
Nikaidoh translocation
nikethamide
Nilandron
nilutamide
Nimbex
Nimbus hemopump
nimesulide
nimodipine
Nimotop
NINDS
    National Institutes of Neurological
    Disorders and Stroke

Ninja FX series over-the-wire coaxial PTCA dilatation balloon catheter
NI-NR
    no infection-no rejection
NIOX nitric oxide breath test system
NIP
    nonspecific chronic interstitial
    pneumonitis
NIPB
    noninvasive blood pressure
nipple
    aortic n.
Nipponese in Honolulu and San Francisco (Ni-Hon-San)
NIPPV
    noninvasive positive pressure ventilation
NIPS
    noninvasive programmed stimulation
NIR
    NIR Elite Monorail system
    NIR Elite OTW stent system
    NIR Primo Monorail coronary stent
NIRflex coronary stent
NIRS, NIS
    near-infrared spectroscopy
Nisocor
nisoldipine
Nissen
    N. 360-degree wrap fundoplication
    N. fundoplication (NF)
niter paper
nitinol
    n. filter
    n. mesh stent
    n. petal
    n. polymeric compound
    n. self-expandable stent
    n. self-expanding coil stent
    n. snare
    n. thermal memory stent
Nit-Occlud device
nitrate
    long-acting n.
    2-nicotinamidoethyl n.
    peroxyacetyl n.
    n. resistance
nitrendipine
nitric
    n. oxide (NO)
    n. oxide analyzer (NOA)
    n. oxide synthase gene therapy
    n. oxide synthase I (NOS, NOS1)
    n. oxide system
nitrite
    amyl n.
    sodium n.
Nitro-Bid Ointment
nitroblue tetrazolium
Nitrocap

Nitro-Dial
Nitro-Dur Patch
nitrofurantoin
Nitrogard Buccal
nitrogen-13 (N-13, N₂)
    n.-13-13 (N-13, N₂)
    n.-13 ammonia
    blood urea n.-13 (BUN)
    n.-13 curve
    n.-13 dioxide (NO₂)
    n.-13 mustard
    n.-13 narcosis
    n.-13 oxide
    n.-13 washout technique
nitroglycerin (NTG)
    n. ointment (NTGO)
    oral n. (ONTG)
nitroglycerin-induced dilation
nitroglycerol
Nitroglyn Oral
nitroimidazole
Nitrolin
Nitrolingual Translingual Spray
Nitrol Ointment
Nitrong SR
Nitropress
nitroprusside
    n. infusion
    sodium n.
    n. sodium
NitroQuick sublingual tablets
nitrosopnea
    childhood n.
nitrosothiol
Nitrospan
Nitrostat Sublingual
nitrotyrosine
nitrous oxide
nitrovasodilator
NIV
    noninvasive ventilation
NIVS
    noninvasive ventilatory support
Nizoral Oral
NK
    natural killer
    NK cell
NKA
    neurokinin A
NL
    neutral lipid

NLDL
    normal low-density lipoprotein
n-LDL
    native LDL
NLHEP
    National Lung Health Education Program
NMBA
    neuromuscular blocking agent
NMDA receptor
N-methyl-D-aspartate
nmol
    nanomole
NMR
    nuclear magnetic resonance
        NMR diffusometry
        NMR relaxometry
        NMR spectroscopy
        NMR topography
NMRI
    nuclear magnetic resonance imaging
NMS
    neurally mediated syncope
NMVS
    neurally mediated vasovagal syncope
NN
    normal-to-normal
    NN interval
N^G-nitro-L-arginine methyl ester (L-NAME)
NNS
    nasal nicotine spray
NNT
    number needed to treat
NNV
    nasal nocturnal ventilation
NO
    nitric oxide
NO₂
    nitrogen dioxide
no
    no added salt (NAS)
    no atrial pacing
    no infection-no rejection (NI-NR)
NOA
    nitric oxide analyzer
Nocardia
    N. asteroides
    N. brasiliensis
    N. transvalensis
nocardiosis
nociceptive threshold
nocturia

N

NOTES

nocturnal
- n. angina
- n. asthma
- n. cardiovascular blunting
- n. desaturation
- n. dyspnea
- n. hypoventilation
- n. oximetry
- n. oximetry screening
- n. oxygenation
- n. polysomnogram (NPSG)
- n. polysomnography
- n. ventilation
- n. walking

nod
- bishop's n.

nodal
- n. arrhythmia
- n. artery
- n. beat
- n. bigeminy
- n. bradycardia
- enhanced atrioventricular n. (EAVN)
- n. escape
- n. escape rhythm
- n. extrasystole
- n. paroxysmal tachycardia
- n. premature beat (NPB)
- n. premature contraction (NPC)
- n. reentrant tachycardia
- n. tissue

nodal-His (NH)

node
- Aschoff-Tawara n.
- atrioventricular n. (AVN)
- A-V n.
- axillary lymph n.'s
- azygos n.
- bifurcation lymph n.
- bronchopulmonary lymph n.
- carinal lymph n.
- compact A-V n.
- Cruveilhier n.'s
- Delphian n.
- dual atrioventricular n.
- Flack n.
- Fraenkel n.
- Heberden n.
- hilar lymph n.
- hilum of lymph n.
- His-Tawara n.
- inferior phrenic lymph n.
- inferior tracheobronchial lymph n.
- jugulodigastric lymph n.
- juxtaesophageal lymph n.
- Keith n.
- Keith-Flack n.
- Koch n.

- lateral jugular lymph n.
- lymph n.
- mediastinal lymph n.'s
- NH region of A-V n.
- Osler n.
- paratracheal lymph n.
- perihilar lymph n.'s
- prelaryngeal lymph n.
- pretracheal lymph n.
- pulmonary lymph n.
- n. of Ranvier
- retropharyngeal lymph n.
- S-A n.
- sentinel n.
- shotty n.'s
- singer's n.
- sinoatrial n. (SAN, SN)
- sinoauricular n. (SAN)
- sinus n. (SN)
- subaortic lymph n.
- subcarinal n.
- superior phrenic lymph n.
- superior tracheobronchial lymph n.
- supraclavicular lymph n.
- Tawara atrioventricular n.
- teacher's n.
- tracheal lymph n.

nodi
- n. lymphoidei bronchopulmonales
- n. lymphoidei juxtaesophageales pulmonales
- n. lymphoidei paratracheales
- n. lymphoidei phrenici inferiores
- n. lymphoidei phrenici superiores
- n. lymphoidei prelaryngeales
- n. lymphoidei pretracheales
- n. lymphoidei retropharyngeales
- n. lymphoidei tracheobronchiales inferiores
- n. lymphoidei tracheobronchiales superiores

nodofascicular

nodohisian (NH)
- n. bypass tract

nodosa
- arteritis n.
- periarteritis n.
- polyarteritis n.

nodose arteriosclerosis

nodosum
- erythema n.

nodoventricular
- n. fiber
- n. tract

nodular
- n. arteriosclerosis
- n. infiltrate
- n. interlobular septal thickening
- n. lymphoid hyperplasia

n. opacity
n. pulmonary amyloidosis
n. sarcoidosis
n. sclerosing Hodgkin lymphoma
n. sclerosis
n. vasculitis
nodularity
nodule
acinar n.
Albini n.
Arantius n.
Aschoff n.
Bianchi n.'s
calcified n.
Caplan n.
centrilobular n.
cold n.
hematogenous n.
interstitial n.
intrapulmonary rheumatoid n.
lung n.
meningotheloid n.
metastatic n.
Morgagni n.
necrobiotic n.
peribronchiolar n.
perilymphatic n.
random n.
rheumatoid n.
round pneumonia n.
solitary pulmonary n. (SPN)
subcutaneous n.
warm n.
Wegener n.
nodus
n. atrioventricularis
n. sinuatrialis
n. sinuatrialis echo
noise
perceived n. (PN)
n. reversion
noise-reversion mode
noisy chest
no-leak technique
Nolvadex tablet
nomifensine maleate
nomogram
Radford n.
nonacute total coronary occlusion
nonagenarian

nonallergic
n. noninfectious perennial rhinitis (NANIPER)
n. rhinitis with eosinophilia (NARES)
nonarticulated stent
nonasthmatic eosinophilic bronchitis
nonatheromatous
n. arterial narrowing
n. arteriosclerosis
n. artery
nonatopic asthma
nonbacteremic
nonbacterial
n. thrombotic endocardial lesion
n. thrombotic endocarditis (NBTE)
n. verrucous endocarditis
nonballoon therapy
noncalcified valve
noncardiac (NC)
n. angiography
n. pulmonary edema (NCPE)
n. surgery
n. syncope
noncardiogenic pulmonary edema
noncaseating granuloma
noncavitary
noncleaved cell lymphoma
noncollagenous pneumoconiosis
noncommitted biphasic shock therapy
noncommunicating air space
noncompensatory pause
noncompliant
n. balloon
n. ventricle
noncontact endocardial mapping
noncontractile area (NCA)
noncoronary
n. cusp (NCC)
n. sinus
noncrushing vascular clamp
nondecremental retrograde ventriculoatrial conduction
nondepolarizing drug
nondipper pattern
nondisjunction
nondominant vessel
nonejection systolic click
nonessential
nonesterified
n. cholesterol (NEC)
n. fatty acid

N

NOTES

nonesterified fatty acid
nonexcitatory signal
nonexertional angina
nonexpansional dyspnea
nonfasting state
nonfatal cardiac event
nonfenestrated endothelium
nonflow-limited
nonfluent aphasia
nongenomic
nonglycoside inotropic agent
nonhemodynamic effect
non-high density lipoprotein (NHDL)
non-Hodgkin lymphoma
nonhomogeneous pulmonary time-
    constant distribution
nonhypercapnic respiratory failure
non-IgE-mediated reaction
nonimmunocompromised host
noninducible
noninfectious complication
noninfective valve endocarditis
noninhalation
Nonin Onyx pulse oximeter
noninsulin-dependent diabetes mellitus
    (NIDDM)
nonintegrated transvenous defibrillation
    lead
nonintubated patient
noninvasive
    n. assessment
    n. blood pressure (NIBP, NIPB)
    n. evaluation
    n. extrathoracic ventilator (NEV)
    n. face mask ventilation
    lower extremity n. (LENI)
    n. mechanical ventilation
    n. monitor
    n. murmur
    n. positive pressure ventilation
        (NIPPV, NPPV)
    n. positive-pressure ventilation
        (NPPV)
    n. positive pressure ventilatory
        support
    n. programmed stimulation (NIPS)
    n. temporary pacemaker
    n. test
    n. transcutaneous cardiac pacing
        (NTCP)
    n. ventilation (NIV)
    n. ventilation with positive pressure
    n. ventilatory support (NIVS)
nonionic
    n. contrast material
    n. contrast medium
nonischemic dilated cardiomyopathy
nonliquefaciens
    Moraxella n.

nonnecrotizing angiitis
nonobstructive valve thrombosis
nonocclusive mesenteric ischemia
nonoperative closure
nonostial plaque
nonpacemaker (NPM)
nonpanting
    n. maneuver
    n. measurement
nonparametric data
nonparoxysmal atrioventricular
    junctional tachycardia (NPJT)
nonpenetrating rupture
nonpharmacologic measure of treatment
nonphasic sinus arrhythmia
nonpitting edema
nonpressor dose
nonprimary
    n. cardiac arrest
    n. lobe
    n. pulmonary hypertension
    n. ventricular fibrillation
nonpyramidal hemimotor syndrome
nonquinolone antibiotic
non-Q-wave myocardial infarction
    (NQMI, NQWMI)
nonrapid eye movement (NREM)
nonrebreather mask
nonrebreathing
    n. mask
    n. valve
nonreset nodus sinuatrialis
nonreversibility
nonrheumatic
    n. AF
    n. valvular aortic stenosis
nonsegmental
    n. disease
    n. perfusion defect
nonselective coronary angiography
nonsense mutation
non-sensing
    atrial n.-s.
nonsinusoidal waveform
nonsmall-cell
    n.-c. lung cancer (NSCLC)
    n.-c. lung carcinoma (NSCLC)
nonspecific
    n. bronchial hyperreactivity
    n. challenge test
    n. chronic interstitial pneumonitis
        (NIP)
    n. climatic change
    n. idiopathic pulmonary fibrosis
    n. interstitial pneumonia (NSIP)
    n. interstitial pneumonitis (NSIP)
    n. intraventricular block
    n. intraventricular conduction delay
        (NSIVCD)

n. irritant
n. lung fibrosis
n. T-wave aberration
n. T-wave abnormality
nonspecific ST and T (NSSTT)
non-ST
n.-ST segment elevation myocardial infarction (NSTEMI)
n.-ST segment myocardial infarction (non-STEMI)
non-STEMI
non-ST segment myocardial infarction
nonstentable lesion
nonsteroidal
n. antiinflammatory agent
n. antiinflammatory drug (NSAID)
nonsuppressible
n. arrhythmia
n. ventricular tachycardia
nonsurgical septal reduction therapy (NSRT)
nonsustained ventricular tachycardia (NSVT)
nonthoracotomy
n. defibrillation lead system
n. lead implantable cardioverter-defibrillator
n. system antitachycardia device (NTS-AICD)
nonthrombogenic
nontransmural myocardial infarction (NTMI)
nontransplanted
nontuberculous mycobacteria (NTM)
nontypeable *Haemophilus influenzae* **(NTHI)**
nonuniform
n. direct cardiac compression
n. rotational defect (NURD)
nonvalved graft
nonvalvular atrial fibrillation (NVAF)
nonvenereal syphilis
nonventilated patient
Noonan syndrome
Noon A-V fistula clamp
no-phase wrap
No Pour Pak suction catheter kit
NoProfile Olbert Catheter system balloon dilatation catheter
noradrenaline
Norcuron

Nordach treatment
no-reflow
n.-r. phenomenon
n.-r. syndrome
norepinephrine (NE)
n. bitartrate
fasting plasma n.
n. uptake 1
norethindrone
norfloxacin
Norisodrine
normal
n. coronary arteries (NCA)
n. electrical axis
n. geometry
n. intravascular pressure
n. low-density lipoprotein (NLDL)
n. saline
n. sinus rhythm (NSR)
n. transvalvular regurgitation (NTVR)
n. triglyceridemia (NTG)
n. vital capacity (NVC)
normalization of inverted T wave
normalized systemic vascular resistance (NSVR)
normal-to-normal (NN)
normobaric environment
normocapnia
normocholesterolemic
Normodyne
N. injection
N. Oral
normokinesia
normolipidemic
normomagnesemia
normonatremic
normoperfused
normotension
normotensive (NT)
n. pneumothorax
normothermic cardioplegia
normovolemia
normovolemic (NV)
n. hemodilution
normoxia
Normozide
Noroxin Oral
Norpace CR
Norpramin
NOR-Q.D.

NOTES

N

Norris
　　N. score
　　N. test
north
　　N. American blastomycosis
　　N. American Cerebral Transluminal
　　　Angioplasty Registration
　　　(NACPTAR)
　　N. American Inoue Balloon
　　　registry
　　N. American Society for Pacing
　　　and Electrophysiology (NAPSE)
northern
　　N. blot
　　N. hybridization analysis
Norton flow-directed Swan-Ganz
　　thermodilution catheter
nortriptyline hydrochloride
Norvasc
norvegicus
　　Rattus n.
norverapamil
Norvir
Norwalk agent
Norwood
　　N. operation
　　N. operation for hypoplastic left-
　　　sided heart
　　N. repair
　　N. univentricular heart procedure
NOS
　　nitric oxide synthase I
NOS1
　　nitric oxide synthase I
nose
　　n. clip
　　respiratory region of tunica mucosa
　　　of n.
Nosema connori
no-sigh period
nosocomial
　　n. aspiration
　　n. disease
　　n. endocarditis
　　n. infection
　　n. pathogen
　　n. pneumonia (NP)
nosocomii
　　angina n.
nosology
　　Berlin n.
Nostrilla
notch
　　anacrotic n.
　　aortic n.
　　atrial n.
　　cardiac n.
　　dicrotic n. (DN)
　　interarytenoid n.

Sibson n.
sternal n.
suprasternal n. (SN)
thyroid n.
notched
　　n. P wave
　　n. S wave
notching
　　midsystolic n.
　　rib n.
note
　　percussion n. (PN)
notha
　　angina n.
　　peripneumonia n.
　　pneumonia n.
no-touch technique
Nottingham
　　N. Extended Activities of Daily
　　　Living scale
　　N. Health profile
　　N. introducer
　　N. Sensory Assessment test
Nova
　　N. II pacemaker
　　N. Microsonics ImageVue system
Novacode serial ECG classification
Novacor
　　N. Diasys cardiac device
　　N. left ventricular assist device
　　N. left ventricular assist system
　　N. LVAD
　　N. mechanical circulatory support
　　　system
Novametrix
　　N. NICO cardiopulmonary
　　　management system
　　N. pulse oximeter
　　N. Tidal Wave handheld
　　　capnograph
Novamoxin
Novantrone
Novasen
Novastan
Novo
novo
　　de n.
Novo-Atenol
Novo-AZT
Novo-Captopril
Novo-Chlorpromazine
Novo-Clonidine
Novo-Cloxin
Novo-Cromolyn
Novo-Digoxin
Novo-Diltazem
Novo-Dipiradol
Novo-Hydrazide
Novo-Hydroxyzine

Novo-Hylazin
Novo-Lexin
Novolin 70/30
Novomedopa
Novo-Metoprolol
Novo-Nifedin
Novo-Pen-VK
Novo-Pindol
Novo-Prazin
Novo-Prednisolone
Novo-Prednisone
Novo-Reserpine
Novo-Rythro Encap
Novo-Salmol
Novo-Semide
NovoSeven
Novo-Spiroton
Novoste catheter
Novo-Tamoxifen
Novo-Thalidone
Novo-Timol
Novo-Triamzide
Novo-Trimel
Novo-Veramil
NOxBOX monitor
Nozovent nasal-valve dilator
NP
    nasopharyngeal
    nosocomial pneumonia
NPB
    Nellcor Puritan Bennett
    nodal premature beat
        NPB-75 handheld capnograph/pulse
        oximeter
NPB-40 handheld pulse oximeter
NPB-75 handheld capnograph/pulse
  oximeter
NPC
    nodal premature contraction
NPH Iletin insulin
NPJT
    nonparoxysmal atrioventricular junctional
    tachycardia
NPM
    nonpacemaker
        NPM cells
NPPE
    negative pressure pulmonary edema
NPPV
    nasal positive pressure ventilation
    noninvasive positive-pressure ventilation
    noninvasive positive pressure ventilation

N-propanol
NPSG
    nocturnal polysomnogram
NPT
    near patient test
NPV
    negative predictive value
    negative pressure ventilation
NQMI
    non-Q-wave myocardial infarction
NQWMI
    non-Q-wave myocardial infarction
NR
        Organidin NR
        Tussi-Organidin DM NR
Nramp
    natural resistance macrophage-associated
    protein
NRDS
    neonate respiratory distress syndrome
NREM
    nonrapid eye movement
        NREM sleep
NRMI
    National Registry of Myocardial
    Infarction
NS
    nasal steroid
        NS echo
NSAID
    nonsteroidal antiinflammatory drug
NSCLC
    nonsmall-cell lung cancer
    nonsmall-cell lung carcinoma
NSCT
    National Society of Cardiovascular
    Technologists
NSE
    neuron-specific enolase
NSIP
    nonspecific interstitial pneumonia
    nonspecific interstitial pneumonitis
NSIVCD
    nonspecific intraventricular conduction
    delay
NSR
    normal sinus rhythm
NSRT
    nonsurgical septal reduction therapy
NSSTT
    nonspecific ST and T
        NSSTT wave

N

NOTES

NSTEMI
non-ST segment elevation myocardial infarction
NSVR
normalized systemic vascular resistance
NSVT
nonsustained ventricular tachycardia
NT
normotensive
NTCP
noninvasive transcutaneous cardiac pacing
N-terminal
N-t. proANF
N-t. proatrial natriuretic factor
N-t. pro brain natriuretic peptide (NT-proBNP)
NTF
nasogastric tube feeding
NTG
nitroglycerin
normal triglyceridemia
NTGO
nitroglycerin ointment
NTHI
nontypeable *Haemophilus influenzae*
NTM
nontuberculous mycobacteria
NTMI
nontransmural myocardial infarction
NT-proBNP
N-terminal pro brain natriuretic peptide
NT-proBNP ELISA enzyme immunoassay
NTS-AICD
nonthoracotomy system antitachycardia device
NTVR
normal transvalvular regurgitation
Nu
Nu-Amoxi
Nu-Ampi
Nu-Atenol
Nu-Capto
Nu-Cephalex
Nu-Clonidine
Nu-Cloxi
Nu-Cotrimox
Nu-Diltiaz
Nu-Hydral
Nu-Iron
Nu-Medopa
Nu-Metop
Nu-Nifedin
Nu-Pen-VK
Nu-Pindol
Nu-Prazo
Nu-Propranolol
Nu-Timolol

Nu-Triazide
Nu-Verap
nuchal rigidity
nuclear
n. factor-kappa-B (NF-kappa-B)
n. magnetic resonance (NMR)
n. magnetic resonance imaging (NMRI)
n. pacemaker
n. perfusion imaging
n. probe
n. stent
nucleatum
Fusobacterium n.
nuclei (*pl. of* nucleus)
nucleic acid direct amplification test
nucleotide
total adenine n. (TAN)
nucleus, pl. **nuclei**
apoptotic n.
caudate n.
suprachiasmatic n.
vein of caudate n.
Nucofed Pediatric Expectorant
Nucotuss
Nuhn gland
null
n. hypothesis
n. point
number
n. needed to treat (NNT)
representative CT (Hounsfield) n.
Reynolds n.
Strouhal n.
Wasserman n.
nummiform
nummular
n. aortitis
n. sputum
nummulation
nun's venous hum murmur
Nuprin
NURD
nonuniform rotational defect
Nurolon suture
nursing
coronary care n. (CCN)
nutcracker esophagus
nutraceutical (*var. of* nutriceutical)
Nutracort
Nu-Trake Weiss emergency airway system
Nutraplus topical
nutriceutical, nutraceutical
nutrient cardioplegia
Nu-Trim dietary fat substitute
nutrition
enteral n.
parenteral n.

Nuvance
Nu-Vois artificial larynx
Nuvolase 660 laser system
NV
   normovolemic
NVAF
   nonvalvular atrial fibrillation
NVC
   normal vital capacity
NVE
   native valve endocarditis
NVP
   nevirapine

Nycore pigtail catheter
Nydrazid injection
NYHA
   NYHA classification of congestive
    heart failure
   NYHA functional classification
    I–IV
Nylex diagnostic catheter
nylon
   Xcelon n.
Nyquist limit
nystatin
Nystat-Rx

NOTES

N

Ω (*var. of* ohm)

O
    oxygen
      O antigen
      O point of cardiac apex pulse

O2, O$_2$
    oxygen
      O2 Advantage oxygen conserving device
      ambulatory O2
      O2 radical
      O2 via nasal cannula

OA
    occipital artery
    occupational asthma
    oral appliance

OAD
    obstructive airway disease

oakridgensis
    Legionella o.

OARS
    Older Americans Resources and Services

Oasis thrombectomy system

oat
    o. cell
    o. cell carcinoma

OB
    obliterative bronchiolitis

obesity
    android o.
    exogenous o.
    female pattern o.
    gynoid o.
    o. hypertension
    o. hypoventilation syndrome (OHS)
    male pattern o.
    morbid o.
    Roux-en-Y o.
    WHR for upper body o.

oblique
    anterior o. (AO)
    o. fissure
    o. fissure of lung
    left anterior o. (LAO)
    right anterior o. (RAO)
    o. sinus

obliterans
    arteriosclerosis o.
    arteritis o.
    bronchiolitis o. (BO)
    bronchiolitis fibrosa o.
    cerebral thromboangiitis o. (CTAO)
    endarteritis o.
    pericarditis o.

    phlebitis o.
    thromboangiitis o.

obliterating
    o. pericarditis
    o. phlebitis

obliteration
    coil o.

obliterative
    o. bronchiolitis (OB)
    o. bronchitis
    o. cardiomyopathy
    o. pericarditis
    o. pleuritis
    o. pulmonary hypertension (OPH)
    o. vascular disease

oblongata
    medulla o.

O'Brien airway needle

obscuration
    aortic o.

Observer's Assessment of Alertness/Sedation Scale

obstructed

obstruction
    airflow o.
    airways o. (AO)
    aortic arch vessel o.
    baffle o.
    chronic airflow o. (CAO)
    chronic thrombotic pulmonary vascular o. (CTPVO)
    chronic upper respiratory o.
    coronary artery o. (CAO)
    dynamic intracavitary o.
    embolic o.
    endobronchial o.
    extracranial carotid o.
    extrathoracic airway o.
    fixed airflow o.
    foreign body airway o. (FBAO)
    hypopharyngeal o.
    infundibular o.
    irreversible airway o.
    left ventricular inflow tract o.
    left ventricular outflow tract o. (LVOTO)
    mechanical o.
    multivessel coronary artery o.
    outflow tract o.
    predilated polytetrafluoroethylene o.
    pulmonary vascular o. (PVO)
    retropalatal o.
    reversible airway o.
    right ventricular inflow o.
    right ventricular outflow o.

O

obstruction *(continued)*
    stop-valve airway o.
    subaortic o.
    subpulmonary o.
    subvalvular o.
    subvalvular aortic o. (SAO)
    superior vena cava o. (SVCO)
    total o. (TO)
    upper airway o. (UAO)
    vena cava o.
    vena caval o.
    ventricular inflow tract o.
    ventricular outflow tract o.
obstructive
    o. airway disease (OAD)
    o. atelectasis
    o. edema
    o. emphysema
    o. hypertrophic cardiomyopathy
    (OHC)
    o. hypopnea
    o. lung disease (OLD)
    o. murmur
    o. pneumonia
    o. shock
    o. sleep apnea (OSA)
    o. sleep apnea-induced
    cardiovascular change
    o. sleep apnea syndrome (OSAS)
    o. thrombus
    o. valve thrombosis
    o. ventilatory defect
    o. ventilatory dysfunction
obturating embolism
obturator
    Check-Flo sheath o.
    Fitch o.
    Hemaflex PTCA sheath with o.
    Hemaquet PTCA sheath with o.
obtuse
    o. marginal (OM)
    o. marginal artery (OMA)
    o. marginal branch (OMB)
    o. marginal coronary artery
    o. marginal lymphatic
    o. margin of heart
occ, occl
    occlusion
    occlusive
occipital artery (OA)
occipitalis
    basilaris ossis o.
occl *(var. of* occ)
occluder
    air clamp inflatable vessel o.
    Amplatzer duct o.
    ASDOS umbrella o.
    o. balloon wash-out technique
    Bard Clamshell septal o.

    catheter-tip o.
    clamshell septal o.
    Crile tip o.
    double-disk o.
    Flo-Rester vascular o.
    Hunter detachable balloon o.
    modified Rashkind PDA o.
    Pediatric Cardiology Devices
    Sideris Buttoned device o.
    PFO-Star o.
    square-shaped o.
    tilting disk o.
    tip o.
occludin
occluding thrombus
occlusion (occ, occl)
    acute coronary o. (ACO)
    angioplasty-related vessel o.
    arterial o.
    balloon o.
    balloon coronary o. (BCO)
    balloon test o. (BTO)
    basilar artery o. (BAO)
    bradycardia after arteriovenous
    fistula o. (BAVFO)
    branch retinal artery o. (BRAO)
    branch retinal vein o. (BRVO)
    branch vein o. (BVO)
    branch vessel o.
    central retinal artery o. (CRAO)
    central vein o. (CVO)
    chronic coronary O.'s
    chronic total o. (CTO)
    coronary artery o.
    coronary branch o.
    femoral artery o.
    femoral vein o.
    iliac artery o.
    inferior mesenteric vascular o.
    inferior vena cava o.
    intermittent aortic o. (IAO)
    intermittent coronary sinus o.
    (ICSO)
    left main coronary o.
    left marginal coronary artery o.
    (LMCAO)
    long iliac artery o.
    mesenteric artery o.
    mesenteric vascular o.
    middle cerebral artery o. (MCAO)
    nonacute total coronary o.
    pressure-controlled intermittent
    coronary sinus o. (PICSO)
    pulmonary artery o. (PAO)
    recurrent mesenteric vascular o.
    side branch o.
    superior mesenteric vascular o.
    temporary unilateral pulmonary
    artery o.

thrombotic o. (ThrO, TO)
transcatheter coil o.
transient spastic o. (TSO)
venous mesenteric vascular o.

occlusive (occ, occl)
o. disease
o. thromboaortopathy
o. thrombus

OCCPR
open chest cardiopulmonary resuscitation

occult
o. cardiogenic shock
o. pericardial constriction
o. pericarditis

occupational
o. asthma (OA)
o. asthmogen
o. health and safety (OHS)
o. lung disease

OCG
omnicardiogram

Ochrobacterium anthropi
ochrometer
ochronosis
Ochsner-Mahorner
O.-M. echocardiogram
O.-M. test

OCR
oculocardiac reflex

OCRG
oxycardiorespirography

OCT
optical coherence tomography
orthotopic cardiac transplantation

octafluoropropane
octapolar catheter
Octocaine
Octopus
O. tissue stabilization system
O. 2+, 3 tissue stabilization system
O. tissue stabilizer
O. tissue stabilizing device

octreotide
oculocardiac reflex (OCR)
oculocraniosomatic disease
oculomucocutaneous syndrome
oculopharyngeal reflex
oculoplethysmography (OPG)
oculopneumoplethysmography
oculovagal reflex

OD
outer diameter

odds ratio (OR)

ODI
oxygen desaturation index

ODN
oligodeoxynucleotide

odorans
Alcaligenes o.

odoratus
Lathyrus o.

odor-triggered panic attack

ODTS
organic dust toxic syndrome

O'Dwyer intubation

odynophagia

OEF
oxygen extraction fraction

Oehler symptoms

Oehl muscle

O_2ER
oxygen extraction ratio

Oertel treatment

off-axis

office
o. angina
o. hypertension

off-pump
o.-p. coronary artery bypass (OPCAB)
o.-p. vascular surgery

ofloxacin

Ogata method

OGTT
oral glucose tolerance test

OHC
obstructive hypertrophic cardiomyopathy

OHCA
out-of-hospital cardiac arrest

OHD
organic heart disease

OHI
operative hypertension indicator

ohm, Ω
O. law

Ohmeda
O. 6200, 6300 CO_2 monitor
O. handheld oximeter
O. pulse oximeter
O. thoracic suction regulator

ohmic heating

ohmmeter

NOTES

O

Ohnell
X wave of O.
OHS
obesity hypoventilation syndrome
occupational health and safety
open heart surgery
OHT
orthotopic heart transplant
OIA
osmotically induced asthma
oil
canola o.
o. embolism
emu o.
fish o.
marine o.'s
MCT O.
o. mist asthma
progesterone O.
rapeseed o.
o. red O stain
trypsin, balsam peru, and castor o.
oil-aspiration pneumonia
ointment
Nitro-Bid O.
nitroglycerin o. (NTGO)
Nitrol O.
Whitfield o.
Xylocaine Topical O.
OKT3
OKT3 antibody
Orthoclone OKT3
OL
open label
open labeled
OLB
open lung biopsy
Olbert
O. balloon
O. balloon catheter
OLBI
overlapping biphasic impulse
Olcott torque device
OLD
obstructive lung disease
Older Americans Resources and Services (OARS)
old myocardial infarction (OMI)
Olean
oleate
ethanolamine o.
oleogomenol
olestra
Oligella urethralis
oligemia
pulmonary o.
oligemic shock
oligodeoxynucleotide (ODN)
antisense o.

oligonucleotide microarray
oliguria
Oliver-Rosalki method
Oliver sign
olive-tipped
o.-t. Magnum wire
o.-t. needle
olivopontocerebellar atrophy
olmesartan medoxomil
olprinone
Olympix II PTCA dilatation catheter
Olympus
O. bioptome
O. echoendoscope
O. One-Step Button tube
OM
obtuse marginal
OM coronary artery
OM-1
first obtuse marginal artery
OM-2
second obtuse marginal artery
OMA
obtuse marginal artery
omapatrilat
OMB
obtuse marginal branch
Omega
O. NV angioplasty catheter
O. stent
omega-3 unsaturated fatty acids
omental wrap
omentopexy
omeprazole
OMI
old myocardial infarction
Omni
O. analyzer
O. Flush catheter
Omnicarbon
O. heart valve prosthesis
O. prosthetic heart valve
omnicardiogram (OCG)
OmniCath atherectomy catheter
Omnicef
OmniCell
O. catheter module
O. supply system
Omnicor Programmer
omnidirectional M-mode
OmniFilter percutaneous guidewire microfilter
Omnipaque
Omniplane TEE
Omniscience single leaflet cardiac valve prosthesis
Omni-Tract system
omnivore

omotracheale
    trigonum o.
omphalitis
omphalocele
Omsk hemorrhagic fever
OMVC
    open mitral valve commissurotomy
Oncaspar
Onchocerca volvulus
oncology mix
Onconase
Oncor ApopTaq kit
oncostatin M
oncotic pressure
Oncovin injection
Ondine
    O. breathing
    O. curse
one-block claudication
one-flight exertional dyspnea
one-hole
    o.-h. angiographic catheter
    o.-h. angioplastic catheter
One Touch blood glucose monitor
one-ventricle heart
one-vessel angioplasty
onion
    o. bulb dilation
    o. scale lesion
onset
    sudden rate o.
Ontak
ONTG
    oral nitroglycerin
On-X
    On-X mechanical bi-leaflet
      prosthetic heart valve
onychograph
oocyte
    Xenopus o.
OOH/CA
    out-of-hospital cardiac arrest
OOH-SCD
    out-of-hospital sudden cardiac death
OOO
    OOO mode
    OOO pacemaker
    OOO pacing
opacification
    alveolar o.
    amorphous parenchymal o.
    faint o.

    ground-glass o.
    selective graft o.
opacify
opacity
    ground-glass o.
    nodular o.
    vitreous o.
opalescent sputum
OPCAB
    off-pump coronary artery bypass
open
    o. atrial disk
    o. bronchus sign
    o. chest cardiac massage
    o. chest cardiac resuscitation
    o. chest cardiopulmonary
      resuscitation (OCCPR)
    o. circuit method
    o. heart surgery (OHS)
    o. label (OL)
    o. labeled (OL)
    o. lung approach
    o. lung biopsy (OLB)
    o. mitral valve commissurotomy
      (OMVC)
    O. Pivot heart valve
    o. pneumothorax
    o. surgery (OS)
    o. tuberculosis
Open-Cath
    Abbokinase O.-C.
opener
    adenosine triphosphate-sensitive
      potassium channel o.
    potassium channel o.
opening
    anodal o. (AO)
    aortic o. (AO)
    aortic valve o. (AVO)
    atrioventricular o. (AVO)
    atrioventricular valve o. (AO)
    esophageal o.
    fistulous o.
    mitral o. (Mo)
    mitral valve o. (MVO)
    o. pressure
    o. snap (OS)
    tricuspid o. (To)
open-label ACE-inhibitor therapy
OpenSail
    O. balloon catheter
    O. coronary dilatation catheter

O

NOTES

operation
- Abbe o.
- Anel o.
- arterial switch o.
- atrial baffle o.
- Babcock o.
- Barnard o.
- Beck I, II o.
- Bentall o.
- Berger o.
- bidirectional Glenn o.
- Blalock-Hanlon o.
- Blalock-Taussig o.
- Brock o.
- cautery-assisted palatal stiffening o. (CAPSO)
- Cox maze o.
- Damus-Kaye-Stansel o.
- David o.
- DKS o.
- electrode catheter ablation o.
- encircling endocardial ventriculotomy o.
- endocardial to epicardial resection o.
- Estlander o.
- fenestrated Fontan o.
- Fontan o.
- Freund o.
- Glenn o.
- Goldsmith o.
- Grondahl-Finney o.
- Guiraudon corridor o.
- Heller-Belsey o.
- Heller-Nissen o.
- hemi-Fontan o.
- Hunter o.
- Konno o.
- laser maze o.
- Lindesmith o.
- multivalve o.
- Mustard atrial switch o.
- Norwood o.
- Palma o.
- Potts o.
- Ransohoff o.
- Rastan o.
- Rastelli o.
- Sawyer o.
- Schede o.
- second-look o.
- Senning o.
- switch o.
- talc o.
- Tanner o.
- transcatheter closure of atrial septal defect o.
- Trendelenburg o.
- triangular resection of leaflet o.
- valve-conserving o.
- Waterston o.

operative hypertension indicator (OHI)

operculum, pl. **opercula**

OPG
- oculoplethysmography

OPH
- obliterative pulmonary hypertension

opiate

opioid

Opisthorchis

Opitz syndrome

OPO
- organ procurement organization

opportunistic
- o. infection
- o. pneumonia

opsoclonia

opsonin

opsonization

opsonophagocytic receptor

Opta
- O. 5 catheter
- O. Pro PTA dilatation catheter

Opti
- O. 1 pH/blood gas analyzer
- O. 1 portable blood analyzer

optic
- o. atrophy
- o. disk
- o. neuritis

optical
- o. coherence tomography (OCT)
- o. fiber catheter

Optical Sensors stand-alone arterial blood gas monitoring system

Opticath oximeter catheter

OptiChamber valved holding chamber

OptiCor digital cardiac communication and storage system

Opti-Flow catheter

OptiHaler drug delivery system

OPTIMAAL

Optima pacemaker

Optimine

Opti-Plast XT balloon catheter

Optiray
- O. 320
- O. contrast
- O. contrast medium

Optison
- O. contrast
- O. contrast agent
- O. injectable suspension

OPTN
- Organ Procurement and Transplantation Network

Optochin
- O. disk test

O. test for *Streptococcus
  pneumoniae*

Optrin

Opus

O. cardiac troponin I assay
O. RM single chamber pacemaker

OR

odds ratio

Oracle

O. Focus imaging catheter
O. Focus PTCA catheter
O. Micro Plus
O. Micro Plus PTCA catheter

oral

Achromycin V O.
o. airflow in liters per second
  (V_O)
Aller-Chlor O.
AllerMax O.
Altace O.
o. anticoagulant therapy
o. appliance (OA)
Apresoline O.
Aristocort O.
Atarax O.
Banophen O.
Benadryl O.
Betapace O.
Betapen-VK O.
Blocadren O.
Brethine O.
Calm-X O.
o. candidiasis
Cartrol O.
Catapres O.
CeeNU O.
Ceftin O.
Celestone O.
Chlor-Trimeton O.
Cipro O.
Cleocin HCl O.
Cleocin Pediatric O.
Compazine O.
o. contraceptive-induced
  hypertension
Cortef O.
Cyklokapron O.
Cytomel O.
Cytoxan O.
Decadron O.
Delta-Cortef O.
Deltasone O.

Demadex O.
Diflucan O.
Dormin O.
Doryx O.
Doxychel O.
Dramamine O.
Dynacin O.
Edecrin O.
E.E.S. O.
E-Mycin O.
Eryc O.
EryPed O.
Ery-Tab O.
Erythrocin O.
Eryzole O.
Flagyl O.
o. flecainide therapy
o. flora
Floxin O.
Flumadine O.
Genahist O.
o. glucose tolerance test (OGTT)
Indocin O.
Kerlone O.
o. L-arginine system
Lasix O.
Lincocin O.
Loniten O.
Maxaquin O.
Medrol O.
Mephyton O.
Meticorten O.
Minocin O.
Monodox O.
Mycobutin O.
o. nitroglycerin (ONTG)
Nitroglyn O.
Nizoral O.
Normodyne O.
Noroxin O.
o. part of pharynx
PCE O.
PediaCare O.
Pediapred O.
Pediazole O.
Phenetron O.
poliovirus vaccine, live,
  trivalent, o.
Prelone O.
Proglycem O.
Provera O.
Retrovir O.

O

NOTES

oral (*continued*)
    Rifadin O.
    Rimactane O.
    Sporanox O.
    Sterapred O.
    Sumycin O.
    Tetralan O.
    Trandate O.
    o. triamcinolone inhalation
    o. tuberculosis
    Vancocin O.
    Vasotec O.
    Veetids O.
    VePesid O.
    Vibramycin O.
    Videx O.
    Vistaril O.
    Xylocaine O.
oral-inhalation dexamethasone
oralis
    Bacteroides o.
Orbenin
orbofiban
orciprenaline sulfate
order
    anodal opening o. (AOO)
Ordrine AT Extended Release Capsule
Oretic
organ
    Golgi tendon o.
    o. procurement organization (OPO)
    O. Procurement and Transplantation
      Network (OPTN)
    o. system failure
    o. transplantation system
organelle
    vesicular-vacuolar o. (VVO)
organic
    o. dust
    o. dust pneumoconiosis
    o. dust toxic syndrome (ODTS)
    o. heart disease (OHD)
    o. murmur
    o. phosphorus
Organidin NR
organism
    Cox o.
    encapsulated o.
    gram-negative o.
    gram-positive o.
    intracellular o. (ICO)
    pleuropneumonia-like o. (PPLO)
organization
    Extracorporeal Life Support O.
      (ELSO)
    International Standards O. (ISO)
    Internation Civil Aviation o.
    organ procurement o. (OPO)
    World Health O. (WHO)

organized thrombus
organizing
    o. empyema
    o. pneumonia
organoid pattern
organophosphate
Orgaran
oriental hemoptysis
orifice
    aortic o.
    aortic valve o. (AVO)
    atrioventricular o.
    cardiac o.
    common atrioventricular o. (CAVO)
    effective regurgitant o. (ERO)
    esophagogastric o.
    flow across o.
    mitral o. (MO)
    mitral valve o. (MVO)
    pulmonary o.
    o. of pulmonary trunk
    regurgitant o.
    stent-jail o.
    o. of superior vena cava
    tricuspid o.
    valvular o.
orificial
    o. stenosis
    o. tuberculosis
origin
    anomalous o.
    myocardial disease of unknown o.
      (MDUO)
    myocardiopathy of unknown o.
      (MUO)
original
    Doan's O.
    O. Pink Tape waterproof adhesive
      tape
Orimune
orlistat
Ornish
    O. diet
    O. theory
ornithosis
oroendotracheal tube
orofiban
oropharyngeal tularemia
oropharynx
    crowded o.
orotracheal
    o. intubation
    o. tube
orphan
    enteric cytopathogenic human o.
      (ECHO)
    enterocytopathogenic human o.
      (ECHO)
    respiratory and enteric o. (REO)

ORPM
>   orthorhythmic pacemaker
Orsi-Grocco method
ORT
>   orthodromic reciprocating tachycardia
orthoarteriotony
orthocardiac reflex
Orthoclone OKT3
orthodeoxia
orthodox sleep
orthodromic
>   o. atrioventricular reciprocating
>   tachycardia
>   o. A-V reentrant tachycardia
>   o. circus movement tachycardia
>   o. conduction
>   o. reciprocating tachycardia (ORT)
orthogonal
>   o. electrocardiogram
>   o. lead system
>   o. plane
>   o. view
orthograde conduction
Orthomyxoviridae virus
orthomyxovirus
orthopercussion
orthopnea
>   three-pillow o.
>   two-pillow o.
orthopneic
orthorhythmic pacemaker (ORPM)
orthosis
>   ankle-foot o. (AFO)
orthostasis autoregulation
orthostatic
>   o. dyspnea
>   o. hypertension
>   o. hypopiesis
>   o. hypotension
>   o. syncope
>   o. tachycardia
orthostatism
>   vasovagal o.
orthotopic
>   o. cardiac transplant
>   o. cardiac transplantation (OCT)
>   o. heart transplant (OHT)
>   o. univentricular artificial heart
Oruvail
oryzae
>   *Aspergillus o.*
>   *Rhizopus o.*

OS
>   opening snap
>   open surgery
OSA
>   obstructive sleep apnea
OSAP appliance
OSAS
>   obstructive sleep apnea syndrome
Osborne (J) wave
Osciflator balloon inflation syringe
oscillating
>   o. balloon inflation
>   o. dilation
>   o. paraboloid
>   o. saw
oscillation
>   external chest wall o.
>   forced o. (FO)
>   high-frequency o. (HFO)
>   high-frequency chest wall o.
>   (HFCWO)
>   o. technique
oscillator
>   Hayek o.
oscillatory afterpotential
oscillometer
oscillometric signal
oscilloscope
Oscor pacing lead
OSD
>   OSD monitor
>   Profilate OSD
oseltamivir phosphate
OSF
>   outlet strut fracture
Osler
>   O. node
>   O. sign
>   O. triad
Osler-Weber-Rendu
>   O.-W.-R. disease
>   O.-W.-R. syndrome
Osmitrol injection
osmolality
osmolarity
osmometer
osmoregulation
osmoregulatory
osmotaxis
osmotic
>   o. challenge

O

NOTES

osmotic (*continued*)
    o. diuretic
    o. pressure
osmotically induced asthma (OIA)
ossification
    pulmonary o.
ossifying pneumonitis
Ossoff-Karlan laryngoscope
osteitis
    caseous o.
    o. deformans
    o. tuberculosa multiplex cystica
osteoarthritis
    hyperplastic o.
osteoarthropathy
    hypertrophic pulmonary o.
    pneumogenic o.
    pulmonary hypertrophic o.
osteochondroma
osteogenesis imperfecta
osteonecrosis
    dysbaric o.
osteoplastica
    tracheopathia o.
osteopontin
    o. messenger ribonucleic acid
    o. mRNA
osteoradionecrosis
osteosarcoma
osteosynthesis
    exit surgical o.
    plastic surgical o.
    surgical o.
osteotomy
    anterior inferior mandibular o.
      (AIMO)
    maxillomandibular o. (MMO)
ostia (*pl. of* ostium)
ostial
    o. lesion
    o. narrowing
    o. stenosis
Ostia stent
ostium, pl. **ostia**
    coronary o.
    o. of coronary sinus (CSO)
    left coronary o. (LCO)
    o. primum
    o. primum defect
    right coronary o. (RCO)
    o. secundum
    o. secundum defect
    solitary coronary o.
    o. trunci pulmonalis
    ostia venarum pulmonalium
Ostwald viscometer
Osypka
    O. atrial lead
    O. rotational angioplasty

otopharyngeal tube
Ototemp 3000
ototoxicity
OTW
    over-the-wire
    OTW HighSail coronary dilatation
      catheter
    OTW perfusion catheter
    OTW thrombolytic brush
ouabain
outer diameter (OD)
outflow
    o. cardiac patch
    left ventricle o. (LVO)
    maximum venous o. (MVO)
    o. murmur
    right ventricular o. (RVO)
    subcostal o. (SCOT)
    o. tract
    o. tract obstruction
outlet strut fracture (OSF)
out-of-hospital
    o.-o.-h. cardiac arrest (OHCA,
      OOH/CA)
    o.-o.-h. sudden cardiac death
      (OOH-SCD)
output
    biliary cholesterol o. (BCO)
    cardiac o. (CO, Q̇, QT, Q-T)
    cardiac minute o. (CMO)
    cardiac power o. (CPO)
    o. circuit
    continuous cardiac o. (CCO)
    Fick cardiac o.
    heart minute o. (HMO)
    impedance cardiac o. (ICO)
    left ventricular o.
    left ventricular systolic o. (LVSO)
    low cardiac o. (LCO)
    measured o.
    minute o.
    pacemaker o.
    postoperative low cardiac o.
      (PLCO)
    predicted cardiac o. (PCO)
    right ventricular stroke o. (RVSO)
    stroke o.
    thermodilution cardiac o. (TDCO)
    ultrasonic cardiac o. (UCO)
outside-in signaling
ovale
    foramen o. (FO)
    patent foramen o. (PFO)
    Plasmodium o.
oval foramen
ovalis
    anulus o.
    fossa o.
overdilation

overdistention
    alveolar o.
overdrive
    o. atrial pacing
    o. mode
    o. suppression
overexpressed protein
overexpression
    beta-2 AR o.
    cardiac-specific o.
    IGF-1 o.
    TIMP-3 o.
    tissue inhibitor of metalloproteinase-3 o.
overflow wave
Overholt procedure
overhydration
overinflation
    congenital lobar o.
overlap
    o. syndrome
    o. vasculitis
overlapping biphasic impulse (OLBI)
overlay
    psychogenic o.
overload
    circulatory o.
    diastolic o.
    left atrial o. (LAO)
    pressure o.
    right ventricular diastolic o. (RVDO)
    right ventricular volume o. (RVVO)
    volume o.
overnight
    o. polysomnography
    o. pulse oximetry
overreactivity
    physiological o.
override
    aortic o.
overriding aorta
oversampling
oversedation
oversensing
    afterpotential o.
    myopotential o.
    o. pacemaker
oversewing
overshoot phenomenon

over-the-needle catheter
over-the-wire (OTW)
    o.-t.-w. balloon dilatation system
    o.-t.-w. pacing lead
    o.-t.-w. PTCA balloon catheter
overventilation
Owens
    O. balloon
    O. balloon catheter
    O. Lo-Profile dilatation catheter
Owren
    O. disease
    O. factor V deficiency
oxacillin sodium
oxalate
    calcium o.
oxalosis
oxamniquine
oxandralone
oxazepam
oxazolidinone
Oxford
    O. Handicap Scale
    O. technique
ox heart
oxidase
    cytochrome c o. (COX)
    diamine o. (DO)
    monoamine o. (MAO)
    postheparin plasma diamine o. (PHD)
    xanthine o.
oxidation
    intraplaque LDL o.
oxidative
    o. metabolism
    o. modification of LDL (oxLDL, ox-LDL)
    o. phosphorylation
    o. stress
oxide
    cadmium o.
    endothelium-derived nitric o. (EDNO)
    exhaled nitric o. (eNO, ENO)
    expired nitric o. (eNO, ENO)
    magnesium o.
    nitric o. (NO)
    nitrogen o.
    nitrous o.
    stannic o.
    tin o.

O

NOTES

oxidized
 o. cellulose
 o. LDL
 o. low-density lipoprotein (OxLDL)
oxidoreductase
 dopachrome o. (DCOR)
Oxilan
OxiLink oximeter probe cover
OxiMax pulse oximetry device
oximeter
 Armstrong handheld pulse o.
 AutoCorr portable pulse o.
 AVOXimeter 1000E whole
  blood o.
 BI-OX III ear o.
 CO o.
 CO_2SMO capnograph/pulse o.
 Cricket pulse o.
 Criticare pulse o.
 Datascope pulse o.
 Dinamap pulse o.
 ear o.
 FingerPrint handheld pulse o.
 8500 handheld pulse o.
 Hewlett-Packard ear o.
 Nellcor N200 pulse o.
 Nellcor Symphony pulse o.
 Nonin Onyx pulse o.
 Novametrix pulse o.
 NPB-40 handheld pulse o.
 NPB-75 handheld
  capnograph/pulse o.
 Ohmeda handheld o.
 Ohmeda pulse o.
 Oxypleth pulse o.
 OxyTemp handheld pulse o.
 Oxytrak pulse o.
 Palco Laboratories Model 300, 400
  pulse o.
 pulse o.
 3800 pulse o.
 Pulsox-5 pulse o.
 Respironics 920P handheld pulse o.
 Respironics 930 pulse o.
 SensorMedics SAT-TRAK pulse o.
 Tidal Wave Sp capnometer/pulse o.
oximetric catheter
Oximetrix 3 System
oximetry
 carbon monoxide o.
 central venous o.
 cerebral o.
 CO o.
 CO_2 o.
 finger o.
 Hb o.
 HbO_2 o.
 N_2 o.
 near-infrared cerebral o.

 nocturnal o.
 overnight pulse o.
 OxiScan overnight pulse o.
 oxygen saturation measured by
  pulse o. (SpO_2)
 PCO_2 o.
 PO_2 o.
 pulse o. (PO)
 reflectance o.
 spectrophotometric o.
OxiScan
 O. overnight pulse oximetry
 O. oximetry program
 O. oximetry recording and
  reporting system
Oxisensor II adult sensor
**Oxismart advanced signal processing
and alarm technology**
oxitropium bromide
OxLDL
 oxidized low-density lipoprotein
oxLDL, ox-LDL
 oxidative modification of LDL
oxolamine
oxothiazolidine
oxotremorine
oxprenolol
Oxsoralen Topical
oxtriphylline
oxycardiorespirography (OCRG)
Oxycel
OxyData Plus oxygen monitor
Oxyfill oxygen refilling system
oxygen (O, O2, O_2)
 o.-15
 aqueous o.
 blood o.
 blow-by o.
 o. capacity
 central venous o. (CVO)
 o. challenge test
 o. consumption (VO_2)
 o. consumption index
 o. consumption per minute (VO_2)
 o. content
 o. cost
 o. cost of breathing
 O. Cost Diagram questionnaire
 cytotoxic singlet o.
 o. debt
 o. delivery (DO_2)
 o. dependence
 o. desaturation index (ODI)
 o. dissociation curve
 o. entrainment
 o. exchange
 o. extraction
 o. extraction fraction (OEF)
 o. extraction ratio (O_2ER)

fraction of inspired o. (FIO$_2$, FiO$_2$)
o. free radical release
humidified o.
hyperbaric o. (HBO)
o. inhalation
o. mask
myocardial o. (MO$_2$)
o. paradox
partial pressure of o. (PO$_2$)
partial pressure of inspiratory o. (P$_{IO_2}$)
o. poisoning
o. radical
o. radical scavenger
o. saturation (So$_2$)
o. saturation of hemoglobin of arterial blood
o. saturation measured by pulse oximetry (SpO$_2$)
o. step-up method
supplemental o.
o. tension
o. tent
o. therapy
o. toxicity
T-piece o.
o. transport
transtracheal o. (TTO)
o. uptake
oxygenated hemoglobin
oxygenation
apneic o.
bubble o.
disk o.
enhanced o.
extracorporeal membrane o. (ECMO)
fetal o.
film o.
hyperbaric o.
nocturnal o.
pump o.
rotating disk o.
screen o.
venoarterial extracorporeal membrane o. (VA-ECMO)
oxygenator
Affinity o.
Biocor 200 high performance o.
bubble o.

disk o.
extracorporeal membrane o.
extracorporeal pump o.
Gambro o.
intravascular o. (IVOX)
Lilliput o.
Maxima Plus plasma resistant fiber o.
Monolyth o.
o. Optima o.
plasma-resistant fiber o. (PRF)
pump o.
Sarns membrane o. (SMO)
oxygen-binding capacity
oxygen-carrying
o.-c. capacity
o.-c. perfluorochemical liquid
oxygen-diffusing capacity
oxygen-free radical
oxygen-induced
o.-i. hypercapnia
o.-i. hypercarbia
oxyhemodynamic index
oxyhemoglobin (HbO$_2$)
o. dissociation curve
o. saturation
Oxy-Hood pressurizer
Oxylator-EM 100 automatic resuscitation and inhalation system
OxyLead interconnect cable
Oxylite ambulatory oxygen system
Oxymatic
O. electronic oxygen conserver
oxymetazoline
Oxypleth pulse oximeter
oxypurinol
OxySAT oxygen saturation meter
oxysterol inhibitor
OxyTemp handheld pulse oximeter
oxytetracycline hydrochloride
OxyTip sensor
oxytoca
Klebsiella o.
Oxytrak pulse oximeter
Oxy-Ultra-Lite ambulatory oxygen system
oyster mass of mucus
ozaenae
Klebsiella pneumoniae subsp. *o.*
ozone

O

NOTES

P
    electrocardiographic wave corresponding
    to a wave of depolarization crossing the
    atria
    partial pressure
    pressure
        P cell
        P congenitale
        P duration
        P loop
        P mitrale
        P pulmonale
        P pulmonale syndrome
        P substance of Lewis
        P synchronous pacing
        P terminal force
        P vector
        P wave
        P wave amplitude
        P wave axis
        P wave triggered ventricular
        pacemaker
P2
    pulmonic second heart sound
P$_{IO_2}$
    partial pressure of inspiratory oxygen
P$_{Emax}$
    maximal expiratory mouth pressure
P$_T$
    total pressure
P$_{Imax}$
    maximal inspiratory mouth pressure
P$_A$
    arterial pressure of arterial fluid
p
    pulse
p24
        p. antigen
        p. antigen test
p22^{phox} protein
p47^{phox} protein
p67^{phox} protein
P-A
PA
    atrial pressure
    partial pressure of arterial fluid
    pressure augmentation
    pulmonary angiography
    pulmonary arterial
    pulmonary artery
    pulmonary atresia
    pulmonary autograft
        Adalat PA
        PA banding
        PA filling pressure

PA-1648
P&A
    percussion and auscultation
Pa
    pascal
    pulmonary arterial
        Pa pressure
pAAT
    plasma alpha-1 antitrypsin
PAB
    premature atrial beat
PABP
    pulmonary artery balloon pump
PABV
    percutaneous aortic balloon valvuloplasty
PAC
    pericarditis, arthropathy, camptodactyly
    phenacetin, aspirin, and caffeine
    premature atrial contraction
    pulmonary artery catheterization
        PAC syndrome
**Paceart complete pacemaker patient
    testing system**
Pace bipolar pacing catheter
paced
        p. cycle length
        p. depolarization integral
        p. rhythm
        p. ventricular evoked response
pacemaker (PM)
        AAI p.
        AAI/AAIR p.
        AAT p.
        Accufix p.
        Activitrax II p.
        Activitrax single-chamber
        responsive p.
        Activitrax variable rate p.
        activity-guided p.
        activity-sensing p.
        Actros p.
        p. adaptive rate
        adaptive-rate p.
        Addvent atrioventricular p.
        Aequitron p.
        Affinity p.
        AFP II p.
        p. afterpotential
        Alcatel p.
        p. amplifier refractory period
        antitachycardia p. (ATP)
        AOO p.
        artificial p.
        Arzco p.
        Astra T4, T6 p.

P

501

pacemaker *(continued)*
atrial asynchronous p.
atrial-based p.
atrial demand inhibited p.
atrial demand triggered p.
atrial synchronous
  noncompetitive p.
atrial synchronous ventricular
  inhibited p.
atrial triggered noncompetitive p.
atrial VOO p.
atrioventricular sequential p.
p. augmentor
Autima II dual-chamber p.
automatic p.
p. automaticity
A-V sequential p.
A-V synchronous p.
Axios 04 p.
Betacel-Biotronik p.
bifocal demand DVI p.
Biorate p.
Biotronik p.
bipolar p.
breathing p.
p. burst pacing
p. can
p. capture
cardiac p.
p. catheter
Chardack-Greatbatch p.
Chardack Medtronic p.
Chronos 04 p.
Circadia dual-chamber rate-
  adaptive p.
circadian p.
p. circus movement tachycardia
  (PCMT)
p. code system
committed mode p.
Contak CD ventricular
  resynchronization p.
Cook p.
Coratomic R wave inhibited p.
Cosmos 283 DDD p.
Cosmos II DDD p.
CPI/Guidant p.
crosstalk p.
p. current (I_F)
Cyberlith p.
Cybertach automatic-burst atrial p.
Cybertach 60 bipolar p.
Dash single-chamber rate-adaptic p.
DDD p.
DDI mode p.
demand p.
Devices, Ltd. p.
Dialog p.
Discovery DDDR p.

Dromos p.
DSI-III screw-in lead p.
dual chamber p. (DCP)
dual-chamber Medtronic Kappa
  400 p.
dual-demand p.
Durapulse p.
DVI p.
Ectocor p.
ectopic p.
electric cardiac p.
p. electrode
Electrodyne p.
electronic p.
Elema p.
Elema-Schonander p.
Elite dual-chamber rate-
  responsive p.
Encor p.
p. endocarditis
end-of-life p.
Endotak p.
Enertrax 7100 p.
Entity p.
escape p.
p. escape interval
external p.
p. failure
fixed-rate p.
fully automatic p.
Guardian p.
Guidant CRM p.
Hancock bipolar balloon p.
p. hysteresis
p. impedance
Integrity AFx DR model 5346 p.
Intermedics atrial antitachycardia p.
Intermedics Marathon dual-chamber
  rate-responsive p.
Intermedics Marathon VVI single-
  chamber p.
Intermedics Stride p.
Intertach II p.
Kairos p.
Kantrowitz p.
Kappa 400 Series p.
p. lead
p. lead fracture
Lillehei p.
lithium-powered p.
Maestro implantable cardiac p.
p. malfunction
Mark IV respiratory p.
Medtronic Activitrax rate-responsive
  unipolar ventricular p.
Medtronic bipolar p.
Medtronic Elite DDDR p.
Medtronic Elite II p.
Medtronic Kappa 400 p.

Medtronic temporary p.
Medtronic Thera DR p.
Medtronic Thera i-series cardiac p.
Meridian p.
Meta DDDR p.
Meta II p.
Meta MV p.
Meta rate-responsive p.
Microlith P p.
Micro Minix p.
Microny II SR+ p.
Microny K SR p.
migrating p.
Momentum DR p.
Multicor II cardiac p.
Nanos 01 p.
noninvasive temporary p.
Nova II p.
nuclear p.
OOO p.
Optima p.
Opus RM single chamber p.
orthorhythmic p. (ORPM)
p. output
p. output reprogramming
p. output voltage
oversensing p.
Pacesetter Trilogy DR p.
Paragon II p.
permanent p. (PPM)
pervenous p.
phantom p.
Philos DR-T p.
physiologic p.
piezoelectric crystal-based p.
Pinnacle p.
p. pocket
p. potential
primary p.
Programalith A-V p.
Programalith II, III p.
programmable p.
programmer p.
Pulsar DDD p.
Pulsar NI implantable p.
P wave triggered ventricular p.
QT interval sensing p.
Quantum p.
rate-adaptive p.
rate-modulated p.
p. reedswitch
reedswitch of p.

Reflex 8220 p.
reflex p.
refractory period of electronic p.
runaway p.
SAVVI p.
p. sensitivity
Sensor p.
Sequicor III p.
shifting p.
Siemens p.
Siemens-Elema p.
smart p.
Sorin p.
p. sound
p. spike
standby p.
Stanicor p.
p. stimulus artifact
subsidiary atrial p.
Symbios 7006 p.
Synchrocor p.
p. syndrome (PS)
Synergyst DDD p.
Synergyst II p.
Telectronics p.
p. telemetry
temperature-sensing p.
temporary p. (TPM)
p. threshold
tined lead p.
transcutaneous p. (TCP, TCPC)
transmural antitachycardia p.
transthoracic p.
transvenous p. (TVP)
Ultra p.
p. undersensing
unipolar atrial p.
unipolar sequential p.
universal p.
VAT p.
VDD p.
Ventak AICD p.
Ventak PRx p.
Ventricor p.
ventricular asynchronous p.
ventricular demand-inhibited p.
ventricular demand-triggered p.
Versatrax II 7000A p.
Vigor DR p.
Vista 4, T, TRS p.
Vitatron Diamond II p.
VOO p.

NOTES

P

503

pacemaker *(continued)*
    VVD p.
    VVI p.
    VVIR p.
    VVT p.
    wandering p.
    wandering atrial p. (WAP)
    p. wires (PMW)
    Zoll NTP 1000 noninvasive p.
pacemaker-mediated tachycardia (PMT)
pacemapping
Paceport catheter
pacer-cardioverter-defibrillator (PCD)
Pacerone tablet
Pacesetter
    P. APS II 3004 programmer
    P. APS pacemaker programmer
    P. Tendril DX steroid-eluting
      active-fixation pacing lead
    P. Trilogy DR pacemaker
Pacesetter/St. Jude lead
pace-terminable
pace-terminate
Pachon
    P. method
    P. test
pachypleuritis
PACI
    partial anterior circulation infarct
pacing
    AAI p.
    AAI-RR p.
    AAT p.
    acceleration-guided activity p.
    activity-guided p.
    antitachycardia p. (ATP)
    AOO p.
    asynchronous p.
    atrial p. (AP)
    atrial incremental p.
    atrial overdrive p.
    atrial septum septal p.
    atrial train p.
    atrioventricular synchronous p.
    autodecremental p.
    biatrial p.
    biventricular p.
    burst atrial p.
    burst of rapid atrial p. (BRAP)
    burst of ventricular p. (BVP)
    cardiac p. (CP)
    p. in cardiomyopathy (PIC)
    cardioventricular p. (CVP)
    p. catheter
    closed-loop p.
    p. code
    p. counter
    coupled atrial p. (CAP)
    p. cycle length (PCL)

DDD p.
DDDR p.
DDI p.
DDIR p.
decremental atrial p.
demand p.
diaphragmatic p.
direct His bundle p. (DHBP)
dual-chamber p.
dual-site right atrial p.
p. duration
DVI p.
endocardial p.
epicardial p.
external high-output ramp p.
high-frequency burst p.
p. hysteresis
implantable cardioverter-
    defibrillator/atrial tachycardia p.
    (ICD-ATP)
p. impulse (PI)
incremental atrial p.
incremental ventricular p.
inhibited p.
intracardiac p.
p. lead impedance
p. modality
p. mode
multisite biventricular p.
no atrial p.
noninvasive transcutaneous
    cardiac p. (NTCP)
OOO p.
overdrive atrial p.
pacemaker burst p.
permanent p.
P synchronous p.
RAMP p.
rapid p.
rapid atrial p. (RAP)
rapid-burst p.
rate modulated p. (RAMP)
rate-responsive ventricular p.
right atrial p.
right ventricular outflow tract p.
right ventricular septal p.
RVOT p.
sequential p.
shock p.
p. spike
p. stimulus
subthreshold p.
suprathreshold p.
SVA p.
p. system analyzer
temporary p.
threshold p.
p. threshold
trains of ventricular p.

transatrial p.
transcutaneous p. (TCP, TCPC)
transesophageal p. (TEP)
transesophageal atrial p. (TAP, TEAP)
transesophageal echocardiography with p. (TEEP)
trichamber p.
triggered p.
underdrive p.
univentricular p.
VAT p.
VDD p.
VDI p.
ventricular p. (VP)
ventricular safety p.
VOO p.
VVD p.
VVI p.
VVIR p.
VVI-RR p.
VVI/VVIR p.
VVT p.

pacing-induced
p.-i. angina
p.-i. heart failure
p.-i. tachycardia (PIT)

Pacis
pack
AeroGear fanny p.
interferon alfa-2b and ribavirin combination p.
RIK fluid-filled head p.

packer
body p.

pack-year smoking history
paclitaxel
PaCO₂
arterial carbon dioxide tension
arterial partial pressure of CO_2

PACP
pulmonary artery counterpulsation
PACS
partial anterior circulation syndrome
postoperative atrial fibrillation in cardiac surgery
PACT
Philadelphia Association of Clinical Trials
Prescription Analyses and Cost
PACU
postanesthesia care unit

PACWP
pulmonary arterial capillary wedge pressure
PAD
peripheral arterial disease
phenacetin, aspirin, and desoxyephedrine
public access defibrillation
public access to defibrillation
public access defibrillator
pulmonary artery diastolic
pulsatile assist device
pad
digitizing p.
electrode p.
Heartstream FR2 AED with attenuated defibrillation p.
Littman defibrillation p.
pericardial fat p.
pharyngoesophageal p.'s
p. sign
Signa P.
SomaSensor p.
PADCAB
perfusion-assisted direct coronary artery bypass
paddle
anteroposterior p.
cardioversion p.
defibrillation p.
defibrillator p.
electrode p.
PADP
pulmonary artery diastolic pressure
PAE
postantibiotic effect
Paecilomyces variotii
PAEDP
pulmonary artery end-diastolic pressure
PAF
paroxysmal atrial fibrillation
platelet activating factor
pulmonary arteriovenous fistula
PAFD
pulmonary artery filling defect
PAFIB
paroxysmal atrial fibrillation
PAG
pulmonary angiography
PAGE
perfluorocarbon-associated gas exchange
Page episodic hypertension
Paget disease of bone

NOTES

P

Paget-von Schrötter
P.-v. S. syndrome
P.-v. S. venous thrombosis
PAGOD
pulmonary hypoplasia, hypoplasia of
pulmonary artery, agonadism,
omphalocele/diaphragmatic defect,
dextrocardia
PAGOD syndrome
PAH
polycyclic aromatic hydrocarbon
pulmonary alveolar hypoventilation
pulmonary artery hypertension
pulmonary artery hypotension
PAHVC
pulmonary alveolar hypoxic
vasoconstrictor
PAI
perforating artery infarct
plasminogen activator inhibitor
PAI-1
plasminogen activator inhibitor-1
pain
anginal p.
atypical chest p.
burning p.
calf p.
chest p. (CP)
crushing chest p.
dream p.
dull p.
functional p.
low-risk chest p. (LRCP)
musculoskeletal p.
phantom p.
pleuritic chest p.
psychogenic p.
pulmonary p.
rest p.
staccato p.
vasoocclusive p. (VOP)
waxing and waning chest p.
paired
p. beats
p. electrical stimulation
p. stimulus
PAK
percutaneous access kit
Pal
Vital-Port Infusion P.
palatal surgery
palate
high arched p.
palatina
tonsilla p.
palatine tonsil
palatini
tensor p.
palatopharyngeal sphincter

palatoplasty
laser-assisted p. (LAP)
palatovaginal canal
Palco Laboratories Model 300, 400
pulse oximeter
pale
p. hypertension
p. thrombus
paleopneumoniae
Peptostreptococcus p.
palestinensis
Acanthamoeba p.
palisading histiocyte
palivizumab
palliation
palliative
p. prognostic index
p. surgery
pallida
asphyxia p.
pallidum
microhemagglutination *Treponema p.*
Treponema p.
pallor
palm
liver p.
tripe p.
Palma operation
palmar
p. arch
carpal arch p.
p. click
p. erythema
p. xanthoma
palmare
xanthoma striatum p.
Palmaz-Schatz (PS)
P.-S. balloon-expandable stent
P.-S. coronary stent
P.-S. Crown stent
P.-S. PS-204 stent
P.-S. stent (PSS)
Palmaz vascular stent
palmi (*pl. of* palmus)
palmic
palmitate
clofazimine p.
colfosceril p.
palmitic acid
palmitoylcarnitine
palmodic
palmoscopy
palmus, pl. **palmi**
palpable A wave
palpation
bimanual precordial p.
palpitatio cordis
palpitation
heart p.'s

paroxysmal p.
premonitory p.
PALS
pediatric life support
palsy
pseudobulbar p.
suprabulbar p.
Palv
alveolar pressure
PAM
pulmonary alveolar microlithiasis
pulse amplitude modulation
2-PAM
2-pralidoxime
PAM2, PAM3 monitor
Pamelor
p-**aminosalicylic acid**
pamoate
pyrantel p.
PAMP
pulmonary artery mean pressure
Panacet
panacinar emphysema
panbronchiolitis
diffuse p. (DPB)
pANCA
perinuclear antineutrophil cytoplasmic
antibody
pancarditis
panchamber enlargement
Pancoast
P. syndrome
P. tumor
panconduction defect
pancreas
Starling curve of p.
pancreatic
p. dornase
p. enzyme
p. extract
p. polypeptide (PP)
pancreaticopleural fistula
pancreatin asthma
pancreatitis
pancreatopleural fistula
pancuronium bromide
pandiastolic
panel
cardiac laboratory p. (CLP)
Cholestech LDX system with TC
and Glucose P.
lipid p.

p. of reactive antibodies (PRA)
South Florida RAST p.
thyroid p.
Triage Cardio ProfilER p.
panel-reactive antibody (PRA)
pang
breast p.
Panhematin
panhyperemia
panhypogammaglobulinemia
panic disorder
paninspiratory
Panje voice button
panlobular emphysema
panniculitis
panniculus
panning
panophthalmitis
pansystolic
p. flow
p. murmur
pantaloon
p. embolism
p. patch
Panther balloon
panting maneuver
pantoprazole sodium
pantothenate synthetase
pantyhose
Glattelast compression p.
panzerherz
PAO
pulmonary artery occlusion
PAO$_2$
alveolar oxygen partial pressure
PAo
ascending aortic pressure
pulmonary artery occlusion pressure
PaO$_2$
arterial oxygen partial pressure
arterial oxygen tension
PAOD
peripheral arterial occlusive disease
peripheral arteriosclerotic occlusive
disease
PAOP
pulmonary artery occlusion pressure
PAP
positive airway pressure
pulmonary artery pressure
papain
Papanicolaou solution

NOTES

P

papaverine hydrochloride
paper
    asthma p.
    niter p.
papilla, pl. **papillae**
    Bergmeister p.
papillary
    p. adenocarcinoma
    p. carcinoma
    p. fibroelastoma (PES)
    p. frond
    p. muscle (PM)
    p. muscle abscess
    p. muscle of conus arteriosus
    p. muscle dysfunction
    p. muscle rupture (PMR)
    p. muscle syndrome
    p. muscle tip
    p. muscle traction
    p. tumor
papilledema
papillitis
papillomatosis
    recurrent respiratory p.
papillomavirus
    human p. (HPV)
papillotome
    Wilson-Cook p.
PAPm
    mean pulmonary artery pressure
Pappenheim stain
papulonecrotic tuberculosis
papulosis
    atrophic p.
pa-pv
    pulmonary arterial pressure, pulmonary
    venous pressure
PAPVC
    partial anomalous pulmonary venous
    connection
PAPVD
    partial anomalous pulmonary venous
    drainage
PAPVR
    partial anomalous pulmonary venous
    return
PAR
    posterior wall or aortic root
    primary angioplasty research
    pulmonary arteriolar resistance
    pulse amplitude ratio
paraaminobenzoic acid
paraaminosalicylate sodium
paraaminosalicylic acid (PAS, PASA)
paraaortic bodies
paraboloid
    oscillating p.
paracentesis
    pericardial p.

    thoracic p.
    p. thoracis
paracetamol sensitivity
parachute
    p. deformity
    p. mitral valve
paracicatricial emphysema
Paracoccidioides brasiliensis
paracoccidioidin skin test
paracoccidioidomycosis
paracorporeal heart
paracrine
    p. factor
    p. signaling
paradigm
paradox
    calcium p.
    early systolic p. (ESP)
    French p.
    p. image
    oxygen p.
    thoracoabdominal p.
paradoxic
    p. embolism
    p. pulse
    p. rocking impulse
    p. split of S_2
    p. wall motion
paradoxical
    p. aberrancy
    p. bronchospasm
    p. cerebral embolism
    p. embolization
    p. embolus
    p. pulse (PP)
    p. respiration
    p. systolic expansion (PSE)
    p. vasoconstriction
paradoxically split S_2 sound
paradoxus
    pulsus p. (PP)
paraesophageal hernia
paraffin block
paraffinoma
PARAflow circulatory support system
paraganglioma tumor
Paragon
    P. coronary stent
    P. II pacemaker
    P. nitinol stent
    P. PAS stent
paragonimiasis
Paragonimus westermani
parahaemolyticus
    Haemophilus p.
    Vibrio p.
parahilar
    p. fibrosis
    p. region

parahisian accessory pathway
parainfluenzae
    Haemophilus p. (HPI)
parainfluenza virus
parallel shunt
paralysis
    diaphragmatic p.
    diphtheric p.
    diphtheritic p.
    hemidiaphragm p.
    hypokalemic periodic p.
    ischemic p.
    periodic p.
    phrenic nerve p.
    respiratory p.
    sleep p.
    tick p.
    vasomotor p.
    Volkmann ischemic p.
paralytica
    dysphagia p.
paralytic chest
paralyticus
    laryngismus p.
    thorax p.
paramagnetic substance
paramedic
parameter
    late potential p.
    portable monitor of respiratory p.'s
      (PMRP)
    systemic hemodynamic p.'s
    ventricular inotropic p. (VIP)
parameterized diastolic filling (PDF)
paramethasone acetate
parametric
    p. image
    p. imaging
Paramyxoviridae virus
Paramyxovirus
paraneoplastic
    p. pemphigus
    p. syndrome
paraoxonase polymorphism
ParaPac ventilator
parapharyngeum
    spatium p.
paraplane echocardiography
Paraplatin
parapneumonic effusion
paraprosthetic leak

parapsilosis
    Candida p.
paraquat
pararrhythmia
parasagittal plane
paraseptal
    p. emphysema
    p. pathway
parasitic
    p. cardiomyopathy
    p. infestation
paraspinal line
parasternal
    p. examination
    p. heave
    p. long axis
    p. long-axis view
    p. long-axis view echocardiogram
    p. short axis
    p. short-axis view
    p. short-axis view echocardiogram
    p. systolic lift
    p. systolic thrill
    p. window
parasympathetic
    p. function
    p. nerve fibers
    p. nervous system
parasympathomimetic
parasynapsis
parasyndesis
parasystole
    atrial p.
    junctional p.
    pure p.
    ventricular p.
parasystolic
    p. beat
    p. ventricular tachycardia
parathyroid hormone
paratracheal
    p. chain
    p. lymph node
    p. region
paratracheales
    nodi lymphoidei p.
Paratrend
    P. 7 continuous blood gas monitor
    P. 7+ multiparameter blood gas
      monitor
paravalvular
ParCA catheter

NOTES

P

parchemin
  bruit de p.
parchment
  p. heart
  p. right ventricle
parenchyma
  pulmonary p.
parenchymal
  p. amyloidosis
  p. asbestosis
  p. aspergillosis
  p. disease
  p. fibrosis
  p. hematoma (PH)
  p. hemorrhage (PH)
  p. laceration
  p. lesion
  p. sarcoidosis
parenchymatous
  p. myocarditis
  p. pneumonia
parenteral
  Coly-Mycin M P.
  P. nutrition
parent radionuclide
paresis
pargyline
  methyclothiazide and p.
Pari
  P. LC Plus reusable nebulizer
  P. LC Star reusable nebulizer
  P. Proneb Ultra nebulizer
paries membranaceus tracheae
parietal
  p. ball
  p. band
  p. endocarditis
  p. pericardiectomy
  p. pericardium (PP)
  p. pleura
  p. pleural damage
  p. pulse (PP)
  p. thrombus
parietalis
  pleura p.
parietooccipital artery
Park
  P. aneurysm
  P. blade septostomy
Parks 800 bidirectional Doppler flowmeter
Parlodel
Parodi catheter
paromomycin sulfate
paroxetine
paroxysmal
  p. atrial fibrillation (PAF, PAFIB)
  p. atrial tachycardia (PAT)
  p. atrial tachycardia with aberrancy

  p. atrioventricular nodal reciprocal tachycardia (PAVNRT)
  p. burst
  p. cough
  p. dyspnea on exertion (PDE)
  p. hypertension
  p. junctional tachycardia (PJT)
  p. nocturnal dyspnea (PND)
  p. nocturnal hemoglobinuria (PNH)
  p. nodal tachycardia
  p. palpitation
  p. pulmonary edema
  p. reentrant supraventricular tachycardia
  p. sinus tachycardia
  p. sleep
  p. supraventricular arrhythmia
  p. supraventricular tachycardia (PST, PSVT)
  p. tachycardia (PT)
  p. ventricular tachycardia (PVT)
paroxysm of coughing
parrot
  p. fever
  P. murmur
pars, pl. partes
  p. abdominalis esophagi
  p. basalis arteriae pulmonalis
  p. cervicalis esophagi
  p. costalis diaphragmatis
  partes intersegmentales
  p. intralobaris intersegmentalis venae posterioris lobi superioris pulmonis dextri
  p. lumbalis diaphragmatis
  p. mediastinalis pulmonis
  p. membranacea
  p. nasalis pharyngis
  p. oralis pharyngis
  p. pharyngea hypophyseos
  p. thoracica esophagi
part
  central apical P. (CAP)
  certified distinct P. (CDP)
  P. per million (ppm)
partial
  p. anomalous pulmonary veins
  p. anomalous pulmonary venous connection (PAPVC)
  p. anomalous pulmonary venous drainage (PAPVD)
  p. anomalous pulmonary venous return (PAPVR)
  p. anterior circulation infarct (PACI)
  p. anterior circulation syndrome (PACS)
  p. atrioventricular canal
  p. autobullectomy

p. A-V canal defect
p. chordal-sparing mitral valve replacement
p. confluens sinuum thrombosis
p. CVID
p. encircling endocardial ventriculotomy
p. heart block
p. intermixed fibrosis
p. liquid ventilation (PLV)
p. occlusion inferior vena cava clip
p. pressure (P, PP)
p. pressure of arterial fluid (PA)
p. pressure of carbon dioxide (PCO$_2$)
p. pressure of carbon monoxide (PCO)
p. pressure of end-tidal CO$_2$ (PETCO$_2$)
p. pressure of inspiratory oxygen (P$_{IO_2}$)
p. pressure of oxygen (PO$_2$)
p. rebreathing mask
p. thromboplastin time (PTT, ptt)

partially coagulated effusion
particle
Amberlite p.'s
Dane p.
PVA foam embolization p.
remnant-like lipoprotein p. (RLP)
particulate respirator
partition
atrial p.
partitioning
left atrial p.
Partuss LA
Parvolex
parvus
pulsus p.
PAS
paraaminosalicylic acid
peripheral access system
persistent atrial standstill
posterior airway space
premature atrial stimulus
pulmonary arterial stenosis
pulmonary artery systolic
PASA
paraaminosalicylic acid
pascal (Pa)
P. principle

PASE
Physical Activity Scale for the Elderly Evaluation
PASG
pneumatic antishock garment
PASP
pulmonary artery systolic pressure
passage
adiabatic fast p.
P. hemostasis valve
Passager stent graft
passivation
pharmacologic plaque p.
plaque p.
passive
p. clot
p. congestion
p. edema
p. hyperemia
p. interval
p. mode
p. smoking
p. tilting
p. vascular exercise (pavex)
passover humidifier
Passy-Muir
P.-M. O2 Adapter
P.-M. tracheostomy speaking valve
paste
electrode p.
Pasteurella
P. aerogenes
P. multocida
pasteurellosis
PASVR
pulmonary anomalous superior venous return
Pasys ST cardiac pacing system
PAT
paroxysmal atrial tachycardia
patch
Acuseal cardiovascular p.
Adcon-C resorbable liquid p.
p. angioplasty
atrial septal defect p.
autologous blood p.
autologous pericardial p.
BioGlue surgical p.
buspirone transdermal p.
cardiac p.
CardioFix pericardium p.
chest wall p.

NOTES

P

patch *(continued)*
    p. closure
    CorRestore implantable p.
    Dacron intracardiac p.
    defibrillation p.
    Deponit P.
    electrodispersive skin p.
    epicardial defibrillator p.
    extrapericardial p.
    Fluoropassiv thin-wall carotid p.
    Gore-Tex cardiovascular p.
    Gore-Tex soft tissue p.
    p. graft reconstruction
    Habitrol P.
    Ionescu-Shiley pericardial p.
    MacCallum p.
    Minitran P.
    Nicoderm P.
    nicotine transdermal p.
    Nicotrol P.
    Nitro-Dur P.
    outflow cardiac p.
    pantaloon p.
    pericardial p.
    Peyer p.
    polypropylene intracardiac p.
    p. repair
    retropectoral p.
    sandwich p.
    Silastic p.
    SJM pericardial p.
    soldier's p.'s
    subcutaneous p.
    Teflon felt p.
    Teflon intracardiac p.
    transanular p.
    transcatheter p.
    Transderm-Nitro P.
patch-coil system
patch-graft
    p.-g. angioplasty
    Dacron onlay p.-g.
patchplasty
patchy
    p. atelectasis
    p. consolidation
    p. hyperintensity
    p. infiltrate
    p. infiltration
PATE
    pulmonary artery thromboembolism
patency
    catheter p.
    coronary bypass graft p.
    epicardial artery p.
    epicardial vessel p.
    heparin and early p.
    infarct artery p.
    probe p.

    p. rate
    stent p.
    TIMI p.
    vein graft p.
    venous coronary graft p.
patent
    p. bronchus sign
    p. ductus (PD)
    p. ductus arteriosus (PDA)
    p. ductus arteriosus flow jet
    p. ductus arteriosus murmur
    p. ductus arteriosus umbrella
    p. foramen ovale (PFO)
Pathfinder mini microcatheter
pathogen
    nosocomial p.
pathogenesis
pathogenicity
pathologic
    p. complete response
    p. murmur
    p. QT (QTU)
    p. trigger
pathology
    coexistent p.
    multivalve p.
pathophysiology
pathostimulation
pathway
    accessory p. (AP)
    antegrade internodal p.
    anterior internodal p.
    atrio-His p.
    atrioventricular p. (AP)
    atrioventricular node p.
    Bachmann p.
    concealed accessory p.
    conduction p.
    diacylglycerate p.
    electrical p.
    Fas-Fas ligand p.
    FasL p.
    fast p.
    final common p.
    free-wall accessory p.
    integrin-dependent p.
    internodal p.
    Jak/STAT p.
    Kent p.
    lipoxygenase p.
    MAPK p.
    mitogen-activated kinase p.
    parahisian accessory p.
    paraseptal p.
    reentrant p.
    retinohypothalamic p.
    retrograde fast p.
    scavenger cell p.
    selective past p.

septal p.
shunt p.
slow A-V node p.
slow and fast A-V nodal p.
surgical ablation of p.
Thorel p.

patient
ABCDE in trauma p.
p. activator mode
p. compliance
intubated p.
p. monitor
multiple-trauma p.
nonintubated p.
nonventilated p.
postinfarct p.
Postural Assessment Scale for
Stroke P.

patient-controlled
p.-c. analgesia (PCA)
p.-c. analgesic (PCA)

patient-triggered recording
Patil stereotactic system
Patriot moderate support guide wire
pattern
abdominal paradox breathing p.
airspace-filling p.
airway p.
alveolar p.
alveolar-filling p.
ballerina-foot p.
butterfly p.
candle flame p.
cephalization of pulmonary flow p.
circadian blood pressure p.
concave p.
contraction p.
crochetage EKG p.
deer-antler vascular p.
diastolic filling p.
dip-and-plateau p.
dipper p.
disturbed circadian blood
pressure p.
eggshell p.
embryonic phenotype p.
fishnet p.
ground-glass p.
honeycomb p.
hourglass p.
impaired relaxation mitral flow p.
interstitial p.

intraventricular conduction p.
juvenile p.
maximum contraction p. (MCP)
miliary p.
military p.
mosaic p.
nondipper p.
organoid p.
QR, QS p.
QS p.
respiratory p.
respiratory alternans breathing p.
restrictive filling p.
restrictive physiology mitral
flow p.
reticular p.
reticulonodular p.
salt and pepper p.
sawtooth p.
scintillating speckle p.
scooped p.
sine wave p.
sinusoidal strut p.
S_1Q_3 p.
$S_1Q_3T_3$ p.
torpedo-shaped p.
upstroke p.
uptake-mismatch p.
vascular p.
ventricular contraction p.
W p.
watershed p.

patty
cottonoid p.

PAU
penetrating aortic ulcer
penetrating atherosclerotic ulcer

pauciimmune glomerulonephritis
Paulin venography technique
pause
compensatory p.
full compensatory p.
noncompensatory p.
postectopic p.
postextrasystolic p.
preautomatic p.
sinus exit p.
ventricular p.

pause-dependent arrhythmia
PAV
percutaneous aortic valvuloplasty
proportional assist ventilation

NOTES

P

Pavcnik Monodisk device
pavementing
Paveral Stanley Syrup With Codeine
Phosphate
pavex
    passive vascular exercise
PAVF
    pulmonary arteriovenous fistula
Pavlov reflex
PAVM
    pulmonary arteriovenous malformation
PAVNRT
    paroxysmal atrioventricular nodal
      reciprocal tachycardia
pAVP
    plasma arginine vasopressin
PAVSD
    pulmonary atresia with ventricular septal
      defect
PAW
    pulmonary artery wedge
PAWP
    pulmonary artery wedge pressure
Paykel scale
PB
    premature beat
PBC
    perfusion balloon catheter
PBF
    peripheral blood flow
    pulmonary blood flow
PBMC
    peripheral blood mononuclear cell
PBMV
    pulmonary blood mixing volume
PBP
    percutaneous balloon pericardiotomy
PBPV
    percutaneous balloon pulmonary
      valvuloplasty
PBS
    phosphate-buffered saline
    pulmonary branch stenosis
PBV
    percutaneous balloon valvuloplasty
    pulmonary balloon valvuloplasty
    pulmonary blood volume
PBZ
    Pyribenzamine
PC
    portacaval
    posterior circulation
    posterior circumflex artery
    precordial
    pressure control
    pulmonary circulation
    pulmonary compliance
    pulmonic closure

PCA
    patient-controlled analgesia
    patient-controlled analgesic
    portacaval anastomosis
    posterior cerebral artery
    precoronary care area
    prehospital cardiac arrest
      fetal-type PCA
      PCA system
PCAD
    progression of coronary artery disease
PCB
    portacaval bypass
    protected catheter brushing
PCBS
    percutaneous cardiopulmonary bypass
      support
PCC
    precoronary care
PCCU
    postcoronary care unit
PCD
    pacer-cardioverter-defibrillator
    primary ciliary dyskinesia
    programmable cardioverter-defibrillator
      PCD ICD generator
      Jewel PCD
      PCD Transvene implantable
        cardioverter-defibrillator system
PCDC
    plasma clot diffusion chamber
PCE Oral
PCF
    peak cough flow
PCG
    phonocardiogram
    pneumocardiogram
PCI
    percutaneous coronary intervention
    prophylactic brain irradiation
PCIRV
    pressure-controlled inverse ratio
      ventilation
PCIS
    postcardiac injury syndrome
PCL
    pacing cycle length
PCMT
    pacemaker circus movement tachycardia
PCNA
    proliferating cell nuclear antigen
PCO
    partial pressure of carbon monoxide
    predicted cardiac output
PCO_2
    partial pressure of carbon dioxide
      PCO_2 oximetry
PCoA
    posterior communicating artery

P-congenitale
PCP
> peripheral coronary pressure
> *Pneumocystis carinii* pneumonia
> postoperative constrictive pericarditis
> pulmonary capillary pressure

PCPB
> percutaneous cardiopulmonary bypass

PCPS
> percutaneous cardiopulmonary support

PCR
> polymerase chain reaction
>> PCR assay
>> PCR test

PCr
> phosphocreatine

PCRA
> percutaneous coronary rotational
> atherectomy

PCS
> portacaval shunt
> postcardiotomy syndrome
> proximal coronary sinus

PCT
> portacaval transposition

PCTI
> penetrating cardiac trauma index

PCV
> pressure-controlled ventilation

PCW
> pulmonary capillary wedge

PCWP
> pulmonary capillary wedge pressure

PD
> patent ductus
> postural drainage
> pulsed diastolic
> pulse duration
> pure dysarthria
>> PD Access with Peel-Away needle
>> introducer
>> PD 123319 AT receptor agonist
>> PD 2000 defibrillator

P/D
> proximal-to-distal
>> P/D vessel

Pd
> diastolic pressure

PDA
> patent ductus arteriosus
> posterior descending artery

> snare-assisted coil occlusion of
> PDA
> PDA umbrella

PD-AB-SAAP
> pulsed diastolic autologous blood
> selective aortic arch perfusion

PDB
> preperitoneal dilator balloon
>> PDB preperitoneal distention
>> balloon system

PDC, PdC
> pediatric cardiology

PD-CSE
> pulsed Doppler cross-sectional
> echocardiography

PDE
> paroxysmal dyspnea on exertion
> phosphodiesterase inhibitor
> pulsed Doppler echocardiography
>> PDE isoenzyme inhibitor

PDE-I
> phosphodiesterase inhibitor

PDE3I
> phosphodiesterase III inhibition

P-dextrocardiale
PDF
> parameterized diastolic filling
> probability density function

PDGF
> platelet-derived growth factor

PD-GXT
> postdischarge graded-exercise test

PDH
> progressive disseminated histoplasmosis
> pyruvate dehydrogenase

PDHRF
> platelet-derived histamine-releasing factor

PDP
> peak diastolic pressure

PD&P
> postural drainage and percussion

PDPV
> postural drainage, percussion and
> vibration

PDR
> proliferative diabetic retinopathy

PDT
> percutaneous dilatational tracheostomy
> percutaneous dilational tracheostomy

PDUFA
> Prescription Drug User Fee Act

NOTES

P

PDV
peak diastolic velocity
PE
cisplatin, etoposide
pericardial effusion
preexcitation
pulmonary edema
pulmonary embolism
pulmonary emphysema
PE balloon
PE-60-I-2 implantable pronged unipolar electrode
PE-60-K-10 implantable unipolar endocardial electrode
PE-60-KB implantable unipolar endocardial electrode
PE-85-I-2 implantable pronged unipolar electrode
PE-85-K-10 implantable unipolar endocardial electrode
PE-85-KB implantable unipolar endocardial electrode
PE-85-KS-10 implantable unipolar endocardial electrode
PEA
pulseless electrical activity
peak
p. A, E velocity
p. airway pressure (Ppeak)
p. cough flow (PCF)
p. diastolic filling rate
p. diastolic pressure (PDP)
p. diastolic velocity (PDV)
p. ejection rate (PER)
p. ejection time (PET)
p. ejection velocity (V_{pe})
p. emptying rate
p. exercise
p. exercise oxygen consumption (VO_2)
p. exercise ventilation (V_E)
p. expiratory flow (PEF)
p. expiratory flow rate (PEFR)
p. expiratory maneuver
p. filling rate (PFR)
p. flow (PF)
p. flowmeter (PFM)
h p.
p. heart rate (PHR)
p. incidence
p. inspiratory flow (PIF)
p. inspiratory flow rate (PIFR)
p. inspiratory pressure (PIP)
p. instantaneous Doppler gradient
p. jet flow rate
p. left ventricular pressure (PLVP)
p. lengthening rate
p. magnitude

p. myocardial video intensity (PMVI)
p. negative pressure (P-min, PNP)
p. oxygen uptake
p. positive pressure (P+max)
p. respiratory ratio (RER)
p. shortening rate
p. systolic aortic pressure (PSAP)
p. systolic gradient (PSG)
p. systolic gradient pressure
p. systolic pressure (PSP)
p. systolic velocity
p. tidal expiratory flow (PTEF)
p. tidal inspiratory flow (PTIF)
p. transaortic flow velocity
p. transaortic valve gradient
p. and trough
p. and trough levels
p. twitch force
p. VO_2
p. workload
p. work rate (Wmax)
peaked P wave
PEAP
positive end-airway pressure
pearl
keratin p.
Laënnec p.
p. sign
string of p.'s
pear-shaped heart
peau d'orange
PEC
pulmonary ejection click
pecorum
Chlamydia p.
pect
pectinate muscle
pectoral
ectopia cordis p.
p. emulation
p. fascia
p. fremitus
p. heart
p. tea
pectoralgia
pectoralis
fascia p.
p. major
p. minor
regio p.
pectoriloquous bronchophony
pectoriloquy
aphonic p.
whispered p.
whispering p.
pectoris
angina p. (ang pect, AP)
angor p.

stable angina p. (SAP)
unstable angina p. (UAP)
variant angina p. (VAP)
pectorophony
pectus
    p. carinatum
    p. deformity
    p. excavatum
    p. gallinatum
    p. recurvatum
pedal
    p. edema
    p. pulse
pedal-mode ergometer
PediaCare Oral
Pediacof
Pediapred Oral
pediatric
    Benylin P.
    p. cardiology (PDC, PdC)
    P. Cardiology Devices Sideris
      Buttoned device occluder
    p. cardiomyopathy
    Cleocin P.
    p. finger clip sensor
    p. hypertension
    p. lead
    P. LifeShirt system
    p. life support (PALS)
    p. pigtail catheter
    Robitussin P.
    p. vascular clamp
Pediazole Oral
pedicle graft
Pedi-Dri
Pedituss
Pedoff continuous wave transducer
pedunculated thrombus
PedvaxHIB
peel
    pericardial p.
    pleural p.
    visceral p.
Peel-Away
    P.-A. banana catheter
    P.-A. introducer set
peel-away sheath
peeling-back mechanism
PEEP
    positive end-expiratory pressure
    PEEP valve

PEEPi
    intrinsic positive end-expiratory pressure
PEF
    peak expiratory flow
    pulmonary edema fluid
%PEF
    percent predicted peak expiratory flow
pefloxacin
PEFR
    peak expiratory flow rate
PEG
    polyethylene glycol
      PEG interleukin-2
      PEG tube
pegademase bovine
pegaspargase
PEG-LES
    polyethylene glycol electrolyte lavage
    solution
pegvisomant
PEJ
    percutaneous endoscopic jejunostomy
      PEJ tube
Pel
    lung elastic recoil pressure
PELA
    peripheral excimer laser angioplasty
PELCA
    percutaneous excimer laser coronary
    angioplasty
      PELCA Registry
Pelger-Huet cell
pellagra
pellet
    Testopel P.
pellucidum
    pineal p.
    septum p.
Pelorus stereotactic system
Pel-V
    elastic pressure-volume
PEM
    precordial electrocardiographic
    monitoring
pemphigus
    paraneoplastic p.
PE-MT balloon dilatation catheter
pen
    Cardioblate surgical ablation p.
    light p.
Penaz volume-clamp method
penbutolol sulfate

NOTES

P

PenChant coronary stent delivery system
penciclovir
pencil percussion
pendelluft
  p. effect
  p. phenomenon
pendulous heart
pendulum
  cor p.
  p. rhythm
  p. test
penetrance
penetrating
  p. aortic ulcer (PAU)
  p. atherosclerotic ulcer (PAU)
  p. cardiac trauma index (PCTI)
  p. chest injury
  p. rupture
  p. thoracic trauma
penetration
penetrator artery
penicillin
  benzathine benzyl p.
  p. G
  p. G benzathine
  p. G benzathine and procaine combined
  p. G procaine
  penicillinase-resistant p.
  p. phenoxymethyl
  semisynthetic p.
  p. VK
  p. V potassium
penicillinase-resistant penicillin
penicilliosis
Penicillium marneffei
penicilloyl polylysine (PPL)
penile-brachial pressure index
penis
  cavernous vein of p.
Penn
  P. Convention criteria
  P. formula
  P. method
  P. State TAH
pentaacetate
  diethylenetriamine p.-a. (DTPA)
pentachloride
  antimony p.
pentachrome
  Movat p.
pentaerythritol tetranitrate (PETN)
pentagastrin
pentalogy
  Cantrell p.
  p. of Fallot
  Fallot p.
Pentalumen catheter

pentamidine
  p. in aerosol form
  aerosolized p.
  p. isethionate
Pentam-300 injection
pentane
pentasaccharide
Pentatrichomonas hominis
Pentax bronchoscope
pentazocine
pentetate
  imciromab p.
pentobarbital
Pentothal Sodium
pentoxifylline
pentraxin
penumbra
  ischemic p.
Pen.Vee K
PEP
  positive expiratory pressure
  preejection period
  PEP mask
PEPA
  peptidase A
PEPc
  corrected pre-ejection period
PEPI
  preejection period index
Pepper
  P. Medical Antidisconnect Device strap
  P. Medical tube neck band
peppermint test
peptic
  p. aspiration pneumonitis
  p. esophagitis
  p. ulcer
peptidase A (PEPA)
peptide
  adrenomedullin p.
  atrial natriuretic p. (ANP)
  brain natriuretic p. (BNP)
  B-type natriuretic p. (BNP)
  calcitonin gene-related p. (CGRP)
  cerebrovascular amyloid p. (CVAP)
  C-type natriuretic p. (CNP)
  Dendroaspis natriuretic p. (DNP)
  human atrial natriuretic p. (hANP)
  immunoreactive atrial natriuretic p. (iANP, IrANP)
  p. mucolytic
  natriuretic p.
  N-20 terminal p.
  N-terminal pro brain natriuretic p. (NT-proBNP)
  procollagen type III aminoterminal p. (PIIIP)
  protegrin antimicrobial p.

rat atrial natriuretic p. (rANP)
TFF-domain p.
tick anticoagulant p.
vasoactive intestinal p. (VIP)
vasoconstrictor p.
vasoinhibitory p. (VIP)
vasorelaxant p.
peptidoglycan
peptidomimetic
Peptococcus constellatus
Peptostreptococcus
    P. anaerobius
    P. asaccharolyticus
    P. evolutus
    P. paleopneumoniae
    P. prevotii
    P. productus
PER
    peak ejection rate
per
    p. primam healing
    p. primam intentionem
    p. secundum healing
    p. secundum intentionem
Per-C-Cath
perceived
    p. exertion
    p. noise (PN)
percent
    p. diameter stenosis (%DS)
    p. of maximum predicted heart rate
    p. predicted peak expiratory flow (%PEF)
perceptual-sensory neglect
perchloric acid
Perclose
    P. vascular closure device
    P. vascular surgical closure system
Percor Stat-DL intra-arotic balloon catheter
PercuCut biopsy needle
PercuGuide lesion marking system
percussion
    auscultation and p. (A&P)
    p. and auscultation (P&A)
    chest p.
    coin p.
    p. dullness
    fist p.
    Goldscheider p.
    Murphy p.

p. note (PN)
pencil p.
piano p.
Plesch p.
postural drainage and p. (PD&P)
p. and postural drainage (P&PD)
slapping p.
p. sound
strip p.
tangential p.
threshold p.
p. wave
percussor
    G5 Neocussor p.
    Vibracare p.
PercuSurge GuardWire
percutaneous
    p. access kit (PAK)
    p. alcohol septal reduction
    p. aortic balloon valvuloplasty (PABV)
    p. aortic valvuloplasty (PAV)
    p. approach
    p. balloon angioplasty
    p. balloon aortic valvuloplasty
    p. balloon mitral valvuloplasty
    p. balloon pericardiotomy (PBP)
    p. balloon pulmonary valvuloplasty (PBPV)
    p. balloon pulmonic valvuloplasty
    p. balloon valvuloplasty (PBV)
    p. brachial sheath
    p. cannulated screw
    p. cardiopulmonary bypass (PCPB)
    p. cardiopulmonary bypass support (PCBS)
    p. cardiopulmonary support (PCPS)
    p. catheter insertion
    p. catheter introducer kit
    p. coronary intervention (PCI)
    p. coronary rotational atherectomy (PCRA)
    p. cutting needle
    p. dilatational tracheostomy (PDT)
    p. dilational tracheostomy (PDT)
    p. endoscopic jejunostomy (PEJ)
    p. excimer laser coronary angioplasty (PELCA)
    p. extrapleural analgesia
    p. femoral
    p. intraaortic balloon counterpulsation (PIBC)

NOTES

P

percutaneous *(continued)*
    p. intraaortic balloon counterpulsation catheter
    p. intracoronary angioscopy
    p. intrapericardial fibrin-glue infusion therapy
    p. laser angioplasty
    p. left heart bypass (PLHB)
    p. mechanical mitral commissurotomy
    p. mechanical thrombectomy (PMT)
    p. mechanical thrombectomy system
    p. mitral annular reduction
    p. mitral balloon commissurotomy (PMBC)
    p. mitral balloon valvotomy (PMBV)
    p. mitral balloon valvuloplasty (PMBV)
    p. mitral commissurotomy (PMC)
    p. mitral valvotomy (PMV)
    p. mitral valvuloplasty (PMV)
    p. myocardial channeling (PMC)
    p. myocardial laser revascularization
    p. myocardial revascularization (PMR)
    p. myocardial revascularization procedure
    p. needle aspiration biopsy
    p. occlusion of ductus
    p. patent ductus arteriosus closure
    p. pericardiocentesis
    p. radiofrequency catheter
    p. radiofrequency catheter ablation
    p. rotational thrombectomy (PRT)
    p. rotational thrombectomy catheter
    p. technique
    p. thrombolytic device (PTD)
    p. tracheotomy
    p. transatrial mitral commissurotomy
    p. transhepatic cardiac catheterization
    p. transluminal
    p. transluminal angioplasty (PTA)
    p. transluminal angioscopy (PTAS)
    p. transluminal balloon angioplasty (PTBA)
    p. transluminal balloon dilatation (PTBD)
    p. transluminal balloon valvuloplasty
    p. transluminal coronary
    p. transluminal coronary angioplasty (PTCA)
    p. transluminal coronary recanalization (PTCR)
    p. transluminal coronary revascularization (PTCR)
    p. transluminal coronary rotational ablation (PTCRA)
    p. transluminal dilatation (PTD)
    p. transluminal myocardial revascularization (PTMR)
    p. transluminal renal angioplasty (PTRA)
    p. transluminal rotational atherectomy (PTRA)
    p. transluminal septal myocardial ablation (PTSMA)
    p. transmyocardial laser revascularization (PMR)
    p. transmyocardial revascularization (PTMR)
    p. transthoracic needle biopsy (PTNB)
    p. transtracheal bronchography
    p. transtracheal jet ventilation (PTJV)
    p. transtracheal needle ventilation
    p. transvenous mitral commissurotomy (PTMC)
    p. tunnel
    p. ventricular assist device

percutaneously introduced

PerDUCER percutaneous pericardial access device

peregrinum
    Mycobacterium p.

perennial allergic rhinitis

Perez sign

Per-fit percutaneous tracheostomy kit

perflenapent injectable emulsion

perflexane lipid microsphere

perflubron

perfluorocarbon (PFC)

perfluorocarbon-associated gas exchange (PAGE)

perfluorocarbon-exposed sonicated dextrose albumin (PESDA)

perflutren
    Definity p.
    p. lipid microspheres

perforating
    p. artery
    p. artery infarct (PAI)

perforation
    cardiac p.
    esophageal p.
    guidewire p.
    myocardial p.
    septal p.
    ventricular p.

perforator
    gaiter p.
    septal p.

Performa diagnostic catheter

performance
    cardiac p. (CP)
    p. index (PI)
    left ventricular systolic p.
    Tei index of myocardial p.
    ventricular p.

perfringens
    Clostridium p.

PerfTrak
    P. display
    P. perfusion waveform display

perfuse

perfusion
    autologous blood selective aortic
      arch p. (AB-SAAP)
    p. balloon catheter (PBC)
    p. balloon PTCA
    p. bed
    blood p.
    bradykinin p.
    cardiac p.
    p. catheter
    cerebral p.
    cool head-warm body p.
    p. defect
    p. imaging MRI
    isolated heat p.
    lung p. (LP, Lp)
    misery p.
    mosaic p.
    myocardial p.
    p. pressure
    pulsed diastolic autologous blood
      selective aortic arch p. (PD-AB-
      SAAP)
    regional p.
    remote access p. (RAP)
    root p.
    p. scan
    p. scintigraphy
    selective aortic arch p. (SAAP)
    splanchnic bed p.
    stuttering of p.
    transcardiac vein p.
    p. via collateral

perfusion-assisted direct coronary artery
bypass (PADCAB)

perfusion-weighted
    p.-w. imaging
    p.-w. MRI (PWI)

Periactin

periaortic
    p. abscess
    p. hematoma

periapical

periarteriolar fibrosis

periarteritis nodosa

peribronchial
    p. cuffing
    p. desquamation
    p. fibrosis
    p. pneumonia
    p. sheath

peribronchiolar
    p. airspace consolidation
    p. granulomatous inflammation
    p. inflammatory infiltrate
    p. layer
    p. metaplasia
    p. nodule

peribronchiolitis

peribronchitis

peribronchovascular
    p. disease
    p. distortion
    p. hemorrhage
    p. thickening

pericarbon
    p. bioprosthesis
    p. pericardial prosthesis

pericardectomy

pericardia (*pl. of* pericardium)

pericardiaca
    pleura p.

pericardiacophrenica
    arteria p.

pericardiac tumor

pericardial
    p. baffle
    p. basket
    p. biopsy
    p. calcification
    p. constraint
    p. cyst
    p. disease
    p. echo
    p. effusion (PE)
    p. fat pad
    p. flap
    p. fluid (PF)
    p. fluid culture (PFC)
    p. fremitus
    p. friction rub

NOTES

P

521

pericardial *(continued)*
    p. friction sound
    p. knock (PK)
    p. lavage
    p. murmur
    p. paracentesis
    p. patch
    p. peel
    p. poudrage
    p. pressure
    p. reflex
    p. sac
    p. sling
    p. symphysis
    p. synechia
    p. tamponade (PT)
    p. tap
    p. teratoma
    p. well
    p. window
pericardicentesis *(var. of*
  pericardiocentesis)
pericardiectomy
    parietal p.
    visceral p.
pericardii
    concretio p.
    hydrops p.
    synechia p.
pericardiocentesis, pericardicentesis
    echo-guided p.
    percutaneous p.
pericardiology
pericardiophrenic artery
pericardiorrhaphy
pericardioscopy
pericardiosternal ligament
pericardiostomy
pericardiotomy
    percutaneous balloon p. (PBP)
    p. scissors
    subxiphoid limited p.
pericarditic
pericarditis
    acute fibrinous p.
    acute idiopathic p. (AIP)
    acute lupus p. (ALP)
    adhesive p.
    amebic p.
    bacterial p.
    calcific p.
    p. calculosa
    p. callosa
    carcinomatous p.
    cholesterol p.
    chronic constrictive p.
    constrictive p. (CP)
    drug-associated p.
    drug-induced p.

    dry p.
    effusive-constrictive p.
    epistenocardiac p.
    p. epistenocardica
    fibrinous p.
    fibrous p.
    gram-negative p.
    hemorrhagic p.
    histoplasmic p.
    idiopathic p.
    infective p.
    inflammatory p.
    internal adhesive p.
    ischemic p.
    localized p.
    meningococcal p.
    neoplastic p.
    p. obliterans
    obliterating p.
    obliterative p.
    occult p.
    postinfarction p.
    postmyocardial injury p.
    postoperative p.
    postoperative constrictive p. (PCP)
    purulent p. (PP)
    radiation-induced p.
    rheumatic p.
    serofibrinous p.
    serous p.
    p. sicca
    Sternberg p.
    subacute p.
    suppurative p.
    transient p.
    traumatic p.
    tuberculous p.
    uremic p.
    p. villosa
    viral p.
    p. with effusion
pericarditis, arthropathy, camptodactyly
  (PAC)
pericarditis-myocarditis syndrome
pericardium, gen. **pericardii**,
  pl. **pericardia**
    absent p.
    adherent p.
    bread-and-butter p.
    calcified p.
    congenital absence of left p.
      (CALP)
    congenitally absent p.
    diaphragmatic p.
    dropsy of p.
    empyema of p.
    p. externum
    p. fibrosum
    fibrous p.

p. internum
parietal p. (PP)
p. serosum
shaggy p.
thickened p.
ventricular p. (VP)
visceral p.
pericentriolar
periciliary fluid
perielectrode fibrosis
periesophageal
Periflow balloon dilation catheter
Periflux PF 1 D blood-flowmeter
perigraft
p. flow
p. thrombosis
perihilar
p. adenopathy
p. haze
p. lymph node
p. marking
periinfarction
p. block
p. conduction defect (PICD)
p. zone
perilymphatic
p. distribution
p. nodule
**perimembranous ventricular septal
defect**
Perimount RSR pericardial bioprosthesis
perimuscular plexus
perimyocarditis
perimyocytic fibrosis
perimyoendocarditis
perindoprilat
perindopril erbumine
perineal artery
perinodal tissue
perinuclear
p. antineutrophil cytoplasmic
antibody (pANCA)
p. cisterna
period
absolute refractory p. (ARP)
accessory pathway effective
refractory p. (APERP)
p. of accommodation
alveolar p.
antegrade refractory p.
atrial effective refractory p.
(AERP)

atrial refractory p.
atrioventricular node functional
refractory p. (AVNFRP)
atrioventricular refractory p.
(AVRP)
blanking p.
canalicular p.
corrected pre-ejection p. (PEPc)
diastolic filling p. (DFP)
effective conduction p. (ECP)
effective refractory p. (ERP)
ejection p.
functional conduction p. (FCP)
functional refractory p. (FRP)
heartbeat p. (HBP)
intersystolic p.
isoelectric p.
isometric p. of cardiac cycle
isometric contraction p.
isometric relaxation p.
isovolumetric relaxation p. (IVRP)
isovolumic relaxation p.
no-sigh p.
pacemaker amplifier refractory p.
postinfarction p.
postsphygmic p.
postventricular atrial refractory p.
(PVARP)
preejection p. (PEP)
presphygmic p.
pulse p.
pulse repetition p. (PRP)
refractory p.
relative refractory p. (RRP)
right ventricular pre-ejection p.
(RVPEP)
right ventricular refractory p.
(RVERP)
saccular p.
sigh p.
systolic ejection p. (SEP)
TAB p.
total atrial blanking p.
total atrial refractory p. (TARP)
ventricular effective refractory p.
(VERP)
p. of ventricular filling
ventriculoatrial effective
refractory p.
vulnerable p.
washout p.
Wenckebach p.

NOTES

P

periodic
  p. breathing
  p. edema
  p. leg movement (PLM)
  p. limb movement disorder (PLMD)
  p. paralysis
  p. polyserositis
  p. respiration
  p. short pulse (PSP)
periodicity
  A-V node Wenckebach p.
  circadian p.
  Wenckebach p.
perioperative
  p. antibiotic
  p. myocardial infarction (PMI)
periorbital edema
periosteotome
  Alexander-Farabeuf p.
periosteum
peripartal
  p. cardiomyopathy
  p. heart disease
  p. heart failure
peripartum
  p. cardiac failure (PPCF)
  p. cardiomyopathy
  p. myocarditis
peripharyngeal space
peripharyngeum
peripheral
  p. access system (PAS)
  p. airspace
  p. AngioJet system
  p. arterial disease (PAD)
  p. arterial occlusive disease (PAOD)
  p. arteriosclerosis
  p. arteriosclerotic occlusive disease (PAOD)
  p. artery
  p. artery bypass
  p. artery tonometry
  p. atherectomy system
  p. atherosclerotic disease
  p. blood eosinophilia
  p. blood flow (PBF)
  p. blood mononuclear cell (PBMC)
  p. blood smear
  p. chemoreceptor
  p. circulation
  p. conduction disease
  p. coronary pressure (PCP)
  p. cyanosis
  p. edema
  p. excimer laser angioplasty (PELA)
  p. interstitial disease

  p. interstitium
  p. laser angioplasty (PLA)
  p. muscle strength
  p. neuropathy
  p. paracicatricial emphysema
  p. pulmonary artery stenosis (PPAS)
  p. pulmonic stenosis
  p. pulse present
  p. pulses palpable both legs (PPPBL)
  p. resistance
  p. resistance unit (PRU)
  p. stigmata
  p. vascular disease (PVD)
  p. vascular resistance (PVR)
  p. vasoconstriction
  p. vasodilation
  p. vasodilator effect
  p. venous pressure (PVP)
  p. zone radioaerosol clearance
peripherally inserted catheter (PIC)
peripneumonia notha
periprosthetic
  p. mitral regurgitation
  p. valve abscess
  p. valve aortic insufficiency
peripylephlebitis
peristalsis
  high-altitude p. (HAP)
peristaltic wave (PW)
peristasis
peristatic hyperemia
Peri-Strips
perisystole
perisystolic
perithelium
  Eberth p.
peritoneal
  continuous cyclic p.
  p. dialysis
peritracheal
Peritrate SA
peritubular capillary (PTC)
perivalvular
  p. leak
  p. leakage (PVL)
perivascular
  p. canal
  p. edema
  p. eosinophilic infiltrate
  p. fibrosis
  p. infiltration (PVI)
  p. lymphocytic infiltrate
  p. rupture
  p. sheath
  p. spaces
periventricular hyperintensity (PVH, PVHI)

Perles
> Tessalon P.

Perma-Flow coronary bypass graft

PermaNeb reusable nebulizer

permanent
> p. atrial tachycardia
> p. cardiac pacing lead
> p. junctional reciprocating
> tachycardia (PJRT)
> p. pacemaker (PPM)
> p. pacemaker placement
> p. pacing

Permapen injection

permeability
> airway p.
> alveolar p. (AP)
> endothelial p.
> microvascular p.

permissive hypercapnia (PHC)

pernio
> lupus p.

peroneal
> p. artery
> p. muscular atrophy

peroxidase
> avidin-biotin p.

peroxide
> dicymyl p.
> hydrogen p.
> lipid p.

peroxisome
> p. proliferator-activated receptor
> (PPAR)
> p. proliferator-activated receptor
> gamma (PPAR-gamma)
> p. proliferator response element
> (PPRE)

peroxyacetyl nitrate

peroxyl radical-trapping potential

peroxynitrite

perpetual arrhythmia

perpetuus
> pulsus irregularis p.

Per-Q-Cath percutaneously inserted central venous catheter

Persantine-isonitrile stress test

Persantine thallium stress test

persistence
> microbubble p.

persistent
> p. atrial standstill (PAS)
> p. common atrioventricular canal

> p. ductus arteriosus
> p. fetal circulation (PFC)
> p. ostium primum
> p. pulmonary hypertension of
> newborn (PPHN)
> p. shunt
> p. truncus arteriosus (PTA)

personal
> P. Best peak flowmeter
> p. heart device (PHD)

personalized aerobics for cardiovascular enhancement

Perspex block

persulfate salt

pertechnetate sodium

Perthes
> P. syndrome
> P. test

perturbation
> autonomic p.

perturbed
> p. autonomic nervous system
> function
> p. carotid baroreceptor

Pertussin CS, ES

pertussis
> *Bordetella p.*
> *Haemophilus p.*
> p. toxin

peruana
> verruga p.

pervenous
> p. catheter
> p. pacemaker

PES
> papillary fibroelastoma
> postextrasystolic
> preexcitation syndrome
> programmed electrical stimulation

PESDA
> perfluorocarbon-exposed sonicated
> dextrose albumin

PESP
> postextrasystolic potentiation

pestis
> *Yersinia p.*

PET
> peak ejection time
> polyethylene terephthalate
> poor exercise tolerance
> positron emission tomography
> progressive exercise test

NOTES

P

PET (*continued*)
    PET balloon atherectomy device
    PET scan
    PET scanning
    PET with C-11 acetate
petal
    nitinol p.
petal-fugal flow
PETCO$_2$
    partial pressure of end-tidal CO_2
petechia, pl. **petechiae**
petechial hemorrhage
Peterson elastic modulus
pethidine
Petit sinus
PETN
    pentaerythritol tetranitrate
Petriellidium boydii
petrified cardiac myxoma
Petrillium
petrosal ganglion
pexelizumab
Peyer patch
Peyrot thorax
PF
    peak flow
    pericardial fluid
    pulmonary function
PFA
    arteria femoris profunda
PFC
    perfluorocarbon
    pericardial fluid culture
    persistent fetal circulation
PFF
    polymer fume fever
PFM
    peak flowmeter
      TruZone PFM
PFO
    patent foramen ovale
PFO-Star occluder
PFR
    peak filling rate
PFS
    Adriamycin PFS
    Idamycin PFS
    Vincasar PFS
PFSDQ
    Pulmonary Functional Status and
    Dyspnea Questionnaire
PFSS
    pulmonary functional status scale
PFT
    pulmonary function test
PG
    post graft

PGCMS
    Philadelphia Geriatric Center Morale
    Scale
PGF
    primary graft failure
PGI$_2$
    prostacyclin
P-glycoprotein
Pg-Ppl
    gastric-intrapleural pressure
PGVS
    postganglionic vagal stimulation
PH
    parenchymal hematoma
    parenchymal hemorrhage
    pulmonary hypertension
P-H
    Purkinje-HIS
      P-H conduction time
      P-H interval
pH
    hydrogen ion concentration
    intramucosal pH
    pH Meter
    scalp pH
phacoma
phage
    luciferase reporter p.
phagocyte
phagocytic
    p. function
    p. pneumonocyte
phagocytose
phagocytosis
phalangis
    corpus p.
phalanx
    body of p.
Phalen stress test
Phanatuss Cough Syrup
phantom
    p. aneurysm
    p. flow artifact
    P. guidewire
    P. nasal mask
    P. nasal mask CPAP
    p. pacemaker
    p. pain
    p. sponge
    p. tumor
    p. V Plus catheter
pharmacodynamics
pharmacoeconomics
pharmacokinetics
pharmacologic
    p. environment
    p. plaque passivation
    p. stress

p. stress echocardiography
p. stress perfusion imaging
pharmacological
p. cardioversion
p. intervention in atrial fibrillation (PIAF)
pharmacology
in vitro p.
Pharmacopeia
United States P. (USP)
pharmacotherapy
pharmomechanical thrombolysis
pharyngalgia
pharyngea
arteria p.
pharyngeae
venae p.
pharyngeal
p. arch
p. branch
p. branch of descending palatine artery
p. branch of glossopharyngeal nerve
p. branch of inferior thyroid artery
p. branch of pterygopalatine ganglion
p. branch of vagus nerve
p. canal
p. collapsibility
p. crisis
p. gland
p. lymphatic ring
p. nervous plexus
p. pouch
p. pouch syndrome
p. raphe
p. reflex
p. ridge
p. space
p. tonsil
p. tracheal lumen (PTL)
p. vein
pharyngeales
glandulae p.
pharyngealis
tonsilla p.
pharynges (*pl. of* pharynx)
pharyngeus
plexus nervosus p.
recessus p.
pharyngis (*gen. of* pharynx)
cavitas p.

cavum p.
globus p.
pars nasalis p.
pars oralis p.
raphe p.
tunica mucosa p.
tunica muscularis p.
pharyngitis
acute p.
arcanobacterial p.
atrophic p.
catarrhal p.
chronic p.
croupous p.
diphtheric p.
diphtheritic p.
follicular p.
gangrenous p.
glandular p.
granular p.
herpangina p.
membranous p.
phlegmonous p.
plague p.
p. sicca
p. ulcerosa
pharyngobranchial duct
pharyngoconjunctival fever
pharyngoepiglottic
pharyngoesophageal
p. cushions
p. pads
p. sphincter
pharyngoglossal
pharyngoglossus
pharyngolaryngeal
pharyngomaxillary space
pharyngometer
Eccovision acoustic p.
pharyngonasal cavity
pharyngooral
pharyngopalatine
pharyngopalatinus
pharyngoparalysis
pharyngoplasty
Hynes p.
pharyngoscopy
pharyngospasm
pharyngostaphylinus
pharyngotracheal lumen airway (PTL, PTLA)

NOTES

P

527

pharyngotympanic groove
pharynx, gen. **pharyngis,** pl. **pharynges**
  constrictor muscle of p.
  inferior constrictor muscle of p.
  lacuna pharyngis
  laryngeal part of p.
  middle constrictor muscle of p.
  nasal part of p.
  oral part of p.
  raphe of p.
phase
  p. angle
  convalescent p.
  ejection p.
  fibrinopurulent p.
  harmonic p. (HARP)
  p. heterophony
  p. image
  p. image analysis
  p. imaging
  Korotkoff p. I–V
  midexpiratory p.
  plateau p.
  supernormal recovery p.
  terminal p.
  upstroke p.
  venous p.
  vulnerable p.
  washout p.
phased
  p. array receiver coil
  p. array sector scanner
  p. array sector transducer
  p. array system
  p. array technology
  p. array ultrasonographic device
phase-encoded velocity image
phasic
  p. excursion
  p. intragraft flow velocity
  p. sinus arrhythmia
PHAVER
  pterygia, heart defects, autosomal
    recessive inheritance, vertebral defects,
    ear anomalies, radial defect
  pterygia, heart defects, autosomal
    recessive inheritance, vertebral defects,
    ear anomalies, radial defects
    PHAVER syndrome
PHC
  permissive hypercapnia
PHD
  personal heart device
  postheparin plasma diamine oxidase
Phemister elevator
phenacetin,
  p. aspirin, and caffeine (PAC)
  p. aspirin, and desoxyephedrine
  (PAD)

phenazopyridine
  sulfisoxazole and p.
Phenergan
  P. injection
  P. With Codeine
Phenetron Oral
Phenhist Expectorant
phenindamine tartrate
phenindione sensitivity
phenobarbital
  theophylline, ephedrine, and p.
phenolformaldehyde
phenomenon, pl. **phenomena**
  AFORMED p.
  Anrep p.
  Aschner p.
  Ashley p.
  Ashman p.
  Austin Flint p.
  blush p.
  Bowditch p.
  cascade p.
  coronary steal p.
  diaphragm p.
  diaphragmatic p.
  dip p.
  Duckworth p.
  Ehret p.
  embolic p.
  Gallavardin p.
  gap conduction p.
  Gärtner vein p.
  Goldblatt p.
  Gregg p.
  Hering p.
  Hill p.
  Katz-Wachtel p.
  Kienbock p.
  Koch p.
  Litten p.
  low-reflow p.
  malperfusion p.
  no-reflow p.
  overshoot p.
  pendelluft p.
  preconditioning p.
  Raynaud p.
  recoil p.
  reentry p.
  R-on-T p.
  Schellong-Strisower p.
  Splendore-Hoeppli p.
  staircase p.
  steal p.
  treppe p.
  Venturi p.
  warm-up p.
  washout p.
  Wenckebach p.

Williams p.
Woodworth p.
zone 1 p.
phenothiazine
phenotype
high-risk p.
large cell carcinoma with
rhabdoid p.
metastatic p.
Pi MM, MZ, SS, SZ, ZZ p.
proteinase inhibitor p. (Pi)
phenoxybenzamine hydrochloride
phenoxymethyl
penicillin p.
phenprocoumon
phentermine
fenfluramine and p. (Fen-Phen)
phentolamine
p. hydrochloride
p. mesylate
p. methanesulfonate
phenyl
p. aminosalicylate
p. salicylate
phenylalanine
formyl methionyl leucyl p. (FMLP)
phenylalkylamine
phenylbutazone sensitivity
phenylephrine
guaifenesin, phenylpropanolamine,
and p.
p. hydrochloride
isoproterenol and p.
p. ramp method
phenylpropanolamine
caramiphen and p.
guaifenesin and p.
p. hydrochloride
hydrocodone and p.
p. toxicity
phenytoin
pheochromocytoma
PHI
pontine hyperintensity
Phialophora verrucosa
Philadelphia
P. Association of Clinical Trials
(PACT)
P. Geriatric Center Morale Scale
(PGCMS)
Philip gland

Philips
P. ACS NT 1.5 Gyroscan MRI
P. Integris 3000 biplane digital
subtraction angiography device
P. Medical Systems Tomoscan
AVE1 CT spiral scanner
P. Medical Systems Tomoscan SR
7000 CT spiral scanner
P. Tomoscan 310 CT scanner
Philos DR-T pacemaker
PHLA
postheparin lipolytic activity
phlebarteriectasia
phlebectomy
transilluminated powered p. (TIPP)
phlebemphraxis
phlebitis
adhesive p.
blue p.
chlorotic p.
descending p.
gouty p.
malignancy-associated p.
migrating p.
p. nodularis necrotisans
p. obliterans
obliterating p.
plastic p.
puerperal p.
sclerosing p.
superficial p.
phlebodynamics
phlebogenous
phlebogram
phlebograph
phlebography
phlebolithiasis
phlebomanometer
phleborrheogram
Cranley-Grass p.
phlebostasis
phlebotomize
phlebotomy
bloodless p.
phlegm
phlegmasia
p. alba dolens
p. cerulea dolens
phlegmonosa
angina p.

NOTES

P

phlegmonous
    p. laryngitis
    p. pharyngitis
phlei
    Mycobacterium p.
phonarteriogram
phonarteriography
Phonate speaking valve
phonoangiography
    carotid p.
phonocardiogram (PCG)
phonocardiograph
    linear p.
    logarithmic p.
    spectral p.
    stethoscopic p.
phonocardiographic transducer
phonocardiography
    spectral p. (SPCG)
phonocatheter
phonoscope
phonoscopy
phosducin
phosgene
phosphatase
    acid p.
    alkaline p. (AP)
    alkaline phosphatase antialkaline p.
    (APAAP)
phosphate
    Aralen P.
    azapetine p.
    p.-buffered saline (PBS)
    chloroquine p.
    Cleocin P.
    codeine p.
    Decadron P.
    dexamethasone sodium p. (DSP)
    disopyramide p.
    etoposide p.
    Hexadrol P.
    histamine acid p.
    hydrocortisone sodium p.
    Hydrocortone P.
    Linctus With Codeine p.
    myocardial creatine p.
    nicotinamide adenine dinucleotide p.
    (NADPH)
    oseltamivir p.
    Paveral Stanley Syrup With
    Codeine P.
    polyribosylribitol p. (PRP)
    primaquine p.
    sodium p.
    triciribine p. (TCN-P)
phosphatidylcholine (PtdCho)
    dipalmitoyl p. (DPPC)
phosphatidylinositol
phosphatidylserine

phosphine
phosphinic acid
phosphocreatine (PCr)
phosphodiesterase
    p. enzyme
    p. III inhibition (PDE3I)
    p. inhibitor (PDE, PDE-I)
    p. isoenzyme inhibitor
    sphingomyelin p.
phosphofructokinase
phosphoinositide
phosphoinositol
phosphokinase
    creatine p. (CPK)
phospholamban
phospholipase
    postheparin p. (PHP)
phospholipid
    surfactant p.
phospholipidosis
    alveolar p.
phosphomonoesterase
phosphorus
    organic p.
    p. tribromide
phosphorus-31 magnetic resonance spectroscopy (^{31}P-MRS)
phosphorylase
    glycogen p.
    p. kinase
    thymidine p.
phosphorylation
    mitochondrial oxidative p.
    oxidative p.
phosphorylcholine
Phospho-Soda
    Fleet P.-S.
photoablation
photoaffinity
photoangioplasty
photobiological response
photochemical air pollution
photocoagulation
PhotoDerm VL device
photodiode
photodisruption
photodynamic therapy (PTD)
Photofrin
PhotoGenica V-Star laser
photohemotachometer
photo-mask and etch-on-a-tube (PMEOAT)
photometer
    HemoCue p.
photometry
    emission flame p.
photomicrography
photomultiplier

photon
    annihilation p.
    P. DR dual-chamber ICD
    P. Micro DR/VR implantable
    cardioverter defibrillator
photopeak
photoplethysmography (PPG)
photoprotection
photoreactivation
photoresection
photosensitizing reaction
photostethoscope
PHP
    postheparin phospholipase
PHR
    peak heart rate
phren
phrenic
    p. artery
    p. nerve
    p. nerve crush injury
    p. nerve paralysis
    p. pleura
phrenica
    pleura p.
phrenicocolic
phrenicocolicum
    ligamentum p.
phrenicocostal sinus
phrenicogastric
phrenicoglottic
phrenicohepatic
phrenicosplenic
phrenocardia
phrenocolic
phrenogastric
phrenohepatic
PHRT
    Public Health Response Team
    PHRT protocol
PHT
    portal hypertension
    pressure half-time
    pulmonary hypertension
**phthalic anhydride irritant-induced
    asthma**
phthinoid
    p. bronchitis
    p. chest
phthisis
    aneurysmal p.
    bacillary p.

    black p.
    collier's p.
    diabetic p.
    fibroid p.
    grinder's p.
    miner's p.
    potter's p.
    pulmonary p.
    stone cutter's p.
phycomycosis
Phylax
    P. AV dual-chamber implantable
    cardioverter-defibrillator
    P. 06 implantable cardioverter-
    defibrillator
phylaxis
phyllosilicate
physical
    P. Activity Scale for the Elderly
    Evaluation (PASE)
    p. inactivity
    p. stimulus
    p. therapy
    P. Work Capacity exercise stress
    test
physicians
    American College of Chest P.
    (ACCP)
physiochemical
**Physio-Control Lifestat
    sphygmomanometer**
physiologic
    p. congestion
    p. dead space
    p. dead space fraction
    p. dead space ventilation (V_D/V_T)
    p. measurement
    p. monitoring
    p. murmur
    p. pacemaker
    p. pattern release (PPR)
    p. shunt fraction
    p. third heart sound
physiological
    p. dead space ventilation per
    minute (V_D)
    p. monitoring
    p. overreactivity
    p. split of S_2
    p. stress
physiologically split S_2 sound

NOTES

P

physiology
    constrictive p.
    Damus-Kaye-Stansel procedure for single ventricle p.
    Eisenmenger p.
    single-ventricle p.

Physios
    P. CTM 01 cardiac transplant monitor
    P. CTM 01 noninvasive cardiac transplant monitoring system
    P. CTM 01 noninvasive telemonitor

physiotherapy
    chest p. (CPT)
    movement science p.

phytanic acid accumulation
Phytis stent
phytoestrogen
    soy p.

phytohemagglutinin
phytonadione
phytopneumoconiosis
PI
    pacing impulse
    performance index
    pontine infarct
    primary infarction
    protease inhibitor
    pulmonary infarction
    pulsatility index
        alpha-1 PI
        PI MRI technique

Pi
    proteinase inhibitor phenotype
        Pi MM, MZ, SS, SZ, ZZ phenotype

PIA
    preinfarction angina

PIAF
    pharmacological intervention in atrial fibrillation
    prognosis in atrial fibrillation

pial collateralization
piano percussion
piaulement
    bruit de p.

PIBC
    percutaneous intraaortic balloon counterpulsation
        PIBC catheter

PIC
    pacing in cardiomyopathy
    peripherally inserted catheter

PICA
    posterior inferior cerebellar artery
    posterior inferior communicating artery

Piccolino
    P. balloon
    P. Monorail catheter

PICD
    periinfarction conduction defect

PICH
    primary intracerebral hemorrhage

Pick
    P. and Go monitor
    P. syndrome

Picker
    P. CS scanner
    P. Dyna Mo collimator
    P. Edge 1.5-T scanner
    P. Magnascanner
    P. PQ 2000 CT scanner
    P. Vista HPQ MRI scanner
    P. Vistar image analysis system
    P. Voxel image analysis system

pickwickian syndrome
Picornaviridae virus
Picovir
picrosirius red stain
PICSO
    pressure-controlled intermittent coronary sinus occlusion

picture
    anodal opening p. (AOP)

PID
    preimplantation diagnosis

PIE
    prosthetic infectious endocarditis
    pulmonary infiltrate with eosinophilia
    pulmonary infiltration with eosinophilia
    pulmonary interstitial emphysema
        PIE syndrome

piechaudii
    Alcaligenes p.

Pie Medical CAAS II analysis system
Pierce-Donachy Thoratec ventricular assist device
Pierre Robin syndrome
piesimeter
    Hales p.

piesis
piezo
    p. electric snore sensor
    p. PLM sensor

piezoelectric
    p. crystal
    p. crystal-based pacemaker
    p. ultrasound transducer

PIF
    peak inspiratory flow

PIFR
    peak inspiratory flow rate

pigeon
    p. breeder's lung

p. chest
p. fancier's lung
pigeon-breast deformity
pigeon-breeder's disease
piggyback
pigment induration of lung
pigskin
pigtail rotation catheter
PIH
pregnancy-induced hypertension
PIIIP
procollagen type III aminoterminal
peptide
PI3-kinase
pilin
22-KDa p. antiadhesion
pill
birth control p.
pillar
tonsillar p.
Pilling
P. bronchoscope
P. Weck Y-stent forceps
pillow-shaped balloon
pilocarpine iontophoresis test
pilot needle
PILP
postinfarction late potential
pilsicainide
Pima
PIMI
predictive index for myocardial infarction
psychophysiological interventions in
myocardial ischemia
pimobendan
PIMS
programmable implantable medication
system
pinacidil
pinchcock mechanism
pincushion distortion
pindolol
pineal pellucidum
pine resin
pinhole
p. balloon rupture
p. VSD
pink
p. sputum
p. tetralogy of Fallot
pinked up
Pinkerton .018 balloon catheter

pink Fallot of tetralogy
Pinnacle
P. introducer sheath
P. pacemaker
pinocytosis
pinocytotic
pinosome
Pins
P. sign
P. syndrome
pioglitazone
PIP
peak inspiratory pressure
plasma cell interstitial pneumonitis
positive inspiratory pressure
pipecuronium bromide
piperacillin and tazobactam sodium
piperazine citrate
pipobroman
Pipracil
pirbuterol
p. acetate
p. acetate inhalation aerosol
pirenzepine
piretanide
pirfenidone
piriform, pyriform
p. sinus
p. thorax
piritrexim isethionate
pirmenol
pirodavir
Pirogoff angle
pirolazamide
piroximone
Pirquet reaction
PIRS
postinfarction risk stratification
PIS
preinfarction syndrome
PISA
proximal isovelocity surface area
Pisces lead
pistol
p. shot femoral sound
p. shot of Traube
piston pulse
PIT
pacing-induced tachycardia
pit
inferior costal p.
Pitie-Salpetriere saphenous vein hook

NOTES

P

Pitressin injection
pitting edema
Pittman IMA retractor system
Pittsburgh
>P. pneumonia
>P. pneumonia agent

pivampicillin
pivot point
pivoxil
>cefditoren p.

pixel
pizza lung
Pizzolatto stain
PJC
>premature junctional contraction

P-J interval
PJRT
>permanent junctional reciprocating
> tachycardia

PJT
>paroxysmal junctional tachycardia

PK
>pericardial knock

PKA
>protein kinase A

PKase
>protein kinase

PKC
>protein kinase C

P13 kinase
PLA
>peripheral laser angioplasty

PLa
>left atrial pressure

PlA
>platelet antigen

Pla
>left atrial pressure

placebo
placement
>carotid angioplasty and stent p.
>catheter-directed thrombolysis and
> endovascular stent p.
>intracoronary stent p.
>lead p.
>permanent pacemaker p.
>prophylactic filter p.
>stent p.
>temporary pacemaker p.
>Thoracoport p.

placental
>p. barrier
>p. circulation
>p. respiration

plague
>bubonic p.
>p. pharyngitis

>p. pneumonia
>pneumonic p.

plain old balloon angioplasty (POBA)
PLA-I platelet antigen
plakoglobin
planar
>p. myocardial imaging
>p. myocardial scintigraphy
>p. thallium imaging
>p. thallium scintigraphy
>p. thallium test
>p. xanthoma

plane
>Addison p.
>apical four-chamber p. (Ap4CH)
>axial p.
>circular p.
>coronal p.
>cove p.
>midsagittal p.
>orthogonal p.
>parasagittal p.
>sagittal p.
>short-axis p.
>sternal p.
>sternoxiphoid p.
>transaxial p.

planigraphy
planimeter
planimetry
>p. method
>TapeMeasure computerized p.
>p. volume

planithorax
plant
>p. sterol
>p. toxicity

plantar ischemia test
plaque
>p. area
>atheromatous p.
>atherosclerotic p. (AP)
>p. burden
>calcified p.
>carcinoid p.
>carotid p.
>complex p.
>disrupted p.
>p. disruption
>echogenic p.
>echolucent p.
>p. embolization
>equistenotic p.
>fibrofatty p.
>fibrous p.
>p. fissure
>p. fissuring
>p. fracture
>glistening yellow coronary p.

heterogeneous p.
Hollenhorst p.
homogeneous p.
intraluminal p.
lipid-laden p.
lipid-rich p.
p. lumen
p. marker
p. motion
myointimal p.
p. neovascularity
nonostial p.
p. passivation
pleural p.
p. prolapse
protuberant p.
p. rupture
senile p.
shelf of p.
p. shift
p. stabilization
p. stabilization therapy
p. strutting
submucosal p.
thoracic aortic atherosclerotic p.
ulcerated p.
unstable p.
p. volume
p. vulnerability
vulnerable p.
white p.
yellow p.
plaque-cracker
LeVeen p.-c.
Plaquenil
plaquing
plasma
p. alpha-1 antitrypsin (pAAT)
p. arginine vasopressin (pAVP)
p. beta-thromboglobulin
p. catecholamine
p. cell interstitial pneumonitis (PIP)
p. cell pneumonia
p. clot diffusion chamber (PCDC)
p. coagulation system
p. colloid osmotic pressure
p. endothelin
p. endothelin concentration
p. erythropoietin
p. exchange column
p. extravasation
p. fibrinogen

fresh frozen p. (FFP)
p. glycocalicin
p. homocysteine
p. homocysteine concentration
p. nicotine level
platelet-poor p. (PPP)
platelet-rich p. (PRP)
p. protein exudation
p. renin
p. renin activity (PRA)
p. retinol
p. skimming
p. thromboplastin antecedent (PTA)
p. thromboplastin component (PTC, PTH)
p. thromboplastin factor (PTF)
p. thyroxine level (PTL)
p. viscosity (PV)
p. volume
p. volume expander
zoster immune p. (ZIP)
plasmagel
plasmahaut
plasmakinin
plasmalemma
Plasma-Lyte A
Plasmanate
plasmapheresis
Plasma-Plex bottle
plasma-resistant fiber oxygenator (PRF)
plasmatic vascular destruction
plasmin
plasminemia
plasminogen
p. activator
p. activator inhibitor (PAI)
p. activator inhibitor-1 (PAI-1)
plasminogen-streptokinase complex
Plasmodium
P. embolism
P. falciparum
P. malariae
P. ovale
P. vivax
plastic
p. bronchitis
p. endocarditis
p. phlebitis
p. pleurisy
p. polymer
p. sewing ring
p. surgical osteosynthesis

NOTES

P

plasticity
    cortical p.
    skeletal muscle p.
plasty
    endoventricular circular patch p.
    sliding p.
plate
    polar p.
    Strasburger cell p.
    tantalum p.
    p. thrombosis
    p. thrombus
    trach p.
    tracheostomy p.
plateau
    h p.
    maximal response p. (MRP)
    p. phase
    p. pressure (Pplat)
    p. pulse
    p. response
    ventricular p.
platelet
    p. activating factor (PAF)
    p. activation
    p. activity
    p. aggregation
    p. aggregation inhibitor
    p. antibody
    p. antigen (PlA)
    p. consumption
    p. factor 4
    gel-filtered p. (GFP)
    p. glycoprotein IIb/IIIa blockade
    p. glycoprotein IIb/IIIa blocker
    p. glycoprotein IIb/IIIa inhibitor
    P. IIb/IIIa Antagonist for the Reduction of Acute Coronary Syndrome Events in a Global Organization Network
    p. IIb/IIIa inhibitor
    p. imaging
    p. membrane glycoprotein
    p. receptor glycoprotein
    p. thrombosis
    p. thrombus
platelet-aggregating factor
platelet-derived
    p.-d. growth factor (PDGF)
    p.-d. histamine-releasing factor (PDHRF)
plateletpheresis
platelet-poor plasma (PPP)
platelet-rich plasma (PRP)
platelets
    hemolysis, elevated liver enzymes, and low p. (HELLP)
platelike atelectasis

platform
    Complete stent delivery p.
    TomTec echo p.
Platinol-AQ
platinum
    p. coil
    salt of p.
    p. wire
platinum-iridium electrode
Platinum Plus guidewire
platypnea
platypnea-orthodeoxia syndrome
platysma
Plavix
PLCO
    postoperative low cardiac output
PLCx
    posterolateral circumflex branch
        PLCx coronary artery
PLE
    protein-losing enteropathy
pledget
    Meadox Teflon felt p.
    p.-supported
    Teflon p.
pledgeted mattress suture
PlegiaGuard pressure relief valve
pleiotropic cytokine
Plendil
plenus
    pulsus p.
pleomorphic
    p. premature ventricular complex
    p. tachycardia
Plesch
    P. percussion
    P. test
PLET
    polymyxin, lysome, EDTA, thallous acetate
Pletal
plethora
plethoric
plethysmograph
    body p.
    BPXG body p.
    MasterScreen BabyBody p.
    MedGraphics model 1085 body p.
    mercury-in-rubber strain gauge p.
    pressure p.
    pressure-compensated flow p.
    respiratory inductance p. (RIP)
    Respitrace p.
    volume-displacement p.
plethysmography
    cuff p.
    digital pulse p. (DPP)
    impedance p. (IPG)
    respiratory inductance p. (RIP)

serial impedance p.
servocontrolled p.
strain-gauge p.
thermistor p.
venous impedance p. (VIP)
venous occlusion p. (VOP)
pleura, pl. **pleurae**
adipose folds of p.
black p.
cavum pleurae
cervical p.
costal p.
p. costalis
costodiaphragmatic recess of p.
costomediastinal recess of p.
cupula of p.
cupula pleurae
diaphragmatic p.
p. diaphragmatica
discission of p.
fibrin bodies of p.
mediastinal p.
p. mediastinalis
parietal p.
p. parietalis
p. pericardiaca
phrenic p.
p. phrenica
p. pulmonalis
pulmonary p.
visceral p.
p. visceralis
pleuracentesis (*var. of* pleurocentesis)
(*See also* thoracentesis)
pleuracotomy
pleural
p. abrasion
p. adhesion
p. amyloidosis
p. aspergillosis
p. biopsy
p. bleb
p. calculus
p. cap
p. cavity
p. crackle
p. cupula
p. disease
p. effusion shunt
p. empyema
p. fibrin ball
p. fluid

p. fluid neutrophilia
p. fremitus
p. friction rub
p. lavage
p. line
p. mass
p. meniscus sign
p. mesothelioma
p. mouse
p. peel
p. plaque
p. poudrage
p. pressure (Ppl)
p. rale
p. reaction
p. recess
p. rings
p. sac
p. scarring
p. sclerosant
p. shock
p. sinus
p. sliding
p. space
p. space evacuation
p. space monitoring
p. suction
p. surface
p. tag
p. tap
p. tent
p. thickening
p. toilet
p. tube
p. villi
pleurales
recessus p.
villi p.
pleuralgia
pleuralis
cavitas p.
pleurectomy
thoracoscopic apical p.
thorascopic apical p.
Pleur-evac
P.-e. autotransfusion system
P.-e. device
P.-e. suction
pleurisy
acute p.
adhesive p.
blocked p.

NOTES

P

pleurisy *(continued)*
- cholesterol p.
- chronic p.
- chyliform p.
- chylous p.
- circumscribed p.
- costal p.
- diaphragmatic p.
- diffuse p.
- double p.
- dry p.
- encysted p.
- exudative p.
- fibrinous p.
- hemorrhagic p.
- ichorous p.
- indurative p.
- interlobar p.
- interlobular p.
- latent p.
- mediastinal p.
- metapneumonic p.
- plastic p.
- primary p.
- productive p.
- proliferating p.
- pulmonary p.
- pulsating p.
- purulent p.
- sacculated p.
- secondary p.
- serofibrinous p.
- serous p.
- single p.
- suppurative p.
- tuberculous p.
- typhoid p.
- visceral p.
- wet p.
- p. with effusion

pleuritic
- p. chest pain
- p. pneumonia
- p. rub

pleuritis
- fibrinous acute p.
- lupus p.
- obliterative p.
- rheumatoid p.
- tuberculous p.

pleuritogenous

pleurocentesis, pleuracentesis

pleurodesis
- chemical p.
- doxycycline p.
- mechanical p.
- talc p.
- thoracoscopic talc p.
- thorascopic talc p.

pleurodynia

pleuroesophageal
- p. fistula
- p. line
- p. muscle

pleuroesophageus
- musculus p.

pleurogenic pneumonia

pleurogenous

pleurography

pleurolith

pleuroparenchymal abnormality

pleuroparietopexy

pleuropericardial
- p. cyst
- p. incision
- p. murmur
- p. rub
- p. window

pleuropericarditis

pleuroperitoneal
- p. canal
- p. cavity
- p. fold
- p. shunt
- p. shunting

pleuropneumonectomy

pleuropneumonia-like organism (PPLO)

pleuropulmonary
- p. blastoma
- p. infection

pleuroscopy

pleurovisceral

Pleurx
- P. pleural catheter
- P. pleural catheter/home drainage kit

plexectomy

plexiform lesion

PlexiPulse compression device

plexogenic pulmonary arteriopathy

plexopathy
- brachial p.

plexus, pl. **plexuses**
- ascending pharyngeal p.
- Batson p.
- brachial p.
- esophageal nervous p.
- Gelweave 3 branch P.
- p. gulae
- Haller p.
- lingual p.
- p. nervosus esophageus
- p. nervosus pharyngeus
- p. periarterialis arteriae lingualis
- p. periarterialis arteriae pharyngeae ascendentis
- perimuscular p.
- pharyngeal nervous p.

p. pulmonalis
pulmonary nervous p.
superior vascular p. (SVP)
PLHB
percutaneous left heart bypass
pliability
PLIC
posterior limb of the internal capsule
plicamycin
plication
PLLA
poly-L-lactic acid
PLM
periodic leg movement
PLMD
periodic limb movement disorder
PLMV
posterior leaf mitral valve
plombage
plop
cardiac tumor p.
tumor p.
plot
box p.
box-and-whisker p.
bull's-eye p.
whisker p.
PLSA
posterolateral segment artery
posterolateral segment [coronary] artery
plug
collagen p.
Ivalon p.
mucus p.
Shiley decannulation p.
Teflon Bardic p.
Traube p.
plugged telescoping catheter
plugging
mucous p.
PlugStation
P. earplug dispenser
P. earplug station
plumb-line sign
Plummer disease
Plummer-Vinson syndrome
plunging goiter
plurilocular
plus
CO₂SMO P.
Duramist P.
2010 P. Holter system

ligand p. 1, 2, 3
Lorcet P.
Nicorette P.
Oracle Micro P.
PLV
left ventricular pressure
partial liquid ventilation
posterior left ventricle
PLVP
peak left ventricular pressure
PM
mean pressure
pacemaker
papillary muscle
posterior mitral
presystolic murmur
Prony method
P+max
peak positive pressure
PMBC
percutaneous mitral balloon
commissurotomy
PMBV
percutaneous mitral balloon valvotomy
percutaneous mitral balloon valvuloplasty
PMC
percutaneous mitral commissurotomy
percutaneous myocardial channeling
premature mitral closure
premotor cortex
PMD
primary myocardial disease
pMDI
pressurized metered-dose inhaler
PM-DM
polymyositis-dermatomyositis
PMEOAT
Photo-Mask and Etch-on-a-Tube
photo-mask and etch-on-a-tube
PMF
progressive massive fibrosis
PMH
pure motor hemiparesis
PMHR
predicted maximal heart rate
PMI
perioperative myocardial infarction
point of maximal impulse
point of maximum impulse
P-min
peak negative pressure

NOTES

P

PMIS
   postmyocardial infarction syndrome
P-mitrale
PML
   posterior mitral leaflet
   progressive multifocal
      leukoencephalopathy
   prolapsing mitral leaflet
PMN
   polymorphonuclear leukocyte
   polymorphonuclear neutrophil
PMR
   papillary muscle rupture
   percutaneous myocardial
      revascularization
   percutaneous transmyocardial laser
      revascularization
PMRP
   portable monitor of respiratory
      parameters
^{31}P-MRS
   phosphorus-31 magnetic resonance
      spectroscopy
PMS
   P.-Amantadine
   P.-Erythromycin
   P.-Hydroxyzine
   P. Isoniazid
   P.-Methylphenidate
   P.-Progesterone
   P.-Pyrazinamide
PMS-Levothyroxine Sodium
PMS-Sodium Cromoglycate
PMT
   pacemaker-mediated tachycardia
   percutaneous mechanical thrombectomy
   PMT AccuSpan tissue expander
   Thrombex PMT
PMV
   percutaneous mitral valvotomy
   percutaneous mitral valvuloplasty
   prolapse of mitral valve
   PMV 2000 series speaking valve
PMVI
   peak myocardial video intensity
PMVL, pMVL
   posterior mitral valve leaflet
PMW
   pacemaker wires
PN
   perceived noise
   percussion note
PNB
   premature nodal beat
PNC
   premature nodal contracture
PND
   paroxysmal nocturnal dyspnea
   postnasal drip

PND-Rh
   postnasal drip due to rhinitis
PNDS
   postnasal drainage syndrome
   postnasal drip syndrome
PND-Si
   postnasal drip due to sinusitis
pneocardiac reflex
pneopneic reflex
PNET
   primitive neuroectodermal tumor
pneumatic
   p. antishock garment (PASG)
   p. compression stockings
   p. cuff
   p. hammer disease
   p. peripheral circulation
      improvement device (PPCID)
   p. tourniquet
   p. trousers
pneumatics
pneumatocardia
pneumatocele
pneumatohemia
pneumatonometer
   Digibind p.
pneumectomy
Pneumo
   P. disposable pneumotachometer
   P. Sleeve
pneumobacillus
   Friedländer p.
pneumobronchotomy
pneumobulbar
pneumocardial
pneumocardiogram (PCG)
pneumocentesis
pneumococcal
   p. empyema
   p. pneumonia
   p. vaccine
pneumococcosis
pneumococcus, pl. **pneumococci**
   Fraenkel p.
pneumoconiosis
   antimony p.
   arc welder's p.
   asbestos p.
   bauxite p.
   coal worker's p. (CWP)
   collagenous p.
   fuller's earth p.
   hard metal p.
   kaolin p.
   limonite p.
   magnetite p.
   mica p.
   mixed-dust p.
   noncollagenous p.

organic dust p.
rheumatoid p.
shale p.
p. siderotica
silicotic p.
talc p.
tungsten carbide p.
pneumocystic
Pneumocystis
    P. carinii
    P. carinii pneumonia (PCP)
Pneumocystis
    P. choroidopathy
    P. pneumonia
    P. pneumonitis
pneumocystosis
pneumocyte
    type II p.
pneumodynamics
pneumogastric
pneumogenic osteoarthropathy
pneumogram
pneumograph
pneumohemia
pneumohemothorax
pneumohydropericardium
pneumohydrothorax
pneumomediastinography
pneumomediastinum
pneumomycosis
pneumonectomy
    extrapleural p. (EPP)
    simultaneously stapled p. (SSP)
Pneumo-Needle reusable instrument
pneumonia (*See also* pneumonitis)
    abortive p.
    acute interstitial p. (AIP)
    adenoviral p.
    p. alba
    alcoholic p.
    amebic p.
    anthrax p.
    antimicrobial-resistant hospital-acquired p.
    apex p.
    apical p.
    p. aposthematosa
    aspiration p.
    atypical p.
    bacillary p.
    bacterial pneumococcal p.
    bilious p.

bronchial p.
bronchiolitis obliterans with organizing p. (BOOP)
Buhl desquamative p.
Candida p.
Carrington p.
caseous p.
catarrhal p.
central p.
cerebral p.
cheesy p.
Chlamydia p.
chronic eosinophilic p. (CEP)
chronic fibrous p.
cold agglutinin p.
community-acquired p. (CAP)
congenital aspiration p.
contusion p.
core p.
Corrigan p.
croupous p.
cryptogenic organizing p. (COP)
deglutition p.
desquamative interstitial p. (DIP)
p. dissecans
double p.
Eaton agent p.
embolic p.
Enterobacter p.
eosinophilic p.
ephemeral p.
ether p.
exogenous lipid p.
fibrinous acute lobar p.
fibrous p.
Friedländer bacillus p.
gangrenous p.
gelatinous acute p.
giant cell p.
Hecht p.
herpes simplex p.
hospital-acquired p. (HAP)
HSV p.
hypersensitivity p.
hypostatic p.
idiopathic acute eosinophilic p.
idiopathic interstitial p.
indurative p.
influenzal p.
influenza virus p.
inhalation p.
p. interlobularis

NOTES

P

pneumonia *(continued)*
    p. interlobularis purulenta
    interstitial plasma cell p.
    intrauterine p.
    Kaufman p.
    Klebsiella p.
    Legionella p.
    Legionnaire p.
    leptospiral p.
    lingular p.
    lipid p.
    lipoid p.
    lobar p.
    lobular p.
    Löffler p.
    Louisiana p.
    lymphoid interstitial p. (LIP)
    massive p.
    measles p.
    metastatic p.
    migratory p.
    mycoplasmal p.
    necrotizing p.
    nonspecific interstitial p. (NSIP)
    nosocomial p. (NP)
    p. notha
    obstructive p.
    oil-aspiration p.
    opportunistic p.
    organizing p.
    parenchymatous p.
    peribronchial p.
    Pittsburgh p.
    plague p.
    plasma cell p.
    pleuritic p.
    pleurogenic p.
    pneumococcal p.
    Pneumocystis p.
    Pneumocystis carinii p. (PCP)
    polymicrobial p.
    postobstructive p.
    primary atypical p.
    primary eosinophilic p.
    primary influenza p.
    progressive p.
    Proteus p.
    purulent p.
    Reisman p.
    rheumatic p.
    rickettsial p.
    Scopulariopsis spp p.
    secondary p.
    segmental p.
    septic p.
    Serratia p.
    P. Severity Index (PSI)
    staphylococcal p.
    Stoll p.

streptococcal p.
superficial p.
suppurative p.
terminal p.
toxemic p.
transplant p.
traumatic p.
Trichosporon beigelii p.
tuberculous p.
tularemic p.
TWAR p.
typhoid p.
unilateral p.
unresolved p.
uremic p.
usual interstitial p. (UIP)
vagus p.
varicella p.
ventilator-associated p. (VAP)
viral p.
walking p.
wandering p.
white p.
woolsorter's p.

pneumoniae
    Bacillus p.
    Chlamydia p.
    Diplococcus p.
    Klebsiella p.
    Legionella p.
    Mycoplasma p.
    Optochin test for *Streptococcus* p.
    Streptococcus p.

pneumonic
    p. fever
    p. plague

pneumonic-type adenocarcinoma

pneumonitis *(See also* pneumonia)
    acute interstitial p. (AIP)
    acute lupus p. (ALP)
    acute radiation p.
    aspiration p.
    bronchiolitis with interstitial p.
      (BIP)
    chemical p.
    cholesterol p.
    CMV p.
    cryptogenic organizing p. (COP)
    cytomegalovirus p.
    desquamative interstitial p. (DIP)
    eosinophilic p.
    giant cell interstitial p. (GIP)
    granulomatous p.
    herpes simplex p.
    hypersensitivity p. (HP)
    interstitial p.
    kerosene p.
    lymphocytic interstitial p. (LIP)
    lymphoid interstitial p. (LIP)

malarial p.
mixed alveolar-interstitial p.
nonspecific chronic interstitial p.
  (NIP)
nonspecific interstitial p. (NSIP)
ossifying p.
peptic aspiration p.
plasma cell interstitial p. (PIP)
Pneumocystis p.
radiation p.
uremic p.
usual interstitial p. (UIP)
varicella p.
pneumonoconiosis
bauxite p.
rheumatoid p.
pneumonocyte
phagocytic p.
pneumonopathy
eosinophilic p.
pneumonoresection
pneumonotherapy
pneumoparotid
pneumopathy
leukemic cell lysis p.
seropositive nonsyphilitic p.
Pneumopent
pneumopericardium (**PPC**)
tension p.
ventilator-induced p.
pneumopexy
pneumophila
  Legionella p.
pneumoplethysmography
pneumopleuritis
pneumopleuroparietopexy
pneumoresection
pneumorrhachis
pneumoscope
pneumosilicosis
pneumosintes
  Bacteroides p.
Pneumotach
p. disposable mouthpiece
MicroTach p.
p. spirometer
pneumotachogram
pneumotachograph
Fleisch p.
flow-sensing p.
Silverman-Lilly p.

pneumotachometer
hot-wire p.
Pneumo disposable p.
pneumotaxic center
pneumotherapy
pneumothorax, pl. **pneumothoraces**
artificial p.
catamenial p.
clicking p.
closed chest p.
extrapleural p.
iatrogenic p.
induced p.
normotensive p.
open p.
pressure p.
primary spontaneous p. (PSP)
pure p.
secondary p.
simultaneous bilateral
  spontaneous p. (SBSP)
spontaneous p. (SP)
tension p.
therapeutic p.
traumatic p.
unilateral p.
valvular p.
ventilator-induced p.
pneumotomy
Pneumovax 23
pneumovirus
pneuPAC
p. resuscitator
p. ventilator
**PneuView ventilator testing and
training system**
PNH
paroxysmal nocturnal hemoglobinuria
PNP
peak negative pressure
PNPB
positive-negative pressure breathing
PNS
posterior nasal spine
PNS Unna boot
**^{31}P nuclear magnetic resonance
spectroscopy**
Pnu-Imune 23
PO
pulse oximetry

NOTES

P

543

PO₂
: partial pressure of oxygen
    PO₂ oximetry

POBA
: plain old balloon angioplasty

POC
: point-of-care
: polyolefin copolymer
    POC Bandit catheter
    POC blood gas test

POCI
: posterior circulation infarct

pocket
: abdominal p.
: generator p.
: pacemaker p.
: regurgitant p.
: retropectoral p.
: p. of Zahn

Pocket-Dop II

Pockethaler
: Vancenase P.

PocketPeak peak flowmeter

POCS
: posterior circulation syndrome

POCT
: point-of-care testing
    POCT device

pod
: rigid p.

podagra

POEMS
: polyneuropathy, organomegaly, endocrinopathy, monoclonal gammopathy and skin changes
    POEMS syndrome

POET
: pulse oximeter/end tidal CO₂

pogonion
: gonion to p. (GO-POG)

POH
: postoperative hemorrhage

poikilocytosis

poikilothermy

point
: Addison p.
: A, D, E, J, Z p.
: p. of Arrhigi
: Boyd p.
: p. of care test
: Castellani p.
: p. of critical stenosis
: cut p.
: de Mussy p.
: equal-pressure p. (EPP)
: Erb p.
: exit p.
: Guéneau de Mussy p.
: hinge p.

: isoelectric p.
: lower infection p.
: p. of maximal impulse (PMI)
: p. of maximum impulse (PMI)
: null p.
: pivot p.
: sella nasion p. A (SNA)
: sella nasion p. B (SNB)
: p. tenderness
: upper infection p.

pointes
: quinidine-induced torsade de p.
: torsade de p. (TDP, TdP)

point-of-care (POC)
: p.-o.-c. analysis
: p.-o.-c. testing (POCT)
: p.-o.-c. testing device

Poiseuille
: P. equation
: P. law
: P. resistance formula

poisoning
: arsenic p.
: arsine gas p.
: fluorocarbon p.
: lead p.
: mercury p.
: oxygen p.

Poisson regression

pokkuri sudden arrhythmia-death syndrome

polacrilex chewing gum

polar
: p. coordinate map
: P. Electro sport tester
: p. plate
: P. Vantage XL heart rate monitor

Polaramine

polarcardiography computing system

Polaris CPAP system

Polaris-DX steerable diagnostic catheter

polarity
: reverse p.

polarization
: electrochemical p.
: fluorescence p.

polarographic method

Polhemus-Schafer-Ivemark syndrome

Polichinelle
: voix de P.

policy
: chest pain p. (CPP)

poliomyelitis

poliovirus
: p. vaccine, live, trivalent, oral

polixus
: *Rhodnius p.*

pollen asthma

pollution
    air p.
    photochemical air p.
poloxamer 188
polyacrylamide gel electrophoresis
polyacrylonitrile membrane
polyamide
polyamidoamine
polyangiitis
    microscopic p. (MPA)
polyanion precipitation procedure
polyarteritis
    disseminated p.
    hypertensive pulmonary p.
    p. nodosa
polyarthritis
polyblennia
polycarbonate urethane
polycardia
polychondritis
    relapsing p.
Polycitra-K
polyclonal gammopathy
polycrotic
polycrotism
polycyclic aromatic hydrocarbon (PAH)
polycystic
    p. kidney
    p. kidney disease
    p. lung
    p. tumor
polycythemia
    compensatory p.
    p. hypertonica
    p. vera
polydactyly
polyene
polyestradiol
polyether alcohol asthma
polyethylene
    p. glycol (PEG)
    p. glycol electrolyte lavage solution
      (PEG-LES)
    p. terephthalate (PET)
    p. terephthalate balloon
Polyflex lead
Polygam S/D
polygenic
    p. hypercholesterolemia
    p. hyperlipidemia
polyglandular autoimmune syndrome
  type II

polyglycolic acid
polygonal arcade
polygraph
    Mackenzie p.
    Night Owl pocket p.
polyhedral surface reconstruction
PolyHeme
Poly-Histine CS
polyhydroxybutyrate polymer
poly-L-lactic
    p.-L-l. acid (PLLA)
    p.-L-l. acid stent
polylysine
    benzylpenicilloyl p. (PPL)
    penicilloyl p. (PPL)
polymer
    p. fume fever (PFF)
    hyaluronic acid p.
    plastic p.
    polyhydroxybutyrate p.
    polyphosphate esters p.
polymerase
    p. chain reaction (PCR)
    Taq DNA p.
polymeric endoluminal paving stent
polymetabolic syndrome
polymicrobial pneumonia
polymorphic
    p. premature ventricular complex
    p. slow wave
    p. ventricular tachycardia
polymorphism
    ACE deletion/insertion p.
    adducin p.
    angiotensin-converting enzyme
      deletion/insertion p.
    gene p.
    paraoxonase p.
    restriction fragment length p.
      (RFLP)
polymorphonuclear
    p. leukocyte (PMN)
    p. neutrophil (PMN)
polymorphous ventricular tachycardia
polymyalgia rheumatica syndrome
polymyositis-dermatomyositis (PM-DM)
polymyxa
    Bacillus p.
polymyxin, lysome, EDTA, thallous
  acetate (PLET)
polyneuritiformis
    heredopathia atactica p.

NOTES

P

polyneuropathy
  ascending p.
  p., organomegaly, endocrinopathy,
    monoclonal gammopathy and skin
    changes (POEMS)
  Roussy-Lévy p.
polyolefin
  p. copolymer (POC)
  p. copolymer balloon
polyorganophosphazene-coated stent
polyostotic fibrous dysplasia
polyp
  bronchial inflammatory p.
  cardiac p.
polypeptide
  atrial natriuretic p. (ANP)
  gastric inhibitory p. (GIP)
  pancreatic p. (PP)
polyphaga
  Acanthamoeba p.
polyphenol
  red wine p.
polyphosphate esters polymer
polyphosphoinositide
polyploidy
polypoidal lesion
polypoid bronchitis
polyposis
  nasal p.
polypous endocarditis
polypropylene
  p. intracardiac patch
  p. stent
polyribosylribitol
  p. phosphate (PRP)
  p. phosphate-diphtheria toxoid
    conjugate (PRP-D)
polysaccharide-iron complex
polysaccharide storage disease
PolySafe A-track lead
polyserositis
  familial paroxysmal p.
  periodic p.
polysomatic
polysome
polysomnogram (PSG)
  Nihon Kohden p.
  nocturnal p. (NPSG)
polysomnographic index
polysomnography (PSG)
  home unattended p.
  nocturnal p.
  overnight p.
  telemonitored p.
polysplenia
Polystan
  P. cardiotomy reservoir
  P. perfusion cannula
  P. venous return catheter

polystyrene latex microsphere
polytef
  p. artificial vessel
  p. implant
polytef-sheathed needle
polytetrafluoroethylene (PTFE)
  p. covered stent
  expanded p. (ePTFE)
  predilated p.
  p. prosthesis
  p. stent graft
polythiazide
  prazosin and p.
polyunsaturated
  p. fat
  p. fatty acid (PUFA)
polyurethane
  p. foam
  p. foam embolus
polyuria
polyvinyl
  p. alcohol (PVA)
  p. chloride (PVC)
  p. chloride balloon
  p. chloride tube
  p. prosthesis
POM
  pulse oximetry monitoring
Pompe disease
ponderal index
ponderance
  ventricular p.
Pondimin
Pondocillin
ponopalmosis
Ponstel
Pontiac fever
pontine
  p. hyperintensity (PHI)
  p. infarct (PI)
  p. ischemic rarefaction
Pontocaine
P-on-T wave
pool
  blood p.
pooling
poor
  p. exercise tolerance (PET)
  p. expiratory effort
  p. R-wave progression
poorly
  p. differentiated carcinoma
  p. reversible asthma
popliteal
  p. aneurysm
  p. artery
  p. pulse
pop-off valve

poppet
>prosthetic p.
>Silastic p.

popping sensation

POPS
>postoperative pacing study

POR
>postocclusive oscillatory response

porcelain aorta

porcine
>p. bioprosthesis
>p. heterograft
>p. prosthesis
>p. prosthetic valve
>p. xenograft

pore
>Kohn p.

porfimer

pork
>p. insulin
>P. NPH Iletin II
>P. Regular Iletin II

porphyria
>acute intermittent p. (AIP)

porphyrin

Porphyromonas gingivalis

Porstmann technique

PORT
>postoperative radiotherapy

port
>p. access technique
>CathLink 20 implanted p.
>chest p.
>Import vascular access p.
>Luer-Lok p.
>Q P.
>SEA p.
>side arm pressure p.

porta, pl. **portae**
>p. hepatis
>p. lienis

portable
>p. aerosol delivery device
>AutoSet P. II
>p. chest radiograph
>p. monitoring device
>p. monitor of respiratory parameters (PMRP)
>Pulsair .5 liquid oxygen p.
>p. volume ventilator

Port-A-Cath
>P.-A.-C. device
>P.-A.-C. implantable catheter system

portacaval (PC)
>p. anastomosis (PCA)
>p. bypass (PCB)
>p. H graft
>p. shunt (PCS)
>p. transposition (PCT)

Port-Access
>P.-A. coronary artery bypass grafting
>P.-A. minimally invasive cardiac surgery
>St. Jude Medical P.-A.

portae (*pl. of* porta)

Portagen diet

portal
>p. circulation
>p. hypertension (PHT)
>p. perfusion pressure (PPP)
>p. pressure gradient (PPG)
>p. pyemia
>p. vein (PV)
>p. vein dilation (PVD)
>p. vein thrombosis (PVT)
>p. venous flow (PVF)

Porta Pulse 3 defibrillator

Porta-Resp monitor

Port Charles influenza

Porter sign

Portex
>P. Per-fit tracheostomy kit
>P. Per-fit tracheostomy tube
>P. Soft-Seal cuff system

portion
>infradiaphragmatic p.
>p. of the segment between the end of the S wave and the beginning of the T wave (S-T)

portogram

portography
>computed tomography angiographic p. (CTAP)
>computed tomography in arterial p. (CTAP)
>splenic p.
>transthoracic p. (THP)

portoportal anastomosis

portopulmonary
>p. hypertension
>p. shunt

NOTES

P

547

portosystemic anastomosis
portovenography
Posadas mycosis
Posadas-Wernicke disease
Posey Cufflator tracheal cuff inflator
 and manometer
position
> Andral decubitus p.
> body p.
> electrical heart p.
> heart p.
> LAO p.
> left anterior oblique p.
> RAO p.
> recovery p.
> right anterior oblique p.
> scalloped subcoronary p.
> semilateral supine p.
> shock p.
> sniffing p.
> Trendelenburg p.
> tricuspid p.

positional obstructive sleep apnea
 syndrome
positioner
> CAS-8000V general angiography p.
> Thornton anterior p. (TAP)

positioning
> prone p.

positive
> p. afterpotential
> p. airway pressure (PAP)
> p. airway pressure ventilation
> p. arterial remodeling
> p. chronotropism
> p. end-airway pressure (PEAP)
> p. end-expiratory pressure (PEEP)
> p. expiratory pressure (PEP)
> false p.
> p. inspiratory pressure (PIP)
> p. predictive value (PPV)
> p. pressure
> p. pressure mechanical ventilation
> p. support ventilator (PSV)
> P. Symptom Distress Index (PSDI)
> p. symptom total (PST)
> p. treppe

positive-negative pressure breathing
 (PNPB)
Positrol II catheter
positron
> p. emission tomography (PET)
> p. emitter

post
> p. balloon angioplasty restenosis
> p. bypass spasm
> p. graft (PG)

postabsorptive state

postanesthesia
> p. care unit (PACU)
> p. pulmonary edema

postangioplasty
postantibiotic effect (PAE)
postbronchodilator
postbypass
postcapillary hypertension
postcardiac injury syndrome (PCIS)
postcardiotomy
> p. psychosis syndrome
> p. syndrome (PCS)

postcardioversion pulmonary edema
postcatheterization
postcoital asthma
postcommissurotomy syndrome
postcontrast echocardiogram
postcoronary care unit (PCCU)
postdiastolic
postdicrotic
postdiphtheritic stenosis
postdischarge graded-exercise test (PD-
 GXT)
postdiuresis scan
postdrive depression
postductal
postectopic pause
posterior
> p. airway space (PAS)
> p. approach
> p. basal segmental artery of right
> lung
> p. branch of right superior
> p. cerebral artery (PCA)
> p. circulation (PC)
> p. circulation infarct (POCI)
> p. circulation syndrome (POCS)
> p. circumflex artery (PC)
> p. communicating artery (PCoA)
> p. cricoarytenoid muscle
> p. descending artery (PDA)
> p. inferior cerebellar artery (PICA)
> p. inferior communicating artery
> (PICA)
> p. isthmus
> p. junction line
> p. leaflet
> p. leaf mitral valve (PLMV)
> p. left ventricle (PLV)
> p. left ventricular wall motion on
> echocardiogram
> p. limb of the internal capsule
> (PLIC)
> p. margin of pulmonary artery
> (PPA)
> p. mitral (PM)
> p. mitral leaflet (PML)
> p. mitral valve leaflet (PMVL,
> pMVL)

p. myocardial infarction
p. nasal spine (PNS)
p. papillary muscle (PPM)
p. pulmonary artery (PPA)
p. pulmonary leaflet (PPL)
p. Q wave
regio p.
regio cruris p.
p. rib fracture
p. right coronary artery (pRCA)
p. tibial pulse
p. tricuspid leaflet (PTL)
p. upper lung zone
p. wall (PW)
p. wall or aortic root (PAR)
p. wall excursion (PWE)
p. wall infarct (PWI)
p. wall of left ventricle (PWLV)
p. wall thickness
posterius
segmentum bronchopulmonale p.
segmentum bronchopulmonale basale p.
posteroinferior dyskinesis
posterolateral
p. circumflex branch (PLCx)
p. segment artery (PLSA)
p. thoracotomy
posteroseptal wall
postesophageal
postexercise
p. echocardiogram
p. scan
postextrasystolic (PES)
p. aberrancy
p. beat
p. pause
p. potentiation (PESP)
p. T wave
postganglionic vagal stimulation (PGVS)
posthemothorax
postheparin
p. lipolytic activity (PHLA)
p. phospholipase (PHP)
p. plasma diamine oxidase (PHD)
posthyperventilation apnea
postictal state
postinfarct
p. cardiosclerosis
p. patient
p. ventricular remodeling

postinfarction
p. angina
p. late potential (PILP)
p. pericarditis
p. period
p. risk stratification (PIRS)
p. syndrome
postinfectious bradycardia
postinfective bradycardia
postinflammatory
postinjury
p. empyema
p. immunosuppression
postintervention
postischemic
p. dysfunction
p. heart
p. myocardium
postmenopausal
postmicturition syncope
postmitotic
postmortem
p. clot
p. thrombus
postmyocardial
p. infarction
p. infarction syndrome (PMIS)
p. injury pericarditis
postnasal
p. catarrh
p. drainage syndrome (PNDS)
p. drip (PND)
p. drip due to rhinitis (PND-Rh)
p. drip due to sinusitis (PND-Si)
p. drip syndrome (PNDS)
postobstructive
p. atelectasis
p. pneumonia
postocclusion hyperemia
postocclusive oscillatory response (POR)
postoperative
p. atrial fibrillation in cardiac surgery (PACS)
p. chest radiograph
p. constrictive pericarditis (PCP)
p. endocarditis
p. hemorrhage (POH)
p. low cardiac output (PLCO)
p. pacing study (POPS)
p. pericarditis
p. radiotherapy (PORT)

NOTES

P

postpartum
    p. cardiomyopathy (PPCM)
    p. hypertension
postperfusion
    p. arrhythmia
    p. lung
    p. psychosis
    p. syndrome
postpericardiotomy syndrome (PPS)
postpharyngeal space
postphlebitic syndrome
postpneumonectomy tuberculous empyema
postpneumonic
postprandial
    p. angina
    p. blood sugar
    p. hypotension
    p. lipemia (PPL)
postprimary tuberculosis
postprocedural management
postpump
    p. image
    p. syndrome
postrandomization
postrema
postrenal azotemia
postresuscitation
postresuscitative death
postrheumatic cusp retraction
postsphygmic
    p. interval
    p. period
poststenosis dilation (PSD)
poststenotic (PST)
    p. dilation
poststreptococcal inflammatory process
poststroke pruritus
postsynaptic cholinergic mechanism
postsystolic shortening
posttest
    Tukey-Kramer p.
postthrombolytic therapy
posttransfusion syndrome
posttransplantation
    p. lymphoproliferative disorder (PTLPD, PTLD)
    p. malignancy
posttraumatic
    p. ARDS
    p. pulmonary pseudocyst
posttussive
    p. emesis
    p. syncope
postural
    P. Assessment Scale for Stroke Patient
    p. drainage (PD)
    p. drainage of infected secretion

    p. drainage and percussion (PD&P)
    p. drainage, percussion and vibration (PDPV)
    p. hypotension
    p. orthostatic tachycardia syndrome (POTS)
    p. syncope
posture
    Stern p.
    p. technique
posturing
    decerebrate p.
    posturing decerebrate p.
postventricular
    p. atrial blanking (PVAB)
    p. atrial refractory period (PVARP)
Potain sign
potassium (K)
    p. aminosalicylate
    amoxicillin and clavulanate p.
    canrenoate p.
    p. channel opener
    p. chloride (KCl)
    p. chloride cardioplegia
    p. citrate and citric acid
    p. gluconate
    glucose, insulin, and p. (GIK)
    p. hydroxide (KOH)
    p. inhibition
    p. iodide
    p. ion
    losartan p.
    penicillin V p.
    ticarcillin and clavulanate p.
    p. wasting
potassium-sparing diuretic
potassium-wasting diuretic
potential
    action p.
    bioelectric p.
    cardiac action p.
    compound motor action p. (CMAP)
    diastolic p. (Vdia)
    electrical p.
    endocardial p. (ECP)
    fibrillation p.
    heart synchronized evoked p. (HSEP)
    His bundle p.
    interpulse p. (Ipp)
    Kent p.
    late diastolic p. (LDP)
    maximum diastolic p. (MDP)
    maximum negative p.
    membrane p.
    monophasic action p. (MAP)
    motor provoked p. (MEP)
    movement-related cortical p. (MRCP)

nerve action p.
pacemaker p.
peroxyl radical-trapping p.
postinfarction late p. (PILP)
putative slow pathway p.
resting membrane p.
right ventricular endocardial p.
  (RVECP)
sensory nerve action p. (SNAP)
sinus node p. (SNP)
somatosensory evoked p. (SSEP)
total peroxyl radical-trapping
  antioxidant p. (TRAP)
transmembrane p.
ventricular late p. (VLP)

potentiated twitch force
potentiation
interval-dependent p.
postextrasystolic p. (PESP)
twitch p.

potentiator
POTS
postural orthostatic tachycardia syndrome

Pott aneurysm
Pottenger sign
potter's
p. asthma
p. phthisis

Potts
P. anastomosis
P. bronchial forceps
P. needle
P. operation
P. procedure
P. shunt

Potts-Cournand needle
Potts-Smith anastomosis
pouch
Cardio-Cool myocardial
  protection p.
p. hematoma
laryngeal p.
pharyngeal p.

poudrage
Beck epicardial p.
pericardial p.
pleural p.
talc p.

pound
p.'s per square inch (psi)
p.'s per square inch gauge (psig)

Pourcelot index

povidone-iodine
powder
Acarosan dust mite p.
budesonide inhalation p.
fluticasone propionate and
  salmeterol inhalation p.
lyophilized p.

powdered tantalum
power
p. Doppler ultrasound
exercise cardiac p. (ECP)
p. failure
P. Grip Over the Wire Stent
  Delivery system
P. Grip stent
p. injector
left ventricular p.
p. motion imaging
resolving p.
spectral p.
p. spectral analysis
p. spectral density (PSD)
p. spectrum of HRV
ventricular p.

Powerflex
P. angioplasty balloon
P. Extreme PTA balloon catheter
P. P3 high pressure balloon
  catheter

Powerheart
P. AECD
P. automatic external cardioverter-
  defibrillator

Powerlink endoluminal graft system
PP
pancreatic polypeptide
paradoxical pulse
parietal pericardium
parietal pulse
partial pressure
pulse pressure
pulsus paradoxus
purulent pericarditis

PPA
posterior margin of pulmonary artery
posterior pulmonary artery
pure pulmonary atresia

Ppa
pulmonary artery pressure

PPACK
D-Phe-L-Pro-L-Arg-chloromethyl ketone

NOTES

P

PPAR
peroxisome proliferator-activated receptor
PPAR-gamma
peroxisome proliferator-activated receptor
gamma
PPAS
peripheral pulmonary artery stenosis
Ppaw
pulmonary artery wedge pressure
PPC
pneumopericardium
PPCF
peripartum cardiac failure
PPCID
pneumatic peripheral circulation
improvement device
PPCID sequential foot compression
device
PPCID slippers
PPCM
postpartum cardiomyopathy
PPD
purified protein derivative
PPD skin test
P&PD
percussion and postural drainage
Ppeak
peak airway pressure
PPG
photoplethysmography
portal pressure gradient
PPH
primary pulmonary hypertension
PPHN
persistent pulmonary hypertension of
newborn
P-P interval
PPL
benzylpenicilloyl polylysine
penicilloyl polylysine
posterior pulmonary leaflet
postprandial lipemia
primary pulmonary non-Hodgkin
lymphoma
PPL skin test
Ppl
pleural pressure
Pplat
plateau pressure
PPLO
pleuropneumonia-like organism
PPM
permanent pacemaker
posterior papillary muscle
pulse position modulated
ppm
part per million
pulses per minute

PPP
platelet-poor plasma
portal perfusion pressure
PPPBL
peripheral pulses palpable both legs
PPR
physiologic pattern release
PPR verapamil
PPRE
peroxisome proliferator response element
PPS
postpericardiotomy syndrome
pPTCA
primary percutaneous transluminal
coronary angioplasty
P-pulmonale
PPV
positive predictive value
Ppw
pulmonary wedge pressure
P-Q, PQ
P-Q interval
P-Q segment depression
P:QRS ratio
P-R
pulmonary regurgitation
pulse rate
pulse repetition
time between the P wave and beginning
of QRS complex
P-R interval
P-R segment
P&R
pulse and respiration
PRA
panel of reactive antibodies
panel-reactive antibody
plasma renin activity
PR-AC measurement
practitioner
respiratory care p. (RCP)
practolol
^{32}P radioactive stent
praecox
ascites p.
lymphedema p.
2-pralidoxime (2-PAM)
pranayama breathing technique
pranlukast
Pravachol
pravastatin sodium
prawn asthma
praxis
praziquantel
prazosin
p. hydrochloride
p. and polythiazide
pRCA
posterior right coronary artery

preamplifier
Arzco p.
preanesthetic
prearteriole
preatheroma
preautomatic pause
pre-beta 1 HDL
precapillary
p. anastomosis
p. arteriole
p. pulmonary hypertension
p. sphincter
precardiac mesoderm
precatheterization
Precedex
Precept lead
precipitation
heparin-induced extracorporeal low-density lipoprotein p. (HELP)
precipitin
precipitous drop in blood pressure
Preclude pericardial membrane
preconditioning
ischemic p. (IPC)
p. phenomenon
p. signal
precordial (PC)
p. A wave
p. bulge
p. catch syndrome
p. electrocardiographic monitoring (PEM)
p. electrocardiography
p. heave
p. honk
p. lead
p. motion
p. movement
p. pulse
p. ST depression
p. ST segment
p. thrill
p. thump
p. whoop
precordialgia
precordium
quiet p.
precoronary
p. angioplasty
p. care (PCC)
p. care area (PCA)

Precose
Predator PTCA catheter
predeposit autologous donation
prediastole
prediastolic murmur
predicrotic
predicted
p. cardiac output (PCO)
p. maximal heart rate (PMHR)
prediction
code excited linear p. (CELP)
predictive
p. index for myocardial infarction (PIMI)
p. survival marker
p. value
predictor
APACHE CV Risk P.
Corazonix P.
predilated
p. polytetrafluoroethylene
p. polytetrafluoroethylene graft
p. polytetrafluoroethylene obstruction
p. polytetrafluoroethylene stent
predischarge test
prednisolone
methyl p.
systemic p.
Prednisol TBA injection
prednisone
predominant emphysema
predose level
preductal
preeclampsia
preejection period (PEP)
preejection period index (PEPI)
preexcitation (PE)
left lateral ventricular p. (LLVP)
left posterior ventricular p. (LPVP)
right posterior ventricular p. (RPVP)
p. syndrome (PES)
ventricular p.
preexcited
preexisting condition
pregnancy
anaphylactoid syndrome of p.
dyspnea of p.
pregnancy-induced hypertension (PIH)
prehospital cardiac arrest (PCA)
preimplantation diagnosis (PID)

NOTES

P

preinfarction
>p. angina (PIA)
>p. syndrome (PIS)

prekallikrein

prelaryngeales
>nodi lymphoidei p.

prelaryngeal lymph node

preload
>cardiac p.
>p. reduction
>p. reserve
>ventricular p.

Prelone Oral

premature
>p. atherosclerosis
>p. atrial beat (PAB)
>p. atrial complex
>p. atrial contraction (PAC)
>p. atrial extrastimulus
>p. atrial stimulus (PAS)
>p. atrioventricular junctional complex
>p. beat (PB)
>p. contraction
>p. diastolic distention
>p. excitation
>p. junctional beat
>p. junctional contraction (PJC)
>p. mitral closure (PMC)
>p. nodal beat (PNB)
>p. nodal contracture (PNC)
>p. stimulus
>p. systole
>p. valve closure
>ventricular p. (VP, Vp)
>p. ventricular beat (PVB)
>p. ventricular complex
>p. ventricular complex-trigger hypothesis
>p. ventricular contraction (PVC)
>p. ventricular depolarization (PVD)
>p. ventricular extrasystole (PVE)
>p. ventricular systole (PVS)

prematurity
>chronic pulmonary insufficiency of p.
>retinopathy of p. (ROP)

premedication

premonitory
>p. palpitation
>p. syndrome

premotor cortex (PMC)

premounted stent

prenalterol hydrochloride

prenylamine

preoperative antibiotic

preparation
>insulin p.

>isometrically contracting myocardial p.
>Langendorff heart p.

preperitoneal
>p. dilator balloon (PDB)
>p. fat

preprandial

prepump image

prerenal azotemia

presacral edema

presaturation pulse

presbycardia

presbyesophagus

presbylaryngia

prescription
>P. Analyses and Cost (PACT)
>P. Drug User Fee Act (PDUFA)
>exercise p.

present
>peripheral pulse p.

presentation
>roentgenographic p.

preservation
>tissue p.

preserved left ventricular systolic function

preshaped catheter

presphygmic
>p. interval
>p. period

Press-mate SAT

pressor
>p. drug
>p. effect

pressoreceptive

pressoreceptor reflex

pressosensitive

pressosensitivity
>reflexogenic p.

pressure (P)
>absolute p.
>active p. (AP)
>airway-esophageal balloon p.
>alveolar p. (Palv)
>alveolar capillary intravascular p.
>alveolar carbon dioxide p.
>alveolar oxygen partial p. (PAO$_2$)
>ambient p.
>ambulatory blood p. (ABP)
>ambulatory venous p. (AVP)
>aortic p. (AOP, AoP, AP)
>aortic blood p. (AoBP)
>aortic dicrotic notch p.
>aortic mean p. (AOMP, AoMP)
>aortic pullback p.
>aortic systolic p. (ASP)
>area diastolic p. (ADP)
>area systolic p. (ASP)
>arterial p. (AP)

arterial blood p. (ABP, aBP)
arterial carbon dioxide p.
arterial dicrotic notch p.
arterial oxygen partial p. (PaO$_2$)
ascending aortic p. (PAo)
ascending aortic blood p.
assisted peak systolic p. (APSP)
atmospheres of p.
atmospheric p.
atrial p. (PA)
atrial filling p.
p. augmentation (PA)
average diastolic p. (AVDP)
average mean p. (AMP)
back p.
balloon aortic end-diastolic p.
  (BAEDP)
barometric p.
beat-to-beat finger arterial p.
bilevel positive airway p. (BiPAP)
blood p. (bl pr, BP, B/P)
brachial artery p. (BrAP)
capillary p. (CP)
capillary hydrostatic p. (CHP)
capillary wedge p.
carbon dioxide p.
cardiovascular p.
central venous p. (CVP)
cerebral perfusion p. (CPP)
chest wall elastic recoil p. (Pth)
coaxial p.
colloid oncotic p. (COP)
colloid osmotic p.
compliance, rate, oxygenation
  and p. (CROP)
continuous positive air p.
continuous positive airway p.
  (CPAP)
p. control (PC)
p. controller
p. conversion
coronary perfusion p. (CorPP,
  CPP)
coronary sinus occlusion p. (CSOP)
coronary venous p.
cricoid p.
p. cycled ventilation
p. cycled ventilator
p. decay
deep venous p. (DVP)
diastolic p. (DP, Pd)
diastolic aortic p. (DAP)

diastolic blood p. (DBP)
diastolic filling p. (DFP)
differential blood p.
distal coronary occlusion p.
  (DCOP)
distal coronary perfusion p.
Donders p.
Doppler p.
downstream venous p. (DSVP)
dynamic p.
effective systolic p. (ESP)
elastic recoil p.
end-diastolic p. (EDP)
end-diastolic left ventricular p.
end-expiratory esophageal p.
endocardial p.
end-systolic p. (ESP)
end-systolic left ventricular p.
erect diastolic blood p. (EDBP)
expiratory positive airway p.
  (EPAP)
external cardiac p. (ECP)
extreme p. (EP)
femoral artery p.
femoral blood p. (FBP)
filling p. (FP)
finger systolic blood p. (FSBP)
gastric-intrapleural p. (Pg-Ppl)
p. gradient
p. guide pressure wire
p. half-time (PHT)
p. half-time technique
high blood p. (HBP)
hyperbaric p.
inferior vena cava p. (ICVP)
inflation p.
p. injector
inspiratory occlusion p.
inspiratory positive airway p.
  (IPAP)
inspiratory resistance and positive
  expiratory p. (IR-PEP)
intermittent positive p. (IPP)
intraalveolar p.
intracardiac p.
intracranial p. (ICP)
intramyocardial p.
intrapericardial p. (IPP)
intrapleural oncotic p.
intrathoracic p.
intravascular p. (IVP)

NOTES

P

pressure *(continued)*

intrinsic positive end-expiratory p. (PEEPi)

Joint National Committee on Prevention, Detection, Evaluation, and Treatment of High Blood P.

jugular venous p. (JVP)

juxtacardiac pleural p.

labile blood p.

left anterior descending arterial p. (LADP)

left atrial p. (LAP, PLa, Pla)

left atrial transmural p. (LATP)

left ventricular p. (LVP, PLV)

left ventricular developed p. (LVDP)

left ventricular diastolic p. (LVDP)

left ventricular end-diastolic p. (LVEDP, LVEP)

left ventricular filling p. (LVFP)

left ventricular systolic p. (LVSP)

low blood p. (LBP)

lower body negative p. (LBNP)

lung elastic recoil p. (Pel)

maximal exercise systolic p. (MESP)

maximal expiratory p. (MEP)

maximal expiratory mouth p. (P_{Emax})

maximal inspiratory p. (MIP)

maximal inspiratory mouth p. (P_{Imax})

maximal sniff-induced esophageal p.

maximal sniff-induced gastric p.

maximal sniff-induced transdiaphragmatic p.

maximum closure p. (MCP)

maximum expiratory p. (MEP)

maximum expiratory airflow-static lung elastic recoil p. (MFSR)

maximum inspiratory p. (MIP)

maximum left ventricular p. (LVPmax)

mean p. (PM)

mean airway p. (MAP)

mean aortic p. (MAP)

mean arterial p. (MAP)

mean arterial blood p. (MABP, MBP)

mean blood p. (MBP)

mean daily erect blood p. (MDEBP)

mean daily supine blood p. (MDSBP)

mean diastolic left ventricular p.

mean intravascular p. (MIP)

mean left atrial p. (MLAP)

mean maternal arterial blood p. (MMAP)

mean pulmonary artery p. (MPAP, PAPm)

mean pulmonary artery wedge p. (MPAWP)

mean pulmonary venous p. (MPVP)

mean resting diastolic blood p. (MDBP)

mean right atrial p. (MRAP)

mean right ventricular p. (MRVP)

mean systemic arterial p. (MSAP)

mean systolic left ventricular p.

p. measurement

minimum audible p. (MAP)

minimum left ventricular p. (LVPmin)

MPA p.

narrowed pulse p.

nasal continuous positive airway p. (NCPAP, nCPAP)

p. necrosis

negative end-expiratory p. (NEEP)

negative expiratory p. (NEP)

negative intrapleural p.

noninvasive blood p. (NIBP, NIPB)

noninvasive ventilation with positive p.

normal intravascular p.

oncotic p.

opening p.

osmotic p.

p. overload

p. overload-induced aortic valve calcific thickening

Pa p.

PA filling p.

partial p. (P, PP)

peak airway p. (Ppeak)

peak diastolic p. (PDP)

peak inspiratory p. (PIP)

peak left ventricular p. (PLVP)

peak negative p. (P-min, PNP)

peak positive p. (P+max)

peak systolic p. (PSP)

peak systolic aortic p. (PSAP)

peak systolic gradient p.

perfusion p.

pericardial p.

peripheral coronary p. (PCP)

peripheral venous p. (PVP)

plasma colloid osmotic p.

plateau p. (Pplat)

p. plethysmograph

pleural p. (Ppl)

p. pneumothorax

portal perfusion p. (PPP)

positive p.

positive airway p. (PAP)

positive end-airway p. (PEAP)

positive end-expiratory p. (PEEP)
positive expiratory p. (PEP)
positive inspiratory p. (PIP)
precipitous drop in blood p.
PSG p.
pullback p.
pulmonary arterial p.
pulmonary arterial capillary
  wedge p. (PACWP)
pulmonary arterial end-diastolic p.
pulmonary arterial pressure,
  pulmonary venous p. (pa-pv)
pulmonary arterial wave p.
pulmonary artery p. (PAP, Ppa)
pulmonary artery diastolic p.
  (PADP)
pulmonary artery end-diastolic p.
  (PAEDP)
pulmonary artery mean p. (PAMP)
pulmonary artery occlusion p.
  (PAo, PAOP)
pulmonary artery occlusive
  wedge p.
pulmonary artery systolic p.
  (PASP)
pulmonary artery wedge p.
  (PAWP, Ppaw)
pulmonary capillary p. (PCP)
pulmonary capillary wedge p.
  (PCWP)
pulmonary hypertension p.
pulmonary vascular p.
pulmonary venous p. (PVP)
pulmonary wedge p. (Ppw, PWP)
p. pulse
pulse p. (PP)
p. pulse differentiation
PW p.
radial artery systolic p. (RASP)
p. recovery
resting p.
resting venous p. (RVP)
right atrial p. (RAP)
right atrial mean p. (RAMP)
right ventricular p. (RVP)
right ventricular diastolic p.
right ventricular end-diastolic p.
  (RVEDP)
right ventricular filling p. (RVFP)
right ventricular peak systolic p.
right ventricular systolic p. (RUSP,
  RVSP)

RVED p.
seated diastolic blood p. (SDBP)
segmental limb p. (SLP)
segmental limb systolic p. (SLP)
self-adjusting nasal continuous
  positive airway p. (APAP)
shunt p. (SP)
p. sling
sniff nasal inspiratory p.
standing diastolic blood p. (SDBP)
standing venous p. (SVP)
p. stasis
stopped flow p. (SFP)
stump p.
supersystemic pulmonary artery p.
supine diastolic blood p. (SDBP)
p. support ventilation (PSV)
p. support ventilator (PSV)
systemic arterial p. (SAP)
systemic blood p. (PSA)
systemic mean arterial p. (SMAP)
systolic p. (Ps, SP)
systolic arterial blood p. (SABP)
systolic atrial p. (SAP)
systolic blood p. (BPS, SBP, SYS-
  BP)
systolic left ventricular p.
systolic pulmonary artery p. (sPAP)
p. time product (PTP)
torr p.
total p. (P_T)
p. tracing
transdiaphragmatic p.
p. transducer
p. transducer airflow sensor
transesophageal p.
transmural p.
transmyocardial perfusion p.
transpulmonary p. (Ptp)
transthoracic p.
twitch esophageal p.
twitch gastric p.
twitch transdiaphragmatic p.
unintended positive end
  expiratory p. (autoPEEP, intrinsic
  PEEP)
upper airway closing p. (UACP)
upper airway opening p. (UAOP)
p. urticaria
variable positive airway p. (VPAP)
venous p. (VP)
venous blood p. (VBP)

NOTES

P

pressure *(continued)*
  venous stop flow p. (VSFP)
  ventricular p. (PV)
  ventricular diastolic p.
  ventricular filling p.
  p. wave (PW)
  p. waveform
  wedge p. (WP)
  widening of pulse p.
  zero diastolic blood p.
  zero end-expiratory p. (ZEEP)
  zero end-inspiratory p.
  zero-flow p. (Pzf, ZFP)
pressure-compensated
  p.-c. flow
  p.-c. flow plethysmograph
pressure-controlled
  p.-c. intermittent coronary sinus
    occlusion (PICSO)
  p.-c. inverse ratio ventilation
    (PCIRV)
  p.-c. respirator
  p.-c. ventilation (PCV)
  p.-c. ventilation technique
pressure-flow relationship
pressurelike
  p. sensation
  p. sensation in chest
pressure-natriuresis curve
pressure-overload hypertrophy
pressure-regulated
  p.-r. volume control (PRVC)
  p.-r. volume control ventilation
pressure-volume
  p.-v. analysis
  p.-v. curve
  p.-v. data
  p.-v. diagram
  elastic p.-v. (Pel-V)
  p.-v. loop
  p.-v. relation
PressureWire-3 sensor
PressureWire guidewire
**pressurized metered-dose inhaler
  (pMDI)**
pressurizer
  Oxy-Hood p.
Pressurometer blood pressure monitor
PresTab
  Glynase P.
presternalis
  regio p.
Presto-Flash spirometry system
Presto spirometry system
presyncopal
  p. episode
  p. medication
  p. spell

presyncope
  iterative p.
presystole
presystolic
  p. gallop (PSG)
  p. murmur (PM, PSM)
  p. pressure and volume
  p. pulsation
  p. thrill
pretibial
  p. edema
  p. myxedema
pretracheales
  nodi lymphoidei p.
pretracheal lymph node
pretreatment
  icatibant p.
Pretz-D
prevalence
Prevel sign
prevention
  mucin clot p. (MCP)
  primary p.
  secondary p.
preventive allergy treatment
preventricular stenosis
Preveon
prevertebral space
Prevotella melaninogenica
prevotii
  Peptostreptococcus p.
PreVue III digitizing system
PRF
  plasma-resistant fiber oxygenator
  pulse repetition frequency
PRHHP
  Puerto Rico Heart Health Program
prickle cell carcinoma
prick-test method
Priftin
Prima
  P. laser guidewire
  P. total occlusion device
  P. total occlusion system
Primacor
primaquine
  p. phosphate
  p. phosphate antimalarial
primary
  p. angioplasty research (PAR)
  p. atelectasis
  p. atypical pneumonia
  p. bronchus
  p. cardiac arrhythmia
  p. cardiac malignancy
  p. ciliary dyskinesia (PCD)
  p. closure
  p. coccidioidomycosis
  p. complex

p. donor (d(A))
p. effusion lymphoma
p. electrical disease
p. endocardial fibroelastosis
p. eosinophilic pneumonia
p. fibroproliferative pulmonary
   vasculopathy
p. graft failure (PGF)
p. hypertension
p. infarction (PI)
p. infection
p. influenza pneumonia
p. intracerebral hemorrhage (PICH)
p. isolated chylopericardium
p. lung carcinoma
p. myocardial disease (PMD)
p. pacemaker
p. percutaneous transluminal
   coronary angioplasty (pPTCA)
p. pleural aspergillosis
p. pleurisy
p. pleuropulmonary disease
p. prevention
p. pulmonary histiocytosis X
p. pulmonary hypertension (PPH)
p. pulmonary hypertension murmur
p. pulmonary non-Hodgkin
   lymphoma (PPL)
p. pulmonary parenchymal disease
p. restrictive cardiomyopathy
p. sensorimotor cortex (SM1)
p. spontaneous pneumothorax (PSP)
p. systemic amyloidosis
p. thrombus
p. tuberculosis
p. ventricular fibrillation (PVF)
p. ventricular tachycardia (PVT)
Primatene Mist
Primaxin
prime
crystalloid p.
P. ECG mapping system
RR p.
primed lymphocyte test
priming
p. dose
retrograde autologous p.
primitive
p. aorta
p. neuroectodermal tumor (PNET)
primordial catheter tube

primum
p. atrial septal defect
ostium p.
persistent ostium p.
septum p.
Principen
principle
Beer-Lambert p.
Castaneda p.
Fick p.
Frank-Straub-Wiggers-Starling p.
hemodynamic p.
Huygens p.
Laplace p.
Pascal p.
Prinivil
PrinterNOx
P. nitric oxide/nitrogen dioxide
   monitor
P. nitric oxide with MKII analyzer
Prinzide
Prinzmetal
P. effect
P. variant angina
Priscoline injection
prism method
privet cough
proaccelerin
proadrenomedullin N-terminal 20
   peptide
Pro-Air
ProAmatine
Pro-Amox
Pro-Ampi
proANF
proatrial natriuretic factor
   N-terminal proANF
proarrhythmia
proarrhythmic effect
proatherosclerotic factor
proatherothrombogenic molecule
proatrial natriuretic factor (proANF)
probability
Cooperman event p.
p. density function (PDF)
intermediate p.
Pro-Bal Protected balloon-tipped
   catheter
proband
probe
acoustic impedance p.

NOTES

P

probe *(continued)*

acridinium ester labeled nucleic acid p.
ambulatory ventricular function p.
AngeLase combined mapping-laser p.
p. balloon catheter
bilateral circumactive p. (BICAP)
blood-flow p.
cardiac p.
Chandler V-pacing p.
coronary artery p.
digoxigenin-labeled DNA p.
DNA p.
Doppler flow p.
Doppler velocity p.
four-beam laser Doppler p.
Hewlett-Packard biplane 5-MHz p.
Hewlett-Packard omniplane 5-MHz p.
high-esophageal pH p.
hot-tip laser p.
low-esophageal pH p.
multielectrode p.
Neo-Therm neonatal skin temperature p.
nuclear p.
p. patency
Radiometer p.
Robicsek vascular p.
scintillation p.
p. shield
Siemens-Elema AB pulse transducer p.
Silverstein stimulator p.
transesophageal echo p.
Vasoscope 3 Doppler p.

Probeta
probing sheath exchange catheter
probucol
procainamide

N-acetyl p. (NAPA)
p. hydrochloride

procaine

p. hydrochloride
penicillin G p.

Procanbid
Procan SR
procarbazine

cyclophosphamide, doxorubicin, methotrexate, p. (CAMP)
p., hydroxyurea, radiotherapy protocol

Procardia XL
procaterol
Procath electrophysiology catheter
procedure

ad hoc p.
Alliston p.
Anderson p.
arachnophlebectomy p.
arterial switch p.
atrial maze p.
Batista left ventricular reduction p.
Batista left ventriculectomy p.
Bentall p.
Bernstein p.
bidirectional Glenn p. (BDG)
Bing-Taussig heart p.
Björk method of Fontan p.
Blalock-Taussig p.
Brock p.
cardiac hybrid revascularization p.
Chamberlain p.
Charles p.
cherry-picking p.
Clagett p.
Cockett p.
compartment p.
corridor p.
Daggett p.
Damian graft p.
Damus-Kaye-Stansel p.
deairing p.
debubbling p.
debulking p.
domino p.
Dor p.
Dotter p.
double switch p.
Effler-Groves mode of Allison p.
esophageal sling p.
fenestrated Fontan p.
Fontan-Baudet p.
Fontan-Kreutzer p.
Fontan modification of Norwood p.
genioglossal advancement p.
Gill-Jonas modification of Norwood p.
Glenn anastomosis p.
hemi-Fontan p.
His-Hass p.
intracardiac amobarbital sodium p.
Jacobaeus p.
Jatene arterial switch p.
Jonas modification of Norwood p.
Junod p.
Karhunen-Loeve p.
Ko-Airan bleeding control p.
Kolmogorov-Smirnov p.
Kondoleon-Sistrunk elephantiasis p.
Konno p.
Lam p.
Langevin updating p.
latissimus dorsi p.
left atrial isolation p.
Lewis-Tanner p.
Luke p.

Lyon-Horgan p.
maxillomandibular advancement p.
maze p.
MIDCAB p.
minimally invasive p. (MIP)
minimally invasive direct coronary
  artery bypass p.
MLR p.
modified Fontan p.
Moore p.
Morrow p.
Mustard p.
Mustard-Senning p.
myocardial laser revascularization p.
Myosplint p.
Nicks p.
Norwood univentricular heart p.
Overholt p.
percutaneous myocardial
  revascularization p.
polyanion precipitation p.
Potts p.
Quaegebeur p.
Rashkind p.
Rastan-Konno p.
Rastelli p.
Ross aortic valve replacement p.
Ross-Konno pediatric
  aortoventriculoplasty p.
Sade modification of Norwood p.
salting-out p.
Schenk-Eichelter vena cava plastic
  filter p.
Schonander p.
Senning-Rastelli p.
Senning transposition p.
septation p.
shunt p. (SP)
Simplate p.
Somnoplasty p.
Sondergaard p.
Stansel p.
Sugiura p.
switch p.
Thal p.
tonsillar Somnoplasty p.
transjugular balloon valvuloplasty p.
Vineberg cardiac
  revascularization p.
Waterston-Cooley p.
Womack p.

process
consolidative p.
costal pit of transverse p.
Grip Technology stent crimping p.
Markov p.
myocardial infiltrative p.
poststreptococcal inflammatory p.
vocal p.
xiphisternal p.
xiphoid p.
process-based criteria
processing
film p.
model-based image p. (MBIP)
signal p.
processor
prochlorperazine
procoagulant
procollagen
p. type III aminoterminal peptide
  (PIIIP)
type I, III p.
proconvertin
p. blood coagulation factor
p. prothrombin conversion
  accelerator
Procort
Procrit
ProCross
P. Rely balloon
P. Rely over-the-wire balloon
  catheter
Procytox
prodromal symptom
prodrome
Prodrox injection
prodrug
combretastatin A4 p. (CA4P)
product
Ad5FGF-4 gene therapy p.
Autoplex Factor VIII inhibitor
  bypass p.
BioBypass gene-based drug
  delivery p.
calcium p.
CFC-free p.
digoxin reduction p. (DRP)
double p.
fibrin degradation p.
fibrinogen degradation p.
fibrinogen-fibrin degradation p.
fibrin split p.

NOTES

product *(continued)*
    gene therapy p.
    heart rate-pressure p.
    heart rate-systolic blood pressure p.
     (RPP)
    lipid peroxidation p.
    pressure time p. (PTP)
    rate-pressure p. (RPP)
    rate pressure p.
production
    carbon dioxide p.
    energy p.
    IL-10 p.
    mucus p.
    sputum p.
    venous carbon dioxide p. (VCO_2)
    ventilation/carbon dioxide p.
     (VE/VCO_2)
productive
    p. bronchitis
    p. cough
    p. pleurisy
    p. sputum
    p. tuberculosis
productus
    Peptostreptococcus p.
profibrinolytic
Profilate OSD
profile
    aortic valve velocity p.
    Astra p.
    BUFUL p.
    coronary risk p.
    deflated p.
    flow p.
    hemodynamic p.
    Hospital Admission Risk P.
     (HARP)
    Nottingham Health p.
    P. Plus balloon dilatation catheter
    risk factor p.
    serum lipid p.
    Sickness Impact p. (SIP)
    sound intensity p.
    ultra low p. (ULP)
profilin
Profilnine heat-treated
Proflex 5 catheter
profound systemic vasodilation
profunda
    arteria femoris p. (PFA)
    p. femoris artery
    p. femoris vein
    reconstitution via p.
    vena circumflexa iliaca p.
profundaplasty
profusion
progeria

Progestasert
progestational agent
progesterone
    continuous p.
    cyclic p.
    micronized p.
    p. oil
progestin
Proglycem Oral
prognosis in atrial fibrillation (PIAF)
Prograf
Prograft bifurcated endograft
Program
program
    Air Wise p.
    APT p.
    azimilide supraventricular
     arrhythmia p.
    cardiac rehabilitation and
     prevention p.
    coronary care training p. (CCTP)
    coronary rehabilitation p. (CRP)
    expedited recovery p.
    ischemic heart disease life stress
     monitoring p.
    lifestyle intervention, food and
     exercise p. (LIFE)
    Linde Walker Oxygen P.
    Minnesota Heart Health P.
     (MHHP)
    multidisciplinary pulmonary
     rehabilitation p.
    myocardial infarction
     rehabilitation p. (MIRP)
    National Asthma Education P.
     (NAEP)
    National Asthma Education and
     Prevention P. (NAEPP)
    National Cholesterol Education P.
     (NCEP)
    National Heart, Lung, Blood
     Institute/National Asthma
     Education Prevention P.
     (NHLBI/NAEPP)
    National High Blood Pressure
     Education P. (NHBPEP)
    National Lung Health Education P.
     (NLHEP)
    OxiScan oximetry p.
    Puerto Rico Heart Health P.
     (PRHHP)
    recurrent coronary prevention p.
     (RCPP)
    Sentry antimicrobial surveillance p.
    SleepGen polysomnography data
     entry p.
    SMILE p.
    smoking cessation p. (SCP)

Programalith
P. II, III pacemaker
P. A-V pacemaker
programmability
programmable
p. cardioverter-defibrillator (PCD)
p. implantable medication system (PIMS)
p. pacemaker
programmed
p. cut-off rate
p. electrical stimulation (PES)
p. ventricular stimulation (PVS)
programmer
Omnicor P.
p. pacemaker
Pacesetter APS II 3004 p.
Pacesetter APS pacemaker p.
progression
p. of coronary artery disease (PCAD)
poor R-wave p.
R-wave p. (RWP)
progressive
p. disseminated histoplasmosis (PDH)
p. dyspnea
p. exercise test (PET)
p. interstitial pulmonary fibrosis
p. massive fibrosis (PMF)
p. multifocal leukoencephalopathy (PML)
p. multiple hyaloserositis
p. parenchymal restriction
p. pneumonia
p. pump failure
p. scanning
p. systemic sclerosis (PSS)
p. thrombus
ProHance
proinflammatory
p. cytokine
p. substance
proiosystole, proiosystolia
proischemic
project
bronchoscopy quality improvement p.
coronary drug p. (CDP)
projection
angiographic area of lateral p. (AL)

angiographic area of left anterior oblique p. (ALAO)
angiographic area of right anterior oblique p. (ARAO)
anterior oblique p.
anteroposterior p.
left anterior oblique p.
left lateral p.
right anterior oblique p.
spider p.
steep left anterior oblique p.
projector
Tagarno 3SD cineangiography p.
prolactin-producing decidual cell
prolapse
aortic valve p.
bileaflet p.
p. coil
idiopathic mitral valve p. (IMVP)
mitral valve p. (MPV, MVP)
p. of mitral valve (PMV)
plaque p.
tricuspid valve p. (TVP)
unileaflet p.
valvular p.
prolapsed
p. middle scallop of posterior leaflet
p. mitral valve syndrome
prolapsing
p. mitral leaflet (PML)
p. mitral valvar leaflet
Prolastin
Proleukin
proliferans
endarteritis p.
proliferating
p. cell nuclear antigen (PCNA)
p. pleurisy
proliferation
in-stent neointimal p.
intimal p.
intimal fibrous p. (IFP)
myxomatous p.
neointimal p.
proliferative
p. bronchiolitis
p. diabetic retinopathy (PDR)
prolongation
p. of expiration
p. of P-R interval

NOTES

P

563

prolonged
>p. pulmonary eosinophilia
>p. Q-T interval syndrome

Proloprim

promethazine
>p. and dextromethorphan
>p. hydrochloride
>p., phenylephrine, and codeine

Promine

prominence
>laryngeal p.
>subcutaneous bursa of the
>laryngeal p.

prominent
>p. pulmonary vein
>p. U wave

prominentia laryngea

Promit

promyelocyte

Proneb Ultra nebulizer

prone positioning

Pronestyl
>P.-SR

prongs
>Allegiance nasal p.
>Invacare nasal p.
>Kendall nasal p.
>nasal p.
>Pro-Tech nasal p.
>Sims nasal p.
>Uno nasal p.

Pronova suture

Prony method (PM)

propafenone hydrochloride

propagated thrombus

propagating thrombosis

propagation
>impulse p.
>p. of R wave
>p. of thrombus

propantheline

Propaq Encore vital signs monitor

Pro/Pel
>P. coating
>P. coating cardiac device

propellant
>halogenated hydrocarbon p.

propensity
>systemic thrombotic p.

propeptide
>aminoterminal p.

property
>chemoattracting p.
>p.'s of lipophilicity
>vagolytic p.

prophylactic
>p. antibiotic
>p. aspirin regimen
>p. brain irradiation (PCI)

>p. filter placement
>p. implantable cardioverter-
>defibrillator implantation
>p. therapy
>p. thoracostomy

prophylaxis
>SBE p.

propidium iodide stain

propionate
>fluticasone p. (FP)
>salmeterol and fluticasone p.

Propionibacterium acnes

propionyl-L-carnitine

Proplex T

propofol

proportional assist ventilation (PAV)

propranolol
>p. hydrochloride
>p. and hydrochlorothiazide

proprius

Propulsid

propylthiouracil (PTU)

prorenin

ProSom

prospective gating

prostacyclin (PGI$_2$)
>p. analog UT-15
>p. metabolite

prostaglandin
>p. D2
>p. E, E1
>p. G$_2$
>p. H$_2$

Prostar
>P. 9F, 11F percutaneous vascular
>surgery system
>P. Plus percutaneous vascular
>surgical device
>P. XL hemostatic puncture closure
>device
>P. XL 8, 10 suture mediated
>closure system

prosthesis, pl. **prostheses**
>Alvarez p.
>Angelchik antireflux p.
>antireflux p.
>aortic p.
>ball-and-cage p.
>ball valve p.
>Barnard mitral valve p.
>Beall disk valve p.
>Beall mitral valve p.
>bifurcated aortofemoral p.
>bifurcation p.
>bileaflet p.
>Björk-Shiley aortic valve p.
>Björk-Shiley convexoconcave 60-
>degree valve p.
>Björk-Shiley floating disk p.

blood vessel p. (BVP)
caged ball valve p.
Carbomedics cardiac valve p.
Carbo-Seal ascending aortic p.
cardiac valve p.
Carpentier-Edwards aortic valve p.
Carpentier-Edwards glutaraldehyde-
  preserved porcine xenograft p.
collar p.
Cooley-Bloodwell mitral valve p.
Cutter aortic valve p.
Cutter-Smeloff aortic valve p.
DeBakey ball valve p.
DeBakey Vasculour-II vascular p.
Delrin frame of valve p.
duckbill voice p.
Duromedics valve p.
esophageal p.
Golaski-UMI vascular p.
Gott-Daggett heart valve p.
Groningen voice p.
Hammersmith mitral p.
Hancock mitral valve p.
heart valve p.
Ionescu-Shiley valve p.
knitted vascular p.
Lillehei-Kaster cardiac valve p.
Lillehei-Kaster mitral valve p.
Meadox woven velour p.
mechanical p.
Medtronic-Hall heart valve p.
Medtronic-Hall tilting-disk valve p.
Microknit vascular graft p.
Milliknit Dacron p.
Milliknit vascular graft p.
mitral p.
Monostrut cardiac valve p.
Neville tracheal p.
Omnicarbon heart valve p.
Omniscience single leaflet cardiac
  valve p.
pericarbon pericardial p.
polytetrafluoroethylene p.
polyvinyl p.
porcine p.
Quattro mitral valve p.
single-disk p.
Sorin Bicarbon bileaflet aortic
  valve p.
Sorin mitral valve p.
Starr-Edwards aortic valve p.
Starr-Edwards ball valve p.

Starr-Edwards cardiac valve p.
Starr-Edwards disk valve p.
Starr-Edwards heart valve p.
Starr-Edwards mitral p.
stentless porcine aortic valve p.
St. Jude heart valve p.
St. Jude Medical valve p.
supraannular p.
Teflon trileaflet p.
Teflon woven p.
tilting disk aortic valve p.
Ultra low resistance voice p.
vascular graft p.
Weavenit p.
woven Teflon p.
woven-tube vascular graft p.

prosthetic
  p. aortic valve
  p. ball valve
  p. cardiac valve
  p. infectious endocarditis (PIE)
  p. mitral valve thrombosis
  p. poppet
  p. ring annuloplasty
  St. Jude composite p.
  p. valve endocarditis (PVE)
  p. valve regurgitation (PVR)
  p. valve sewing ring
  p. valve sound
  p. valve stenosis (PVS)
  p. valve vegetation
Prostin VR Pediatric injection
prostration
protamine sulfate
protease
  p. inhibitor (PI)
  mast cell p.
protease-antiprotease imbalance
Pro-Tech nasal prongs
protected
  p. catheter brushing (PCB)
  p. specimen brush (PSB)
  p. specimen brushing (PSB)
protection
  airway p.
  automated boundary p. (ABP)
  myocardial p.
  short transitional edge p. (STEP)
protective
  p. block
  p. ventilation
  p. zone

NOTES

P

protector
    pulse-oximetry p.
Protegra
protegrin antimicrobial peptide
protein
    p. A
    activator p. (AP)
    alpha-B-crystallin p.
    amyloid A p.
    amyloid precursor p. (APP)
    apolipoprotein regulatory p. (APR)
    p. B
    bone morphogenetic p. type 2
      (BMP-2)
    BvgS p.
    cardiac gap junction p.
    CD45 cell surface p.
    p. C deficiency
    cholesteryl ester transfer p. (CETP)
    Clara cell secretory p.
    coagulation p.
    contractile p.
    C-reactive p. (CRP)
    CTLA4Ig p.
    cytosolic p.
    p. electrophoresis
    enhanced green fluorescent p.
      (eGFP)
    eosinophil cationic p. (ECP)
    fatty acid binding p. (FABP)
    G p.
    G_i p.
    Gc p.
    glycosylation of intracellular p.'s
    $gp91^{phox}$ p.
    heat shock p. (HSP, Hsp, hsp)
    high-density lipoprotein binding p.
      (HDLBP)
    high-sensitivity C-reactive p.
    45-kilodalton p.
    p. kinase (PKase)
    p. kinase A (PKA)
    p. kinase C (PKC)
    lipoprotein receptor-related p. (LRP)
    M p.
    macrophage inflammatory p. (MPI)
    melanoma inhibitory activity p.
    MIA p.
    microsomal triglyceride transfer p.
      (MTP)
    mitogen-activated p. (MAP)
    M-line p.
    monocyte chemoattractant p. (MCP)
    myosin-binding p. C (MyBP-C)
    natural resistance macrophage-
      associated p. (Nramp)
    NF-ATc p.
    overexpressed p.
    $p22^{phox}$ p.

    $p47^{phox}$ p.
    $p67^{phox}$ p.
    protooncogenic p.
    rat urine p.
    recognition p.
    p. S
    p. S-100B
    p. S deficiency
    secretory leukoprotease inhibitor p.
    soy p.
    STAT4 p.
    STAT6 p.
    sterol regulatory element-binding p.
      (SREBP)
    surfactant p. (SP)
    Tamm-Horsfall p.
    thrombus precursor p. (TpT)
    ToxR p.
    p. tyrosine phosphatase-gamma
      (PTP-gamma)
    tyrosine phosphorylated p.
    underexpressed p.
protein-1
    macrophage inflammatory p.-1
      (MIP-1)
    monocyte chemoattractant p.-1
      (MCP-1)
    monocyte chemotactic p.-1 (MCP-1)
proteinase
    p. inhibitor phenotype (Pi)
protein-calorie
    p.-c. deficiency
    p.-c. malnutrition
protein-losing enteropathy (PLE)
proteinosis
    alveolar p.
    pulmonary alveolar p.
proteinuria
proteoglycan
proteolysis
    quantum p.
proteolytic enzyme
Proteus
    P. mirabilis
    P. pneumonia
    P. syndrome
    P. vulgaris
Protex swivel adapter
prothrombin
    p. activity (PTA)
    p. complex (PTC)
    p. G20210A mutated allele
    p. time (PT, PTT)
    p. time fixing agent (PTFA)
    p. time/partial thromboplastin time
      (PT/PTT)
    p. time ratio (PTR)
prothrombinase complex

prothrombosis
 systemic p.
prothrombotic state
protocol
 ABC p.
 Astrand-Rhyming p.
 Balke treadmill p.
 Balke-Ware treadmill p.
 Bruce treadmill p.
 cardiac rehabilitation p.
 CEqual Lite cardiac
  rehabilitation p.
 CEqual Plus cardiac
  rehabilitation p.
 chronotropic exercise assessment p.
  (CAEP)
 continuous ramp p.
 Cornell exercise p.
 Cornell modification of the
  Bruce p.
 Ellestad p.
 exsanguination p.
 high-ramp p.
 James exercise p.
 Kattus treadmill p.
 LITE p.
 low-ramp p.
 MacNamara p.
 Mayo exercise treadmill p.
 McHenry p.
 McNamara p.
 moderate-ramp p.
 modified Bruce p.
 modified Ellestad p.
 Naughton treadmill p.
 PHRT p.
 procarbazine, hydroxyurea,
  radiotherapy p.
 RAMP antitachycardia p.
 RAMP-based p.
 RAMP treadmill p.
 Reeves treadmill p.
 reinjection p.
 resident assessment p. (RAP)
 rest metabolism/stress perfusion p.
 Sheffield modification of Bruce
  treadmill p.
 Sheffield treadmill p.
 standard Bruce p.
 Stanford treadmill exercise p.
 step treadmill p.
 TAMI p.

 therapist-driven p. (TDP)
 USAFSAM treadmill exercise p.
 weaning p.
 Weber-Janicki cardiopulmonary
  exercise p.
 Westminster drug-free p.
protodiastolic
 p. gallop
 p. murmur
 p. rumble
protofibril
protokylol hydrochloride
proton
 p. density
 p. pump inhibitor
 p. spectroscopy
proton-beam radiotherapy
Protonix
protooncogene
protooncogenic
 p. effect
 p. protein
 p. protein kinase
protoplasmic block
protoporphyrin
 erythrocyte p.
 free p.
 p. IX
 zinc p.
protoveratrine A, B
protozoal myocarditis
protozoan
protriptyline hydrochloride
protruding atheroma
protuberantia laryngea
protuberant plaque
prourokinase
 recombinant p.
Pro-Vent
 P.-V. arterial blood gas kit
 P.-V. arterial blood sampling kit
Proventil HFA
Provera Oral
Providencia
Provigil
provocation
 bronchial p.
 histamine p.
 p. test
Provocholine
provoking agent
Provox speaking valve

NOTES

P

prowazekii
    Rickettsia p.
proxetil
    cefpodoxime p.
proximal
    p. convoluted tubule
    p. coronary sinus (PCS)
    p. and distal portion of vessel
    p. flow convergence method
    p. isovelocity surface area (PISA)
    p. segment
    p. stenosis
proximal-to-distal (P/D)
PRP
    platelet-rich plasma
    polyribosylribitol phosphate
    pulse repetition period
PRP-D
    polyribosylribitol phosphate-diphtheria
    toxoid conjugate
    PRP-D vaccine
PRP-OMPC vaccine
PRR
    pulmonary reimplantation response
    pulse repetition rate
PR/RP ratio
PRS wave
PRT
    percutaneous rotational thrombectomy
PRU
    peripheral resistance unit
prudent diet
Pruitt-Inahara carotid shunt
prune
    p. juice expectoration
    p. juice sputum
pruning
    branch vessel p.
pruritus
    poststroke p.
Prussian helmet sign
PRVC
    pressure-regulated volume control
    PRVC ventilation
**PRx implantable cardioverter-
  defibrillator**
PS
    pacemaker syndrome
    Palmaz-Schatz
    pulmonary sequestration
    pulmonary stenosis
    pulmonic stenosis
    PS 153 stent
Ps
    systolic pressure
PSA
    systemic blood pressure
    PSA stationary oxygen system
psammoma bodies

psammosarcoma
PSAP
    peak systolic aortic pressure
PSB
    protected specimen brush
    protected specimen brushing
PSC
    pulse synchronized contractions
PSD
    poststenosis dilation
    power spectral density
PSDI
    Positive Symptom Distress Index
PSE
    paradoxical systolic expansion
P-selectin
    P.-s. cell adhesion molecule
    P.-s. expression
P-Series sleep monitoring system
Pseudallescheria
    P. boydii
    P. maltophilia
    P. stutzeri
pseudallescheriasis
pseudangina, pseudoangina
pseudo
    p. R', S wave
pseudoalternating current
pseudoaneurysm
    arterial p.
    femoral p.
pseudoangina (*var. of* pseudangina)
pseudoapoplexy
pseudoasthma
pseudo-A-V block
pseudobronchiectasis
pseudobulbar palsy
Pseudo-Car DM
pseudocavitation
pseudocholinesterase deficiency
pseudochylothorax
pseudocirrhosis
pseudocoarctation of aorta
pseudocomplication
pseudocroup
pseudocylindrical bronchiectasis
pseudocyst
    posttraumatic pulmonary p.
    pulmonary p.
pseudodextrocardia
pseudodiastolic
pseudodiphtheriticum
    Bacillus p.
pseudodisappearance criterion
pseudoejection sound
pseudoephedrine
    acetaminophen, dextromethorphan, p.
    acrivastine and p.
    carbinoxamine and p.

chlorpheniramine and p.
p. and dextromethorphan
guaifenesin and p.
p. HCl
hydrocodone and p.
p. and ibuprofen
triprolidine and p.
pseudoexudate
pseudofusion beat
pseudoheart disease (PsHD)
pseudohypoparathyroidism
pseudohypotension
pseudoinfarction
pseudo-Kaposi sarcoma
pseudolumen
pseudolupus
pseudo-Mahaim fiber
pseudomalfunction
pseudomallei
  Pseudomonas p.
pseudomembranous
  p. angina
  p. *Aspergillus* tracheobronchitis
  p. bronchitis
  p. croup
  p. tracheobronchial aspergillosis
pseudomonad
Pseudomonas
  P. aeruginosa
  P. cepacia
  P. elastase
  P. exotoxin
  P. maltophilia
  P. pseudomallei
  P. stutzeri
pseudomucinous
pseudonormalization
  p. of T wave
  T-wave p.
pseudoparalytica
  myasthenia gravis p.
pseudopericarditis
pseudopneumonia
pseudopodia
pseudo-P pulmonale
pseudothrombocytopenia
pseudotruncus arteriosus
pseudotuberculosis
  Yersinia p.
pseudotumor
  inflammatory p. (IPT)
pseudotumoral mediastinal amyloidosis

Pseudovent
pseudoxanthoma
  p. elasticum
  p. elasticum syndrome
PSG
  peak systolic gradient
  polysomnogram
  polysomnography
  presystolic gallop
  full PSG
  PSG LOC guidewire extension
  PSG pressure
PsHD
  pseudoheart disease
PSI
  Pneumonia Severity Index
psi
  pounds per square inch
psig
  pounds per square inch gauge
P-sinistrocardiale
psittaci
  Chlamydia p.
psittacosis inclusion bodies
PSM
  presystolic murmur
PSP
  peak systolic pressure
  periodic short pulse
  primary spontaneous pneumothorax
PSS
  Palmaz-Schatz stent
  progressive systemic sclerosis
  pure sensory syndrome
PST
  paroxysmal supraventricular tachycardia
  positive symptom total
  poststenotic
PSV
  positive support ventilator
  pressure support ventilation
  pressure support ventilator
PSVT
  paroxysmal supraventricular tachycardia
psychic akinesia
psychocardiac reflex
psychogenic
  p. cough
  p. dyspnea
  p. overlay
  p. pain
  p. syncope

NOTES

P

psychological
> p. factor
> p. stimulus

psychophysiological interventions in myocardial ischemia (PIMI)

psychosis
> postperfusion p.

Psychosocial
> P. Adjustment to Illness Scale
> P.'s factor

psychostimulant

psychotherapy

psychotropic agent

psyllium

PT
> paroxysmal tachycardia
> pericardial tamponade
> prothrombin time
> pulmonary thrombosis
> thromboplastin

PTA
> percutaneous transluminal angioplasty
> persistent truncus arteriosus
> plasma thromboplastin antecedent
> prothrombin activity

PTAS
> percutaneous transluminal angioscopy

PTB
> pulmonary tuberculosis

PTBA
> percutaneous transluminal balloon angioplasty

PTBD
> percutaneous transluminal balloon dilatation

PTC
> peritubular capillary
> plasma thromboplastin component
> prothrombin complex

PTCA
> percutaneous transluminal coronary angioplasty
>> perfusion balloon PTCA
>> rescue PTCA

PTCR
> percutaneous transluminal coronary recanalization
> percutaneous transluminal coronary revascularization

PTCRA
> percutaneous transluminal coronary rotational ablation

PTD
> percutaneous thrombolytic device
> percutaneous transluminal dilatation
> photodynamic therapy

PtdCho
> phosphatidylcholine

PTED
> pulmonary thromboembolic disease

PTEF
> peak tidal expiratory flow

pteronyssinus
>> Dermatophagoides p.

pterygia, heart defects, autosomal recessive inheritance, vertebral defects, ear anomalies, radial defects (PHAVER)

pterygoid chest

pterygopalatine ganglion

PTF
> plasma thromboplastin factor

PTFA
> prothrombin time fixing agent

PTFE
> polytetrafluoroethylene
>> PTFE closure
>> PTFE stent graft

PTFE-covered stent

PTH
> plasma thromboplastin component

Pth
> chest wall elastic recoil pressure

PTIF
> peak tidal inspiratory flow

PTJV
> percutaneous transtracheal jet ventilation

PTL
> pharyngeal tracheal lumen
> pharyngotracheal lumen airway
> plasma thyroxine level
> posterior tricuspid leaflet

PTLA
> pharyngotracheal lumen airway

PtL airway

PTLPD, PTLD
> posttransplantation lymphoproliferative disorder
>> intrathoracic PTLPD

PTM
> pulse time modulation

PTMC
> percutaneous transvenous mitral commissurotomy

PTMR
> percutaneous transluminal myocardial revascularization
> percutaneous transmyocardial revascularization

PTNB
> percutaneous transthoracic needle biopsy

PTP
> pressure time product

Ptp
> transpulmonary pressure

PTP-gamma
> protein tyrosine phosphatase-gamma

PT/PTT
  prothrombin time/partial thromboplastin
    time
PTR
  prothrombin time ratio
PTRA
  percutaneous transluminal renal
    angioplasty
  percutaneous transluminal rotational
    atherectomy
PTSMA
  percutaneous transluminal septal
    myocardial ablation
PTT
  partial thromboplastin time
  prothrombin time
  pulse transmission time
ptt
  partial thromboplastin time
PTU
  propylthiouracil
public
  p. access defibrillation (PAD)
  p. access to defibrillation (PAD)
  p. access defibrillator (PAD)
  P. Health Response Team (PHRT)
puerile respiration
puerperal
  p. phlebitis
  p. thrombosis
**Puerto Rico Heart Health Program
  (PRHHP)**
PUFA
  polyunsaturated fatty acid
puff
  p. of smoke
  veiled p.
puffball
puffer
puffing sound
Puig
  P. Massana annuloplasty ring
  P. Massana-Shiley annuloplasty ring
  P. Massana-Shiley annuloplasty
    valve
pullback
  aortic p.
  p. atherectomy device
  p. pressure
pulley
pull-through
  station p.-t.

Pulmanex resuscitator
Pulmicort
  P. Respules
  P. Turbuhaler
pulmo
  p. dexter
  p. sinister
Pulmo-Aide
  P.-A. aerosol compressor/nebulizer
  P.-A. nebulizer
  P.-A. Traveler
pulmoaortic canal
Pulmocare
Pulmo-Graph
pulmolith
PulmoMate aerosol compressor/nebulizer
Pulmo-Mist compressor
pulmonale
  acute cor p.
  acutely decompensated cor p.
  atrium p.
  chronic cor p.
  cor p. (CP)
  glomus p.
  ligamentum p.
  P p.
  pseudo-P p.
pulmonales
  nodi lymphoidei
    juxtaesophageales p.
  venae p.
pulmonalis
  arteria p.
  ostium trunci p.
  pars basalis arteriae p.
  pleura p.
  plexus p.
  sinus trunci p.
  sulcus p.
  truncus p.
  valva trunci p.
pulmonalium
  ostia venarum p.
pulmonary
  p. acid aspiration syndrome
  p. acinus
  p. actinomycosis
  p. adenomatosis
  p. agenesis
  p. air embolism
  p. alveolar hemorrhage
  p. alveolar hypoventilation (PAH)

NOTES

P

pulmonary (*continued*)

p. alveolar hypoxic vasoconstrictor (PAHVC)
p. alveolar microlithiasis (PAM)
p. alveolar proteinosis
p. alveolus
p. amebiasis
p. amyloidosis
p. angiogram
p. angiography (PA, PAG)
p. angiotensin I converting enzyme
p. anomalous superior venous return (PASVR)
p. anthrax
p. aplasia
p. arch
p. arterial (PA, Pa)
p. arterial capillary wedge pressure (PACWP)
p. arterial end-diastolic pressure
p. arterial pressure
p. arterial pressure, pulmonary venous pressure (pa-pv)
p. arterial stenosis (PAS)
p. arterial system
p. arterial wave pressure
p. arterial web
p. arteriolar resistance (PAR)
p. arterioplasty
p. arteriovenous fistula (PAF, PAVF)
p. arteriovenous malformation (PAVM)
p. arteritides
p. artery (PA)
p. artery balloon pump (PABP)
p. artery band
p. artery banding
p. artery catheterization (PAC)
p. artery counterpulsation (PACP)
p. artery diastolic (PAD)
p. artery diastolic pressure (PADP)
p. artery end-diastolic pressure (PAEDP)
p. artery filling defect (PAFD)
p. artery flotation catheter
p. artery homograft
p. artery hypertension (PAH)
p. artery hypotension (PAH)
p. artery mean pressure (PAMP)
p. artery occlusion (PAO)
p. artery occlusion pressure (PAo, PAOP)
p. artery occlusive wedge pressure
p. artery pressure (PAP, Ppa)
p. artery rupture
p. artery sling
p. artery steal
p. artery stenosis

p. artery systolic (PAS)
p. artery systolic pressure (PASP)
p. artery thromboembolism (PATE)
p. artery wedge (PAW)
p. artery wedge pressure (PAWP, Ppaw)
p. aspergillosis
p. atresia (PA)
p. atresia with ventricular septal defect (PAVSD)
p. autograft (PA)
p. autograft valve
p. A-V O_2 difference
p. balloon valvuloplasty (PBV)
p. barotrauma
basal part of left and right inferior p.
p. bed gradient
p. blastoma
p. blood flow (PBF, Qp)
p. blood mixing volume (PBMV)
p. blood volume (PBV)
p. botryomycosis
p. branch of autonomic
p. branch stenosis (PBS)
p. bulla
p. calcification
p. capillary blood flow (Qc, Qpc)
p. capillary blood volume (Vc)
p. capillary pressure (PCP)
p. capillary wedge (PCW)
p. capillary wedge pressure (PCWP)
p. cavitation
p. cavity
p. circulation (PC)
p. coccidioidomycosis
p. coin lesion
p. compliance (PC)
p. component of second heart sound
p. cone
p. congestion
p. consolidation
p. contusion
p. conus
p. cryptococcosis
p. cyanosis
p. DCS
p. diffusion capacity (D_{CO})
p. disease anemia syndrome
p. dysmaturity syndrome
p. dyspnea
p. edema (PE)
p. edema fluid (PEF)
p. effusion
p. ejection click (PEC)
p. embolectomy
p. embolism (PE)

p. embolization
p. embolus
p. emphysema (PE)
p. epithelium
p. failure
p. fat embolism syndrome
p. fever
p. fibrosis
p. function (PF)
P. Functional Status and Dyspnea Questionnaire (PFSDQ)
p. functional status scale (PFSS)
p. function status
p. function test (PFT)
p. gas exchange
p. glomangiosis
p. hamartoma
p. heart
p. hematoma
p. hemodynamics
p. hemosiderosis
p. hilum
p. hyalinizing granuloma
p. hyperinfection syndrome
p. hypertension (PH, PHT)
p. hypertension pressure
p. hypertrophic osteoarthropathy
p. hypoplasia, hypoplasia of pulmonary artery, agonadism, omphalocele/diaphragmatic defect, dextrocardia (PAGOD)
p. hypostasis
p. incompetence
p. infarct
p. infarction (PI)
p. infarction syndrome
p. infiltrates with eosinophilia syndrome
p. infiltrate with eosinophilia (PIE)
p. infiltration with eosinophilia (PIE)
p. insufficiency
p. interstitial edema
p. interstitial emphysema (PIE)
p. Langerhans cell histiocytosis
p. leukostasis
p. ligament
p. lobule
p. lymphangioleiomyomatosis
p. lymphangiomyomatosis
p. lymph node
p. lymphoma

p. meniscus sign
p. metastasectomy
p. microthromboembolism
p. mucormycosis
p. murmur
p. mycosis
p. nervous plexus
p. notch sign
p. oligemia
p. orifice
p. ossification
p. outflow tract
p. pain
p. parenchyma
p. parenchymal injury
p. parenchymal window
p. phthisis
p. pleura
p. pleurisy
p. pseudocyst
p. pulse
p. rale
p. reexpansion
p. regurgitation (P-R)
p. reimplantation response (PRR)
p. resistance
p. restriction
p. ridge
p. sarcoidosis
p. scintigraphy
p. sequestration (PS)
p. shunt
p. sinus
p. sling syndrome
p. stenosis (PS)
p. sulcus
p. surfactant
p. systemic blood flow ratio
p. target sign
p. thromboembolic disease (PTED)
p. thromboembolism
p. thrombosis (PT)
p. toilet
p. transpiration
p. trunk
p. tuberculosis (PTB)
p. valve (PV)
p. valve anomaly
p. valve area
p. valve disease
p. valve echocardiography
p. valve gradient (PVG)

NOTES

P

pulmonary *(continued)*
p. valve repair (PVR)
p. valve replacement (PVR)
p. valve restenosis
p. valve stenosis
p. valve vegetation
p. valvotomy
p. valvular regurgitation
p. valvular stenosis (PVS)
p. valvuloplasty
p. vascular bed
p. vascular disease (PVD)
p. vascular marking
p. vascular obstruction (PVO)
p. vascular obstructive disease
(PVOD)
p. vascular pressure
p. vascular reactivity
p. vascular redistribution
p. vascular resistance (PVR)
p. vascular resistance index (PVRI)
p. vasculature
p. vasculitis
p. vasoconstriction
p. vasodilation
p. vein (PV)
p. venoocclusive disease (PVOD)
p. venous atrial (PVa)
p. venous atrium
p. venous confluence (PVC)
p. venous congestion (PVC)
p. venous connection
p. venous connection anomaly
p. venous drainage
p. venous flow (PVF)
p. venous hypertension (PVH,
PVHI)
p. venous pressure (PVP)
p. venous return
p. venous return anomaly
p. venous systolic (PVs)
p. ventilation
p. wedge (PW)
p. wedge angiography
p. wedge pressure (Ppw, PWP)
pulmonary-to-systemic
p.-t.-s. flow ratio (Qp:Qs)
p.-t.-s. vascular resistance (Rp:Rs)
pulmonic
aortic end p.
p. area
p. closure (PC)
p. endocarditis
p. incompetence
p. insufficiency
p. murmur
p. regurgitation
p. second heart sound (P2)
p. stenosis (PS)

p. tricuspid
p. valve
p. valve closure sound
p. valve stenosis
pulmonic-to-systemic flow ratio (Qp:Qs)
pulmonis
alveoli p.
apex p.
basis p.
facies costalis p.
facies interlobares p.
facies medialis p.
facies mediastinalis p.
fissura obliqua p.
hilum p.
impressio cardiaca p.
ligamentum latum p.
margo anterior p.
margo inferior p.
pars mediastinalis p.
pulmonitis
pulmonocoronary reflex
pulmonologist
PulmoSonic nebulizer
PulmoSphere
PulmoTrack respiratory sound analyzer
Pulmowrap
Pulmozyme
Pulsair .5 liquid oxygen portable
Pulsar
P. DDD pacemaker
P. Max sensor
P. NI implantable pacemaker
pulsate
pulsatile
p. assist device (PAD)
p. flow
pulsatility index (PI)
pulsating
p. empyema
p. pleurisy
pulsation
ascending aorta synchronized p.
(AASP)
intraaortic balloon p. (IABP)
presystolic p.
suprasternal p.
pulsations
jugular venous p. (JVP)
Pulsator
P. dry heparin arterial blood gas
kit
P. syringe
pulse (p) *(See also* pulsus)
abdominal p.
abrupt p.
alternating p.
p. amplitude
amplitude of p.

p. amplitude modulation (PAM)
p. amplitude ratio (PAR)
anacrotic p.
anadicrotic p.
apical p. (AP)
arterial p.
atrial liver p.
atrial venous p.
p. average intensity (Ipa)
Bamberger bulbar p.
bigeminal bisferious p.
bisferious p.
blood pressure and p. (BP&P)
blood volume p. (BVP)
bounding p.
brachial p.
bulbar p.
cannonball p.
capillary p.
carotid p.
catacrotic p.
catadicrotic p.
catatricrotic p.
centripetal venous p.
collapsing p.
cordy p.
Corrigan p.
coupled p.
C point of cardiac apex p.
p. curve
CV wave of jugular venous p.
C wave of jugular venous p.
p. deficit
dicrotic p.
digitalate p.
dorsalis pedis p.
p. duration (PD)
elastic p.
entoptic p.
filiform p.
formicant p.
F point of cardiac apex p.
funic p.
f wave of jugular venous p.
gaseous p.
p. generator
guttural p.
hard p.
hyperkinetic p.
hypokinetic p.
I_{sata} p.
I_{sapt} p.

I_{sa} p.
incisura p.
intermittent p.
p. inversion harmonic imaging
irregularly irregular p.
Isp p.
Ita p.
Itp p.
jerky p.
jugular vein p. (JVP)
jugular venous p.
Kussmaul paradoxical p.
labile p.
long p.
maximum digital p. (MDP)
p. method
Monneret p.
monocrotic p.
monophasic p.
mousetail p.
movable p.
myurous p.
nail p.
O point of cardiac apex p.
p. oximeter
3800 p. oximeter
p. oximeter/end tidal CO_2 (POET)
p. oximetry (PO)
p. oximetry device
p. oximetry monitoring (POM)
paradoxic p.
paradoxical p. (PP)
parietal p. (PP)
pedal p.
p. period
periodic short p. (PSP)
piston p.
plateau p.
popliteal p.
p. position modulated (PPM)
posterior tibial p.
precordial p.
presaturation p.
p. pressure (PP)
pressure p.
P. Pro heart rate monitor
P. Pro heart rate monitor watch
pulmonary p.
quadrigeminal p.
quick p.
Quincke p.
radial p. (RP)

NOTES

P

pulse *(continued)*

p. rate (P-R)
p. repetition (P-R)
p. repetition frequency (PRF)
p. repetition period (PRP)
p. repetition rate (PRR)
p. and respiration (P&R)
respiratory p.
reversed paradoxical p.
Riegel p.
SF wave of cardiac apex p.
soft p.
spatial average p. average (I_{sapa})
spike-and-dome p.
standard temperature and p. (STP)
sustained p.
p. synchronized contractions (PSC)
temperature and p. (T&P, T+P)
tense p.
thready p.
tibial p.
tidal wave p.
p. time modulation (PTM)
p. tracing
p. transmission time (PTT)
trigeminal p.
triphammer p.
triple-humped pressure p.
p. trisection
ulnar p.
undulating p.
unequal p.
vagus p.
venous p.
vermicular p.
p. volume recording (PVR)
V peak of jugular venous p.
water hammer p.
p. wave
p. wave duration
p. wave velocity (PWV)
p. width
wiry p.
p. with modulation (PWM)
X depression of jugular venous p.
X descent of jugular venous p.
Y depression of jugular venous p.
Y descent of jugular venous p.

pulsed

p. diastolic (PD)
p. diastolic autologous blood
  selective aortic arch perfusion
  (PD-AB-SAAP)
p. Doppler cross-sectional
  echocardiography (PD-CSE)
p. Doppler echocardiography (PDE)
p. Doppler flowmetry
p. Doppler tissue imaging
p. dye laser

p. laser ablation
p. wave (PW)

PulseDose

P. EX2000D oxygen conserver
P. oxygen delivery technology
P. portable compressed oxygen
  system

**pulsed-spray pharmomechanical
thrombolysis**
pulsed-wave

p.-w. Doppler (PWD)
p.-w. Doppler mapping
p.-w. tissue Doppler (PWTD)

2-MHz pulsed-wave Doppler transducer
pulse-height analyzer
pulseless

p. bradycardia
p. disease
p. electrical activity (PEA)
p. idioventricular rhythm

pulse-oximetry protector
pulses per minute (ppm)
PulseSpray infusion system
**pulse-spray pharmomechanical
thrombolysis**
pulsimeter, pulsometer
Pulsox-5 pulse oximeter
PulStar pneumatic wrap system
pulsus *(See also* pulse)

p. alternans
p. anadicrotus
p. bigeminus
p. bisferiens
p. caprisans
p. catacrotus
p. celer
p. celerrimus
p. cordis
p. debilis
p. differens
p. duplex
p. durus
p. filiformis
p. fluens
p. formicans
p. fortis
p. frequens
p. heterochronicus
p. inaequalis
p. incongruens
p. infrequens
p. intercidens
p. intercurrens
p. irregularis
p. irregularis perpetuus
p. magnus
p. mollis
p. monocrotus
p. myurus

p. paradoxus (PP)
p. parvus
p. parvus et tardus
p. plenus
p. quadrigeminus
p. rarus
p. tremulus
p. trigeminus
p. vacuus
p. venosus
p. vibrans

pultaceous debris
Pulvinal
Pulvules

Cinobac P.
Seromycin P.

Pumactant
pumilus

Bacillus p.

pump

Abbott infusion p.
abdominothoracic p.
Acat 1 intraaortic balloon p.
Affinity blood p.
AutoCat intraaortic balloon p.
AVCO balloon p.
Axiom double sump p.
balloon p.
Bio-Medicus p.
blood p.
BVS p.
CADD-Plus intravenous infusion p.
cardiopulmonary bypass p.
centrifugal p.
Cormed ambulatory infusion p.
p. current
Datascope System 90 intraaortic
  balloon p.
DeBakey VAD continuous-axial-
  flow p.
ECMO p.
Emerson p.
p. failure
p. failure death
Flowtron DVT p.
p. function
Gomco thoracic drainage p.
Harvard p.
heart p.
HeartMate p.
Imed Gemini PCI-IV p.
Imed infusion p.

impeller p.
Infusaid infusion p.
Infuse-A-Port p.
intraaortic balloon p. (IABP)
ion p.
Jobst extremity p.
KAAT II Plus intraaortic
  balloon p.
Kangaroo p.
Kontron intraaortic balloon p.
left ventricular assist system
  implantable p.
left ventricular bypass p. (LVBP)
Life Care P.
Lindbergh p.
p. lung
Master Flow Pumpette p.
Medtronic SynchroMed p.
muscular venous p.
Neuroperfusion p.
p. oxygenation
p. oxygenator
pulmonary artery balloon p.
  (PABP)
Quest Medical MPS cardioplegia
  fluid delivery p.
Reitan catheter p.
respiratory p.
roller p.
sodium-potassium p. (NaK-ATPase)
sump p.
SynchroMed programmable p.
Thoratec p.
TransAct intraaortic balloon p.
Travenol infusion p.
volumetric infusion p.

pump-assisted coronary hemoperfusion
Pumpette

Stat 2 P.

pumping

intraaortic balloon p. (IABP, IBP)
venoarterial bypass p. (VABP)

pumpkin-seeding
punch

Abrams pleural biopsy p.
p. biopsy
Goosen vascular p.

punctate

p. hyperintensity
p. mucosal lesion

puncture

apical left ventricular p.

NOTES

P

puncture *(continued)*
    computer-assisted pericardial p. (CASPER)
    direct cardiac p.
    left ventricular p.
    tracheoesophageal p.
    transcricothyroid p.
    transseptal p.
    venous p.
    ventricular p.
pup cell
pupil
    Argyll Robertson p.
Pura-Vario-AL stent
Pura-Vario-AS stent
Pura-Vario-A stent
Pura-Vario stent
pure
    p. dysarthria (PD)
    p. flutter
    p. motor hemiparesis (PMH)
    p. motor stroke
    p. parasystole
    p. pneumothorax
    p. pulmonary atresia (PPA)
    p. sensorimotor stroke
    p. sensory stroke
    p. sensory syndrome (PSS)
purified
    p. protein derivative (PPD)
    p. protein derivative test
    p. protein derivative of tuberculin
purifier
    Air Supply wearable air p.
    Bemis air p.
purine nucleotides adenosine triphosphate
purinergic action
purinoceptor
    endothelial p.
Puritan
    P. all purpose compressor
    P. Bennett Aeris 590 oxygen concentrator
    P. Bennett 7250 metabolic monitor
    P. Bennett ventilator
Purkinje
    P. cell
    P. conduction
    P. disease
    P. fiber
    P. image tracker
    P. network
    P. system
    P. tumor
Purkinje-HIS (P-H)
Purmann method
puromucous
purple grape juice

purpose
    low energy all-P. (LEAP)
purpura
    allergy p.
    anaphylactoid p.
    p. fulminans
    Henoch-Schönlein p.
    idiopathic thrombocytopenic p. (ITP)
    thrombotic thrombocytopenic p. (TTP)
purpurea
    Digitalis p.
purr
purring thrill
pursed-lip breathing
pursestring suture
pursing
    lip p.
Pursuit balloon angioplasty catheter
purulent
    p. effusion
    p. pericarditis (PP)
    p. pleurisy
    p. pneumonia
    p. sputum
purulenta
    pneumonia interlobularis p.
pushability
pusher wire
putative slow pathway potential
putrid
    p. bronchitis
    p. empyema
    p. sputum
PV
    plasma viscosity
    portal vein
    pulmonary valve
    pulmonary vein
    ventricular pressure
PVA
    polyvinyl alcohol
    PVA foam embolization particle
PVa
    pulmonary venous atrial
PVAB
    postventricular atrial blanking
pVAD
    TandemHeart p.
PVARP
    postventricular atrial refractory period
PVB
    premature ventricular beat
PVC
    polyvinyl chloride
    premature ventricular contraction
    pulmonary venous confluence
    pulmonary venous congestion

PVD
    peripheral vascular disease
    portal vein dilation
    premature ventricular depolarization
    pulmonary vascular disease
PVE
    premature ventricular extrasystole
    prosthetic valve endocarditis
PVF
    portal venous flow
    primary ventricular fibrillation
    pulmonary venous flow
PVF K tablet
PVG
    pulmonary valve gradient
PVH, PVHI
    periventricular hyperintensity
    pulmonary venous hypertension
PVI
    perivascular infiltration
PVL
    perivalvular leakage
PVO
    pulmonary vascular obstruction
PVOD
    pulmonary vascular obstructive disease
    pulmonary venoocclusive disease
PVP
    peripheral venous pressure
    pulmonary venous pressure
PVR
    peripheral vascular resistance
    prosthetic valve regurgitation
    pulmonary valve repair
    pulmonary valve replacement
    pulmonary vascular resistance
    pulse volume recording
PVRI
    pulmonary vascular resistance index
PVS
    premature ventricular systole
    programmed ventricular stimulation
    prosthetic valve stenosis
    pulmonary valvular stenosis
PVs
    pulmonary venous systolic
PVT
    paroxysmal ventricular tachycardia
    portal vein thrombosis
    primary ventricular tachycardia
PV-Tussin

PW
    peristaltic wave
    posterior wall
    pressure wave
    pulmonary wedge
    pulsed wave
      PW pressure
P-wave duration
PWD
    pulsed-wave Doppler
PWE
    posterior wall excursion
PWI
    perfusion-weighted MRI
    posterior wall infarct
PWLV
    posterior wall of left ventricle
PWM
    pulse with modulation
PWP
    pulmonary wedge pressure
PWTD
    pulsed-wave tissue Doppler
PWV
    pulse wave velocity
pycnogenol
pyemia
    arterial p.
    portal p.
pyemic embolism
pyknosis
pylori
    Helicobacter p.
pyloric incompetence
pyocyanine
pyogenes
    Streptococcus p.
pyogenic infection
Pyopen
pyopneumopericardium
pyopneumothorax
pyothorax-associated lymphoma
PYP
    pyrophosphate
    PYP imaging
    PYP scan
pyramid
    Food Guide p.
    Mediterranean Diet p.
    p. method

NOTES

pyrantel pamoate
pyrazinamide (PZA)
    rifampin, isoniazid, and p.
pyrexia
Pyribenzamine (PBZ)
pyridazinone dinitrile
pyridoxalated
    stroma-free hemoglobin p. (SFHb)
    p. stroma-free hemoglobin (SFHb)
pyridoxine hydrochloride
pyriform (*var. of* piriform)
pyrimethamine
    sulfadoxine and p.
pyrogenic mediator
pyrogen reaction

pyrolytic carbon
pyrophosphate (PYP)
    p. imaging
    p. scan
    p. scintigram
    p. scintigraphy
    technetium p.
    technetium-99m p.
pyruvate dehydrogenase (PDH)
pyruvic acid
PZA
    pyrazinamide
Pzf
    zero-flow pressure

Q
- Q fever
- Q Port
- Q wave
- Q wave regression

Q̇
- cardiac output

QALY
- quality-adjusted life-years

QAR
- quantitative autoradiography

Qc
- pulmonary capillary blood flow

QCA
- quantitative coronary angiography
- quantitative coronary arteriography

Q-cath
- Q-c. catheterization recording system

QC 253 CO-oximetry control
QCS
- quick confusion scale

QCT
- quantitative computed tomography

QCU
- qualitative coronary ultrasound

Q-H interval
QMC
- quadricusp mitral valve

QMI
- Q-wave myocardial infarction

Q-M interval
QMV
- quadricusp mitral valve

QOM
- quality of movement

Qp
- pulmonary blood flow

Qpc
- pulmonary capillary blood flow

Q-Plex metabolic cart and pulmonary function unit
Qp:Qs
- pulmonary-to-systemic flow ratio
- pulmonic-to-systemic flow ratio

Q_s/Q_t
- intrapulmonary shunt fraction

QQ, QR, TT genotype
QR, Q-R
- QR interval

QRB interval
QR, QS pattern
QRS
- complex of Q, R, S, waves corresponding to depolarization of ventricles

- QRS alternans
- QRS axis
- QRS change
- QRS complex
- QRS complex configuration
- QRS complex duration
- QRS contour
- fusion QRS
- QRS interval
- QRS loop
- QRS morphology
- QRS synchronous atrial defibrillation shocks
- QRS vector

QRS-ST junction
QRS-T
- angle between QRS and T vectors
- QRS-T angle
- QRS-T complex
- QRS-T interval
- QRS-T value

QS
- monophasic negative QRS complex
- QS complex
- QS deflection
- QS pattern
- QS wave

QS_2
- total electromechanical systole
- $Q-S_2$ interval

Qs
- systemic blood flow

QSQT
- shunted blood to total blood flow
- QSQT ratio

Q-Stress
- Q-S. treadmill
- Q-S. treadmill stress test

Q-switched Nd:YAG laser
QT, Q-T
- cardiac output
- QT dispersion (QTd)
- QT interval
- QT interval corrected for heart rate (QTc, Q-Tc)
- QT interval dispersion
- QT interval duration
- QT interval sensing pacemaker
- long QT (LQT)
- QT syndrome
- QT ventilation

Q-T
- corrected Q-T

QT1
- long QT1 (LQT1)

QT2
    long Q. (LQT2)
QTc, Q-Tc
    QT interval corrected for heart rate
    QTc interval
QTd
    QT dispersion
QTI:QT index
QTL
    quantitative trait locus
QTp/QTe
    ratio of QTp/QTe
QT/QTc dispersion
Q-TRAK IAQ monitor
QTU
    pathologic QT
    QTU prolongation
QU, Q-U
    QU interval
quad
    q. coughing
    q. screen format
QuadPolar electrode
quadrangular resection
quadratum
    foramen q.
quadrature
    q. birdcage coil
    q. head coil
quadricusp
    q. mitral valve (QMC, QMV)
    q. mitral valve bioprosthesis
    q. stentless mitral bioprosthetic
    valve
quadricuspid
quadrigeminal
    q. pulse
    q. rhythm
quadrigeminus
    pulsus q.
quadrigeminy
quadriparesis
quadriplegia
quadripolar
    q. diagnostic catheter
    q. Itrel 2 pulse generator
    q. pacing catheter
    q. Quad electrode
    q. steerable electrode catheter
    q. steerable mapping/ablation
    catheter
    q. thermocouple-equipped ablation
    catheter
quadruple rhythm
quadruplet
Quaegebeur procedure

Quain
    Q. fatty degeneration
    Q. fatty heart
qualitative coronary ultrasound (QCU)
quality
    q. control
    q. enhancement research initiative
    (QUERI)
    indoor air q. (IAQ)
    q. of life
    q. of movement (QOM)
    Q. of Well-Being Index
    Q. of Well-Being Scale
    questionnaire
quality-adjusted life-years (QALY)
quality-of-care indicator
QuantiFeron-TB test
quantification
    acoustic q. (AQ)
    digital echo q. (DEQ)
    shunt q.
quantify
Quantison contrast agent
quantitative
    q. arteriography
    q. autoradiography (QAR)
    q. computed tomography (QCT)
    q. coronary angiographic analysis
    q. coronary angiography (QCA)
    q. coronary angiography caliper
    measurement
    q. coronary arteriography (QCA)
    q. Doppler
    q. edge-detection angiography
    q. left ventriculography
    q. trait locus (QTL)
    q. two-dimensional echocardiography
    q. wall motion score (QWMS)
quantum
    q. mottling
    Q. pacemaker
    q. proteolysis
    Q. PSV
    Q. TTC balloon dilator
Quartet system
quartile range
quartisternal
quartz transducer
quasisinusoidal waveform
**quaternary ammonium atropine
derivative**
Quattro mitral valve prosthesis
Queckenstedt sign
Queensland
    Q. fever
    Q. tick typhus
quellung reaction
Queltuss
Quénu-Muret sign

quercetin
QUERI
> quality enhancement research initiative
>> IHD QUERI
>>> ischemic heart disease quality
>>> enhancement research initiative

query fever
Quest
> Q. Medical
> Q. Medical delivery set
> Q. Medical microplegia system
> Q. Medical MPS cardioplegia fluid
> delivery pump
> Q. Medical MPS console
> Q. MPS myocardial protection
> system

questionnaire
> Asthma Quality of Life Q.
> (AQLQ)
> Childhood Asthma Q. (CAQ)
> Chronic Respiratory Q. (CRQ)
> Cognitive Failures Q. (CFQ)
> Coping Strategies q.
> cough-specific quality of life q.
> Dyspnea Scale q.
> Fagerstrom tolerance q. (FTQ)
> Functional Outcomes of Sleep Q.
> (FOSQ)
> Karolinska quality of life q.
> Kellner q.
> LIHFE q.
> London School of Hygiene
> Cardiovascular Rose Q.
> Mahler Baseline Dyspnea Index q.
> MAQOL q.
> McGill-Melzack Pain Q.
> McGill Pain Q.
> Medical Research Council q.
> Minnesota Leisure Time Physical
> Activity Q.
> Minnesota Living with Heart
> Failure q.
> Oxygen Cost Diagram q.
> Pulmonary Functional Status and
> Dyspnea Q. (PFSDQ)
> Quality of Well-Being Scale q.
> Rose Q.
> Seattle Angina Q.
> Sickness Impact Profile q.
> St. George Respiratory Q. (SGRQ)
> Veterans Specific Activity Q.
> (VSAQ)

Questran Light
Quetelet index
Quibron
quick
> q. confusion scale (QCS)
> Q. intravenous liver function test
> Q. prothrombin time test
> q. pulse

QuickDraw venous cannula
QuickFlash arterial catheter
QuickFlow
> Q. DPS
> Q. DPS distal perfusion system

QuickFurl SL balloon
QuicKlamp hemostasis device
QuickSeal femoral arterial closure
> **system**

quiet
> q. breath sounds
> q. chest
> q. heart sounds
> q. precordium

Quik-Chek external pacer tester
Quik-Coff electrical cough stimulator
Quik-Prep electrode
quinacrine
Quinaglute Dura-Tabs
quinapril
> q. hydrochloride
> q. and hydrochlorothiazide

quinaprilat
Quinatime
Quincke
> Q. disease
> Q. edema
> Q. pulse
> Q. sign

quinestrol
quinethazone
Quinidex Extentabs
quinidine
> q. gluconate
> q. sulfate
> q. syncope syndrome

quinidine-induced torsade de pointes
quinine sulfate
quinolone
Quinones
> method of Q.

quinsy
> lingual q.

NOTES

Quinton
    Q. PermCath catheter
    Q. Synergy cardiac information
       management system
Quinton-Scribner shunt
quinupristin
quotient
    intelligence q. (IQ)

    respiratory q. (RQ)
    V̇/Q̇ q.
Q-wave myocardial infarction (QMI)
QWIKLoad
    CardioSEAL septal occlusion
       system with Q.
QWMS
    quantitative wall motion score

R

first positive deflection during the QRS
complex
gas constant
roentgen
    R axis
    R on T ventricular premature
      contraction
    R unit
    R′ wave
    R wave amplitude
    R wave gating
    R wave upstroke

R3

ReoPro Readministration Registry

R′

second positive deflection during QRS
complex

**R1 rapid exchange balloon dilatation
catheter**

**R2L rapid exchange balloon dilatation
catheter with extended pressure
range**

RIII reflex

RA

rheumatoid arthritis
right atrium
right auricle
rotational atherectomy
    RA 523 blood gas/CO-oximetry
      control
    RA cell
    Integris 3D RA

RAA

right atrial appendage

RAAS

renin-angiotensin-aldosterone system

rAAT

recombinant alpha-1 antitrypsin

rabbit

r. antithymocyte globulin
r. aorta-contracting substance (RCS)
r. fever

rabbit-ear sign

rabies

Rabinov venography technique

RACAT

rapid acquisition computed axial
tomography

racemic

r. epinephrine
r. warfarin sodium

racemose aneurysm

Rackley method

racquet incision

RAD

reactive airways disease
regional alveolar damage
right atrium diameter
right axis deviation
    RAD airway laryngeal blade

rad

radiation absorbed dose

radarkymography

Radford nomogram

radial

r. approach
r. artery
r. artery graft
r. artery systolic pressure (RASP)
r. pulse (RP)

radiant heat device (RHD)

radiata

corona r.

radiation

r. absorbed dose (rad)
biological effects of ionizing r.
r. equivalent in man (rem)
extended field r. (EFR)
r. fibrosis
gamma r.
hyperfractionated r. (HRT)
intracoronary artery r.
ionizing r. (IR)
r. lung disease
mitogenic r.
r. pneumonitis
r. safety
scatter r.
secondary r.
r. therapy

radiation-induced

r.-i. atherosclerosis
r.-i. heart disease (RIHD)
r.-i. pericarditis

radical

free r.
hydroxyl r.
O2 r.
oxygen r.
oxygen-free r.

radicle

radiculitis

cervical r.

Radifocus

R. catheter guidewire
R. Glidewire
R. wire

radii (*pl. of* radius)

Radii-T catheter

R

radio
    LDL/HDL r.
radioactive
    r. iodinated serum albumin (RISA)
    r. stent
    r. tantalum
    r. xenon test
radioallergosorbent test (RAST)
radiocardiogram (RKG)
radiocardiography
radiocontrast dye
radiodense
radiodermatitis
radioelectrocardiography (RCG, RECG)
radiofrequency (RF)
    r. ablation (RFA)
    r. ablator
    r. catheter ablation
    r. current (RFC)
    r. electrophrenic respiration
    r. energy
    r. hot balloon
    r. percutaneous myocardial
      revascularization (RF-PMR)
radiofrequency-assisted valvotomy
radiograph
    chest r. (CXR, CxR)
    portable chest r.
    postoperative chest r.
radiographic
    r. cephalometry
    r. technique
radiography
    digital r.
    dual-energy digital r.
radioimmunoassay (RIA)
    Coat-a-Count r.
    Insulin Riabead II r.
    Mallinckrodt r.
radioimmunotherapy
radioisotope
radiolabeled
    r. fibrinogen
    r. gallium
    r. iodine
    r. microsphere
radioligand binding assay
radiologic scimitar syndrome
radiologist
    thoracic r.
radiology
    interventional r.
    Society of Cardiovascular and
      Interventional R. (SCVIR)
radiolucent
Radiometer probe
radiometry
    BACTEC r.
radionecrosis injury

Radionics
    R. radiofrequency generator
    R. RFG-35
radionuclide
    r. angiocardiography
    r. angiography (RNA)
    r. cineangiocardiography
    daughter r.
    r. generator
    gold-195m r.
    r. imaging
    parent r.
    r. perfusion lung scanning
    r. superior cavography (RNSC)
    r. technique
    r. venography (RNV)
    r. ventriculography (RNV, RNVG)
radiopacity
radiopaque
    r. end marker
    r. ERCP catheter
    r. tantalum stent
radiopharmaceutical imaging
radiotelemetry
radiotherapy (XRT)
    continuous hyperfractionated
      accelerated r. (CHART)
    postoperative r. (PORT)
    proton-beam r.
radiotracer
RadiStop radial compression system
radius, pl. **radii**
    thrombocytopenia-absent r. (TAR)
Radius self-expanding stent
radix linguae
radon
RADS
    reactive airways disease syndrome
    reactive airways dysfunction syndrome
RAE
    right atrial enlargement
    RAE endotracheal tube
Raeder-Harbitz syndrome
RAF
    repetitive atrial firing
Raff-Glantz derivative method
RAFW
    right atrial free wall
ragpicker's disease
ragsorter's disease
RAH
    right atrial hypertrophy
Rahn-Otis sample
RAI
    right atrial inversion
    right atrial involvement
railroad track sign
RAITI
    right atrial inversion time index

rake retractor
rale
> amphoric r.
> atelectatic r.
> basilar r.
> bibasilar r.
> border r.
> bronchial r.
> bronchiectatic r.
> bubbling r.
> cavernous r.
> cellophane r.
> clicking r.
> coarse r.
> collapse r.
> consonating r.
> crackling r.
> crepitant r.
> r. de retour
> dry r.
> extrathoracic r.
> gurgling r.
> guttural r.
> r. indux
> inspiratory r.
> laryngeal r.
> marginal r.
> metallic r.
> moist r.
> mucous r.
> musical r.
> pleural r.
> pulmonary r.
> r. redux
> r.'s and rhonchi
> sibilant r.
> Skoda r.
> snoring r.
> sonorous r.
> subcrepitant r.
> tracheal r.
> Velcro r.
> ventricular r. (VR)
> vesicular r.
> wet r.
> whistling r.

Raman
> R. spectography
> R. spectroscopy

rami (*pl. of* ramus)
ramipril
Ramond sign

RAMP
> rate modulated pacing
> right atrial mean pressure
>> RAMP antitachycardia protocol
>> RAMP-based protocol
>> RAMP pacing
>> RAMP treadmill protocol

RAMT
> right atrial mobile thrombi

ramus, pl. **rami**
> r. anterior descendens
> r. anterior lateralis
> rami bronchiales
> rami bronchiales segmentorum
> r. communicans cum nervo glossopharyngeo
> rami esophageales
> rami esophageales aortae thoracicae
> rami esophageales arteriae gastricae sinistrae
> rami esophageales arteriae thyroideae inferioris
> rami esophagei
> rami esophagei nervi laryngei recurrentis
> rami esophagei nervi vagi
> r. intermedius
> r. intermedius artery
> r. internus nervi laryngei superioris
> rami isthmi faucium nervi lingualis
> r. lobi medii arteriae pulmonalis dextrae
> r. medianus
> r. posterior descendens
> r. posterior venae pulmonalis dextrae superioris
> rami pulmonales systematis autonomici

Randall-Baker Soucek (RBS)
Rand appropriateness selection criteria
randomized trials
random nodule
random-zero sphygmomanometer
Ranfac needle
range
> D2L OTW balloon dilatation catheter with extended pressure r.
> dynamic r.
> heart rate r. (HRR)
> interquartile r.
> logarithmic dynamic r.
> quartile r.

R

NOTES

range *(continued)*
    R2L rapid exchange balloon
    dilatation catheter with extended
    pressure r.
range-alternating current
range-gated transducer
Ranger
    R. balloon
    R. over-the-wire balloon catheter
ranging
    echo r.
ranine artery
Ranke complex
Rankin Disability Scale
ranolazine
rANP
    rat atrial natriuretic peptide
Ransohoff operation
Ranvier
    node of R.
RAO
    right anterior oblique
    RAO angulation
    RAO position
    RAO view
RAP
    rapid atrial pacing
    remote access perfusion
    resident assessment protocol
    right atrial pressure
    RAP cannula
rapamycin
rape
    bruit de scie ou de r.
rapeseed oil
raphe
    r. linguae
    pharyngeal r.
    r. pharyngis
    r. of pharynx
rapid
    r. acquisition computed axial
    tomography (RACAT)
    r. antigen-detection test
    r. atrial pacing (RAP)
    r. atrial stimulation (RAS)
    r. depolarization
    r. early action in coronary
    treatment (REACT)
    r. eye movement (REM)
    r. filling
    r. filling wave
    r. fluid loading
    r. nonsustained ventricular
    tachycardia
    r. pacing
    r. plasma test
    r. platelet function assay (RPFA)
    r. sequence induction (RSI)

    r. shallow breathing index (RSBI)
    r. troponin T
    r. Y descent
rapid-burst pacing
Rapidlab 800 Critical Care system
RapidMist metered dose spray
    applicator
Rapidpoint
    R. access
    R. Coag
rapid-sequence intubation
Rappaport-Sprague stethoscope
rappel
    bruit de r.
Raptor PTCA balloon
rarefaction
    pontine ischemic r.
rarus
    pulsus r.
RAS
    rapid atrial stimulation
    renal artery stenosis
    rotational atherectomy system
rash
    erythematous maculopapular r.
    maculopapular r.
Rashkind
    R. balloon atrial septostomy
    R. balloon technique
    R. double umbrella
    R. double umbrella device
    R. procedure
    R. septostomy balloon catheter
Ras mitogen-activated protein kinase
Rasmussen
    R. aneurysm
    R. syndrome
Rasor blood pumping system (RBPS)
RASP
    radial artery systolic pressure
raspatory
    rib r.
rasping murmur
RAST
    radioallergosorbent test
Rastan-Konno procedure
Rastan operation
Rastelli
    R. operation
    R. procedure
rat
    r. atrial natriuretic peptide (rANP)
    borderline hypertensive r. (BHR)
    r. urine protein
rate
    atrial r. (AR)
    atrial heart r. (AHR)
    atrial overdrive stimulation r.
    (AST)

R

atrial tachycardia detection r. (ATDR)
basal fetal heart r. (BFHR)
basal heart r. (BHR)
baseline fetal heart r.
baseline variability of fetal heart r.
beat-to-beat variability of fetal heart r.
beginning-of-life r.
blood flow r. (BFR)
body acceleration synchronous with heart r. (BASH)
complication r.
count r.
critical r.
diastolic descent r. (DDR)
disintegration r.
ejection r. (ER)
end-of-life r.
erythrocyte sedimentation r. (ESR)
expiratory flow r.
fetal heart r. (FHR)
flow r.
glomerular filtration r. (GFR)
heart r. (HR, HRT)
highest equivalent heart r. (HEHR)
r. hysteresis
r. immunonephelometry
indocyanine green plasma disappearance r. (ICG-PDR)
inspiratory flow r.
intrinsic heart r. (IHR)
key pulse r. (KPR)
left ventricular peak filling r. (LVPFR)
low flow r.
magnet r.
maternal heart r. (MHR)
maximal expiratory flow r. (MEFR)
maximal heart r. (Hrmax, MHR)
maximal inspiratory flow r. (MIFR)
maximal midexpiratory flow r. (MMEFR)
maximal ventilation r. (MVR)
maximum determined heart r. (MDHR)
maximum flow r.
maximum midexpiratory flow r. (MMEF, MMF)
maximum predicted heart r. (MPHR)

maximum pulse r. (MPR)
maximum sensory r.
mean atrial r.
mean circumferential fiber-shortening r. (MCFSR)
mean midexpiratory flow r. ($FEF_{25-75\%}$)
mean normalized systolic ejection r.
mean systolic ejection r. (MSER)
miss r.
r. modulated pacing (RAMP)
r. modulation
mortality r. (MR)
myocardial metabolic r. (MMR)
pacemaker adaptive r.
patency r.
peak diastolic filling r.
peak ejection r. (PER)
peak emptying r.
peak expiratory flow r. (PEFR)
peak filling r. (PFR)
peak heart r. (PHR)
peak inspiratory flow r. (PIFR)
peak jet flow r.
peak lengthening r.
peak shortening r.
peak work r. (Wmax)
percent of maximum predicted heart r.
predicted maximal heart r. (PMHR)
r. pressure product
programmed cut-off r.
pulse r. (P-R)
pulse repetition r. (PRR)
QT interval corrected for heart r. (QTc, Q-Tc)
relative slow sinus r. (RSSR)
relative survival r.
repetition r.
respiratory r. (RR)
resting heart r. (RHR)
resting metabolic r. (RMR)
r. and rhythm (R&R)
right ventricular peak filling r. (RVPFR)
slew r. (SR)
r. smoothing
stroke ejection r.
ST segment divided by heart r. (ST/HR)
submaximal heart r. (HRSUB)

NOTES

rate *(continued)*

submaximum heart r.
Svedberg flotation r.
systolic ejection r. (SER)
target heart r. (THR)
time forced expiratory r.
time-to-peak filling r.
transvalvular flow r.
vasoconstriction r. (VCR)
ventilator r.
ventricular heart r. (VHR)
Westergren erythrocyte
  sedimentation r.
Wintrobe sedimentation r.
work r.

rate-adaptive

r.-a. device
r.-a. pacemaker

rate-dependent

r.-d. angina
r.-d. bundle branch block

rate-drop

r.-d. response (RDR)
r.-d. response mode
r.-d. sensing

rate-modulated pacemaker
rate-pressure product (RPP)
rate-responsive

dual-chamber r.-r.
r.-r. pulse generator
single-chamber r.-r.
r.-r. ventricular pacing

Rathke pouch tumor
rating

Borg dyspnea r.
r. of perceived breathing difficulty
  (RPBD)
r. of perceived exertion (RPE)

ratio *(See also* relation)

AH:HA r.
ankle-brachial blood pressure r.
aorta-left atrium r.
aortic root r.
cardiothoracic r. (CT, CTR)
conduction r.
contrast r.
C/P r.
C/PL r.
C/TG r.
dead space gas volume to tidal
  gas volume r. (V_{DS}/V_T)
dead space:tidal volume r.
early to late diastolic filling r.
  (E/A, E:A)
E/A wave r.
E:I r.
embolus-to-blood r. (EBR)
end-systolic volume r.

r. of expiration time and total
  time of breathing cycle (tE/tTOT)
flow r.
forced expiratory volume timed to
  forced vital capacity r.
  (FEV/FVC)
I:E r.
r. of ingested saturated fat and
  cholesterol to calories
r. of inspiration time and total
  time of breathing cycle (tI/tTOT)
inspiratory to expiratory r. (I:E)
r. of inspiratory time to total
  breathing cycle time (T_I/T_{TOT})
international normalized r. (INR)
La:A r.
LA/Ao r.
L/H r.
L/S r.
murmur/energy r. (MER)
odds r. (OR)
oxygen extraction r. (O_2ER)
peak respiratory r. (RER)
P:QRS r.
prothrombin time r. (PTR)
PR/RP r.
pulmonary systemic blood flow r.
pulmonary-to-systemic flow r.
  (Qp:Qs)
pulmonic-to-systemic flow r.
  (Qp:Qs)
pulse amplitude r. (PAR)
QSQT r.
r. of QTp/QTe
renal vein renin r.
residual volume/total lung
  capacity r.
resistance r.
respiratory exchange r. (RER)
R/Q wave r.
RV/TLC r.
S/A r.
segmental venous capacitance r.
  (SVCR)
sex r.
shunt r.
signal-to-noise r.
subendocardial to epicardial resting
  perfusion r.
systolic velocity r.
TC/HDL r.
r. of tidal expiratory flow at 25%
  of tidal volume and peak tidal
  expiratory flow ($TEF_{25}/PTEF$)
r. of tidal expiratory and
  inspiratory flow at 50% of tidal
  volume (TEF_{50}/TIF_{50})
transmitral Doppler E:A r.
transmitral E:A r.

trough-to-peak r.
V/C r.
velocity r. (VR)
venous diameter r. (VDR)
ventilation/perfusion r.
waist-to-hip r. (WHR)
rationalization
rattle of return
Rattus
 R. *norvegicus*
 R. *norvegicus* allergen
Rauchfuss triangle
Raulerson syringe
Rautaharju ECG criteria
Rauwolfia
 R. alkaloid
 R. extract
 Rauwolfia serpentina
rauwolscine
RAVC
 retrograde atrioventricular conduction
RAW
 right atrial wall
Raw
 airways resistance
ray
 beta r.
 gamma r.
 r. sum
 x-r.
Rayleigh scattering
Raynaud
 R. disease
 R. gangrene
 R. phenomenon
 R. sign
 R. syndrome
RB
 respiratory bronchiolitis
 right bundle
Rb
 rubidium
Rb-82
 rubidium-82
 Rb-82 PET
RBA
 right brachial artery
RBB
 right bundle branch
RBBB
 right bundle-branch block

RBBsB
 right bundle branch system block
RBC
 red blood cell
RBCD
 right border cardiac dullness
RBD
 right border of dullness
 right brain damage
RBPS
 Rasor blood pumping system
RBS
 Randall-Baker Soucek
 RBS face mask
RBV
 right brachial vein
RCA
 right coronary artery
 rotational coronary atherectomy
RCBF
 renal cortical blood flow
rCBF
 regional cerebral blood flow
RCC
 right coronary cusp
RCCA
 right common carotid artery
RCD
 relative cardiac dullness
RCFR
 relative coronary flow reserve
RCG
 radioelectrocardiography
RCHF
 right congestive heart failure
RCM
 right costal margin
RCO
 right coronary ostium
RCP
 respiratory care practitioner
RCPP
 recurrent coronary prevention program
RCS
 rabbit aorta-contracting substance
 right coronary sinus
RCT
 cutting balloon RCT
RCVA
 right cerebrovascular accident
RCVR
 renal cortical vascular resistance

R

NOTES

RDF
  Adriamycin RDF
RDI
  respiratory disturbance index
rDNA
  recombinant deoxyribonucleic acid
  lepirudin r.
RDR
  rate-drop response
  RDR mode
RDS
  respiratory distress syndrome
RDX coronary radiation catheter delivery system
reabsorbable suture
REACT
  rapid early action in coronary treatment
reaction
  allergic r.
  anaphylactoid r.
  Arthus-type r.
  cholera vaccine r.
  egg-yellow r.
  Eisenmenger r.
  Fernandez r.
  fibrinolytic r.
  fight-or-flight r.
  Haber-Weiss r.
  hemoclastic r.
  hexokinase r.
  hunting r.
  inflammatory r.
  Kveim r.
  ligase chain r. (LCR)
  local r.
  Maillard r.
  methacholine r.
  monocytic leukemoid r.
  non-IgE-mediated r.
  photosensitizing r.
  Pirquet r.
  pleural r.
  polymerase chain r. (PCR)
  pyrogen r.
  quellung r.
  reverse transcriptase polymerase chain r. (RT-PCR)
  smallpox vaccine r.
  vagal r.
  vasovagal r.
  Weil-Felix r.
  xanthine oxidase r.
reactivation tuberculosis
reactive
  r. airways disease (RAD)
  r. airways disease syndrome (RADS)
  r. airways dysfunction syndrome (RADS)
  r. dilation
  r. hyperemia
  r. mesothelial hyperplasia
  r. upper airways dysfunction syndrome (RUDS)
reactivity
  cerebrovascular r. (CVR)
  digital vascular r. (DVR)
  methacholine r.
  pulmonary vascular r.
  vascular r.
reader
  Fisher Micro-capillary Tube R.
Read test
reagin
Rea-Lo
real-time
  r.-t. perfusion imaging
  r.-t. position management (RPM)
  r.-t. position management tracking system
  r.-t. telemetry
  r.-t. three-dimensional echocardiography
  r.-t. ultrasound
reassessment
Reaven syndrome
Rebar-18 micro catheter
Rebetron
rebound angina
rebreathing
  r. bag
  r. mask
  r. method
  r. technique
recainam
recalcitrant
  r. hypertension
  r. obstructive airways disease
recall antigen
recalled
  spoiled gradient r. (SPGR)
recanalization
  balloon occlusive intravascular lysis enhanced r.
  coronary r.
  excimer vascular r.
  percutaneous transluminal coronary r. (PTCR)
  r. versus recannulization
recannulization
  recanalization versus r.
Recath bypass graft marker
receiver
  Medtronic radiofrequency r.
recent myocardial infarction (RMI)
receptive aphasia
receptor
  A_{2A} adenosine r.

adrenergic r. (ADR, AR)
A-II r.
alpha r.
alpha 1A adrenergic r. (ADRA1A)
alpha-1-adrenergic r.
alpha-2-adrenergic r. (ADRAR)
alpha 2C adrenergic r. (ADRA2C)
beta r.
beta-1,-2 r.
beta-adrenergic r. (βAR, BAR)
beta-1B adrenergic r. (ADRA1B)
bone morphogenetic protein r. (BMPR)
cholinergic r.
chylomicron remnant r.
dopamine D2 r. (DD2R)
endothelin A, B r.'s
epithelial 5′-nucleotide r.
factor II r. (F2R)
Fas r.
Fc r.'s
FMLP r.
glycoprotein IIb/IIIa r.
H1 r.
r. for hyaluronan-mediated motility (RHAMM)
imidazoline r. (I-receptor)
irritant r.
juxtacapillary r.
juxtapulmonary-capillary r.
low-density lipoprotein r. (LDLR, LDL-R)
melanocortin-4 r. (MC4-R)
muscarinic r.
myocardial beta adrenergic r. (MBAR)
NMDA r.
opsonophagocytic r.
peroxisome proliferator-activated r. (PPAR)
peroxisome proliferator-activated r. gamma (PPAR-gamma)
ryanodine r.
stretch r.
tachykinin r.
toll-like r. (TLR)
very low density lipoprotein r. (VLDLR)

β_2-receptor
receptor-operated calcium channel
recess
costodiaphragmatic r.
pleural r.
Rosenmüller r.
subphrenic r.
superior omental r.
supratonsillar r.

recessed balloon septostomy catheter
recessus
r. pharyngeus
r. pleurales

RECG
radioelectrocardiography

Rechtschaffen scoring method
recipient heart
reciprocal
r. beat
r. bigeminy
r. regulation
r. rhythm
r. ST depression

reciprocating
r. macroreentry orthodromic tachycardia
r. rhythm
r. tachycardia (RT)

reciprocity
reclosure
recoarctation of aorta
recognition protein
recoil
elastic r.
luminal r.
lung elastic r.
r. phenomenon
r. wave

recombinant
r. alpha-1 antitrypsin (rAAT)
r. alteplase
r. deoxyribonucleic acid (rDNA)
r. desulfatohirudin
r. hirudin (r-hirudin)
r. human antithrombin III (rhATIII)
r. human IL-10 (rhuIL-10)
r. human relaxin
r. human vascular endothelial growth factor (rhVEGF)
r. lys-plasminogen
r. polyethylene glycol (r-PEG)
r. prourokinase
r. reteplase
r. tissue plasminogen activator (rt-PA)

NOTES

recombinant *(continued)*
    r. tissue-type plasminogen activator
    r. urokinase (r-UK)
Recombinate
recompression
reconstitution
    r. via collateral
    r. via profunda
reconstruction
    aortic r.
    arterial r.
    bifurcated vein graft for
      vascular r.
    inferior vena cava r. (IVCR)
    patch graft r.
    polyhedral surface r.
    right ventricular outflow tract r.
    Sheen airway r.
    stent r.
recorder
    blood pressure r. (BPR)
    cardiac event r.
    cardiac output r. (COR)
    circadian event r.
    Del Mar Avionics three-channel r.
    DM-400 Holter ECG cassette r.
    event r.
    HeartCard 3X cardiac event r.
    24-hour ambulatory
      electrocardiographic r.
    implantable loop r.
    King of Hearts Express 3X cardiac
      event r.
    Marquette Holter r.
    Medilog 4000 ambulatory ECG r.
    Mingograf 82 r.
    Narco Biosystems r.
    Narco Physiograph-6B r.
    Reveal Plus insertable loop r.
    videotape r.
recording
    bipolar esophageal r.
    cardiopneumographic r. (CPG)
    Doppler r.
    intracardiac catheter r. (ICR)
    long-time r.
    M-mode strip chart r.
    patient-triggered r.
    pulse volume r. (PVR)
    2120 R. Spirometer
    time-based event r.
    transtelephonic r.
    X, Y, Z r.'s
recovery
    corrected time of sinoatrial node
      function r. (CTSNFR)
    fluid-attenuated inversion r.
      (FLAIR)
    r. from inactivation

    functional r.
    heart rate r. (HRR)
    r. position
    pressure r.
recrossability
recrudescence
recruitable collateral vessel
recruitment
    alveolar r.
    capillary r.
    eosinophil r.
    host-generated neutrophils r.
rectification
    anomalous r.
    inward-going r.
rectilinear
    r. biphasic shock
    r. biphasic waveform
    r. scan
    r. ST-segment depression
rectivirgula
    Saccharopolyspora r.
rectocardiac reflex
rectus abdominis muscle
recurrence
    early ischemic r. (EIR)
    familial r.
    r. risk
recurrent
    r. coronary prevention program
      (RCPP)
    r. glioblastoma multiforme (RGM)
    r. infective exacerbation
    r. lobar hemorrhage (RLH)
    r. mesenteric ischemia
    r. mesenteric vascular occlusion
    r. myocardial infarction
    r. respiratory infection (RRI)
    r. respiratory papillomatosis
recurrentis
    rami esophagei nervi laryngei r.
recurring
    R. Figures test for short-term
      memory
    r. venous thromboembolism (RVTE)
    R. Words test for short-term
      memory
recursion
    Levinson-Durbin r.
recurvatum
    pectus r.
red
    r. atrophy
    r. blood cell (RBC)
    r. cedar asthma
    r. coronary thrombus
    r. hepatization
    r. hypertension
    r. induration

r. infarct
r. light therapy (RLT)
r. soft coral asthma
R. system
r. wine polyphenol
Redha-cut catheter
redilation
redistribution
r. imaging
pulmonary vascular r.
vascular r.
red-streaked sputum
reduced
r. afterload
r. signal intensity
r. vascular response (RVR)
reducer
reducing
r. event
r. valve
reductase
3-hydroxy-3-methylglutaryl coenzyme A r.
r. inhibitor
methylenetetrahydrofolate r. (MTHFR)
reduction
absolute risk r. (ARR)
afterload r.
alcohol septal r.
gradient r.
left ventricular r. (LVR)
percutaneous alcohol septal r.
percutaneous mitral annular r.
preload r.
relative risk r. (RRR)
stapled lung r.
redundant cusp syndrome
reduplication murmur
redux
rale r.
REE
resting energy expenditure
reedswitch
pacemaker r.
r. of pacemaker
reelevation
ST r.
ST-segment r.
Reel syndrome
reendothelialization

reentrant
r. atrial tachycardia
r. circuit
r. excitation
r. loop
r. mechanism
r. pathway
r. supraventricular tachycardia
r. tachycardia (RT)
r. ventricular arrhythmia (RVA)
r. ventricular tachyarrhythmia
reentry
anatomical r.
anisotropic r.
atrial r.
atrioventricular nodal r. (AVNR)
A-V nodal r.
bundle branch r. (BBR)
dual-loop intraatrial r.
figure-of-eight intraatrial r.
r. phenomenon
Schmitt-Erlanger model of r.
sinoatrial nodal r. (SANDR)
sinus nodal r.
r. theory
ventricular r.
r. waveform
wavelength of r.
Reeves treadmill protocol
reexpansion
lung r.
pulmonary r.
reexploration
surgical r.
REF
ejection fraction at rest
right ventricular ejection fraction
refeeding syndrome
reference
r. catheter
r. electrode
r. phantom CT
r. value
r. vessel diameter (RVD)
REFI
regional ejection fraction image
refill
transcapillary r.
refined grain
reflectance oximetry
reflected pressure waveform
reflecting level

NOTES

reflection
    guidewire r.
reflex
    abdominocardiac r.
    Abrams heart r.
    r. angina
    aortic r.
    Aschner r.
    Aschner-Dagnini r.
    r. asthma
    atriopressor r.
    auriculopressor r.
    Babinski r.
    Bainbridge r.
    baroreceptor r.
    Bezold-Jarisch r.
    bregmocardiac r.
    Breuer-Hering inflation r.
    cardiac depressor r.
    carotid sinus r.
    chemoreceptor r.
    Churchill-Cope r.
    coronary r.
    r. cough
    cough r.
    r. cough test
    craniocardiac r.
    Cushing r.
    depressor r.
    diving r.
    Erben r.
    esophagosalivary r.
    exercise pressor r.
    eyeball compression r.
    eyeball-heart r.
    gag r.
    gasp r.
    Head paradoxical r.
    heart r.
    hepatojugular r.
    Hering-Breuer r.
    Hoffman r.
    hypochondrial r.
    inflation r.
    jaw r. (JR)
    Kisch r.
    Kocher-Cushing r.
    laryngeal r.
    Livierato r.
    Loven r.
    McDowall r.
    mute r.
    nasobronchial r.
    oculocardiac r. (OCR)
    oculopharyngeal r.
    oculovagal r.
    orthocardiac r.
    r. pacemaker
    R. 8220 pacemaker

    Pavlov r.
    pericardial r.
    pharyngeal r.
    pneocardiac r.
    pneopneic r.
    pressoreceptor r.
    psychocardiac r.
    r. pulmonary arterial vasoconstriction
    pulmonocoronary r.
    rectocardiac r.
    respiratory r.
    RIII r.
    sinus r.
    sneeze r.
    somatic nociceptive flexion r.
    spinal nociceptive flexion r.
    R. steerable guidewire
    r. stimulation
    suck r.
    r. sympathetic dystrophy
    r. sympathoexcitation
    r. tachycardia
    vagal r.
    r. vagal bronchoconstriction
    vascular r.
    r. vasoconstriction
    vasoconstrictive r.
    r. vasodilation
    vasopressor r.
    venorespiratory r.
    viscerocardiac r.
Re/Flex filter
reflexogenic pressosensitivity
Reflotron bedside theophylline test
Refludan injection
reflux
    abdominojugular r.
    cardioesophageal r.
    erosive r.
    esophageal r.
    r. esophagitis
    extraesophageal r.
    gastroesophageal r. (GER)
    hepatojugular r. (HJR)
    mitral r. (MR)
    nasopharyngeal r.
    transvalvular r.
    valvular r.
    venous r. (VR)
reform
    capacitor r.
refractoriness
    dispersion of r.
refractory
    r. congestive heart failure
    r. hypoxemia
    r. to medical therapy
    r. period

r. period of electronic pacemaker
r. shock
r. tachycardia
refrigeration
thermoacoustic r.
Ref-Star EP catheter
Refsum
R. disease
R. syndrome
Regency SR, SR+ pulse generator
regimen
antithrombotic r.
dosage r.
exercise r.
prophylactic aspirin r.
stepped-care antihypertensive r.
titration r.
regio
r. axillaris
r. cruris anterior
r. cruris posterior
r. inguinalis
r. nasalis
r. pectoralis
r. posterior
r. presternalis
r. respiratoria tunicae mucosae nasi
region
AN r.
DiGeorge chromosome r. (DGCR)
DiGeorge critical r. (DGCR)
DiGeorge syndrome critical r.
(DGSCR)
r. of interest (ROI)
N r.
NH r.
parahilar r.
paratracheal r.
r. of respiratory mucosa
watershed r.
regional
r. alveolar damage (RAD)
r. cerebral blood flow (rCBF)
r. dyssynergy
r. ejection fraction image (REFI)
r. ischemia
r. myocardial blood flow (RMBF)
r. oxygen saturation (rS_{02})
r. perfusion
r. vasodilation
r. wall motion (RWM)

r. wall motion abnormality
(RWMA)
r. wall motion index
registration
flow-time r.
North American Cerebral
Transluminal Angioplasty R.
(NACPTAR)
registry
balloon valvuloplasty r. (BVR)
Cardiac Ablation R.
International Cooperative Pulmonary
Embolism R.
Long Bare Stent R.
Mansfield Valvuloplasty R.
North American Inoue Balloon r.
PELCA R.
ReoPro Readministration R. (R3)
regression
arteriographic r.
coronary plaque r.
r. equation
Poisson r.
Q wave r.
xanthoma r.
regular
R. Iletin II
r. purified pork insulin
r. rate and rhythm (RRR, RR&R)
r. sinus rhythm (RSR, rSR′)
regularly irregular rhythm
regulation
reciprocal r.
regulator
aluminum oxygen r.
Boehringer suction R.
cystic fibrosis transmembrane r.
(CFTR)
cystic fibrosis transmembrane
conductance r.
Easy Dial Reg oxygen r.
Ohmeda thoracic suction r.
regulon
BvgAS r.
regurgitant
r. fraction
r. jet
r. jet area
r. murmur
r. orifice
r. orifice area (ROA)
r. pocket

NOTES

R

regurgitant *(continued)*
    r. volume (RV, RVol)
    r. wave
regurgitation
    aortic r. (AR)
    aortic valve r.
    atrioventricular valve r.
    commissural mitral r.
    faint pulmonary r.
    functional mitral r.
    homograft insertion for
      pulmonary r.
    ischemic mitral r.
    mitral r. (MR)
    mitral valve r.
    normal transvalvular r. (NTVR)
    periprosthetic mitral r.
    prosthetic valve r. (PVR)
    pulmonary r. (P-R)
    pulmonary valvular r.
    pulmonic r.
    Sellers classification of mitral r.
    semilunar valve r.
    tricuspid r. (TR)
    tricuspid valve r. (TVR)
    valvular r.
rehabilitation
    American Association of
      Cardiovascular and Pulmonary R.
      (AACVPR)
    cardiac r. (CR)
    r. exercise
    home-based cardiac r.
    vocational r.
    work r.
rehalation
Reich-Nechtow clamp
Reid
    R. classification
    R. index
    R. index measurement
Reil
    ball of R.
    band of R.
reinfarction
reinfection tuberculosis
reinfusion
reinjection protocol
reinnervation in transplanted heart
Reisman
    R. myocardosis
    R. pneumonia
Reisseisen muscle
Reitan catheter Pump
Reiter
    R. disease
    R. syndrome
reject control

rejection
    acute r. (AR)
    acute allograft r.
    acute cellular xenograft r.
    acute lung r.
    allograft r.
    r. cardiomyopathy
    r. cardiomyopathy transplant
    delayed xenograft r. (DXR)
    graft r.
    hyperacute r.
    no infection-no r. (NI-NR)
rejection-associated pulmonary fibrosis
relapsing
    r. fever
    r. polychondritis
relation *(See also* ratio)
    concentration-effect r.
    diastolic pressure-volume r.
    end-systolic pressure-volume r.
    end-systolic stress-dimension r.
    force-frequency r.
    force-length r.
    force-velocity r.
    force-velocity-length r.
    force-velocity-volume r.
    interval-strength r.
    length-resting tension r.
    length-tension r.
    pressure-volume r.
    resting length-tension r.
    tension-length r.
    ventilation/perfusion r.
    ventricular end-systolic pressure-
      volume r.
relationship
    diastolic pressure-flow r. (DPFR)
    end-systolic force-length r. (ESFL)
    end-systolic pressure-volume r.
      (ESPVR)
    Fick r.
    Laplace r.
    pressure-flow r.
    stress-shortening r.
relative
    r. cardiac dullness (RCD)
    r. cardiac volume
    r. coronary flow reserve (RCFR)
    r. heart rate variability (RHRV)
    r. humidity
    r. incompetence
    r. inspiratory effort (RIE)
    r. lymphocyte count
    r. mitral stenosis
    r. refractory period (RRP)
    r. risk (RR)
    r. risk reduction (RRR)
    r. slow sinus rate (RSSR)
    r. survival rate

r. vessel diameter (RVD)
r. wall thickness (RWT)
relaxant
muscle r.
smooth muscle r.
relaxation
r. atelectasis
atrial r.
diastolic r.
dynamic r.
early diastolic r. (EDR)
endothelium-dependent vascular r.
endothelium-independent vascular r.
endothelium-mediated r.
isovolumetric r.
isovolumic r.
left ventricular r.
left ventricular diastolic r.
r. loading
smooth muscle r.
stress r.
r. technique
r. time
r. time index
r. training
ventricular r.
relaxin
recombinant human r.
relaxometry
NMR r.
release
Acutrim Precision R.
allergen-induced mediator r.
catecholamine r.
oxygen free radical r.
physiologic pattern r. (PPR)
sustained r. (SR)
Relenza
reliever
Arthritis Foundation Pain R.
Medtronic Pulsor Intrasound pain r.
REM
rapid eye movement
REM sleep
REM sleep-related hypoxemia
rem
radiation equivalent in man
Remac system
remedial psychological stressor
remedy
R. sleep therapy
R. sleep therapy system

Remicade
remifentanil
remission
Legroux r.
remnant
chylomicron r. (CMR)
r. lipoprotein (RLP)
remnant-like
r.-l. lipoprotein particle (RLP)
r.-l. particle lipoprotein
remodeling
adverse ventricular r.
airway r.
arterial r.
atrial reverse r.
Batista ventricular r.
cardiac r.
concentric r.
coronary r.
flow-responsive r.
heart chamber r.
myocardial r.
negative r.
positive arterial r.
postinfarct ventricular r.
reverse r.
vascular r.
ventricular r.
Remodulin
remote
r. access perfusion (RAP)
r. access perfusion cannula
remotely monitored ICD
removal
extracorporeal carbon dioxide r.
REMstar CPAP system
Renaissance spirometry system
renal
r. angiography
r. arteriography
r. artery
r. artery bypass graft
r. artery disease
r. artery forceps
r. artery-reverse saphenous vein
bypass
r. artery stenosis (RAS)
r. azotemia
r. blood vessel
r. cortical blood flow (RCBF)
r. cortical necrosis

R

NOTES

renal *(continued)*
    r. cortical vascular resistance (RCVR)
    r. cyst
    r. dialysis
    r. diet
    r. dyspnea
    r. failure
    r. fistula
    r. function
    r. hypertension
    r. insufficiency
    r. juxtaglomerular cell
    r. kallikrein-kinin system
    r. parenchymal disease
    r. plasma flow (RPF)
    r. tuberculosis
    r. vein
    r. vein renin ratio
    r. venography
renal-splanchnic steal
Rendell-Baker face mask
Rendu-Osler-Weber
    R.-O.-W. disease
    R.-O.-W. syndrome
Renese
renin
    r. angiotensin
    r. inhibitor
    r. level
    plasma r.
renin-angiotensin
    r.-a. blocker
    r.-a. system
renin-angiotensin-aldosterone
    r.-a.-a. cascade
    r.-a.-a. system (RAAS)
Renografin-76
renography
    captopril r.
renomedullary lipid
renoprival hypertension
renopulmonary
Renormax
renovascular
    r. angiography
    r. hypertension (RVH)
Renovist
Rentamine
Rentrop
    R. catheter
    R. classification
REO
    respiratory and enteric orphan
    REO virus
reocclusion
reoperation
ReoPro Readministration Registry (R3)
Reovirus

repair
    Alfieri r., Alfieri-plasty
    Allison hiatal hernia r.
    Boerema hernia r.
    Brom r.
    cap r.
    DeBakey-Creech aneurysm r.
    Effler hiatal hernia r.
    endovascular r. (EVR)
    Fontan r.
    Hatafuku fundus onlay patch esophageal r.
    minimally invasive valve r. (MIVR)
    Mustard atrial r.
    Norwood r.
    patch r.
    pulmonary valve r. (PVR)
    Senning atrial baffle r.
reparative cardiac surgery
repeat
    r. balloon mitral valvotomy
    r. revascularization
repeated ultrasound-guided needle thoracocentesis
Repel-CV bioresorbable adhesion-barrier film
reperfused myocardium
reperfusion (RP)
    r. arrhythmia
    r. catheter
    emergency r.
    facilitated r.
    r. injury
    late r.
    r. pulmonary edema
    r. therapy
reperfusion-induced hemorrhage
reperfusion/occlusion
repetition
    pulse r. (P-R)
    r. rate
    r. time (TR)
repetitive
    r. atrial firing (RAF)
    r. monomorphic ventricular tachycardia
    r. paroxysmal ventricular tachycardia
    r. stunning
    r. ventricular response (RVR)
rephasing
    even-echo r.
replacement
    aortic root r. (ARR)
    aortic valve r. (AVIR, AVR)
    battery elective r.
    blood r.
    composite valve graft r.

double valve r. (DVR)
extended aortic root r. (EARR)
minimally invasive valve r.
 (MIVR)
mitral and aortic valve r. (MAVR)
mitral valve r. (MVR)
partial chordal-sparing mitral
 valve r.
pulmonary valve r. (PVR)
supraannular mitral valve r.
 (SMVR)
total chordal-sparing mitral valve r.
tricuspid valve r. (TVR)
valve r. (VR)

repletion

replication

repolarization

benign early r. (BER)
early r. (ER)
early rapid r.
final rapid r.
myocardial r.

representative CT (Hounsfield) number

repression

reprogramming

pacemaker output r.

reptilase

RER

peak respiratory ratio
respiratory exchange ratio

Rescaps-D Capsule

Rescriptor

ReSCU

respiratory special care unit

rescue

r. angioplasty
citrovorum r.
r. PTCA
r. shock
r. stent implantation

ResCue Key

rescu PAC ventilator

research

Agency for Health Care Policy
 and R. (AHCPR)
R. Pneumotach System
 instrumentation module
primary angioplasty R. (PAR)

resection

activation map-guided surgical r.
atrial septal r.
bronchial sleeve r.

r. clamp
endocardial r.
endocardial-to-endocardial r.
infundibular wedge r.
lesser r.
myotomy-myectomy-septal r.
quadrangular r.
segmental lung r.
septal r.
Torek r. of thoracic esophagus

Resectisol Irrigation Solution

reserpine

chlorothiazide and r.
hydralazine, hydrochlorothiazide,
 and r.
hydrochlorothiazide and r.
hydroflumethiazide and r.

reserve

r. air
blood flow r.
breathing r. (BR)
cardiac r.
cardiopulmonary r. (CPR)
r. cell carcinoma
contractile r.
coronary arterial r.
coronary flow r. (CFR)
coronary flow velocity r. (CFVR,
 CVR)
coronary vascular r.
coronary vasodilator r.
diastolic r.
extraction r.
flow r.
fractional flow r. (FFR)
fractional velocity r. (FVR)
Frank-Starling r.
heart rate r. (HRR)
limited ventricular r.
myocardial r.
myocardial fractional flow r.
 (FFR_{myo})
preload r.
relative coronary flow r. (RCFR)
respiratory r.
stenotic flow r. (SFR)
systolic r.
vasodilator r.
ventricular r.

reservoir

Biocor softshell venous r.
cardiotomy r.

R

NOTES

reservoir *(continued)*
    Intersept cardiotomy r.
    Jostra cardiotomy r.
    Polystan cardiotomy r.
    William Harvey cardiotomy r.
reset
    r. nodus sinuatrialis
    sinus node r.
resident assessment protocol (RAP)
residual
    r. air
    r. deep vein thrombosis
    r. DVT
    r. gradient
    r. jet
    r. lung capacity
    r. pleural thickening
    r. shunt
    r. stenosis
    r. volume (RV)
    r. volume fraction (RVF)
    r. volume/total lung capacity
      (RV/TLC)
    r. volume/total lung capacity ratio
residue
    fucose r.
resin
    anion exchange r.
    bile acid binding r.
    cholestyramine r.
    epoxy r.
    pine r.
    thermosetting r.
resistance
    afterload r.
    airways r. (Raw)
    aortic valve r.
    cerebrovascular r. (CVR)
    coronary vascular r.
    diaphragmatic fatigue r.
    elastic r.
    expiratory r.
    glucocorticoid r.
    hydraulic r.
    insulin r.
    minimal vascular r. (MVR)
    r. to movement of lung tissue
      (Rti)
    multidrug r.
    nitrate r.
    normalized systemic vascular r.
      (NSVR)
    peripheral r.
    peripheral vascular r. (PVR)
    pulmonary r.
    pulmonary arteriolar r. (PAR)
    pulmonary-to-systemic vascular r.
      (Rp:Rs)
    pulmonary vascular r. (PVR)

    r. ratio
    renal cortical vascular r. (RCVR)
    respiratory r. (Rrs)
    stenosis r.
    systemic arterial r. (Rsa)
    systemic vascular r. (SVR)
    total airway r. (Rtot)
    total peripheral r.
    total peripheral vascular r. (TPVR)
    total pulmonary r.
    total pulmonary vascular r. (TPVR)
    total systemic vascular r. (TSVR)
    total vascular r. (TVR)
    r. training (RT)
    valve r.
    vascular r. (VR)
    vascular peripheral r.
    r. to venous return (RVR)
    r. vessel
resistant
    high-altitude pulmonary edema r.
      (HAPE-r)
    r. hypertension
resistive heating
resistor
    fixed orifice r.
    magnetic valve r.
    spring-loaded r.
    threshold r.
    underwater seal r.
    water column r.
    weighted ball r.
resolution
    energy r.
    high spatial r.
    spatial r.
    ST segment r.
    temporal r.
resolving power
resonance
    bandbox r.
    bell-metal r.
    cardiovascular magnetic r. (CMR)
    cough r.
    cracked-pot r.
    nuclear magnetic r. (NMR)
    shoulder-strap r.
    skodaic r.
    tympanitic r.
    whispering r.
    wooden r.
resonant frequency
resorption
    r. atelectasis
    bulla r.
Respa DM
Respa-GF
Respaire-60 SR
Respaire-120 SR

Respalor
Respa-1st
RespiGam
Respihaler
    Dexacort Phosphate in R.
RespiPac
    Zagam R.
respirable aerosol
Respiradyne pulmonary function device
respiration
    abdominal r.
    absent r.
    accelerated r.
    accessory muscles of r.
    aerobic r.
    agonal r.
    amphoric r.
    anaerobic r.
    apneustic r.
    artificial r.
    assisted r.
    asthmoid r.
    Austin Flint r.
    Biot r.
    Bouchut r.
    bronchial r.
    bronchocavernous r.
    r. bronchoscope
    bronchovesicular r.
    cavernous r.
    cell r.
    central r.
    cerebral r.
    Cheyne-Stokes r.
    cogwheel r.
    collateral r.
    controlled diaphragmatic r.
    Corrigan r.
    costal r.
    cyclic r.
    decreased r.
    diaphragmatic r.
    diffusion r.
    direct r.
    divided r.
    electrophrenic r.
    external r.
    forced r.
    granular r.
    harsh r.
    internal r.
    interrupted r.

    intrauterine r.
    jerky r.
    Kussmaul r.
    Kussmaul-Kien r.
    labored r.
    meningitic r.
    metamorphosing r.
    mitochondrial r.
    mouth-to-mouth r.
    nervous r.
    paradoxical r.
    periodic r.
    placental r.
    puerile r.
    pulse and r. (P&R)
    radiofrequency electrophrenic r.
    rude r.
    Schafer method of artificial r.
    Seitz metamorphosing r.
    shallow r.
    sighing r.
    slow r.
    sonorous r.
    stertorous r.
    stridulous r.
    supplementary r.
    suppressed r.
    temperature, pulse, and r.
    thoracic r.
    transitional r.
    tubular r.
    unlabored r.
    vesiculocavernous r.
    vicarious r.
    wavy r.
respiratometer
    Collins r.
respirator
    BABYbird r.
    Bragg-Paul r.
    cuirass r.
    Drinker r.
    Emerson cuirass r.
    r. lung
    Monaghan r.
    Morch r.
    particulate r.
    pressure-controlled r.
    tank r.
    volume-controlled r.
    volumetric diffusive r. (VDR)

R

NOTES

respiratoria
>glottis r.
>rima r.

respiratorium
>systema r.

respiratorius
>apparatus r.

respiratory
>r. acidosis
>r. activity
>r. airways
>r. alkalosis
>r. alternans
>r. alternans breathing pattern
>r. apparatus
>r. arousal scoring
>r. arrest
>r. arrhythmia
>r. artifact
>r. bronchiole
>r. bronchiolitis (RB)
>r. burst
>r. capacity
>r. care practitioner (RCP)
>r. center
>r. collapse
>r. compromise
>r. cycle
>r. dead space
>r. depressant action
>r. depression
>r. distress
>r. distress syndrome (RDS)
>r. distress syndrome of the newborn
>r. disturbance index (RDI)
>r. drive
>r. effort-related arousal
>r. embarrassment
>r. and enteric orphan (REO)
>r. event
>r. exchange
>r. exchange ratio (RER)
>r. excursion
>r. failure
>r. feedback (RFb)
>r. flora
>r. frequency (f)
>r. function
>r. gas analysis
>r. gated MRCA
>r. gated three-dimensional gradient-echo sequence
>r. gating
>r. glycoconjugate (RGC)
>r. inductance plethysmograph (RIP)
>r. inductance plethysmography (RIP)
>r. insufficiency

>r. irritant
>r. metabolism
>r. minute volume
>r. mucosa
>r. murmur
>r. muscle fatigue
>r. ordered phase encoding (ROPE)
>r. paralysis
>r. pattern
>r. pulse
>r. pump
>r. quotient (RQ)
>r. rate (RR)
>r. reflex
>r. region of tunica mucosa of nose
>r. reserve
>r. resistance (Rrs)
>r. sinus arrhythmia (RSA)
>r. sound
>r. special care unit (ReSCU)
>r. standstill
>r. stridor
>r. support
>r. swing
>r. syncytial virus (RSV)
>r. syncytial virus conduit
>r. syncytial virus immunoglobulin (RSV-IG)
>r. syncytial virus IV immune globulin
>r. system
>Taiwan acute r. (TWAR)
>r. toilet
>r. tract
>r. tract infection
>r. tract lining fluid (RTLF)
>r. triggering
>r. waveform variation

respiratory-gated 2 D segmented-FLASH MRCA image

Respirgard II nebulizer

respirometer
>Dräger r.
>Fraser Harlake r.
>Haloscale r.
>Wright r.

Respironics
>R. BIPAP bilevel ventilator
>R. CPAP machine
>R. Oasis humidifier
>R. 920P handheld pulse oximeter
>R. 930 pulse oximeter

Respitrace
>R. machine
>R. plethysmograph

responder
>isolated volume r. (IVR)
>r. ventilator

response
  acute r.
  atrial flutter r. (AFR)
  atrial tachycardic r.
  autonomic r.
  biphasic r.
  blunted exercise r.
  bronchodilator r.
  cell-mediated immune r.
  cephalic vasomotor r. (CVR)
  chemotactic r.
  cholinergic r.
  chronotropic r.
  controlled ventricular r.
  Cushing pressure r.
  double ventricular r. (DVR)
  dynamic frequency r.
  dysfunctional airway immune r.
  electrocardiographic r. (ECR)
  R. electrophysiology catheter
  endothelium-dependent dilator r. to
    substance P
  fetal ventricular myocyte
    proliferative r.
  fight-or-flight r.
  frequency r.
  giving-in/giving-up r.
  hemodynamic mental stress r.
  Henry-Gauer r.
  hypercapnic ventilatory r.
  hypoxic ventilatory r. (HVR)
  implantation r.
  incrementing r.
  local thrombotic r.
  metaboreflex r.
  methacholine r.
  neointimal hyperplastic r.
  paced ventricular evoked r.
  pathologic complete r.
  photobiological r.
  plateau r.
  postocclusive oscillatory r. (POR)
  pulmonary reimplantation r. (PRR)
  rate-drop r. (RDR)
  reduced vascular r. (RVR)
  repetitive ventricular r. (RVR)
  sensor-driven r.
  sequential vascular r. (SVR)
  slow r.
  square wave r.
  sympathoexcitatory r.
  sympathoinhibitory r.

  thyrotropin-releasing hormone r.
  vagal r.
  vagotonic baroreceptor r.
  vasodilatory r.
  vasomotor r. (VMR)
  ventilatory r.
  ventricular r.
  vigilance r.
  visually evoked flow r. (VEFR)
response-to-injury
  r.-t.-i. hypothesis
  r.-t.-i. hypothesis of atherogenesis
  r.-t.-i. theory
responsiveness
  adenosine airways r.
  bronchial r. (BR)
  myofilament calcium r.
Respule
  Pulmicort R.
Res-Q
  R.-Q ACD implantable cardioverter-
    defibrillator
  R.-Q arrhythmia control device
  R.-Q Micron ICD
  R.-Q Micron implantable
    cardioverter-defibrillator
rest
  r. angina
  r. dyspnea
  r. ejection fraction
  ejection fraction at r. (REF)
  r. and exercise gated nuclear
    angiography
  r. hypoxemia
  r. metabolism/stress perfusion
    protocol
  r. pain
  r. radionuclide angiography
rested state contraction (RSC)
Resten-NG
restenosis
  aortic valve r.
  computer-assisted evaluation of
    stenosis and r. (CAESAR)
  coronary artery descriptors and r.
    (CADR)
  diffuse in-stent r.
  in-stent r. (ISR)
  intralesion r.
  intrastent r. (IR)
  r. lesion
  mitral r.

NOTES

R

restenosis *(continued)*
>   post balloon angioplasty r.
>   pulmonary valve r.
>   r. risk
>   rotablator and r. (R&R)
>   tricuspid r.

restenotic narrowing
rest-exercise equilibrium radionuclide ventriculography
resting
>   r. energy expenditure (REE)
>   r. heart rate (RHR)
>   r. hypertension
>   r. length-tension relation
>   r. membrane potential
>   r. metabolic rate (RMR)
>   r. parasternal long-axis view
>   r. parasternal short-axis view
>   r. pressure
>   r. sinus tachycardia
>   r. stroke volume
>   r. systolic function
>   r. tidal breathing
>   r. tidal volume
>   r. value
>   r. vascular tone
>   r. venous pressure (RVP)

Reston subtype of Ebola
restoration
>   r. of spontaneous circulation (ROSC)
>   surgical ventricular r. (SVR)

restored cycle
Restoril
rest-redistribution thallium-201 imaging
restriction
>   r. endonuclease
>   r. fragment length polymorphism (RFLP)
>   progressive parenchymal r.
>   pulmonary r.

restrictive
>   r. airways defect
>   r. airways disease
>   r. cardiomyopathy
>   r. filling pattern
>   r. functional impairment
>   r. heart disease
>   r. lung disease
>   r. physiology mitral flow pattern
>   r. ventilatory defect
>   r. ventilatory dysfunction

restrictus
>   *Aspergillus r.*

result
>   stent-like r. (SLR)
>   true-negative test r.
>   true-positive test r.

resuscitate
>   do not r. (DNR)

resuscitation
>   active compression-decompression cardiopulmonary r. (ACD-CPR)
>   albumin r.
>   bystander cardiac pulmonary r. (ByCPR)
>   bystander cardiopulmonary r. (BCPR)
>   cardiac r. (CR)
>   cardiopulmonary r. (CPR)
>   cardiopulmonary cerebral r. (CPCR)
>   r. cart
>   closed chest cardiac r. (CCCR)
>   closed chest cardiopulmonary r. (CCPR)
>   crystalloid r.
>   do not attempt r. (DNAR)
>   external cardiopulmonary r. (ECPR)
>   family-witnessed r.
>   heart-lung r. (HLR)
>   high-impulse cardiopulmonary r. (HI-CPR)
>   high-impulse compression cardiopulmonary r. (HIC-CPR)
>   International Liaison Committee on R. (ILCOR)
>   interposed abdominal compression cardiopulmonary r. (IAC CPR)
>   mechanical cardiopulmonary r.
>   mouth-to-mouth r.
>   open chest cardiac r.
>   open chest cardiopulmonary r. (OCCPR)
>   standard cardiopulmonary r. (SCPR)
>   volume r.

resuscitator
>   active compression-decompression r.
>   Ambu Spur disposable r.
>   BagEasy disposable manual r.
>   First Response manual r.
>   Hope r.
>   Hudson Lifesaver r.
>   infant Ambu r.
>   Laerdal r.
>   NeoVO2R infant volume control r.
>   pneuPAC r.

resveratrol
resynchronizer
>   HFCWO ventricular r.
>   high-frequency chest wall oscillation ventricular r.

retained lung fluid (RLF)
retard
>   expiratory r.

retardation
>   fragile X-mental r. (FRAX-MR)

Retavase

retention
>   r. cyst
>   mucus r.
>   secretion r.
>   sodium r.
>   sputum r.
>   tracer r.
>   water r.

reteplase (RPA, r-PA)
reteplase-abciximab
rethoracotomy
reticula (*pl. of* reticulum)
reticularis
>   livedo r.

reticular pattern
reticulation
reticuloendothelial system
reticulonodular
>   r. infiltrate
>   r. pattern

reticulum, pl. **reticula**
>   agranular endoplasmic r. (AER)
>   endoplasmic r.
>   sarcoplasmic r.

retina, pl. **retinas, retinae**
>   cyanosis retinae

retinal
>   r. artery
>   r. vessel

retinohypothalamic pathway
retinoic acid
retinol
>   plasma r.
>   serum r.

retinopathy
>   diabetic r.
>   hypertensive r.
>   r. of prematurity (ROP)
>   proliferative diabetic r. (PDR)

retour
>   rale de r.

retraction
>   intercostal r.
>   postrheumatic cusp r.
>   r. wave

retractor
>   abdominal vascular r.
>   Ablaza-Blanco aortic wall r.
>   Adson r.
>   Allison lung r.
>   Andrews r.

>   Bookwalter r.
>   Cooley atrial r.
>   Cosgrove r.
>   Davidson scapular r.
>   DeBakey chest r.
>   Finochietto r.
>   Finochietto-Geissendorfer rib r.
>   Gelpi r.
>   IMA r.
>   inferior mesenteric artery r.
>   Lilienthal-Sauerbruch r.
>   Lukens thymus r.
>   lung r.
>   malleable r.
>   Meyerding r.
>   rake r.
>   Theis rib r.
>   Zalkind lung r.

Retract-O-Tape
retraining
>   computerized diaphragmatic
>   breathing r. (CDBR)

retransplantation
retrieval
>   intravascular foreign body r.

retriever
retrocardiac space
retroconduction
retrocrural adenopathy
retroesophageal aorta
retrognathia
retrograde
>   r. aortography
>   r. arterial capture
>   r. atrial activation mapping
>   r. atrioventricular conduction
>   (RAVC)
>   r. autologous priming
>   r. beat
>   r. block
>   r. catheter insertion
>   r. catheterization
>   r. embolism
>   r. fast pathway
>   r. femoral approach
>   r. filling
>   r. hypertension
>   r. P wave
>   r. translaryngeal intubation
>   r. VA conduction

retrolingual

NOTES

retropalatal
r. airways
r. obstruction
retropectoral
r. patch
r. pocket
retroperfusion
coronary sinus r.
synchronized r. (SRP)
retroperitoneal hematoma
retropharyngeal
r. abscess
r. lymph node
r. space
retropharyngeales
nodi lymphoidei r.
retropharyngeum
spatium r.
retropharyngitis
retropharynx
retrosternal
r. air space
r. thyroid
retrotracheal space
Retrovir
R. injection
R. Oral
retroviral vector
retrovirus
return
anomalous pulmonary venous r.
r. extrasystole
hemi-anomalous pulmonary
venous r. (HAPVR)
partial anomalous pulmonary
venous r. (PAPVR)
pulmonary anomalous superior
venous r. (PASVR)
pulmonary venous r.
rattle of r.
resistance to venous r. (RVR)
r. of spontaneous circulation
(ROSC)
systemic venous r.
total anomalous pulmonary
venous r. (TAPVR)
venous r. (VR)
returning cycle
Retzius veins
reuptake blockade
Reuter tip deflecting wire guide
revascularization
Biosense-guided laser myocardial r.
catheter-based r.
coronary r.
direct myocardial r. (DMR)
heart laser r.
Helionetics/Acculase excimer laser
transmyocardial r.

hybrid r.
ischemia-driven r.
laser r.
myocardial r. (MR)
myocardial laser r. (MLR)
percutaneous myocardial r. (PMR)
percutaneous myocardial laser r.
percutaneous transluminal
coronary r. (PTCR)
percutaneous transluminal
myocardial r. (PTMR)
percutaneous transmyocardial r.
(PTMR)
percutaneous transmyocardial
laser r. (PMR)
radiofrequency percutaneous
myocardial r. (RF-PMR)
repeat r.
surgical r.
r. system
target lesion r. (TLR)
target vessel r. (TVR)
transmyocardial r. (TMR)
transmyocardial laser r. (TMLR)
Reveal Plus insertable loop recorder
Revelation
R. endocardial microcatheter
R. microcatheter for EP mapping
R. Tx microcatheter for RF
ablation
reverberation
r. artifact
echo r.
reversal
atrial r. (AR)
holodiastolic flow r.
lead r.
r. speed of bronchoconstriction in
response to methacholine (r-Sm)
systolic r.
venous flow r. (VR)
reverse
r. differential cyanosis
r. polarity
r. remodeling
r. saphenous vein
r. squeeze
r. transcriptase polymerase chain
reaction (RT-PCR)
r. transcriptase polymerase chain
reaction test
reversed
r. arm leads
r. bypass
r. coarctation
r. ductus arteriosus
r. paradoxical pulse
r. reciprocal rhythm
r. saphenous vein graft

R

r. shunt
r. three sign
reversibility
reversible
r. airway obstruction
r. bronchospasm
r. ischemic neurologic defect
(RIND)
r. left ventricular dysfunction
r. obstructive airways disease
(ROAD)
reversion
noise r.
Reversol injection
Revex
reviparin
revision
International Classification of
Diseases, Ninth R. (ICD-9)
rewarming
continuous arteriovenous r. (CAVR)
Reye syndrome
Rey Figure Copy test
Reynolds number
RF
radiofrequency
rheumatic fever
RF catheter ablation
RF Marinr catheter
RF wave
RFA
radiofrequency ablation
RFb
respiratory feedback
RfB
RfB System-I for controlled
diaphragmatic breathing
RFC
radiofrequency current
RFG-35
Radionics RFG-35
RF-generated thermal balloon catheter
RFLP
restriction fragment length polymorphism
RF-PMR
radiofrequency percutaneous myocardial
revascularization
RGC
respiratory glycoconjugate
RGEA
right gastroepiploic artery

RGM
recurrent glioblastoma multiforme
RH
right heart
Rh
rhesus
Rh antibody
Rh factor
Mini-Gamulin Rh
rhabdomyolysis
rhabdomyoma
rhabdomyosarcoma
RHAMM
receptor for hyaluronan-mediated motility
rhamnolipid mucus secretion
rhATIII
recombinant human antithrombin III
RHB
right heart bypass
RHC
right heart catheterization
RHD
radiant heat device
rheumatic heart disease
right hemisphere damage
rheocardiography
rheography
light reflexion r.
rheologic
r. change
r. therapy
rheology
rheolytic
r. coronary thrombectomy
rheolytic thrombectomy catheter
Rheomacrodex
rhesus (Rh)
rheumatic
r. AF
r. aortitis
r. arteritis
r. carditis
r. endocarditis
r. fever (RF)
r. heart disease (RHD)
r. mitral insufficiency
r. mitral stenosis (RMS)
r. mitral valve stenosis
r. myocarditis
r. pericarditis
r. pneumonia

NOTES

rheumatic *(continued)*
r. valvular heart disease (RVHD)
r. valvulitis
rheumatica
angina r.
rheumatism
r. of heart
tuberculous r.
rheumatoid
r. arteritis
r. arthritis (RA)
r. factor
r. lung
r. nodule
r. pleuritis
r. pneumoconiosis
r. pneumonoconiosis
Rheumatrex
RHF
right heart failure
rhinitis
allergic r.
irritant r.
r. medicamentosa
nonallergic noninfectious
perennial r. (NANIPER)
perennial allergic r.
postnasal drip due to r. (PND-Rh)
seasonal allergic r.
vasomotor r.
rhinocerebral infection
rhinoconjunctivitis
Rhinocort Aqua
rhinomanometer
rhinopharyngeal
rhinopharynx
rhinoscleroma
rhinoscleromatis
Klebsiella r.
rhinoscopy
fiberoptic r.
Rhinosyn
R.-DMX
R. Liquid
Rhinosyn-PD Liquid
rhinovirus (RV)
r-hirudin
recombinant hirudin
Rhizopus oryzae
RHMV
right heart mixing volume
rhodesiense
Trypanosoma r.
Rho(D) immune globulin
Rhodnius polixus
Rhodococcus equi
RhoGAM

rhoGDI
RhoGDP-dissociation inhibitor 1
RhoGDP-dissociation inhibitor 1 (rhoGDI)
Rho-kinase
rhonchal fremitus
rhonchus, pl. **rhonchi**
expiratory rhonchi
rales and rhonchi
sibilant rhonchi
sonorous rhonchi
Rhotral
RHR
resting heart rate
RHRV
relative heart rate variability
rhuIL-10
recombinant human IL-10
rhVEGF
recombinant human vascular endothelial growth factor
rhysodes
Acanthamoeba r.
rhythm
accelerated atrioventricular junctional r.
accelerated A-V junctional r.
accelerated idioventricular r. (AIVR)
accelerated ventricular r. (AVR)
agonal r.
artificial pacemaker-induced ventricular r. (APIVR)
atrial escape r.
atrioventricular junction r. (AVJR)
atrioventricular junctional r.
atrioventricular nodal r., A-V nodal r.
A-V atrioventricular junctional r.
baseline r.
bigeminal r.
cantering r.
cardiac r. (CR)
R. catheter
chaotic r.
circadian r.
concealed r.
coronary nodal r.
coronary sinus r.
coupled r.
r. disturbance
diurnal r.
ectopic r.
embryocardia r.
escape r.
fetal heart r.
fibrillation r.
force and r. (F and R)
gallop r.

idiojunctional r.
idionodal r.
idioventricular r. (IVR)
irregular r.
irregularly irregular cardiac r.
junctional r. (JR)
junctional escape r. (JER)
lower nodal r.
midnodal r.
mu r.
nodal escape r.
normal sinus r. (NSR)
paced r.
pendulum r.
pulseless idioventricular r.
quadrigeminal r.
quadruple r.
rate and r. (R&R)
reciprocal r.
reciprocating r.
regularly irregular r.
regular rate and r. (RRR, RR&R)
regular sinus r. (RSR, rSR′)
reversed reciprocal r.
sinus r. (SR)
slow escape r.
r. strip
systolic gallop r.
tic-tac r.
trainwheel r.
trigeminal r.
triple r.
underlying heart r. (UHR)
ventricular r. (VR)
ventricular paced r. (VPR)
wide complex r.
rhythmicity
Rhythmin
Rhythmonorm
rhythmophone
RhythmScan
RI
Röhrer body mass index
RIA
radioimmunoassay
rib
r. approximator
r. cage
r. cutter
r. elevator
r. fracture
r. guillotine

lower r.
r. margin
middle r.
r. notching
r. raspatory
r. shears
r. spreader
upper r.
ribavirin
Ribbert thrombosis
ribbon
r. muscle
safety r.
ribonucleic acid (RNA)
riboprobe
CMV IE-2 r.
HIV-1 r.
IE-2 r.
riboside
AICA r.
ribosome
RIC
right interventricular coronary
RIC artery
Richet aneurysm
Richter transformation
Ricketts-Abrams technique
Rickettsia
R. australis
R. prowazekii
rickettsial
r. endocarditis
r. myocarditis
r. pneumonia
ridge
eustachian r.
neointimal r.
pharyngeal r.
pulmonary r.
supraortic r. (SAR)
riding
r. embolism
r. embolus
RIE
relative inspiratory effort
Riedel
R. struma
R. thyroiditis
Riegel pulse
Rienhoff-Finochietto rib spreader
Rienhoff thoracic scissors

NOTES

RIF
rifampin
rifabutin
Rifadin
R. injection
R. Oral
rifalazil
Rifamate
rifampicin
rifampin (RIF)
r. and isoniazid
rifampin, isoniazid, and pyrazinamide
rifamycin
rifapentine
Rifater
Rift Valley fever virus
right
r. ankle index
r. anterior oblique (RAO)
r. anterior oblique equivalent
r. anterior oblique position
r. anterior oblique projection
r. aortic arch
r. arm (VR)
r. atrial appendage (RAA)
r. atrial enlargement (RAE)
r. atrial free wall (RAFW)
r. atrial hypertrophy (RAH)
r. atrial inversion (RAI)
r. atrial inversion time index
  (RAITI)
r. atrial involvement (RAI)
r. atrial mean pressure (RAMP)
r. atrial mobile thrombi (RAMT)
r. atrial myxoma
r. atrial pacing
r. atrial pressure (RAP)
r. atrial thrombus
r. atrial wall (RAW)
r. atrium (RA)
r. atrium diameter (RAD)
r. auricle (RA)
r. auricle of heart
r. axis deviation (RAD)
r. border cardiac dullness (RBCD)
r. border of dullness (RBD)
r. brachial artery (RBA)
r. brachial vein (RBV)
r. brain damage (RBD)
r. bundle (RB)
r. bundle branch (RBB)
r. bundle-branch block (RBBB)
r. bundle branch system block
  (RBBsB)
r. cardiac work index (RWCI)
r. cerebrovascular accident (RCVA)
r. common carotid artery (RCCA)
r. congestive heart failure (RCHF)
r. coronary artery (RCA)

r. coronary catheter
r. coronary cusp (RCC)
r. coronary ostium (RCO)
r. coronary sinus (RCS)
r. costal margin (RCM)
r. crus of diaphragm
r. gastroepiploic artery (RGEA)
r. heart (RH)
r. heart bypass (RHB)
r. heart catheter
r. heart catheterization (RHC)
r. heart failure (RHF)
r. heart mixing volume (RHMV)
r. hemidiaphragm height
r. hemisphere damage (RHD)
r. hemisphere stroke
r. inferior pulmonary vein
r. inferior vena cava (RIVC)
r. internal mammary artery (RIMA)
r. internal mammary artery graft
r. internal thoracic artery (RITA)
r. internal thoracic artery graft
r. interventricular coronary (RIC)
r. Judkins catheter
r. lower lobe (RLL)
r. lower pulmonary vein (RLPV)
r. main bronchus
r. margin of heart
r. middle cerebral artery (R-MCA)
r. middle lobe (RML)
r. parasternal impulse
r. portal vein (RPV)
r. posterior ventricular preexcitation
  (RPVP)
r. pulmonary artery (RPA)
r. pulmonary vein (RPV)
r. recurrent laryngeal nerve
r. septum (RS)
r. single lung transplant (RSLTx)
r. superior pulmonary vein
r. superior vena cava (RSVC)
r. triangular ligament of liver
r. upper lobe (RUL)
r. upper pulmonary vein (RUPV)
r. ventricle (RV)
r. ventricle activation (RVA)
r. ventricle anterior wall (RVAW)
r. ventricle infarction (RVI)
r. ventricular (RV)
r. ventricular apex (RVA)
r. ventricular assist device (RVAD)
r. ventricular cardiomyopathy
r. ventricular copulsation balloon
  (RVCB)
r. ventricular diastolic collapse
  (RVDC)
r. ventricular diastolic overload
  (RVDO)
r. ventricular diastolic pressure

r. ventricular diastolic volume (RVDV)
r. ventricular dimension (RVD)
r. ventricular dysplasia
r. ventricular ejection fraction (REF, RVEF)
r. ventricular ejection time (RVET)
r. ventricular end-diastolic (RVED)
r. ventricular end-diastolic diameter (RVEDD)
r. ventricular end-diastolic pressure (RVEDP)
r. ventricular end-diastolic volume (RVEDV)
r. ventricular end-diastolic volume index (RVEDVI)
r. ventricular end-flow (RVEF)
r. ventricular endocardial potential (RVECP)
r. ventricular end-systolic volume (RVESV)
r. ventricular end-systolic volume index (RVESVI)
r. ventricular enlargement (RVE)
r. ventricular failure (RVF)
r. ventricular filling pressure (RVFP)
r. ventricular function
r. ventricular heave
r. ventricular hypertrophy (RVH)
r. ventricular hypoplasia
r. ventricular infarction
r. ventricular inflow obstruction
r. ventricular inflow tract (RVIT)
r. ventricular internal dimension (RVID)
r. ventricular isovolumic relaxation time (RV-IVRT)
r. ventricular mean (RVM)
r. ventricular myxoma
r. ventricular outflow (RVO)
r. ventricular outflow obstruction
r. ventricular outflow tract (RVOT)
r. ventricular outflow tract pacing
r. ventricular outflow tract reconstruction
r. ventricular outflow tract tachycardia
r. ventricular peak filling rate (RVPFR)
r. ventricular peak systolic pressure

r. ventricular pre-ejection period (RVPEP)
r. ventricular pressure (RVP)
r. ventricular refractory period (RVERP)
r. ventricular septal pacing
r. ventricular stroke output (RVSO)
r. ventricular stroke volume (RVSV)
r. ventricular stroke work (RVSW)
r. ventricular stroke work index (RVSWI)
r. ventricular systolic pressure (RUSP, RVSP)
r. ventricular systolic time interval
r. ventricular volume (RVV)
r. ventricular volume overload (RVVO)
r. ventricular wall (RVW)
r. ventricular wall motion
r. ventricular wall thickness (RVWT)
r. vertebral artery (RVA)
right-angle chest tube
right-left shunt (R-Lsh)
right middle cerebral artery (R-MCA)
right-sided
    r.-s. endocarditis
    r.-s. heart failure
right-to-left shunt (RLS)
right-ventricle afterload
rightward axis
rigid
    r. bronchoscopy
    r. monopolar loop
    r. pod
    r. thoracoscope
rigidity
    nuchal r.
Rigiflex TTS balloon catheter
rigor
    calcium r.
RIHD
    radiation-induced heart disease
RIK fluid-filled head pack
Riley-Cournand equation
Riley-Day syndrome
Riley needle
rilmenidine
riluzole

NOTES

RIMA
　　right internal mammary artery
　　RIMA graft
rima
　　r. respiratoria
　　r. vestibuli
　　r. vocalis
Rimactane Oral
rimantadine hydrochloride
rimiterol
RIND
　　reversible ischemic neurologic defect
Rindfleisch fold
ring
　　r. abscess
　　AnnuloFlex flexible annuloplasty r.
　　AnnuloFlo annuloplasty r.
　　annuloplasty r.
　　aortic r.
　　atrial r.
　　atrioventricular valve r.
　　cardiac lymphatic r.
　　Carpentier r.
　　Carpentier-Edwards Physio
　　　annuloplasty r.
　　circumaortic venous r.
　　coronary r.
　　double-flanged valve sewing r.
　　Duran annuloplasty r.
　　r. electrode
　　esophageal contraction r.
　　fibrous r.
　　knitted sewing r.
　　left ventricular cavity obstruction r.
　　Lower r.'s
　　metal sewing r.
　　pharyngeal lymphatic r.
　　plastic sewing r.
　　pleural r.'s
　　prosthetic valve sewing r.
　　Puig Massana annuloplasty r.
　　Puig Massana-Shiley annuloplasty r.
　　Schatzki esophageal r.
　　Sculptor annuloplasty r.
　　Seguin annuloplasty r.
　　sewing r.
　　r. shadow
　　r. sign
　　SJM Seguin annuloplasty r.
　　SJM Tailor annuloplasty r.
　　supraannular suture r.
　　supraortic r. (SAR)
　　tantalum r.
　　tonsillar r.
　　tracheal r.
　　vascular r.
　　Waldeyer throat r.
　　Waldeyer tonsillar r.

Ringer
　　R. lactate
　　R. solution
RinoFlow ENT wash unit
Riolan
　　anastomosis of R.
RIP
　　respiratory inductance plethysmograph
　　respiratory inductance plethysmography
　　RIP portable sleep monitor
RISA
　　radioactive iodinated serum albumin
risk
　　r. calculator
　　competing r.'s
　　r. factor
　　r. factor profile
　　Goldman index of r.
　　r. index
　　modified multifactorial index of
　　　cardiac r.
　　recurrence r.
　　relative r. (RR)
　　restenosis r.
　　stochastic r.
　　r. stratification
　　surgical r.
　　r. threshold
RITA
　　right internal thoracic artery
　　RITA graft
Ritalin
Ritalin-SR
Ritchie Articular Index
ritodrine
ritonavir
Riva-Rocci sphygmomanometer
RIVC
　　right inferior vena cava
Rivermead
　　R. Behavioral Memory Test
　　R. Motor Assessment Arm score
Rivero-Carvallo
　　R.-C. effect
　　R.-C. sign
Rivetti-Levinson IntraLuminal shunt
Riviere sign
Rivinus
　　R. canals
　　R. gland
Rizaben
RKG
　　radiocardiogram
R-lactate enzyme monotest
RLF
　　retained lung fluid
RLH
　　recurrent lobar hemorrhage

RLL
  right lower lobe
RLP
  remnant-like lipoprotein particle
  remnant lipoprotein
    RLP lipoprotein
RLPV
  right lower pulmonary vein
RLS
  right-to-left shunt
R-Lsh
  right-left shunt
RLT
  red light therapy
RMBF
  regional myocardial blood flow
R-MCA
  right middle cerebral artery
RMI
  recent myocardial infarction
    RMI antegrade cardioplegia catheter
RML
  right middle lobe
RMR
  resting metabolic rate
rMRGlu
  glucose metabolism
RMS
  rheumatic mitral stenosis
RNA
  radionuclide angiography
  ribonucleic acid
    RNA glycosidase toxin
RNSC
  radionuclide superior cavography
RNV
  radionuclide venography
  radionuclide ventriculography
RNVG
  radionuclide ventriculography
ROA
  regurgitant orifice area
ROAD
  reversible obstructive airways disease
Roadmapper
roadmapping
    coronary r.
Roadrunner extra-support wire guide
Robafen
    R. AC
    R. CF
    R. DM

Robertshaw tube
Robertson sign
Robicsek vascular probe
Robinson index
Robinul Forte
Robiscek technique
Robitussin
    R. A-C
    R. Cough Calmers
    R. DM
    R. Pediatric
    R. Severe Congestion Liqui-Gels
Rocephin IM
Rochalimaea
Rocha-Lima inclusion
Roche-Microwell plate hybridization method
Rochester
    R. Kocher clamp
    R. needle
    R. Péan clamp
rocker
rocket immunoelectrophoretic method of Laurell
Rockey ventricular cannula
Rocky Mountain spotted fever
rocuronium
rodhaini
    Babesia r.
Rodrigo equation
Rodriguez aneurysm
roentgen (R)
    r. knife
roentgenogram
    apical lordotic r.
    chest r. (CR)
roentgenographically occult lung cancer (ROLC)
roentgenographic presentation
roentgenography
    chest r. (CR)
Roesler-Bressler infarction
RoEzIt skin moisturizer
Rofact
Roferon-A
Rogaine topical
Roger
    R. bruit
    bruit de R.
    R. disease

R

NOTES

Roger *(continued)*
    maladie de R.
    R. murmur
Rogitine
Roho mattress
Rohrer
    R. body mass index (RI)
    R. equation
ROI
    region of interest
Rokitansky disease
ROLC
    roentgenographically occult lung cancer
role
    cardioprotective r.
roller pump
Rolleston rule
rolling hernia
Romana sign
Romhilt-Estes
    R.-E. point score criteria
    R.-E. point scoring system
    R.-E. score
ROMI
    rule out myocardial infarction
romied
    ruled out for myocardial infarction
Rondamine-DM drops
Rondec
    R.-DM
    R. Drops
    R. Filmtabs
    R. Syrup
rongeur
    aortic valve r.
    Bailey aortic valve r.
R-on-T
    R-o.-T arrhythmia susceptibility
    R-o.-T phenomenon
    R-o.-T premature ventricular
      complex
R-on-T-initiated
    R-o.-T-i. nonsustained VT
    R-o.-T-i. VF
roof of left atrium
room
    cardiovascular recovery r. (CVRR)
Roos test
root
    anterior wall of aortic r. (AWAR)
    aortic r.
    free r.
    r. inclusion method
    r. injection
    r. of lung
    r. perfusion
    posterior wall or aortic r. (PAR)
    r. tailoring
root-mean-square voltage

ROP
    retinopathy of prematurity
ROPE
    respiratory ordered phase encoding
ropy sputum
Rosai-Dorfman disease
Rosalki technique
ROSC
    restoration of spontaneous circulation
    return of spontaneous circulation
rose
    r. hips asthma
    R. Questionnaire
    r. spot
    R. tamponade
Rosenbach syndrome
Rosenberg syndrome
Rosenmüller recess
rosette
    acinar r.
rosiglitazone
Ross
    R. aortic valve replacement
      procedure
    R. needle
    R. River virus
Rossetti modification of Nissen
fundoplication
Ross-Konno pediatric
aortoventriculoplasty procedure
Rostan asthma
rostral
    r. ventrolateral medulla (RVLM)
    r. ventromedial medulla (RVMM)
rosuvastatin
ROTA
    rotablator atherectomy
rotablator
    r. atherectomy (ROTA)
    r. and restenosis (R&R)
Rotacaps
    Ventolin R.
ROTACS
    rotational angioplasty catheter system
Rotadisk
    Flovent R.
RotaGlide lubricant
Rotahaler
RotaLink rotational atherectomy device
rotary
    r. atherectomy device
    r. vertigo
rotating
    r. blades
    r. disk oxygenation
rotation
    cardiac r.
    clockwise r.

counterclockwise r.
shoulder r.

rotational
r. ablation
r. angioplasty catheter system (ROTACS)
r. atherectomy (RA)
r. atherectomy device
r. atherectomy system (RAS)
r. coronary atherectomy (RCA)
r. dynamic angioplasty catheter

RotaWire Floppy Gold guide wire
Rotch sign
Rotex needle
Rothbarth
R. Uni-Flo infusion catheter
R. Uni-Flo infusion set

Rothia dentocariosa
Rothschild sign
Roth spot
Rotoslide
rotundum
foramen r.

Roubac
Roubin infusion catheter
Rougnon-Heberden disease
rouleau formation
round
r. foramen
r. heart
r. hematoma
r. pneumonia nodule

rounded atelectasis
round-robin classification
roundworm
Rous sarcoma virus (RSV)
Roussy-Lévy
R.-L. disease
R.-L. polyneuropathy
R.-L. syndrome

route of insertion
routine
cardiac ambulation r. (CAR)

Roux-en-Y obesity
Rovamycine
roxithromycin
royal
R. Flush Plus high-flow angiographic flush catheter
r. jelly-induced asthma

RP
radial pulse
reperfusion

RPA
reteplase
right pulmonary artery

r-PA
reteplase

RPBD
rating of perceived breathing difficulty

RPE
rating of perceived exertion

r-PEG
recombinant polyethylene glycol

RPF
renal plasma flow

RPFA
rapid platelet function assay

R-P interval
RPM
real-time position management
RPM tracking system
RPM tracking system/catheter

RPP
heart rate-systolic blood pressure product
rate-pressure product

Rp:Rs
pulmonary-to-systemic vascular resistance

RPV
right portal vein
right pulmonary vein

RPVP
right posterior ventricular preexcitation

RQ
respiratory quotient

R/Q wave ratio
RR
relative risk
respiratory rate
RR cycle
RR interval dynamics
RR interval stability
RR prime

R&R
rate and rhythm
rotablator and restenosis

RRI
recurrent respiratory infection

R-R′ interval
R-R interval

NOTES

RRP
relative refractory period
RRR
regular rate and rhythm
relative risk reduction
RR&R
regular rate and rhythm
Rrs
respiratory resistance
RS
right septum
RS complex
RS deflection
rS$_{02}$
regional oxygen saturation
RSA
respiratory sinus arrhythmia
Rsa
systemic arterial resistance
RSBI
rapid shallow breathing index
RSC
rested state contraction
RSI
rapid sequence induction
RSI orotracheal intubation
RSLTx
right single lung transplant
r-Sm
reversal speed of bronchoconstriction in
response to methacholine
RSR, rSR′
regular sinus rhythm
rSr
electrocardiographic complex
rsr prime (rSR′)
RSSR
relative slow sinus rate
RS-T
RS-T interval
RS-T segment
R-Stent stent
RSV
respiratory syncytial virus
Rous sarcoma virus
RSVA
ruptured sinus of Valsalva aneurysm
RSVC
right superior vena cava
RSV-IG
respiratory syncytial virus
immunoglobulin
RT
reciprocating tachycardia
reentrant tachycardia
resistance training
RT3D echo
R-Test Evolution

Rti
resistance to movement of lung tissue
RTLF
respiratory tract lining fluid
Rtot
total airway resistance
rt-PA
recombinant tissue plasminogen activator
catabolism of rt-PA
double-chain rt-PA
RT-PCR
reverse transcriptase polymerase chain
reaction
rub
centripetal r. (CPR)
friction r.
gallop, murmur, r. (GMR)
pericardial friction r.
pleural friction r.
pleuritic r.
pleuropericardial r.
saddle leather friction r.
rubbery sputum
rubella syndrome
rubeola
Rubex
rubidium (Rb)
rubidium-81
rubidium-82 (Rb-82)
rubidium-82 imaging
rubidium-82 positron emission
tomography
Rubinstein-Taybi syndrome
Rubinul
rubitecan
rubor
dependent r.
rubs, gallops, murmurs
Rubulavirus
ruby laser
rude respiration
rudimentary chamber
Rudolph Full Face mask
RUDS
reactive upper airways dysfunction
syndrome
Ruel aorta clamp
r-UK
recombinant urokinase
RUL
right upper lobe
rule
r. of bigeminy
Gibson r.
Liebermeister r.
r. out myocardial infarction
(ROMI)

R

Rolleston r.
shorthand r.
ruled out for myocardial infarction (romied)
rumble
    Austin Flint r.
    booming r.
    diastolic r.
    filling r.
    middiastolic r.
    protodiastolic r.
    third sound r.
rumbling diastolic murmur
Rumel
    R. clamp
    R. tourniquet
Rumpel-Leede test
run
    second pump r.
runaway pacemaker
runoff
    aortofemoral arterial r.
    aortogram with distal r.
    arterial r.
    r. arteriogram
    digital r.
    distal r.
    venous r.
rupture
    aortic r.
    balloon r.
    blunt cardiac r.
    cardiac r.
    chamber r.
    chordae tendineae r.
    chordal r.
    coronary plaque r.
    diaphragmatic r.
    esophageal r.
    IEM r.
    internal elastic membrane r.
    interventricular septal r.
    intraperitoneal r.
    intrapleural r.
    membrane r.
    myocardial free wall r.
    nonpenetrating r.
    papillary muscle r. (PMR)
    penetrating r.
    perivascular r.
    pinhole balloon r.
    plaque r.

    pulmonary artery r.
    thoracic aortic r. (TAR)
    traumatic r.
    r. trigger
    valve r.
    ventricular septal r.
ruptured
    r. aortic aneurysm
    r. sinus of Valsalva
    r. sinus of Valsalva aneurysm (RSVA)
RUPV
    right upper pulmonary vein
Ruschelit polyvinyl chloride endotracheal tube
RUSP
    right ventricular systolic pressure
Russian influenza
rusty sputum
Ru-Tuss
    r.-t. DE
    r.-t. Expectorant
RV
    regurgitant volume
    residual volume
    rhinovirus
    right ventricle
    right ventricular
RVA
    reentrant ventricular arrhythmia
    right ventricle activation
    right ventricular apex
    right vertebral artery
RVAD
    right ventricular assist device
RVAW
    right ventricle anterior wall
RVCB
    right ventricular copulsation balloon
RVD
    reference vessel diameter
    relative vessel diameter
    right ventricular dimension
RVDC
    right ventricular diastolic collapse
RVDO
    right ventricular diastolic overload
RVDV
    right ventricular diastolic volume
RVE
    right ventricular enlargement

NOTES

RVECP
right ventricular endocardial potential
RVED
right ventricular end-diastolic
RVED pressure
RVEDD
right ventricular end-diastolic diameter
RVEDP
right ventricular end-diastolic pressure
RVEDV
right ventricular end-diastolic volume
RVEDVI
right ventricular end-diastolic volume
index
RVEF
right ventricular ejection fraction
right ventricular end-flow
RVERP
right ventricular refractory period
RVESV
right ventricular end-systolic volume
RVESVI
right ventricular end-systolic volume
index
RVET
right ventricular ejection time
RVF
residual volume fraction
right ventricular failure
RVFP
right ventricular filling pressure
RVH
renovascular hypertension
right ventricular hypertrophy
RVHD
rheumatic valvular heart disease
RVI
right ventricle infarction
RVID
right ventricular internal dimension
RVIT
right ventricular inflow tract
RV-IVRT
right ventricular isovolumic relaxation
time
RVLM
rostral ventrolateral medulla
RVM
right ventricular mean
RVMM
rostral ventromedial medulla
RVO
right ventricular outflow
RVol
regurgitant volume
RVOT
right ventricular outflow tract
RVOT pacing

RVP
resting venous pressure
right ventricular pressure
RVPEP
right ventricular pre-ejection period
RVPFR
right ventricular peak filling rate
RVR
reduced vascular response
repetitive ventricular response
resistance to venous return
RVSO
right ventricular stroke output
RVSP
right ventricular systolic pressure
RVSV
right ventricular stroke volume
RVSW
right ventricular stroke work
RVSWI
right ventricular stroke work index
RVTE
recurring venous thromboembolism
RV/TLC
residual volume/total lung capacity
RV/TLC ratio
RVV
right ventricular volume
RVVO
right ventricular volume overload
RVW
right ventricular wall
RVWT
right ventricular wall thickness
R-wave progression (RWP)
RWCI
right cardiac work index
RWM
regional wall motion
RWMA
regional wall motion abnormality
RWP
R-wave progression
RWT
relative wall thickness
RX
RX CrossSail coronary dilatation
catheter
Folgard RX
RX Streak balloon catheter
ryanodine receptor
Ryna-C Liquid
Rynacrom
Ryna-CX
Ryna Liquid
Rynatan
Rynatuss Pediatric Suspension
Rythmodan
Rythmodan-LA

NOTES

R

S
negative deflection that follows an R
wave
septum
systole
S′ wave
S660
S660 small vessel coronary stent
S660 with Discrete Technology
coronary stent system
S670
S670 coronary stent
S670 with Discrete Technology
coronary stent system
S₁
first heart sound
S₂
second heart sound
S2 allele
S₃
third heart sound
S₃ gallop
S₄
fourth heart sound
S₄ gallop
S₇
summation gallop
S₇ gallop
S7 coronary stent
SA
salvage angioplasty
secondary arrest
sinoatrial
sinus arrest
sinus arrhythmia
stable angina
Peritrate SA
S-A
sinoatrial
S-A nodal reentrant tachycardia
S-A node
S/A
stent-to-artery
S/A ratio
SAA
serum amyloid type A
SAAP
selective aortic arch perfusion
SAB
sinoatrial block
Sabin-Feldman dye test
Sable PTCA balloon catheter
sabot
coeur en s.
s. heart

SABP
systolic arterial blood pressure
Sabulin
SAC
serial autocorrelation
SAC data acquisition technology
sac
air s.
alveolar s.
aneurysmal s.
aortic s.
Hilton s.
Lap S.
lateral s.
pericardial s.
pleural s.
sacchari
Thermoactinomyces s.
Saccharomonospora
Saccharomyces anginae
Saccharopolyspora rectivirgula
Saccomanno
S. fixative
S. morphologic criteria
saccular
s. aneurysm
s. bronchiectasis
s. period
sacculated
s. empyema
s. pleurisy
sacculation
localized s.
saccule of larynx
sacculus
s. alveolares
s. alveolaris
s. laryngis
saccus endolymphaticus
sacral edema
sacrococcygeal aorta
SACS
secondary anticoagulation system
SACT
sinoatrial conduction time
SAD
sinoaortic denervation
saddle
s. embolism
s. embolus
s. leather friction rub
s. thrombus
**Sade modification of Norwood
procedure**

SADS
sudden arrhythmic death syndrome
SAEB
sinoatrial entrance block
SAECG
signal-averaged electrocardiogram
signal-averaged electrocardiography
SAED
semiautomatic external defibrillator
Safar bronchoscope
safe
S. Step blood-collection needle
S. Tussin 30
Safe-Steer
S.-S. guidewire
S.-S. support catheter
S.-S. system
Safe-T Tube
Montgomery S.-T T.
SafeTway pediatric mouthpiece
safety
s. guidewire
occupational health and s. (OHS)
radiation s.
s. ribbon
sag
ST s.
sagittal
s. cut
s. plane
s. view
SAH
subarachnoid hemorrhage
SAHS
sleep apnea/hypopnea syndrome
saht
sail sound
saint (St.)
Sala cell
salbutamol
Salflex
salicylate
carbazochrome s.
choline s.
magnesium s.
phenyl s.
sodium s.
saline
Broncho S.
half-normal s.
heparinized s.
hypertonic s.
iced s.
s. jet
s. loading
normal s.
phosphate-buffered s. (PBS)
s. slush
salivagram

salivaris
caruncula s.
salivarius
Streptococcus s.
salivation, lacrimation, urination, and defecation (SLUD)
Salkowski test
salmeterol
s. and fluticasone propionate
s. xinafoate
Salmonella choleraesuis
salmon skin
salol
saloon door parasternal approach
salsalate
salt
dietary s.
ethylenediaminetetraacetic acid disodium s.
gold s.
s. of nickel
no added s. (NAS)
s. and pepper pattern
persulfate s.
s. of platinum
salt and pepper appearance
salt and water dependent hypertension
s. wasting
saltans
thrombophlebitis s.
salt-depletion syndrome
salt-free diet
salting-out procedure
Salubria biomaterial
saluresis
saluretic agent
salute
allergic s.
Salutensin-Demi
saluting
salvage
s. angioplasty (SA)
s. balloon angioplasty
intraoperative cell s.
limb s.
myocardial s.
salves
tachycardia en s.
salvo
s. of beats
s. of ventricular tachycardia
SAM
surface adherent monocyte
systolic anterior motion
SAM system
Sam Levine sign
sample
end-tidal s.

Haldane-Priestley s.
Rahn-Otis s.
sampler
continuous ambulatory blood s.
(CABS)
sampling
bioptic s.
blood s.
chorionic villus s.
Samsoon-Young
S.-Y. airway class I-IV
S.-Y. modification of Mallampati
airway classification
Samuels
S. forceps
S. hemoclip
SAN
sinoatrial node
sinoauricular node
San
S. Joaquin Valley disease
S. Joaquin Valley fever
Sanchez-Cascos cardioauditory syndrome
Sanders bed
Sandhoff disease
Sandifer syndrome
Sandler-Dodge area-length method
Sandman system
Sandoglobulin
Sandostatin LAR
SANDR
sinoatrial nodal reentry
Sandrock test
sandwich
s. enzyme-linked immunosorbent
assay
s. patch
Sanfilippo syndrome
sanguinis
fragilitas s.
ictus s.
Sansert
Sansom sign
SANWS
sinoatrial node weakness syndrome
SAO
subvalvular aortic obstruction
SaO₂
arterial oxygen saturation
SAP
stable angina pectoris

systemic arterial pressure
systolic atrial pressure
SAPD
signal-averaged P-wave duration
saphenofemoral
s. junction
s. system
saphenous
s. vein (SV)
s. vein bypass (SVB)
s. vein bypass graft angiography
s. vein bypass grafting (SVBG)
s. vein cannula
s. vein cutdown (SVC)
s. vein graft (SVG)
s. vein harvesting (SVH)
s. vein patch closure
s. vein varicosity
SAPH Finder surgical balloon dissector
SAPHtrak balloon dissector
saprophytic
SAPS
Simplified Acute Physiology Score
SAQLI
Sleep Apnea Quality of Life Index
saquinavir mesylate
SAR
supraortic ridge
supraortic ring
saralasin
sarcoglycan
sarcoid
Boeck s.
s. granuloma
sarcoidosis
bronchial s.
fibrocystic s.
nodular s.
parenchymal s.
pulmonary s.
sarcolemmal
s. bleb
s. calcium channel
s. glucose
s. level
s. membrane
sarcolemma lipid
sarcoma
cardiac s.
Kaposi s. (KS)
metastatic s.
pseudo-Kaposi s.

S

NOTES

sarcoma *(continued)*
soft tissue s.
synovial s.
sarcomatoid mesothelioma
sarcomatous tumor
sarcomere
Sarcophaga
sarcoplasmic
s. reticulum
s. reticulum-associated glycolytic
enzymes
sarcosporidiosis
sarcotubular system
Sarns
S. aortic arch cannula
S. electric saw
S. intracardiac suction tube
S. membrane oxygenator (SMO)
S. soft-flow aortic cannula
S. two-stage cannula
S. ventricular assist device
S. wire-reinforced catheter
Sarot bronchus clamp
SARS
severe acute respiratory syndrome
SART
sinoatrial recovery time
saruplase
SAS
small aorta syndrome
subaortic stenosis
subarachnoid space
supravalvular aortic stenosis
synchronous atrial stimulation
SAST
selective arterial secretin injection test
SAT
subacute thrombosis
systolic acceleration time
Press-mate SAT
satellite lesion
Satinsky clamp
sativa
Vicia s.
Satterthwaite method
saturated
s. fatty acid (SFA)
s. solution of potassium iodide
(SSKI)
saturation
arterial s.
arterial oxygen s. (SaO$_2$)
s. index
mean nocturnal s.
mixed venous oxygen s. (SvO$_2$)
oxygen s. (So$_2$)
oxyhemoglobin s.
regional oxygen s. (rS$_{02}$)
step-up in oxygen s.

s. time
venous s.
saucerize
Sauerbruch-Herrmannsdorfer-Gerson diet
sausaging of vein
SAV
sequential atrioventricular
Savary-Gilliard esophageal dilator
Saventrine Intravenous
Saver
Cell S.
Haemonetics Cell S.
SAVVI pacemaker
Savvy PTA dilatation catheter
saw
oscillating s.
Sarns electric s.
sternum s.
Stryker s.
sawtooth
s. pattern
s. P wave
Sawyer operation
SAX
short axis
SAX-MV
short-axis mitral valve
SAX-PM
short-axis plane, papillary muscle
SB
shortness of breath
sinus bradycardia
S-100B
protein S-100B
SBE
shortness of breath on exertion
subacute bacterial endocarditis
SBE prophylaxis
SBF
systemic blood flow
SBI
silent brain infarction
SBP
systolic blood pressure
SBS
sick building syndrome
SBSE
supine bicycle stress echocardiography
SBSP
simultaneous bilateral spontaneous
pneumothorax
SBT
serum bactericidal titer
SC
semilunar valve closure
systolic click
SC-210 sidestream capnograph
SC-300 portable capnograph

SCA
> sudden cardiac arrest
> superior cerebellar artery

scabbard trachea

SCABG
> single coronary artery bypass graft

SCAD, sCAD
> spontaneous coronary artery disease
> spontaneous coronary artery dissection

scaffolding

SCAI
> Society for Cardiac Angiography and
> Interventions

scalar
> s. electrocardiogram
> s. lead

scale
> Abbreviated Injury S. (AIS)
> activity s.
> ADL s.
> Ashworth S.
> Behavioral Dyscontrol S. (BDCS)
> Berg Balance S.
> Borg s. (1-20)
> Borg numerical s.
> Borg rating of perceived
>   exertion s.
> Borg treadmill exertion s.
> cardiac adjustment s. (CAS)
> Centers for Epidemiologic Studies
>   Depression s. (CES-D)
> Cook-Medley hostility s.
> Cook multiple-assessment s.
> Delirium Rating S.
> dyspnea s.
> Epworth sleepiness s. (ESS)
> European Stroke S. (ESS)
> Fagerstrom tolerance s.
> French s.
> Fugl-Meyer motor test s.
> Gaffky s.
> Geriatric Depression S.
> Glasgow Coma S. (GCS)
> gray s.
> Grossman s.
> Health Locus of Control S.
> Holmes-Rahe s.
> Hospital Anxiety and Depression S.
>   (HADS)
> Karnofsky rating s.
> Lawton Instrumental Activities of
>   Daily Living s.

> Likert s. (LS)
> Likert 5-point s.
> mechanical visual analogue s.
> Montgomery-Asberg Depression
>   Rating S. (MADRS)
> Motor Assessment S. (MAS)
> National Institutes of Health
>   Stroke S. (NIHSS)
> Nottingham Extended Activities of
>   Daily Living s.
> Observer's Assessment of
>   Alertness/Sedation S.
> Oxford Handicap S.
> Paykel s.
> Philadelphia Geriatric Center
>   Morale S. (PGCMS)
> Psychosocial Adjustment to
>   Illness S.
> pulmonary functional status s.
>   (PFSS)
> quick confusion s. (QCS)
> Rankin Disability S.
> Sickness Impact Profile s.
> SIP s.
> Spielberger Anger Expression s.
> Stroke Impact S. (SIS)
> subject's treatment-emergent
>   symptom s. (STRESS)
> Tennant distress s.
> Toronto Alexithymia S.
> visual analog s. (VAS)
> voxel gray s.
> Wigle s.

scalene
> s. fat pad biopsy
> s. lymph node biopsy

scalenectomy

scalenotomy
> Adson-Coffey s.

scalenus
> s. anterior syndrome
> s. anticus syndrome

scalloped
> s. commissure
> s. subcoronary position

scalloping

scalp
> s. electrode
> s. pH
> s. vein needle

SCAN
> systolic coronary artery narrowing

NOTES

S

scan

apical hypoperfusion on thallium s.
Cardiolite s.
Cardiotec s.
carotid duplex s.
cine s.
computed tomographic s.
s. converter
coronary artery s. (CAS)
CT s.
dipyridamole thallium-201 s.
duplex Doppler s.
dynamic CT s.
four-hour s.
gallium s.
gallium-67 s.
gated cardiac s.
HRCT s.
lung s.
milk s.
MUGA cardiac blood pool s.
multiple gated acquisition cardiac
  blood pool s.
perfusion s.
PET s.
postdiuresis s.
postexercise s.
PYP s.
pyrophosphate s.
rectilinear s.
scintillation s.
scout s.
sector s.
septal hyperperfusion on thallium s.
sestamibi s.
spiral CT s.
TCT s.
teboroxime s.
technetium-99m hexamibi s.
thin-slice CT s.
transmission s.
ultrafast computed tomography s.
ultrafast CT s.
ventilation/perfusion lung s.
V̇/Q̇ lung s.

scanner

computed tomography s.
Corometrics Doppler s.
Del Mar Avionics S.
Evolution s.
GE 9800 CT s.
GE Lightspeed CT s.
GE Signa Horizon SR 120 whole-
  body s.
Hewlett-Packard 77020 A phased-
  array sector s.
Imatron CT s.
Konica KFDR-S laser film s.
phased array sector s.

Philips Medical Systems Tomoscan
  AVE1 CT spiral s.
Philips Medical Systems Tomoscan
  SR 7000 CT spiral s.
Philips Tomoscan 310 CT s.
Picker CS s.
Picker Edge 1.5-T s.
Picker PQ 2000 CT s.
Picker Vista HPQ MRI s.
Siemens Somatom DR CT s.
Siemens Somatom Plus 4A s.
SonoHeart s.
SONOS 1500, 2500 s.
Toshiba s.
ultrafast computed tomographic s.
ultrafast CT s.

scanning

coronary calcium s.
duplex s.
electronic s.
s. electron microscope (SEM)
fluorodopamine positron emission
  tomographic s.
s. format
gated blood-pool s.
helical CT s.
interlaced s.
lung s.
MUGA s.
PET s.
progressive s.
thallium s.
venous duplex s. (VDS)

scanning-beam digital x-ray

scar

s. cancer
s. carcinoma
s. emphysema
fibrotic s.
infarct s.
myocardial fibrous s.
zipper s.

scarlatinosa

angina s.

scarlet fever

Scarpa

S. fascia
S. method

scarring

apical s.
pleural s.

scatter

Compton s.
s. radiation

scattered echo

scattergram

scattering

Rayleigh s.

scatterplot smoothing technique

scavenger
> s. cell pathway
> free-radical s.
> lysophosphatidylcholine s.
> oxygen radical s.

scavenging tube
SCD
> sequential compression device
> subacute coronary disease
> sudden cardiac death
> sudden coronary death

SCE
> serious cardiac event

Scedosporium apiospermum
SCF
> stem cell factor

Schafer method of artificial respiration
Schapiro sign
Schapiro-Wilks test
Schatzki esophageal ring
Schatz-Palmaz intravascular stent
Schaumann
> S. disease
> S. syndrome

Schede
> S. operation
> S. thoracoplasty

Scheie syndrome
Schellong-Strisower phenomenon
Schellong test
schenckii
> *Sporothrix s.*

Schenk-Eichelter vena cava plastic filter procedure
Schepelmann sign
Schick sign
Schiff test
Schiller method
Schindler esophagoscope
Schistosoma
> *S. haematobium*
> *S. japonicum*
> *S. mansoni*

schistosomiasis
schistothorax
Schlesinger solution
Schlichter test
Schmidt-Lanterman cleft
Schmidt syndrome
Schmitt-Erlanger model of reentry
Schmitz-Rode catheter
Schmorl furrow

Schneider
> S. index
> S. Speedy stent
> S. Wallstent

schneiderian respiratory membrane
Schneider-Meier-Magnum system
Scholten
> S. biopsy forceps
> S. endomyocardial bioptome

Schonander
> S. procedure
> S. technique

Schoonmaker-King single catheter technique
Schott treatment
Schuco nebulizer
Schueler Model 200 Aspirator
Schüller method
Schultz angina
Schultze test
Schumacher aorta clamp
schwannoma
Schwarten LP guidewire
SCI
> silent cerebral infarct
> silent cerebral infarction

scie
> bruit de s.

Scimed
> S. angioplasty catheter
> S. stent

scimitar
> s. sign
> s. syndrome

scintigram
> pyrophosphate s.

scintigraphic perfusion defect
scintigraphy
> AMA-Fab s.
> antimyosin infarct-avid s.
> diethylenetriamine pentaacetate aerosol inhalation lung s.
> dipyridamole thallium-201 s.
> dobutamine perfusion s.
> DTPA aerosol inhalation lung s.
> exercise thallium s.
> exercise thallium-201 s.
> gallium-67 s.
> gastroesophageal s.
> gated blood-pool s.
> GBP s.
> indium-111 s.

S

scintigraphy *(continued)*
  infarct-avid hot-spot s.
  infarct-avid myocardial s.
  iodine-131 MIBG s.
  labeled FFA s.
  MAA perfusion lung s.
  macroaggregated albumin perfusion lung s.
  microsphere perfusion s.
  milk s.
  myocardial cold-spot perfusion s.
  myocardial perfusion s. (MPS)
  myocardial stress perfusion s. (MSPS)
  myocardial viability s.
  perfusion s.
  planar myocardial s.
  planar thallium s.
  pulmonary s.
  pyrophosphate s.
  single-photon gamma s.
  SPECT s.
  stress perfusion s.
  stress thallium s.
  ^{99m}Tc sestamibi s.
  thallium myocardial s. (TMS)
  thallium-201 perfusion s.
  thallium-201 planar s.
  thallium rest-redistribution s.
  thallium-201 SPECT s.
  ventilation s.
scintillating speckle pattern
scintillation
  s. camera
  s. cocktail
  s. probe
  s. scan
scintiphotography
scintiscan
  technetium-99m stannous pyrophosphate s.
scintiscanner
scintiview
scirrhous carcinoma
scissors
  bandage s.
  Beall circumflex artery s.
  Crafoord lobectomy s.
  De Martel s.
  Dennis dissecting s.
  Duffield cardiovascular s.
  Jabaley-Stille Super Cut S.
  Jorgenson thoracic s.
  Karmody venous s.
  Metzenbaum s.
  pericardiotomy s.
  Rienhoff thoracic s.
SCL
  sinus cycle length

SCLC
  small cell lung carcinoma
sclera, pl. **sclerae**
  blue s.
scleredema
  s. adultorum
  s. of Buschke
sclerodactyly
scleroderma
  diffuse cutaneous s.
  s. lung
ScleroLaser
Scleromate
sclerosant
  pleural s.
sclerosing
  s. agent
  s. cholangitis
  s. hemangioma
  s. phlebitis
  variceal s.
sclerosis, pl. **scleroses**
  amyotrophic lateral s. (ALS)
  aortic s.
  arterial s.
  arteriocapillary s.
  arteriolar s.
  coronary s. (CS)
  endocardial s.
  Mönckeberg s.
  multiple s.
  nodular s.
  progressive systemic s. (PSS)
  subendocardial s.
  systemic s. (SS)
  tuberous s.
  valvular s.
  vascular s.
  venous s.
Sclerosol intrapleural aerosol
sclerotherapy
  endoscopic variceal s. (EVS)
  variceal s.
sclerotic
SCN5A mutation
Scoop 1, 2 catheter
scooped pattern
scooping
  ST s.
Scopulariopsis **spp pneumonia**
score
  Acute Physiology and Chronic Health Evaluation s.
  Agatston s.
  Aldrich ST elevation s.
  Anderson phasing s.
  Anderson-Wilkins acuteness s.
  APACHE s.
  asthma severity s. (ASS)

AW acuteness s.
Barthel ADL s.
Berning and Steensgaard-Hansen s.
Brasfield chest radiograph s.
Brush electrocardiographic s.
calcium s.
Califf s.
Canadian Cardiovascular Society
  angina s. (CCSAS)
Cardiac Infarction Injury S.
cardiovascular and respiratory
  elements of trauma s. (CVRS)
clinical pulmonary infection s.
  (CPIS)
Detsky s.
Dripps-American Surgical
  Association s.
Duke treadmill exercise s.
Duke treadmill prognostic s.
Dundee rank factor s. (DRFS)
echo s.
Estes s.
extent of pleural carcinomatosis s.
  (EPC)
Fugl-Meyer motor test s.
Gensini s.
Goldman cardiac risk index s.
Hollenberg treadmill exercise s.
Injury Severity S. (ISS)
jeopardy s.
Katz activities of daily living s.
Ladder of Life s.
lung injury s. (LIS)
Mallampati s.
Murray s.
Norris s.
quantitative wall motion s.
  (QWMS)
Rivermead Motor Assessment
  Arm s.
Romhilt-Estes s.
Selvester complete 32-point QRS s.
Selvester simplified QRS s.
Simplified Acute Physiology S.
  (SAPS)
total coronary s. (TCS)
treadmill s. (TS)
VAMC prognostic s.
wall motion s.
Wilkins echocardiographic s.
Yesavage s.

scoring
  microarousal s.
  respiratory arousal s.
scorpion venom
SCOT
  subcostal outflow
scotoma, pl. **scotomata**
Scot-Tussin
  S.-T. DM Cough Chasers
  S.-T. Senior Clear
scout
  s. film
  s. scan
  s. view
SCP
  smoking cessation program
SCPR
  standard cardiopulmonary resuscitation
sCRAG
  serum cryptococcal antigen
SCRAM face mask
scratch
  Lerman-Means s.
scratchy murmur
screening
  nocturnal oximetry s.
  spirometric s.
screen oxygenation
screw
  percutaneous cannulated s.
screw-in
  s.-i. epicardial electrode
  s.-i. lead
  s.-i. sutureless myocardial electrode
screw-on lead
screw-thread stent
scrofulaceum
  Mycobacterium s.
scroll reentrant wave
scrub typhus
SCS
  spinal cord stimulation
  systolic click syndrome
Sculptor annuloplasty ring
scurvy
SCV-CPR
  simultaneous compression-ventilation
  CPR
SCVIR
  Society of Cardiovascular and
  Interventional Radiology

NOTES

S

SD
   septal defect
   spreading depression
   systolic discharge

S/D
   systolic/diastolic
      Polygam S/D

SDB
   sleep-disordered breathing

SDBP
   seated diastolic blood pressure
   standing diastolic blood pressure
   supine diastolic blood pressure

SDH
   subdural hematoma

SDHD
   sudden death heart disease

SDIHD
   sudden death ischemic heart disease

SDS
   stent delivery system

SDS-PAGE
   sodium dodecylsulfate polyacrylamide gel electrophoresis

SDS-polyacrylamide gel

SE
   early systolic wave
   spin-echo
      SE image

SEA
   side-entry access
      SEA port

sea frond

seagull
   s. bruit
   s. murmur

seal
   Asherman chest s.
   Ultimate Seal CPAP mask s.
   watertight s.

sealant
   CoSeal resorbable synthetic s.
   FloSeal Matrix hemostatic s.
   FocalSeal-L surgical s.

seal-bark cough

sealing
   collagen vascular s. (CVS)

Sealy-Laragh technique

Seaquence stent

searcher
   Allport-Babcock s.

seasonal
   s. allergic rhinitis
   s. allergy

seated diastolic blood pressure (SDBP)

Seattle Angina Questionnaire

Sebastiani syndrome

SEC
   spontaneous echo contrast

SECG
   stress electrocardiography

Sechrist IV-100 infant ventilator

second
   beat per s. (BPS)
   breaths per s. (BPS)
   dyne s.'s
   forced expiratory volume in 1 s. (FEV_1)
   s. gas effect
   s. harmonic imaging (SHI)
   s. harmonic imaging ultrasound technique
   s. heart sound (S_2)
   s. messenger
   meter per s. (m/s, m/sec)
   s. mitral sound
   s. obtuse marginal artery (OM-2)
   oral airflow in liters per s. (V_O)
   s. positive deflection during QRS complex (R')
   s. pump run
   s. through fifth shock count

secondary
   s. anticoagulation system (SACS)
   s. aortic area
   s. arrest (SA)
   s. asphyxia
   s. atelectasis
   s. bronchitis
   s. bronchus
   s. cardiomyopathy
   s. chemoprophylaxis
   s. dextrocardia
   s. infection
   s. pleurisy
   s. pneumonia
   s. pneumothorax
   s. prevention
   s. pulmonary hypertension
   s. pulmonary lobule
   s. radiation
   s. septal hypertrophy
   s. thrombus
   s. tuberculosis

second-degree
   s.-d. A-V block
   s.-d. heart block

second-generation cephalosporin

secondhand smoke

second-look operation

second-phase tilt

second-wind angina

secretagogue

secretion
   airway s.
   altered airway s.
   chloride s.
   constitutive s.

continuous aspiration of
   subglottic s.'s (CASS)
infected s.
s. mobilization
mucus s.
nasopharyngeal s.
postural drainage of infected s.
s. retention
rhamnolipid mucus s.
specialized CC-chemokine s.
subglottic s.
secretor
   gene s.
secretory
   s. leukocyte protease inhibitor
      (SLPI)
   s. leukoprotease inhibitor (SLPI)
   s. leukoprotease inhibitor protein
   s. leukoproteinase inhibitor (SLPI)
   s. sphingomyelinase (S-SMase)
sector
   s. scan
   s. scan echocardiography
   s. transducer
Sectral
secundum
   s. atrial septal defect (ASD2)
   foramen s.
   ostium s.
   septum s.
secundum-type atrial septal defect
Securcut aspiration biopsy needle
Securon SR
sedation
   conscious s.
sedative administration
sedative-hypnotic drug
sedentary lifestyle
seeding
   cell s.
   graft s.
   pumpkin-s.
Seeker guidewire
seesaw murmur
segment
   abnormal ST s.
   akinetic s.
   anterolateral s.
   anteroseptal s.
   apical bronchopulmonary s.
   apicoposterior bronchopulmonary s.
   bronchopulmonary s.

depressed ST s. (DEP ST SEG)
downsloping ST s.
downstream s.
dyskinetic s.
dyssynergic myocardial s.
flail s.
horizontal ST s.
inferior lingular
   bronchopulmonary s.
inferolateral s.
inferoseptal s.
isoelectric ST s.
lateral basal bronchopulmonary s.
s. length, septal (SLS)
s. length, systolic (SLS)
malperfused s.
midcoronary s.
P-R s.
precordial ST s.
proximal s.
RS-T s.
ST s.
subapical s.
subsuperior s.
Ta s.
TP s.
T-P-Q s.
TQ s.
upsloping ST s.
upstream s.
segmental
   s. arterial disorganization
   s. atelectasis
   s. bronchus
   s. limb pressure (SLP)
   s. limb systolic pressure (SLP)
   s. lung resection
   s. pneumonia
   s. pressure index
   s. stenosis
   s. venous capacitance (SVC)
   s. venous capacitance ratio (SVCR)
   s. wall motion (SWM)
   s. wall motion analysis (SWMA)
segmentalis
   bronchus s.
segmentation
   k-space s.
   time-resolved imaging by automatic
      data s. (TRIADS)
segmentectomy

S

NOTES

segmented
    s. hyalinizing vasculitis
    s. K-space approach
    s. neutrophils
    s. ring tripolar (SRT)
    s. ring tripolar lead
segmentorum
    rami bronchiales s.
    stratum s.
segmentum
    s. bronchopulmonale
    s. bronchopulmonale apicale
    s. bronchopulmonale apicoposterius
    s. bronchopulmonale basale anterius
    s. bronchopulmonale basale laterale
    s. bronchopulmonale basale mediale
    s. bronchopulmonale basale
      posterius
    s. bronchopulmonale lingulare
      superius
    s. bronchopulmonale posterius
    s. cardiacum
    s. subapicale
    s. subsuperius
Seguin annuloplasty ring
SEI
    subendocardial infarction
Seiler cartilage
seismic wave
seismocardiogram
seismocardiography
Seitz
    S. metamorphosing respiration
    S. sign
seizure
SELCA
    smooth excimer laser coronary
    angioplasty
Seldinger
    S. needle
    S. percutaneous technique
    S. sheath
selectin blocker
selective
    s. angiography
    s. aortic arch perfusion (SAAP)
    s. aortography
    s. arterial secretin injection test
      (SAST)
    s. arteriography
    s. cardiac catheterization
    s. estrogen receptor modulator
      (SERM)
    s. graft opacification
    s. intracoronary thrombolysis
      (SICT)
    s. past pathway
    s. septal branch injection of
      ethanol

    s. shunt (SS)
    s. transvenous approach
    s. venous catheterization (SVC)
selenium
    s. deficiency
    s. dioxide
    s. sulfide
self-adjusting nasal continuous positive airway pressure (APAP)
self-expandable metallic stent
self-expanding
    s.-e. microporous stent (SEMS)
    s.-e. stent
self-guiding catheter
self-positioning balloon catheter
self-powered treadmill
self-terminating tachycardia
sella
    s. nasion point A (SNA)
    s. nasion point B (SNB)
sellae
    foramen diaphragmatis s.
Sellers
    S. classification of mitral
      regurgitation
    S. criteria
    S. grade
    S. mitral regurgitation classification
Sellick maneuver
Selute Picotip steroid-eluting device
Selvester
    S. complete 32-point QRS score
    S. simplified QRS score
SEM
    scanning electron microscope
    systolic ejection murmur
sematilide hydrochloride
Semb apicolysis
SEMI
    subendocardial myocardial infarction
semiautomatic external defibrillator (SAED)
semidirect lead
semihorizontal heart
semiinvasive aspergillosis
semilateral supine position
semilunar
    s. valve
    s. valve closure (SC)
    s. valve regurgitation
    s. valve stenosis
semiquantitation
semiquantitative index
semirigid catheter
semispinal muscle of thorax
semisynthetic penicillin
semivertical heart
Semliki Forest virus
Semmes-Weinstein monofilaments

Semon sign
Semprex-D
SEMS
   self-expanding microporous stent
Sendai virus
SenDx 100 blood gas and electrolyte analysis system
senescent
   s. aortic stenosis
   s. heart
   s. myocardium
senile
   s. amyloidosis
   s. arrhythmia
   s. arteriosclerosis
   s. emphysema
   s. plaque
senilis
   arcus s.
   circus s.
senility
Senning
   S. atrial baffle repair
   S. operation
   S. transposition procedure
Senning-Rastelli procedure
sensation
   elephant-on-the-chest s.
   popping s.
   pressurelike s.
   Sensation intraaortic balloon catheter
   thermal s.
sensing
   afterpotential s.
   s. circuit
   far-field R-wave s.
   integrated bipolar s.
   rate-drop s.
   s. spike
sensitivity
   s. analysis
   atrial s.
   aureomycin s.
   baroreceptor s.
   baroreceptor reflex s. (BRS)
   baroreflex s. (BRS)
   chlortetracycline s.
   digitalis s.
   pacemaker s.
   paracetamol s.
   phenindione s.

   phenylbutazone s.
   sulfonamide s.
   ventricular s.
sensitization
   baroreceptor s.
sensitized cell
sensor
   activity s.
   BioZtect s.
   s. blending
   blood gas s.
   Capnostat CO_2 s.
   catheter-based s.
   ClipTip reusable s.
   Dymedix sleep s.
   FilterWatch s.
   flat tube pressure s.
   Handi oxygen s.
   ImPressure ultrasound pressure s.
   infant airflow and effort s.
   Oxisensor II adult s.
   OxyTip s.
   S. pacemaker
   pediatric finger clip s.
   piezo electric snore s.
   piezo PLM s.
   pressure transducer airflow s.
   PressureWire-3 s.
   S. PTFE-nitinol guidewire with hydrophilic tip
   Pulsar Max s.
   SpiroSense flow s.
   Stat-Shell disposable pulse oximeter s.
   VTI oxygen monitor with disposable polarographic oxygen s.
sensor-driven response
sensorimotor
   s. cortex (SMC)
   s. stroke
sensorium
   clouded s.
SensorMedics
   S. generator
   S. mass flow sensor heated wire flowmeter
   S. 2900 metabolic cart
   S. SAT-TRAK pulse oximeter
sensory
   s. cross-checking
   s. nerve
   s. nerve action potential (SNAP)

S

NOTES

sensory *(continued)*
  s. nerve conduction velocity
    (SNCV)
sentinel
  S. ICD device
  S. 2010 implantable cardioverter-
    defibrillator
  s. node
  S. seal pleural drainage unit
Sentry antimicrobial surveillance
  program
SEP
  systolic ejection period
separation
  aortic cusp s.
  E point to septal s. (EPSS)
  maximum aortic cusp s. (MACS)
Sephadex G24 chromatography
Sepracoat coating solution
Sepracor
SEPS
  subfascial endoscopic perforator surgery
sepsis
  alcoholism, leukopenia,
    pneumococcal s. (ALPS)
  Capnocytophaga canimorsus s.
  endotoxic s.
  line s.
sepsis-related organ failure assessment
  (SOFA)
septa, pl. **septae**
septal
  s. ablation
  s. akinesia
  s. annuloplasty
  s. arcade
  s. artery embolization
  s. cell
  s. collateral
  s. defect (SD)
  s. dip
  s. dropout
  s. hyperperfusion on thallium scan
  s. hypertrophy
  s. isthmus
  s. line
  s. myectomy
  s. myotomy
  s. pathway
  s. perforating artery
  s. perforation
  s. perforator
  s. perforator branch
  s. resection
  segment length, s. (SLS)
  s. thickening
  s. wall motion

septation
  s. of heart
  s. procedure
septectomy
  atrial s.
  Blalock-Hanlon atrial s.
  Edwards s.
septi
septic
  s. embolization
  s. endocarditis
  s. fever
  s. pneumonia
  s. pulmonary edema (SPE)
  s. shock
  s. thromboembolism
septicemia
  anthrax s.
  s. sputum
septicum
  Clostridium s.
septomarginalis
  trabecula s.
septoplasty
  balloon atrial s.
  bedside balloon atrial s.
  Brockenbrough atrial s.
septostomy
  atrial s.
  atrial balloon s.
  balloon s.
  balloon atrial s. (BAS)
  blade atrial s.
  Mullins blade and balloon s.
  Park blade s.
  Rashkind balloon atrial s.
Septra DS
septum (S)
  aneurysm of atrial s. (AAS)
  atrial s. (AS)
  conal s.
  interalveolar s.'s
  interatrial s. (IAS)
  interpulmonary s.
  interventricular s. (IVS)
  left s. (LS)
  s. linguae
  s. mediastinale
  membranous s.
  s. pellucidum
  s. primum
  right s. (RS)
  s. secundum
  sigmoid s.
  s. spurium
  Swiss cheese interventricular s.
  tissue s.'s
  ventricular s. (VS)
sequela, pl. **sequelae**

Sequel compression system
sequence
>activation s.
>analyzer of interrated s.'s (AIS)
>anaplerotic s.
>2D gradient-echo s.
>DiGeorge s. (DGS)
>direct mapping s.
>3D segmented-FLASH imaging s.
>3D time-of-flight magnetic
>   resonance angiographic s.
>FLASH s.'s
>intraatrial activation s.
>intracardiac atrial activation s.
>inversion spin-echo pulse s. (ISE)
>Kozak s.
>missed ostium s. (MOS)
>respiratory gated three-dimensional
>   gradient-echo s.
>spin-echo imaging s.

sequencing
>DNA s.

sequential
>s. atrioventricular (SAV)
>s. compression device (SCD)
>s. dilation
>s. organ failure assessment (SOFA)
>s. pacing
>s. vascular response (SVR)
>s. ventriculoatrial (SVA)

sequestrant
>bile acid s.
>low-dose bile-acid s.

Sequestra 1000 system
sequestration
>s. bronchopneumonia
>pulmonary s. (PS)

sequestrectomy
Sequicor III pacemaker
SER
>systolic ejection rate

sera (*pl. of* serum)
Serafini hernia
seratrodast
Seretide
Serevent Diskus
serial
>s. autocorrelation (SAC)
>s. autocorrelation data acquisition
>   technology
>s. blood gas
>s. change

>s. cut films
>s. dilation
>s. ECG tracing
>s. electrocardiogram tracing
>s. impedance plethysmography
>s. thrombin time (STT)

series
>800 s. blood gas and critical
>   analyte system
>s. elastic element
>S. 7900 mouth breathing face
>   mask
>S. 8900 nasal and mouth breathing
>   face mask

serine kinase
serious cardiac event (SCE)
SERM
>selective estrogen receptor modulator

seroconversion
serofibrinous
>s. pericarditis
>s. pleurisy

serological test
Seroma-Cath catheter
Seromycin Pulvules
seronegative
>CMV s.
>s. spondyloarthropathy

seropneumothorax
seropositive
>CMV s.
>s. nonsyphilitic pneumopathy

serosanguineous effusion
serosum
>pericardium s.

serothorax
serotonin
serotype
>M-protein s.

serotyping
serous
>s. effusion
>s. membrane
>s. pericarditis
>s. pleurisy

serpentina
>*Rauwolfia s.*

serpentine aneurysm
serpiginous
Serpula lacrymans
serrated catheter

NOTES

Serratia
    S. liquefaciens
    S. marcescens
    S. pneumonia
serraticus
    stridor s.
serratus anterior muscle
sertraline hydrochloride
serum, pl. **sera**
    s. albumin
    s. amylase
    s. amyloid type A (SAA)
    antilymphocyte s.
    s. bactericidal titer (SBT)
    brain-heart infusion and rabbit s.
      (BHIRS)
    s. cholesterol
    s. creatine kinase
    s. cryptococcal antigen (sCRAG)
    ERIG s.
    s. glutamic-oxaloacetic transaminase
      (SGOT)
    s. glutamic-pyruvic transaminase
      (SGPT)
    s. IgE
    s. iron
    s. KL-6
    s. lipid profile
    s. magnesium
    s. marker
    s. myoglobin (S-Mgb)
    s. neopterin
    s. prothrombin conversion
      accelerator (SPCA)
    s. renin level
    s. reserve cholesterol binding
      capacity (SRCBC)
    s. retinol
    s. shock
    s. sickness
    s. thrombotic accelerator (STA)
    s. triglyceride
service
    National Health S. (NHS)
    Older Americans Resources
      and s.'s (OARS)
    vascular access s. (VAS)
Servo
    S. Screen 390 ventilator monitoring
      device
    S. Ventilator 300
servocontrolled plethysmography
SES
    sirolimus-eluting stent
sesquioxide
    germanium s.
sestamibi
    s. perfusion imaging
    s. scan

    s. SPECT
    s. stress test
    ^{99m}Tc s.
    s. technetium-99m SPECT with
      dipyridamole stress test
    thallium s. (^{201}Tl sestamibi)
    ^{201}Tl s.
      thallium sestamibi
SET
    shredding embolectomy thrombectomy
set
    Acland-Banis arteriotomy s.
    Arrow Hi-flow infusion s.
    Borst side-arm introducer s.
    Dotter intravascular retrieval s.
    Flexor Check-Flo introducer s.
    Masimo S.
    micropuncture introducer s.
    minimum data s. (MDS)
    multi-sideport catheter infusion s.
    Neff percutaneous access s.
    Neo-Sert umbilical vessel catheter
      insertion s.
    Peel-Away introducer s.
    Quest medical MPS delivery s.
    Rothbarth Uni-Flo infusion s.
    Shuttle-SL Flexor Tuohy Borst
      side-arm introducer s.
    Tissomat application device and
      spray s.
    U-Mid-O$_2$ Jet S.
    Wylie endarterectomy s.
S.E.T. thrombectomy system catheter
seven-pinhole tomography
severe
    s. acute respiratory syndrome
      (SARS)
    s. refractory neurocardiogenic
      syncope
Severinghaus electrode
severity
    stenosis s.
sevoflurane
Sewall technique
sewing
    s. ring
    s. ring area (SRA)
    s. ring loop
sew-on electrode
sex
    s. ratio
    s. steroid
sexual
    s. angina
    s. asthma
    s. syncope
SF
    shunt flow

spontaneous fibrillation
SF wave of cardiac apex pulse

SF$_6$
sulfur hexafluoride

SF-36 Health Survey

SFA
saturated fatty acid
subclavian flap aortoplasty
superficial femoral artery
superior femoral artery

SFHb
pyridoxalated stroma-free hemoglobin
stroma-free hemoglobin pyridoxalated

SFP
stopped flow pressure

SFR
stenotic flow reserve

SG
stent graft

SGOT
serum glutamic-oxaloacetic transaminase

SGPT
serum glutamic-pyruvic transaminase

SGRQ
St. George Respiratory Questionnaire

SGS
stroke guidance system

SH
spontaneously hypertensive
standard heparin

shadow
acoustic s.
S. balloon
bat wing s.
butterfly s.
cardiac s.
mediastinal s.
S. over-the-wire balloon catheter
ring s.
snowstorm s.
summation s.

shadow-free laryngoscope

shadowing
acoustic s.

shaft
Adante monorail catheter s.
UniTrack s.

shaggy pericardium

Shaher-Puddu classification

shake test

shaking sound

shale pneumoconiosis

shallow
s. breathing
s. pathologic Q wave
s. respiration
s. T wave inversion
s. water blackout

shallow-water blackout syndrome

shape
echo-signal s.
spheroid left ventricular s.

shaping behavioral technique

Shapshay-Healy laryngoscope

sharing
United Network for Organ S.
(UNOS)

Shaver disease

SHD
structural heart disease
sudden heart death

shear
atrial s.
s. force
s. rate of blood
s. stress
s. thinning

shears
Bethune-Corylloss.
Coryllos-Bethune rib s.
Coryllos-Shoemaker rib s.
Duval-Coryllos rib s.
Frey-Sauerbruch rib s.
Giertz-Shoemaker rib s.
Gluck rib s.
rib s.
Shoemaker rib s.

sheath
Arrow s.
arterial s.
blue Cook s.
cardiogenic s.
carotid s.
chronic s.
compensated s.
Cordis Bioptome s.
Daig s.
Desilets-Hoffman s.
s. and dilator system
excimer s.
femoral venous s.
French s.
GlideCath s.
Hemaflex s.

NOTES

sheath *(continued)*
    Hemaquet s.
    hemostatic s.
    Introducer II s.
    Klein transseptal introducer s.
    Mullins transseptal catheterization s.
    peel-away s.
    percutaneous brachial s.
    peribronchial s.
    perivascular s.
    Pinnacle introducer s.
    Seldinger s.
    short monorail polyethylene
      imaging s.
    SL1 s.
    sonolucent distal imaging s.
    Spectranetics laser s. (SLS)
    subclavian peel-away s.
    Super ArrowFlex catheterization s.
    Teflon s.
    Terumo Pinnacle s.
    Terumo Radiofocus s.
    transseptal s.
    vascular s.
    venous s.
sheath-based IVUS catheter
sheath/dilator
    Mullins s./d.
sheathing
    halo s.
Sheehan and Dodge technique
Sheen airway reconstruction
sheep
    s. antidigoxin Fab antibody
    s. blowfly asthma
sheepskin boot
sheet
    cellular s.
    chest pain order s. (CPOS)
    mucous s.'s
    s. sign
Sheffield
    S. exercise stress test
    S. modification of Bruce treadmill
      protocol
    S. Screening Test for Acquired
      Language Disorders (STALD)
    S. treadmill protocol
Shekelton aneurysm
shelf
    apical s.
    s. of plaque
shell
    chest s.
shellfish asthma
shelving edge
Shenstone tourniquet
shepherd's crook deformity
Sherpa guiding catheter

SHI
    second harmonic imaging
    SHI ultrasound technique
Shibley sign
shield
    Cath-Gard catheter contamination s.
    chest s.
    face s.
    probe s.
shift
    axis s.
    baseline s.
    chloride s.
    Doppler s.
    fluid s.
    mediastinal s.
    midline s.
    plaque s.
shifter
    frequency s.
shifting
    isovolume s.
    s. pacemaker
Shigella
shiitake mushroom extract
Shiley
    S. catheter
    S. convexoconcave heart valve
    S. decannulation plug
    S. Phonate speaking valve
    S. tracheostomy tube
Shimadzu
    S. cardiac ultrasound
    S. DAR-2400 coronary
      arteriographic analyzer
Shimazaki area-length method
shiner
    allergic s.
Shinobi steerable guidewire
SHJL4 catheter
SHJR4 catheter
SHJR4s
    side-hole Judkins curve right 4 short
      SHJR4s catheter
shock
    biphasic s.
    s. blocks
    burst s.
    cardiac output s.
    cardiogenic s. (CGS, CS)
    chronic s.
    circulatory s.
    compensated s.
    s. count
    DC electric s.
    declamping s.
    decompensated s.
    defibrillation s.
    diastolic s.

direct current electric s.
distributive s.
double external direct current s.
endotoxin s.
high-energy transthoracic s.
hyperdynamic septic s.
hypovolemic s.
s. index
infarction with S.
insulin s.
irreversible s.
s. lung
obstructive s.
occult cardiogenic s.
oligemic s.
s. pacing
pleural s.
s. position
QRS synchronous atrial
   defibrillation s.'s
rectilinear biphasic s.
refractory s.
rescue s.
septic s.
serum s.
synchronized s.
systolic s.
s. therapy
toxic s.
vasodilatory s.
vasogenic s.
s. waveform
shocky
shoddy fever
Shoemaker rib shears
Shone
S. anomaly
S. complex
short
s. axis (SAX)
s. coupling interval
s. monorail imaging catheter
s. monorail polyethylene imaging
   sheath
side-hole Judkins curve right 4 s.
   (SHJR4s)
s. stent
s. tapers
s. transitional edge protection
   (STEP)
short-axis
s.-a. image

s.-a. mitral valve (SAX-MV)
s.-a. parasternal view
s.-a. plane
s.-a. plane mitral valve
s.-a. plane, papillary muscle (SAX-
   PM)
s.-a. slice
s.-a. tomogram
shortening
circumferential fiber s.
endocardial s.
fiber s.
s. fraction
fractional myocardial s.
long-axis fractional s. (LAFS)
midwall s.
myocardial fiber s.
postsystolic s.
s. of P-R interval
telomeric s.
s. velocity
velocity of circumferential fiber s.
   (VCF)
ventricular wall s.
**Short-Form 36 Health Survey (SF-36
   Health Survey)**
shorthand rule
short-long-short cycle
shortness
s. of breath (SB, SOB)
s. of breath on exertion (SBE,
   SOBOE)
short-term
flow-assisted s.-t. (FAST)
short-winded
Shoshin disease
shot
fast low-angle s. (FLASH)
sinus s.
shotty node
shoulder
s. horizontal flexion
s. rotation
shoulder-hand syndrome
shoulder-strap resonance
shower
embolic s.
shredding
s. embolectomy thrombectomy
   (SET)
s. embolectomy thrombectomy
   catheter

S

NOTES

shrinkage
  arterial s.
shrinker
  Juzo s.
SHT
  symptomatic hemorrhage
SHU-454 contrast medium
shudder
  carotid s.
shunt
  Allen-Brown s.
  Anastaflo s.
  aorta to pulmonary artery s.
  aorticopulmonary s.
  aortofemoral artery s.
  aortopulmonary s.
  arteriopulmonary s.
  arteriovenous s. (AVS)
  ascending aorta to pulmonary
    artery s.
  atrial ventricular s.
  atriopulmonary s.
  balloon s.
  bidirectional cavopulmonary s.
  Blalock-Taussig s. (BTS)
  BT s.
  Buselmeier s.
  cardiac s.
  carotid artery s.
  cavocaval s.
  cavopulmonary s.
  Cimino arteriovenous s.
  ClearView intracoronary s.
  ClearView intravascular
    arteriotomy s.
  coronary anastomotic s.
  s. cyanosis
  Denver pleural effusion s.
  s. detection
  distal splenorenal s.
  Drapanas mesocaval s.
  emergency portocaval s. (EPCS)
  extracardiac s.
  Flo-Thru s.
  s. flow (SF)
  Glenn s.
  Gore-Tex s.
  Gott s.
  interarterial s.
  intracardiac s.
  intrapulmonary s.
  Javid s.
  s. leak
  left-to-right s.
  LeVeen peritoneovenous s.
  Marion-Clatworthy side-to-end vena
    caval s.
  mesoatrial s. (MAS)
  mesocaval s.

  modified Blalock-Taussig s.
    (MBTS)
  parallel s.
  s. pathway
  persistent s.
  pleural effusion s.
  pleuroperitoneal s.
  portacaval s. (PCS)
  portopulmonary s.
  Potts s.
  s. pressure (SP)
  s. procedure (SP)
  Pruitt-Inahara carotid s.
  pulmonary s.
  s. quantification
  Quinton-Scribner s.
  s. ratio
  residual s.
  reversed s.
  right-left s. (R-Lsh)
  right-to-left s. (RLS)
  Rivetti-Levinson IntraLuminal s.
  selective s. (SS)
  side-to-side portacaval s. (SSPS)
  splenorenal s.
  Sundt carotid endarterectomy s.
  systemic to pulmonary s.
  T-AnastoFlo s.
  Thomas s.
  total cavopulmonary s. (TCPS)
  transjugular intrahepatic
    portosystemic s. (TIPS)
  Uresil Vascu-Flo carotid s.
  USCI s.
  Vascu-Flo carotid s.
  ventriculoatrial s. (VAS)
  Waterston s.
shunt-dependent lesion
shunted
  s. blood
  s. blood to total blood flow
    (QSQT)
shunting
  s. circuit
  interatrial s. (IAS)
  intraatrial s.
  intrapulmonary s.
  pleuroperitoneal s.
  venoarterial s.
shuttle
  s. test
  s. test walk
shuttlemaker's disease
Shuttle-SL Flexor Tuohy Borst side-arm
  introducer set
Shwachman
  S. score of clinical well-being
  S. syndrome
Shy-Drager syndrome

SI
> stroke index

Si
> silicon
>> Si Carbide

SIAD
> syndrome of inappropriate antidiuresis

SIADH
> syndrome of inappropriate antidiuretic
> hormone

sialic acid

SIBD
> silent ischemic brain damage

sibilance

sibilant
> s. rale
> s. rhonchi

Sibson
> S. aponeurosis
> S. notch
> S. vestibule

sibutramine

sICAM
> soluble intracellular adhesion molecule

Sicar sign

sicca
> bronchiectasia s.
> bronchitis s.
> laryngitis s.
> pericarditis s.
> pharyngitis s.
> s. syndrome

SICH
> spontaneous intracerebral hemorrhage

Sicilian Gambit formulation

sick
> s. building syndrome (SBS)
> s. sinus syndrome (SSS)

sickle
> s. cell anemia
> s. cell crisis
> s. cell disease
> s. cell thalassemia
> s. cell trait

Sickledex test

sicklemia

sickling

sickness
> African sleeping s.
> cardiopulmonary decompression s.
> (the chokes)
> cave s.

> compressed-air s.
> decompression s. (DCS)
> S. Impact profile (SIP)
> S. Impact Profile questionnaire
> s. Impact Profile scale
> mountain s.
> serum s.
> sleeping s.

SICOR recording system

SICT
> selective intracoronary thrombolysis

SICU
> surgical intensive care unit

side
> s. arm adapter
> s. arm pressure port
> s. biting clamp
> s. branch
> s. branch compromise
> s. branch occlusion
> s. lobe
> s. lobe artifact
> s. stretching

side-entry access (SEA)

side-hole
> s.-h. Judkins curve right 4
> s.-h. Judkins curve right 4 short
> (SHJR4s)

sideport

Sideris
> S. adjustable buttoned device
> S. clamp

sideropenic dysphagia

siderophage

siderophore

siderosis
> welder's s.

siderotica
> pneumoconiosis s.

sidestream
> s. $ETCO_2$
> S. high-efficiency nebulizer

side-to-side portacaval shunt (SSPS)

**sidewinder percutaneous intra-aortic
balloon catheter**

SIDS
> sudden infant death syndrome

Siemens
> S. biplane Neurostar digital
> subtraction angiography system
> S. Evolution electron beam CT
> S. Magnetom 1.5-T MRI

S

NOTES

Siemens *(continued)*
   S. open heart table
   S. Orbiter gamma camera
   S. pacemaker
   S. SI 400 ultrasound
   S. Somatom DR CT scanner
   S. Somatom Plus 4A scanner
   S. Sonoline CD echograph
   S. ventilator

Siemens-Elema
   S.-E. AB pulse transducer probe
   S.-E. AG bicycle ergometer
   S.-E. pacemaker

SIESTA
   snooze-induced excitation of sympathetic
   triggered activity

sieve
   Mobin-Uddin s.

Sievers model 280 nitric oxide analyzer

sigh
   s. function
   s. period

sighing
   s. dyspnea
   s. respiration

sigma
   S. I monoplace hyperbaric therapy
   system
   S. II Dualplace hyperbaric oxygen
   therapy system
   S. method
   S. Plus monoplace hyperbaric
   oxygen therapy system
   unipolar Pisces S.

sigmoid septum

sign
   Abrahams s.
   ace of spades s.
   air bronchogram s.
   air crescent s.
   antler s.
   applesauce s.
   Aschner s.
   atrioseptal s.
   Auenbrugger s.
   Aufrecht s.
   auscultatory s.
   Baccelli s.
   bagpipe s.
   Bamberger s.
   Bamberger-Pins-Ewart s.
   Bard s.
   B6 bronchus s.
   Béhier-Hardy s.
   bent bronchus s.
   Bethea s.
   Biermer s.
   Biot s.
   Bird s.

black pleura s.
Bouillaud s.
Boyce s.
Bozzolo s.
Branham s.
Braunwald s.
bread-and-butter textbook s.
breathing bag s.
Broadbent inverted s.
Brockenbrough s.
Brockenbrough-Braunwald s.
Brockenbrough-Braunwald-Morrow s.
bronchial meniscus s.
calcium s.
Carabello s.
Cardarelli s.
cardiorespiratory s.
Carvallo s.
Castellino s.
Cegka s.
Charcot s.
Cheyne-Stokes s.
Chvostek s.
clenched fist s.
comet s.
comet tail s.
cooing s.
Corrigan s.
Cruveilhier s.
Cruveilhier-Baumgarten s.
cuff s.
D'Amato s.
Davis s.
de la Camp s.
Delbet s.
Delmege s.
Demarquay s.
de Musset s. (aortic aneurysm)
de Mussy s. (pleurisy)
d'Espine s.
Dew s.
Dieuaide s.
Dorendorf s.
double-lumen s.
doughnut s.
Drummond s.
Duchenne s.
Duroziez s.
E s.
Ebstein s.
Ellis s.
epicardial fat pad s.
Erni s.
Ewart s.
Ewing s.
Faget s.
failing lung s.
fallen lung s.
Federici s.

Fischer s.
fissure s.
flying W s.
Friedreich s.
Glasgow s.
gloved finger s.
Golden S s.
Gowers s.
Grancher s.
Greene s.
Griesinger s.
Grocco s.
Grossman s.
Gunn crossing s.
Hall s.
halo s.
Hamman s.
Heim-Kreysig s.
Heimlich s.
Hill s.
hilum convergence s.
hilum overlay s.
Homans s.
Hoover s.
Hope s.
Horner s.
hot nose s.
Huchard s.
hyperdense middle cerebral
  artery s. (HMCAS)
inferior triangle s.
intrapericardial s.
intravascular fetal air s.
Jaccoud s.
Jackson s.
Karplus s.
Kellock s.
knuckle s.
Korányi s.
Kreysig s.
Kussmaul s.
Laënnec s.
Lancisi s.
Landolfi s.
Levine s.
Liebermeister s.
Litten diaphragm s.
Livierato s.
Lombardi s.
Löwenberg cuff s.
Macewen s.
Mahler s.

Mannkopf s.
McCort s.
McGinn-White s.
s. mechanism for ventilator
  breathing
Meltzer s.
Moschcowitz s.
Moses s.
Müller s.
Murat s.
Musset s.
mute toe s.'s
Nicoladoni s.
Nicoladoni-Branham s.
Oliver s.
open bronchus s.
Osler s.
pad s.
patent bronchus s.
pearl s.
Perez s.
Pins s.
pleural meniscus s.
plumb-line s.
Porter s.
Potain s.
Pottenger s.
Prevel s.
Prussian helmet s.
pulmonary meniscus s.
pulmonary notch s.
pulmonary target s.
Queckenstedt s.
Quénu-Muret s.
Quincke s.
rabbit-ear s.
railroad track s.
Ramond s.
Raynaud s.
reversed three s.
ring s.
Rivero-Carvallo s.
Riviere s.
Robertson s.
Romana s.
Rotch s.
Rothschild s.
Sam Levine s.
Sansom s.
Schapiro s.
Schepelmann s.
Schick s.

NOTES

S

sign *(continued)*
    scimitar s.
    Seitz s.
    Semon s.
    sheet s.
    Shibley s.
    Sicar s.
    silhouette s.
    Skoda s.
    Smith s.
    snake-tongue s.
    square root s.
    steeple s.
    Steinberg thumb s.
    Sterles s.
    Sternberg s.
    stretched bronchus s.
    string s.
    stripe s.
    superior triangle s.
    T s.
    tail s.
    tenting s.
    thumbprint bronchus s.
    tilt vital s.'s
    trapezius ridge s.
    Traube s.
    Trimadeau s.
    tripod s.
    Troisier s.
    Trunecek s.
    Unschuld s.
    vital s.'s
    Walker-Murdoch wrist s.
    water lily s.
    Weill s.
    Wenckebach s.
    Westermark s.
    Williams s.
    Williamson s.
    windsock s.
    Wintrich s.

Signa
    S. EXCITE 3.0T MRI system
    S. Pad

signal
    s. amplitude
    s. averaging
    Doppler s.
    gating s.
    high-intensity transient s. (HITS)
    hyperintense heterogeneous s.
    intracranial microembolic s.
    isointense heterogeneous s.
    s. loss
    magnetic resonance s.
    microembolic s. (MES)
    mosaic jet s.'s
    navigator echo s.

    nonexcitatory s.
    oscillometric s.
    preconditioning s.
    s. processing
    spin echo s.
    terminal filtered QRS s.
    s. transducer and activator of transcription (STAT, Stat)
    s. transducer and activator of transcription protein family
    ventricular far-field s.

signal-averaged
    s.-a. echocardiogram
    s.-a. echocardiography
    s.-a. electrocardiogram (SAECG)
    s.-a. electrocardiography (SAECG)
    s.-a. P-wave duration (SAPD)

signaling
    autocrine s.
    integrin s.
    myocardial adrenergic s.
    outside-in s.
    paracrine s.
    transmembrane s.

signal-loss cloud
signal-to-noise ratio
signal-void jet
signet-ring cell carcinoma
Sigvaris compression stockings
Silafed Syrup
Silastic
    S. catheter
    S. electrode casing
    S. patch
    S. poppet
    S. strain gauge
    S. tape

sildenafil citrate
Sildicon-E
silence
    ECG s.
silent
    s. angina
    s. brain infarction (SBI)
    s. cerebral infarct (SCI)
    s. cerebral infarction (SCI)
    s. coronary artery fistula
    s. electrode
    s. embolism
    s. gap
    s. ischemic brain damage (SIBD)
    s. mitral stenosis
    s. myocardial infarction (SMI)
    s. myocardial ischemia
    S. Night diagnostic and screening device
    s. pericardial effusion
    s. stroke
    s. trace leak

silhouette
  cardiac s.
  cardiomediastinal s.
  egg-on-a-string s.
  immediate s.
  late s.
  s. sign
  s. sign of Felson
silica
silicatosis
silicoanthracosis
silicon (Si)
silicone lead
silicoproteinosis
silicosis
silicosis-CWP-berylliosis
silicotic pneumoconiosis
silicotuberculosis
silk guidewire
silo-filler's
  s.-f. disease
  s.-f. lung
Silphen
  S. Cough
  S. DM
Siltussin DM
silver (Ag)
  s. bead electrode
  Grocott methenamine s. (GMS)
  s. polisher's lung
  S. Speed hydrophilic guidewire
  s. sulfadiazine
  S. syndrome
Silverman-Lilly pneumotachograph
silver-methenamine stain
silver-silver chloride electrode
Silverstein stimulator probe
silver-wire effect
silver-wiring of retinal artery
Silvester method
SIMA
  single internal mammary artery
simiae
  Mycobacterium s.
simian virus 40 (SV40)
Simmons II, III catheter
Simmons-type sidewinder catheter
Simon
  S. foci
  S. nitinol inferior vena cava filter
  S. nitinol IVC filter
Simplate procedure

simple chronic bronchitis
simplex
  angina s.
  carcinoma s.
  herpes s.
Simplicity Spirometer
Simplified Acute Physiology Score
  (SAPS)
Simpson
  S. atherectomy catheter
  S. AtheroCath catheter
  S. AtheroCath system
  S. peripheral AtheroCath
  S. PET balloon
  S. positron emission tomography
    balloon
  S. rule for ventricular volume
Simpson-Golabi-Behmel syndrome
Simpson-Robert
  S.-R. catheter
  S.-R. vascular dilation system
Simron
Sims nasal prongs
simulator
  single lung PneuView s.
Simulect
simultaneous
  s. bilateral spontaneous
    pneumothorax (SBSP)
  s. catheter mapping
  s. compression-ventilation CPR
    (SCV-CPR)
simultaneously stapled pneumonectomy
  (SSP)
SIMV
  synchronized intermittent mandatory
    ventilation
simvastatin
Sindbis virus
sine
  s. wave
  s. wave pattern
sinensis
  Clonorchis s.
Sinequan
Sinex Long-Acting
singer's node
Singh-Vaughan-Williams arrhythmia
  classification
single
  s. atrium

NOTES

single (*continued*)
    s. chain urokinase-type plasminogen activator
    s. chamber cardiac pacing system
    s. coronary artery bypass graft (SCABG)
    s. extrastimulus
    s. internal mammary artery (SIMA)
    s. lumen
    s. lung PneuView stimulator
    s. papillary muscle syndrome
    s. pleurisy
    s. premature atrial beat
    s. premature extrastimulation
    s. ventricle
    s. ventricle malposition
single-balloon
    s.-b. valvotomy
    s.-b. valvuloplasty
single-breath
    s.-b. carbon monoxide test
    s.-b. diffusion
    s.-b. nitrogen curve
    s.-b. nitrogen elimination
    s.-b. nitrogen washout test
single-chamber
    s.-c. Maximo remote monitoring ICD
    s.-c. pulse generator
    s.-c. rate-responsive
single-crystal gamma camera
single-disk prosthesis
single-gene disorder
single-lung transplant (SLT)
single-pass lead
single-patient use manometer
single-photon
    s.-p. detection
    s.-p. emission
    s.-p. emission computed tomographic imaging
    s.-p. emission computed tomography (SPECT)
    s.-p. emission tomography
    s.-p. emission tomography imaging
    s.-p. gamma scintigraphy
single-plane aortography
single-stage exercise stress test
single-ventricle physiology
single-vessel
    s.-v. coronary stenosis
    s.-v. disease (SVD)
Singulair
singultus
sinister
    bronchus principalis s.
    pulmo s.
sinistra
    arteria pulmonalis s.

    vena obliqua atrii s.
    vena pulmonalis inferior s.
    vena pulmonalis superior s.
sinistrae
    rami esophageales arteriae gastricae s.'s
sinistri
    incisura cardiaca pulmonis s.
    lingula pulmonis s.
sinistrocardia
sinistrum
    atrium s.
    atrium cordis s.
    cor triatriatum s.
Sin Nombre virus (SNV)
sinoaortic
    s. baroreflex activity
    s. denervation (SAD)
sinoatrial, sinuatrial (SA, S-A)
    s. arrest
    s. ball
    s. baroreflex
    s. block (SAB)
    s. bradycardia
    s. conduction time (SACT)
    s. entrance block (SAEB)
    s. exit block
    s. nodal artery
    s. nodal reentry (SANDR)
    s. node (SAN, SN)
    s. node dysfunction
    s. node weakness syndrome (SANWS)
    s. recovery time (SART)
sinoauricular
    s. block
    s. node (SAN)
sinoauricular block
sinobronchial syndrome
sinobronchitis
sinogram
sinopulmonary
sinospiral fiber
sinotubular junction
sinoventricular
    s. conduction
    s. tachycardia (SVT)
Sintrom
sinuatrial (*var. of* sinoatrial)
sinuatrialis
    nodus s.
    nonreset nodus s.
    reset nodus s.
Sinumist-SR Capsulets
sinus
    aortic s.
    s. arrest (SA)
    s. arrhythmia (SA)
    basilar s.

s. bradycardia (SB)
carotid s.
s. catarrh
cavernous s. (CS)
s. coronarius
coronary s. (CS)
costophrenic s.
s. cycle length (SCL)
distal coronary s. (DCS)
s. exit block
s. exit pause
left coronary s. (LCS)
s. mechanism
s. nodal automaticity
s. nodal reentrant tachycardia
s. nodal reentry
s. node (SN)
s. node artery
s. node/AV conduction abnormality
s. node cycle length (SNCL)
s. node disease
s. node dysfunction (SND)
s. node electrogram (SNE)
s. node formation (SNF)
s. node function
s. node potential (SNP)
s. node recovery time (SNRT, SRT)
s. node recovery time, direct measuring (SNRTd)
s. node recovery time, indirect measuring (SNRTi)
s. node reset
noncoronary s.
oblique s.
ostium of coronary s. (CSO)
Petit s.
phrenicocostal s.
piriform s.
pleural s.
proximal coronary s. (PCS)
pulmonary s.
s. reflex
s. rhythm (SR)
right coronary s. (RCS)
s. shot
s. standstill
superior sagittal s. (SSS)
s. tachycardia (ST)
s. thrombosis
transverse s. (TS)
transverse/sigmoid s. (TS/SS)

s. trunci pulmonalis
Valsalva s.
s. of Valsalva
s. of Valsalva aneurysm
s. of Valsalva aortography
s. venosus
s. venosus atrial septal defect
s. x-ray
SinuScope system
sinusitis
irritant s.
postnasal drip due to s. (PND-Si)
sinusoid
intramyocardial s.
myocardial s.
sinusoidal strut pattern
SIP
Sickness Impact profile
SIP scale
siphon
carotid s.
Siri equation
Sirius red stain
sirolimus-eluting stent (SES)
SIRS
systemic inflammatory response syndrome
SIS
Stroke Impact Scale
SISA
stenting in small arteries
sitaxsentan
site
arrhythmogenic s.
arterial entry s.
entry s.
exit s.
extrapulmonary s.
gene transfer injection s.
glycine s.
lysine-binding s.
target s.
site-specific surgery
Sitophilus granarius
sitostanol ester margarine
sitting-up view
situ
carcinoma in s.
situation
bailout s.
situational syncope

NOTES

S

situs
- s. ambiguus
- cardiac s.
- s. inversus
- s. solitus
- s. transversus

sivelestat

six-minute walk test (6MWT, 6-MWT)

size
- aerodynamic s.
- enzymatic infarct s.
- French catheter s. 3-34

sizer
- Björk-Shiley heart valve s.
- Meadox graft s.

sizing balloon

SJM

St. Jude Medical
- SJM Masters Series heart valve
- SJM mechanical heart valve
- SJM pericardial patch
- SJM Quattro mitral valve
- SJM Regent mechanical heart valve
- SJM Rosenkranz pediatric retractor system
- SJM Seguin annuloplasty ring
- SJM Tailor annuloplasty ring

Sjögren syndrome

SK

streptokinase

skein

skeletal
- s. alpha-actin mRNA
- s. muscle
- s. muscle plasticity

skeleton
- cardiac s.
- fibrous s.
- s. of heart
- Teflon-coated wire s.

skeletonization

skewer technique

skilled nursing facility (SNF)

Skimmer laryngeal blade tip

skimming

plasma s.

skin
- s. button
- s. change
- s. heart
- nail-fold s.
- salmon s.
- tenting of s.
- s. test anergy
- s. turgor

skin-fold thickness

skip graft

skipped beat

Skoda
- S. rale
- S. sign

skodaic resonance

SK-Pramine

SL

systolic wave, latent

SL1 sheath

Slalom
- S. balloon
- S. PTA dilatation catheter

slant
- s. hole collimator
- s. hole tomography

slapping percussion

slaved programmed electrical stimulation

SLB

surgical lung biopsy

SLD

Spatz-Lindenberg disease

SLE

systemic lupus erythematosus

sleep
- s. apnea
- s. apnea/hypopnea syndrome (SAHS)
- S. Apnea Quality of Life Index (SAQLI)
- s. architecture
- crescendo s.
- D s.
- deep s.
- s. deprivation
- desynchronized s.
- s. diagnostic
- s. diary
- s. disturbance
- diurnal s.
- dreaming s.
- fast wave s.
- s. fragmentation
- s. hypoxia
- S. Multimedia 2.6 computerized textbook
- NREM s.
- orthodox s.
- s. paralysis
- paroxysmal s.
- REM s.
- slow-wave s. (SWS)
- s. spindle
- synchronized s. (S-sleep)

sleep-disordered
- s.-d. breathing (SDB)
- s.-d. breathing event

SleepGen polysomnography data entry program

sleepiness
　　excessive daytime s. (EDS)
sleeping
　　s. sickness
　　s. tachycardia
Sleepscan
　　S. Airflow Pressure Transducer
　　S. Traveler ambulatory
　　　polysomnography system
　　S. Traveler home monitoring
　　　system
sleeve
　　s. lobectomy
　　LocalMed catheter infusion s.
　　Pneumo S.
sleuth
　　carbon monoxide s.
　　CO S.
　　ETO S.
slew rate (SR)
SL-GXT
　　symptom-limited graded exercise test
slice
　　canthomeatal s.
　　coronal s.
　　short-axis s.
　　transaxial s.
sliding
　　s. filament theory
　　s. hiatal hernia
　　lung s.
　　s. plasty
　　pleural s.
　　s. rail catheter
　　s. scale method
slim disease
sling
　　cardiac s.
　　pericardial s.
　　pressure s.
　　pulmonary artery s.
　　s. ring complex
　　vascular s.
slippers
　　PPCID s.
　　WalkCare s.
slipping rib syndrome
slit ventricle syndrome (SVS)
Slo-Niacin
slope
　　closing s.
　　diastolic s.

　　disappearance s.
　　D-to-E s.
　　E-to-F s.
　　flat diastolic s.
　　mitral E-to-F s.
　　ST/HR s.
Slo-Phyllin Gyrocaps
slot blot
slotted
　　s. needle
　　s. tube articulated stent
slough
sloughed bronchial epithelium
slow
　　s. A-V node pathway
　　s. channel
　　s. escape rhythm
　　s. and fast A-V nodal pathway
　　S. fe
　　s. paroxysmal atrial tachycardia
　　　(SPAT)
　　s. respiration
　　s. response
　　s. tissue
　　s. vital capacity (SVC)
　　s. wave
　　s. zone
slow-channel blocker
slow-fast tachycardia
slowing
　　conduction s.
　　diffuse paroxysmal s.
　　junctional s. (JS)
slow-pathway ablation
slow-reacting substance of anaphylaxis
　　(SRS-A)
slow-wave sleep (SWS)
SLP
　　segmental limb pressure
　　segmental limb systolic pressure
SLPI
　　secretory leukocyte protease inhibitor
　　secretory leukoprotease inhibitor
　　secretory leukoproteinase inhibitor
SLR
　　stent-like result
SLS
　　segment length, septal
　　segment length, systolic
　　Spectranetics laser sheath
SLT
　　single-lung transplant

NOTES

S

SLUD
salivation, lacrimation, urination, and
defecation
sludged blood
sludging
slurred
s. R wave
s. speech
slurring of QRS, ST
slurry
gelatin sponge s.
talc s.
slush
saline s.
Sly disease
SM
sonomicrometry
systolic motion
systolic murmur
SM1
primary sensorimotor cortex
Sm
speed of bronchoconstriction in response
to methacholine
SMA
smooth muscle actin
superior mesenteric artery
supplemental motor area
small
s. airways disease
s. aorta syndrome (SAS)
s. carcinoma
s. cell lung carcinoma (SCLC)
s. low-density lipoprotein
s. lung carcinoma
s. P wave
small-lung emphysema
small-particle aerosol generator (SPAG)
smallpox vaccine reaction
small-vessel infarction (SVI)
small-volume
s.-v. aspiration
s.-v. nebulizer (SNV, SVN)
SMAP
systemic mean arterial pressure
smart
s. defibrillator
s. pacemaker
S. Trigger
S. Trigger Bear 1000 ventilator
SmartFlow multiple lesion device
SmartKard digital Holter system
SmartMist
S. asthma management system
S. respiratory management system
SmartNeedle
SMC
sensorimotor cortex
smooth muscle cell

smear
bronchoscopic s.
buffy coat s.
lower respiratory tract s.
peripheral blood s.
sputum s.
smearing artifact
smear-negative tuberculosis
smear-positive tuberculosis
Smec balloon catheter
smegmatis
Mycobacterium s.
Smeloff-Cutter ball-cage prosthetic valve
Smeloff heart valve
SMG
supramarginal gyrus
S-Mgb
serum myoglobin
S-Mgb assay
SMI
silent myocardial infarction
sustained maximal inspiration
SMILE
So Much Improvement with a Little
Exercise
SMILE program
Smith
S. clip
S. sign
Smith-Lemli-Opitz syndrome
SMO
Sarns membrane oxygenator
smoke
cigarette s. (CS)
echocardiographic s.
environmental tobacco s. (ETS)
puff of s.
secondhand s.
wood s.
smokelike echoes
smoker's
s. bronchitis
s. cough
s. tongue
smoking
s. cessation
s. cessation program (SCP)
cigarette s.
s. history
passive s.
smoking-induced angina
smooth
s. coronary artery
s. excimer laser coronary
angioplasty (SELCA)
s. lesion
s. muscle actin (SMA)
s. muscle cell (SMC)
s. muscle relaxant

s. muscle relaxation
s. pseudo-Winger-Ville distribution (SPWVD)

smoothing
digital s.
rate s.

smoothness index

SMVR
supraannular mitral valve replacement

SMVT
sustained monomorphic ventricular tachycardia

SMX/TMP
sulfamethoxazole/trimethoprim

SN
sinoatrial node
sinus node
suprasternal notch

SNA
sella nasion point A
sympathetic nerve activity

snack
meat, eggs, dairy, invisible fat, condiments, s.'s (MEDICS)

snake
s. graft
s. venom

snake-tongue sign

SNAP
sensory nerve action potential

snap
aortic second sound opening s. (A2-OS)
closing s.
mitral opening s. (MOS)
opening s. (OS)
tricuspid opening s.

snare
s. catheter
caval s.
s. device
gooseneck s.
Microvena goose neck s.
Needle's Eye s.
nitinol s.
s. technique
transvenous nitinol s.

snare-assisted coil occlusion of PDA

snare-drum effect

SNB
sella nasion point B

SNCL
sinus node cycle length

SNCV
sensory nerve conduction velocity

SND
sinus node dysfunction

SNE
sinus node electrogram

Sneddon syndrome

sneeze
s. reflex
s. syncope

SNF
sinus node formation
skilled nursing facility

Snider match test

sniff
s. nasal inspiratory pressure
s. test

sniffing position

sniffling bronchophony

Sniper hydrophilic Nitinol guidewire

S-nitrosoglutathione (GSNO)

S-nitrosothiol

SNM
Society of Nuclear Medicine

SNOAR appliance

snooze-induced excitation of sympathetic triggered activity (SIESTA)

Snore-Ezzer oral appliance

Snorex, Snor-X
S. Mouthguard
S. oral appliance

snoring
heroic s.
s. rale

snowman
s. abnormality
s. configuration
s. heart

snowplow effect

snowstorm shadow

SNP
sinus node potential

SNRT
sinus node recovery time

SNRTd
sinus node recovery time, direct measuring

S

NOTES

SNRTi
sinus node recovery time, indirect measuring
SNS
sympathetic nervous system
Snuggle Warm convective warming system
SNV
Sin Nombre virus
small-volume nebulizer
SO₂
sulfur dioxide
⁸²So
strontium-82
So₂
oxygen saturation
soap curd
SOB
shortness of breath
SOBOE
shortness of breath on exertion
sobria
  Aeromonas s.
  Aeromonas hydrophila biovar s.
society
American Cancer S. (ACS)
American Roentgen Ray S.
British Cardiac S. (BCS)
Canadian Cardiovascular S. (CCS)
S. for Cardiac Angiography and Interventions (SCAI)
S. of Cardiovascular and Interventional Radiology (SCVIR)
S. for Cardiovascular Surgery (SVS)
S. of Nuclear Medicine (SNM)
S. of Thoracic Surgeons (STS)
sock array
sodium
s. acetate
s. aminosalicylate
aminosalicylate s.
ardeparin s.
s. ascorbate
beraprost s. (BPS)
s. bicarbonate
brequinar s.
cefazolin s.
cefmetazole s.
cefonicid s.
cefoperazone s.
cefotaxime s.
cefoxitin s.
ceftizoxime s.
ceftriaxone s.
cephalothin s.
cephapirin s.
cerivastatin s.
s. channel

s. channel blockade
s. channel gene
s. chloride
cloxacillin s.
colistimethate s.
s. content of food
s. cromoglycate
cromolyn s.
s. current (I_{Na})
dalteparin s.
danaparoid s.
dantrolene s.
dextrothyroxine s.
s. dichloroacetate
dicloxacillin s.
dietary s.
s. dodecylsulfate polyacrylamide gel electrophoresis (SDS-PAGE)
enoxaparin s.
epoprostenol s.
ertapenem s.
s. ferric gluconate complex
fondaparinux s.
fosinopril s.
s. ion
ioxaglate s.
s. lactate
Luminal S.
meclofenamate s.
s. meglumine diatrizoate
s. meglumine ioxaglate
mercaptomerin s.
metam s.
methicillin s.
s. methylprednisolone
mezlocillin s.
montelukast s.
morrhuate s.
nafcillin s.
nedocromil s.
s. nitrite
s. nitroprusside
nitroprusside s.
oxacillin s.
pantoprazole s.
paraaminosalicylate s.
S. P.A.S.
Pentothal S.
pertechnetate s.
s. pertechnetate Tc-99m
s. phosphate
piperacillin and tazobactam s.
PMS-Levothyroxine S.
s. polystyrene sulfonate
s. polystyrene sulfonate enema
pravastatin s.
racemic warfarin s.
s. retention
s. salicylate

stibogluconate s.
s. tetradecyl sulfate
thiamylal s.
thiopental s.
thiopentone s.
s. thiosulfate
tinzaparin s.
treprostinil s.
warfarin s.

sodium-channel blocker
sodium-potassium
s.-p. adenotriphosphatase (NaK-ATPase)
s.-p. exchange
s.-p. pump (NaK-ATPase)

Soemmerring
arterial vein of S.

SOFA
sepsis-related organ failure assessment
sequential organ failure assessment

soft
s. event
s. pulse
s. thoracoport
s. tissue calcification
s. tissue sarcoma

Softclix lancet device
Softech endotracheal tube
Softip
S. catheter
S. oxygen nasal cannula

Softouch diagnostic catheter
Soft-Vu Omni flush catheter
software
ADOPT-like s.
Clarity s.
3-dimensional MSPECT s.
Image-Measure morphometry s.
ImageVue s.
MedGraphics Breeze PF s.
Solaris FLOW image analysis s.
SPSS s.
Stat View s.
Tachyarrhythmia Detection S.
TrakPro data analysis s.
VISTA s.

SOH
sympathetic orthostatic hypotension

Sokolow-Lyon
S.-L. voltage
S.-L. voltage criteria

SolAiris
S. III, V oxygen concentrator

solani
Fusarium s.

Solarcaine topical
Solaris FLOW image analysis software
Solcotrans autotransfusion unit
soldered bond
soldering
s. flux
s. fumes

soldier's
s. heart
s. patch

Solera thrombectomy catheter
solid angle concept
solitary
s. coronary ostium
s. pulmonary arteriovenous fistula
s. pulmonary nodule (SPN)

solitus
situs s.
ventricular situs s.
visceroatrial situs s.

Solo
S. balloon
S. catheter

solubility
lipid s.

soluble
s. adhesion molecule
s. intracellular adhesion molecule (sICAM)

Solu-Cortef Injection
Soludrast contrast material
Solu-Medrol injection
Solurex L.A.
Soluspan
Celestone S.

solution
agitated saline s.
albuterol sulfate inhalation s.
Atrovent Inhalation S.
Belzer s.
Bretschneider-HTK cardioplegic s.
Brompton s.
Burow s.
Cafcit oral s.
caffeine citrate oral s.
cardioplegic s.
cardioplegic perfusion s. (CPS)
Carnoy s.

S

NOTES

solution *(continued)*
    Celsior s.
    Collins s.
    coronary perfusate s. (CPS)
    cromolyn sodium inhalation s.
    crystalloid cardioplegic s.
    Dakin s.
    Denhardt s.
    dextran s.
    Duration Nasal S.
    ECS cardioplegic s.
    Euro-Collins s.
    extracellular-like, calcium-free s.
     (ECS)
    Fowler s.
    Gey fixative s.
    hand agitated s.
    Hank's balanced salt s.
    Hartmann s.
    ICS cardioplegic s.
    Intal Nebulizer S.
    intracellular-like, calcium-bearing
     crystalloid s. (ICS)
    iseganan HCl oral s.
    Isoetharine Inhalation S. USP 1%
    Krebs s.
    Krebs-Henseleit s.
    LET s.
    levalbuterol HCl inhalation s.
    low-chloride St. Thomas s.
    Lugol s.
    Massier s.
    Melrose s.
    Myers S.
    Nasalcrom Nasal S.
    Neo-Synephrine 12 Hour Nasal S.
    Papanicolaou s.
    polyethylene glycol electrolyte
     lavage s. (PEG-LES)
    Resectisol Irrigation S.
    Ringer s.
    Schlesinger s.
    Sepracoat coating s.
    Sporicidin sterilizing s.
    stroma-free hemoglobin s.
    St. Thomas s.
    TOBI Inhalation S.
    Twice-A-Day Nasal S.
    Tyrode s.
    University of Wisconsin s.
    4-Way Long Acting Nasal S.
    Xopenex inhalation s.
    Xylocaine Topical S.
solvent vapor
SOM
    sustained outward movement
SomaSensor
    S. device
    S. pad

somatic
    s. cell therapy
    s. nociceptive flexion reflex
somatomedin
Somatom Volume Zoom computed
   tomography system
somatosensory
    s. evoked potential (SSEP)
    s. evoked potential test
somatostatin
Somavert
somnambulism
somniloquism
somniloquy
Somnoplasty
    S. procedure
    S. system
Somnus Somnoplasty system
So Much Improvement with a Little
   Exercise (SMILE)
Sonazoid
Sondergaard procedure
Sones
    S. coronary catheter
    S. Hi-Flow catheter
    S. selective coronary arteriography
    S. technique
    S. woven Dacron catheter
sonicated
    s. albumin-dextrose contrast
    s. contrast agent
    s. dextrose albumin
sonication technique
sonicator
Sonix 2000 ultrasonic nebulizer
sonogram
sonography
    Acuson computed s.
    carotid B-mode s.
    contrast-enhanced transcranial color-
     coded real-time s. (CE-TCCS)
    Doppler s. (DS)
    extracranial Doppler s. (ECD)
    functional transcranial Doppler s.
     (fTCD)
    TCD s.
    transcranial color-coded s. (TCCS)
    two-dimensional transcranial color-
     coded s. (2D-TCCS)
SonoHeart
    S. hand-carried echocardiography
    S. handheld, all digital
     echocardiography system
    S. scanner
SonoHeart Elite Ultrasound System
sonolucency
sonolucent
    s. distal imaging sheath
    s. zone

sonomicrometer piezoelectric crystal
sonomicrometry (SM)
sonorous
    s. rale
    s. respiration
    s. rhonchi
SONOS
    S. 4500 echocardiography system
    S. 500 imaging system
    S. 1500, 2500 scanner
    S. 2000, 5500 ultrasound imager
SonoVue ultrasound contrast media
Sopha Medical gamma camera
Sorbitrate
Sorin
    S. Bicarbon bileaflet aortic valve
      prosthesis
    S. Carbostent stent
    S. heart valve
    S. lead
    S. mitral valve prosthesis
    S. pacemaker
    S. prosthetic valve
Sorivudine
soroche
sorter
    cell s.
    fluorescence-activated cell s.
      (FACS)
SOS guidewire
Sotacor
sotalol
    s. HCl
    s. hydrochloride
Sotradecol injection
Soucek
    Randall-Baker S. (RBS)
souffle
    cardiac s.
    fetal s.
    funic s.
    mammary s.
soufflet
    bruit de s.
sound
    absent breath s.'s
    adventitious breath s.'s
    adventitious heart s.'s
    anodal closure s. (ACS)
    anodal opening s. (AOS)
    aortic s. (AS)
    aortic closure s.

aortic ejection s. (AES)
aortic first s. (A1)
aortic second sound, pulmonary
  second s. (A2P2)
aortic tunica adventitious
  breath s.'s
atrial s.
auscultatory s.
bandbox s.
Beatty-Bright friction s.
bell s.
bellows s.
bottle s.
breath s.
bronchial breath s.'s
bronchovesicular breath s.'s
cannon s.
cardiac s.
coarse breath s.'s
coin s.
cracked-pot s.
crowing breath s.'s
crunching s.
decreased breath s.'s
distant breath s.'s
distant heart s.'s
double-shock s.
eddy s.
ejection s. (ES)
esophageal adventitious breath s.'s
FBPM spectral analysis of
  heart s.'s
fetal heart s. (FHS)
fifth Korotkoff s. (K5)
first heart s. (S_1)
flapping s.
fourth heart s. (S_4)
fourth Korotkoff s. (K4)
friction s.
gallop s.
heart s.'s (HS)
heart s.'s S_1, S_2, S_3, S_4
hippocratic s.
s. intensity profile
mammary souffle s.
metallic breath s.'s
mitral s.'s (MS)
mitral first s. (M_1)
mitral second s. (M_2)
muffled heart s.'s
pacemaker s.
paradoxically split S_2 s.

NOTES

S

sound *(continued)*
    percussion s.
    pericardial friction s.
    physiologically split S_2 s.
    physiologic third heart s.
    pistol shot femoral s.
    prosthetic valve s.
    pseudoejection s.
    puffing s.
    pulmonary component of second
      heart s.
    pulmonic second heart s. (P2)
    pulmonic valve closure s.
    quiet breath s.'s
    quiet heart s.'s
    respiratory s.
    sail s.
    second heart s. (S_2)
    second mitral s.
    shaking s.
    splitting of heart s.
    squeaky-leather s.
    succussion s.'s
    tambour s.
    third heart s. (S_3)
    tic-tac s.'s
    to-and-fro s.
    tracheal s.
    tricuspid first s. (T1)
    tricuspid valve closure s. (T1)
    tubular breath s.'s
    tumor plop s.
    tympanitic s.
    vesicular breath s.'s
    waterwheel s.
    s. wave cycle
    widely split second s.
    xiphisternal crunching s.
source
    germanium-68 external s.
south
    S. Beach diet
    S. Florida RAST panel
southern
    S. blot
    S. blot analysis
Souttar tube
soy
    s. phytoestrogen
    s. protein
soybean lecithin asthma
SP
    shunt pressure
    shunt procedure
    spontaneous pneumothorax
    surfactant protein
    systolic pressure
    SP-A,-B,-C.-D
Spirovit SP-1,-10 portable spirometer

SP-10 spirometer
space
    air s.
    alveolar dead s.
    anatomic dead s.
    antecubital s.
    anterior clear s.
    Bogros s.
    Böttcher s.
    s. of Burns
    Cotunnius s.
    cystic s.
    dead s.
    echo-free s.
    extrapleural s.
    H s.
    Henke s.
    His perivascular s.
    Holzknecht s.
    intercostal s.
    interelectrode s.
    interpleural s.
    interstitial s.
    intrapleural s.
    Larrey s.
    lateral pharyngeal s.
    mediastinal s.
    noncommunicating air s.
    peripharyngeal s.
    perivascular s.'s
    pharyngeal s.
    pharyngomaxillary s.
    physiologic dead s.
    pleural s.
    posterior airway s. (PAS)
    postpharyngeal s.
    prevertebral s.
    respiratory dead s.
    retrocardiac s.
    retropharyngeal s.
    retrosternal air s.
    retrotracheal s.
    subarachnoid s. (SAS)
    subphrenic s.
    Talairach s.
    Traube semilunar s.
    Virchow-Robin s.
    Westberg s.
    Zang s.
Spacehaler
SpaceLabs Holter monitor
Spacemaker balloon dissector
space-occupying
    s.-o. effect
    s.-o. lesion
spacer
    ACE MDI s.
    Ellipse compact s.
    MDI s.

spacing
spadelike configuration
SPAF
> spontaneous paroxysmal atrial fibrillation

SPAG
> small-particle aerosol generator

spalling effect
SPAMM
> spatial modulation of magnetization
> > SPAMM technique

sPAP
> systolic pulmonary artery pressure

spare tire bulge
sparfloxacin
sparing
> myocardial s.

spark erosion
Sparks mandrel technique
spasm
> arterial s.
> bronchial s.
> bronchopulmonary s.
> carpopedal s.
> catheter-induced s. (CIS)
> catheter-induced coronary artery s.
> catheter-related peripheral vessel s.
> catheter-tip s.
> coronary s.
> coronary artery s. (CAS)
> diffuse esophageal s. (DES)
> epicardial arterial s.
> ergonovine-induced s.
> esophageal s.
> post bypass s.
> vascular s.
> venous s.
> vessel s.

spasmodic
> s. asthma
> s. croup

spastica
> dysphagia s.

spasticity
SPAT
> slow paroxysmal atrial tachycardia

spatial
> s. average intensity (I_{sa})
> s. average pulse average (I_{sapa})
> s. average, temporal average intensity (I_{sata})
> s. modulation of magnetization (SPAMM)

> s. modulation of magnetization technique
> s. peak intensity (I_{sp})
> s. peak pulse average intensity (I_{sppa})
> s. peak, temporal average intensity (I_{sapt})
> s. resolution
> s. tracking
> s. vector
> s. vectorcardiogram (SVCG)
> s. vectorcardiography

spatium, pl. spatia
> s. intercostale
> s. lateropharyngeum
> s. parapharyngeum
> s. pharyngeum laterale
> s. retropharyngeum
> s. suprasternale

Spatz-Lindenberg disease (SLD)
Spaulding classification system
SPCA
> serum prothrombin conversion accelerator

SPCG
> spectral phonocardiography

SPE
> septic pulmonary edema
> sustained physical exercise

speaking valve
Spearman coefficient
Spears laser balloon
special
> Lasix S.

specialized CC-chemokine secretion
specific
> s. bronchial challenge test
> s. compliance

specificity
speckle
> Doppler s.

speckling
SPECT
> single-photon emission computed tomography
> > adenosine ^{99m}Tc sestamibi SPECT
> > gated SPECT
> > SPECT imaging
> > MIBI SPECT
> > SPECT scintigraphy
> > sestamibi SPECT

S

NOTES

SPECT *(continued)*
>> stress perfusion and rest function by sestamibi-gated SPECT
>> technetium-99m sestamibi SPECT
>> technetium-sestamibi SPECT

spectacular shrinking deficit

spectography
>> magnetic resonance s.
>> Raman s.

spectra (*pl. of* spectrum)

Spectracef-TAP

Spectral
>> S. Cardiac STATus CK-MB/myoglobulin panel test
>> S. Cardiac STATus rapid format troponin I panel test

spectral
>> s. analysis
>> s. Doppler
>> s. Doppler velocity measurement
>> s. envelope
>> s. leakage
>> s. peak velocity
>> s. phonocardiograph
>> s. phonocardiography (SPCG)
>> s. power
>> s. temporal mapping
>> s. turbulence mapping
>> s. waveform

Spectranetics
>> S. C rapid-exchange laser catheter
>> S. Extreme catheter
>> S. laser
>> S. laser sheath (SLS)
>> S. Prima laser guidewire

spectrometer
>> Amis 2000 respiratory mass s.
>> Burker Avance s.
>> InSpectra tissue s.

spectrometry
>> atomic absorption s.
>> gas chromatography-mass s. (GC-MS)

spectrophotometer
>> Cary 118C s.
>> Hitachi U-2000 s.
>> liquid scintillation s.

spectrophotometric oximetry

spectrophotometry
>> time of flight and absorbance s.
>> TOFA s.

spectroscopy
>> electron paramagnetic resonance s.
>> flame emission s. (FES)
>> fluorescence s.
>> graphite furnace atomic absorption s.
>> magnetic resonance s. (MRS)
>> near-infrared s. (NIRS, NIS)
>> NMR s.
>> phosphorus-31 magnetic resonance s. (^{31}P-MRS)
>> ^{31}P nuclear magnetic resonance s.
>> proton s.
>> Raman s.

spectroscopy-directed laser

spectrum, pl. **spectra**

SpectRx test

specular echo

speculum, pl. **specula**
>> Yankauer pharyngeal s.

speech
>> alaryngeal s.
>> esophageal s.
>> s. mental stress test
>> slurred s.

speed of bronchoconstriction in response to methacholine (Sm)

spell
>> blackout s.
>> grayout s.
>> hypercyanotic s.
>> hypoxic s.
>> presyncopal s.
>> syncopal s.
>> Tet s.
>> tetrad s.
>> tetralogy of Fallot s.

Spembly cryoprobe

Spencer plication of vena cava

Spens syndrome

SPET imaging

SPF
>> standard perfusion fluid
>> systemic pulmonary fistula

SPGR
>> spoiled gradient recalled

sphaericus
>> *Bacillus* s.

Sphaerophorus necrophorus

sphenoidal fissure

sphere
>> attraction s.

sphericity index

spheroid left ventricular shape

spheroplast

sphincter
>> cardioesophageal s.
>> esophageal s.
>> gastroesophageal s.
>> hepatic s.
>> inferior esophageal s.
>> palatopharyngeal s.
>> pharyngoesophageal s.
>> precapillary s.

Sphingobacterium

sphingolipidosis

sphingomyelinase
  secretory s. (S-SMase)
sphingomyelin phosphodiesterase
Sphrintzen syndrome
sphygmic interval
sphygmocardiograph
sphygmocardioscope
sphygmochronograph
sphygmocorder
SphygmoCor non-invasive aortic blood pressure system
sphygmogram
sphygmograph
sphygmographic
sphygmography
sphygmoid
sphygmomanometer, sphygmometer
  Ayers s.
  Baumanometer standard mercury s.
  Erlanger s.
  Faught s.
  Hawksley random zero mercury s.
  Janeway s.
  London School of Hygiene and Tropical medicine s.
  Mosso s.
  Physio-Control Lifestat s.
  random-zero s.
  Riva-Rocci s.
sphygmomanometry
sphygmometroscope
sphygmooscillometer
sphygmopalpation
sphygmophone
sphygmoscope
  Bishop s.
sphygmoscopy
sphygmosystole
sphygmotonograph
sphygmotonometer
sphygmoviscosimetry
spider
  s. angioma
  arterial s.
  s. burst
  S. embolic protection device
  s. projection
  vascular s.
  s. venom
  s. x-ray view
Spielberger Anger Expression scale

SPIH
  superimposed pregnancy-induced hypertension
spike
  s. activity
  atrial s.
  H s.
  pacemaker s.
  pacing s.
  sensing s.
  wave s.
  s. wave (SW, S/W)
spike-and-dome
  s.-a.-d. configuration
  s.-a.-d. pulse
spike-wave stupor (SWS)
SPI-Lite sleep position indicator
spill
  chylous s.
spillover
  jugular venous catechol s.
spin
  s. density
  s. echo signal
  s. tagging
spinal
  s. cord stimulation (SCS)
  s. embolism
  s. muscle of thorax
  s.nociceptive flexion reflex
spindle
  aortic s.
  s. cell carcinoma
  s. fiber
  His s.
  sleep s.
spine
  posterior nasal s. (PNS)
spin-echo (SE)
  s.-e. imaging
  s.-e. imaging sequence
  s.-e. MRI
Spinhaler
spin-lattice time
spinocerebellar
  s. ataxia
  s. degeneration
spinothalamic tract
spin-spin time
spiral
  s. computed tomography
  s. CT scan

S

NOTES

spiral *(continued)*
    Curschmann s.
    s. dissection
    s. hypertrophic cardiomyopathy
    s. reentrant wave
spiral-embedded tube
spiralis
    Trichinella s.
spiramycin
spirapril hydrochloride
Spiriva
spirochetal
    s. disease
    s. infection
    s. myocarditis
spirochete
Spir-O-Flow peak flowmeter
spirogermanium
spirogram
    forced expiratory s. (FES)
spirograph
spirography
spiro-index
Spirolite 201 spirometer
spirometer
    Benedict-Roth s.
    Calculair s.
    chain-compensated s.
    closed-circuit s.
    Coach incentive s.
    Collins Survey s.
    Compact II desktop s.
    Discovery handheld s.
    Eagle s.
    Flash portable s.
    flow-sensing s.
    Gould Instrument Systems s.
    Horizon PFT s.
    incentive s.
    Inspiron incentive s.
    Krogh apparatus s.
    MasterLab Pro pneumotachograph s.
    MedicAIR Plus s.
    Micro DiaryCard s.
    MicroLab ML3500 desktop
      diagnostic s.
    MicroLoop II handheld s.
    MicroLoop pocket s.
    Micro Plus s.
    Pneumotach s.
    2120 Recording S.
    Simplicity S.
    SP-10 s.
    Spirolite 201 s.
    SpiroVision-3+ s.
    Spirovit SP-1,-10 portable s.
    Stead-Wells water-seal type s.
    Tissot s.

    Vitalograph 2120 handheld
      recording s.
    Vitalor incentive s.
    volume-displacement s.
    water-sealed s.
    wedge s.
    Welch Allyn Pneumocheck s.
    Wright s.
spirometric screening
spirometry
    DX-Portable s.
    incentive s.
    MultiSPIRO computerized s.
    MultiSPIRO DX-Portable Plus s.
    stacked inspiratory s.
    SX/DX computerized s.
    Tri-flow incentive s.
    Welch Allyn/Schiller SP-1
      budget s.
    Welch Allyn/Schiller SP-10
      diagnostic s.
2170 Spirometry Software system
spironolactone
    hydrochlorothiazide and s.
Spiros
    S. DPI
    S. dry powder inhaler
    S. inhalation system
spiroscope
SpiroSense
    S. flow sensor
    S. system
SpiroVision-3 spirometry system
SpiroVision-3+ spirometer
Spitzer theory
SPL
    superior parietal lobule
splanchnic
    s. bed perfusion
    s. blood flow
    s. vessel
splanchnicotomy
splash
    succussion s.
splayed
    carina not s.
Splendore-Hoeppli phenomenon
splenic
    s. anemia
    s. flexure syndrome
    s. perfusion measurement
    s. portography
    s. venoconstriction
splenomegaly
splenopneumonia
splenoportal hypertension
splenoportography
splenorenal shunt

splenosis
> thoracic s.

splice

splint
> wrist positioning s.

splinter hemorrhage

splinting

split
> s. fused commissure
> paradoxic s. of S_2
> physiological s. of S_2

split-function lung test

split-lung ventilation

split-sheath introducer

splitter
> beam s.

splitting
> commissural s.
> s. of heart sound

SPN
> solitary pulmonary nodule

SpO_2
> oxygen saturation measured by pulse oximetry

spoiled gradient recalled (SPGR)

spondylitis
> ankylosing s.

spondyloarthropathy
> seronegative s.

sponge
> absorbable gelatin s.
> collagen s.
> Collostat hemostatic s.
> gelatin s.
> Gelfoam s.
> Ivalon s.
> laparotomy s.
> phantom s.

spongy myocardium

spontaneous
> s. cervical artery dissection (sCAD)
> s. closure of fistula
> s. coronary artery disease (SCAD, sCAD)
> s. coronary artery dissection (SCAD, sCAD)
> s. echo contrast (SEC)
> s. extrasystole
> s. fibrillation (SF)
> s. intracerebral hemorrhage (SICH)
> s. lysis

> s. paroxysmal atrial fibrillation (SPAF)
> s. pneumothorax (SP)
> s. reentrant sustained ventricular tachycardia
> s. ventilation

spontaneously hypertensive (SH)

Sporanox Oral

Sporicidin sterilizing solution

Sporothrix schenckii

sporotrichosis

sport
> isometric s.

spot
> Brushfield s.
> café-au-lait s.
> Campbell De Morgan s.
> cold s.
> cotton-wool s.
> De Morgan s.'s
> Horder s.'s
> hot s.
> Koplik s.
> s. lesion
> milk s.'s
> rose s.
> Roth s.
> tendinous s.
> ventricular milk s.'s
> s. welding
> white s.

spot-film fluorography

spotty
> s. coronary calcium
> s. predicted stenosis

spray
> Astelin nasal s.
> Hurricaine s.
> metered-dose s.
> nasal nicotine s. (NNS)
> nicotine nasal s.
> Nicotrol NS nasal s.
> Nitrolingual Translingual S.

spread
> lymphangitic s.
> venous s.

spreader
> Bailey rib s.
> Burford-Finochietto rib s.
> DeBakey rib s.
> Favaloro-Morse rib s.
> Finochietto rib s.

NOTES

S

spreader *(continued)*
    Harken rib s.
    Lilienthal-Sauerbruch rib s.
    Medicon rib s.
    Miltex rib s.
    rib s.
    Rienhoff-Finochietto rib s.
spreading depression (SD)
spring
    S. catheter
    s. coil
    disk s.
spring-loaded
    s.-l. resistor
    s.-l. vascular stent
springwater cyst
sprinkle
    Humibid S.
Sprint Model 6942, 6943
  tachyarrhythmia lead
SPSS software
S-P-T
SPTI
    systolic pressure time index
spuria
    angina s.
spurious aneurysm
spurium
    septum s.
sputum, pl. **sputa**
    s. aerogenosum
    albuminoid s.
    s. analysis
    blood-tinged s.
    bloody s.
    brown s.
    s. coctum
    copious s.
    s. crudum
    s. cruentum
    currant jelly s.
    s. cytology
    egg-yolk s.
    s. elastase
    elastic fibers in s.
    s. expectoration
    fetid s.
    frothy s.
    gelatinous s.
    globular s.
    green s.
    hemorrhagic s.
    icteric s.
    s. induction
    moss-agate s.
    mucoid s.
    mucopurulent s.
    nummular s.
    opalescent s.

    pink s.
    s. production
    productive s.
    prune juice s.
    purulent s.
    putrid s.
    red-streaked s.
    s. retention
    ropy s.
    rubbery s.
    rusty s.
    septicemia s.
    s. smear
    tenacious s.
    s. tenacity
    viscid s.
    s. viscoelasticity
    s. viscosity and elasticity
    s. volume
    white s.
    yellow s.
    yellowish-green s.
sputum-epithelium interface
SPV
    stentless porcine valve
SPWVD
    smooth pseudo-Winger-Ville distribution
Spyglass angiography catheter
S_1Q_3 pattern
S-QRS interval
$S_1Q_3T_3$ pattern
squamous
    s. alveolar cell
    s. cell bronchogenic carcinoma
square
    s. root sign
    s. wave response
    s. wave stimulus
squared
    kilogram per meter s. (kg/m^2)
    liter per minute per meter s.
     (Lpm/m^2)
    meter per second s. (m/s^2)
square-shaped occluder
squeak
squeaky-leather sound
squeeze
    s. effect
    face s.
    reverse s.
    thoracic s.
    tussive s.
squeezer
SR
    sinus rhythm
    slew rate
    sustained release
     bupropion SR
     Calan SR

SR calcium ATPase
Cardene SR
Cardizem SR
Deconamine SR
Isoptin SR
Nitrong SR
Procan SR

SRA
sewing ring area

Sramek formula

SRCBC
serum reserve cholesterol binding
capacity

Src kinase

SREBP
sterol regulatory element-binding protein

SRP
synchronized retroperfusion

SRS-A
slow-reacting substance of anaphylaxis

SRT
segmented ring tripolar
sinus node recovery time
SRT lead

SRVT
sustained reentrant ventricular
tachyarrhythmia

SS
selective shunt
subaortic stenosis
systemic sclerosis

S-Scort New-Duet suction unit

S-segment airway conductance

SSEP
somatosensory evoked potential

S-Series sleep system

SSI
surgical site infection

S_1-S_2 interval

SSKI
saturated solution of potassium iodide

S-sleep
synchronized sleep

S-SMase
secretory sphingomyelinase

SSP
simultaneously stapled pneumonectomy

SSPS
side-to-side portacaval shunt

SS-QOL
stroke-specific quality of life

SSS
sick sinus syndrome
superior sagittal sinus

SSS-58

S-sulfate

ST
sinus tachycardia
stent thrombosis
stress test
systolic time
ST alteration
ST deviation
ST interval
ST junction
ST reelevation
ST sag
ST scooping
ST segment
ST segment alternans
ST segment changes
ST segment coving
ST segment depression (STD)
ST segment divided by heart rate
(ST/HR)
ST segment elevation
ST segment resolution
ST wave

S-T
portion of the segment between the end
of the S wave and the beginning of the
T wave

St.
saint
St. George Respiratory
Questionnaire (SGRQ)
St. Joseph Adult Chewable Aspirin
St. Joseph Cough Suppressant
St. Jude bileaflet prosthetic valve
St. Jude cardiac device
St. Jude composite prosthetic
St. Jude composite prosthetic valve
St. Jude heart valve prosthesis
St. Jude Medical (SJM)
St. Jude Medical bileaflet tilting-
disk aortic valve
St. Jude Medical Biocor valve
St. Jude Medical bioImplant valve
St. Jude Medical Port-Access
St. Jude Medical Port-Access
mechanical heart valve
St. Jude Medical valve prosthesis
St. Jude mitral valve

NOTES

S

665

St. *(continued)*
    St. Jude prosthetic aortic valve
    St. Thomas Hospital cardioplegia
    St. Thomas solution
    St. Vitus dance
ST3 amplified stethoscope
STA
    serum thrombotic accelerator
stab
    s. electrode
    s. incision
    s. wound
stability
    circulatory s.
    hemodynamic s.
    RR interval s.
stabilization
    internal pneumatic s.
    membrane s.
    plaque s.
stabilizer
    Axius vacuum 2 s.
    S. balanced performance guidewire
    Cohn cardiac s.
    S. marker wire
    S. marker wire steerable guidewire
    Octopus tissue s.
    S. Plus steerable guidewire
    S. XS steerable guidewire
stab-in epicardial electrode
stable
    s. angina (SA)
    s. angina pectoris (SAP)
staccato pain
Stachrom PAI chromogenic assay
Stachybotrys atra
Stack
    S. autoperfusion balloon
    S. perfusion catheter
stacked inspiratory spirometry
stacking
    breath s.
Stadie-Riggs microtome
stadiometer
STAE
    subsegmental transcatheter arterial
    embolization
Stagesic
staging
    TNM s.
    videothoracoscopic operator s.
    (VOS)
stagnant
    s. anoxia
    s. hypoxia
stagnation
    contrast s.
STAI
    State-Trait Anxiety Inventory

stain, staining
    acetoorcein s.
    Alcian blue-PAS s.
    Azan-Mallory s.
    calcofluor s.
    Coomassie blue s.
    Dieterle s.
    Diff-Quik s.
    direct immunofluorescent s.
    endocardial s.
    Giemsa s.
    GMS s.
    Goldner trichrome s.
    Gomori methenamine silver s.
    Gram s.
    Grocott s.
    H&E s.
    hematotylin-eosin s.
    immunoperoxidase s.
    Kinyoun s.
    Mallory s.
    Masson trichrome s.
    May-Grünwald-Giemsa s.
    Miller elastic s.
    Movat s.
    mucicarmine s.
    oil red O s.
    Pappenheim s.
    picrosirius red s.
    Pizzolatto s.
    propidium iodide s.
    silver-methenamine s.
    Sirius red s.
    toluidine blue s.
    TTC s.
    TUNEL s.
    van Gieson s.
    Verhoeff elastica s.
    Verhoeff tissue elastin s.
    Weigert-van Gieson s.
    Wright s.
    Wright-Giemsa s.
    Ziehl-Neelsen s.
stainless
    s. steel balloon expandable stent
    s. steel guidewire
    s. steel mesh stent
staircase phenomenon
STALD
    Sheffield Screening Test for Acquired
    Language Disorders
Stamey test
stand-alone
    s.-a. balloon angioplasty
    s.-a. laser treatment
standard
    s. atmosphere
    Boehringer Mannheim s.
    s. Bruce protocol

s. cardiopulmonary resuscitation (SCPR)
s. deviation
s. heparin (SH)
hypertension s.
s. Lehman catheter
s. limb lead
s. needle
s. perfusion fluid (SPF)
s. temperature and pressure, dry
s. temperature and pulse (STP)
standardization wave
standby
s. pacemaker
s. pulse generator
Stand Displacement Amplification test
standing
s. diastolic blood s. (SDBP)
s. venous pressure (SVP)
standstill
atrial s.
auricular s.
cardiac s.
persistent atrial s. (PAS)
respiratory s.
sinus s.
ventricular s.
Stanford
S. biopsy method
S. bioptome
S. treadmill exercise protocol
S. type A,B aortic dissection
Stanicor pacemaker
stannic oxide
Stannius ligature
stannosis
stanozolol anabolic steroid
Stansel procedure
staphyledema
staphylococcal
s. bronchitis
s. endocarditis
s. infection
s. pneumonia
Staphylococcus
S. aureus
S. epidermidis
staphylokinase
staphylopharyngorrhaphy
stapled lung reduction
stapler
Androsov vascular s.

CEEA s.
Endo GIA s.
Endopath EZ45 thoracic linear s.
Ethicon Endopath EZ45 s.
stapling
bleb s.
starch
hydroxyethyl s.
STARFlex device
Starling
S. curve
S. curve of pancreas
S. equation
S. force
S. law
S. mechanism
Starr-Edwards
S.-E. aortic valve prosthesis
S.-E. ball-and-cage valve
S.-E. ball valve prosthesis
S.-E. cardiac valve prosthesis
S.-E. disk valve prosthesis
S.-E. heart valve prosthesis
S.-E. mitral prosthesis
S.-E. mitral valve
S.-E. prosthetic valve
S.-E. Silastic valve
Stary
S. histology classification
S. histology grading
stasis, pl. **stases**
s. cirrhosis
s. dermatitis
s. edema
pressure s.
s. ulcer
venous s.
STAT
signal transducer and activator of transcription
STAT protein family
Stat
signal transducer and activator of transcription
Stat 2 Pumpette
Stat View software
STAT4 protein
STAT6 protein
state
acute confusional s. (ACS)
cardiovascular steady s.
glycometabolic s.

NOTES

S

state *(continued)*
    gradient recalled acquisition in a steady s. (GRASS)
    hypercoagulable s.
    hyperdynamic s.
    hyperinsulinemic euglycemic clamp metabolic s.
    hyperkinetic s.
    myocardial contraction s.
    nonfasting s.
    postabsorptive s.
    postictal s.
    prothrombotic s.
State-Trait Anxiety Inventory (STAI)
stathmokinesis
static
    s. dilation technique
    s. lung compliance
    s. lung volume
statin therapy
station
    analog video acquisition s.
    DICOM acquisition s.
    MedicAIR Plus spirometry s.
    PlugStation earplug s.
    s. pull-through
stationary
    s. arterial wave
    s. bicycle
Stat-Shell disposable pulse oximeter sensor
status
    acute-on-chronic s.
    s. anginosus
    s. asthmaticus
    battery s.
    cardiac s.
    s. epilepticus
    functional s.
    IND s.
    investigational new drug s.
    mental s.
    neurologic s.
    pulmonary function s.
    work s.
staurosporine
stave cell
stavudine
stay
    length of s. (LOS)
STD
    ST segment depression
Stead-Wells water-seal type spirometer
steady Doppler
steady-state method
steal
    coronary s.
    endoperoxide s.
    iliac s.

    s. mechanism
    s. phenomenon
    pulmonary artery s.
    renal-splanchnic s.
    subclavian s.
    transmural s.
stealth angioplasty balloon
steam-fitter's asthma
STEAMI
    ST-elevation acute myocardial infarction
steam tent
stearothermophilus
    Bacillus s.
steatorrhea
steatosis
    s. cardiaca
    s. cordis
steel
Steell murmur
steel-winged butterfly needle
steep left anterior oblique projection
steeple sign
steepling
    s. of trachea
    tracheal s.
steerable
    s. angioplastic guidewire
    s. decapolar electrode catheter
    s. guidewire catheter
    s. over-the-wire angioplasty technique
Steerocath-A ablation catheter
Steerocath-Dx special procedure octa catheter
Steerocath-T temperature ablation catheter
Stegemann-Stalder method
Steidele complex
Steinberg thumb sign
Steinert
    S. disease
    S. myotonic dystrophy
ST-elevation acute myocardial infarction (STEAMI)
stellate
    s. ganglion
    s. ganglion blockade
stem
    s. bronchus
    s. cell factor (SCF)
    left main s. (LMS)
    transposition of arterial s.
STEMI
    ST-segment elevation myocardial infarction
sten
    stenosed
    stenosis
stenocardia

stenosal murmur
stenosed (sten)
stenosis, pl. **stenoses (sten)**
  acute mitral s. (AMS)
  airway s.
  aortic s.
  aortic valve s. (AVS)
  area of s. (AS)
  atrial s. (AS)
  bottle neck s.
  branch pulmonary artery s.
  bronchial s.
  buttonhole s.
  buttonhole mitral s.
  calcific aortic s. (CAS)
  calcific mitral s.
  calcific nodular aortic s.
  caroticovertebral s.
  carotid s.
  carotid artery s. (CAS)
  chronic aortic s.
  cicatricial s.
  congenital aortic s.
  congenital mitral s.
  coronary artery s.
  coronary luminal s.
  coronary ostial s.
  critical aortic s.
  critical coronary s.
  critical valvular s.
  diameter s. (DS)
  discrete subaortic s. (DSAS, DSS)
  discrete subvalvular aortic s.
   (DSAS)
  distal s.
  Dittrich s.
  double aortic s.
  dynamic s.
  eccentric s.
  enucleation of subaortic s.
  fibrous subaortic s.
  filiform s.
  fish-mouth mitral s.
  flow-limiting s.
  focal eccentric s.
  geometry of s.
  granulation s.
  hemodynamically significant s.
  high-grade s.
  hourglass s.
  hypertrophic muscular subaortic s.
   (HMSAS)

  hypertrophic subaortic s. (HSAS,
   HSS)
  idiopathic hypertrophic subaortic s.
   (IHSS)
  infundibular s.
  infundibular pulmonary s. (IPS)
  left main coronary s.
  linear s.
  long axis-discrete subaortic s.
   (LAX-DSS)
  mitral s. (MS)
  muscular subaortic s. (MSS)
  myocardial infundibular s.
  napkin-ring s.
  nonrheumatic valvular aortic s.
  orificial s.
  ostial s.
  percent diameter s. (%DS)
  peripheral pulmonary artery s.
   (PPAS)
  peripheral pulmonic s.
  point of critical s.
  postdiphtheritic s.
  preventricular s.
  prosthetic valve s. (PVS)
  proximal s.
  pulmonary s. (PS)
  pulmonary arterial s. (PAS)
  pulmonary artery s.
  pulmonary branch s. (PBS)
  pulmonary valve s.
  pulmonary valvular s. (PVS)
  pulmonic s. (PS)
  pulmonic valve s.
  relative mitral s.
  renal artery s. (RAS)
  residual s.
  s. resistance
  rheumatic mitral s. (RMS)
  rheumatic mitral valve s.
  segmental s.
  semilunar valve s.
  senescent aortic s.
  s. severity
  silent mitral s.
  single-vessel coronary s.
  spotty predicted s.
  subaortic s. (SAS, SS)
  subinfundibular s.
  subpulmonary s.
  subpulmonic s.
  subvalvar s.

S

NOTES

stenosis *(continued)*

    subvalvular aortic s.
    subvalvular mitral s.
    supravalvar aortic s. (SVAS)
    supravalvular aortic s. (SAS)
    supraventricular aortic s. (SVAS)
    tight s.
    tricuspid s. (TS)
    valvular aortic s.
    valvular pulmonic s.
    vascular s.
    Waterston anastomosis for
      congenital pulmonary s.
    X-linked aqueductal s. (XLAS)

stenothorax

stenotic

    s. flow reserve (SFR)
    s. jet
    s. lesion
    s. valvular heart disease

Stenotrophomonas maltophilia

stent

    access by radial artery multilink s.
      (ARMS)
    Acculink self-expanding s.
    ACS Multi-Link coronary s.
    ACS Multi-Link Duet s.
    ACS Multi-Link RX Ultra s.
    ACS Multi-Link Tristar s.
    ACS RX Multi-Link s.
    activated balloon expandable
      intravascular s.
    ACT-ONE s.
    AneuRx s.
    angiopeptin-eluting s.
    antirestenotic s.
    s. apposition
    aSpire covered s.
    autologous vein graft-coated s.
      (AVGCS)
    AVE Microstent II s.
    AVE S540, S670 s.
    balloon-expandable flexible coil s.
    balloon-expandable intravascular s.
    Bard XT coronary s.
    bare-metal s.
    BeStent 2 coronary s.
    BeStent Rival s.
    bifurcated s.
    biocompatible s.
    biodegradable s.
    BioDiamond F s.
    BioDiamond Micro s.
    BiodivYsio added support s.
    BiodivYsio AS PC-coated s.
    BiodivYsio OC over-the-wire s.
    BiodivYsio open cell s.
    BiodivYsio PC s.
    BiodivYsio small vessel s.

    BiodivYsio SV PC-coated s.
    CardioCoil coronary s.
    carotid s.
    cell-coated s.
    cell-seeded s.
    coil s.
    Cook intracoronary s.
    Cordis CrossFlex coronary s.
    Cordis tantalum coil s.
    Corinthian s.
    s. creep
    CrossFlex coil s.
    CrossFlex LC-stainless steel, laser-
      cut coronary s.
    Crown s.
    cutting balloon before s.
      (CBBEST)
    Cypher sirolimus-eluting coronary s.
    s. delivery system (SDS)
    s. deployment
    diaphragm of s.
    DNA-coated s.
    double-J s.
    s. dressing
    Driver coronary s.
    drug-eluting s. (DES)
    drug-loaded biodegradable
      polymer s.
    Dumon endobronchial silicone s.
    Dumon tracheobronchial s.
    Dynamic Y s.
    Elastalloy Ultraflex Strecker
      nitinol s.
    Elgiloy s.
    eluting s.
    s. embolization
    emergency bailout s.
    Enforcer SDS coronary s.
    Expander s.
    s. expansion
    flat wire coil s.
    Flex s.
    flexible coil s.
    fork s.
    Freitag s.
    Genus s.
    GFX Micro s. III
    GFX over-the-wire coronary s.
    Gianturco expandable wire s.
      (GEWS)
    Gianturco-Roubin Flex II s.
    Gianturco-Roubin Flex-Stent
      coronary s.
    Gianturco Z s.
    Global Therapeutics V-Flex s.
    gold-coated Inflow coronary s.
    s. graft (SG)
    Guidant s.

S

heat-activated recoverable
  temporary s. (HARTS)
helical coil s.
Hepacoat s.
Hood stoma s.
Igaki-Tamai s.
s. implantation
InStent VascuCoil s.
IntraCoil self expanding nitinol s.
intravascular s.
INX s.
Iris coronary s.
Iris II s.
Isostent s.
s. jail
J & J s.
Johnson & Johnson coronary s.
Johnson and Johnson Interventional
  Systems s.
Jomed s.
Jostent coronary s.
kissing s.'s
LP s.
Mac s.
Magic Wallstent s.
Medex coronary C1 s.
Medinol NIR s.
Medivent self-expanding coronary s.
Medivent vascular s.
Medtronic AVE S660 coronary s.
Medtronic BeStent s.
Medtronic interventional vascular s.
Med-Xcor s.
Memotherm s.
mesh s.
Micro II s.
s. migration
MINI Crown s.
MS-CIS SV s.
multicellular s.
Multi-Link Ascent s.
Multi-Link Duet s.
Multi-Link Solo s.
Neville s.
NexStent carotid s.
Nexus coronary s.
NIRflex coronary s.
NIR Primo Monorail coronary s.
nitinol mesh s.
nitinol self-expandable s.
nitinol self-expanding coil s.
nitinol thermal memory s.

nonarticulated s.
nuclear s.
Omega s.
Ostia s.
Palmaz-Schatz s. (PSS)
Palmaz-Schatz balloon-expandable s.
Palmaz-Schatz coronary s.
Palmaz-Schatz Crown s.
Palmaz-Schatz PS-204 s.
Palmaz vascular s.
Paragon coronary s.
Paragon nitinol s.
Paragon PAS s.
s. patency
Phytis s.
s. placement
poly-L-lactic acid s.
polymeric endoluminal paving s.
polyorganophosphazene-coated s.
polypropylene s.
polytetrafluoroethylene covered s.
Power Grip s.
^{32}P radioactive s.
predilated polytetrafluoroethylene s.
premounted s.
PS 153 s.
PTFE-covered s.
Pura-Vario s.
Pura-Vario-A s.
Pura-Vario-AL s.
Pura-Vario-AS s.
radioactive s.
radiopaque tantalum s.
Radius self-expanding s.
s. reconstruction
R-Stent s.
Schatz-Palmaz intravascular s.
Schneider Speedy s.
Scimed s.
S7 coronary s.
S670 coronary s.
screw-thread s.
Seaquence s.
self-expandable metallic s.
self-expanding s.
self-expanding microporous s.
  (SEMS)
short s.
sirolimus-eluting s. (SES)
slotted tube articulated s.
Sorin Carbostent s.
spring-loaded vascular s.

NOTES

stent (*continued*)

S660 small vessel coronary s.
stainless steel balloon
  expandable s.
stainless steel mesh s.
Strecker balloon-expandable s.
Strecker tantalum s.
s. strut
STS s.
Supra G coronary s.
s. or surgery
Symphony nitinol s.
T s.
tantalum s.
Tenax-XR Trinity s.
Terumo s.
thermal memory s.
thermoexpandable s.
s. thrombosis (ST)
T-shaped s.
tubular slotted s.
T-Y s.
UltraCross s.
Ultraflex self-expanding s.
Ultraflex tracheobronchial s.
VascuCoil peripheral vascular s.
Velocity s.
V-Flex FMJ s.
V-Flex Plus s.
Wallgraft s.
Wallstent flexible, self-expanding
  wire-mesh s.
Wallstent Magic s.
Wallstent spring-loaded s.
Westaby tracheobronchial silicone s.
Wiktor balloon expandable
  coronary s.
Wiktor GX coronary s.
Wiktor-I implantable s.
wire mesh self-expandable s.
XT radiopaque coronary s.
X-Trode s.
Y, Z s.
zigzag s.

stentable

s. disease
s. lesion

stent-anchoring device
stent-assisted coiling of basilar fusiform aneurysm
stented bioprosthetic valve
stent-graft

Ancure s.-g.
Inoue endovascular s.-g.
Lifepath s.-g.
transluminally placed Inoue
  endovascular s.-g.
Viabahn endoprosthesis s.-g.

stenting

airway s.
bailout s.
Brockenbrough atrial s.
carotid angioplasty and s. (CAS)
carotid artery s.
coronary s.
endoluminal s.
femoropopliteal s.
high-pressure balloon s.
intracoronary s.
kissing s.
s. in small arteries (SISA)
transradial primary s.
Y s.

stent-jail orifice
stentless

s. porcine aortic valve
s. porcine aortic valve prosthesis
s. porcine bioprosthesis
s. porcine valve (SPV)
s. porcine xenograft

stent-like result (SLR)
stent-mounted

s.-m. allograft valve
s.-m. heterograft valve

stent/system
stent-to-artery (S/A)
STEP

short transitional edge protection

step-down therapy
Step-One Diet
stepped bur approach
stepped-care antihypertensive regimen
step treadmill protocol
Step-Two Diet
step-up in oxygen saturation
stepwise
Sterapred Oral
stercoralis

Strongyloides s.

stereoauscultation
stereolithography
stereoscopic interrogation
Steri-Cath catheter
Steri-Neb
Sterles sign
sternad
sternal

s. border
s. compression
s. dehiscence
s. extremity of clavicle
s. fracture
s. notch
s. part of diaphragm
s. plane
s. synchondrosis
s. wiring

S

sternalgia
sternal-splitting incision
Sternberg
S. myocardial insufficiency
S. pericarditis
S. sign
Sterneedle tuberculin test
sternochondral junction
sternoclavicular angle
sternocleidomastoid artery
sternocostal triangle
sternodynia
sternomastoid
sternotomy
median s.
sternotracheal
sternoxiphoid plane
Stern posture
sternum
s. saw
wiring of s.
steroid
s. aerosol
anabolic s.
s. elution
high-dose s.
nasal s. (NS)
sex s.
stanozolol anabolic s.
steroid-dependent
s.-d. asthma
s.-d. asthmatic
steroid-eluting
s.-e. electrode
s.-e. pacemaker lead
steroidogenesis
steroid-resistant asthma
steroid-sparing agent
sterol
plant s.
s. regulatory element-binding
protein (SREBP)
stertor
hen-cluck s.
stertorous respiration
Stertzer
S. brachial catheter
S. guiding catheter
STET
submaximal treadmill exercise test
stethoscope
Acoustascope esophageal s.

bell s.
Cardiology II s.
Classic II s.
differential s.
Doppler fetal s.
double-headed s.
Harvey Elite s.
Labtron s.
Littman class II pediatric s.
Rappaport-Sprague s.
ST3 amplified s.
stethoscopic phonocardiograph
Stevens-Johnson syndrome
**Stewart-Hamilton cardiac output
technique**
STG
superior temporal gyrus
sthenic fever
ST/HR
ST segment divided by heart rate
ST/HR index
ST/HR slope
STI
systolic time interval
stibogluconate sodium
stick
arterial s.
Vaxcel mini s.
Stifcore
S. aspiration needle
S. biopsy injection needle
stiff
s. heart
s. heart syndrome
s. left atrium syndrome
s. lung
stiffness
active dynamic s.
chamber s.
diastolic s.
elastic s.
end-diastolic chamber s. (EDCS)
s. index
muscle s.
myocardial s.
vascular s.
ventricular systolic s.
volume s.
stigma, pl. **stigmata**
peripheral stigmata

NOTES

Still
    S. disease
    S. murmur
Stilphostrol
stimulant
    adrenergic s.
stimulated acoustic emission
stimulation
    alpha-adrenergic s.
    beta-adrenergic s. (BAS)
    beta-1,-2 adrenergic s.
    beta adrenoceptor s.
    blood monocyte s.
    carotid sinus s.
    chest wall s. (CWS)
    direct s.
    functional magnetic s.
    muscarinic s.
    noninvasive programmed s. (NIPS)
    paired electrical s.
    postganglionic vagal s. (PGVS)
    programmed electrical s. (PES)
    programmed ventricular s. (PVS)
    rapid atrial s. (RAS)
    reflex s.
    slaved programmed electrical s.
    spinal cord s. (SCS)
    subthreshold s.
    supramaximal tetanic s.
    synchronous atrial s. (SAS)
    s. threshold
    transcutaneous electrical s. (TES)
    transesophageal atrial s. (TRAS)
    ultrarapid subthreshold s.
    vagal s.
    vagus nerve s.
    ventricular-programmed s.
stimulator
    Atrostim phrenic nerve s.
    BioZ.sim ICG S.
    Bloom programmable s.
    Grass S88 muscle s.
    InSync multisite cardiac s.
    Quik-Coff electrical cough s.
stimulus, pl. **stimuli**
    chemical s.
    chemoattracting stimuli
    heterotopic s.
    hypercapnic s.
    ischemic-type preconditioning s.
    neurohumoral s.
    pacing s.
    paired s.
    physical s.
    premature s.
    premature atrial s. (PAS)
    psychological s.
    square wave s.

    thrombogenic s.
    triple s.
stimulus-T interval
Stinger S ablation catheter
stippling of lung field
stochastic risk
stocking-glove distribution
stockings
    Bellavar medical support s.
    Carolon life support
      antiembolism s.
    compression s.
    elastic s.
    Fast-Fit vascular s.
    Florex medical compression s.
    graduated compression s. (GCS)
    Jobst Vairox gradient compression
      vascular s.
    Juzo s.
    Medi-Strumpf s.
    pneumatic compression s.
    Sigvaris compression s.
    TED antiembolism s.
    thigh-high antiembolic s.
    Vairox high compression
      vascular s.
    VenES II Medical s.
    venous pressure gradient support s.
      (VPGSS)
    Zimmer antiembolism support s.
stocking-seam incision
stoichiometric fashion
Stokes
    S.-Adams attack
    S.-Adams disease
    S.-Adams syndrome
    collar of S.
Stokes-Adams
    S.-A. attack
    S.-A. disease
    S.-A. syndrome
Stokvis-Talma syndrome
Stoll pneumonia
stoma
    tracheostomy s.
stomach
    s. cough
    left coronary artery of s.
Stomatococcus
stone
    cholesterol s. (CS)
    s. cutter's phthisis
    s. heart
    s. like myxoma
    lung s.
    s. stripper's asthma
stool
    melenic s.

stop
 S. at Ring lead
 S. at Tip lead
stopcock
 three-way s.
stopped flow pressure (SFP)
stop-valve airway obstruction
storage
 tracer s.
store
 myocyte magnesium s.
stored electrocardiogram
storm
 electric s.
 thyroid s.
Stormer balloon catheter
Storz bronchoscope
Storz-Hopkins laryngoscope
STP
 standard temperature and pulse
straddling
 s. aorta
 s. atrioventricular valve
 s. embolism
 s. thrombus
 s. tricuspid valve
 s. of valve
straight
 s. back syndrome
 s. blade
 s. flush percutaneous catheter
 s. hemostat
 s. sinus thrombosis
 s. stylet
 s. tipped catheter
 s. tube graft
straight-line ECG
StraightShot arterial cannula
0157-H7 strain
strain
 carer s.
 cell s.
 0157-H7 s.
 left heart s. (LHS)
 left ventricular s. (LVS)
strain-gauge plethysmography
stramonium
strand
 iridium s.
stranding effusion
strandy infiltrate

strap
 hook-and-loop fastener s.
 s. muscle
 Pepper Medical Antidisconnect
 Device s.
Strasburger cell plate
stratification
 postinfarction risk s. (PIRS)
 risk s.
stratified thrombus
stratigraphy
Stratus cardiac troponin I test
Strauss method
strawberry tongue
streak
 fatty s.
streaking
 basophilic vascular s.
streaky infiltrate
Strecker
 S. balloon-expandable stent
 S. tantalum stent
strength
 Allerest Maximum S.
 Bayer Low Adult S.
 double s. (DS)
 peripheral muscle s.
 s. training
strenuous exercise
Streptase
streptavidin
Streptobacillus moniliformis
streptococcal
 s. antibody
 s. bacteremia
 s. bronchitis
 s. carditis
 s. empyema
 s. endocarditis
 s. infection
 s. pneumonia
Streptococcus
 S. agalactiae
 S. anginosus
 S. faecalis
 S. milleri
 S. mitis
 S. pneumoniae
 S. pyogenes
 S. pyogenes infection
 S. salivarius
 S. viridans

NOTES

S

675

streptodornase
streptogramin antibiotic
streptokinase (SK)
   s. antibody
   intracoronary s. (ICSK)
streptokinase-plasminogen complex
streptokinase-streptodornase
streptokinase-urokinase myocardial
  infarct test (SUMIT)
streptolysin O
Streptomyces tsukubaensis
streptomycin sulfate
streptozocin
STRESS
   subject's treatment-emergent symptom
   scale
stress
   adenosine s.
   circumferential end-systolic s.
    (cESS)
   circumferential wall s. (CWS)
   dipyridamole s.
   S. Echo bed
   s. echocardiography
   s. electrocardiography (SECG)
   emotional s.
   end-diastolic circumferential s.
    (EDCS)
   end-systolic s. (ESS)
   end-systolic circumferential wall s.
   end-systolic left ventricular s.
    (ESS)
   end-systolic wall s. (ESWS)
   handgrip s.
   left ventricular end-systolic s.
   left ventricular wall s.
   mental s.
   meridional wall s.
   s. MUGA electrocardiogram
   oxidative s.
   s. perfusion and rest function
   s. perfusion and rest function by
    sestamibi-gated SPECT
   s. perfusion scintigraphy
   pharmacologic s.
   physiological s.
   s. relaxation
   shear s.
   s. SPECT perfusion imaging
   tend-and-befriend response to s.
   tensile s.
   s. test (ST)
   s. thallium-201 myocardial
    perfusion imaging
   s. thallium scintigraphy
   ventricular end-systolic wall s.
   wall s.
   s. washout myocardial perfusion
    image

stress-injected sestamibi-gated SPECT
  with echocardiography
stressor
   remedial psychological s.
stress-redistribution-reinjection thallium-
  201 imaging
stress-related
   s.-r. arrhythmia
   s.-r. hypertension
stress-shortening relationship
stretch
   atrial s.
   s. receptor
stretched
   s. bronchus sign
   s. diameter
stretch-induced cardiomyocyte
  hypertrophy
stretching
   side s.
   s. syncope
stria, gen. and pl. striae
   striae cutis distensae
striation
   tabby cat s.
   tigroid s.
striatocapsular infarction
stricture
   anastomotic s.
   esophageal s.
   Wickwitz esophageal s.
strident
stridor
   biphasic s.
   congenital laryngeal s.
   inspiratory s.
   laryngeal s.
   respiratory s.
   s. serraticus
stridulosa
   laryngitis s.
stridulous respiration
stridulus
   laryngismus s.
strike
   heel s.
string
   s. of pearls
   s. sign
strip
   bovine pericardium s.
   Breathe Right nasal s.
   cardiac monitor s.
   Cover-Strip wound closure s.'s
   ECG monitor s.
   felt s.
   s. percussion
   rhythm s.
stripchart tracing

stripe
> s. sign
> subepicardial fat s.

stripper
> Alexander rib s.
> Dorian rib s.
> hydraulic vein s.
> Kurten vein s.
> Linton vein s.
> Matson-Alexander rib s.
> thrombus s.
> Trace vein s.
> Zollinger-Gilmore intraluminal vein s.

stroke
> acute caudate s.
> acute hemispheric s.
> acute ischemic s. (AIS)
> atheroembolic s.
> atherothrombotic s.
> s. belt
> brain stem s.
> cardioembolic s. (CES)
> cardiogenic s.
> caudate hemorrhagic s.
> caudate ischemic s.
> cortical s.
> crude s.
> cryptogenic s.
> early progressing s. (EPS)
> s. ejection rate
> embolic s.
> s. guidance system (SGS)
> heart s.
> heat s.
> hemorrhagic s.
> S. Impact Scale (SIS)
> s. index (SI)
> ipsilateral s.
> ischemic s.
> lacunar s.
> late progressing s. (LPS)
> left hemisphere s. (LCVA)
> light s.
> migraine s.
> mini s.
> MRI-identified s.
> National Institutes of Neurological Disorders and S. (NINDS)
> s. output
> pure motor s.
> pure sensorimotor s.

> pure sensory s.
> right hemisphere s.
> sensorimotor s.
> silent s.
> subcortical s.
> thromboembolic s.
> undetermined pathological-type s.
> s. unit (SU)
> s. volume (SV)
> s. volume index (SVI)
> s. work (SW)
> s. work index (SWI)

stroke-specific quality of life (SS-QOL)
stroma-free
> s.-f. hemoglobin pyridoxalated (SFHb)
> s.-f. hemoglobin solution

strong
> Thyroid S.
> S. unbridling of celiac artery axis

Strongyloides stercoralis
strongyloidiasis
strontium-82 (^{82}So)
Stroop color word conflict test
Strophanthus gratus
Strouhal number
structural
> s. heart disease (SHD)
> s. valve deterioration (SVD)

structure
> chordal s.
> echodense s.
> tubuloreticular s.
> wall s.

structured interview
struma, pl. **strumae**
> Riedel s.

strut
> central bridging s.
> George Washington s.
> stent s.
> tricuspid valve s.

strutting
> plaque s.

Stryker saw
STS
> Society of Thoracic Surgeons
> STS stent

ST-segment
> ST-s. elevation myocardial infarction (STEMI)
> ST-s. reelevation

S

NOTES

ST-T
>ST-T. deviation
>ST-T. segment changes
>ST-T. wave
>ST-T. wave changes

STT
>serial thrombin time

ST, T vector

Stuart-Prower factor

study (*See also* trial, program, protocol)
>postoperative pacing s. (POPS)

stuffer

stump
>bronchial s.
>cardiac s.
>s. pressure

stunned
>s. atrium
>s. myocardium

stunning
>left atrial appendage s.
>myocardial s.
>repetitive s.

stupor
>spike-wave s. (SWS)

Sturge-Weber syndrome

stuttering
>s. myocardial infarction
>s. of perfusion

stutzeri
>*Pseudallescheria s.*
>*Pseudomonas s.*

stylet
>Bing s.
>Cook locking s.
>K s.
>Liberator locking s.
>lighted s.
>locking s.
>straight s.
>TFX Medical catheter s.
>transmyocardial pacing s.
>transthoracic pacing s.
>wire s.

styrene asthma

SU
>stroke unit

Sub-4 small vessel balloon dilatation catheter

subacute
>s. bacterial endocarditis (SBE)
>s. bronchopneumonia
>s. care
>s. coronary disease (SCD)
>s. infective endocarditis
>s. myocardial infarction
>s. pericarditis
>s. tamponade
>s. thrombosis (SAT)

>s. unit
>s. ventricular free wall

subannular mattress suture

subantihypertensive dose

subaortic
>s. lymph node
>s. obstruction
>s. stenosis (SAS, SS)

subapicale
>segmentum s.

subapical segment

subarachnoid
>s. hemorrhage (SAH)
>s. space (SAS)

subcarinal node

subclavian
>s. approach for cardiac catheterization
>s. arteriovenous fistula
>s. artery
>s. artery bypass graft
>s. flap
>s. flap aortoplasty (SFA)
>s. lymphatic
>s. murmur
>s. peel-away sheath
>s. steal
>s. steal syndrome
>s. triangle
>s. vein
>s. vein catheterization (SVC)
>s. vein thrombosis (SVT)
>s. vessel

subclavian-carotid bypass

subclavian-subclavian bypass

subclavicular murmur

subclinical
>s. asthma
>s. hypothyroidism

subcortical
>s. junctional infarct
>s. stroke
>s. vascular encephalopathy (SVE)

subcostal
>s. outflow (SCOT)
>s. right ventricle view
>s. zone

subcrepitant rale

subcutanea
>bursa s.

subcutaneous
>s. bursa of the laryngeal prominence
>s. emphysema
>s. nodule
>s. patch
>s. patch electrode
>s. suture
>s. tunneling device

subcuticular suture
subdiaphragmatic
subdiastolic
subdural hematoma (SDH)
subendocardial
> s. to epicardial resting perfusion
> ratio
> s. fibrosis
> s. infarction (SEI)
> s. ischemia
> s. layer
> s. myocardial infarction (SEMI)
> s. sclerosis
> s. zone

subendocardium
subendothelial matrix
subendothelium
subepicardial
> s. fat stripe
> s. fatty infiltration

suberosis
subeustachian isthmus
subfascial endoscopic perforator surgery
(SEPS)
subglottic
> s. laryngitis
> s. secretion

subinfundibular stenosis
subjective fremitus
subject's treatment-emergent symptom
scale (STRESS)
subjunctional heart block
sublethal
Sublimaze Injection
sublingual
> S. artery
> S. bursa
> S. caruncula
> S. crescent
> S. gland
> Nitrostat S.
> S. vein

sublingualis
> bursa s.
> caruncula s.
> glandula s.
> vena s.

submassive pulmonary embolism
submaximal
> s. effort tourniquet test
> s. heart rate (HRSUB)

> s. maneuver
> s. treadmill exercise test (STET)

submaximum heart rate
Sub-Microinfusion catheter
submucosa
> airway s.

submucosal
> s. gland
> s. gland hypertrophy
> s. plaque

submucous
suboptimally visualized
suboptimal visualization
subpectoral
> s. implantation of cardioverter-
> defibrillator
> s. implantation of pulse generator

subpharyngeal
subphrenic
> s. abscess
> s. recess
> s. space

subpleural
> s. edema
> s. honeycombing

subpulmonary
> s. obstruction
> s. stenosis

subpulmonic
> s. effusion
> s. stenosis

Sub-Q-Set subcutaneous continuous
infusion device
Subramanian clamp
subsalicylate
> bismuth s.

subsarcolemmal cisterna
subsartorial tunnel
subscript
subsegmental
> s. atelectasis
> s. bronchus
> s. transcatheter arterial embolization
> (STAE)

subsidiary atrial pacemaker
substance
> digoxin-like immunoreactive s.
> (DLIS)
> myocardial depressant s. (MDS)
> neurotransmitter s.
> s. P
> paramagnetic s.

S

NOTES

substance *(continued)*
    proinflammatory s.
    rabbit aorta-contracting s. (RCS)
    thiobarbituric acid reactive s.
      (TBARS)
    vasoactive s.
    vasoconstrictor s. (VCS)
    vasodepressor s.
    vasodilator s. (VDS)
substernal thyroid
substitute
    Hemolink investigational hemoglobin
      product or blood s.
    Nu-Trim dietary fat s.
substitutional cardiac surgery
substrate
    arrhythmogenic s.
    exogenous s.
    s. gel zymography
    s. metabolism
    tachyarrhythmic s.
subsuperior segment
subsuperius
    segmentum s.
subthreshold
    s. pacing
    s. stimulation
subthyroid tracheostomy
subtilis
    Bacillus s.
subtraction
    s. angiography
    digital s.
    functional s.
    intraoperative digital s. (IDIS)
    mask-mode s.
subtype
    Sudan s.
    Zaire s.
subvalvar stenosis
subvalvular
    s. aortic obstruction (SAO)
    s. aortic stenosis
    s. apparatus
    s. mitral stenosis
    s. obstruction
    s. thickening (SVTh)
subventricular (SV)
subxiphoid
    s. area
    s. limited pericardiotomy
    s. window
succinate
    cifenline s.
    hydrocortisone hydrogen s.
    hydrocortisone sodium s.
    methylprednisolone s.
    metoprolol s.
succinylcholine chloride

succussion
    hippocratic s.
    s. sounds
    s. splash
sucker
    intracardiac s.
sucking chest wound
suck reflex
Sucquet anastomosis
Sucquet-Hoyer anastomosis
Sucrets Cough Calmers
suction
    diastolic s.
    hydrostatic s.
    nasotracheal s.
    pleural s.
    Pleur-evac s.
suctioning
    cuff s.
Sudafed
    S. Cold & Cough Liquid Caps
    S. Severe Cold
Sudan subtype
sudden
    s. arrhythmic death syndrome
      (SADS)
    s. cardiac arrest (SCA)
    s. cardiac death (SCD)
    s. coronary death (SCD)
    s. death heart disease (SDHD)
    s. death ischemic heart disease
      (SDIHD)
    s. heart death (SHD)
    s. infant death syndrome (SIDS)
    s. rate onset
    s. unexplained death
    s. unexplained death syndrome
      (SUDS)
    s. unexplained nocturnal death
      (SUND)
    s. unexplained nocturnal death
      syndrome
SUDS
    sudden unexplained death syndrome
sufentanil citrate
suffocate
suffocating gas
suffocation
suffocative
    s. bronchitis
    s. catarrh
    s. goiter
sugar
    capillary blood s. (CBS)
    S. clip
    fasting blood s.
    postprandial blood s.
    s. tumor
Sugarbaker staging system

Sugita clip
Sugiura procedure
suicide ventricle
suis
    Actinobacillus s.
    bronchus s.
suit
    antigravity s., anti-G s.
    Life S.
    MAST s.
Sular
sulbactam
    ampicillin and s.
sulcus, pl. **sulci**
    atrioventricular s.
    bulboventricular s.
    coronary s.
    costophrenic s.
    interventricular s.
    intraparietal s. (IPS)
    s. pulmonalis
    pulmonary s.
    s. terminalis
sulfadiazine
    silver s.
sulfadiazine, sulfamethazine, and
  sulfamerazine
sulfadoxine and pyrimethamine
sulfamerazine
    sulfadiazine, sulfamethazine, and s.
sulfamethoxazole/trimethoprim
  (SMX/TMP)
sulfasalazine
sulfate
    amikacin s.
    amphetamine s.
    atropine s.
    bleomycin s.
    Capastat S.
    capreomycin s.
    cholesterol s. (CS)
    chondroitin s.
    debrisoquine s.
    dermatan s.
    dextran s.
    dextroamphetamine s.
    dimethyl s.
    ephedrine s.
    ferrous s.
    gentamicin s.
    guanadrel s.

    guanethidine s.
    hydroxychloroquine s.
    isoprenaline s.
    isoproterenol s.
    lobeline s.
    magnesium s.
    metaproterenol s.
    neomycin s.
    netilmicin s.
    orciprenaline s.
    paromomycin s.
    penbutolol s.
    protamine s.
    quinidine s.
    quinine s.
    sodium tetradecyl s.
    streptomycin s.
    terbutaline s.
    trimethoprim s.
    trospectomycin s.
    vinblastine s.
    vincristine s.
    Wyamine S.
Sulfatrim DS
sulfhydryl depletion hypothesis
sulfide
    hydrogen s.
    selenium s.
sulfinpyrazone
sulfisoxazole
    erythromycin and s.
    s. and phenazopyridine
sulfonamide sensitivity
sulfonate
    sodium polystyrene s.
sulfonylurea
sulfosalicylic acid
sulfoxide
    albendazole s.
    dimethyl s.
sulfur
    s. dioxide (SO_2)
    s. hexafluoride (SF_6)
sulindac
Sullivan
    S. bubble cushion
    S. HumidAire heated humidifier
    S. III CPAP
    S. Mirage nasal mask
    S. nasal variable positive airway
    pressure unit

S

NOTES

Sullivan (*continued*)
    S. V Elite Real Time Clock
      CPAP machine
    S. VPAP II
sulmazole
Sulphan Blue
sum
    ray s.
sumatriptan
SUMIT
    streptokinase-urokinase myocardial
      infarct test
summation
    s. beat
    s. gallop (S_7)
    impulse s.
    s. shadow
sump pump
Sumycin Oral
SunBox light box
SUND
    sudden unexplained nocturnal death
      SUND syndrome
sundowning
Sundt carotid endarterectomy shunt
sunflower asthma
super
    S. ArrowFlex catheterization sheath
    s. stress test
    S. Torque Plus catheter
Super-4 catheter ablation system
superdicrotic
superdominant artery
superficial
    s. circumflex iliac vein
    s. external pudendal artery
    s. femoral artery (SFA)
    s. medial artery of foot
    s. phlebitis
    s. pneumonia
superficialis
    esophagitis dissecans s.
    vena circumflexa iliaca s.
superimposed
    s. echodensity
    s. pregnancy-induced hypertension
    (SPIH)
    s. thrombosis
superimposition
superinfection
    bacterial s.
superior
    arteria glutealis s.
    arteria laryngea s.
    s. articular facet of atlas
    s. carotid artery
    s. cerebellar artery (SCA)
    s. costal facet
    s. femoral artery (SFA)

    fovea costalis s.
    s. laryngeal artery
    s. laryngeal cavity
    s. laryngeal vein
    s. lobe of right/left lung
    s. mesenteric artery (SMA)
    s. mesenteric artery bypass
    s. mesenteric artery syndrome
    s. mesenteric vascular occlusion
    s. mesenteric vein
    s. omental recess
    s. parietal lobule (SPL)
    s. phrenic lymph node
    posterior branch of right s.
    s. pulmonary sulcus tumor
    s. pulmonary vein
    s. pulmonary vein ablation
    s. QRS axis
    s. sagittal sinus (SSS)
    s. temporal gyrus (STG)
    s. thalamostriate vein
    s. thyroid artery
    s. tracheobronchial lymph node
    s. triangle sign
    s. vascular mediastinum
    s. vascular plexus (SVP)
    s. vena cava (SVC)
    s. vena cava compression syndrome
    (SVCCS)
    s. vena cava obstruction (SVCO)
    s. vena cava syndrome (SVCS)
    vena laryngea s.
superiores
    nodi lymphoidei phrenici s.
    nodi lymphoidei
      tracheobronchiales s.
superioris
    ramus internus nervi laryngei s.
    ramus posterior venae pulmonalis
      dextrae s.
superius
    segmentum bronchopulmonale
      lingulare s.
    tuberculum thyroideum s.
supernatant
supernormal
    s. conduction
    s. recovery phase
supernumerary bronchus
superoinferior heart
superoxide
    s. anion
    s. catalase
    s. dismutase
supersaturation
    tissue s.
supersensitivity
    denervation s.
SuperStitch device

supersystemic pulmonary artery pressure
supertension
supine
    s. bicycle ergometry
    s. bicycle stress echocardiography (SBSE)
    s. diastolic blood pressure (SDBP)
    s. exercise
    s. hypotension syndrome
    s. rest gated equilibrium image
supplement
    high cholesterol and tocopherol s. (HCTS)
    Vivonex Plus nutritional s.
supplemental
    s. air
    s. motor area (SMA)
    s. oxygen
supplementary respiration
supplementation
    magnesium s.
supply
    adequate blood s.
    energy s.
    myocardial oxygen s.
support
    Abee s.
    advanced cardiac life s. (ACLS)
    advanced life s. (ALS)
    advanced trauma life s. (ATLS)
    basic cardiac life s. (BCLS)
    basic life s. (BLS)
    biventricular s. (BVS)
    bradycardia pacing s.
    cardiopulmonary s. (CPS)
    esophageal-directed pressure s. (EDPS)
    extracorporeal life s. (ECLS)
    inotropic s.
    life s.
    mechanical ventilatory s.
    noninvasive positive pressure ventilatory s.
    noninvasive ventilatory s. (NIVS)
    pediatric life s. (PALS)
    percutaneous cardiopulmonary s. (PCPS)
    percutaneous cardiopulmonary bypass s. (PCBS)
    respiratory s.
    vasopressor s.

    ventilatory s.
    volume-assured pressure s. (VAPS)
support-defibrillation
    basic life s.-d. (BLS-D)
supported angioplasty
suppressant
    cough s.
    St. Joseph Cough S.
suppressed respiration
suppressible ventricular tachycardia
suppression
    s. of arrhythmia
    overdrive s.
suppuration
suppurative
    s. bronchiectasis
    s. necrotizing aspergillosis
    s. pericarditis
    s. pleurisy
    s. pneumonia
Supra
    S. G coronary stent
    Lipidil S.
supraannular
    s. constriction
    s. mitral valve replacement (SMVR)
    s. prosthesis
    s. suture ring
suprabulbar palsy
suprachiasmatic nucleus
supraclavicular
    s. examination
    s. fossa
    s. lymph node
    s. lymph node biopsy
supracoronary
supracristal ventricular septal defect
supradiaphragmatic
supraglottoplasty
suprahepatic caval clamp
suprahisian block
supramarginal gyrus (SMG)
supramaximal tetanic stimulation
Suprane
supranormal
    s. conduction
    s. excitability
    s. excitation
supraortic
    s. ridge (SAR)
    s. ring (SAR)

S

NOTES

suprapleural membrane
suprasellar aneurysm
suprasternal
    s. examination
    s. notch (SN)
    s. pulsation
    s. view
suprasternale
    spatium s.
suprasystolic
supratentorial
    s. ICH
    s. intracerebral hemorrhage
suprathreshold pacing
supratonsillar recess
supratrochleares
    venae s.
supravalvar, supravalvular
    s. aortic stenosis (SVAS)
    s.'s aortic stenosis (SAS)
    s. aortic stenosis-infantile
      hypercalcemia syndrome
    s. aortic stenosis syndrome
    s. aortography
supraventricular
    s. aortic stenosis (SVAS)
    s. arrhythmia
    s. crest
    s. ectopy
    s. extrasystole (SVC)
    s. premature beat (SVPB)
    s. premature complex (SVPC)
    s. premature contraction
    s. tachyarrhythmia (SVT)
    s. tachycardia (SVT)
supraventricularis
    crista s.
Suprax
Supreme electrophysiology catheter
surcingle
surdocardiac syndrome
SureGrip breathing bag
SureStepPro professional blood glucose
  management system
SureTemp electronic thermometer
surface
    s. adherent monocyte (SAM)
    Carmeda BioActive S.
    diaphragmatic s.
    high-density lipoprotein-cell s.
    (HDL-c)
    pleural s.
surfactant
    aerosolized s.
    bovine lavage extract s. (BLES)
    s. deficiency
    heterologous s.
    hydrolysis of s.
    s. phospholipid

    s. protein (SP)
    pulmonary s.
    s. replacement therapy
Surfaxin
surf test
surgeon
    Society of Thoracic s.'s (STS)
    thoracic s.
surgery
    ablative cardiac s.
    antiarrhythmic s.
    bypass s.
    cardiac s. (CAS)
    cardiothoracic s. (CTS)
    cardiovascular s. (CVS)
    cervical plexus block for carotid
      endarterectomy s.
    computer-assisted pericardial s.
      (CASPER)
    conservative s. (CS)
    coronary artery bypass s. (CABS)
    coronary artery bypass graft s.
      (CABGS)
    coronary artery bypass grafting s.
    endoscopic vascular s. (ESVS)
    excisional cardiac s.
    extracranial/intracranial bypass s.
    keyhole s.
    lung volume reduction s. (LVRS)
    maze III s.
    MICAB s.
    MIDCAB s.
    noncardiac s.
    off-pump vascular s.
    open s. (OS)
    open heart s. (OHS)
    palatal s.
    palliative s.
    Port-Access minimally invasive
      cardiac s.
    postoperative atrial fibrillation in
      cardiac s. (PACS)
    reparative cardiac s.
    site-specific s.
    Society for Cardiovascular S.
      (SVS)
    stent or s.
    subfascial endoscopic perforator s.
      (SEPS)
    substitutional cardiac s.
    valve-preserving s.
    ventricular reduction s.
    video-assisted thoracic s. (VATS)
    video-assisted thoracoscopic s.
      (VATS)
surgical
    s. ablation
    s. ablation of pathway
    s. embolectomy

s. emphysema
s. intensive care unit (SICU)
s. lung biopsy (SLB)
s. osteosynthesis
s. reexploration
s. revascularization
s. risk
s. site infection (SSI)
s. tuberculosis
s. ventricular restoration (SVR)

Surgicel gauze
Surgiclip
Auto Suture S.
Surgilase 150 laser
Surgilon suture
Surg-I-Loop
Surgitool prosthetic valve
Surgitron unit
Surmontil
Surpasse balloon
Surpass PTCA perfusion catheter
Survanta
surveillance
S. angiography
S. bronchoscopy
National Nosocomial Infection S.
survey
environmental s.
Jenkins Activity S.
National Health and Nutrition
Examination S. I
SF-36 Health S.
Short-Form 36 Health Survey
Short-Form 36 Health S. (SF-36
Health Survey)
Surveyor recording device
survival
s. time
survivor
susceptibility
s. artifact
R-on-T arrhythmia s.
susceptible
high-altitude pulmonary edema s.
(HAPE-s)
suspended
s. heart
s. heart syndrome
suspension
Aristocort Intralesional S.
budesonide inhalation s.
calfactant intratracheal s.

CellCept oral s.
Children's Motrin S.
Curosurf intratracheal s.
hyoid s.
s. laryngoscopy
mycophenolate mofetil oral s.
Optison injectable s.
Rynatuss Pediatric S.

suspensory ligament of esophagus
suspicion
index of s.
sustained
s. maximal inspiration (SMI)
s. monomorphic ventricular
tachycardia (SMVT)
s. outward movement (SOM)
s. physical exercise (SPE)
s. pulse
s. rate duration
s. reentrant ventricular
tachyarrhythmia (SRVT)
s. release (SR)
s. tachycardia
s. ventricular tachycardia (SVT)

Sustiva
susurrus
Sutterella wadsworthensis
Sutton law
suture
absorbable s.
Cardioflon s.
chromic catgut s.
Cooley U s.'s
Deklene II cardiovascular s.
Dermalon s.
Dexon Plus s.
Endoknot s.
end-to-side s.
ePTFE vascular s.'s
Ethibond s.
everting mattress s.
figure-of-eight s.
Gabbay-Frater valve s.
interrupted pledgeted s.
mattress s.
Mersilene braided nonabsorbable s.
Micrins microsurgical s.
monofilament absorbable s.
monofilament polypropylene s.
Nurolon s.
pledgeted mattress s.
Pronova s.

S

NOTES

suture *(continued)*
    pursestring s.
    reabsorbable s.
    subannular mattress s.
    subcutaneous s.
    subcuticular s.
    Surgilon s.
    Techstar percutaneous s.
    through-and-through continuous s.
    through-the-wall mattress s.
    Ti-Cron s.
    traction s.
    transfixion s.
    U s.'s

sutured plaque electrode
suturing
    coupled s.
suxamethonium
SV
    saphenous vein
    stroke volume
    subventricular
SV40
    simian virus 40
SVA
    sequential ventriculoatrial
        SVA pacing
SVAS
    supravalvar aortic stenosis
    supraventricular aortic stenosis
SVB
    saphenous vein bypass
SVBG
    saphenous vein bypass grafting
SVC
    saphenous vein cutdown
    segmental venous capacitance
    selective venous catheterization
    slow vital capacity
    subclavian vein catheterization
    superior vena cava
    supraventricular extrasystole
        SVC lead
        SVC syndrome
SVCCS
    superior vena cava compression
        syndrome
SVCG
    spatial vectorcardiogram
SVCO
    superior vena cava obstruction
SVCR
    segmental venous capacitance ratio
SVCS
    superior vena cava syndrome
SVD
    single-vessel disease
    structural valve deterioration

SVE
    subcortical vascular encephalopathy
Svedberg flotation rate
SVG
    saphenous vein graft
SVH
    saphenous vein harvesting
SVI
    small-vessel infarction
    stroke volume index
    systolic velocity integral
SVM
    syncytiovascular membrane
SVN
    small-volume nebulizer
SvO$_2$
    mixed venous oxygen saturation
        continuous cardiac output with
          SvO$_2$
SVP
    standing venous pressure
    superior vascular plexus
SVPB
    supraventricular premature beat
SVPC
    supraventricular premature complex
SVR
    sequential vascular response
    surgical ventricular restoration
    systemic vascular resistance
SVRI
    systemic vascular resistance index
SVS
    slit ventricle syndrome
    Society for Cardiovascular Surgery
SVT
    sinoventricular tachycardia
    subclavian vein thrombosis
    supraventricular tachyarrhythmia
    supraventricular tachycardia
    sustained ventricular tachycardia
SVTh
    subvalvular thickening
SW
    spike wave
    stroke work
S/W
    spike wave
swallow
    barium s.
    s. syncope
    wet s.
swallowing
    fiberoptic endoscopic evaluation
        of s. (FEES)
Swan-Ganz
    S.-G. balloon flotation catheter
    S.-G. bipolar pacing catheter
    S.-G. flow-directed catheter

S.-G. Pacing TD catheter
S.-G. syndrome
S-warfarin
sweat chloride test
sweating
sweep
Sweet Tip bipolar lead
swelling
    ventricular mural s.
SWI
    stroke work index
swimmer's view
swimming
    hypoxic lap s.
swing
    respiratory s.
    s. test
swinging heart
Swiss
    S. cheese defect
    S. cheese interventricular septum
switch
    DNA s.
    internal reed s.
    isoactin s.
    isomyosin s.
    late arterial s.
    mode s.
    s. operation
    s. procedure
switching
    automatic mode s. (AMS)
    mode s.
SWM
    segmental wall motion
SWMA
    segmental wall motion analysis
SWS
    slow-wave sleep
    spike-wave stupor
Swyer-James syndrome
SX/DX computerized spirometry
Sydenham
    S. chorea
    S. cough
sydowi
    Aspergillus s.
Sylvest disease
Sylvian fissure
Sylvius
    valve of S.

Symbicort
    S. 100/6 Turbuhaler
    S. 200/6 Turbuhaler
Symbion
    S. cardiac device
    S. Jarvik-7 artificial heart
    S. J-7 70-mL ventricle total
        artificial heart
Symbios 7006 pacemaker
Symmetrel
symmetric
    s. asphyxia
    s. dimethylarginine
symmetrical
    bilateral s. (BS)
    s. phased array
sympathectomy, sympathetectomy
    cervicothoracic s.
    lumbar s.
sympathetic
    s. nerve
    s. nerve activity (SNA)
    s. nervous system (SNS)
    s. nervous system activity
    s. neurotransmission
    s. orthostatic hypotension (SOH)
sympathoadrenal system
sympathoexcitation
    reflex s.
sympathoexcitatory response
sympathoinhibition
sympathoinhibitory response
sympatholytic
sympathomimetic
    s. amine
    s. drug
sympathovagal
    s. balance
    s. imbalance
    s. transition
Symphony
    S. nitinol stent
    S. patient monitoring system
symphysis, pl. **symphyses**
    cardiac s.
    pericardial s.
symptom
    Baumes s.
    Burghart s.
    cardinal s.
    Duroziez s.
    Fischer s.

S

NOTES

symptom *(continued)*
    Kussmaul s.
    Oehler s.'s
    prodromal s.
    Trunecek s.
symptomatic
    s. asthma
    s. hemorrhage (SHT)
    s. therapy
symptomaticity
symptom-free interval
symptom-limited
    s.-l. graded exercise test (SL-GXT)
    s.-l. maximal treadmill test
    s.-l. treadmill exercise test
Synacol CF
Synagis
synaptene
synaptic
SYNBIAPACE
    synchronous biatrial pacing therapy
Syn-Captopril
synchondrosis
    sternal s.
Synchrocor pacemaker
SynchroMed programmable pump
synchronization
synchronized
    s. DC cardioversion
    s. direct current cardioversion
    s. intermittent mandatory
    s. intermittent mandatory ventilation
      (SIMV)
    s. retroperfusion (SRP)
    s. shock
    s. sleep (S-sleep)
synchronizer
    CardioSync cardiac s.
synchronous
    s. airway lesions
    s. atrial contraction
    s. atrial stimulation (SAS)
    s. biatrial pacing therapy
      (SYNBIAPACE)
    s. endobronchial disease
synchrony
    atrial s.
    atrioventricular s.
    A-V s.
    S. II, III DDDR pulse generator
    ventricular contractile s.
synchrotron-based transvenous
  angiography
syncopal
    s. migraine
    s. migraine headache
    s. spell
syncope
    Adams-Stokes s.

    s. anginosa
    cardiac s.
    cardiogenic s.
    cardioinhibitory vasovagal s.
    cardioneurogenic s.
    carotid sinus s.
    cerebrovascular s.
    cough s.
    defecation s.
    deglutition s.
    diver's s.
    exertional s.
    factitious s.
    head-up tilt-induced s.
    hypoglycemic s.
    hypoxic s.
    hysterical s.
    isoproterenol-induced vasovagal s.
    laryngeal s.
    local s.
    metabolic s.
    micturition s.
    migraine s.
    mixed neurally mediated s.
    Morgagni-Adams-Stokes s.
    near s.
    neurally mediated s. (NMS)
    neurally mediated vasovagal s.
      (NMVS)
    neurocardiac s.
    neurocardial s.
    neurocardiogenic s.
    neurologic s.
    neuromediated s.
    noncardiac s.
    orthostatic s.
    postmicturition s.
    posttussive s.
    postural s.
    psychogenic s.
    severe refractory
      neurocardiogenic s.
    sexual s.
    situational s.
    sneeze s.
    stretching s.
    swallow s.
    toilet-seat s.
    transient s.
    tussive s.
    vasodepressor s.
    vasodepressor-cardioinhibitory s.
    vasomotor s.
    vasovagal s. (VVS)
    visceral s.
syncytial virus
syncytiovascular membrane (SVM)
syndactyly
Syn-Diltiazem

syndrome

abdominal compartment s. (ACS)
acquired immunodeficiency s.
  (AIDS)
acquired valvular heart s. (AVHS)
acute brain s.
acute chest s. (ACS)
acute coronary s. (ACS)
acute ischemic coronary s. (AICS)
acute respiratory distress s.
  (ARDS)
acute retroviral s.
acute right heart s. (ARHS)
acute sickle cell chest s.
acute sickle chest s. (ASCS)
Adams-Stokes s.
adrenogenital s.
adult respiratory distress s. (ARDS)
advanced sleep phase s.
AFA s.
agitation s.
Albright s.
ALCAPA s.
Alport s.
ALPS s.
Alstrom s.
amniotic fluid s.
Andersen s.
anomalous first rib thoracic s.
anomalous origin of left coronary
  artery from pulmonary artery s.
antiphospholipid s.
aortic arch s. (AAS)
aortic arteritis s.
aortocaval compression s.
apallic s.
Apert s.
Ardystil s.
arteriohepatic dysplasia s.
Asherson s.
Ask-Upmark s.
Austrian s.
Ayerza s.
Babinski s.
Babinski-Vasquez s.
ballooning mitral cusp s.
ballooning mitral valve s.
ballooning posterior leaflet s.
Bamberger-Marie s.
bangungot s.
Bannwarth s.
Barlow s.

Barsony-Polgar s.
Barth s.
Bartter s.
Bauer s.
Beau s.
beer and cobalt s.
Behçet s.
Bernheim s.
Besnier-Boeck-Schaumann s.
Beuren s.
billowing mitral leaflet s. (BMLS)
billowing mitral valve s.
Blackfan-Diamond s.
Bland-Garland-White s.
Bloom s.
blue finger s.
blue toe s.
blue velvet s.
Boerhaave s.
brachial s.
Bradbury-Eggleston s.
bradycardia-tachycardia s.
brady-tachy s. (BTS)
Brett s.
Brock s.
bronchiolitis obliterans s. (BOS)
Brugada s.
bubbly lung s.
Budd-Chiari s.
Bürger-Grütz s.
busulfan lung s.
capillary leak s. (CLS)
Caplan s.
carcinoid s.
cardiac disturbance s.
cardioauditory s.
cardiofacial s.
cardiofaciocutaneous s. (CFC)
carotid sinus hypersensitivity s.
carotid steal s.
Carpenter s.
CATCH-22 s.
cat cry s.
cauda equina s.
Ceelen-Gellerstedt s.
central sleep apnea s. (CSAS)
Cepacia s.
cervical rib s.
Char s.
Charcot s.
Charcot-Weiss-Baker s.
CHARGE s.

S

NOTES

syndrome *(continued)*

Chédiak-Higashi s.
chemoreceptor s.
chest pain s. (CPS)
Chiari s.
Chiari-Budd s.
Chinese restaurant asthma s.
cholesterol emboli s.
chronic fatigue s. (CFS)
chronic hyperventilation s.
Churg-Strauss s. (CSS)
chylomicronemia s.
Clarke-Hadfield s.
CLH s.
click s.
click-murmur s.
Cockayne s.
Cogan s.
compartment s.
compensatory antiinflammatory
  response s. (CARS)
complete form of DiGeorge s.
  (cDGS)
congenital central hypoventilation s.
congenital long QT interval s.
Conn s.
Conradi-Hünermann s.
Cornelia de Lange s.
coronary slow flow s. (CSFS)
coronary-subclavian steal s.
costochondral s.
costoclavicular rib s.
costosternal s.
cranio-cerebello-cardiac s. (3C,
  CCC)
CREST s.
cricopharyngeal achalasia s.
cri du chat s.
Crow-Fukase s.
cryptophthalmos s.
Cushing s.
cutis laxa s.
Cyriax s.
DaCosta s.
deadly quartet s.
declamping shock s.
defects s.
de Lange s.
delayed pulmonary toxicity s.
  (DPTS)
Determann s.
DG/VCF s.
diffuse obstructive pulmonary s.
  (DOPS)
DiGeorge s. (DG, DGS)
disturbance of function occlusion s.
  (DOFOS)
Down s. (DS)
Dressler s.

drowned newborn s.
drug-induced lupus s.
Duncan s.
dysarthria-clumsy hand s. (DCHS)
dyskinesia s.
dyslipidemic hypertension s.
early repolarization s.
early ventricular repolarization s.
  (EVRS)
Eaton-Lambert s.
economy class s.
effort s.
Ehlers-Danlos s.
Eisenmenger s.
elfin facies s.
Ellis-van Creveld s.
eosinophilia-myalgia s. (EMS)
eosinophilic lung s.
eosinophilic pulmonary s.
epibronchial right pulmonary
  artery s.
euthyroid sick s.
familial atrial myxoma s.
familial cholestasis s.
familial chylomicronemia s.
fat embolism s. (FES)
fear of food s.
Fechtner s.
fetal alcohol s. (FAS)
fetal aspiration s.
fibrinogen-fibrin conversion s.
flapping valve s.
Fleischner s.
floppy valve s.
Foix-Cavany-Marie s.
folded-lung s.
Forney s.
Forrester s.
four-day s.
FRAX-MR s.
Gaisböck s.
gastrocardiac s.
Gerhardt s.
Goldenhar s.
Goodpasture s.
Gorlin s.
Gowers s.
Grönblad-Strandberg s.
Guillain-Barré s.
Gulf War s.
Halbrecht s.
Hamman s.
Hamman-Rich s. (HRS)
hantavirus pulmonary s.
Hare s.
heart-hand s.
heart and hand s.
Hegglin s.
Heiner s.

HELLP s.
hemangioma-thrombocytopenia s.
hemolysis, elevated liver function
  tests and low platelets s.
Henoch-Schönlein s.
heparin-induced thrombosis-
  thrombocytopenia s. (HITTS)
hepatopulmonary s. (HPS)
Hermansky-Pudlak s.
Herner s.
heterotaxy s.
high-altitude hypertrophic
  cardiomyopathy s. (HHCS)
high-pressure neurologic s. (HPNS)
HO s.
holiday heart s.
Holt-Oram s. (HOS)
homocystinuria s.
Horner s.
Howel-Evans s.
Hughes-Stovin s.
Hunter s.
Hunter-Hurler s.
Hurler s.
hyperabduction s.
hyperapolipoprotein B s.
hypercalcemia s.
hypereosinophilia s.
hypereosinophilic s.
hyperkinetic heart s. (HHS)
hyperlucent lung s.
hyperperfusion s.
hypersensitive carotid sinus s.
hyperventilation s. (HVS)
hyperviscosity s.
hyponatremic-hypertensive s.
hypoplastic left heart s. (HLHS)
hypoplastic left ventricle s. (HLVS)
idiopathic hypereosinophilic s.
  (IHES)
idiopathic hyperkinetic heart s.
  (IHHS)
idiopathic long Q-T interval s.
immotile cilia s.
s. of inappropriate antidiuresis
  (SIAD)
s. of inappropriate antidiuretic
  hormone (SIADH)
incontinentia pigmenti s.
infant respiratory distress s. (IRDS)
insulin resistance s.
intermediate coronary s.

Ivemark s.
Jackson s.
Janus s.
Jervell and Lange-Nielsen s.
Jeune s.
Job s.
Kallmann s.
Kartagener s.
Kasabach-Merritt s.
Kawasaki s.
Kearns-Sayre s.
Kimmelstiel-Wilson s.
Klein-Waardenburg s.
Klinefelter s.
Klippel-Feil s.
Klippel-Trenaunay-Weber s.
Kostmann s.
Kugelberg-Welander s.
Kussmaul s.
Labbe neurocirculatory s.
lacunar s. (LACS)
LAMB s.
Lambert-Eaton myasthenic s.
Landouzy-Dejerine s.
Landry-Guillain-Barré s.
Laron s. (LS)
Laubry-Soulle s.
Laurence-Moon-Bardet-Biedl s.
Laurence-Moon-Biedl s.
Leitner s.
Lemierre s.
Lenègre s.
Lenz s.
LEOPARD s.
Leredde s.
Leriche s.
Lev s.
Libman-Sacks s.
Liddle s.
Löffler s.
Löfgren s.
long QT s. (LQTS)
long QTU s.
low cardiac output s. (LCOS,
  LOS)
Lown-Ganong-Levine s.
low-salt s.
low-sodium s.
LQT s.
Lutembacher s.
Macleod s.
malignant carcinoid s.

NOTES

syndrome (*continued*)

malignant superior vena caval s.
malignant SVC s.
malignant vasovagal s.
Mallory-Weiss s.
Marfan s.
Marie s.
Marie-Bamberger s.
Maroteaux-Lamy s.
Martorell s.
mastocytosis s.
Maugeri s.
McArdle s.
Meadows s.
meconium aspiration s. (MAS)
Meigs s.
Mendelson s.
Ménière s.
metabolic s.
metastatic carcinoid s.
middle lobe s.
midsystolic click s.
milk-alkali s.
Miller Fisher variant of Guillain-Barré s.
mirror-image lung s.
mitral valve prolapse s. (MVPS)
Mönckeberg s.
Mondor s.
Morestin s.
Morgagni-Adams-Stokes s.
Morquio s.
Mounier-Kuhn s.
Moynahan s.
mucocutaneous lymph node s.
multiple cholesterol emboli s. (MCES)
multiple lentigines s.
multiple-organ dysfunction s. (MODS)
myocardial ischemic s.
NAME s.
neonate respiratory distress s. (NRDS)
nephrotic s.
Netherton s.
neurally mediated syncopal s.
nonpyramidal hemimotor s.
Noonan s.
no-reflow s.
obesity hypoventilation s. (OHS)
obstructive sleep apnea s. (OSAS)
oculomucocutaneous s.
Opitz s.
organic dust toxic s. (ODTS)
Osler-Weber-Rendu s.
overlap s.
PAC s.
pacemaker s. (PS)

Paget-von Schrötter s.
PAGOD s.
Pancoast s.
papillary muscle s.
paraneoplastic s.
partial anterior circulation s. (PACS)
pericarditis-myocarditis s.
Perthes s.
pharyngeal pouch s.
PHAVER s.
Pick s.
pickwickian s.
PIE s.
Pierre Robin s.
Pins s.
platypnea-orthodeoxia s.
Plummer-Vinson s.
POEMS s.
pokkuri sudden arrhythmia-death s.
Polhemus-Schafer-Ivemark s.
polyglandular autoimmune s. type II
polymetabolic s.
polymyalgia rheumatica s.
positional obstructive sleep apnea s.
postcardiac injury s. (PCIS)
postcardiotomy s. (PCS)
postcardiotomy psychosis s.
postcommissurotomy s.
posterior circulation s. (POCS)
postinfarction s.
postmyocardial infarction s. (PMIS)
postnasal drainage s. (PNDS)
postnasal drip s. (PNDS)
postperfusion s.
postpericardiotomy s. (PPS)
postphlebitic s.
postpump s.
posttransfusion s.
postural orthostatic tachycardia s. (POTS)
P pulmonale s.
precordial catch s.
preexcitation s. (PES)
preinfarction s. (PIS)
premonitory s.
prolapsed mitral valve s.
prolonged Q-T interval s.
Proteus s.
pseudoxanthoma elasticum s.
pulmonary acid aspiration s.
pulmonary disease anemia s.
pulmonary dysmaturity s.
pulmonary fat embolism s.
pulmonary hyperinfection s.
pulmonary infarction s.

pulmonary infiltrates with
  eosinophilia s.
pulmonary sling s.
pure sensory s. (PSS)
QT s.
quinidine syncope s.
radiologic scimitar s.
Raeder-Harbitz s.
Rasmussen s.
Raynaud s.
reactive airways disease s. (RADS)
reactive airways dysfunction s.
  (RADS)
reactive upper airways
  dysfunction s. (RUDS)
Reaven s.
redundant cusp s.
Reel s.
refeeding s.
Refsum s.
Reiter s.
Rendu-Osler-Weber s.
respiratory distress s. (RDS)
Reye s.
Riley-Day s.
Rosenbach s.
Rosenberg s.
Roussy-Lévy s.
rubella s.
Rubinstein-Taybi s.
salt-depletion s.
Sanchez-Cascos cardioauditory s.
Sandifer s.
Sanfilippo s.
scalenus anterior s.
scalenus anticus s.
Schaumann s.
Scheie s.
Schmidt s.
scimitar s.
Sebastiani s.
severe acute respiratory s. (SARS)
shallow-water blackout s.
shoulder-hand s.
Shwachman s.
Shy-Drager s.
sicca s.
sick building s. (SBS)
sick sinus s. (SSS)
Silver s.
Simpson-Golabi-Behmel s.
single papillary muscle s.

sinoatrial node weakness s.
  (SANWS)
sinobronchial s.
Sjögren s.
sleep apnea/hypopnea s. (SAHS)
slipping rib s.
slit ventricle s. (SVS)
small aorta s. (SAS)
Smith-Lemli-Opitz s.
Sneddon s.
Spens s.
Sphrintzen s.
splenic flexure s.
Stevens-Johnson s.
stiff heart s.
stiff left atrium s.
Stokes-Adams s.
Stokvis-Talma s.
straight back s.
Sturge-Weber s.
subclavian steal s.
sudden arrhythmic death s. (SADS)
sudden infant death s. (SIDS)
sudden unexplained death s.
  (SUDS)
sudden unexplained nocturnal
  death s.
SUND s.
superior mesenteric artery s.
superior vena cava s. (SVCS)
superior vena cava compression s.
  (SVCCS)
supine hypotension s.
supravalvar aortic stenosis s.
supravalvar aortic stenosis-infantile
  hypercalcemia s.
surdocardiac s.
suspended heart s.
SVC s.
Swan-Ganz s.
Swyer-James s.
systemic inflammatory response s.
  (SIRS)
systolic click s. (SCS)
systolic click-late systolic
  murmur s.
systolic click-murmur s.
tachybrady s.
tachycardia-bradycardia s.
tachycardia-polyuria s.
Takayasu s.
TAR s.

S

NOTES

syndrome *(continued)*
    Taussig-Bing s.
    Taybi s.
    telangiectasia s.
    thoracic compressive s.
    thoracic endometriosis s. (TES)
    thoracic outlet s. (TOS)
    thoracic outlet compression s.
    thrombocytopenia-absent radius s.
    thromboembolic s.
    Tietze s.
    total anterior circulation s. (TACS)
    Townes-Brocks s.
    toxic oil s. (TOS)
    Treacher Collins s.
    Trousseau s.
    Turner s.
    twiddler's s.
    TWISTED s.
    Uhl s.
    Ulick s.
    Ullmann s.
    unroofed coronary sinus s.
    upper airways resistance s. (UARS)
    Urbach-Wiethe s.
    V_1-like ambulatory lead s.
    V_5-like ambulatory lead s.
    VACTERL s.
    vascular leak s. (VLS)
    vasovagal s.
    VATER association s.
    VCF s.
    velocardiofacial s. (VCFS)
    vena cava s.
    venolobar s.
    venous insufficiency s. (VIS)
    Vernet s.
    Villaret s.
    Vogt-Koyanagi-Harada s.
    Waardenburg s.
    Wallenberg s.
    Ward-Romano s.
    wasting s.
    Watson s.
    Weber-Osler-Rendu s.
    Werner s.
    West s.
    white clot s.
    Willebrand-Jurgens s.
    Williams s.
    Williams-Campbell s.
    Wilson-Mikity s.
    Wiskott-Aldrich s.
    Wolff-Parkinson-White s.
    WPW s.
    s. X
    XO s.
    XXXX s.
    XXXY s.

    yellow nail s. (YNS)
    Yentl s.
    Young s.
synechia, pl. **synechiae**
    bronchial s.
    pericardial s.
    s. pericardii
Synercid
synergism
synergistic
SynerGraft
    S. implant
    S. pulmonary heart valve
    S. tissue-engineered heart valve
Synergyst
    S. DDD pacemaker
    S. II pacemaker
Syngamus laryngeus
syngenesioplastic transplant
Syn-Nadolol
Synox fractal pacemaker lead
synpneumonic empyema
Syntel
    S. latex-free embolectomy catheter
    S. latis graft cleaning catheter
synthase
    constitutive nitric oxide s. (cNOS)
    endothelial constitutive nitric
      oxide s. (ecNOS, eNOS)
    endothelial nitric oxide s. (eNOS)
    glycogen s.
    inducible nitric oxide s. (iNOS)
    nitric oxide s. I (NOS, NOS1)
synthesis
    cytokine-induced endothelial s.
    leukotriene s.
    matrix s.
    thromboxane s.
synthetase
    inducible nitric oxide s. (iNOS)
    pantothenate s.
Synthroid
synvinolin
syphilis
    cardiovascular s.
    nonvenereal s.
    tertiary s.
syphilitic
    s. aortic aneurysm
    s. aortic valvulitis
    s. aortitis
    s. arteritis
    s. endarteritis
    s. endocarditis
    s. laryngitis
    s. myocarditis
Syracol-CF
syringe
    anaerobic Pulsator s.

Angioject s.
Gas-Lyte ABG s.
GlideCath s.
Lyo-Ject s.
Namic angiographic s.
Osciflator balloon inflation s.
Pulsator s.
Raulerson s.
Ultraject prefilled s.

syrup
albuterol sulfate s.
Allerphed S.
Ambenyl Cough S.
Amgenal Cough S.
Aprodine S.
Benylin Cough S.
Bromanyl Cough S.
Bromotuss w/Codeine Cough S.
Cardec-S S.
Decofed S.
Deconamine S.
Histalet S.
Phanatuss Cough S.
Rondec S.
Silafed S.
Tusstat S.

sys
systolic

SYS-BP
systolic blood pressure

syst
systole
systolic

system
Abiomed biventricular support s.
ABI Vest Airway Clearance s.
ABL 625 s.
ABL 520 blood gas
measurement s.
Access MV s.
AccuNet embolic protection s.
Achieve Off-Pump s.
ACIST injection s.
ACS Concorde over-the-wire
catheter s.
ACS Multi-Link coronary s.
ACS Multi-Link RX Ultra
coronary stent s.
Active Can defibrillator lead s.
ACT MicroCoil delivery s.
Acuson cardiovascular s.

Acuson XP-128
echocardiographic s.
Acuson-XP 128
echocardiographic s.
adrenergic nervous s.
Advanced Cardiovascular S.'s
(ACS)
Advantx LC+ cardiovascular
imaging s.
Aegis ICD s.
AeroNOx nitric oxide delivery and
analysis s.
AeroNOx nitric oxide transport s.
AeroView optical intubation s.
AirSep OxiScan Oximetry
recording, reporting, and
archiving s.
Aladdin Infant Flow s.
Aladdin nasal CPAP s.
Albert Grass Heritage digital
PSG s.
Albert Grass Heritage EEG s.
Albert Grass neurodata s.
Alcon Closure S.
AlereNet s.
Alice4 Sleep Diagnostic s.
Alveolus stent technology s.
Anaconda device and delivery s.
ANCOR imaging s.
Ancure s.
Androderm Transdermal s.
AneuRx fully supported modular s.
AneuRx stent graft s.
AngeCool RF catheter ablation s.
AngioJet and Merk rheolytic
thrombectomy s.
AngioJet rapid thrombectomy s.
Angiomat Illumena contrast
delivery s.
AngioRad Afterloader s.
AngioRad radiation s.
AnnuloFlo annuloplasty ring s.
anular phased array s. (APAS)
Aortic Connector s.
Apollo Light S.'s
Argyle-Turkel safety thoracentesis s.
Aria LX CPAP s.
arrhythmia mapping s.
artificial heart energy s. (AHES)
Artrek cineangiographic analysis s.
Atakr s.
ATL UltraMark 9 ultrasound s.

S

NOTES

system *(continued)*
atrial septal defect occlusion s. (ASDOS)
atrial septum defect occluder s. (ASDOS)
atrioventricular conduction s. (AVCS)
AutoCapture pacing s.
autologous blood management s.
automated cervical cell screening s.
automatic exposure s.
autonomic nervous s. (ANS)
AutoSet Portable II CPAP s.
Autotrans s.
autotransfusion s.
Autovac LF autotransfusion s.
Axcis percutaneous myocardial revascularization s.
Axcis PMR s.
BACTEC s.
Balloon-on-a-Wire dilatation s.
Bard percutaneous cardiopulmonary support s.
Baylor autologous transfusion s.
Beckman ICS Nephelometer s.
BeStent Rival coronary stent s.
BeStent 2 with Discrete Technology coronary stent s.
Beta-Cath s.
BiliBlanket phototherapy s.
Biodex S.
bionic baroreflex s.
Biosense NOGA catheter-based endocardial mapping s.
Biosound Genesis II scanning s.
biotin/streptavidin s.
BioZ hemodynamic monitoring s.
BioZ noninvasive cardiac function monitoring s.
BioZ.pc s.
BiPAP duet s.
BiPAP S/T-D 30 s.
BiPAP S/T-D ventilatory support s.
BiPAP Vision s.
brachiocephalic s.
BRAT s.
Breeze E150 ventilation s.
Bridge X3 renal stent s.
Burette multiple patient delivery s.
BVS-5000 biventricular support s.
Bx Velocity stent with Raptor OTW delivery s.
Bx Velocity with Hepacoat on Raptor stent s.
Cadence tiered therapy defibrillator s.
CAESAR analysis s.
CapnoProbe sublingual CO_2 s.
CARDEA data management s.

cardiac conduction s.
cardiac surgery reporting s. (CSRS)
Cardioblate BP, RF surgical ablation s.
CardioGenesis TMR s.
CardioLab 2000 single monitor EP s.
CardioTek electrophysiologic tracer s.
cardiovascular s. (CVS)
Cardiovascular Angiography Analysis S. (CAAS)
cardiovascular imaging s. (CVIS)
cardiovascular measurement s. (CMS)
cardiovascular reflex conditioning s. (CRCS)
CardoSEAL septal occlusion s.
CARTO EP navigation s.
CARTO magnetic mapping s.
CARTO XP s.
CASE computerized exercise ECG s.
CATHCOR LX hemodynamic recording s.
catheter-snare s.
catheter-tip micromanometer s.
Cath-Finder catheter tracking s.
CDI 2000 blood gas monitoring s.
Cell Saver autologous blood recovery s.
Cell Saver Haemonetics Autotransfusion s.
Cenflex central monitoring s.
CFC-free delivery s.
CGR biplane angiographic s.
CH 2000 cardiac diagnostic s.
Checkmate gamma brachytherapy s.
Chilli cooled ablation s.
Cholestech LDX s.
cholesterol monitoring s.
cineangiographic s.
cineless recording s.
cine-pulse s.
CineView Plus Freeland s.
Circulaire aerosol drug delivery s.
circulatory support s.
Clarity multiparameter monitoring s.
CLeaRS cardiac lead removal s.
CMS AccuProbe 450 s.
CoaguChek aPTT testing s.
codominant s.
COER-24 delivery s.
ColorZone Management s.
CompAire Elite compressor nebulizer s.
complement s.
complete pacemaker patient testing s. (CPPTS)

computerized sleep analysis s.
conduction s.
conductive s.
Contak CD CRTD Easytrak s.
Contak Renewal 3 CRTD s.
coordinate s.
coordinate reduction time
  encoding s. (CORTES)
Cordis LC Multipurpose stent s.
Cordis Mini stent s.
coronary implant s. (CIS)
CorRestore s.
Cosgrove-Edwards annuloplasty s.
CoumaCare Coumadin
  management s.
CoumaCare patient management s.
CPS s.
Cryocare cardiac surgical s.
CryoCor cryoablation s.
C-Vest radiation detector s.
cytochrome P450 s.
Dallas Classification S.
DAR breathing s.
da Vinci robotic surgical s.
DCI-S automated coronary
  analysis s.
demand oxygen delivery s.
  (DODS)
Desai VectorCath mapping s.
Diameter Index Safety S. (DISS)
Digital Cardiac Imaging s.
digital vascular imaging s. (DVIS)
dilator-sheath s.
Dinamap s.
distal perfusion s. (DPS)
2D TEE s. Ultra-Neb 99
Duct-Occlud s.
Duke University
  quantitative/qualitative evaluation s.
  (DUQUES)
DUPEL drug delivery s.
Dymer excimer delivery s.
Dynalink biliary self-expanding
  stent s.
Dynasty delivery s.
Eagle portable ventilation s.
EasyOne spirometry s.
echocardiographic automated
  boundary detection s.
echocardiographic scoring s.
EchoFlow blood velocity meter s.
Echovar Doppler s.

Eclipse PTMR s.
edge-detection s.
Elecsys troponin T immunoassay s.
electroanatomical mapping s.
electrode s.
Electronic HouseCall s.
Embol-X arterial cannula and
  filter s.
endocrine s.
Endosaph vein harvest s.
Endotak lead s.
Ensite 3000 s.
EnSite NavX intracardiac
  nonfluoroscopic navigation s.
EPT-1000 XP cardiac ablation s.
Equinox digital EEG s.
Equinox occlusion balloon s.
Erie S.
ES 300-Cardiac T ELISA troponin
  T immunoassay s.
Estes point s.
Estes-Romhilt ECG point-score s.
event-link data s.
EVS vascular closure s.
factor XII-kallikrein-kinin s.
FemoStop femoral compression s.
fiberoptic catheter delivery s.
fibrinolytic s.
FilterWire EX embolic
  protection s.
Finger Phantom pulse oximeter
  testing s.
fixed-wire balloon dilatation s.
Flowtron DVT pump s.
Frank ECG lead placement s.
Frank XYZ orthogonal lead s.
Freezor CryoAblation s.
Galaxy IVUS imaging s.
Galileo intravascular radiotherapy s.
gamma radiation therapy s.
gated s.
GE Advantx s.
GE CT Advantage high-speed
  CT s.
Gem SensiCath blood gas
  monitoring s.
GenBank information s.
GenESA closed-loop delivery s.
Genic coronary stent delivery s.
GE Signa 1.5-T MRI s.
GFX 2 coronary stent s.

S

NOTES

697

system *(continued)*

GoodKnight 418A, 418G, 418P CPAP s.

GS Modular pulmonary testing s.

Guardwire angioplasty s.

Guardwire emboli containment s.

GuardWire Plus s.

Guidant Heart Rhythm Technologies Linear Ablation s.

Guidant Multi-Link Tetra coronary stent s.

Guidant TRIAD three-electrode energy defibrillation s.

Gyroscan HP Philips 15S whole-body s.

Haemolite autologous blood recovery s.

Haemonetics Cell Saver s.

Heart Laser s.

HeartMate implantable pneumatic left ventricular assist s.

HeartMate vented electric left ventricular assist s.

Heartport catheter s.

Heartport Port-Access s.

hematopoietic s.

hemoglobin-based therapeutic s.

Hemopump cardiac assist s.

HEPAtech air purification s.

Hewlett-Packard 5 MHz phased-array TEE s.

Hewlett-Packard SONOS 1000, 1500, 2500 ultrasound s.

hexaxial reference s.

Hi-Care closed suction and pulmonary hygiene s.

HICOR s.

His-Purkinje s.

Hitachi PCT-3600W PET s.

HomMed monitoring s.

Horizon AutoAdjust CPAP s.

Horizon LT CPAP s.

Horizon nasal CPAP s.

Housecall transtelephonic monitoring s.

hub and spoke referral s.

Hunt and Hess grades I through V aneurysm grading s.

HydroDot neuromonitoring s.

hypoxia warning s.

iliofemoral venous s.

ImageView s.

implantable left ventricular assist s. (IPLVAS)

INCA s.

Incardia valve s.

indirect blood pressure measuring s. (IBPMS)

Infant Flow noninvasive nasal CPAP s.

Infant Resuscitation s.

Infiniti catheter introducer s.

infrahisian conduction s.

Inhale deep lung delivery s.

Innervasc expandable vascular access s.

INOvent delivery s.

integrated lead s.

Integris cardiac imaging s.

Integris H5000 digital x-ray imaging s.

Integrity AFx AutoCapture pacing s.

IntraLuminal Safe-Steer s.

Invacare Venture HomeFill complete home oxygen s.

IRMA blood gas analysis s.

Irri-Cath suction s.

isocenter s.

Jinotti closed suctioning s.

Johnson & Johnson Interventional S.'s

kallikrein-bradykinin s.

Karl Storz D-LIGHT AF autofluorescence s.

King double umbrella closure s.

KK s.

KnightStar 335 respiratory-support s.

lead extraction s.

left ventricular assist s. (LVAS)

Leocor hemoperfusion s.

Leukotrap red cell storage s.

LIFE-Lung S.

Lifepath AAA endovascular graft s.

Liposorber LA-15 s.

Lown grading s.

Luxtec fiberoptic s.

lymphohematogenous drainage s.

Lyra laser s.

Mallinckrodt Hi-Care Pulmonary Hygiene s.

Mark V ProVis injection s.

Marquette Case-12 electrocardiographic s.

Marquette Case-12 exercise s.

Mason-Likar 12-lead ECG s.

M/D 4 defibrillator s.

MDS s.

MedGraphics Cardio O2 s.

medication monitoring event s. (MEMS)

Medi-Facts s.

Medi-Tech catheter s.

MedNova NeuroShield cerebral protection s.

Medos mechanical circulatory
support s.
Medtronic Cardiorhythm Atakr II
RF ablation s.
Medtronic Hemopump s.
Medtronic Interactive Tachycardia
Terminating s.
Medtronic Octopus 2+ tissue
stabilizing s.
Meier-Magnum s.
Metrix atrial defibrillation s.
MicroAir ultrasonic nebulizer s.
Micro Delta/Max Delta s.
MicroGas 7650 transcutaneous
monitoring s.
MicroLysus s.
micromanometer catheter s.
microwave cardiac ablation s.
MIDCAB s.
minimum data set s.
mobile artery and vein imaging s.
(MAVIS)
Mobin-Uddin filter s.
modular electrocardiogram
analysis s. (MEANS)
Monaldi drainage s.
Monovial drug delivery s.
MT-100 ECG Holter s.
mucociliary s.
Mullins sheath s.
MULTIFIT computer-based chronic
illness management s.
Multi-Link coronary stent s.
Multi-Link Frontier coronary
stent s.
Multi-Link Penta coronary stent s.
Multi-Link Pixel stent s.
Multi-Link Tetra coronary stent s.
Multi-Link Tristar stent s.
Multi-Link Zeta coronary stent s.
Multitest cell-mediated immunity s.
Myocardial Infarction Data
Acquisition S.
myocardial protection s. (MPS)
MyoSIGHT dedicated nuclear
cardiology camera s.
MYOtherm XP cardioplegia
delivery s.
nasal CPAP s.
Neotrend s.
nervous s.
Neurostar angiography s.

Neurotrac II neurologic
monitoring s.
Nihon Kohden polygraph s.
NIOX nitric oxide breath test s.
NIR Elite Monorail s.
NIR Elite OTW stent s.
nitric oxide s.
nonthoracotomy defibrillation
lead s.
Novacor left ventricular assist s.
Novacor mechanical circulatory
support s.
Novametrix NICO cardiopulmonary
management s.
Nova Microsonics ImageVue s.
Nu-Trake Weiss emergency
airway s.
Nuvolase 660 laser s.
Oasis thrombectomy s.
Octopus tissue stabilization s.
Octopus 2+, 3 tissue
stabilization s.
OmniCell supply s.
Omni-Tract s.
Optical Sensors stand-alone arterial
blood gas monitoring s.
OptiCor digital cardiac
communication and storage s.
OptiHaler drug delivery s.
oral L-arginine s.
organ transplantation s.
orthogonal lead s.
over-the-wire balloon dilatation s.
Oximetrix 3 S.
OxiScan oximetry recording and
reporting s.
Oxyfill oxygen refilling s.
Oxylator-EM 100 automatic
resuscitation and inhalation s.
Oxylite ambulatory oxygen s.
Oxy-Ultra-Lite ambulatory
oxygen s.
Paceart complete pacemaker patient
testing s.
pacemaker code s.
PARAflow circulatory support s.
parasympathetic nervous s.
Pasys ST cardiac pacing s.
patch-coil s.
Patil stereotactic s.
PCA s.

S

NOTES

system *(continued)*

PCD Transvene implantable cardioverter-defibrillator s.

PDB preperitoneal distention balloon s.

Pediatric LifeShirt s.

Pelorus stereotactic s.

PenChant coronary stent delivery s.

Perclose vascular surgical closure s.

PercuGuide lesion marking s.

percutaneous mechanical thrombectomy s.

peripheral access s. (PAS)

Peripheral AngioJet s.

peripheral atherectomy s.

phased array s.

Physios CTM 01 noninvasive cardiac transplant monitoring s.

Picker Vistar image analysis s.

Picker Voxel image analysis s.

Pie Medical CAAS II analysis s.

Pittman IMA retractor s.

plasma coagulation s.

Pleur-evac autotransfusion s.

2010 Plus Holter s.

PneuView ventilator testing and training s.

polarcardiography computing s.

Polaris CPAP s.

Port-A-Cath implantable catheter s.

Portex Soft-Seal cuff s.

Power Grip Over the Wire Stent Delivery s.

Powerlink endoluminal graft s.

Presto-Flash spirometry s.

Presto spirometry s.

PreVue III digitizing s.

Prima total occlusion s.

Prime ECG mapping s.

programmable implantable medication s. (PIMS)

Prostar 9F, 11F percutaneous vascular surgery s.

Prostar XL 8, 10 suture mediated closure s.

PSA stationary oxygen s.

P-Series sleep monitoring s.

pulmonary arterial s.

PulseDose portable compressed oxygen s.

PulseSpray infusion s.

PulStar pneumatic wrap s.

Purkinje s.

Q-cath catheterization recording s.

Quartet s.

Quest Medical microplegia s.

Quest MPS myocardial protection s.

QuickFlow DPS distal perfusion s.

QuickSeal femoral arterial closure s.

Quinton Synergy cardiac information management s.

RadiStop radial compression s.

Rapidlab 800 Critical Care s.

Rasor blood pumping s. (RBPS)

RDX coronary radiation catheter delivery s.

real-time position management tracking s.

Red s.

Remac s.

Remedy sleep therapy s.

REMstar CPAP s.

Renaissance spirometry s.

renal kallikrein-kinin s.

renin-angiotensin s.

renin-angiotensin-aldosterone s. (RAAS)

respiratory s.

reticuloendothelial s.

revascularization s.

Romhilt-Estes point scoring s.

rotational angioplasty catheter s. (ROTACS)

rotational atherectomy s. (RAS)

RPM tracking s.

Safe-Steer s.

SAM s.

Sandman s.

saphenofemoral s.

sarcotubular s.

Schneider-Meier-Magnum s.

secondary anticoagulation s. (SACS)

SenDx 100 blood gas and electrolyte analysis s.

Sequel compression s.

Sequestra 1000 s.

800 series blood gas and critical analyte s.

sheath and dilator s.

SICOR recording s.

Siemens biplane Neurostar digital subtraction angiography s.

Sigma II Dualplace hyperbaric oxygen therapy s.

Sigma I monoplace hyperbaric therapy s.

Sigma Plus monoplace hyperbaric oxygen therapy s.

Signa EXCITE 3.0T MRI s.

Simpson AtheroCath s.

Simpson-Robert vascular dilation s.

single chamber cardiac pacing s.

SinuScope s.

SJM Rosenkranz pediatric retractor s.

Sleepscan Traveler ambulatory polysomnography s.
Sleepscan Traveler home monitoring s.
SmartKard digital Holter s.
SmartMist asthma management s.
SmartMist respiratory management s.
Snuggle Warm convective warming s.
Somatom Volume Zoom computed tomography s.
Somnoplasty s.
Somnus Somnoplasty s.
SonoHeart Elite Ultrasound S.
SonoHeart handheld, all digital echocardiography s.
SONOS 500 imaging s.
Spaulding classification s.
SphygmoCor non-invasive aortic blood pressure s.
2170 Spirometry Software s.
SpiroSense s.
Spiros inhalation s.
SpiroVision-3 spirometry s.
S-Series sleep s.
stent delivery s. (SDS)
stroke guidance s. (SGS)
Sugarbaker staging s.
Super-4 catheter ablation s.
SureStepPro professional blood glucose management s.
S660 with Discrete Technology coronary stent s.
S670 with Discrete Technology coronary stent s.
sympathetic nervous s. (SNS)
sympathoadrenal s.
Symphony patient monitoring s.
System Five echocardiogram s.
T s.
Talent LPS endoluminal stent-graft s.
Talos stent delivery s.
TAM s.
TBird ventilator s.
TCD100M digital transcranial Doppler s.
TCI Heartmate mechanical circulatory support s.
TEC atherectomy s.
Technos ultrasound s.

Techstar XL 6F percutaneous vascular surgical s.
Techstar XL 6F PVS s.
Telectronics Pacing S.'s
Terumo telescoping catheter s.
Testoderm Transdermal s.
ThAIRapy vest airway clearance s.
The Closer suture-mediated closure s.
TheraPEP positive expiratory pressure therapy s.
Therapeutic Intervention Scoring S. (TISS)
ThermoChem-HT s.
ThermoFlo s.
TherOx Aqueous Oxygen s.
Thora-Klex chest drainage s.
Thoraseal chest tube drainage s.
Thoratec VAD s.
Thrombex PMT s.
Thrombolytic Assessment S. (TAS)
Thumper 1007 CPR s.
TMS 1000 tachyarrhythmia monitoring s.
TomTec Imaging S.'s
tonsillar Somnoplasty s.
Total O_2 delivery s.
Total O_2/Oxilite oxygen s.
Total O_2 supplementary oxygen s.
Total Synchrony S.
TRAKE-fit s.
Tranquility Quest CPAP S.
transesophageal pacing s.
transluminal lysing s.
transtelephonic ambulatory monitoring s.
Trap cardiovascular filtration s.
Trap neurovascular filtration s.
Trap vascular filtration s.
Traveler portable oxygen s.
TriActiv balloon-protected flush extraction s.
Triad defibrillator s.
Triage cardiac rapid diagnostic test s.
triaxial reference s.
TriVex s.
TrueMax 2400 metabolic measuring s.
Trufill n-BCA liquid embolic s.
TruTrak data sampling s.
turbine-powered ICU ventilator s.

S

NOTES

system *(continued)*
two-bottle thoracic drainage s.
Ultraflex esophageal stent s.
Unified Medical Language s.
(UMLS)
Unilink s.
Unistep Plus delivery s.
Univision echocardiographic s.
USCI Probe balloon-on-a-wire
dilatation s.
vacuum-assisted venous return s.
Vanguard modular endograft s.
Vapor-Phase heated
humidification s.
Vapotherm oxygen delivery s.
Vario s.
vascular s.
VasoView Uniport endoscopic
saphenous vein harvesting s.
VDD pacing s.
VenaFlow compression s.
VenaFlow DVT prophylaxis s.
Venodyne EPS-410 external
pneumatic compression s.
venous arterial blood management
protection s. (VAMP)
Ventak Prizm 2 s.
Ventak PRx defibrillation s.
Ventak PRx III/Endotak s.
840 ventilator s.
Ventritex TVL s.
VersaStep laparoscopy s.
vessel occlusion s.
Veterans Affairs Medical Center
scoring s.
Viagraph ECG s.
video s.
videodensitometric analysis s.
Vigilance monitoring s.
Vingmed CFM 800
echocardiographic s.
Virtuoso LX Smart CPAP s.
Visa Iris s.
Vision blood cardioplegia s.
Vitatron pacing s.
VNUS Closure S.
VPAP II ST ventilatory support s.
Wallstent endoprosthesis with
Unistep Plus delivery s.
wall tracking s.
WaveMap intracoronary blood
pressure measurement s.
WaveWire intracoronary blood
pressure measurement s.
Welch Allyn/Schiller AT-10
Exercise Testing s.
White s.
Wiktor GX Hepamed coated
coronary stent s.

Wiktor GX Hepamed coronary
stent s.
Wiktor Prime coronary stent s.
Xillix ACCESS s.
Xillix LIFE-Lung s.
X-PRESS vascular closure s.
X-Scribe stress testing s.
X-Sizer single-use catheter s.
XYZ lead s.
Yellow IRIS s.
Zenith AAA endovascular graft s.

systema
s. cardiovasculare
s. conducens cordis
s. respiratorium

system/catheter
RPM tracking s./c.

systemic
s. arterial air embolism
s. arterial catheter
s. arterial pressure (SAP)
s. arterial resistance (Rsa)
s. betamethasone
s. blood flow (Qs, SBF)
s. blood pressure (PSA)
s. circulation
s. collateral
dexamethasone s.
s. erythromycin
s. granulomatous vasculitis
s. heart
s. hemodynamic parameters
s. hemodynamics
s. hydration
s. hydrocortisone
s. infection
s. inflammatory response syndrome
(SIRS)
s. lupus erythematosus (SLE)
s. mean arterial pressure (SMAP)
s. necrotizing vasculitis
s. prednisolone
s. prothrombosis
s. to pulmonary artery anastomosis
s. to pulmonary connection
s. pulmonary fistula (SPF)
s. to pulmonary shunt
s. sclerosis (SS)
s. thromboembolism
s. thrombotic propensity
triamcinolone (s.)
s. vascular hypertension
s. vascular resistance (SVR)
s. vascular resistance index (SVRI)
s. venous atrium
s. venous hypertension
s. venous return

systole (S, syst)
aborted s.

s. alternans
anticipated s.
atrial s.
auricular s.
cardiac s.
duration of s. (DS)
electrical s.
electromechanical s.
frustrate s.
hemic s.
isovolumic s.
late s.
premature s.
premature ventricular s. (PVS)
total electromechanical s. (QS_2)
ventricular s.
ventricular ectopic s.
systolic (sys, syst)
s. acceleration time (SAT)
s. anterior motion (SAM)
s. apical impulse
s. apical murmur
s. arterial blood pressure (SABP)
s. atrial pressure (SAP)
basal s.
s. blood pressure (BPS, SBP, SYS-BP)
s. bruit
s. bulging
s. click (SC)
s. click-late systolic murmur syndrome
s. click-murmur syndrome
s. click syndrome (SCS)
s. coronary artery narrowing (SCAN)
s. current
s. current of injury
s. discharge (SD)
s. doming
s. ejection murmur (SEM)
s. ejection period (SEP)

s. ejection rate (SER)
s. function
s. gallop
s. gallop rhythm
s. gradient
s. heart failure
s. honk
s. hypertension
s. left ventricular pressure
s. motion (SM)
s. murmur (SM)
s. pressure (Ps, SP)
s. pressure time index (SPTI)
pulmonary artery s. (PAS)
s. pulmonary artery pressure (sPAP)
pulmonary venous s. (PVs)
s. pulmonary venous velocity
s. reflection wave
s. regurgitant murmur
s. reserve
s. reversal
segment length, s. (SLS)
s. shock
s. S wave
s. thrill
s. time (ST)
s. time interval (STI)
s. trough
s. upstroke time
s. velocity integral (SVI)
s. velocity ratio
s. wall motion velocity (Vsys)
s. wave, latent (SL)
s. whipping
s. whoop
systolic/diastolic (S/D)
systolometer
SyvekPatch
szulgai
Mycobacterium s.

S

NOTES

T
  electrocardiographic wave corresponding
    to the repolarization of the ventricles
  temperature
  thrombus
    T artifact
    T cell
    T cell defect
    T graft
    T loop
    T lymphocyte
    T sign
    T stent
    T system
    T technique
    T tube
    T wave
    T wave alternans (TWA)
    T wave change
    T wave flattening
    T wave inversion
T1
  tricuspid first sound
  tricuspid valve closure sound
T$_4$
  thyroxine
T$_E$
  duration of expiration
  expiratory time
T$_I$
  duration of inspiration
  inspiratory time
T$_b$
  buildup time
T1-weighted image
T2 relaxation time
T2-weighted MRI
TA
  arterial tension
  tantalum
  transposition of aorta
  tricuspid atresia
  truncus arteriosus
T + A
  ticlopidine plus aspirin
^{178}TA
  tantalum-178
TAA
  thoracic aortic aneurysm
  transcoronary alcohol ablation
  transverse aortic arch
  triamcinolone acetonide
TAB
  total atrial blanking
    TAB period

tabacosis
tabby
    t. cat heart
    t. cat striation
tabetic cuirass
table
    Akron tilt t.
    anterior t.
    t. binding
    decompression t.
    Diamond-Forrester t.
    Siemens open heart t.
tablet
    Afrin T.
    Aprodine T.
    Aristocort T.
    Atacand Plus t.
    Avelox t.
    Betapace AF t.
    Cardizem T.
    CellCept t.
    Cenafed Plus T.
    cerivastatin sodium t.
    Deconamine T.
    diltiazem HCl extended-release t.
    Genac T.
    Mevacor lovastatin t.
    moxifloxacin HCl t.
    mycophenolate mofetil t.
    NitroQuick sublingual t.
    Nolvadex t.
    Pacerone t.
    Taztia XT extended-release t.
    Triposed T.
    Wobenzym t.
tabourka
    bruit de t.
TAC
    truncus arteriosus communis
Tac-3 injection
tach
    V t.
        ventricular tachycardia
tache
    t. blanche
    t. laiteuse
tachometer
tachy
    tachycardia
tachyarrhythmia
    T. Detection Software
    double ectopic t.
    malignant ventricular t.
    multifocal supraventricular t.
    reentrant ventricular t.

T

tachyarrhythmia *(continued)*
 supraventricular t. (SVT)
 sustained reentrant ventricular t.
  (SRVT)
 triple ectopic t.
 ventricular t. (VTA)
tachyarrhythmic substrate
tachybrady
 t. arrhythmia
 t. syndrome
tachycardia (tachy)
 accelerated idioventricular t.
 accessory pathway mediated t.
 alternating bidirectional t.
 antidromic circus movement t.
 antidromic reciprocating t.
 artificial circus movement t.
  (ACMT)
 atrial t. (AT)
 atrial chaotic t.
 atrial ectopic t. (AET)
 atrial paroxysmal t.
 atrial ventricular nodal reentry t.
 atrial ventricular reciprocating t.
  (AVRT)
 atriofascicular Mahaim reentrant t.
 atrioventricular junctional
  reciprocating t.
 atrioventricular nodal t. (AVNT)
 atrioventricular nodal reentrant t.
  (AVNRT)
 atrioventricular nodal reentry t.
  (AVNRT)
 atrioventricular reciprocating t.
  (AVRT)
 atrioventricular reentrant t. (AVRT)
 atypical atrioventricular nodal
  reentrant t. (AAVNRT)
 auricular t.
 automatic atrial t. (AAT)
 automatic ectopic t.
 A-V junctional t.
 A-V nodal reentry t.
 A-V node reentrant t.
 A-V reciprocating t.
 Belhaussen t.
 bidirectional ventricular t.
 bundle branch reentrant t.
 burst of ventricular t.
 chaotic atrial t.
 chronic ectopic atrial t. (CEAT)
 circus movement t. (CMT)
 Coumel t.
 t. cycle length
 double t. (DT)
 drug-refractory t.
 ectopic atrial t. (EAT)
 ectopic junctional t.
 endless loop t. (ELT)

 endocardial mapping of
  ventricular t.
 t. en salves
 entrainment of t.
 essential t.
 exercise-induced ventricular t.
 t. exophthalmica
 familial t.
 fascicular t.
 fetal t.
 idiopathic ventricular t. (IVT)
 idioventricular t.
 inappropriate sinus t. (IST)
 incessant atrial t.
 incessant ventricular t.
 inducible polymorphic ventricular t.
 intraatrial reentrant t.
 intraatrial reentry t. (IART)
 junctional t. (JT)
 junctional ectopic t. (JET)
 junctional reciprocating t.
 macroreentrant atrial t.
 Mahaim-type t.
 malignant ventricular t.
 monoform t.
 monomorphic ventricular t. (MVT)
 multifocal atrial t. (MAT, MFAT,
  MFT)
 multiform t.
 narrow-complex t.
 nodal paroxysmal t.
 nodal reentrant t.
 nonparoxysmal atrioventricular
  junctional t. (NPJT)
 nonsuppressible ventricular t.
 nonsustained ventricular t. (NSVT)
 orthodromic atrioventricular
  reciprocating t.
 orthodromic A-V reentrant t.
 orthodromic circus movement t.
 orthodromic reciprocating t. (ORT)
 orthostatic t.
 pacemaker circus movement t.
  (PCMT)
 pacemaker-mediated t. (PMT)
 pacing-induced t. (PIT)
 parasystolic ventricular t.
 paroxysmal t. (PT)
 paroxysmal atrial t. (PAT)
 paroxysmal atrioventricular nodal
  reciprocal t. (PAVNRT)
 paroxysmal junctional t. (PJT)
 paroxysmal nodal t.
 paroxysmal reentrant
  supraventricular t.
 paroxysmal sinus t.
 paroxysmal supraventricular t. (PST,
  PSVT)
 paroxysmal ventricular t. (PVT)

t. pathway mapping
permanent atrial t.
permanent junctional reciprocating t.
  (PJRT)
pleomorphic t.
polymorphic ventricular t.
polymorphous ventricular t.
primary ventricular t. (PVT)
rapid nonsustained ventricular t.
reciprocating t. (RT)
reciprocating macroreentry
  orthodromic t.
reentrant t. (RT)
reentrant atrial t.
reentrant supraventricular t.
reflex t.
refractory t.
repetitive monomorphic
  ventricular t.
repetitive paroxysmal ventricular t.
resting sinus t.
right ventricular outflow tract t.
salvo of ventricular t.
S-A nodal reentrant t.
self-terminating t.
sinoventricular t. (SVT)
sinus t. (ST)
sinus nodal reentrant t.
sleeping t.
slow-fast t.
slow paroxysmal atrial t. (SPAT)
spontaneous reentrant sustained
  ventricular t.
suppressible ventricular t.
supraventricular t. (SVT)
sustained t.
sustained monomorphic
  ventricular t. (SMVT)
sustained ventricular t. (SVT)
torsade de pointes ventricular t.
ventricular t. (V tach, VT)
ventricular fibrillation/ventricular t.
  (VF/VT)
wide QRS t.
t. window
Wolff-Parkinson-White reentrant t.
tachycardia-bradycardia syndrome
tachycardiac
tachycardia-dependent aberrancy
tachycardia-induced
t.-i. cardiomyopathy

t.-i. heart failure
t.-i. myopathy
tachycardia-polyuria syndrome
tachycardic
tachycrotic
tachydysrhythmia
tachykinin
t. receptor
t. receptor antagonist
tachypacing
tachyphylactic
tachyphylaxis
tachypnea
happy t.
nervous t.
tachyrhythmia
tachysystole
TACI
total anterior circulation infarct
tacrolimus
TACS
total anterior circulation syndrome
Tactilaze angioplasty
tactile fremitus
TADcath temporary transvenous
  defibrillation catheter
TAE
transcatheter arterial embolization
tag
emergency medical t. (EMT)
epicardial fat t.
pleural t.
two-dimensional t.
Tagarno 3SD cineangiography projector
tagged
t. acquisition
expression sequence t. (EST)
t. magnetic resonance imaging
tagging
spin t.
TAH
total artificial heart
  Berlin TAH
  CardioWest TAH
  Penn State TAH
  University of Akron TAH
  Utah TAH
  Vienna TAH
tailoring
root t.
tail sign
Taiwan acute respiratory (TWAR)

T

NOTES

Takayasu
> T. aortitis
> T. arteritis
> T. disease
> idiopathic arteritis of T.
> T. syndrome

Takayasu-Onishi disease
Take Control
Talairach space
talc
> t. granulomatosis
> t. operation
> t. pleurodesis
> t. pneumoconiosis
> t. poudrage
> t. slurry

talcosis
Talent
> T. bifurcated endograft
> T. graft
> T. LPS endoluminal stent-graft
>   system

tall
> t. oil asthma
> t. T wave

Talon balloon dilatation catheter
Talos stent delivery system
TAM
> transtelephonic ambulatory monitoring
> tricuspid annular motion
> TAM system

Tambocor
tambour
> bruit de t.
> t. sound

TAMI
> transmural anterior myocardial infarction
> TAMI protocol

Tamiflu
Tamm-Horsfall protein
Tamofen
Tamone
tamoxifen
tamponade, tamponage
> acute t.
> atypical t.
> balloon t.
> cardiac t. (CT)
> chronic t.
> esophageal t.
> esophagogastric t.
> heart t.
> low-pressure t.
> pericardial t. (PT)
> Rose t.
> subacute t.
> traumatic t.

TAN
> total adenine nucleotides

T-AnastoFlo shunt
tandem
> T. cardiac device
> t. lesion
> t. needle approach

TandemHeart pVAD
tangential
> t. flow filtration (TFF)
> t. percussion

Tangier disease
TANI
> total axial node irradiation

tank respirator
tannate
> methyclothiazide and
>   cryptenamine t.

Tanner operation
tantalum (TA)
> t. bronchogram
> t. mesh
> t. plate
> powdered t.
> radioactive t.
> t. ring
> t. stent
> t. wire

tantalum-178 (^{178}TA)
> t.-178 generator

TAO
> troleandomycin

TAP
> Thornton anterior positioner
> transesophageal atrial pacing
> transluminal angioplasty

tap
> bloody t.
> mitral t.
> pericardial t.
> pleural t.

TAPE
> temporary atrial pacemaker electrode

tape
> T. Based inhaler
> B101 ET Tape II adhesive t.
> ColorZone t.
> Hy-Tape waterproof adhesive t.
> Original Pink Tape waterproof
>   adhesive t.
> Silastic t.
> twill t.
> umbilical t.
> vascular t.

TapeMeasure computerized planimetry
taper
> short t.

tapered
> t. movable core curved wire guide
> T. Torque guidewire

tapering
    airway t.
Taperseal hemostatic device
tapotage
taprostene
TAPVC
    total anomalous pulmonary venous
      connection
TAPVD
    total anomalous pulmonary venous
      drainage
TAPVR
    total anomalous pulmonary venous return
Taq
    T. DNA polymerase
    T. extender
TAQW
    transient abnormal Q wave
TAR
    thoracic aortic rupture
    thrombocytopenia-absent radius
    TAR syndrome
tar
    coal t.
tardive cyanosis
tardus
    pulsus parvus et t.
target
    dyspnea t.
    t. heart rate (THR)
    t. INR
    t. lesion
    t. lesion revascularization (TLR)
    t. organ disease/clinical
      cardiovascular disease (TOD/CCD)
    t. site
    T. Therapeutics Stealth angioplasty
      balloon
    T. Tip lead
    t. vessel
    t. vessel revascularization (TVR)
Tarka
Taro-Ampicillin
Taro-Atenol
Taro-Cloxacillin
TARP
    total atrial refractory period
TARTI
    total apexcardiographic relaxation time
      index
tartrate
    metoprolol t.

    phenindamine t.
    vinorelbine t.
    zolpidem t.
tartrazine asthma
TAS
    Thrombolytic Assessment System
Ta segment
TASH
    transcoronary ablation of septal
      hypertrophy
task
    bean-spooning t.
    metabolic equivalent of t. (MET)
tasosartan
TAT
    thrombin-antithrombin
    turnaround time
Tatlockia micdadei
taurinum
    cor t.
Taussig-Bing
    T.-B. anomaly
    T.-B. complex
    T.-B. disease
    T.-B. heart
    T.-B. malformation
    T.-B. syndrome
TAV
    transvenous aortovelography
TAVB
    total atrioventricular block
Tawara atrioventricular node
Ta wave
taxane
Taxol
taxonomic
taxonomy
Taxotere
Taybi syndrome
Taylor dispersion
Tay-Sachs disease
Tazicef
Tazidime
Taztia XT extended-release tablet
TB
    tuberculosis
TBARS
    thiobarbituric acid reactive substance
TBB, TBBX, TBBx
    transbronchial biopsy
TBFV
    tidal breathing flow-volume

T

NOTES

TBI
    thrombotic brain infarction
    total body irradiation
TBird ventilator system
TBLB
    transbronchial lung biopsy
TBNA
    transbronchial needle aspiration
TBP
    total bypass
TBV
    total blood volume
TC
    total cholesterol
3TC
    lamivudine
Tc
    tricuspid closure
^{99m}Tc, Tc-99^m, Tc-99m
    technetium-99m
        ^{99m}Tc MIBI-SPECT
        ^{99m} sestamibi
        ^{99m}Tc sestamibi scintigraphy
TCA
    total circulatory arrest
TCABG
    triple coronary artery bypass graft
TCAD
    transplant coronary artery disease
TCAG
    triple coronary artery graft
TCB
    total cardiopulmonary bypass
    transcatheter biopsy
TCC
    transcatheter closure
TCCS
    transcranial color-coded sonography
TCD
    transverse cardiac diameter
        Multigon 500M non-contrast-
        enhanced TCD
        TCD sonography
        TCD ultrasonography
        TCD ultrasound
TCD100M digital transcranial Doppler system
Tc-diethylenetriamine pentaacetic acid
TCF
    total coronary flow
TCG
    time compensation gain
T-channel
TC/HDL
    total cholesterol/high-density lipoproteins
        TC/HDL ratio
TCI Heartmate mechanical circulatory support system
Tc-99m (*var. of* ^{99m}Tc)

TCM30 transcutaneous oxygen monitor
Tc-mercaptoacetyltriglycine
TCN-P
    triciribine phosphate
TCOM
    transcutaneous oxygen monitor
TCP, TCPC
    total cavopulmonary connection
    transcutaneous pacemaker
    transcutaneous pacing
TCPS
    total cavopulmonary shunt
TCS
    total coronary score
TCT
    thoracic computed tomography
    thrombin clotting time
    transcardial catheter therapy
    transcatheter therapy
    trunk control test
        TCT scan
tcu-PA
    two-chain urokinase plasminogen
    activator
TDCO
    thermodilution cardiac output
        TDCO measurement
TDD
    thoracic duct drainage
    transpulmonary thermal-dye dilution
TDI
    tissue Doppler imaging
    toluene diisocyanate
        TDI M-mode echocardiography
TDP
    therapist-driven protocol
    torsade de pointes
TdP
    torsade de pointes
TdT-mediated dUTP nick-end labeling (TUNEL)
TE
    tracheoesophageal
        TE fistula
TE
    echo delay time
    thromboembolism
    treadmill exercise
TEA
    thromboendarterectomy
    transluminal extraction atherectomy
tea
        black t.
        pectoral t.
        t. taster's cough
teacher's node
team
        Bimodality Lung Oncology T.
        (BLOT)

cardiac resuscitation T. (CRT)
code blue T. (CBT)
code response T. (CRT)
Public Health Response T. (PHRT)

TEAP
transesophageal atrial pacing

tear
Boerhaave t.
great vessel t.
intimal t.
Mallory-Weiss t.
medial t.
neointimal t.

teardrop heart

tear gas, teargas

TEB
thoracic electrical bioimpedance

teboroxime
t. imaging
t. scan
technetium-99m t.

Tebrazid

TEC
thromboembolic complication
transluminal endarterectomy catheter
transluminal extraction catheter
TEC atherectomy device
TEC atherectomy system
TEC extraction catheter

TECAB
totally endoscopic coronary artery bypass

TEC-guide catheter

technetium
t. depreotide
t. glucarate
t. hexakis 2-methoxyisobutyl
isonitrile
t. pyrophosphate
t. (Tc)-99m sestamibi tomographic
imaging

technetium-99m-labeled annexin-V

technetium-99m (^{99m}Tc, Tc-99^m, Tc-99m)
t. furofosmin
t. hexakis 2-methoxyisobutyl
isonitrile
t. hexamibi scan
t. methoxyisobutyl isonitrile
t. methylene diphosphonate
t. MIBI
t. MIBI imaging
t. pyrophosphate

t. sestamibi single-photon emission
computed tomography
t. sestamibi SPECT
t. sestamibi stress test
sodium pertechnetate t.
t. stannous pyrophosphate scintiscan
t. teboroxime
t. tetrofosmin

**technetium-99m-sestamibi single-photon
emission computed tomography**

technetium-99m-tetrofosmin imaging

technetium-sestamibi
t.-s. SPECT
t.-s. stress test

technetium-teboroxime

Technicare Omega 500 CT

technique
ablative t.
airway occlusion t.
Amplatz t.
Angus t.
antegrade double balloon/double
wire t.
antegrade/retrograde cardioplegia t.
anterior sandwich patch t.
anterograde transseptal t.
antialiasing t.
Araki-Sako t.
atrial-well t.
background subtraction t.
Bentall inclusion t.
Bergstrom needle biopsy t.
black-white interface t.
blood oxygenation level-
dependent t.
BOLD t.
bootstrap two-vessel t.
breathing t.
Brecher and Cronkite t.
Brockenbrough t.
button t.
Carrie coronary stent placement t.
catheterization t.
chloramine-T t.
Ciaglia serial dilatation t.
clearance t.
clonogenic t.
Collins chain compensated
gasometer t.
Colombo inverted Y t.
Copeland t.
coronary flow reserve t.

NOTES

T

711

technique *(continued)*
    cough CPR t.
    crash t.
    Crawford graft inclusion t.
    Creech t.
    cryosurgical t.
    CT-guided stereotaxic t.
    culotte coronary stenting t.
    cutdown t.
    Davies t.
    DCA debulking t.
    digital subtraction t.
    dilator and sheath t.
    direct insertion t.
    directional atherectomy debulking t.
    Doppler auto-correlation t.
    Dotter t.
    Dotter-Judkins t.
    double-balloon t.
    double-balloon (9-11) t.
    double-dummy t.
    double-syringe t.
    double-wire t.
    Douglas bag t.
    dye dilution t.
    ECG signal-averaging t.
    en bloc no-touch t.
    endocardial mapping t. (EMT)
    entangling t.
    exchange t.
    Exorcist t.
    Fick t.
    Finapres t.
    first-pass t.
    flotation catheter t.
    flow mapping t.
    flush and bathe t.
    forced expiratory t.
    forced oscillation t. (FOT)
    fork stenting t.
    forward triangle t.
    Fourier-acquired steady-state t.
      (FAST)
    gated t.
    George-Lewis t.
    gloved fist t.
    Goris background subtraction t.
    grabbing t.
    Grüntzig t.
    guidewire t.
    harmonic imaging ultrasound t.
    Heartport t.
    high-pressure inflation t.
    hydrogen inhalation t.
    immunofluorescent t.
    immunostaining t.
    indicator dilution t.
    indocyanine green indicator
      dilution t.

    inhaled radioaerosol t.
    Inoue balloon t.
    Inoue single-balloon t.
    inverted V t.
    Jatene t.
    J-loop t.
    Judkins t.
    Judkins-Sones t.
    Kern t.
    kissing balloon t.
    LocaLisa t.
    long-leg venography t.
    Lown t.
    Marbach-Weil t.
    McGoon t.
    Merendino t.
    minimal leak t.
    modified brachial t.
    modified Seldinger t.
    Mullins blade t.
    multibreath nitrogen washout t.
    multiplanar reconstruction t.
    nasal pool t.
    Nikaidoh-Bex t.
    nitrogen washout t.
    no-leak t.
    no-touch t.
    occluder balloon wash-out t.
    oscillation t.
    Oxford t.
    Paulin venography t.
    percutaneous t.
    PI MRI t.
    Porstmann t.
    port access t.
    posture t.
    pranayama breathing t.
    pressure-controlled ventilation t.
    pressure half-time t.
    Rabinov venography t.
    radiographic t.
    radionuclide t.
    Rashkind balloon t.
    rebreathing t.
    relaxation t.
    Ricketts-Abrams t.
    Robiscek t.
    Rosalki t.
    scatterplot smoothing t.
    Schonander t.
    Schoonmaker-King single catheter t.
    Sealy-Laragh t.
    second harmonic imaging
      ultrasound t.
    Seldinger percutaneous t.
    Sewall t.
    shaping behavioral t.
    Sheehan and Dodge t.
    SHI ultrasound t.

skewer t.
snare t.
Sones t.
sonication t.
SPAMM t.
Sparks mandrel t.
spatial modulation of
  magnetization t.
static dilation t.
steerable over-the-wire
  angioplasty t.
Stewart-Hamilton cardiac output t.
T t.
telescoping anastomotic t.
T-graft configuration t.
thermal dilution t.
thermodilution t.
track-ball t.
Trusler aortic valve t.
TurboFLASH t.
two-patch t.
upgated t.
velocity catheter t.
video-assisted diagnostic
  thoracoscopic t.
Waldhausen subclavian flap t.
wax-matrix t.
xenon washout t.
Y t.
Zavala t.

technologist
cardiovascular t. (CVT)
National Alliance of
  Cardiovascular T.'s (NACT)
National Society of
  Cardiovascular T.'s (NSCT)

technology
acquisition zoom t.
AZ t.
BioZ impedance cardiography t.
CardioFix pericardium with
  PhotoFix t.
Coblation t.
FilterLine sampling t.
Focus Angioplasty Catheter T.
Lingraphica system treatment t.
Oxismart advanced signal
  processing and alarm t.
phased array t.
PulseDose oxygen delivery t.
SAC data acquisition t.

serial autocorrelation data
  acquisition t.
vein-to-vein t.

Technos ultrasound system
Techstar
T. device
T. percutaneous suture
T. XL 6F percutaneous vascular
  surgical system
T. XL 6F PVS system

TECSAC
telecollaboration for signal analysis in
  cardiology

Teczem
TED
thromboembolic disease
  TED antiembolism stockings
  TED hose

TEDD
total end-diastolic diameter

tedisamil
Tedlar bag
TEE
transesophageal echocardiography

TEE-DSE
transesophageal echocardiography-
  dobutamine stress echocardiography

Teejel
TEEP
transesophageal echocardiography with
  pacing

TEF
tracheoesophageal fistula

TEF$_{25}$
tidal expiratory flow at 25% of tidal
  volume

TEF$_{25}$/PTEF
ratio of tidal expiratory flow at 25% of
  tidal volume and peak tidal expiratory
  flow

TEF$_{50}$
tidal expiratory flow at 50% of tidal
  volume

TEF$_{50}$/TIF$_{50}$
ratio of tidal expiratory and inspiratory
  flow at 50% of tidal volume

TEF$_{75}$
tidal expiratory flow at 75% of tidal
  volume

**Tefcor movable core straight wire
guide**

T

NOTES

Teflon
T. Bardic plug
T. catheter
T. coating
T. felt bolster
T. felt patch
T. graft
T. intracardiac patch
T. pledget
T. pledget suture buttress
T. sheath
T. trileaflet prosthesis
woven T.
T. woven prosthesis
Teflon-coated
T.-c. guidewire
T.-c. wire skeleton
TEG
thromboelastogram
thromboelastography
tegafur and uracil (UFT)
TEH
theophylline, ephedrine, and hydroxyzine
Teichholz
T. correction
T. ejection fraction
T. equation
T. formula
teichoic acid antibody
teicoplanin
glycopeptide t.
Tei index of myocardial performance
telangiectasia
calcinosis, Raynaud phenomenon,
esophageal involvement,
sclerodactyly, t. (CREST)
hemorrhagic hereditary t.
hereditary hemorrhagic t. (HHT)
t. syndrome
telbermin
telecardiogram
telecardiophone
telecollaboration for signal analysis in cardiology (TECSAC)
Telectronics
T. Accufix pacing lead
T. ATP implantable cardioverter-defibrillator
T. Guardian ATP 4210 device
T. Guardian ATP II ICD
T. pacemaker
T. Pacing Systems
telecurietherapy
telediastolic
telelectrocardiogram
telemetry
cardiac t.
multiple-parameter t. (MPT)

pacemaker t.
real-time t.
telemonitor
Physios CTM 01 noninvasive t.
telemonitored polysomnography
teleradiology
telescope
telescoping anastomotic technique
telesystolic
Tele-thermometer
YSI 4000 T.-t.
telithromycin
telmisartan
telomere
telomeric shortening
telopeptide
type I collagen t. (ICTP)
TEM
transtelephonic exercise monitor
temafloxacin
temazepam
tempeh
temperature (T)
central venous t. (CVT)
core t.
esophageal t.
t. and pulse (T&P, T+P)
t., pulse, and respiration
temperature-sensing pacemaker
Tempo diagnostic catheter
temporal
t. arteritis
t. average intensity (I_{ta})
t. dispersion
t. peak intensity (I_{tp})
t. resolution
temporary
t. atrial pacemaker electrode (TAPE)
t. filter
t. pacemaker (TPM)
t. pacemaker placement
t. pacing
t. pervenous lead
t. unilateral pulmonary artery occlusion
tenacious
t. mucus
t. sputum
tenacity
sputum t.
tenascin-C
Tenax-XR
T.-XR Complete
T.-XR Trinity stent
tend-and-befriend response to stress
tenderness
point t.

tendinea
> macula t.

tendineae
> chordae t.

tendinosum
> xanthoma t.

tendinous
> t. spot
> t. xanthoma
> t. zones of heart

tendo
> t. cricoesophageus
> t. infundibuli

tendon
> t. of conus
> coronary t.
> cricoesophageal t.
> false t.
> t. of infundibulum
> t. of Todaro, Todaro t.
> trefoil t.

tendophony

Tendril
> T. DX implantable pacing lead
> T. DX steroid-eluting active-fixation pacing lead
> T. SDX model 1688 active-fixation pacing lead

tenecteplase (TNKase, TNK-tPA)

Tenex

Tenif

teniposide

Tennant distress scale

tenonometer

tenophony

Tenoretic

Tenormin

Tenox

tense
> t. edema
> t. pulse

tensile stress

Tensilon injection

tension
> alveolar-arterial oxygen t. (A-a 02)
> alveolar carbon dioxide t.
> alveolar oxygen t.
> arterial t. (TA)
> arterial carbon dioxide t. ($PaCO_2$)
> arterial oxygen t. (PaO_2)
> carbon dioxide t.
> isometric systolic t. (IST)

> left ventricular t. (LVT)
> myocardial t.
> oxygen t.
> t. pneumopericardium
> t. pneumothorax
> wall t.

tension-length relation

tension-time index

tensor palatini

Tensys T-line blood pressure monitor

tent
> croup t.
> Croupette child t.
> mist t.
> oxygen t.
> pleural t.
> steam t.

tenting
> t. of hemidiaphragm
> t. sign
> t. of skin

tenuis
> *Alternaria t.*

TEP
> transesophageal pacing

Teq-Paq

Tequin

teratoma
> pericardial t.
> t. tumor

terazosin hydrochloride

terbutaline sulfate

tercile value

terconazole

terephthalate
> polyethylene t. (PET)

terfenadine

terikalant

terminal
> t. aorta
> t. bronchiole
> t. cisterna
> t. edema
> t. endocarditis
> t. filtered QRS signal
> t. groove
> t. internal carotid artery (TICA)
> t. phase
> t. pneumonia
> t. Purkinje fibers
> t. respiratory unit (TRU)

T

NOTES

terminal *(continued)*
    t. weaning
    Wilson central t.
terminalis
    bronchiolus t.
    crista t.
    sulcus t.
termination
    exercise t.
    underdrive t.
terminus
terodiline
Terox RV lead
terpin
    t. hydrate
    t. hydrate and codeine
terrae
    Mycobacterium t.
Terramycin I.M. injection
terreus
    Aspergillus t.
terror
    night t.'s
tertiary
    t. bronchus
    t. contraction
    t. syphilis
Terumo
    T. Crosswire PTCA guidewire
    T. dialyzer
    T. Pinnacle sheath
    T. Radifocus Glidewire
    T. Radiofocus sheath
    T. SP coaxial catheter
    T. SP hydrophilic-polymer-coated
      microcatheter
    T. stent
    T. telescoping catheter system
TES
    thoracic endometriosis syndrome
    transcutaneous electrical stimulation
TESD
    total end-systolic diameter
tesla
Teslac
Tessalon Perles
test
    Aachener Aphasie T.
    abdominal jugular t.
    ABG point-of-care t.
    Acarex-t.
    ACB t.
    Access AccuTnI troponin I t.
    AccuMeter theophylline t.
    AccuTnI troponin I t.
    acetylcholine t.
    acid infusion t.
    Action Research Arm T.
    adenosine thallium t.

Adson t.
Advanced Care cholesterol t.
aerobic exercise stress t.
aerosol challenge t.
ajmaline t.
AlaSTAT latex allergy t.
albumin cobalt binding t.
alertness t.
Allen t.
alternans t.
Amplicor *Mycobacterium*
  tuberculosis t.
amplified *Mycobacterium*
  tuberculosis direct t. (AMTDT)
Anderson t.
angiotensin sensitivity t. (AST)
ankle-brachial index t.
anoxemia t.
antistreptozyme t.
apoE t.
Apt t.
arginine tolerance t. (ATT)
Arloing-Courmont t.
arm exercise stress t.
arm-tongue time t.
arterial blood gas point-of-care t.
  (ABG PCT)
Astrand bicycle exercise stress t.
atrial pacing stress t.
atropine t.
Balke exercise stress t.
Balke-Ware t.
balloon distention t.
Benton Lines T.
Bernstein t.
bicycle ergometer exercise stress t.
bile solubility t.
Blake exercise stress t.
blanch t.
blot t.
Blumenau t.
Bordet-Gengou t.
brachial plexus tension t.
breath excretion t.
breath holding t.
breath pentane t.
Brodie-Trendelenburg tourniquet t.
bronchial challenge t.
bronchoprovocation t.
broth t.
Bruce exercise stress t.
Bruce maximum stress t. (BMST)
Brunnstrom-Fugl-Meyer Scale for
  motor t.
CAMP t.
carbachol provocation t.
carbohydrate utilization t.
Cardiac STATus CK-MB t.

Cardiac STATus CK-MB/myoglobin panel t.
Cardiac STATus rapid format troponin I panel t.
cardiac stress t. (CST)
cardiolipin flocculation t. (CFT)
cardiolipin microflocculation t. (CMFT)
Cardiolite stress t.
cardiopulmonary exercise t. (CPET)
Caregiver Strain T.
carotid sinus t.
Casoni t.
ChemTrak AccuMeter theophylline t.
CLA for infusion of catecholamine in heart stress t.
coccidioidin t.
coin t.
cold pressor t.
complement-fixation t.
Coombs t.
CPX t.
cuff t.
cuff-leak t.
Davidson protocol exercise t.
D-dimer t.
Dehio t.
dexamethasone suppression t.
digit span memory t.
dipalmitoyl phosphatidylcholine t.
dipyridamole echocardiography t. (DET)
dipyridamole handgrip t.
dipyridamole thallium stress t.
direct amplification t. (DAT)
dobutamine stress t.
double simultaneous stimulation t.
DPPC t.
DR-70 tumor marker t.
duodenal string t.
electrophysiologic t.
Elispot t.
Ellestad exercise stress t.
ergonovine provocation t.
Escherich t.
ether t.
euglycemic hyperinsulinemic glucose clamp t.
exercise t. (ET)
exercise stress t. (EST)
exercise tolerance t. (ETT)

exercise treadmill t. (ETT)
extrastimulus t.
Farr t.
fetal heart rate nonstress t. (FHRNST)
flashing checkerboard t.
fluorescent treponemal antibody absorption t.
foam stability t.
Fowler single-breath t.
Frenchay Aphasia Screening T. (FAST)
FTA-ABS t.
GenESA system for radionuclide imaging stress t.
Gibbon-Landis t.
Goethlin t.
goodness-of-fit t.
gradational step exercise stress t.
graded exercise t. (GXT)
Griess t.
guidewire traversal t.
Hallion t.
Ham t.
Hamburger t.
handgrip apexcardiographic t. (HAT)
head-down tilt t.
head-up tilt t.
head-up tilt-table t. (HUTTT)
Heaf t.
Heart Failure Knowledge T.
heart rate variability t.
Heartscan heart attack prediction t.
Henle-Coenen t.
hepatojugular reflux t.
Hess capillary t.
high-altitude simulation t. (HAST)
Hines-Brown t.
Hitzenberg t.
HIVAGEN t.
Hosmer-Lemeshow Goodness-of-Fit t.
Hotelling T2 t.
Howell t.
HRV t.
hypoxemia t.
IgG avidity t.
implantation t. (IT)
incremental shuttle walking t. (ISWT)
inhalation challenge t.

T

NOTES

test *(continued)*

intravenous glucose tolerance t. (IVGTT)
isometric handgrip t.
isoproterenol stress t.
isoproterenol tilt-table t.
Jaeger body t.
Jebsen Hand Function T.
Kattus exercise stress t.
Kleihauer t.
Kleihauer-Betke t.
Kveim antigen skin t.
Kveim-Siltzbach t.
laryngeal cough reflex t. (LCR)
LDL direct blood t.
left atrial transesophageal pacing t. (LATPT)
lepromin t.
Levy Chimeric Faces T.
Lewis-Pickering t.
Liebermann-Burchard t.
Lignieres t.
limited treadmill t. (LTT)
liver function t. (LFT)
Livierato t.
loaded breathing t. (LBT)
low-range heparin management t. (LHMT)
lymphocyte transformation t.
Machado-Guerreiro t.
Mantoux t.
Master exercise stress t.
Master two-step exercise t.
Matas t.
maximal exercise t. (MET)
maximal treadmill t.
maximal treadmill stress t. (MTST)
maximum exercise tolerance t. (METT)
methacholine challenge t.
MHA-TP t.
MIBI stress t.
microneutralization t.
6-minute corridor walk t.
10-minute supine/30-minute tilt t.
6-minute walking t. (6MWT, 6-MWT)
modified shuttle t.
modified treadmill exercise t. (MTET)
Moschcowitz t.
MTD t.
MUGA exercise stress t.
Müller t.
multiple sleep latency t. (MSLT)
multistage exercise t. (MET)
multistage maximal effort exercise stress t.

MycoAKT latex bead agglutination t.
myoglobulin cardiac diagnostic t.
Nagle exercise stress t.
Nathan t.
Naughton cardiac exercise treadmill t.
Naughton graded exercise stress t.
near patient t. (NPT)
N-geneous automated HDL cholesterol t.
Nickerson-Kveim t.
noninvasive t.
nonspecific challenge t.
Norris t.
Nottingham Sensory Assessment t.
nucleic acid direct amplification t.
Ochsner-Mahorner t.
Optochin disk t.
oral glucose tolerance t. (OGTT)
oxygen challenge t.
Pachon t.
p24 antigen t.
paracoccidioidin skin t.
PCR t.
pendulum t.
peppermint t.
Persantine-isonitrile stress t.
Persantine thallium stress t.
Perthes t.
Phalen stress t.
Physical Work Capacity exercise stress t.
pilocarpine iontophoresis t.
planar thallium t.
plantar ischemia t.
Plesch t.
POC blood gas t.
point of care t.
postdischarge graded-exercise t. (PD-GXT)
PPD skin t.
PPL skin t.
predischarge t.
primed lymphocyte t.
progressive exercise t. (PET)
provocation t.
pulmonary function t. (PFT)
purified protein derivative t.
Q-Stress treadmill stress t.
QuantiFeron-TB t.
Quick intravenous liver function t.
radioactive xenon t.
radioallergosorbent t. (RAST)
rapid antigen-detection t.
rapid plasma t.
Read t.
Recurring Figures t. for short-term memory

Recurring Words t. for short-term memory
reflex cough t.
Reflotron bedside theophylline t.
reverse transcriptase polymerase chain reaction t.
Rey Figure Copy t.
Rivermead Behavioral Memory T.
Roos t.
Rumpel-Leede t.
Sabin-Feldman dye t.
Salkowski t.
Sandrock t.
Schapiro-Wilks t.
Schellong t.
Schiff t.
Schlichter t.
Schultze t.
selective arterial secretin injection t. (SAST)
serological t.
sestamibi stress t.
sestamibi technetium-99m SPECT with dipyridamole stress t.
shake t.
Sheffield exercise stress t.
shuttle t.
single-breath carbon monoxide t.
single-breath nitrogen washout t.
single-stage exercise stress t.
six-minute walk t. (6MWT, 6-MWT)
Snider match t.
sniff t.
somatosensory evoked potential t.
specific bronchial challenge t.
Spectral Cardiac STATus CK-MB/myoglobulin panel t.
Spectral Cardiac STATus rapid format troponin I panel t.
SpectRx t.
speech mental stress t.
split-function lung t.
Stamey t.
Stand Displacement Amplification t.
Sterneedle tuberculin t.
Stratus cardiac troponin I t.
streptokinase-urokinase myocardial infarct t. (SUMIT)
stress t. (ST)
Stroop color word conflict t.
submaximal effort tourniquet t.

submaximal treadmill exercise t. (STET)
super stress t.
surf t.
sweat chloride t.
swing t.
symptom-limited graded exercise t. (SL-GXT)
symptom-limited maximal treadmill t.
symptom-limited treadmill exercise t.
technetium-99m sestamibi stress t.
technetium-sestamibi stress t.
thallium-201 exercise stress t.
thallium stress t.
The Cambridge Heart T-Wave Alternans T.
TheoFAST t.
thermodilution t.
thyroid function t.
tilt t.
tilt-table t. (TTT)
tine t.
tiptoe t.
tolazoline t.
treadmill t. (TT)
treadmill exercise t. (TET, TMET)
treadmill exercise stress t.
treadmill performance t. (TPP)
treadmill stress t. (TMST, TST)
Trendelenburg t.
treponemal t.
Triage BNP t.
Tris-buffer infusion t.
true positive stress t. (TPST)
trunk control t. (TCT)
Tuberculin Purified Protein Derivative Tine t.
Tuffier t.
two-step exercise t.
Tzanck t.
Valsalva t.
vasodilator plus exercise treadmill t.
VDRL t.
venous occlusion t.
ventricular accommodation t. (VAT)
VEX treadmill t.
Visov t.
Vitalometer t.

NOTES

test *(continued)*
 Vitalor screening pulmonary
  function t.
 in vitro allergy t.
 Vollmer t.
 volume-challenge t.
 von Recklinghausen t.
 Wada t.
 walk distance t.
 walking ventilation t.
 water-gurgle t.
 Weinberg t.
 whiff t.
 Widal t.
 Wideroe t.
 Wilks-Schapiro t.
 William t.
 Winslow t.
 Wolf Motor Function T. (WMFT)
 word association t. (WAT)
 worksite challenge t.
 X-Scribe stress t.
 Youman-Parlett t.
 Zwenger t.
tester
 IRMA SL blood glucose strip t.
 Polar Electro sport t.
 Quik-Chek external pacer t.
testing *(See also* test)
 Bactec MGIT 960 System for
  Mycobacteria t.
 immediate exercise treadmill t.
  (IETT)
 maximal treadmill t. (MTT)
 methylcholine challenge t. (MCT)
 point-of-care t. (POCT)
Testoderm Transdermal system
testolactone
Testopel Pellet
testosterone
Testred
TET
 total ejection time
 treadmill exercise test
Tet, tet
 tetralogy of Fallot
tetani
 Clostridium t.
tetanus
 anodal closure t. (ACTe)
 anodal duration t. (ANDTE,
  AnDTe)
 anodal opening t. (AOT, AOTe)
 cathodal closure t. (CCTe)
 cathodal opening t. (COTe)
 cathode duration t. (CDTe)
tethered leaflet
tethering

tetracaine
 t. hydrochloride
 lidocaine, epinephrine and t. (LET)
tetrachloride
 zirconium t.
tetracrotic
tetracycline
tetrad
 Fallot t.
 t. spell
tetraethylammonium chloride
tetrahedron chest
tetrahydrobiopterin
tetrahydrochloride
 diaminobenzidine t.
Tetralan Oral
tetralogy
 Eisenmenger t.
 Fallot t. (FT)
 t. of Fallot (Tet, tet, TF, TOF,
  TOF, T of F)
 t. of Fallot spell
 pink Fallot of t.
tetranitrate
 erythrityl t.
 pentaerythritol t. (PETN)
tetrapolar esophageal catheter
tetrazolium
 nitroblue t.
tetrodotoxin
tetrofosmin
 technetium-99m t.
Tet spell
tE/tTOT
 ratio of expiration time and total time of
  breathing cycle
Teutleben ligament
Teveten
texaphyrin
 lutetium t.
Texas
 T. Heart Institute (THI)
 T. influenza
textbook
 Sleep Multimedia 2.6
  computerized t.
tezosentan
TF
 tetralogy of Fallot
 Thomsen-Friedenreich
  TF antigen
TFA
 trans fatty acids
TFF
 tangential flow filtration
TFF-domain peptide
TFPI
 tissue factor pathway inhibitor

TFT
thrombus formation time
TFVL
tidal flow-volume loop
TFX Medical
T. M. catheter stylet
T. M. safety needle with introducer
TG
triglyceride
TGA
transposition of great arteries
TGC
time-gain compensation
time-gain control
time-varied gain control
T-Gesic
TGF
transforming growth factor
TGFA
triglyceride fatty acid
TGI
tracheal gas insufflation
TGL
triglyceride
T-graft configuration technique
TGV
thoracic gas volume
transposition of great vessels
ThA
thoracic aorta
ThAIRapy
T. vest
T. vest airway clearance system
thalamic dementia
thalassemia
sickle cell t.
thalidomide
Thalitone
thallium (Tl)
t. electrocardiogram
t. myocardial scintigraphy (TMS)
t. perfusion imaging
t. rest-redistribution scintigraphy
t. scanning
t. sestamibi (^{201}Tl sestamibi)
t. SPECT imaging
t. stress test
t. tomography
t. uptake
t. uptake defect
t. washout

thallium-201
t.-201 exercise stress test
t.-201 perfusion scintigraphy
t.-201 planar scintigraphy
t.-201 SPECT scintigraphy
thallous chloride Tl-201
Thal procedure
Tham
THB
total heart beats
tHcy
total homocysteine
total homocysteine level
THC:YAG laser
THD
transverse heart diameter
the
T. Cambridge Heart T-Wave Alternans Test
T. Closer suture-mediated closure system
T. Sports Breather
thebesian
t. circulation
t. foramina
t. valve
t. vein
Thebesius
vein of T.
theca cordis
Theden method
Theis rib retractor
Theo-24
Theobid
theobromine
Theochron
Theo-Dur
TheoFAST test
Theo-G
Theolair
Theolate
theophyllinate
choline t.
theophylline
t., ephedrine, and hydroxyzine (TEH)
t., ephedrine, and phenobarbital
t. ethylenediamine
t. and guaifenesin
t. sodium glycinate
theorem
Ba t.

NOTES

T

theorem *(continued)*
    Bayes t.
    Bernoulli t.
theory
    Bayliss t.
    Cannon t.
    chaos t.
    cross-linkage t.
    dipole t.
    immunological t.
    Melzack-Wall gate t.
    myogenic t.
    neuroendocrine t.
    neurogenic t.
    Ornish t.
    reentry t.
    response-to-injury t.
    sliding filament t.
    Spitzer t.
Theo-Sav
TheraCys
TheraKair mattress
TheraPEP
    T. positive expiratory pressure
      therapy system
    T. prerespiratory therapy treatment
therapeutic
    t. angiogenesis
    t. bronchoscopy
    t. dissection
    t. efficacy
    t. endpoint
    t. exercise (ther ex, ther ex)
    T. Intervention Scoring System
      (TISS)
    t. modality
    t. pneumothorax
therapist-driven protocol (TDP)
therapy
    AAV-CF t.
    ACE antisense gene t.
    amiodarone t.
    angina-guided t.
    angiotensin-converting enzyme
      antisense gene t.
    antiaggregant t.
    antialdosterone t.
    antiarrhythmic t.
    anticlot t.
    anticoagulant t. (ACT)
    antiendotoxin t.
    antihypertensive diuretic t.
    antiischemic t.
    antimicrobial t.
    antiplatelet t.
    antireflux t.
    antituberculous t.
    augmentation t.
    behavioral t.

beta-blocker t.
bretylium t.
bronchodilator t.
cardiac resynchronization t.
cardiac shock wave t. (CSWT)
cardiac shockwave t. (CSWT)
cerebral protective t.
chest physical t. (CPT)
chimeric-7E3 atiplatelet t.
CI t.
circulator boot t.
Clinitron air-fluidized t.
collapse t.
constraint-induced movement t.
Contak Renewal 3 system cardiac
  resynchronization t.
continuous nebulization t. (CNT)
coronary radiation t.
corrective t. (CT)
corticosteroid t.
cytotoxic gene t.
deep chest t.
device t.
directly observed t. (DOT)
diuretic t.
ECMO t.
efficacy of drug t.
electroconvulsive t.
embolization t.
empiric t.
endobronchial laser t.
endolaser venous t. (ELVT)
endovascular radiation t.
enoxaparin bridge t.
estrogen replacement t. (ERT)
extracorporeal cardiac shock
  wave t.
extracorporeal membrane
  oxygenation t.
fibrinolytic t.
first-line t.
fluid t.
gene t.
HBO t.
highly active antiretroviral t.
  (HAART)
high-output extended aerosol
  respiratory t.
Holter-guided antiarrhythmic drug t.
hormone replacement t. (HRT)
12-hour antiplatelet t.
hyperbaric oxygen t. (HBOT)
hypertensive hypervolemic t. (HHT)
immunosuppression t.
inhalation t.
intracoronary radiation t. (ICRT,
  IRT)
intraoperative intraarterial
  fibrinolytic t. (IIFT)

intravascular red light t. (IRLT)
intravenous immunoglobulin t.
ischemia-guided medical t.
kinetic t.
lipid-lowering t.
long-term oxygen t. (LTOT)
Lymphapress compression t.
maximum medical t.
monophasic shock t.
mucoactive t.
NCPAP t.
nebulized Ig t.
nitric oxide synthase gene t.
nonballoon t.
noncommitted biphasic shock t.
nonsurgical septal reduction t.
  (NSRT)
open-label ACE-inhibitor t.
oral anticoagulant t.
oral flecainide t.
oxygen t.
percutaneous intrapericardial fibrin-
  glue infusion t.
photodynamic t. (PTD)
physical t.
plaque stabilization t.
postthrombolytic t.
prophylactic t.
radiation t.
red light t. (RLT)
refractory to medical t.
Remedy sleep t.
reperfusion t.
rheologic t.
shock t.
somatic cell t.
statin t.
step-down t.
surfactant replacement t.
symptomatic t.
synchronous biatrial pacing t.
  (SYNBIAPACE)
thoracic radiation t. (TRT)
thrombolytic t. (TT)
transcardial catheter t. (TCT)
transcatheter t. (TCT)
transtracheal oxygen t. (TTOT)
TriaDyne II kinetic t.
TTO t.
VEGF gene t.
warfarin t.
zone t.

TheraSnore oral appliance
ther ex
  therapeutic exercise
thermal
  t. angiography
  t. dilution curve
  t. dilution technique
  t. dysregulation
  t. injury
  t. memory stent
  t. sensation
Thermedics cardiac device
thermic fever
thermistor
  t. plethysmography
thermoacoustic refrigeration
Thermoactinomyces
  T. candidus
  T. sacchari
  T. viridis
  T. vulgaris
Thermocardiosystems left ventricular
  assist device
ThermoChem-HT system
thermocouple, thermocoupler
thermodilution
  t. balloon catheter
  cardiac output by t. (COTD)
  t. cardiac output (TDCO)
  coronary sinus t.
  t. curve
  t.-derived
  Kim-Ray t.
  t. measurement
  t. method
  t. Swan-Ganz catheter
  t. technique
  t. test
thermoexpandable stent
ThermoFlo
  T. humidifier
  T. system
thermography
  infrared t.
thermometer
  infrared t.
  SureTemp electronic t.
  Thermoscan Pro-1-Instant t.
thermoplastic head mask
thermoresistible
  Mycobacterium t.
Thermoscan Pro-1-Instant thermometer

NOTES

thermosetting resin
ThermoVent heat and moisture
  exchanger
TherOx Aqueous Oxygen system
thesaurosis
    hairspray t.
THI
    Texas Heart Institute
    THI needle
thiabendazole
thiacetazone
thiamine deficiency
thiamylal sodium
thiazide diuretic
thiazolidinedione derivative
thickened pericardium
thickening
    cardiac wall t.
    diffuse intimal t.
    endocardial t.
    intimal t.
    intimal-medial t.
    leaflet t.
    mediastinal t.
    neointimal t.
    nodular interlobular septal t.
    peribronchovascular t.
    pleural t.
    pressure overload-induced aortic
      valve calcific t.
    residual pleural t.
    septal t.
    subvalvular t. (SVTh)
    valvular t.
    wall t.
thickness
    cap t.
    common carotid artery intima-
      media t. (CCA-IMT)
    end-diastolic t. (EDT)
    end-diastolic wall t. (EDWTH)
    interventricular septal t. (IVS)
    intimal-medial t. (IMT)
    left ventricular wall t. (LVWT)
    media t.
    myocardial wall t. (MWT)
    posterior wall t.
    relative wall t. (RWT)
    right ventricular wall t. (RVWT)
    skin-fold t.
    wall t. (WT)
thick and sticky mucus
thienopyridine
thigh-high antiembolic stockings
thimble valvotomy
ThinLine
    T. EZ bipolar pacemaker lead
    T. EZ pacing lead

thinning
    infarct t.
    shear t.
    ventricular wall t.
thin-section CT
thin-slice CT scan
thin-walled
    t.-w. catheter
    t.-w. needle
thioamide
thiobarbituric
    t. acid-reactive
    t. acid reactive substance (TBARS)
thiocarlide
thiocyanate
thiolprotease
thionamide
thiopental sodium
thiopentone sodium
Thioplex
thioridazine hydrochloride
thiosemicarbazide
thiosemicarbazone
thiosulfate
    sodium t.
thiotepa
thioxanthene
third
    t. heart sound (S₃)
    t. sound rumble
third-degree
    t.-d. atrioventricular block
    t.-d. A-V block
    t.-d. heart block
third-generation cephalosporin
third-order Butterworth filter
thixotropy
Thoma ampulla
Thomas
    T. LT endotracheal tube holder
    T. Quick Block endotracheal tube
      holder
    T. shunt
Thom flap laryngeal reconstruction
  method
Thompson-Hatina method
Thomsen disease
Thomsen-Friedenreich (TF)
    T.-F. antigen
thoracalgia
thoracalis
    aorta t.
thoracentesis
    Argyle-Turkel t.
    blind t.
    t. needle
thoraces (*pl. of* thorax)
thoracic
    t. actinomycosis

t. aorta (ThA)
t. aortic aneurysm (TAA)
t. aortic atherosclerotic plaque
t. aortic dissection
t. aortic rupture (TAR)
t. arch aortography
t. asphyxiant dystrophy
t. axis
t. cage
t. compliance
t. compressive syndrome
t. computed tomography (TCT)
t. crisis
t. crush injury
t. duct
t. duct drainage (TDD)
t. duct ligation
t. electrical bioimpedance (TEB)
t. empyema
t. endometriosis syndrome (TES)
t. esophagus
t. expanding action
t. gas
t. gas volume (TGV, V_{TG})
t. impedance
t. inferior vena cava (TIVC)
t. inlet
t. limb
t. nerve
t. outlet compression syndrome
t. outlet syndrome (TOS)
t. paracentesis
t. part of esophagus
t. percutaneous needle aspiration (TPNA)
t. radiation therapy (TRT)
t. radiologist
t. respiration
t. splenosis
t. squeeze
t. stent graft
t. surgeon
t. trauma
t. vertebral body
t. vessel

thoracica
aorta t.
thoracicae
rami esophageales aortae t.
thoracic-pelvic-phalangeal dystrophy
thoracicus
ductus t.

thoracis
paracentesis t.
thoracoabdominal
t. aortic aneurysm
t. dyssynchrony
t. paradox
thoracocardiography
thoracocentesis
repeated ultrasound-guided needle t.
thoracodorsal artery
thoracodynia
thoracolumbar
thoracopagus twin
thoracophrenolaparotomy
thoracoplasty
apical tailoring t.
costoversion t.
Delorme t.
Fowler t.
Schede t.
Wilms t.
thoracoport
t. placement
Soft t.
thoracoschisis
thoracoscope
rigid t.
thoracoscopic
t. apical pleurectomy
t. talc insufflation
t. talc pleurodesis
thoracoscopy
video-assisted t. (VAT, VATS)
thoracosternotomy
transverse t.
thoracostomy
closed chest t.
closed-tube t.
needle t.
prophylactic t.
tube t.
t. tube
thoracotome
Bettman-Fovash t.
thoracotomy
anterior t.
emergent t.
t. incision
Lewis t.
posterolateral t.
Thora-Drain III chest drainage

T

NOTES

Thora-Klex
    T.-K. chest drainage system
    T.-K. chest tube
Thora-Port
thorascopic
    t. apical pleurectomy
    t. talc pleurodesis
Thoraseal chest tube drainage system
Thora-Seal III chest drainage unit
Thoratec
    T. biventricular assist device
    T. cardiac device
    T. pump
    T. right ventricular assist device
    T. VAD system
thorax, pl. **thoraces**
    amazon t.
    t. asthenicus
    barrel-shaped t.
    cholesterol t.
    compages t.
    empyema t.
    frozen t.
    muscle of t.
    t. paralyticus
    Peyrot t.
    piriform t.
    semispinal muscle of t.
    spinal muscle of t.
    transverse muscle of t.
Thorazine
Thorel
    T. bundle
    T. pathway
Thornell microlaryngoscopy
Thornton anterior positioner (TAP)
Thorotrast
Thorpe flowmeter
THP
    transthoracic portography
THR
    target heart rate
thread
    mucous t.
thready pulse
threatened
    t. closure
    t. myocardial infarction (TMI)
three-block claudication
three-chambered heart
three-channel
    t.-c. electrocardiogram
    t.-c. Holter monitor
three-dimensional (3D)
    t.-d. echocardiography (3DE)
    t.-d. Fourier transform (3DFT)
    t.-d. helical computed tomography
    t.-d. intravascular ultrasound

    t.-d. spoiled gradient-recalled
      acquisition image
    t.-d. tagged magnetic resonance
      imaging
    t.-d. time-of-flight (3DTF)
    t.-d. time-of-flight magnetic
      resonance angiography
three-pillow orthopnea
three-turn epicardial lead
three-vessel coronary disease
three-way stopcock
threonine protein kinase
thresher's lung
threshing fever
threshold
    aerobic t.
    anaerobic t. (AT)
    anginal perceptual t.
    atrial capture t.
    atrial defibrillation t.
    atrial fibrillation t.
    backscatter t.
    capture t.
    cardioversion t.
    cough t.
    defibrillation t. (DFT, DT)
    t. dose
    fibrillation t.
    flicker fusion t.
    ischemic t.
    lactate t.
    lead t.
    nociceptive t.
    pacemaker t.
    pacing t.
    t. pacing
    T. PEP device
    t. percussion
    t. resistor
    risk t.
    stimulation t.
    t. trend
    t. value
    ventilation t.
    ventilatory t.
    ventilatory anaerobic t. (VAT)
    ventricular capture t.
    ventricular premature contraction t.
      (VPCT)
    work t.
threw an embolus
thrill
    aneurysmal t.
    aortic t.
    arterial t.
    coarse t.
    dense t.
    diastolic t.
    parasternal systolic t.

precordial t.
presystolic t.
purring t.
systolic t.
ThrO
thrombotic occlusion
throm, thromb
thrombosis
thrombasthenia
Glanzmann t.
Thrombate III
thrombectomize
thrombectomy
catheter t.
intracoronary aspiration t. (ICAT)
mechanical t.
percutaneous mechanical t. (PMT)
percutaneous rotational t. (PRT)
rheolytic coronary t.
shredding embolectomy t. (SET)
Thrombex
T. PMT
T. PMT system
thrombi (*pl. of* thrombus)
thrombin
clot-bound t.
t. clotting time (TCT)
t. generation
t. time (TT)
topical t.
thrombin-antithrombin (TAT)
t.-a. III complex
thrombin-soaked Gelfoam
thromboangiitis obliterans
thromboaortopathy
occlusive t.
thromboarteritis
thromboaspiration
thromboclasis
thromboclastic
thrombocystis
thrombocytapheresis
thrombocythemia
thrombocytopenia
t.-absent radius (TAR)
t.-absent radius syndrome
drug-induced t.
essential t.
heparin-associated t. (HAT)
heparin-induced t. (HIT)
idiopathic t.
immune t.

lipopolysaccharide-induced t.
malignant t.
thrombocytosis
thromboelastogram (TEG)
thromboelastograph
thromboelastography (TEG)
thromboembolectomy
thromboembolic
t. complication (TEC)
t. disease (TED)
t. pulmonary hypertension
t. stroke
t. syndrome
thromboembolism (TE)
pulmonary t.
pulmonary artery t. (PATE)
recurring venous t. (RVTE)
septic t.
systemic t.
venous t. (VTE)
thromboendarterectomy (TEA)
thromboendarteritis
thromboendocarditis
Thrombogen
thrombogenic
t. component
t. stimulus
thrombogenicity
coil t.
thromboglobulin
beta t.
thromboid
thrombolic
thrombolizer
Angiocor rotational t.
Thrombolizer catheter
thrombolus
thrombolysis
coronary t.
t. in myocardial infarction flow
t. in myocardial infarction frame
count
pharmomechanical t.
pulsed-spray pharmomechanical t.
pulse-spray pharmomechanical t.
selective intracoronary t. (SICT)
**thrombolysis-related intracranial
hemorrhage (TICH)**
thrombolytic
t. agent
T. Assessment System (TAS)

T

NOTES

727

thrombolytic *(continued)*
    t. predictive instrument (TPI)
    t. therapy (TT)
thrombomodulin (TM)
thrombophilia
thrombophilic factor V Leiden mutation
thrombophlebitis (TP)
    t. migrans (TPM)
    t. saltans
thromboplastin (PT)
    partial t. time (PTT, ptt)
    t. time (TT)
thrombopoietin (TPO)
thrombosed
thrombosis, pl. **thromboses (throm, thromb)**
    abacterial t.
    t. activation
    acute t. (AT)
    acute occlusive t. (AOT)
    agonal t.
    aortic t.
    aortoiliac t.
    arterial t.
    atrophic t.
    brachial artery t.
    cardiac t.
    catheter-induced t.
    cavernous sinus t.
    central splanchnic venous t. (CSVT)
    cerebral t.
    cerebral venous t. (CVT)
    cerebrovascular t.
    coagulation t.
    compression t.
    coronary t. (CT)
    coronary artery t.
    cortical vein t.
    creeping t.
    deep venous t. (DVT)
    dilation t.
    effort-induced t.
    embolic t.
    femoral artery t.
    femoral venous t.
    heparin-associated thrombocytopenia and t. (HATT)
    heparin-induced thrombocytopenia and t. (HITT)
    iliac vein t.
    incomplete t.
    infective t.
    inferior vena cava t. (IVCT)
    in situ t.
    in-stent t.
    intraarterial t.
    intramural t.
    IVC t.

    t. of jugular bulb
    jumping t.
    laser-induced t.
    marantic t.
    marasmic t.
    mural t. (MT)
    nonobstructive valve t.
    obstructive valve t.
    Paget-von Schrötter venous t.
    partial confluens sinuum t.
    perigraft t.
    plate t.
    platelet t.
    portal vein t. (PVT)
    t. prevention trial (TPT)
    propagating t.
    prosthetic mitral valve t.
    puerperal t.
    pulmonary t. (PT)
    residual deep vein t.
    Ribbert t.
    sinus t.
    stent t. (ST)
    straight sinus t.
    subacute t. (SAT)
    subclavian vein t. (SVT)
    superimposed t.
    traumatic t.
    venous t.
thrombospondin-1,-2
thrombostasis
Thrombostat
Thrombotest
thrombotic
    t. brain infarction (TBI)
    t. endocarditis
    t. microangiopathy (TMA)
    t. occlusion (ThrO, TO)
    t. thrombocytopenic purpura (TTP)
Thrombo-Wellcotest method
thromboxane
    t. A_2
    t. receptor antagonist
    t. synthesis
    t. synthetase inhibitor
thrombus, pl. **thrombi (T)**
    acute occlusive t. (AOT)
    adherent mobile t.
    adherent mural t.
    agglutinative t.
    agonal t.
    antemortem t.
    anular t.
    atrial t.
    ball valve t.
    blood plate t.
    blood platelet t.
    calcified t.
    capillary thrombi

coral t.
currant jelly t.
fibrin t.
t. formation time (TFT)
free-floating t. (FFT)
free-floating vena caval t.
globular t.
t. grade
hyaline t.
infective t.
intracardiac t. (ICT)
intragraft t.
intraluminal t.
intramural t.
intravascular t.
LAA thrombi
laminated t.
lateral t.
left atrial t. (LAT)
marantic t.
marasmic t.
massive t.
migratory t.
mixed t.
mural t. (MT)
mural thrombi
obstructive t.
occluding t.
occlusive t.
organized t.
pale t.
parietal t.
pedunculated t.
plate t.
platelet t.
postmortem t.
t. precursor protein (TpT)
T. Precursor Protein immunoassay
primary t.
progressive t.
propagated t.
propagation of t.
red coronary t.
right atrial t.
right atrial mobile thrombi
  (RAMT)
saddle t.
secondary t.
straddling t.
stratified t.
t. stripper
traumatic t.

valvular t.
ventricular t.
white coronary t.
thrombus-filled cavity
through-and-through
  t.-a.-t. continuous suture
  t.-a.-t. myocardial infarction
through-the-balloon ultrasound
through-the-needle catheter
through-the-wall mattress suture
throw an embolus
thrush
  t. breast
  t. breast heart
thrust
  cardiac t.
thryotrophin
thulium
  t.-holmium-chromium:yttrium-
    aluminum-garnet laser
  t.-holmium:YAG laser
  t.:YAG laser angioplasty
thumbprint bronchus sign
thump
  chest t.
  precordial t.
Thumper 1007 CPR system
thumpversion
thymectomy
  video-assisted thoracoscopic t.
thymic
  t. asthma
  t. cyst
thymidine phosphorylase
thymoma
thymopentin
thymostimuline
thymusectomy
Thyro-Block
thyrocardiac disease
thyrocervicalis
  truncus t.
thyroid
  aberrant t.
  accessory t.
  t. antibody
  Armour T.
  t. bruit
  t. cachexia
  t. disease
  t. extract
  t. function test

T

NOTES

thyroid *(continued)*
　　t. gland
　　intrathoracic t.
　　t. isthmus
　　lingual t.
　　t. notch
　　t. panel
　　retrosternal t.
　　t. storm
　　T. Strong
　　substernal t.
　　t. tumor
thyroideae
　　musculus levator glandulae t.
thyroidectomy
thyroiditis
　　chronic lymphocytic t.
　　de Quervain t.
　　Hashimoto t.
　　Riedel t.
　　woody t.
thyroid-stimulating hormone (TSH)
thyrointoxication
Thyrolar
thyrolaryngeal
thyrolingual duct
thyromegaly
thyropalatine
thyropharyngeal
thyroprival
thyrotoxic heart disease
thyrotoxicosis
thyrotoxin radioisotope assay
thyrotropin-releasing hormone response
thyroxine, thyroxin (T₄)
D-thyroxine
L-thyroxine
TI
　　tricuspid incompetence
　　tricuspid insufficiency
TIA
　　transient ischemic attack
　　　　crescendo TIA
　　　　vertebrobasilar TIA
TIA + CE
　　transient ischemic attack plus carotid
　　　　endarterectomy
TIAH
　　total implantation of artificial heart
tiamenidine
tiapamil
Tiazac extended-release capsule
Tibbs arterial cannula
tibial
　　t. artery
　　t. pulse
tibioperoneal vessel angioplasty
TICA
　　terminal internal carotid artery

Ticar
ticarcillin
　　t. and clavulanate potassium
　　t. and clavulanic acid
　　t. disodium
TICH
　　thrombolysis-related intracranial
　　　　hemorrhage
tick
　　t. anticoagulant peptide
　　t. paralysis
Ticlid
ticlopidine
　　t. hydrochloride
　　t. plus aspirin (T + A)
Ti-Cron suture
tic-tac
　　t.-t. rhythm
　　t.-t. sounds
TICU
　　trauma intensive care unit
TID
　　transient ischemic dilation
Tidal
　　T. balloon catheter
　　T. Wave handheld capnograph
　　T. Wave Sp capnometer/pulse
　　　　oximeter
tidal
　　t. air
　　t. breathing
　　t. breathing flow-volume (TBFV)
　　t. expiratory flow at 25% of tidal
　　　　volume (TEF₂₅)
　　t. expiratory flow at 50% of tidal
　　　　volume (TEF₅₀)
　　t. expiratory flow at 75% of tidal
　　　　volume (TEF₇₅)
　　t. expiratory volume (TV_E)
　　t. flow
　　t. flow-volume loop (TFVL)
　　t. inspiratory flow at 50% of tidal
　　　　volume (TIF₅₀)
　　t. inspiratory volume (TV_I)
　　t. loop
　　t. volume (TV, V_T)
　　t. wave
　　t. wave pulse
TIE
　　transient ischemic episode
　　transient ischemic event
tiered-therapy
　　t.-t. antiarrhythmic device
　　t.-t. implantable cardioverter-
　　　　defibrillator
　　t.-t. programmable cardioverter-
　　　　defibrillator
Tietze syndrome

TIF$_{50}$
    tidal inspiratory flow at 50% of tidal
    volume
tiger
        t. heart
        t. lily heart
tight
        t. asthmatic
        t. junction
        t. stenosis
tightness
        chest t.
tigroid striation
TIJ lead
Tikosyn
Tilade Inhalation Aerosol
Tildiem
tilt
        first-phase t.
        head-up t. (HUT)
        second-phase t.
        t. test
        t. vital signs
tilting
        t. disk aortic valve prosthesis
        t. disk heart valve
        t. disk occluder
        t. disk prosthetic valve
        passive t.
tilt-table test (TTT)
TIM
        tissue-infiltrating macrophage
        transthoracic intracardiac monitoring
Tim-AK
time
        acceleration t.
        acquisition t.
        activated clotting t. (ACT)
        activated coagulation t. (ACT)
        activated partial thromboplastin t.
            (APTT, aPTT)
        AH conduction t.
        arm-tongue t.
        arteriovenous passage t. (AVP)
        aspirin tolerance t. (ATT)
        atrioventricular t.
        t. in bed
        t. between the P wave and
            beginning of QRS complex (P-R)
        bleeding t. (BLT, Blx, BT)
        blood-clot lysis t. (BLT)
        buildup t. (T$_b$)

        bypass t.
        capacitor forming t.
        carotid ejection t.
        central motor conduction t.
            (CMCT)
        cerebral transit t. (cTT)
        charge t.
        circulation t.
        clot lysis t. (CLT)
        clot retraction t.
        clotting t. (CLT, CT)
        coagulation t. (CT)
        cold ischemic t. (CIT)
        t. compensation gain (TCG)
        conduction t.
        corrected ejection t. (ETc)
        corrected sinus node recovery t.
            (CNRT)
        cross-clamp t.
        dead t.
        deceleration t.
        detect t.
        direct sinoatrial conduction t.
            (DSACT, D-SACT)
        t. domain
        t. domain signal-averaged
            electrocardiogram
        t. domain signal-averaged
            electrocardiography
        donor organ ischemic t.
        door-to-balloon t.
        door-to-needle t.
        doubling t.
        Duke bleeding t.
        echo delay t. (TE)
        ejection t. (ET)
        esophageal transit t.
        euglobulin clot lysis t.
        expiratory t. (T$_E$)
        extubation t.
        t. of flight (TOF)
        t. of flight and absorbance
            (TOFA)
        t. of flight and absorbance
            spectrophotometry
        flushing t.
        forced expiratory t. (FET)
        t. forced expiratory rate
        His-ventricle conduction t.
        H-R conduction t.
        H-V conduction t.
        hydrogen appearance t.

NOTES

T

time *(continued)*

    inspiratory t. (T_I)
    interatrial conduction t.
    intraatrial conduction t.
    intubation t.
    isovolumetric t. (IVT)
    isovolumic relaxation t. (IVRT)
    Ivy bleeding t.
    junctional recovery t. (JRT)
    kaolin-cephalin clotting t. (KCCT)
    kaolin partial thromboplastin t. (KPTT)
    left ventricular ejection t. (LVEJT, LVET)
    longitudinal relaxation t.
    lung-to-finger circulation t. (LFCT)
    lysis t.
    magnetic relaxation t.
    maximum walking t.
    median survival t. (MST)
    partial thromboplastin t. (PTT, ptt)
    peak ejection t. (PET)
    t. to peak expiratory flow (tPTEF)
    t. to peak inspiratory flow (tPTIF)
    P-H conduction t.
    prothrombin t. (PT, PTT)
    prothrombin time/partial thromboplastin t. (PT/PTT)
    pulse transmission t. (PTT)
    quick prothrombin t.
    ratio of inspiratory time to total breathing cycle t. (T_I/T_{TOT})
    relaxation t.
    repetition t. (TR)
    right ventricular ejection t. (RVET)
    right ventricular isovolumic relaxation t. (RV-IVRT)
    saturation t.
    serial thrombin t. (STT)
    sinoatrial conduction t. (SACT)
    sinoatrial recovery t. (SART)
    sinus node recovery t. (SNRT, SRT)
    spin-lattice t.
    spin-spin t.
    survival t.
    systolic t. (ST)
    systolic acceleration t. (SAT)
    systolic upstroke t.
    thrombin t. (TT)
    thrombin clotting t. (TCT)
    thromboplastin t. (TT)
    thrombus formation t. (TFT)
    time to peak expiratory flow and total expiration t. (tPTEF/tE)
    total ejection t. (TET)
    total sleep t. (TST)
    transmitral E-wave deceleration t.
    T2 relaxation t.

    turnaround t. (TAT)
    venous clotting t. (VCT)
    ventilator t.
    ventricular activation t. (VAT)
    ventricular ejection t. (VET)
    wake after sleep onset t. (WASO)

time-activity curve
time-averaged peak velocity
time-based
    t.-b. counter
    t.-b. event recording
time-compensated gain
time-cycled ventilation
time-cycling
timed
    t. forced expiratory volume
    t. vital capacity
time-domain analysis
time-gain
    t.-g. compensation (TGC)
    t.-g. control (TGC)
Timentin
time-of-flight
    t.-o.-f. effect
    t.-o.-f. magnetic resonance angiography (TOF MRA)
time-resolved imaging by automatic data segmentation (TRIADS)
time-to-peak
    t.-t.-p. contrast
    t.-t.-p. filling rate
time-triggered
time-varied
    t.-v. gain (TVG)
    t.-v. gain control (TGC, TVGC)
TIMI
    transmural inferior myocardial infarction
    TIMI classification
    TIMI criteria
    TIMI flow
    TIMI flow grade 0–3
    TIMI frame count
    TIMI frame count index
    TIMI myocardial perfusion grade
    TIMI patency
timing circuit
Timolide
timolol maleate
timori
    Brugia t.
TIMP
    tissue inhibitor of metalloproteinase
TIMP-3
    tissue inhibitor of metalloproteinase-3
    TIMP-3 overexpression
Timpe and Runyon *Mycobacteria* classification
Tina-quant immunoturbidimetric assay

tined
    t. lead pacemaker
    t. ventricular electrode
tine test
tinidazole
tinkle
    Bouillaud t.
    metallic t.
tin oxide
TintElize PAI-1 ELISA kit
tinzaparin
    t. sodium
    t. sodium injection
tiotropium bromide
tip
    t. extrasystole
    Luer-Lok needle t.
    Medtronic t.
    mitral leaflet t.
    t. occluder
    papillary muscle t.
    Sensor PTFE-nitinol guidewire with
      hydrophilic t.
    Skimmer laryngeal blade t.
    Tricut laryngeal blade t.
tip-deflecting wire
TIPP
    transilluminated powered phlebectomy
tiprenolol hydrochloride
TIPS
    transjugular intrahepatic portosystemic
    shunt
tiptoe test
tirilazad mesylate
tirofiban
TISS
    Therapeutic Intervention Scoring System
**Tissomat application device and spray
set**
Tissot spirometer
tissue
    t. ablation
    adipose t.
    atrioventricular conduction t.
    autodigestion of connective t.
    t. bank
    bronchopulmonary t.
    bronchus-associated lymphoid t.
      (BALT)
    caseated t.
    connective t.
    dissected t.

    t. Doppler imaging (TDI)
    t. engineering
    extrathoracic soft t.
    exuberant granulation t. (EGT)
    t. factor
    t. factor pathway inhibitor (TFPI)
    fast t.
    t. fissure
    granulation t.
    gut-associated lymphoid t. (GALT)
    His-Purkinje t.
    t. hypoperfusion
    t. inhibitor of metalloproteinase
      (TIMP)
    t. inhibitor of metalloproteinase-3
      (TIMP-3)
    t. inhibitor of metalloproteinase-3
      overexpression
    interfascicular fibrous t.
    laminated connective t.
    myocardial t.
    myocardial scar t.
    t. necrosis
    neointimal t.
    nodal t.
    perinodal t.
    t. plasminogen activator (tPA)
    t. plasminogen activator inhibitor
      (tPAI)
    t. plasminogen activator release
      deficiency
    t. preservation
    resistance to movement of lung t.
      (Rti)
    t. septa
    slow t.
    t. supersaturation
    t. valve
tissue-infiltrating macrophage (TIM)
tissue-specific antibody
tissue-type plasminogen activator
titanium cage
**Titan mega XL PTCA dilatation
catheter**
titer
    antiheart antibody t.
    anti-Rho(D) t.
    bactericidal t.
    Lyme t.
    serum bactericidal t. (SBT)
titration regimen
titrator

NOTES

tI/tTOT
>ratio of inspiration time and total time of breathing cycle

TIVC
>thoracic inferior vena cava

tizanidine hydrochloride

Tl
>thallium

Tl-201
>Tl-201 perfusion tracer
>thallous chloride Tl-201

²⁰¹Tl
>²⁰¹Tl sestamibi

TLA
>translumbar aortogram
>transluminal angioplasty

TLC
>total lung capacity

TLC-II portable VAD driver

TLCO, TLco
>carbon monoxide transfer factor

TLI
>total lymphoid irradiation

TLR
>target lesion revascularization
>toll-like receptor

TM
>thrombomodulin
>transatrial membranotomy

TMA
>thrombotic microangiopathy

TMC
>Tokyo Medical College
>transmyocardial mechanical channeling
>>TMC needle

TMET
>treadmill exercise test

TMI
>threatened myocardial infarction
>transmural myocardial infarction

TMLR
>transmyocardial laser revascularization

TMP-SMX
>trimethoprim-sulfamethoxazole

TMR
>transmyocardial revascularization
>>Heart Laser for TMR

TMS
>thallium myocardial scintigraphy
>>TMS 1000 tachyarrhythmia monitoring system

TMST
>treadmill stress test

TMZ
>trimetazidine 1

TNB
>transthoracic needle biopsy

TNF
>tumor necrosis factor

TNF-alpha
>tumor necrosis factor-alpha

TNKase, TNK-tPA
>tenecteplase

TNM
>tumor, node, metastasis
>>TNM classification
>>TNM staging

TnT
>troponin C, I, T

TO
>thrombotic occlusion
>total obstruction

To
>tricuspid opening

to-and-fro
>t.-a.-f. murmur
>t.-a.-f. sound

tobacco heart

TOBI Inhalation Solution

toborinone

tobramycin
>nebulized t.
>t. solution for inhalation

tocainide hydrochloride

Todaro
>tendon of T.
>T. tendon
>T. triangle

TOD/CCD
>target organ disease/clinical cardiovascular disease

Todd
>T. Hewitt broth
>T. units

toes
>clubbing of t.

TOF
>tetralogy of Fallot
>time of flight
>>TOF MRA
>>>time-of-flight magnetic resonance angiography

TOFA
>time of flight and absorbance
>>TOFA spectrophotometry

Tofranil

TOF, T of F
>tetralogy of Fallot

tofu

Togaviridae virus

toilet, toilette
>bronchial t.
>pleural t.
>pulmonary t.
>respiratory t.
>tracheobronchial t.

toilet-seat
    t.-s. angina
    t.-s. syncope
Tokyo Medical College (TMC)
tolazamide
tolazoline
    t. hydrochloride
    t. test
tolbutamide
tolerance
    exercise t.
    hemodynamic t.
    impaired glucose t. (IGT)
    poor exercise t. (PET)
Tolinase
toll-like receptor (TLR)
toluene diisocyanate (TDI)
toluidine blue stain
Tolu-Sed DM
Tomcat PTCA guidewire
tomogram
    horizontal long-axis t.
    short-axis t.
    vertical long-axis t.
tomograph
    ECAT III positron t.
tomographic
    high-resolution thin section
      computed t.
    t. radionuclide imaging
    t. radionuclide ventriculography
tomography
    adaptive current t. (ACT)
    adenosine triphosphate single-photon
      emission computed t. (ATP-
      SPECT)
    atrial bolus dynamic computer t.
    axial computed t. (ACT)
    biplanar t.
    Cardiac Protect t.
    cardiovascular computed t. (CVCT)
    cine computed t.
    computed t. (CT)
    computerized axial t. (CAT)
    dual-isotope simultaneous acquisition
      single-photon emission
      computed t. (DISA-SPECT)
    electrical impedance t. (EIT)
    electron beam computed t. (EBCT)
    gated computed t.
    high-resolution computed t. (HRCT)

intravenously enhanced computed t.
    (IVCT)
methoxyisobutyl isonitrile single-
    photon emission computed t.
    (MIBI-SPECT)
multidetector computed t. (MDCT)
multislice spiral computed t.
    (MSCT)
myocardial single photon
    emission t. (MSPECT)
N-13 ammonia positron emission t.
optical coherence t. (OCT)
positron emission t. (PET)
quantitative computed t. (QCT)
rapid acquisition computed axial t.
    (RACAT)
rubidium-82 positron emission t.
seven-pinhole t.
single-photon emission t.
single-photon emission computed t.
    (SPECT)
slant hole t.
spiral computed t.
technetium-99m sestamibi single-
    photon emission computed t.
technetium-99m-sestamibi single-
    photon emission computed t.
thallium t.
thoracic computed t. (TCT)
three-dimensional helical
    computed t.
ultrafast computed t. (UFCT)
ultrafast contrast-enhanced chest
    computed t.
xenon-enhanced computed t.
    (XECT)
x-ray cine computed t.
TomTec
    T. echo platform
    T. Imaging Systems
tone
    bronchial smooth muscle t.
    cardiac vagal t.
    fetal heart t. (FHT)
    heart t.'s (ht)
    resting vascular t.
    Traube double t.
    vagal t.
    vasomotor t.
    Williams tracheal t.
tongs
    Trippi-Wells t.

T

NOTES

tongue
    smoker's t.
    strawberry t.
    t. traction
tongue-jaw lift
tongue-retaining device
tongue-rolling effect
Tonocard
tonometer
    air-puff t.
    Gärtner t.
    Linear KGT t.
tonometered whole blood
tonometry
    applanation t.
    peripheral artery t.
tonoscillograph
tonsil
    Gerlach t.
    kissing t.'s
    laryngeal t.
    lingual t.
    Luschka t.
    palatine t.
    pharyngeal t.
tonsilla
    t. lingualis
    t. palatina
    t. pharyngealis
tonsillar
    t. pillar
    t. ring
    t. Somnoplasty procedure
    t. Somnoplasty system
tonsillaris
    angina t.
tonsillitis
    caseous t.
    chronic catarrhal t.
    diphtherial t.
tonsilloadenoidectomy
tonus
    vasomotor t. (VMT)
tool
    cardiovascular self-assessment t.
    (CST)
    congestive heart failure data t.
    (CHFDT)
    LIMA-Lift t.
    LIMA-Loop t.
    vascular anatomy teaching t.
    (VATT)
Top-Hat supraannular aortic valve
topical
    Aquacare t.
    Bactroban T.
    Benadryl T.
    Carmol t.
    t. cooling

    Efudex T.
    Fluoroplex T.
    Gelfoam T.
    t. hypothermia
    Lanaphilic t.
    Mycostatin T.
    Nutraplus t.
    Oxsoralen T.
    Rogaine t.
    Solarcaine t.
    t. thrombin
    Ultra Mide t.
topography
    NMR t.
Toposar injection
topotecan
Toprol XL
Torcon
    T. NB Advantage coronary
    angiographic catheter
    T. NB selective angiographic
    catheter
Torek resection of thoracic esophagus
toremifene
Tornado embolization coil
Tornalate
Tornwaldt cyst
toroidal valve
Toronto
    T. Alexithymia Scale
    T. SPV aortic valve
    T. SPV bioprosthesis
    T. SPV stentless porcine heart
    valve
torpedo-shaped pattern
Torq-Flex wire guide
torque
    clockwise t.
    t. control
    t. control balloon catheter
    t. tube catheter
    t. vise
torquer
    Clip On t.
torquing ability
torr
    t. pressure
    t. unit
Torricelli
    T. law
    T. model
    T. orifice equation
torsade
    t. de pointes (TDP, TdP)
    t. de pointes ventricular tachycardia
torsemide
tortuosity
tortuous
    t. right coronary artery

t. veins
t. vessel
Torula histolytica
Torulopsis glabrata
torulosis
torus aorticus
TOS
thoracic outlet syndrome
toxic oil syndrome
Toshiba
T. biplane transesophageal transducer
T. electrocardiography machine
T. MRT 200 MRI
T. scanner
T. Sonolayer SSH-140A ultrasound
tosylate
bretylium t.
total
t. absence of circulation on four-vessel angiography
t. acidity
t. adenine nucleotides (TAN)
t. airway resistance (Rtot)
t. alternans
t. anomalous pulmonary venous connection (TAPVC)
t. anomalous pulmonary venous drainage (TAPVD)
t. anomalous pulmonary venous return (TAPVR)
t. anterior circulation infarct (TACI)
t. anterior circulation syndrome (TACS)
t. apexcardiographic relaxation time index (TARTI)
t. artificial heart (TAH)
t. atrial blanking (TAB)
t. atrial blanking period
t. atrial refractory period (TARP)
t. atrioventricular block (TAVB)
t. axial node irradiation (TANI)
t. blood volume (TBV)
t. body irradiation (TBI)
t. bypass (TBP)
t. cardiopulmonary bypass (TCB)
t. cavopulmonary anastomosis
t. cavopulmonary connection (TCP, TCPC)
t. cavopulmonary shunt (TCPS)
t. cholesterol (TC)

cholesterol, t. (CT)
t. cholesterol/high-density lipoproteins (TC/HDL)
t. chordal-sparing mitral valve replacement
t. circulatory arrest (TCA)
t. coronary flow (TCF)
t. coronary score (TCS)
T. Cross balloon catheter
t. ejection time (TET)
t. electromechanical systole (QS_2)
t. end-diastolic diameter (TEDD)
t. end-systolic diameter (TESD)
t. heart beats (THB)
t. homocysteine (tHcy)
t. homocysteine level (tHcy)
t. implantation of artificial heart (TIAH)
t. lung capacity (TLC)
t. lung compliance
t. lymphoid irradiation (TLI)
t. obstruction (TO)
T. O_2 delivery system
T. O_2/Oxilite oxygen system
T. O_2 supplementary oxygen system
t. patient shock count
t. peripheral resistance
t. peripheral resistance index (TPRI)
t. peripheral vascular resistance (TPVR)
t. peroxyl radical-trapping antioxidant potential (TRAP)
t. plasma cholesterol (TPC)
positive symptom t. (PST)
t. pressure (P_T)
t. pulmonary blood flow (TPBF)
t. pulmonary resistance
t. pulmonary vascular resistance (TPVR)
t. repair of tetralogy of Fallot
t. revascularization off pump by coronary artery bypass (TROPCAB)
t. right ventricular volume (TRVV)
t. sleep time (TST)
T. Synchrony System
t. systemic vascular resistance (TSVR)
t. vascular resistance (TVR)

T

NOTES

totally endoscopic coronary artery bypass (TECAB)
touch shock count
Toupet hemifundoplication
Tourguide guiding catheter
tourniquet
    Esmarch t.
    pneumatic t.
    Rumel t.
    Shenstone t.
Touro
    T. Ex
    T. LA
TOVA
    trigger of ventricular arrhythmia
Tovell tube
Townes-Brocks syndrome
toxemia
toxemic pneumonia
toxic
    t. agent
    t. delirium
    t. epidermal necrolysis
    t. fume inhalation
    t. myocarditis
    t. oil syndrome (TOS)
    t. shock
toxicity
    amphetamine t.
    anthracycline t.
    antimony t.
    cobalt t.
    dextroamphetamine t.
    digitalis t.
    digoxin t.
    doxorubicin-induced cardiac t.
    emetine t.
    fluoride t.
    hydrocarbon t.
    oxygen t.
    phenylpropanolamine t.
    plant t.
toxicosis
    Aspergillus t.
toxin
    adenylate cyclase t.
    t. exposure
    pertussis t.
    RNA glycosidase t.
toxin-insensitive current
Toxocara canis
toxoid
    diphtheria and tetanus t.
Toxoplasma gondii
toxoplasmosis
ToxR protein
TP
    thrombophlebitis
    TP baseline

    TP interval
    TP segment
T&P, T+P
    temperature and pulse
TPA
    alteplase
tPA
    tissue plasminogen activator
tPAI
    tissue plasminogen activator inhibitor
TPBF
    total pulmonary blood flow
TPC
    total plasma cholesterol
TPG
    transpulmonary gradient
    transvalvular pressure gradient
T-Phyl
TPI
    thrombolytic predictive instrument
T-piece
    Ayers T-p.
    T-p. oxygen
    T-p. weaning
tpl
    transplantation
    transplanted
TPLV
    transient pulmonary vascular lability
TPM
    temporary pacemaker
    thrombophlebitis migrans
TPNA
    thoracic percutaneous needle aspiration
TPO
    thrombopoietin
TPP
    treadmill performance test
T-P-Q segment
TPRI
    total peripheral resistance index
TPST
    true positive stress test
TPT
    thrombosis prevention trial
TpT
    thrombus precursor protein
tPTEF
    time to peak expiratory flow
tPTEF/tE
    time to peak expiratory flow and total expiration time
tPTIF
    time to peak inspiratory flow
TPVR
    total peripheral vascular resistance
    total pulmonary vascular resistance
TQ segment

TR
 repetition time
 tricuspid regurgitation
trabecula, pl. **trabeculae**
 trabeculae carneae
 t. septomarginalis
trabecular hypertrophy
trabeculation
 muscle t.
trace
 t. metal
 T. vein stripper
tracer
 carbon-11 palmitic acid
  radioactive t.
 t. distribution
 frequency t.
 t. homogeneity
 iodine-123 heptadecanoic acid
  radioactive t.
 t. retention
 t. storage
 Tl-201 perfusion t.
 t. uptake
trach, trake
 tracheostomy
 trach plate
TrachCare
 neonatal Y T.
trachea, pl. **tracheae**
 anular ligament of t.
 bifurcatio tracheae
 bifurcation of t.
 carina of t.
 carina tracheae
 membranous wall of t.
 muscular coat of t.
 paries membranaceus tracheae
 scabbard t.
 steepling of t.
 tunica mucosa tracheae
 tunica muscularis tracheae
tracheal
 t. aspirate
 t. bifurcation
 t. branch
 t. bronchus
 t. button
 t. cartilage
 t. deviation
 t. gas insufflation (TGI)
 t. gland

 t. intubation
 t. lymph node
 t. mucosa
 t. mucus velocity
 t. rale
 t. ring
 t. sound
 t. steepling
 t. triangle
 t. tube
 t. tug
 t. vein
 t. wall injury with intermittent
  stoppage of tracheostomy and
  episodes of dyspnea (TWISTED)
tracheales
 cartilagines t.
 glandulae t.
 venae t.
trachealia
 ligamenta anularia t.
trachealis
 angina t.
 t. muscle
tracheitis
tracheobiliary
tracheobronchial
 t. amyloidosis
 t. angle
 t. aspirate
 t. clearance
 t. collapse
 t. diverticulum
 t. dyskinesia
 t. flora
 t. foreign body
 t. lavage
 t. toilet
 t. tree
 t. tuberculosis
tracheobronchitis
 Aspergillus t.
 influenza t.
 pseudomembranous *Aspergillus* t.
tracheobronchomalacia
tracheobronchomegaly
tracheobronchoscopy
tracheoesophageal (TE)
 t. fistula (TEF)
 t. junction
 t. puncture
tracheofissure

NOTES

T

tracheolaryngeal
Tracheolife HME
tracheomalacia
tracheopathia osteoplastica
tracheopharyngeal
tracheophonesis
tracheophony
tracheoscope
tracheostenosis
tracheostomized
tracheostomy (trach, trake)
    t. button
    t. cuff
    flap t.
    Great Ormond Street t.
    Griggs t.
    Montgomery t.
    percutaneous dilatational t. (PDT)
    percutaneous dilational t. (PDT)
    t. plate
    t. stoma
    subthyroid t.
    T. T.O.M. anatomical model
    t. tube
tracheotome
tracheotomy
    percutaneous t.
Trach-Mist Aerosol Drainage Bay
trachomatis
    Chlamydia t.
Trach-Talk trachesostomy tube
trachyphonia
tracing
    carotid pulse t.
    diamond-shaped t.
    fetal heart monitor t.
    jugular venous pulse t. (JVPT)
    pressure t.
    pulse t.
    serial ECG t.
    serial electrocardiogram t.
    stripchart t.
    venous pressure t.
    venous pulse t.
track
    tram t.
trackability
track-ball technique
tracker
    T. microcatheter
    Purkinje image t.
Tracker-18 Soft Stream side-hole
  microinfusion catheter
tracking
    bolus t.
    spatial t.
    wall t.
Tracleer
Tracrium

tract
    atriodextrofascicular t.
    atriofascicular t.
    atrio-His bypass t.
    atrionodal bypass t.
    bronchopulmonary t.
    bypass t.
    concealed bypass t.
    inflow t.
    James accessory t.'s
    left ventricular outflow t. (LVOT)
    lower respiratory t.
    nodohisian bypass t.
    nodoventricular t.
    outflow t.
    pulmonary outflow t.
    respiratory t.
    right ventricular inflow t. (RVIT)
    right ventricular outflow t. (RVOT)
    spinothalamic t.
    Wolff-Parkinson-White bypass t.
traction
    t. aneurysm
    bilateral carotid artery t. (BiCAT)
    t. bronchiectasis
    t. bronchiolectasis
    Crego t.
    papillary muscle t.
    t. suture
    tongue t.
tragacanth asthma
trailing edge
train
    drive t.
    t.'s of ventricular pacing
trainer
    CardioGrip cardiovascular t.
training
    CDBR respiratory muscle t.
    t. effect
    relaxation t.
    resistance t. (RT)
    strength t.
trainwheel rhythm
trait
    sickle cell t.
Trak Back pullback device
trake (var. of trach)
TRAKE-fit system
TrakPro data analysis software
Trakstar balloon catheter
tram
    t. line
    t. tracks
Trandate
    T. injection
    T. Oral
trandolapril and verapamil
tranexamic acid

tranilast
Tranquility
    T. Bilevel airway patency
      maintenance device
    T. Bilevel CPAP unit
    T. Bilevel positive airway pressure
      therapy device
    T. Quest CPAP device
    T. Quest CPAP System
tranquilizer
trans
    t. fat
    t. fatty acids (TFA)
TransAct intraaortic balloon pump
transaminase
    glutamic-oxaloacetic t. (GOT)
    serum glutamic-oxaloacetic t.
      (SGOT)
    serum glutamic-pyruvic t. (SGPT)
transaminitis
transanular patch
transaortic
    t. valve gradient
transatrial
    t. membranotomy (TM)
    t. pacing
transaxial
    t. plane
    t. slice
transaxillary apical bullectomy
transbrachial aortography
transbronchial
    t. biopsy (TBB, TBBX, TBBx)
    t. lung biopsy (TBLB)
    t. needle aspiration (TBNA)
transcapillary refill
transcardiac
    t. gradient
    t. monocyte
    t. vein perfusion
transcardial catheter therapy (TCT)
transcarotid balloon valvuloplasty
transcatheter
    t. ablation
    t. arterial embolization (TAE)
    t. biopsy (TCB)
    t. closure (TCC)
    t. closure of atrial defect
    t. closure of atrial septal defect
      operation
    t. coil occlusion
    t. device

    t. embolization
    t. embolotherapy
    t. occlusion of atrial septal defect
    t. patch
    t. therapy (TCT)
    t. umbrella
    t. valve implantation
    t. valvotomy
Transcop
transcoronary
    t. ablation of septal hypertrophy
      (TASH)
    t. alcohol ablation (TAA)
    t. chemical ablation
transcranial color-coded sonography
  (TCCS)
transcricothyroid puncture
transcription
    gene t.
    Janus kinase/signal transducer and
      activator of t.
    signal transducer and activator
      of t. (STAT, Stat)
transcutaneous
    t. echo
    t. electrical stimulation (TES)
    t. extraction catheter
    t. lead
    t. oxygen monitor (TCOM)
    t. pacemaker (TCP, TCPC)
    t. pacing (TCP, TCPC)
transdermal
    t. 17-beta-estradiol
    Catapres-TTS T.
    Duragesic T.
Transderm-Nitro Patch
transdiaphragmatic pressure
transducer
    Acuson V5M multiplane
      transesophageal
      echocardiographic t.
    Aloka model SSD-830 2.5- and
      3.5-MHz t.
    anular array t.
    t. aperture
    arterial line t.
    ATL UltraMark IV 7.5-MHz linear
      array t.
    Bentley t.
    charge-coupled device t.
    Deltran disposable t.
    diaphragm t.

T

NOTES

transducer *(continued)*
    Diasonics t.
    differential pressure t.
    Doppler t.
    echocardiographic t.
    footprint of t.
    Gould Statham pressure t.
    HP SONOS 2500 t.
    Medex t.
    2-MHz pulsed-wave Doppler t.
    Mikro-Tip t.
    Millar Mikro-Tip catheter
     pressure t.
    Millar TCB-500 t.
    M-mode t.
    Pedoff continuous wave t.
    phased array sector t.
    phonocardiographic t.
    piezoelectric ultrasound t.
    pressure t.
    quartz t.
    range-gated t.
    sector t.
    Sleepscan Airflow Pressure T.
    Toshiba biplane transesophageal t.
    ultrasound t.
    variomatrix t.
    V510B biplane TEE t.
    Vingmed CFM 750 t.
    V5M multiplane t.
transendothelial
transesophageal
    t. atrial pacing (TAP, TEAP)
    t. atrial stimulation (TRAS)
    t. contrast echocardiography
    t. dobutamine stress
     echocardiography
    t. echo
    t. echocardiography (TEE)
    t. echocardiography-dobutamine
     stress echocardiography (TEE-
     DSE)
    t. echocardiography with pacing
     (TEEP)
    t. echo probe
    t. pacing (TEP)
    t. pacing system
    t. pressure
transfection
    gene t.
transfemoral endoaortic occlusion
  catheter
transfer
    adenovirus-mediated gene t.
    Akt gene t.
    cholesterol-ester t. (CET)
    chordal t.
    ex vivo gene t.
    intraarterial gene t.

    intravascular gene t.
    vascular gene t.
    in vivo gene t.
transferase
    chloramphenicol t.
transfixion suture
transform
    fast Fourier t. (FFT)
    Fourier t.
    gradient field t. (GFT)
    Karhunen-Loéve t. (KLT)
    three-dimensional Fourier t. (3DFT)
transformation
    epicardial-mesenchymal t.
    Haldane t.
    hemorrhagic t. (HT)
    Richter t.
transformer
    vesicular monoamine t. (VMAT)
transforming
    t. growth factor (TGF)
    t. growth factor-beta
transfusion
    autologous t.
    Baylor rapid autologous t. (BRAT)
    donor-specific t.
    exchange t.
    t. factor
transfusional hemosiderosis
transgenesis
transient
    t. abnormal Q wave (TAQW)
    t. asystole
    calcium t.
    t. depolarization
    t. entrainment
    t. heart block
    t. inward current
    t. ischemic attack (TIA)
    t. ischemic attack plus carotid
     endarterectomy (TIA + CE)
    t. ischemic dilation (TID)
    t. ischemic episode (TIE)
    t. ischemic event (TIE)
    t. leukocytosis
    t. mesenteric ischemia
    t. pericarditis
    t. pulmonary vascular lability
     (TPLV)
    t. response imaging (TRI)
    t. spastic occlusion (TSO)
    t. spontaneous circulation (TSC)
    t. ST segment elevation
    t. syncope
    t. tachypnea of newborn (TTNB)
    t. wall motion abnormality
transilluminated powered phlebectomy
  (TIPP)

transition
    forced ischemia-reperfusion t.
    sympathovagal t.
transitional
    t. cell
    t. cell carcinoma
    t. cell zone
    t. respiration
transjugular
    t. balloon valvuloplasty procedure
    t. intrahepatic portosystemic shunt
    (TIPS)
translesional spectral flow velocity
translocation
    Nikaidoh t.
translocator
    adenine nucleotide t.
    adenosine nucleotide t. (ANT)
translumbar
    t. aortogram (TLA)
    t. aortography
transluminal
    t. angioplasty (TAP, TLA)
    t. angioplasty catheter
    t. coronary angioplasty
    t. endarterectomy
    t. endarterectomy catheter (TEC)
    t. extraction atherectomy (TEA)
    t. extraction catheter (TEC)
    t. extraction coronary atherectomy
    t. lysing system
    percutaneous t.
transluminally
    t. placed endovascular branched
    stent graft
    t. placed Inoue endovascular stent-
    graft
transmembrane
    t. calcium flux
    t. potential
    t. signaling
    t. voltage
transmission
    airborne t.
    electrotonic t.
    genetic t.
    t. imaging
    mitral E-wave t.
    t. scan
transmitral
    t. Doppler E:A (ratio)
    t. E:A (ratio)

    t. E-wave deceleration time
    t. flow velocity
    t. gradient
transmitted murmur
transmucosal
    Actiq Oral T.
transmural
    t. anterior myocardial infarction
    (TAMI)
    t. antitachycardia pacemaker
    t. channel
    t. inferior myocardial infarction
    (TIMI)
    t. myocardial infarction (TMI)
    t. pressure
    t. steal
transmyocardial
    t. laser channel
    t. laser revascularization (TMLR)
    t. mechanical channeling (TMC)
    t. pacing stylet
    t. perfusion pressure
    t. revascularization (TMR)
transnexus channel
Transonic flowmeter
transPac ventilator
transpiration
    pulmonary t.
transpl
   transplantation
   transplanted
transplant (TSPL, Tx) *(See also*
  transplantation)
    allogeneic t.
    bilateral lung t. (BLT)
    bilateral sequential single lung t.
    bone marrow t.
    cardiac t.
    t. coronary artery disease (TCAD,
    TxCAD)
    double lung t. (DLT)
    en bloc bilateral lung t.
    heart t. (HT)
    heart-lung t. (HLT, HLTx)
    heterologous cardiac t.
    heterotopic cardiac t.
    heterotopic heart t. (HHT)
    homologous cardiac t.
    living related t. (LRT)
    Lower-Shumway cardiac t.
    lung t. (LT, LTx)
    orthotopic cardiac t.

T

NOTES

transplant *(continued)*
    orthotopic heart t. (OHT)
    t. pneumonia
    rejection cardiomyopathy t.
    right single lung t. (RSLTx)
    single-lung t. (SLT)
    syngenesioplastic t.
transplantation (tpl, transpl, TX, Tx)
    (See also transplant)
    cardiac t. (CTx)
    heart t. (HT)
    heart-lung t. (HLT)
    heterotropic heart t. (HHT)
    International Society for Heart T. (ISHT)
    International Society for Heart and Lung T. (ISHLT)
    orthotopic cardiac t. (OCT)
transplanted (tpl, transpl)
transpleural
transport
    active t.
    T. dilatation balloon catheter
    T. drug delivery catheter
    lactic acid t.
    mucociliary t.
    mucus t.
    oxygen t.
transportability
    cough t.
transportation
    air medical t. (AMT)
transporter
    monocarboxylate t.
transposition
    t. of aorta (TA)
    t. of arterial stem
    t. assessment
    t. complex
    corrected t. (CT)
    t. of great arteries (TGA)
    t. of great vessels (TGV)
    portacaval t. (PCT)
transprosthetic
    t. flow velocity
    t. gradient
transpulmonary
    t. gradient (TPG)
    t. pressure (Ptp)
    t. thermal-dye dilution (TDD)
transradial
    t. approach
    t. cardiac catheterization
    t. coronary angioplasty
    t. primary stenting
transsarcolemmal
    t. calcium current
    t. calcium entry
    t. calcium influx

transseptal
    t. angiocardiography
    t. catheter
    t. conduction
    t. left heart catheterization
    t. needle
    t. puncture
    t. sheath
transstenotic
    t. pressure gradient
    t. pressure gradient measurement
transtelephonic
    t. ambulatory monitoring (TAM)
    t. ambulatory monitoring system
    t. arrhythmia monitoring (TTM)
    t. cardiac event monitoring
    t. exercise monitor (TEM)
    t. recording
transthoracic
    t. acoustic window
    t. color Doppler echocardiography
    t. contrast echocardiography
    t. direct current electrical cardioversion
    t. echocardiogram (TTE)
    t. echocardiography (TTE)
    t. impedance
    t. implantable cardioverter-defibrillator
    t. intracardiac monitoring (TIM)
    t. needle aspiration (TTNA)
    t. needle aspiration biopsy
    t. needle biopsy (TNB)
    t. pacemaker
    t. pacing stylet
    t. portography (THP)
    t. pressure
transthoracically implanted ICD
transtracheal
    t. aspiration
    t. oxygen (TTO)
    t. oxygen catheter
    t. oxygen therapy (TTOT)
transudate
transudation
transudative pleural effusion
transvalensis
    Nocardia t.
transvalvular
    t. aortic gradient
    t. E velocity
    t. flow
    t. flow rate
    t. hemodynamics
    t. pressure gradient (TPG)
    t. reflux
Transvene
    T. lead

T. nonthoracotomy implantable cardioverter-defibrillator
T. tripolar electrode

transvenous (TV)
t. ablation
t. aortovelography (TAV)
t. biopsy
t. cardioversion (TVCV)
t. catheter extraction
t. defibrillator lead
t. device
t. electrode
t. implantable defibrillator
t. internal cardioversion
t. nitinol snare
t. pacemaker (TVP)

transventricular
t. closed valvotomy
t. mitral valve commissurotomy

transverse
t. aortic arch (TAA)
t. artery of face
t. artery of neck
t. cardiac diameter (TCD)
t. cervical artery
t. costal facet
t. fissure of right lung
t. heart diameter (THD)
t. incision
t. muscle of nape
t. muscle of thorax
t. section of heart
t. sinus (TS)
t. thoracosternotomy
t. tubule

transverse/sigmoid sinus (TS/SS)
transversi
fovea costalis processus t.

transversus
t. nuchae muscle
situs t.

transxiphoid approach
tranylcypromine
TRAP
total peroxyl radical-trapping antioxidant potential
TRAP assay

Trap
T. cardiovascular filtration system
T. neurovascular filtration system
T. vascular filtration system

trap
VEGF T.'s
trap-door approach
TrapEase permanent vena cava filter
trapezius ridge sign
trapidil
trapped
t. gas volume
t. lung
Trapper catheter exchange device
trapping
air t.
gas t.
TRAS
transesophageal atrial stimulation
trash foot
Trasicor
trastuzumab
Trasylol
Traube
T. bruit
T. curve
T. double tone
T. dyspnea
T. heart
T. murmur
pistol shot of T.
T. plug
T. semilunar space
T. sign
trauma
American Association for the Surgery of T. (AAST)
blunt chest t.
blunt thoracic t.
t. intensive care unit (TICU)
mechanical t.
penetrating thoracic t.
thoracic t.
truncal t.
vessel t.
traumatic
t. aortic aneurysm
t. aortic disruption
t. aortography
t. apnea
t. asphyxia
t. chylothorax
t. emphysema
t. fistula
t. heart disease
t. hemopericardium

T

NOTES

traumatic *(continued)*
    t. hemorrhage
    t. pericarditis
    t. pneumonia
    t. pneumothorax
    t. rupture
    t. tamponade
    t. thrombosis
    t. thrombus
traveler
    T. portable oxygen system
    Pulmo-Aide T.
Travenol infusion pump
tray
    lock pericardiocentesis set and t.
trazodone hydrochloride
Treacher Collins syndrome
treadmill
    arm ergometry t.
    t. echocardiography
    t. electrocardiogram
    t. exercise (TE)
    exercise t. (ET)
    t. exercise stress test
    t. exercise test (TET, TMET)
    t. incline
    Marquette t.
    t. performance test (TPP)
    Q-Stress t.
    t. score (TS)
    self-powered t.
    t. stress test (TMST, TST)
    t. test (TT)
treadmill-induced angina
treatment
    Albertini t.
    antianginal t.
    arrest-and-reversal t. (ART)
    atherosclerosis prevention and t.
    Brehmer t.
    coronary artery risk assessment
      and t.
    Cosgrove-Edwards annuloplasty
      system with Duraflo t.
    Debove t.
    directly observed t. (DOT)
    efficacy of t.
    emergency medical t. (EMT)
    Forlanini t.
    Frankel t.
    Karell t.
    Lingraphica aphasic t.
    McPheeters t.
    Nauheim t.
    nonpharmacologic measure of t.
    Nordach t.
    Oertel t.
    preventive allergy t.

    rapid early action in coronary t.
      (REACT)
    Schott t.
    stand-alone laser t.
    TheraPEP prerespiratory therapy t.
    Tuffnell t.
Trecator-SC
Tredex powered bicycle
tree
    bronchial t.
    coronary t.
    endobronchial t.
    tracheobronchial t.
tree-in-winter appearance
trefoil
    t. balloon catheter
    t. Schneider balloon
    t. tendon
tremor
    flapping t.
tremulus
    pulsus t.
trench lung
trend
    threshold t.
Trendelenburg
    T. operation
    T. position
    T. test
Trental
trepidatio cordis
treponemal
    t. antibody
    t. test
Treponema pallidum
trepopnea
treppe
    negative t.
    t. phenomenon
    positive t.
treprostinil sodium
TRI
    transient response imaging
Triacin-C
**TriActiv balloon-protected flush
  extraction system**
triad
    acute compression t.
    adrenomedullary t.
    Andersen t.
    t. asthma
    atherogenic metabolic t.
    Beck t.
    Carney t.
    Cushing t.
    T. defibrillator system
    Fallot t.
    Grancher t.
    Hull t.

Kartagener t.
lipid t.
Osler t.
Virchow t.
Widal-Abrami-Lermoyez t.
triadic junction
TRIADS
time-resolved imaging by automatic data
segmentation
TriaDyne II kinetic therapy
Triage
T. BNP test
T. cardiac rapid diagnostic test
system
T. Cardio ProfilER panel
trial (*See also* study, program, protocol)
Emory Angioplasty versus
Surgery T. (EAST)
Philadelphia Association of
Clinical T.'s (PACT)
randomized t.'s
thrombosis prevention t. (TPT)
Zwolle t. (ZT)
Triam-A Injection
triamcinolone
t. acetonide (TAA)
t. diacetate
t. inhalation, nasal
t. (systemic)
Triam Forte Injection
Triaminic
T. AM Decongestant Formula
T. DM
Triamonide injection
triamterene
hydrochlorothiazide and t.
triangle
aortic t.
axillary t.
Burger scalene t.
Calot t.
cardiohepatic t.
carotid t.
clavipectoral t.
Einthoven t.
endocardial t.
Gerhardt t.
infraclavicular t.
Jackson safety t.
Koch t.
t. of Koch
Rauchfuss t.

sternocostal t.
subclavian t.
Todaro t.
tracheal t.
triangular resection of leaflet operation
Triatoma infestans
triatrial heart
triatriatum
cor t.
triaxial
t. accelerometer
t. reference system
triazolam
tribromide
phosphorus t.
tribromide
trichamber pacing
Trichinella spiralis
trichinosis
trichinous embolism
trichiura
Trichuris t.
trichloride
antimony t.
trichlormethiazide
Trichosporon
T. *asahii*
T. *beigelii*
T. *beigelii* pneumonia
trichosporonosis
Trichuris trichiura
triciribine phosphate (TCN-P)
Tricor capsule
tricrotic, tricrotous
tricrotism
tricuspid
t. annular motion (TAM)
t. aortic valve
t. atelectasis
t. atresia (TA)
t. closure (Tc)
t. commissurotomy
t. first sound (T1)
t. incompetence (TI)
t. insufficiency (TI)
t. murmur
t. opening (To)
t. opening snap
t. orifice
t. position
pulmonic t.
t. regurgitant jet

NOTES

tricuspid *(continued)*
    t. regurgitation (TR)
    t. restenosis
    t. stenosis (TS)
    t. valve (TV)
    t. valve annuloplasty
    t. valve anulus
    t. valve area
    t. valve closure sound (T1)
    t. valve disease
    t. valve doming
    t. valve endocarditis
    t. valve flow
    t. valve prolapse (TVP)
    t. valve regurgitation (TVR)
    t. valve replacement (TVR)
    t. valve strut
    t. valve vegetation
    t. valvular leaflet
    t. valvuloplasty
tricuspidalis
    cuspis anterior valvae t.
tricuspid-inferior vena cava isthmus
Tricut laryngeal blade tip
tricyclic antidepressant
Tridil injection
triethiodide
    gallamine t.
trifascicular block
Tri-flow incentive spirometry
triflupromazine
trig
    triglyceride
trigeminal
    t. cough
    t. nerve
    t. pulse
    t. rhythm
trigeminus
    pulsus t.
trigeminy
trigger
    asthma t.
    pathologic t.
    rupture t.
    Smart T.
    t. of ventricular arrhythmia (TOVA)
triggered
    t. activity
    atrial t.
    atrial demand t. (AAT)
    t. harmonic power Doppler imaging
    t. mode
    t. pacing
    ventricular t. (VVT)

triggering
    t. mechanism
    respiratory t.
triglyceride (TG, TGL, trig)
    t. fatty acid (TGFA)
    t. level
    medium chain t.'s
    t. rich lipoprotein (TRL, TRLP)
    serum t.
triglyceridemia
    normal t. (NTG)
trigone
    anterior fibrous t.
    vertebrocostal t.
trigonum omotracheale
Tri-Hydroserpine
triiodothyronine
Tri-Kort injection
trilazad mesylate
trileaflet
trilinear cylindric interpolation algorithm
Trilisate
triloculare
    cor t.
trilocular heart
Trilog Injection
Trilogy
    T. DC, DR, SR pulse generator
trilogy
    t. of Fallot
    Fallot t.
Trilone injection
Trimadeau sign
trimazosin
trimellitic
    t. anhydride
    t. anhydride asthma
trimetazidine 1 (TMZ)
trimethaphan camsylate
trimethoprim-sulfamethoxazole (TMP-SMX)
trimethoprim sulfate
trimetrexate glucoronate
trimipramine maleate
Trimox
Trimpex
trinitrate
    glyceryl t.
trinucleotide
    cytosine-thymine-guanine T.
triolet
    bruit de t.
Triostat injection
Tripedia
tripelennamine
tripe palm
triphammer pulse

triphenyl
    t. tetrazolium chloride
    t. tetrazolium staining method
triphosphatase
    adenosine t. (ATPase)
triphosphate
    adenosine t. (AT, ATP)
    guanosine t. (GTP)
    inositol t.
    purine nucleotides adenosine t.
    uridine t. (UTP)
triple
    t. coronary artery bypass graft
     (TCABG)
    t. coronary artery graft (TCAG)
    t. ectopic tachyarrhythmia
    t. extrastimulus
    t. rhythm
    t. stimulus
triple-balloon valvuloplasty
triple-bandpass filter
triple-humped pressure pulse
triplet
tripod sign
tripolar
    t. defibrillation coil electrode
    t. lead
    segmented ring t. (SRT)
    t. with Damato curve catheter
triport cannula
TriPort hemostasis introducer sheath kit
Triposed Tablet
Trippi-Wells tongs
triprolidine
    t. and pseudoephedrine
triprolidine, pseudoephedrine, and codeine
trisalicylate
    choline magnesium t.
Tris-buffer infusion test
trisection
    pulse t.
tris(hydroxymethyl)aminomethane
trisomy
    t. 13, 18, 21
Tritace
TriTrac-R3D accelerometer
TriVex system
TRL, TRLP
    triglyceride rich lipoprotein
Trocal

trocar
    Axiom thoracic t.
    B-D Potain thoracic t.
    Davidson thoracic t.
    Entree thoracoscopy t.
    Hunt angiographic t.
    large-bore t.
trochleae
    vagina synovialis t.
trochocardia
trochorizocardia
troglitazone
Troisier sign
troleandomycin (TAO)
trolley
tromethamine
Trooper floppy moderate support guide wire
TROPCAB
    total revascularization off pump by
    coronary artery bypass
Tropheryma whipplei
trophic changes
trophoblastic tumor
tropical
    t. endomyocardial fibrosis
    t. pulmonary eosinophilia
tropicalis
    Xenopus t.
tropomyosin
troponin
    t. C, I, T (TnT)
trospectomycin sulfate
trough
    t. dosing
    peak and t.
    t. and peak levels
    systolic t.
    X-descent t.
    Y-descent t.
trough-to-peak ratio
trousers
    military antishock t. (MAST)
    pneumatic t.
Trousseau syndrome
trovafloxacin
Trovan
TR-R9 antithrombin receptor polyclonal antibody
TRT
    thoracic radiation therapy

NOTES

TRU
terminal respiratory unit
Tru-Cut biopsy needle
true
t. aortic aneurysm
t. asthma
t. cyst
t. positive stress test (TPST)
T. Sheathless intraaortic balloon catheter
t. versus false aneurysm aortography
t. vocal cord
TrueMax 2400 metabolic measuring system
true-negative test result
true-positive test result
Trufill n-BCA liquid embolic system
trumpet
angel's t.
truncal
t. distribution of body fat
t. trauma
truncoconal area
truncus, pl. trunci
t. arteriosus (TA)
t. arteriosus communis (TAC)
bifurcatio trunci
t. brachiocephalicus
t. celiacus
t. costocervicalis
t. fascicularis atrioventricularis
t. linguofacialis
t. lymphaticus bronchiomediastinalis
t. pulmonalis
t. thyrocervicalis
Trunecek
T. sign
T. symptom
trunk
bifurcation of pulmonary t.
brachiocephalic t.
bronchomediastinal lymphatic t.
t. control test (TCT)
t. forward flexion
left-sided innominate t.
orifice of pulmonary t.
pulmonary t.
valve of pulmonary t.
Trusler
T. aortic valve technique
T. rule for pulmonary artery banding
T. technique of aortic valvuloplasty
TruTrak data sampling system
TruZone
T. asthma action plan wallet card
T. peak flowmeter
T. PFM

TRVV
total right ventricular volume
Trypanosoma
T. brucei
T. cruzi
T. gambiense
T. rhodesiense
trypanosomiasis
American t.
trypsin balsam peru, and castor oil
TS
transverse sinus
treadmill score
tricuspid stenosis
TSC
transient spontaneous circulation
TSH
thyroid-stimulating hormone
T-shaped stent
TSO
transient spastic occlusion
TSPL
transplant
TS/SS
transverse/sigmoid sinus
TST
total sleep time
treadmill stress test
tsukubaensis
Streptomyces t.
TSVR
total systemic vascular resistance
TT
thrombin time
thrombolytic therapy
thromboplastin time
treadmill test
TT form of MTP gene
T_I/T_{TOT}
ratio of inspiratory time to total breathing cycle time
TTC stain
TTE
transthoracic echocardiogram
transthoracic echocardiography
TTM
transtelephonic arrhythmia monitoring
TTNA
transthoracic needle aspiration
TTNB
transient tachypnea of newborn
TTO
transtracheal oxygen
TTO therapy
TTOT
transtracheal oxygen therapy
TTP
thrombotic thrombocytopenic purpura

TTT
    tilt-table test
T-tubule
T-type calcium channels
Tubasal
Tubbs dilator
tube, tubing
    AccuMark calibrated infant
      feeding t.
    air t.
    Aire-Cuf tracheostomy t.
    American tracheotomy t.
    Andrews-Pynchon t.
    Arm-a-Med endotracheal t.
    Atkins-Cannard tracheal t.
    Bivona Fome-Cuff t.
    Bivona TTS tracheostomy t.
    Blue Line cuffed endotracheal t.
    bronchial t.
    Broncho-Cath double-lumen
      endotracheal t.
    bulboventricular t.
    Caluso PEG t.
    Carabelli t.
    Carlen double-lumen endotracheal t.
    Celestin esophageal t.
    Chaussier t.
    chest t. (CT)
    Cooley sump t.
    cuffed endotracheal t.
    cuffed tracheostomy t.
    Dale-Schwartz t.
    decompressive chest t.
    double-lumen endobronchial t.
    Dow Corning t.
    Durham t.
    endobronchial t.
    endocardial t.
    endotracheal t. (ETT)
    Endotrol endotracheal t.
    Endotrol tracheal t.
    esophageal combination t. (ETC)
    Ewald t.
    fenestrated tracheostomy t.
    Flex DIC tracheostomy t.
    fluffy-cuffed t.
    Fome-Cuf tracheostomy t.
    glutaraldehyde-tanned bovine
      collagen t.
    Gore-Tex t.
    Haldane-Priestley t.
    high pressure connecting t.

    Hi-Lo Evac endotracheal t.
    Hi-Lo Jet tracheal t.
    Holter t.
    Hyperflex tracheostomy t.
    interposition of Dacron t.
    intratracheal t.
    J-shaped t.
    Kamen-Wilkinson endotracheal t.
    Kuhn t.
    Lanz low-pressure cuff
      endotracheal t.
    large-bore chest t.
    large-caliber chest t.
    Laryngoflex reinforced
      endotracheal t.
    laser t.
    Lindholm tracheal t.
    Lo-Pro tracheal t.
    Lore-Lawrence trachea t.
    Luer tracheal t.
    Mackler t.
    Magill Safety Clear Plus
      endotracheal t.
    Mallinckrodt cuffed endotracheal t.
    Montgomery Safe-T-T.
    Mosher life-saving tracheal t.
    Nachlas t.
    nasogastric t.
    nasotracheal t.
    Olympus One-Step Button t.
    oroendotracheal t.
    orotracheal t.
    otopharyngeal t.
    PEG t.
    PEJ t.
    pleural t.
    polyvinyl chloride t.
    Portex Per-fit tracheostomy t.
    primordial catheter t.
    RAE endotracheal t.
    right-angle chest t.
    Robertshaw t.
    Ruschelit polyvinyl chloride
      endotracheal t.
    Sarns intracardiac suction t.
    scavenging t.
    Shiley tracheostomy t.
    Softech endotracheal t.
    Souttar t.
    spiral-embedded t.
    T t.
    t. thoracostomy

T

NOTES

tube *(continued)*
    thoracostomy t.
    Thora-Klex chest t.
    Tovell t.
    tracheal t.
    tracheostomy t.
    Univent t.
    UTTS endotracheal t.
    Vacutainer t.
    Venturi t.
    Vivonex Moss t.
    water-seal chest t.
    wire-wound endotracheal t.
    x-ray t.

tube]
    lidocaine, atropine, naloxone,
      epinephrine [drugs that may be
      administered via endotracheal t.
      (LANE)

**TubeChek esophageal intubation
  detector**

tubercle
    corniculate t.
    cuneiform t.
    Ghon t.

tuberculin
    Koch old t.
    purified protein derivative of t.
    T. Purified Protein Derivative Tine
      Test

tuberculocidal
tuberculoid myocarditis
tuberculoma
tuberculosilicosis
tuberculosis (TB)
    active t.
    acute miliary t.
    adult t.
    aerogenic t.
    Amplicor assay for
      Mycobacterium t.
    anthracotic t.
    arrested t.
    atypical t.
    avian t.
    basal t.
    t. of bones and joints
    cerebral t.
    cestodic t.
    childhood t.
    childhood-type t.
    disseminated t.
    endobronchial t.
    ESAT-6 protein *mycobacterium t.*
    extrapulmonary t.
    exudative t.
    generalized t.
    healed t.
    hematogenous t.

    hilus t.
    inactive t.
    inhalation t.
    t. of larynx
    t. lichenoides
    t. of lung
    miliary t.
    multidrug-resistant t. (MDR-TB)
    mycobacteria other than t. (MOTT)
    Mycobacterium t. (MTB)
    open t.
    oral t.
    orificial t.
    papulonecrotic t.
    postprimary t.
    primary t.
    productive t.
    pulmonary t. (PTB)
    reactivation t.
    reinfection t.
    renal t.
    secondary t.
    smear-negative t.
    smear-positive t.
    surgical t.
    tracheobronchial t.
    t. vaccine

tuberculostat
tuberculostatic
tuberculous
    t. arteritis
    t. bronchopneumonia
    t. caseation
    t. chemotherapy
    t. empyema
    t. empyesis
    t. endocarditis
    t. laryngitis
    t. lymphadenitis
    t. mycotic aneurysm of aorta
    t. nephritis
    t. pericarditis
    t. pleurisy
    t. pleuritis
    t. pneumonia
    t. rheumatism

tuberculum
    t. thyroideum inferius
    t. thyroideum superius

tuberoeruptive xanthoma
tuberous
    t. sclerosis
    t. xanthoma

Tubersol
tubing *(var. of* tube)
tubocurarine chloride
tubular
    t. breath sounds
    t. necrosis

t. respiration
t. slotted stent
tubule
distal convoluted t.
proximal convoluted t.
transverse t.
tuboreticular structure
Tuffier test
Tuffnell treatment
tug, tugging
tracheal t.
Tukey-Kramer posttest
tularemia
oropharyngeal t.
tularemic pneumonia
tularensis
    Francisella t.
tumor
adenomatoid t.
anaplastic t.
Askin t.
t. blush
bronchopulmonary carcinoid t.
carcinoid t.
cardiac t.
carotid body t.
chromaffin cell t.
clear cell t.
congenital peribronchial
  myofibroblastic t.
craniopharyngeal duct t.
desmoplastic small round cell t.
t. embolism
extrathoracic t.
germ cell t.
glomus t.
Godwin t.
granular cell t.
Hürthle cell t.
inflammatory myofibroblastic t.
intracardiac t.
intravascular bronchoalveolar t.
t. marker
mesenchymal-derived t.
mesodermal t.
mesothelial t.
migrated t.
myxoma t.
t. necrosis factor (TNF)
t. necrosis factor-alpha (TNF-alpha)
neuroendocrine t.
neurogenic t.

t., node, metastasis (TNM)
Pancoast t.
papillary t.
paraganglioma t.
pericardiac t.
phantom t.
t. plop
t. plop sound
polycystic t.
primitive neuroectodermal t.
  (PNET)
Purkinje t.
Rathke pouch t.
sarcomatous t.
sugar t.
superior pulmonary sulcus t.
t. suppressor gene inactivation
teratoma t.
thyroid t.
trophoblastic t.
tumorigenic
tumorlet
tumultus cordis
tunable pulsed dye laser
TUNEL
  TdT-mediated dUTP nick-end labeling
  TUNEL assay
  TUNEL method
  TUNEL stain
tungsten
t. carbide pneumoconiosis
t. microelectrode
tunic
Bichat t.
vascular t.
tunica
t. mucosa bronchi
t. mucosa esophagi
t. mucosa laryngis
t. mucosa linguae
t. mucosa pharyngis
t. mucosa tracheae
t. muscularis bronchiorum
t. muscularis esophagi
t. muscularis pharyngis
t. muscularis tracheae
tunnel
aortic and left ventricular t.
  (ALVT)
Kawashima intraventricular t.
percutaneous t.
subsartorial t.

NOTES

T

753

tunneler
Tunturi EL400 bicycle ergometer
Tuohy-Borst
    T.-B. adapter
    T.-B. introducer
tuple-1 gene
turbinate
turbine-powered ICU ventilator system
Turboaire Challenger cold-air bronchial provocation device
TurboFLASH technique
Turbohaler
    Bricanyl T.
Turbuhaler
    Pulmicort T.
    Symbicort 100/6 T.
    Symbicort 200/6 T.
turbulence
    heart rate t.
turbulent
    t. diastolic mitral inflow
    t. jet
turgor
    coronary vascular t.
    skin t.
turnaround time (TAT)
Turner syndrome
Tuss
    HycoClear T.
Tussafed drops
Tuss-Allergine Modified T.D. Capsule
Tussigon
Tussionex
Tussi-Organidin DM NR
tussive
    t. fremitus
    t. squeeze
    t. syncope
Tussogest Extended Release Capsule
Tusstat Syrup
Tuttle thoracic forceps
TV
    tidal volume
    transvenous
    tricuspid valve
TV$_I$
    tidal inspiratory volume
TV$_E$
    tidal expiratory volume
TVCV
    transvenous cardioversion
TVG
    time-varied gain
TVGC
    time-varied gain control
TVP
    transvenous pacemaker
    tricuspid valve prolapse

TVR
    target vessel revascularization
    total vascular resistance
    tricuspid valve regurgitation
    tricuspid valve replacement
TWA
    T wave alternans
TWAR
    Taiwan acute respiratory
    TWAR agent
    TWAR disease
    TWAR pneumonia
T-wave pseudonormalization
Twice-A-Day Nasal Solution
twiddler's syndrome
twill tape
twin
    Bennett t.
    T. Jet nebulizer
    thoracopagus t.
    VersaLab APM2 for t.'s
TWISTED
    tracheal wall injury with intermittent stoppage of tracheostomy and episodes of dyspnea
    TWISTED syndrome
Twisthaler
TwistLock
    T. Cath-Gard
    Hands-Off infusion port heparin-coated thermodilution catheter with T.
twitch
    t. esophageal pressure
    t. force
    t. gastric pressure
    t. potentiation
    t. transdiaphragmatic pressure
two-block claudication
two-bottle thoracic drainage system
two-chain urokinase plasminogen activator (tcu-PA)
two-chamber
    apical t.-c.
    t.-c. view
two-dimensional (2D)
    t.-d. transcranial color-coded sonography (2D-TCCS)
    t.-d. echocardiography (2DE)
    t.-d. integrated backscatter
    t.-d. tag
two-flight exertional dyspnea
two-flights-of-stairs claudication
two-kidney Goldblatt
two-patch technique
two-piece bifurcated intraluminal graft
two-pillow orthopnea

two-stage
>t.-s. cannula
>ultrathin-walled t.-s. (UTTS)

two-step exercise test
two-turn epicardial lead
TX
>transplantation

Tx
>transplant
>transplantation

TxCAD
>transplant coronary artery disease

Tylenol Cold No Drowsiness
tylosin tartrate asthma
tyloxapol
tympanitic
>t. resonance
>t. sound

tympany
>bell t.

type
>t. A, B aortic dissection
>t. A, B behavior
>Ambrose plaque t.
>cardioinhibitory t.
>cell t.
>t. I collagen telopeptide (ICTP)

>t. 1-4 dextrocardia
>t. II cell hyperplasia
>t. III antiarrhythmic agent
>t. I, II dip
>t. I, III procollagen
>t. II pneumocyte
>t. I-VIII glycogen storage disease
>t. Va, Vb, Vc lesion

typhoid
>t. fever
>t. pleurisy
>t. pneumonia

typhus
>African tick t.
>Queensland tick t.
>scrub t.

typical small cell
typing
>human lymphocyte antigen t.

tyramine
Tyrode solution
tyrosine phosphorylated protein
Tyshak
>T. balloon
>T. balloon valvuloplasty catheter

T-Y stent
Tzanck test

T

NOTES

U

U loop
U suture
U virus
U wave
U wave alternans
U wave inversion

UA
ultrasonic arteriography
unstable angina

UACP
upper airway closing pressure

UAE
unsupported arm exercise

UA/NQMI
unstable angina/non-Q-wave myocardial infarction

UAO
upper airway obstruction

UAOP
upper airway opening pressure

UAP
unstable angina pectoris

UAPA
unilateral absence of pulmonary artery

UARS
upper airways resistance syndrome

ubiquinol

ubiquinone

ubiquitin

UCA
ultrasound contrast agent

UCAD
unstable coronary artery disease

UCG
ultrasonic cardiography

UCI-Barnard aortic valve

UCO
ultrasonic cardiac output

UFA
unesterified fatty acid

UFCT
ultrafast computed tomography

UFH
unfractionated heparin

UFT
tegafur and uracil

UGNB
ultrasonically guided needle biopsy

UHFV
ultrahigh frequency ventilation

Uhl
U. anomaly
U. disease

U. malformation
U. syndrome

UHR
underlying heart rhythm

UIP
usual interstitial pneumonia
usual interstitial pneumonitis

UK
urokinase

ulcer
decubitus u.
diabetic u.
foot u.
penetrating aortic u. (PAU)
penetrating atherosclerotic u. (PAU)
peptic u.
stasis u.
venous u.

ulcerans
Mycobacterium u.

ulcerated
u. lesion
u. plaque

ulcerative endocarditis

ulcerogangrenous

ulceromembranous

ulcerosa
angina u.
pharyngitis u.

Uldall subclavian hemodialysis catheter

Ulick syndrome

Ullmann syndrome

ULM
unprotected left main

ulnar
u. nerve
u. pulse

ULP
ultra low profile
ULP catheter

ULPE
upper lobe pulmonary edema

Ultegra
U. rapid platelet function assay
U. RPFA-TRAP

Ultimate
U. nasal mask
U. Seal CPAP mask seal
U. Seal gel interface

Ultimum hemostasis introducer

ultimum moriens

ultra
U. 8 balloon catheter
Cutting Ballon U. 2
U. ICE catheter

U

ultra *(continued)*
    u. low profile (ULP)
    u. low profile fixed-wire balloon dilation catheter
    U. low resistance voice prosthesis
    U. Mide topical
    U. pacemaker
Ultracef
ultracentrifugation
UltraCision ultrasonic knife
UltraCross
    U. profile imaging catheter
    U. stent
ultrafast
    u. computed tomographic scanner
    u. computed tomography (UFCT)
    u. computed tomography scan
    u. contrast-enhanced chest computed tomography
    u. CT scan
    u. CT scanner
ultrafiltration
    continuous arteriovenous u. (CAVU)
Ultraflex
    U. esophageal stent system
    U. self-expanding stent
    U. tracheobronchial stent
UltraFuse
    U. balloon
    U. infusion catheter
ultrahigh frequency ventilation (UHFV)
Ultraject prefilled syringe
Ultra-Lite portable aspirator
Ultramark 9 echocardiograph
Ultramax woven velour vascular graft
ultrarapid subthreshold stimulation
Ultra-Select nitinol PTCA guidewire
UltraSom computerized sleep analyzer
ultrasonic
    u. arteriography (UA)
    u. cardiac output (UCO)
    u. cardiography (UCG, USCG)
    u. integrated backscatter imaging
    u. nebulizer (USN)
ultrasonically guided needle biopsy (UGNB)
ultrasonographer
ultrasonography
    B-mode u.
    compression u.
    Doppler u.
    duplex pulsed-Doppler u.
    endobronchial u. (EBUS)
    high-resolution B-mode u.
    intracaval endovascular u. (ICEUS)
    intracoronary u.
    TCD u.

ultrasonoscope
    Acuson XP-5,-10,-128 u.
ultrasound
    u. ablation catheter
    ADR Ultramark 4 u.
    Aloka u.
    u. angiography
    Biosound 2000 II s.a. high-resolution u.
    B-mode u.
    bronchoscopic u.
    cardiac u.
    u. cardiography
    colorvascular Doppler u.
    continuous-wave Doppler u.
    u. contrast agent (UCA)
    contrast-enhanced u. (CEU)
    U. Contrast Microsphere
    coronary intravascular u.
    Doppler u.
    duplex u.
    echo-guided u.
    endobronchial u. (EBUS)
    gray-scale u.
    Hewlett-Packard 2500 SONOS u.
    high-resolution deep penetration 2D intracardiac u.
    u. holography
    InterTherapy intravascular u.
    intracoronary u. (ICUS)
    intracoronary vascular u. (IVUS)
    intraluminal u. (ILUS)
    intravascular u. (IVUS)
    Irex Exemplar u.
    negative-contrast intravascular u.
    power Doppler u.
    qualitative coronary u. (QCU)
    real-time u.
    Shimadzu cardiac u.
    Siemens SI 400 u.
    TCD u.
    three-dimensional intravascular u.
    through-the-balloon u.
    Toshiba Sonolayer SSH-140A u.
    u. transducer
ultrasound-guided bronchoscopy
ultrasound-tipped catheter
ultrastructure
Ultra-Thin balloon catheter
ultrathin-walled two-stage (UTTS)
ultraviolet laser
Ultravist
    U. contrast
    U. injection
umbilical
    u. artery
    u. tape
    u. vein

umbilicalis
  arteritis u.
umbrella
  ASDOS u.
  atrial septal defect u.
  Bard Clamshell septal u.
  Clamshell septal u.
  u. closure
  double u.
  u. filter
  patent ductus arteriosus u.
  PDA u.
  transcatheter u.
UMI
  UMI catheter
  UMI transseptal Cath-Seal catheter
    introducer
U-Mid-O₂ Jet Set
UMLS
  Unified Medical Language system
unassisted spontaneous ventilation
Unasyn
underdrive
  u. pacing
  u. termination
underexpressed protein
underlying heart rhythm (UHR)
underperfused myocardium
underperfusion
undersedation
undersensing
  atrial u.
  functional u.
  pacemaker u.
undertreatment
underventilation
underwater
  u. seal drainage
  u. seal resistor
undetermined pathological-type stroke
undifferentiated small-cell carcinoma
undulating
  u. deflection that follows T wave
  u. pulse
unequal pulse
unesterified fatty acid (UFA)
unfractionated heparin (UFH)
uniaxial accelerometer
unicommissural
unicuspid aortic valve
unidirectional block

unifascicular block
Unified Medical Language system (UMLS)
unifocal ventricular ectopic beat (UVEB)
UniHeart IV universal nebulizer
unilateral
  u. absence of pulmonary artery (UAPA)
  u. emphysema
  u. hyperlucency of lung
  u. hyperlucent lung
  u. nonfunctioning lung
  u. pneumonia
  u. pneumothorax
  u. spatial neglect (USN)
unileaflet prolapse
Unilink
  U. anastomotic device
  U. system
unilocular
  u. cyst
  u. hydatid disease
unintended positive end expiratory pressure (autoPEEP, intrinsic PEEP)
unintubated
Uniphyl
unipolar
  u. atrial pacemaker
  u. connector
  u. defibrillation coil electrode
  u. electrocardiogram
  u. limb lead on left leg in electrocardiography (aVF, aVL)
  u. limb lead on right arm in electrocardiography (aVR)
  u. limb leads
  u. Pisces Sigma
  u. precordial lead
  u. sequential pacemaker
Uniprost
Uniretic
Uni-Silicone lead
Unisperse blue dye
Unistasis valve
Unistep Plus delivery system
unit (*See also* device)
  Acrodisc u.
  acute coronary care u.
  Aqua-Seal chest drainage u.
  ATA u.
  BCD Plus cardioplegic u.

U

NOTES

unit *(continued)*
 BICAP u.
 Biosound 2000 II ultrasound u.
 Biosound 3000 ultrasound u.
 BiPAP u.
 cardiac u. (CU)
 cardiac care u. (CCU)
 cardiac diagnostic u. (CDU)
 cardiac intensive care u. (CICU)
 cardiac observation u. (COU)
 cardiac rehabilitation u. (CRU)
 cardiac surgical intensive care u. (CSICU)
 cardiac-thoracic u. (CTU)
 cardiothoracic intensive care u. (CTICU)
 cardiovascular intensive care u. (CVICU)
 chest pain observation u. (CPOU)
 clinical research u. (CRU)
 comprehensive cardiac care u. (CCCU)
 coronary care u. (CCU)
 critical care u.
 defibrillator u.
 digital fluoroscopic u.
 ECG triggering u.
 enhanced external counterpulsation u.
 FreeDop portable Doppler u.
 high-dependency u. (HDU)
 Hounsfield u. (HU)
 hybrid u.
 intensive coronary care u. (ICCU)
 intrapleural sealed drainage u.
 kallidinogenase inactivator u.
 kallikrein inactivating u. (KIU)
 Karmen u.'s
 Kreiselman u.
 life change u.
 lung u.
 medical coronary intensive care u. (MCICU)
 medical intensive care u. (MICU)
 million international u.'s (MIU)
 mobile coronary care u. (MCCU)
 myocardial infarction research u. (MIRU)
 peripheral resistance u. (PRU)
 postanesthesia care u. (PACU)
 postcoronary care u. (PCCU)
 Q-Plex metabolic cart and pulmonary function u.
 R u.
 respiratory special care u. (ReSCU)
 RinoFlow ENT wash u.
 Sentinal seal pleural drainage u.
 Solcotrans autotransfusion u.
 S-Scort New-Duet suction u.
 stroke u. (SU)
 subacute u.
 Sullivan nasal variable positive airway pressure u.
 surgical intensive care u. (SICU)
 Surgitron u.
 terminal respiratory u. (TRU)
 Thora-Seal III chest drainage u.
 Todd u.'s
 torr u.
 Tranquility Bilevel CPAP u.
 trauma intensive care u. (TICU)
 Wood u.

united
 U. Network for Organ Sharing (UNOS)
 U. States Air Force School of Aerospace Medicine (USAFSAM)
 U. States Catheter and Instrument, Inc. (USCI)
 U. States Pharmacopeia (USP)
UniTrack shaft
Uni-tussin DM
Univasc
univentricular
 u. atrioventricular connection
 u. heart
 u. pacing
Univent tube
Uni-Vent ventilator
universal
 u. ACE
 u. aerosol cloud enhancer
 AV u. (DDD)
 u. pacemaker
universalis
 adiposis u.
university
 U. of Akron TAH
 U. of Wisconsin solution
Univision echocardiographic system
unlabored respiration
unloading
 left ventricular u.
Uno nasal prongs
UNOS
 United Network for Organ Sharing
unpotentiated twitch force
unprotected
 u. artery
 u. left main (ULM)
unrelated donor (URD)
unresolved pneumonia
unroofed coronary sinus syndrome
Unschuld sign
unstability
unstable
 u. angina (UA)

u. angina/non-Q-wave myocardial
infarction (UA/NQMI)
u. angina pectoris (UAP)
u. coronary artery disease (UCAD)
u. plaque
unstented xenograft valve
unsupported arm exercise (UAE)
up
pinked up
uPA
urokinase plasminogen activator
updraft
albuterol nebulizer u.
U. handheld nebulizer
Ventolin u.
upgated technique
upgoing Babinski
UPP
uvulopalatoplasty
upper
u. airway closing pressure (UACP)
u. airway obstruction (UAO)
u. airway opening pressure
(UAOP)
u. airways
u. airways resistance syndrome
(UARS)
u. infection point
u. lobe bronchus
u. lobe of lung
u. lobe pulmonary edema (ULPE)
u. lung zone
u. nodal extrasystole
u. respiratory infection (URI)
u. ribs
UPPGP
uvulopalatopharyngoglossoplasty
UPPP
uvulopalatopharyngoplasty
up-regulation
upright
u. exercise
u. T wave
upsloping
u. ST elevation
u. ST segment
u. ST segment depression
upstairs-downstairs heart
upstream
u. airway conductance
u. airways
u. segment

upstroke
carotid u.
diastolic u.
u. and falloff
u. pattern
u. phase
R wave u.
u. velocity
uptake
cardiac antimyosin antibody u.
glucose u.
I-123 MIBG u.
insulin-mediated glucose u. (IMGU)
iodine-123
metaiodobenzylguanidine u.
lung u.
maximum oxygen u.
myocardial oxygen u.
myocardial substrate u. (MSU)
N-13 ammonia u.
norepinephrine u. 1
oxygen u.
peak oxygen u.
thallium u.
tracer u.
uptake-mismatch pattern
uracil
tegafur and u. (UFT)
urapidil
urate
Urbach-Wiethe syndrome
URD
unrelated donor
urea
ureae
Actinobacillus u.
Ureaphil Injection
Ureaplasma urealyticum
Urecholine
ureidopenicillin
uremia
uremic
u. lung
u. pericarditis
u. pneumonia
u. pneumonitis
Uremol
Uresil
U. radiopaque silicone band vessel
loops
U. Vascu-Flo carotid shunt

NOTES

U

urethane
    polycarbonate u.
urgency
    hypertensive u.
URI
    upper respiratory infection
uric acid
uridine triphosphate (UTP)
Uridon
urinary
    u. catheter
    u. equol excretion
urine
    brown u.
    u. volume
urinothorax
Urisec
Uritol
urocanic acid
Urografin-76 contrast medium
urokinase (UK)
    recombinant u. (r-UK)
urokinase plasminogen activator (uPA)
Uro-Mag
urorosein
Urozide
urticaria
    aquagenic u.
    pressure u.
USAFSAM
    United States Air Force School of
    Aerospace Medicine
        USAFSAM treadmill exercise
           protocol
USCG
    ultrasonic cardiography
USCI
    United States Catheter and Instrument,
    Inc.
        USCI catheter
        USCI Goetz bipolar electrode

        USCI introducer
        USCI NBIH bipolar electrode
        USCI Probe balloon-on-a-wire
           dilatation system
        USCI shunt
use
    amount of u. (AOU)
    u. dependence
U-shaped catheter loop
USN
    ultrasonic nebulizer
    unilateral spatial neglect
USP
    United States Pharmacopeia
ustus
    Aspergillus u.
usual
    u. interstitial pneumonia (UIP)
    u. interstitial pneumonia of Liebow
    u. interstitial pneumonitis (UIP)
usurpation
UT-15
    prostacyclin analog UT-15
Utah
    U. TAH
    U. total artificial heart
utilization
    MO2 u.
UTP
    uridine triphosphate
UTTS
    ultrathin-walled two-stage
        UTTS endotracheal tube
UVEB
    unifocal ventricular ectopic beat
**uvulopalatopharyngoglossoplasty
(UPPGP)**
uvulopalatopharyngoplasty (UPPP)
    laser-assisted u. (LAUPPP)
uvulopalatoplasty (UPP)
    laser-assisted u. (LAUP)

V

ventricular
volt
volume
    V lead
    V peak of jugular venous
    V tach
    V wave
V6
V$_E$

minute ventilation
peak exercise ventilation
V$_{MAX}$

maximal velocity
maximum velocity
V$_O$

oral airflow in liters per second
V$_{pe}$

peak ejection velocity
V$_T$

tidal volume
V$_{TG}$

thoracic gas volume
V-A

venoarterial
ventriculoatrial
    V-A conduction
    V-A interval
VA

alveolar volume
variant angina
vasodilator agent
ventricular aneurysm
ventricular arrhythmia
ventriculoatrial
ventroanterior
Veterans Administration
V$_A$

alveolar ventilation per minute
VABP

venoarterial bypass pumping
VAC, V-AC

ventriculoatrial conduction

vaccine

ActHIB v.
Bacillus Calmette-Guérin v.
BCG v.
diphtheria, tetanus toxoids, and
    acellular pertussis v.
diphtheria, tetanus toxoids, and
    whole-cell pertussis v.

diphtheria, tetanus toxoids, and
    whole-cell pertussis vaccine and
    Haemophilus type b conjugate v.
Haemophilus type b conjugate v.
HbOC v.
Imovax v.
inactivated poliovirus v.
influenza virus v.
lipopolysaccharide v.
meningococcal v.
pneumococcal v.
PRP-D v.
PRP-OMPC v.
tuberculosis v.
14-valent v.
vaccinia
Vaccinium myrtillus
Vac-Pak-II ultra-lite portable aspirator
VACTERL

vertebral, vascular, anal, cardiac,
    tracheoesophageal, renal, and limb
    anomalies
    VACTERL syndrome
Vacu-Aide home-use aspirator
vacuolated cell
Vacutainer tube
vacuum

v. controller
high v. (HV)
vacuum-assisted venous return system
vacuus

pulsus v.
VAD

venous access device
ventricular assist device
    DeBakey VAD
    HeartSaver VAD
VAE

venous air embolism
VA-ECMO

venoarterial extracorporeal membrane
    oxygenation
VAF

viral-free antigen
VAG

v. atrial fibrillation
v. attack
v. block
v. body
v. bradycardia
v. escape
v. neural crest
v. reaction

V

763

vagal (*continued*)
    v. reflex
    v. response
    v. stimulation
    v. tone
vagectomy
vagi (*pl. of* vagus)
vagina synovialis trochleae
vagolytic
    v. agent
    v. property
vagomimetic intervention
vagotonic baroreceptor response
vagus, pl. **vagi**
    v. arrhythmia
    ganglion inferius nervi vagi
    v. nerve
    v. nerve stimulation
    v. pneumonia
    v. pulse
    rami esophagei nervi vagi
Vairox high compression vascular stockings
Vak
    atrial volume constant
valacyclovir
14-valent vaccine
valgus
    cubitus v.
VALI
    ventilator-associated lung injury
validity
    face v.
vallecula, pl. **valleculae**
vallecular dysphagia
valley fever
Valleylab Force 2 electrosurgical device
valrubicin
Valsalva
    Gelweave V.
    V. maneuver (VS)
    ruptured sinus of V.
    V. sinus
    sinus of V.
    V. test
valsalviana
    dysphagia v.
valsartan and hydrochlorothiazide
Valstar
value
    Astrup blood gas v.
    index v.
    negative predictive v. (NPV)
    positive predictive v. (PPV)
    predictive v.
    QRS-T v.
    reference v.
    resting v.

    tercile v.
    threshold v.
valva trunci pulmonalis
valve
    abnormal cleavage of cardiac v.
    Abrams-Lucas flap heart v.
    absent pulmonary v.
    Access-9 large bore hemostasis v.
    Angell-Shiley bioprosthetic v.
    Angell-Shiley xenograft prosthetic v.
    Angiocor prosthetic v.
    anterior leaflet of the mitral v. (ALMV)
    aortic v. (AOV, AoV, AV)
    aortic bioprosthetic v.
    artificial cardiac v.
    atretic pulmonary v.
    atrial v.
    atrioventricular v. (AVV)
    ATS Open Pivot heart v.
    ATS standard aortic v.
    ATS standard mitral v.
    ball-and-cage prosthetic v.
    ball heart v.
    ball-occluder v.
    Beall prosthetic v.
    Beall-Surgitool ball-cage prosthetic v.
    Bianchi v.
    Bicarbon Sorin v.
    Bicer-Val prosthetic v.
    bicommissural aortic v. (BAV)
    bileaflet tilting-disk prosthetic v.
    Biocor porcine v.
    biological aortic v.
    bioprosthetic v. (BPV)
    bioprosthetic heart v.
    Bio-Vascular prosthetic v.
    Björk-Shiley convexoconcave disk prosthetic v.
    Björk-Shiley mitral v.
    Björk-Shiley monostrut v.
    Blom-Singer v.
    bovine heart v.
    bovine pericardial v.
    B-S v.
    BSCC heart v.
    butterfly heart v.
    caged ball v.
    calcification of tips of the mitral v.
    calcified aortic v.
    Capetown prosthetic v.
    Carbomedics bileaflet prosthetic heart v.
    Carbomedics top-hat supra-annular v.
    cardiac v.

Carpentier-Edwards mitral annuloplasty v.
Carpentier-Edwards pericardial v.
Carpentier-Edwards Perimount mitral v.
Carpentier-Edwards porcine prosthetic v.
Carpentier-Edwards porcine supraannular v.
Carpentier pericardial v.
caval v.
C-C heart v.
CirKuit-Guard pressure relief v.
cleft mitral v.
v. commissure
congenital anomaly of mitral v.
Cooley-Bloodwell-Cutter v.
Cooley-Cutter disk prosthetic v.
CPHV OptiForm mitral v.
crisscross atrioventricular v.
Cross-Jones disk prosthetic v.
Cross-Jones mitral v.
cryopreserved homograft v.
Cutter-Smeloff disk v.
Cutter-Smeloff mitral v.
DeBakey-Surgitool prosthetic v.
v. debris
Delrin heart v.
diastolic fluttering aortic v.
disk-cage v.
Double Play large bore double Y hemostasis v.
Duostat rotating hemostatic v.
Duromedics mitral v.
dysplastic v.
early opening v.
Ebstein malformed v.
echodense v.
Edmark mitral v.
Edwards-Duromedics bileaflet heart v.
Edwards heart v.
eustachian v.
flail mitral v.
floppy aortic v. (FAV)
floppy mitral v. (FMV)
four-legged cage v.
Freestyle bioprosthetic heart v.
Freestyle stentless aortic heart v.
glutaraldehyde-tanned bovine heart v.

glutaraldehyde-tanned porcine heart v.
Gott butterfly heart v.
Guangzhou GD-1 prosthetic v.
Hall-Kaster prosthetic v.
Hall prosthetic heart v.
Hancock II tissue v.
Hancock modified orifice v.
Hancock M.O. II bioprosthesis porcine v.
Hans Rudolph nonbreathing v.
Harken ball v.
heart v.
Heimlich chest drainage v.
Heimlich heart v.
hemostasis v.
hockey-stick tricuspid v.
Hufnagel prosthetic v.
impedance threshold v. (ITV)
Inspector large bore in-line hemostasis v.
intact v.
Ionescu-Shiley pericardial v.
Ionescu trileaflet v.
Kay-Shiley caged-disk v.
left atrial ball v. (LABV)
LeVeen v. (LVV)
Lillehei-Kaster pivoting-disk prosthetic v.
Lillehei-Nakib toroidal v.
Liotta-BioImplant low profile bioprosthesis prosthetic v.
Magovern-Cromie ball-cage prosthetic v.
Malteno v.
v. mapper Steerocath-Dx mapping catheter
MBA hemostasis v.
mechanical v.
Medtronic-Hall monocuspid tilting-disk v.
Medtronic-Hall prosthetic heart v.
Medtronic Hancock II tissue v.
Medtronic Intact bioprosthetic v.
Medtronic Mosaic bioprosthetic v.
midsystolic buckling of mitral v.
midsystolic closure of aortic v.
Mitroflow Synergy PC stented pericardial v.
Montgomery speaking v.
Mosaic porcine bioprosthetic heart v.

NOTES

valve (*continued*)
native v.
noncalcified v.
nonrebreathing v.
Omnicarbon prosthetic heart v.
On-X mechanical bi-leaflet
  prosthetic heart v.
Open Pivot heart v.
v. orifice area
parachute mitral v.
Passage hemostasis v.
Passy-Muir tracheostomy
  speaking v.
PEEP v.
Phonate speaking v.
PlegiaGuard pressure relief v.
PMV 2000 series speaking V.
pop-off v.
porcine prosthetic v.
posterior leaf mitral v. (PLMV)
prolapse of mitral v. (PMV)
prosthetic aortic v.
prosthetic ball v.
prosthetic cardiac v.
Provox speaking v.
Puig Massana-Shiley
  annuloplasty v.
pulmonary v. (PV)
pulmonary autograft v.
v. of pulmonary trunk
pulmonic v.
quadricusp mitral v. (QMC, QMV)
quadricusp stentless mitral
  bioprosthetic v.
reducing v.
v. replacement (VR)
v. resistance
v. rupture
semilunar v.
Shiley convexoconcave heart v.
Shiley Phonate speaking v.
short-axis mitral v. (SAX-MV)
short-axis plane mitral v.
SJM Masters Series heart v.
SJM mechanical heart v.
SJM Quattro mitral v.
SJM Regent mechanical heart v.
Smeloff-Cutter ball-cage
  prosthetic v.
Smeloff heart v.
Sorin heart v.
Sorin prosthetic v.
speaking v.
Starr-Edwards ball-and-cage v.
Starr-Edwards mitral v.
Starr-Edwards prosthetic v.
Starr-Edwards Silastic v.
stented bioprosthetic v.
stentless porcine v. (SPV)

stentless porcine aortic v.
stent-mounted allograft v.
stent-mounted heterograft v.
St. Jude V. (SJM)
St. Jude bileaflet prosthetic v.
St. Jude composite prosthetic v.
St. Jude Medical bileaflet tilting-
  disk aortic v.
St. Jude Medical Biocor v.
St. Jude Medical bioImplant v.
St. Jude Medical Port-Access
  mechanical heart v.
St. Jude mitral v.
St. Jude prosthetic aortic v.
straddling of v.
straddling atrioventricular v.
straddling tricuspid v.
Surgitool prosthetic v.
v. of Sylvius
SynerGraft pulmonary heart v.
SynerGraft tissue-engineered
  heart v.
thebesian v.
tilting disk heart v.
tilting disk prosthetic v.
tissue v.
Top-Hat supraannular aortic v.
toroidal v.
Toronto SPV aortic v.
Toronto SPV stentless porcine
  heart v.
tricuspid v. (TV)
tricuspid aortic v.
UCI-Barnard aortic v.
unicuspid aortic v.
Unistasis v.
unstented xenograft v.
Vascor porcine prosthetic v.
v. vegetation
ventilator speaking v.
Vieussens v.
v. of Vieussens
Wessex prosthetic v.
Xenotech prosthetic v.
valve-conserving operation
valvectomy
valved holding chamber (VHC)
valve-preserving surgery
valvopathy (*var. of* valvuopathy)
valvoplasty (*var. of* valvuloplasty)
valvotomy, valvulotomy
aortic v.
balloon aortic v. (BAV)
balloon pulmonary v.
balloon tricuspid v.
double-balloon v.
Inoue balloon mitral v.
v. knife
Longmire v.

mitral v.
mitral balloon v. (MBV)
mitral valve v.
percutaneous mitral v. (PMV)
percutaneous mitral balloon v. (PMBV)
pulmonary v.
radiofrequency-assisted v.
repeat balloon mitral v.
single-balloon v.
thimble v.
transcatheter v.
transventricular closed v.
valvula, pl. **valvulae**
    v. coronaria dextra valvae aortae
    v. semilunaris dextra
valvular
    v. aortic stenosis
    v. calcification
    v. cardiomyopathy
    v. disease of heart (VDH)
    v. dysfunction
    v. endocarditis
    v. function
    v. heart disease (VHD)
    v. incompetence
    v. insufficiency
    v. leaflet
    v. morphology
    v. orifice
    v. pneumothorax
    v. prolapse
    v. pulmonic stenosis
    v. reflux
    v. regurgitation
    v. sclerosis
    v. thickening
    v. thrombus
    v. vegetation
valvulitis
    aortic v.
    chronic v.
    mitral v.
    rheumatic v.
    syphilitic aortic v.
valvuloplasty, valvoplasty
    aortic v.
    bailout v.
    balloon v. (BV)
    balloon aortic v. (BAV)
    balloon mitral v. (BMV)
    balloon pulmonary v. (BPV)

Carpentier tricuspid v.
catheter balloon v. (CBV)
double-balloon v.
intracoronary thrombolysis
  balloon v.
mitral v.
multiple-balloon v.
percutaneous aortic v. (PAV)
percutaneous aortic balloon v. (PABV)
percutaneous balloon v. (PBV)
percutaneous balloon aortic v.
percutaneous balloon mitral v.
percutaneous balloon pulmonary v. (PBPV)
percutaneous balloon pulmonic v.
percutaneous mitral v. (PMV)
percutaneous mitral balloon v. (PMBV)
percutaneous transluminal balloon v.
pulmonary v.
pulmonary balloon v. (PBV)
single-balloon v.
transcarotid balloon v.
tricuspid v.
triple-balloon v.
Trusler technique of aortic v.
valvulotome
    angioscopic v.
    Hall v.
valvulotomy (*var. of* valvotomy)
valvuopathy, valvopathy
VAM
    ventricular arrhythmia monitor
VAMC
    Veterans Affairs Medical Center
    VAMC prognostic score
VAMP
    venous arterial blood management
    protection system
vampire bat salivary plasminogen activator (DSPA)
van
    v. Andel catheter
    v. Capelle-Durrer (VCD)
    v. den Bergh disease
    v. Gieson stain
    v. Helmont mirror
    v. Horne canal
    V. Slyke method
    V. Tassel catheter
vanadium

V

NOTES

vanadiumism
Vancenase
    V. AQ Inhaler
    V. Pockethaler
Vanceril Oral Inhaler
Vancocin
    V. CP
    V. injection
    V. Oral
Vancoled injection
vancomycin hydrochloride
vancomycin-resistant enterococcus
Vanguard
    V. device
    V. endograft
    V. III endovascular aortic graft
    V. modular endograft system
vanishing lung
Vantex central venous catheter
Vantin
VAP
    variant angina pectoris
    ventilator-associated pneumonia
Vaponefrin
vapor
    inorganic acid v.
    v. massage
    mercury v.
    solvent v.
vaporizer
    Fluotec v.
    Maxi-Myst v.
**Vapor-Phase heated humidification
  system**
vapotherapy
Vapotherm
    V. 2000i
    V. oxygen delivery system
VAPS
    volume-assured pressure support
Va/Q
    alveolar ventilation/perfusion
Vaquez disease
Varco thoracic forceps
variability
    baseline v.
    beat-to-beat v.
    cardiac v.
    diurnal peak flow v.
    heart rate v. (HRV)
    interlead QT v.
    relative heart rate v. (RHRV)
variable
    v. coupling
    v. deceleration
    impedance v.
    v. positive airway pressure (VPAP)

    v. stiffness wire guide
    v. threshold angina
variance cardiography (VC)
variant
    v. angina (VA)
    v. angina pectoris (VAP)
variation
    circadian v.
    diurnal v.
    respiratory waveform v.
variceal
    v. ligation
    v. sclerosing
    v. sclerotherapy
varicella
    v. pneumonia
    v. pneumonitis
varicella-zoster
    v.-z. immunoglobulin (VZIG)
    v.-z. infection
    v.-z. virus (VZV, VZ)
varices (*pl. of* varix)
varicose
    v. vein
    v. vein stripping and ligation
varicosity
    saphenous vein v.
Variflex catheter catheter
**Vari-Lase endovenous laser procedure
  kit**
variomatrix transducer
Vario system
variotii
    Paecilomyces v.
**Varivas R denatured homologous vein
  graft**
varix, pl. varices
    cirsoid v.
    downhill esophageal v.
    esophageal varices
VAS, pl. vasa
    vascular
    vascular access service
    vasculotropin
    ventriculoatrial shunt
    visual analog scale
        horizontal VAS
        mechanical VAS
        vertical VAS
vas
    v.'s afferentia
    v.'s nervorum
    v.'s vasorum
VASC, vasc
    vascular
Vascoray
Vascor porcine prosthetic valve
VascuClamp vascular clamp
VascuCoil peripheral vascular stent

Vascu-Flo carotid shunt
Vascugel device
vascular (VAS, VASC, vasc)
    v. access catheter
    v. access service (VAS)
    v. acoustic emission
    v. anatomy teaching tool (VATT)
    v. attenuation
    v. bed
    v. brachytherapy
    v. bundle
    v. cadherin
    v. cell adhesion molecule-1
     (VCAM-1)
    v. change (VC)
    v. choir
    v. clamp
    v. clip
    v. compromise
    v. death
    v. dementia
    v. depression
    v. disease (VD)
    v. ectasia
    v. endothelial growth factor
     (VEGF)
    v. funnel
    v. gene transfer
    v. graft prosthesis
    v. groove
    v. hemostatic device (VHD)
    v. impedance
    v. incident
    v. injury
    v. insult
    v. leak syndrome (VLS)
    v. marking
    v. matrix
    v. murmur
    v. pattern
    v. peripheral resistance
    v. permeability factor (VPF)
    v. reactivity
    v. redistribution
    v. reflex
    v. remodeling
    v. resistance (VR)
    v. resistance index
    v. ring
    v. ring division
    v. sclerosis
    v. sealing device

    v. sheath
    v. sling
    v. smooth muscle cell (VSMC)
    v. spasm
    v. spider
    v. stenosis
    v. stiffness
    v. system
    v. tape
    v. tunic
    v. wall (VW)
    v. zone
vascularity
vascularization
vasculature
    coronary v.
    pulmonary v.
VascuLink vascular access graft
vasculitic neuropathy
vasculitis, pl. **vasculitides**
    allergic v.
    cardiac v.
    Churg-Strauss v.
    consecutive v.
    Henoch-Schönlein v.
    hypersensitivity v.
    immune-mediated v.
    leukocytoblastic v.
    livedo v.
    lymphoreticular granulomatous v.
    necrotizing granulomatous v.
    nodular v.
    overlap v.
    pulmonary v.
    segmented hyalinizing v.
    systemic granulomatous v.
    systemic necrotizing v.
vasculocardiac syndrome of
  hyperserotonemia
vasculogenesis
vasculogenic impotence
vasculopathy
    allograft v.
    cardiac allograft v. (CAV)
    cerebral v.
    graft v.
    hypertensive v.
    primary fibroproliferative
     pulmonary v.
vasculotropin (VAS)
Vascutek
    V. Gelseal vascular graft

NOTES

V

Vascutek *(continued)*
    V. knitted vascular graft
    V. woven vascular graft
Vaseretic
vasinfectum
vasoactive
    v. drug
    v. intestinal peptide (VIP)
    v. mediator
    v. substance
vasoactivity
vasoconstriction (VC)
    coronary microcirculatory v.
    delayed cerebral v. (DCV)
    hypoxic v.
    hypoxic pulmonary v. (HPV)
    microcirculatory v.
    paradoxical v.
    peripheral v.
    pulmonary v.
    v. rate (VCR)
    reflex v.
    reflex pulmonary arterial v.
vasoconstrictive reflex
vasoconstrictor
    v. center (VCC)
    v. peptide
    pulmonary alveolar hypoxic v. (PAHVC)
    v. substance (VCS)
vasodepression
vasodepressor
    v. lipid (VDL)
    v. material (VDEM, VDM)
    v. substance
    v. syncope
vasodepressor-cardioinhibitory syncope
Vasodilan
vasodilation (VD)
    coronary v.
    endothelium-dependent v.
    flow-mediated v.
    myocardial v. (MVD)
    peripheral v.
    profound systemic v.
    pulmonary v.
    reflex v.
    regional v.
vasodilator (VD)
    v. agent (VA)
    v. center (VDC)
    v. effect
    v. plus exercise treadmill test
    v. reserve
    v. substance (VDS)
vasodilatory
    v. hypotension

    v. response
    v. shock
vasoexcitor material (VEM)
vasofactive cell
vasogenic
    v. edema
    v. shock
vasoinhibitor
vasoinhibitory
    v. center (VIC)
    v. peptide (VIP)
vasomotion
    coronary v.
vasomotor (VM)
    v. angina
    v. center (VMC)
    v. flushing (VMF)
    v. paralysis
    v. response (VMR)
    v. rhinitis
    v. syncope
    v. tone
    v. tonus (VMT)
vasomotoria
    angina pectoris v.
vasoneuronal coupling
vasoocclusive pain (VOP)
vasopeptidase inhibitor (VPI)
vasopressin (VP)
    abnormal v. (AVP)
    aqueous v. (AVP)
    arginine v. (ARVP, AVP)
    1-deamine-4-valine-D-arginine v. (dVDAVP)
    intraarterial v. (IAV)
    intravenous v. (IVV)
    plasma arginine v. (pAVP)
vasopressor
    v. deficiency
    v. reflex
    v. support
vasoreactivity
vasoregulatory asthenia
vasorelaxant peptide
vasorelaxation
vasoresponse
vasorum
    aortic vasa v.
    vasa v.
Vasoscope 3 Doppler probe
VasoSeal
    V. vascular hemostasis device
    V. VHD
vasospasm
    cerebral v. (CVS)
    coronary v.
    diffuse v.
    ergonovine-induced coronary v.
    focal v.

vasospastic
    v. angina (VSA)
    v. disease
Vasotec
    V. IV
    V. Oral
vasotocin
    arginine v. (AVT)
vasotonic angina
Vasotrax handheld monitor
vasovagal
    v. attack
    v. episode
    v. hypotension
    v. orthostatism
    v. reaction
    v. syncope (VVS)
    v. syndrome
VasoView
    V. balloon dissection device
    V. Uniport endoscopic saphenous
    vein harvesting system
VAT
    ventilatory anaerobic threshold
    ventricular accommodation test
    ventricular activation time
    video-assisted thoracoscopy
    VAT pacemaker
    VAT pacing
VATER
    vertebral defects, imperforate anus,
    transesophageal fistula, and radial and
    renal dysplasia
    VATER association syndrome
    VATER complex
VATS
    video-assisted thoracic surgery
    video-assisted thoracoscopic surgery
    video-assisted thoracoscopy
VATT
    vascular anatomy teaching tool
Vaughan-Williams
    V.-W. antiarrhythmic drug
    classification
    V.-W. class effect
Vaxcel
    V. catheter
    V. mini stick
VB
    venous blood
    virtual bronchoscopy

V510B biplane TEE transducer
VBG
    venous bypass graft
VBI
    vertebrobasilar territory ischemia
VBP
    venous blood pressure
    ventricular premature beat
VC
    variance cardiography
    vascular change
    vasoconstriction
    vena cava
    venous capacitance
    venous dilatation
    ventricular contraction
    vital capacity
    volume control
V/C
    ventilation-to-circulation
    V/C ratio
Vc
    pulmonary capillary blood volume
VCA
    viral capsid antigen
VCAM-1
    vascular cell adhesion molecule-1
VCC
    vasoconstrictor center
VCD
    van Capelle-Durrer
    vocal cord dysfunction
    VCD model of cardiac cell
    depolarization-repolarization
VCDF
    volume-cycled decelerating-flow
    ventilation
VCF
    velocardiofacial
    velocity of circumferential fiber
    shortening
    VCF syndrome
V$_{cf}$
    fiber shortening velocity
VCFS
    velocardiofacial syndrome
VCG
    vectorcardiogram
    vectorcardiography
VCO$_2$
    venous carbon dioxide production

V

NOTES

VCPC
vindesine, cisplatin, lomustine,
cyclophosphamide
VCR
vasoconstriction rate
VCS
vasoconstrictor substance
VCT
venous clotting time
VCV
ventricular conduction velocity
volume-controlled ventilation
VD
vascular disease
vasodilation
vasodilator
ventricular dilator
V$_D$
physiological dead space ventilation per
minute
VDC
vasodilator center
VDD
atrial synchronous ventricular inhibited
VDD mode
VDD pacemaker
VDD pacing
VDD pacing system
V-Dec-M
VDEM
vasodepressor material
VDF
ventricular diastolic fragmentation
VDH
valvular disease of heart
VDI
both ventricles inhibited
venous disability index
VDI pacing
VDI pacing mode
Vdia
diastolic potential
VDL
vasodepressor lipid
VDM
vasodepressor material
VDR
venous diameter ratio
volumetric diffusive respirator
VDRL
Venereal Disease Research Laboratory
VDRL test
VDS
vasodilator substance
venous duplex scanning
VDV
ventricular end-diastolic volume
VE
venous extension

ventricular elasticity
ventricular extrasystole
VEA
ventricular ectopic activity
VEB
ventricular ectopic beat
VECG
vector electrocardiogram
VE-cMRI
velocity-encoded cine-magnetic
resonance imaging
vector
adeno-associated viral v.
adenoviral v.
angle between QRS and T v.'s
(QRS-T)
v. cardiography
electric heart v. (EHV)
v. electrocardiogram (VECG)
instantaneous v.
v. loop
magnetic heart v. (MHV)
v. magnetocardiogram (VMCG)
manifest v.
mean manifest v.
P v.
v. phased-array ultrasound tipped
catheter
QRS v.
retroviral v.
spatial v.
ST, T v.
viral v.
vectorcardiogram (VCG)
spatial v. (SVCG)
vectorcardiography (VCG)
left foot electrode in v.
spatial v.
Vector-X coronary guiding catheter
vecuronium
VED
ventricular ectopic depolarization
Veetids Oral
VEF
ventricular ejection fraction
VEFR
visually evoked flow response
vegetal bronchitis
vegetarian diet
vegetation
aortic valve v.
bacterial v.
endocardial v.
leaflet v.
mobile v.
prosthetic valve v.
pulmonary valve v.
tricuspid valve v.
valve v.

valvular v.
ventricular septal defect v.
verrucous v.
vegetative
v. endocarditis
v. lesion
VEGF
vascular endothelial growth factor
VEGF gene therapy
VEGF TRAP
veiled puff
veiling glare
Veillonella
vein
accessory saphenous v.
allantoic v.
anomalous pulmonary v.
antecubital v.
aortocoronary saphenous v. (ACSV)
arrhythmogenic pulmonary v.
autogenous v.
autologous saphenous v. (ASV)
axillary v.
azygos v.
basilic v.
Boyd perforating v.
brachial v.
brachiocephalic v.
bronchial v.
Burow v.
cardiac v.
cardinal v.
v. of caudate nucleus
central v.
cephalic v.
common femoral v.
coronary v.
cryopreserved v.
deep lingual v.
Dodd perforating v.
esophageal v.
external jugular v.
external pudendal v.
facial v.
femoral v.
v. graft
v. graft cannula
v. graft patency
v. graft ring marker
great cardiac v. (GCV)
hemiazygos v.
hepatic v.

human umbilical v. (HUV)
iliac v.
inferior laryngeal v.
inferior thyroid v.
infrasegmental v.
innominate v.
internal cerebral v. (ICV)
internal jugular v.
internal pudendal v.
internal thoracic v.
intersegmental part of pulmonary v.
interventricular v.
intrapulmonary v. (IPV)
jugular v. (JV)
Kohlrausch v.
Krukenberg v.
Kuhnt postcentral v.
laryngeal v.
left inferior pulmonary v.
left internal jugular v.
left lower pulmonary v. (LLPV)
left median v.
left pulmonary v.'s (LPV)
left superior pulmonary v.
left upper pulmonary v. (LUPV)
levoatriocardinal v.
lingual v.
main portal v. (MPV)
main renal v.
Marshall oblique v.
nest of v.'s
partial anomalous pulmonary v.'s
pharyngeal v.
portal v. (PV)
profunda femoris v.
prominent pulmonary v.
pulmonary v. (PV)
renal v.
Retzius v.'s
reverse saphenous v.
right brachial v. (RBV)
right inferior pulmonary v.
right lower pulmonary v. (RLPV)
right portal v. (RPV)
right pulmonary v. (RPV)
right superior pulmonary v.
right upper pulmonary v. (RUPV)
saphenous v. (SV)
sausaging of v.
subclavian v.
sublingual v.
superficial circumflex iliac v.

V

NOTES

vein *(continued)*
    superior laryngeal v.
    superior mesenteric v.
    superior pulmonary v.
    superior thalamostriate v.
    thebesian v.
    v. of Thebesius
    tortuous v.'s
    tracheal v.
    umbilical v.
    varicose v.
    ventricular v.
vein-to-vein technology
Velban
Velbe
Velcro rale
Veletri
velocardiofacial (VCF)
    v. syndrome (VCFS)
velocimeter
    FloMap v.
velocimetry
    Doppler v.
velocity
    airflow v.
    aortic flow v. (AFV)
    aortic jet v.
    aortic pulse-wave v.
    A-peak v.
    average peak v. (APV)
    basal average peak v. (BAPV)
    baseline average peak v. (BAPV)
    blood flow v. (BFV)
    blunted systolic v.
    v. catheter technique
    cerebral blood flow v. (CBFV)
    v. of circumferential fiber
      shortening (VCF)
    conduction v.
    coronary blood flow v. (CBFV)
    coronary flow v.
    detachment v.
    Doppler peak flow v. (Vmax)
    ejection v.
    v. encoding
    end-diastolic v.
    E-peak v.
    E-wave v.
    fiber shortening v. (V_{cf})
    field flow v.
    flow v.
    forward flow of v.
    high regional wall motion v.
      (Vhigh)
    hyperemic v.
    instantaneous spectral peak v.
    jet v.
    left atrial appendage flow v.
    left ventricular outflow tract v.

    long-axis shortening v.
    maximal v. (V_{MAX}, Vmax)
    maximum v. (V_{MAX}, Vmax)
    myocardial Doppler v. (MDV)
    nerve conduction v. (NCV)
    peak A, E v.
    peak diastolic v. (PDV)
    peak ejection v. (V_{pe})
    peak systolic v.
    peak transaortic flow v.
    phasic intragraft flow v.
    pulse wave v. (PWV)
    v. ratio (VR)
    sensory nerve conduction v.
      (SNCV)
    shortening v.
    spectral peak v.
    V. stent
    systolic pulmonary venous v.
    systolic wall motion v. (Vsys)
    time-averaged peak v.
    v. time integral
    tracheal mucus v.
    translesional spectral flow v.
    transmitral flow v.
    transprosthetic flow v.
    transvalvular E v.
    upstroke v.
    ventricular conduction v. (VCV)
    wall motion v.
velocity-encoded cine-magnetic resonance imaging (VE-cMRI)
Velogene rapid TB assay
velopharyngeal
    v. endoscope
    v. insufficiency
Velosef
Velosulin Human
velour collar graft
Velpeau hernia
Velstretch/Velcro headgear
VEM
    vasoexcitor material
vena, pl. venae
    agger valvae venae
    venae bronchiales
    venae cardiacae anteriores
    venae cardiacae minimae
    v. cava (VC)
    v. caval foramen
    v. caval obstruction
    venae circumflexae femoris laterales
    v. circumflexa humeri anterior
    v. circumflexa iliaca profunda
    v. circumflexa iliaca superficialis
    v. contracta
    venae cordis
    venae cordis minimae
    venae dorsales linguae

venae esophageales
v. laryngea inferior
v. laryngea superior
v. lingularis
v. obliqua atrii sinistra
venae pharyngeae
v. profunda linguae
venae pulmonales
v. pulmonalis inferior dextra
v. pulmonalis inferior sinistra
v. pulmonalis superior dextra
v. pulmonalis superior sinistra
v. sublingualis
venae supratrochleares
venae tracheales
vena cava, pl. **venae cavae (VC)**
v. c. cannula
v. c. clip
v. c. filter
foramen venae cavae
inferior v. c. (IVC)
v. c. obstruction
Spencer plication of v. c.
v. c. syndrome
venacavogram
venacavography
inferior v. (IVCV)
venae (*pl. of* vena)
venae cavae (*pl. of* vena cava)
VenaFlow
V. compression system
V. DVT prophylaxis system
Venaport coronary sinus guiding catheter
Vena Tech LGM filter
venectasia
Venereal Disease Research Laboratory (VDRL)
venereum
lymphogranuloma v. (LGV)
venesection (VS, Vs)
VenES II Medical stockings
Venflon needle
venipuncture
contrast-guided v.
venoarterial (V-A)
v. bypass pumping (VABP)
v. extracorporeal membrane oxygenation (VA-ECMO)
v. shunting
venoatrial junction

venoconstriction
splenic v.
venodilation
Venodyne EPS-410 external pneumatic compression system
Venoglobulin-S
venogram
venography
contrast v.
helical CT v.
magnetic resonance v. (MRV)
radionuclide v. (RNV)
renal v.
venolobar syndrome
venom
arthropod v.
bee v.
black widow spider v.
scorpion v.
snake v.
spider v.
venoocclusive disease (VOD)
venopressor
venorespiratory reflex
Venoscope
venosinal
venosity
venostasis
venosus
ductus v.
pulsus v.
sinus v.
venous
v. access
v. access device (VAD)
v. admixture
v. air embolism (VAE)
v. arterial blood management protection system (VAMP)
v. blood (VB)
v. blood pressure (VBP)
v. bypass graft (VBG)
v. cannula
v. capacitance (VC)
v. capacitance bed
v. carbon dioxide production (VCO_2)
central v. (CV)
v. clotting time (VCT)
v. collateral
v. congestion
v. coronary graft patency

NOTES

V

venous *(continued)*
   v. Corrigan wave
   v. cutdown
   v. diameter ratio (VDR)
   v. digital angiogram
   v. dilatation (VC)
   v. disability index (VDI)
   v. duplex scanning (VDS)
   v. embolism
   v. engorgement
   v. extension (VE)
   v. filling index (VFI)
   v. flow controller (VFC)
   v. flow measurement
   v. flow reversal (VR)
   v. graft myringoplasty (VGM)
   v. groove
   v. heart
   v. hum
   v. hyperemia
   v. hypertension
   v. impedance plethysmography (VIP)
   v. insufficiency syndrome (VIS)
   v. intravasation
   v. lakes
   v. mesenteric vascular occlusion
   v. murmur
   v. occlusion plethysmography (VOP)
   v. occlusion test
   v. phase
   v. plasma norepinephrine concentration
   v. pressure (VP)
   v. pressure gradient support stockings (VPGSS)
   v. pressure tracing
   v. pulse
   v. pulse tracing
   v. puncture
   v. reflux (VR)
   v. return (VR)
   v. return curve
   v. runoff
   v. saturation
   v. sclerosis
   v. sheath
   v. smooth muscle
   v. spasm
   v. spread
   v. stasis
   v. stop flow pressure (VSFP)
   v. thromboembolism (VTE)
   v. thrombosis
   v. ulcer
   v. valvular insufficiency
   v. volume (VV, VVol)
   v. web

venovenostomy
venovenous (VV)
   v. access
   v. double-lumen (VVDL)
   v. dye dilution curve
vent
   ventricle
   ventricular
   Heartport endopulmonary vent
Ventak
   V. AICD
   V. AICD pacemaker
   V. A-V III DR automatic implantable cardioverter-defibrillator
   V. ECD
   V. Mini II and III automatic implantable cardioverter-defibrillator
   V. Prizm 2 automatic implantable cardioverter-defibrillator
   V. Prizm dual-chamber implantable defibrillator
   V. Prizm 2 system
   V. PRx cardioverter-defibrillator
   V. PRx defibrillation system
   V. PRx III/Endotak system
   V. PRx pacemaker
VentCheck handheld respiratory monitor
vented-electric HeartMate LVAD
vent fib
   ventricular fibrillation
ventilate
ventilated alveoli
ventilation
   adaptive support v. (ASV)
   airway pressure release v. (APRV)
   alveolar v.
   artificial v.
   assist/control v. (ACV)
   assist/control mode v.
   assisted v.
   assisted mechanical v. (AMV)
   backup v. (BUV)
   bag-mask v.
   bag-valve-mask v.
   v. bronchoscope
   BVM v.
   v. collateralization
   continuous-flow v.
   continuous mandatory v.
   continuous positive pressure v.
   controlled mechanical v.
   control-mode v.
   conventional v. (CV)
   dead space v.
   v. episode
   v. equivalent

forced mandatory intermittent v. (FMIV)
high-frequency v. (HFV)
high-frequency jet v. (HFJV)
high-frequency oscillatory v.
high-frequency percussive v.
high-frequency positive pressure v. (HFPPV)
intermittent demand v. (IDV)
intermittent mandatory v. (IMV)
intermittent mechanical v. (IMV)
intermittent percussive v. (IPV)
intermittent positive pressure v. (IPPV)
intrapulmonary percussive v. (IPV)
inverse-ratio v. (IRV)
jet v.
manual v.
v. mask
maximal v. (MV)
maximum voluntary v. (MVV)
mechanical v. (MV)
v. meter
minute v. (V_E)
mouth-to-face shield v.
mouth-to-mask v.
mouth-to-mouth v.
mouth-to-nose v.
mouth-to-stoma v.
nasal nocturnal v. (NNV)
nasal positive pressure v. (NPPV)
negative pressure v. (NPV)
nocturnal v.
noninvasive v. (NIV)
noninvasive face mask v.
noninvasive mechanical v.
noninvasive positive pressure v. (NIPPV, NPPV)
noninvasive positive pressure v. (NIPPV, NPPV)
partial liquid v. (PLV)
peak exercise v. (V_E)
percutaneous transtracheal jet v. (PTJV)
percutaneous transtracheal needle v.
physiologic dead space v. (V_D/V_T)
positive airway pressure v.
positive pressure mechanical v.
pressure-controlled v. (PCV)
pressure-controlled inverse ratio v. (PCIRV)
pressure cycled v.

pressure-regulated volume control v.
pressure support v. (PSV)
proportional assist v. (PAV)
protective v.
PRVC v.
pulmonary v.
QT v.
v. scintigraphy
split-lung v.
spontaneous v.
synchronized intermittent mandatory v. (SIMV)
v. threshold
time-cycled v.
ultrahigh frequency v. (UHFV)
unassisted spontaneous v.
volume-controlled v. (VCV)
volume-cycled decelerating-flow v. (VCDF)
wasted v.

ventilation/carbon dioxide production (VE/VCO$_2$)

ventilation/perfusion (V/Q)
alveolar v. (Va/Q)
v. defect
v. imaging
v. lung scan
v. matching
v. mismatch
v. ratio
v. relation

ventilation-to-circulation (V/C)

ventilator
740 V.
Adult Star 1010, 2000 ultra-high-frequency v.
Aequitron v.
AirMed v.
Avian transport v.
babyPac v.
Bear 1000 v.
Bear 1, 2 adult volume v.
Bear Cub infant v.
Bennett MA-1, PR-2 v.
3100B high-frequency oscillatory v.
Bio-Med MVP-10 pediatric v.
Bird Ascension v.
Bird VDR v.
blow-by v.
Bourns-Bear v.
Bourns infant v.
compPac v.

V

NOTES

ventilator *(continued)*
    Critical Care V.
    cuirass v.
    v. dependency
    Dräger v.
    E-150 Breeze v.
    Emerson postoperative v.
    Esprit v.
    Galileo v.
    Hamilton v.
    high-frequency chest wall v.
      (HFCWO)
    high-frequency jet v.
    high-frequency oscillation v.
    Infant Star 100, 200 v.
    Infant Star V. 500/950
    Lifecare PLV-100 v.
    v. management
    MicroVent v.
    Monaghan 300 v.
    Newport E100M v.
    Newport Wave V200 v.
    noninvasive extrathoracic v. (NEV)
    ParaPac v.
    pneuPAC v.
    portable volume v.
    positive support v. (PSV)
    pressure cycled v.
    pressure support v. (PSV)
    Puritan Bennett v.
    v. rate
    rescu PAC v.
    Respironics BIPAP bilevel v.
    responder v.
    Sechrist IV-100 infant v.
    Servo V. 300
    Siemens v.
    Smart Trigger Bear 1000 v.
    v. speaking valve
    840 v. system
    v. time
    transPac v.
    Uni-Vent v.
    ventiPAC v.
    Venturi v.
    volume v.
    volume-cycled v.
    Wave VM200 v.
    v. weaning
ventilator-associated
    v.-a. lung injury (VALI)
    v.-a. pneumonia (VAP)
ventilator-induced
    v.-i. lung injury (VILI)
    v.-i. pneumopericardium
    v.-i. pneumothorax
ventilatory
    v. anaerobic threshold (VAT)
    v. assistance

    v. capacity
    v. compliance
    v. equivalent
    v. failure
    v. function
    v. response
    v. support
    v. threshold
Venti mask
ventiPAC ventilator
Ventolin
    V. HFA
    V. Nebules
    V. Rotacaps
    V. updraft
VenTrak respiratory mechanics monitor
ventral
    v. lead 1, 2, 3, 4, 5, 6 (V1-V6)
ventricle (vent)
    AIS model of a beating v.
    anterior papillary muscle of left v.
    anterior right v. (ARV)
    anteroventral third v. (Av3V)
    atrialized v.
    banana-shaped left v.
    calcified papillary muscle in the
      right v.
    double-inlet left v.
    double-outlet left v. (DOLV)
    double-outlet right v. (DORV)
    effective refractory period of
      left v. (ERPLV)
    hypoplasia of right v.
    hypoplastic left v. (HLV)
    indeterminate single v.
    ischemic contracture of left v.
    laryngeal v.
    left v. (LV)
    L-looping of the v.
    Mary Allen Engle v.
    noncompliant v.
    parchment right v.
    posterior left v. (PLV)
    posterior wall of left v. (PWLV)
    right v. (RV)
    single v.
    suicide v.
    volume-overloaded left v.
ventricles
    electrocardiographic wave
      corresponding to the repolarization
      of the v. (T)
Ventricor pacemaker
ventricular (V, vent)
    v. aberration
    v. accommodation test (VAT)
    v. activation time (VAT)
    v. afterload
    v. aneurysm (VA)

v. angiography
v. apex
v. arrhythmia (VA)
v. arrhythmia monitor (VAM)
v. assist device (VAD)
v. asynchronous (VOO)
v. asynchronous pacemaker
v. atresia
atrial carotid v. (ACV)
v. autocapture
v. band of larynx
bidirectional v.
v. bigeminy
v. biopsy
v. block
v. bradycardia
v. canal
v. capture
v. capture beat
v. capture threshold
v. cavity
v. complex
v. conduction
v. conduction velocity (VCV)
v. contour
v. contractile synchrony
v. contraction (VC)
v. contraction pattern
v. couplet
v. demand-inhibited pacemaker
v. demand-triggered (VVD)
v. demand-triggered pacemaker
v. depolarization abnormality
v. diastole
v. diastolic fragmentation (VDF)
v. diastolic pressure
v. dilation
v. dilator (VD)
v. distensibility
v. drive
v. dysfunction
v. dyssynergy
v. echo
v. ectopic activity (VEA)
v. ectopic beat (VEB)
v. ectopic depolarization (VED)
v. ectopic systole
v. ectopy
v. effective refractory period
 (VERP)
v. ejection fraction (VEF)
v. ejection time (VET)

v. elasticity (VE)
v. end-diastolic volume (VDV)
v. endoaneurysmorrhaphy
v. end-systolic pressure-volume
 relation
v. end-systolic wall stress
v. escape
v. escape beat
v. extrasystole (VE)
v. failure
v. far-field signal
v. fibrillation (vent fib, VF)
v. fibrillation arrest
v. fibrillation/ventricular tachycardia
 (VF/VT)
v. filling
v. filling pressure
v. fluid (VF)
v. flutter (VF)
v. function (VF)
v. function curve (VFC)
v. fusion beat
v. gallop (VG)
v. geometry
v. gradient
v. heart rate (VHR)
v. hypertrophy (VH)
v. impedance
v. implantable cardioverter-
 defibrillator (V-ICD, VICD)
v. inflow anomaly
v. inflow tract obstruction
v. inhibited (VVI)
v. inhibited pulse generator
v. inlet
v. inotropic parameter (VIP)
v. interdependence
v. inversion
v. late potential (VLP)
v. lead
left v. (LV)
v. ligament
v. mapping
v. mass
v. milk spots
v. mural swelling
v. myxoma
v. outflow tract obstruction
v. paced rhythm (VPR)
v. pacing (VP)
v. parasystole
v. pause

NOTES

ventricular *(continued)*
- v. perforation
- v. performance
- v. perfusion index (VQI)
- v. pericardium (VP)
- v. plateau
- v. ponderance
- v. power
- v. preexcitation
- v. preload
- v. premature (VP, Vp)
- v. premature beat (VBP, VPB)
- v. premature complex (VPC)
- v. premature contraction (VPC)
- v. premature contraction threshold (VPCT)
- v. premature depolarization (VPD)
- v. pressure (PV)
- v. pressure-volume loop
- v. pulse amplitude
- v. pulse width
- v. puncture
- v. radial dysplasia (VRD)
- v. rale (VR)
- v. reduction surgery
- v. reentry
- v. relaxation
- v. remodeling
- v. reserve
- v. residual volume (VRV)
- v. response
- v. rhythm (VR)
- right v. (RV)
- v. safety pacing
- v. sensing configuration
- v. sensitivity
- v. septal defect (VSD)
- v. septal defect murmur
- v. septal defect vegetation
- v. septal heart defect (VSHD)
- v. septal rupture
- v. septum (VS)
- v. situs solitus
- v. standstill
- v. stroke work (VSW)
- v. stroke work index
- v. synchronous pulse generator
- v. systole
- v. systolic impairment
- v. systolic stiffness
- v. tachyarrhythmia (VTA)
- v. tachycardia (V tach, VT)
- v. tachycardia cycle length (VTCL)
- v. tachycardia event (VTE)
- v. tachycardia/ventricular fibrillation (VT/VF)
- v. thrombus
- v. triggered (VVT)

- v. triggered pulse generator
- v. vein
- v. volume
- v. volume constant (vvk)
- v. wall contractility
- v. wall motion (VWM)
- v. wall shortening
- v. wall thinning
- v. wave

ventricularization
ventricular-programmed stimulation
ventriculoarterial
- v. concordance
- v. coupling
- v. discordance

ventriculoatrial (V-A, VA)
- v. conduction (VAC, V-AC)
- v. effective refractory period
- sequential v. (SVA)
- v. shunt (VAS)
- v. shunt catheter

ventriculocyte
ventriculogram-derived ejection fraction
ventriculographic ejection fraction
ventriculography
- biplane v.
- v. catheter
- contrast v. (CV)
- contrast left v.
- equilibrium multigated radionuclide v.
- left v.
- quantitative left v.
- radionuclide v. (RNV, RNVG)
- rest-exercise equilibrium radionuclide v.
- tomographic radionuclide v.

ventriculojugular (VJ)
ventriculojugulocardiac (VJC)
ventriculomegaly (VM, VML)
ventriculometry (VM)
ventriculophasic
ventriculopuncture
ventriculoradial dysplasia
ventriculorrhaphy
ventriculoscopy
ventriculoseptal defect (VSD)
ventriculotomy
- encircling endocardial v.
- endocardial v. (ECV)
- partial encircling endocardial v.

ventriculus laryngis
Ventritex
- V. Angstrom MD implantable cardioverter-defibrillator
- V. Cadence ICD
- V. Cadence implantable cardioverter-defibrillator

V. Contour
V. TVL system
ventroanterior (VA)
ventrolateral medulla (VLM)
Venture demand oxygen delivery device
Venturi
V. effect
V. exhalation assist
V. force
V. jet adapter
V. mask
V. phenomenon
V. tube
V. ventilator
V. Venti-mask Mark 2
V. wave
venule
venulitis
cutaneous necrotizing v.
VePesid
V. injection
V. Oral
vera
polycythemia v.
verapamil
v. HCl
v. hydrochloride
PPR v.
trandolapril and v.
verapamil-sensitive
veratridine
verbal amnesia
Verhoeff
V. elastica stain
V. tissue elastin stain
Veriflex cardiac device
Veripath peripheral guiding catheter
vermicular pulse
verminous
v. aneurysm
v. bronchitis
Vermizine
Vermox
vernal edema of lung
Vernet syndrome
Verneuil canal
veronii
Aeromonas v.
VERP
ventricular effective refractory period
verruca, pl. **verrucae**

verrucosa
arteritis v.
Phialophora v.
verrucous
v. carcinoma
v. carditis
v. endocarditis
v. vegetation
verruga peruana
Versacaps
VersaLab APM2 for Twins
VersaStep laparoscopy system
Versatrax II 7000A pacemaker
Versed
versicolor
Aspergillus v.
version
Ferrans and Powers Quality of
Life Index, cardiac v.
Verstraeten bruit
vertebra, pl. **vertebrae**
cervical v. (CV)
vertebral
v. artery bypass graft
v. defects, imperforate anus,
transesophageal fistula, and radial
and renal dysplasia (VATER)
v. endarterectomy
v. part of the costal surface of
lung
v. part of diaphragm
v., vascular, anal, cardiac,
tracheoesophageal, renal, and limb
anomalies (VACTERL)
vertebrobasilar
v. occlusive disease
v. territory ischemia (VBI)
v. TIA
vertebrocostal trigone
vertical
v. deceleration
v. deceleration mechanism
v. heart
v. integration
v. long axis
v. long-axis tomogram
v. long-axis view
v. VAS
vertigo
laryngeal v.
rotary v.

V

NOTES

very
>v. high density lipoprotein (VHDL)
>v. long-chain fatty acid (VLCFA)
>v. low-calorie diet (VLCD)
>v. low density lipoprotein (VLDL)
>v. low density lipoprotein receptor (VLDLR)
>v. low density lipoprotein-triglyceride complex (VLDL-TG)

ves
>vessel

vesicle
>air v.
>brush border membrane v. (BBMV)
>intermediary v.
>malpighian v.

vesicular
>v. breath sounds
>v. bronchiolitis
>v. bronchitis
>v. emphysema
>v. fluid
>v. monoamine transformer (VMAT)
>v. murmur
>v. rale

vesicular-vacuolar organelle (VVO)
vesiculobronchial
vesiculobullous
vesiculocavernous respiration
vesnarinone
Vesprin
vessel (ves)
>absorbent v.
>aortic arch v.
>blood v. (BV)
>bouquet of v.'s
>capacitance v.
>v. clamp
>codominant v.
>collateral v.
>collateralizing v.
>conductance v.
>congenitally corrected transposition of great v.'s (CC-TGA)
>coronary resistance v.
>corrected transposition of great v.'s
>v. dilator
>feeder v.
>femoral v.
>ghost v.
>great v.
>infarct-related v.
>intercostal mammary v.
>internal mammary v.
>intramyocardial v.
>large v.
>v. lumen
>native v.

>nondominant v.
>v. occlusion system
>P/D v.
>polytef artificial v.
>proximal and distal portion of v.
>recruitable collateral v.
>renal blood v.
>resistance v.
>retinal v.
>v. spasm
>splanchnic v.
>subclavian v.
>target v.
>thoracic v.
>tortuous v.
>transposition of great v.'s (TGV)
>v. trauma
>v. wall movement

Vesseloops rubber band
vessel-sizing catheter
VEST
>VEST ambulatory nuclear detector
>VEST ambulatory ventricular function monitor
>VEST left ventricular function detector

vest
>Bremer AirFlo V.
>cardiac v.
>Mark VII cooling v.
>ThAIRapy v.

vestibula (*pl. of* vestibulum)
vestibular
>v. fold
>v. laryngitis
>v. ligament

vestibule
>esophagogastric v.
>gastroesophageal v.
>v. of larynx
>Sibson v.

vestibulum, pl. vestibula
>v. laryngis
>rima vestibuli

vestigial fold
VET
>ventricular ejection time

Veterans
>V. Administration (VA)
>V. Affairs Medical Center (VAMC)
>V. Affairs Medical Center scoring system
>V. Affairs Non-Q-Wave Infarction Strategies in Hospital
>V. Specific Activity Questionnaire (VSAQ)

VE/VCO$_2$
>ventilation/carbon dioxide production

VEX treadmill test
VF
    left leg
    ventricular fibrillation
    ventricular fluid
    ventricular flutter
    ventricular function
        VF electrode
        R-on-T-initiated VF
VFA
    volatile fatty acid
VFC
    venous flow controller
    ventricular function curve
        Actis VFC
VFI
    venous filling index
V-Flex
        V-F. FMJ stent
        V-F. Plus stent
VF/VT
    ventricular fibrillation/ventricular
      tachycardia
VG
    ventricular gallop
VGM
    venous graft myringoplasty
VH
    ventricular hypertrophy
VHC
    valved holding chamber
        AeroChamber VHC
VHD
    valvular heart disease
    vascular hemostatic device
        VasoSeal VHD
VHDL
    very high density lipoprotein
Vhigh
    high regional wall motion velocity
V-H interval
VHR
    ventricular heart rate
Viabahn endoprosthesis stent-graft
viability
        v. identification with dipyridamole-
        dobutamine administration (VIDA)
        v. index
        myocardial v.
viable myocardium
Viagra
Viagraph ECG system

vial
Viamonte-Hobbs dye injector
Vibracare percussor
Vibramycin
        V. injection
        V. Oral
vibrans
        pulsus v.
Vibra-Tabs
vibration
        chest percussion and v.
        v. disease
        postural drainage, percussion
        and v. (PDPV)
vibrational angioplasty
Vibrio
        V. cholerae
        V. parahaemolyticus
vibrissa, pl. **vibrissae**
vibroarthrography (VAG)
vibrocardiogram
VIC
    vasoinhibitory center
vicarious respiration
VICD
    ventricular implantable cardioverter-
      defibrillator
V-ICD
    ventricular implantable cardioverter-
      defibrillator
Vicia
        V. sativa
        V. sativa asthma
Vickers Ventimask Mark 2 mask
Vicks
        V. 44D Cough & Head
        Congestion
        V. Formula 44
        V. Formula 44 Pediatric Formula
        V. Pediatric Formula 44E
Vicodin
Victoria influenza
VIDA
    viability identification with dipyridamole-
      dobutamine administration
      myocardial VIDA
      VIDA stress echocardiography
video
        v. camera
        v. densitometry
        v. imaging
        v. loop

V

NOTES

video *(continued)*
    v. monitor
    v. system
videoangiography
    digital v.
video-assisted
    v.-a. diagnostic thoracoscopic technique
    v.-a. thoracic surgery (VATS)
    v.-a. thoracic surgical lung biopsy
    v.-a. thoracic surgical non-rib-spreading lobectomy (VNSSL)
    v.-a. thoracoscopic surgery (VATS)
    v.-a. thoracoscopic thymectomy
    v.-a. thoracoscopy (VAT, VATS)
videobronchoscope
videodensitometric
    v. analysis system
    v. myocardial textural analysis
videodensitometry
videohydrothoracoscope
videointensity
videomorphometry
videotape recorder
videothoracoscopic
    v. operator staging (VOS)
    v. pericardial window
videothoracoscopy
Videx Oral
Vienna
    V. TAH
    V. total artificial heart
Vieussens
    circle of V.
    valve of V.
    V. valve
view
    A2C, A4C v.
    apical four-chamber v.
    apical two-chamber v.
    Baltaxe v.
    caudocranial hemiaxial v.
    cine v.
    coned-down v.
    craniocaudal v.
    Doppler four-chamber v. (D4CV)
    Doppler two-chamber v. (D2CV)
    en bloc face v.
    en face v.
    expiratory v.
    field of v. (FOV)
    first pass v.
    five-chamber v.
    four-chamber v.
    gated v.
    hemiaxial v.
    horizontal long-axis v.
    ice-pick v.

    inspiratory v.
    laid-back v.
    lateral v.
    left portal v. (LPV)
    long axial oblique v.
    long-axis v.
    orthogonal v.
    parasternal long-axis v.
    parasternal short-axis v.
    RAO v.
    resting parasternal long-axis v.
    resting parasternal short-axis v.
    sagittal v.
    scout v.
    short-axis parasternal v.
    sitting-up v.
    spider x-ray v.
    subcostal right ventricle v.
    suprasternal v.
    swimmer's v.
    two-chamber v.
    vertical long-axis v.
    weeping willow v.
view-aliasing artifact
Viggo Spectramed catheter
vigilance
    care v. (CV)
    V. monitoring system
    v. response
Vigilon dressing
Vigor DR pacemaker
Viking
    V. Bard catheter
    V. coronary guiding catheter
VILI
    ventilator-induced lung injury
Villaret syndrome
villosa
    pericarditis v.
villus, pl. **villi**
    pleural villi
    villi pleurales
Vim-Silverman needle
vinblastine sulfate
Vincasar
    V. PFS
    V. PFS injection
Vincent angina
vincristine
    cyclophosphamide, doxorubicin, v. (CAV)
    v. sulfate
vinculum linguae
vindesine, cisplatin, lomustine, cyclophosphamide (VCPC)
Vineberg cardiac revascularization procedure

Vingmed
    V. CFM 800 echocardiographic
      system
    V. CFM 750 transducer
vinorelbine tartrate
vinyl chloride
viomycin
VIP
    vasoactive intestinal peptide
    vasoinhibitory peptide
    venous impedance plethysmography
    ventricular inotropic parameter
V.I.P. Bird volume monitor
Viprinex
Viracept
viral
    v. bronchiolitis
    v. capsid antigen (VCA)
    v. cardiomyopathy
    v. hepatitis
    v. myocarditis (VM)
    v. pericarditis
    v. pneumonia
    v. respiratory infection
    v. vector
viral-free antigen (VAF)
Viramune
Virazole Aerosol
Virchow-Robin space
Virchow triad
Virgo anticardiolipin screening ELISA test kit
viridans
    Aerococcus v.
    v. endocarditis
    Streptococcus v.
viridis
    Thermoactinomyces v.
Virilon
Viringe vascular access flush device
Virtis blender
virtual bronchoscopy (VB)
Virtuoso LX Smart CPAP system
virulence
virus
    adeno-associated v. (AAV)
    Amapari v.
    Andes v.
    Arenaviridae v.
    Astroviridae v.
    avian influenza A (H5N1) v.
    Bayou v.

    Black Creek Canal v.
    v. bronchopneumonia
    CA v.
    Calciviridae v.
    Coe v.
    Columbia S.K. v.
    Coronaviridae v.
    coxsackie A, B, B3, B4 v.
    croup-associated v.
    Ebola v.
    ECHO v.
    EMC v.
    encephalomyocarditis v.
    enteric cytopathogenic human orphan v.
    Epstein-Barr v. (EBV)
    Filoviridae v.
    Hantaan v.
    herpes simplex v. (HSV)
    human immunodeficiency v. (HIV)
    human T-cell lymphotropic v. (HTLV)
    influenza A, B, C v.
    Juquitiba v.
    Kotonkan v.
    Laguna Negra v.
    Lassa v.
    Lipovnik v.
    Marburg v.
    Mayaro v.
    Moloney murine leukemia v.
    Muerto Canyon v.
    Orthomyxoviridae v.
    parainfluenza v.
    Paramyxoviridae v.
    Picornaviridae v.
    REO v.
    respiratory syncytial v. (RSV)
    Rift Valley fever v.
    Ross River v.
    Rous sarcoma v. (RSV)
    Semliki Forest v.
    Sendai v.
    Sindbis v.
    Sin Nombre v. (SNV)
    syncytial v.
    Togaviridae v.
    U v.
    varicella-zoster v. (VZV, VZ)
    West Nile v.
VIS
    venous insufficiency syndrome

V

NOTES

Visa
V. II ST PTCA balloon catheter
V. Iris system
viscera (*pl. of* viscus)
visceral
v. heterotaxy
v. larva migrans
v. peel
v. pericardiectomy
v. pericardium
v. pleura
v. pleurisy
v. syncope
visceralis
pleura v.
visceroatrial
v. situs ambiguus
v. situs inversus
v. situs solitus
viscerobronchial cardiovascular anomaly
viscerocardiac reflex
visceropleural
viscid mucus
viscidosis
viscid sputum
viscoelastic fluid
viscoelasticity
sputum v.
viscometer
Brookfield v.
Ostwald v.
viscosity
blood v. (BlV)
mucus v.
plasma v. (PV)
viscous
viscus, pl. **viscera**
hollow v.
vise
hemodynamic v.
torque v.
Vision
V. blood cardioplegia system
V. PTCA catheter
Visipaque
Visken
Visov test
Vista
V. Brite Tip IG introducer guide
V. Brite Tip large lumen guiding
catheter
V. 4, T, TRS pacemaker
Vistaril
V. Injection
V. Oral
VISTA software
Vistide

visual
v. amnesia
v. analog scale (VAS)
visualization
far-field v.
fluoroscopic v.
near-field v.
suboptimal v.
visualized
suboptimally v.
visually evoked flow response (VEFR)
visuospatial neglect
Vitacuff device
Vitagraft vascular graft
vital
v. capacity (VC)
v. exhaustion
v. signs
VitalCare 506DX monitor
Vitallium
Vitalograph
V. Bacterial/Viral Filter
V. BreathCO Monitor
V. 2120 handheld recording
spirometer
V. pulmonary monitor
vitalography
Vitalometer test
Vitalor
V. incentive spirometer
V. screening pulmonary function
test
Vital-Port Infusion Pal
Vital-Ryder microvascular needle holder
vitamin
v. B, B_1, B_6, B_{12}, C, D, E, K
v. K antagonist
Vitatron
V. catheter electrode
V. Diamond ICD
V. Diamond II pacemaker
V. lead
V. pacing system
vitellogenin
Vitesse
V. C catheter
V. Cos laser catheter
V. E catheter
V. E2 rapid-exchange catheter
V. PrimaFx catheter
vitiated air
Vitrasert
Vitravene
vitrector
vitreous opacity
vitro
in v.
vitronectin

Viva
> Air V.
> V. Primo balloon catheter

Vivactil

Vivalan

vivax
> Plasmodium v.

vivo
> ex v.
> in v.

Vivonex
> V. Moss tube
> V. Plus nutritional supplement

VixOne small-volume nebulizer

VJ
> ventriculojugular

VJC
> ventriculojugulocardiac

VL
> left arm
> VL electrode

VLCD
> very low-calorie diet

VLCFA
> very long-chain fatty acid

VLDL
> very low density lipoprotein

VLDLR
> very low density lipoprotein receptor

VLDL-TG
> very low density lipoprotein-triglyceride complex

V$_5$-like ambulatory lead syndrome

V$_1$-like ambulatory lead syndrome

VLM
> ventrolateral medulla

VLP
> ventricular late potential

VLS
> vascular leak syndrome

VM
> vasomotor
> ventriculomegaly
> ventriculometry
> viral myocarditis

VMap dynamic flow-based image

VMAT
> vesicular monoamine transformer

Vmax
> Doppler peak flow velocity
> maximal velocity
> maximum velocity

V-max

VMC
> vasomotor center

VMCG
> vector magnetocardiogram

VMF
> vasomotor flushing

VML
> ventriculomegaly

V5M multiplane transducer

VMR
> vasomotor response

VMT
> vasomotor tonus

VNSSL
> video-assisted thoracic surgical non-rib-spreading lobectomy

VNUS
> VNUS Closure catheter/radiofrequency generator
> VNUS Closure System

VO$_2$
> aerobic capacity
> oxygen consumption
> oxygen consumption per minute
> peak exercise oxygen consumption
> volume oxygen consumption
> VO$_2$ max
> peak VO$_2$

VOC
> volatile organic compound

vocal
> v. cord
> v. cord dysfunction (VCD)
> v. fremitus
> v. process

vocalis
> chorda v.
> rima v.

vocational rehabilitation

VOD
> venoocclusive disease

Vogt-Koyanagi-Harada syndrome

voice
> amphoric v.
> cavernous v.
> double v.
> eunuchoid v.
> hot potato v.

voix de Polichinelle

NOTES

V

volatile
>v. fatty acid (VFA)
>v. organic compound (VOC)

Volkmann ischemic paralysis

Vollmer test

Volmax

volt (V)
>electron v. (eV)
>kiloelectron v. (keV)
>megaelectron v. (MeV)

voltage
>battery v.
>Cornell v.
>v. criteria
>v. equilibrium
>Gubner-Ungerleider v.
>pacemaker output v.
>root-mean-square v.
>Sokolow-Lyon v.
>transmembrane v.

voltage-dependent
>v.-d. block
>v.-d. calcium channel

voltage-gated channel

voltage-sensitive calcium channel (VSCC)

volume (V)
>alveolar v. (VA)
>aortic valve stroke v. (AVSV)
>blood v. (BLV, BlV)
>cardiac v. (CV)
>cardiopulmonary blood v. (CPBV)
>central blood v. (CBV)
>central circulating blood v. (CCBV)
>cerebral red blood cell v. (CRCV)
>circulating blood v. (CBV)
>circulation v.
>closing v.
>compressible v.
>conductance stroke v.
>consolidated lung v.
>v. contraction
>v. control (VC)
>v. controller
>corrected blood v. (CBV)
>v. depletion
>v. of distribution
>v. of distribution effect
>dP/dt_{MAX} end-diastolic v.
>effective arterial blood v. (EABV)
>effective blood v. (EBV)
>effective circulating blood v. (ECBV)
>effort-independent lung v.
>ejected v. (EV)
>elastic equilibrium v. (EEV)
>end-diastolic v. (EDV)
>end-expiratory lung v. (EELV)

end-inspiratory lung v. (EILV)
end-systolic v. (ESV)
estimated blood v. (EBV)
v. expansion
expectorated sputum v.
expiratory reserve v. (ERV)
extracorporeal v. (ECV)
forced expiratory v. (FEV)
forward stroke v. (FSV)
frequency to tidal v. (f/V_t)
heart v. (HV)
v. heating
high lung v.
v. infusion
inspiratory reserve v. (IRV)
intravascular v.
left atrial active emptying v.
left atrial end diastolic v. (LAEDV)
left atrial end systolic v. (LAESV)
left atrial maximal v.
left atrial minimal v.
left heart blood v. (LHBV)
left ventricular v. (LVV)
left ventricular diastolic v. (LVDV)
left ventricular end-diastolic v. (LVEDV)
left ventricular end-systolic v. (LVESV)
left ventricular infarct v. (LVIV)
left ventricular stroke v. (LVSV)
v. load hypertrophy
v. loading
v. loss
lung v.
lung blood v. (LBV)
mandatory minute v. (MMV)
maximal expiratory flow v. (MEFV)
mean corpuscular v. (MCV)
minute v.
v. overload
v. oxygen consumption (VO_2)
planimetry v.
plaque v.
plasma v.
presystolic pressure and v.
pulmonary blood v. (PBV)
pulmonary blood mixing v. (PBMV)
pulmonary capillary blood v. (Vc)
ratio of tidal expiratory inspiratory flow at 50% of tidal v. (TEF_{50}/TIF_{50})
regurgitant v. (RV, RVol)
relative cardiac v.
residual v. (RV)
respiratory minute v.
resting stroke v.

resting tidal v.
v. resuscitation
right heart mixing v. (RHMV)
right ventricular v. (RVV)
right ventricular diastolic v.
  (RVDV)
right ventricular end-diastolic v.
  (RVEDV)
right ventricular end-systolic v.
  (RVESV)
right ventricular stroke v. (RVSV)
Simpson rule for ventricular v.
sputum v.
static lung v.
v. stiffness
stroke v. (SV)
v. thickness index (VTI)
thoracic gas v. (TGV, V_{TG})
tidal v. (TV, V_T)
tidal expiratory v. (TV_E)
tidal expiratory flow at 25% of
  tidal v. (TEF_{25})
tidal expiratory flow at 50% of
  tidal v. (TEF_{50})
tidal expiratory flow at 75% of
  tidal v. (TEF_{75})
tidal inspiratory v. (TV_I)
tidal inspiratory flow at 50% of
  tidal v. (TIF_{50})
timed forced expiratory v.
total blood v. (TBV)
total right ventricular v. (TRVV)
trapped gas v.
urine v.
venous v. (VV, VVol)
v. ventilator
ventricular v.
ventricular end-diastolic v. (VDV)
ventricular residual v. (VRV)
volume to peak expiratory flow
  and total expiratory v.
  (VPTEF/VT)
**volume-assured pressure support
  (VAPS)**
volume-challenge test
volume-controlled
  v.-c. respirator
  v.-c. ventilation (VCV)
volume-cycled
  v.-c. decelerating-flow ventilation
    (VCDF)
  v.-c. ventilator

volume-displacement
  v.-d. plethysmograph
  v.-d. spirometer
volume-overloaded left ventricle
volumeter
volume-time curve
volumetric
  v. capnogram
  v. diffusive respirator (VDR)
  v. infusion pump
  v. lung depth (Vp)
volumic
  v. ejection
  v. mass
volutrauma
volvulus
  Onchocerca v.
von
  v. Claus chronometric method
  v. Recklinghausen disease
  v. Recklinghausen test
  v. Reyn criteria
  v. Willebrand disease
  v. Willebrand protein (vWP)
VOO
  ventricular asynchronous
  VOO pacemaker
  VOO pacing
voodoo death
Voorhees bag
VOP
  vasoocclusive pain
  venous occlusion plethysmography
voriconazole
Vorse-Webster clamp
vortex
  v. cordis
  v. effect catheter
  v. flow
VOS
  videothoracoscopic operator staging
VoSpire ER
voxel gray scale
Voyager Aortic IntraClusion device
VP
  vasopressin
  venous pressure
  ventricular pacing
  ventricular pericardium
  ventricular premature
    VP beat

NOTES

Vp
    ventricular premature
    volumetric lung depth
V-Pace transluminal pacing lead
VPAP
    variable positive airway pressure
        VPAP II ST-A bilevel flow
          generator
        VPAP II ST ventilatory support
          system
VPB
    ventricular premature beat
VPC
    ventricular premature complex
    ventricular premature contraction
VPCT
    ventricular premature contraction
      threshold
VPD
    ventricular premature depolarization
VPF
    vascular permeability factor
VPGSS
    venous pressure gradient support
      stockings
VPI
    vasopeptidase inhibitor
VPR
    ventricular paced rhythm
VPTEF/VT
    volume to peak expiratory flow and total
      expiratory volume
V/Q
    ventilation/perfusion
        $\dot{V}/\dot{Q}$ defect
        $\dot{V}/\dot{Q}$ lung scan
        $\dot{V}/\dot{Q}$ mismatch
        $\dot{V}/\dot{Q}$ quotient
VQI
    ventricular perfusion index
VR
    right arm
    valve replacement
    vascular resistance
    velocity ratio
    venous flow reversal
    venous reflux
    venous return
    ventricular rale
    ventricular rhythm
        VR electrode
VRD
    ventricular radial dysplasia
Vroman effect
VRV
    ventricular residual volume
VS
    Valsalva maneuver

    venesection
    ventricular septum
Vs
    venesection
VSA
    vasospastic angina
VSAQ
    Veterans Specific Activity Questionnaire
VSCC
    voltage-sensitive calcium channel
VSD
    ventricular septal defect
    ventriculoseptal defect
      Eisenmenger VSD
      pinhole VSD
VSFP
    venous stop flow pressure
VSHD
    ventricular septal heart defect
V-slope method
VSMC
    vascular smooth muscle cell
VSW
    ventricular stroke work
Vsys
    systolic wall motion velocity
VT
    ventricular tachycardia
      VT Mercury Vac organic mercury
        vacuum cleaner
      VT 1000 neonatal workstation
      R-on-T-initiated nonsustained VT
VTA
    ventricular tachyarrhythmia
VTCL
    ventricular tachycardia cycle length
VTE
    venous thromboembolism
    ventricular tachycardia event
VTI
    volume thickness index
      VTI oxygen monitor with
        disposable polarographic oxygen
        sensor
VT/VF
    ventricular tachycardia/ventricular
      fibrillation
Vueport balloon-occlusion guiding
** catheter**
vulgaris
    Proteus v.
    Thermoactinomyces v.
vulnerability
    plaque v.
vulnerable
    v. myocardium
    v. period
    v. phase
    v. plaque

Vumon injection
VV
> venous volume
> venovenous

V1-V6
> ventral lead 1, 2, 3, 4, 5, 6
>> V1-V6 EKG leads

V_D/V_T
> physiologic dead space ventilation

V_{DS}/V_T
> dead space gas volume to tidal gas
> volume ratio

V-Vac suction apparatus
VVD
> ventricular demand-triggered
>> VVD mode
>> VVD pacemaker
>> VVD pacing

VVDL
> venovenous double-lumen
>> VVDL catheter

VVI
> ventricular inhibited
>> VVI pacemaker
>> VVI pacing

VVIR
>> V. pacemaker
>> V. pacing

VVI-RR pacing
VVI/VVIR pacing
vvk
> ventricular volume constant

VVO
> vesicular-vacuolar organelle

VVol
> venous volume

VVS
> vasovagal syncope

VVT
> ventricular triggered
>> VVT mode
>> VVT pacemaker
>> VVT pacing

VW
> vascular wall

VWM
> ventricular wall motion

vWP
> von Willebrand protein

VZIG
> varicella-zoster immunoglobulin

VZV, VZ
> varicella-zoster virus

NOTES

V

W

W pattern
W pattern on right atrial waveform
W wave on echocardiogram

Waardenburg syndrome
Wada test
wadsworthensis
Sutterella w.
wadsworthii
Legionella w.
waist
cardiac w.
w. of catheter
w. of heart
hypertriglyceridemic w.
waisting of balloon
waist-to-hip ratio (WHR)
wake after sleep onset time (WASO)
Waldenström macroglobulinemia
Waldeyer
W. throat ring
W. tonsillar ring
Waldhausen subclavian flap technique
walk
w. distance test
shuttle test w.
Walkabout oxygen conserver
WalkCare slippers
Walker-Murdoch wrist sign
walking
nocturnal w.
w. pneumonia
w. ventilation test
walk-through angina
wall
w. amplitude
anterior w. (AW)
anterior aortic w. (AAW)
anterobasal w.
aortic posterior w. (AOPW, AoPW)
chest w.
free w.
friable w.
inferobasal w.
inner w. (IW)
lateral w. (LW)
left atrial w. (LAW)
left atrial posterior w. (LAPW)
left ventricular w. (LVW)
left ventricular posterior w. (LVPW)
w. motion (WM)
w. motion abnormality (WMA)
w. motion analysis (WMA)
w. motion index (WMI)
w. motion score
w. motion score index (WMSI)
w. motion velocity
posterior w. (PW)
posteroseptal w.
right atrial w. (RAW)
right atrial free w. (RAFW)
right ventricle anterior w. (RVAW)
right ventricular w. (RVW)
w. stress
w. structure
subacute ventricular free w.
w. tension
w. thickening
w. thickness (WT)
w. tracking
w. tracking system
vascular w. (VW)
Wallace Flexihub central venous pressure cannula
Wallenberg syndrome
Wallerian degeneration (WD)
Wallgraft
W. stent
W. tracheobronchial endoprosthesis
Wallstent
W. endoprosthesis with Unistep Plus delivery system
W. flexible, self-expanding wire-mesh stent
Magic W.
W. Magic stent
Schneider W.
W. spring-loaded stent
Walter Reed classification
wand
light w.
wandering
w. atrial pacemaker (WAP)
w. baseline
w. goiter
w. heart
w. pacemaker
w. pneumonia
Wangiella
Wang transbronchial needle
waning
waxing and w.
WAP
wandering atrial pacemaker
ward
general w.
Ward-Romano syndrome
Wardrop method

W

WARF
>warfarin

warfarin (WARF)
>w. dose index (WDI)
>w. sodium
>w. therapy

warfarin-aspirin symptomatic intracranial disease (WASID)

Warfilone

warm
>w. heparinized saline flush
>w. nodule

warmer
>blood w.

warm-up
>w.-u. angina
>w.-u. phenomenon

warning arrhythmia

Warthin-Starry-staining bacillus

wash
>w. bath
>ENT w.
>nasopharyngeal w.

washings
>bronchial w.
>bronchoalveolar w.
>bronchopulmonary w.
>w. and brushings
>lung w.

washout
>w. cannula
>helium w.
>w. period
>w. phase
>w. phenomenon
>thallium w.

WASID
>warfarin-aspirin symptomatic intracranial disease

WASO
>wake after sleep onset time

Wasserman
>W. needle
>W. number

Wasserman-positive pulmonary infiltrate

wasted ventilation

wasting
>potassium w.
>salt w.
>w. syndrome

WAT
>word association test

watch
>Pulse Pro heart rate monitor w.

watch-crystal fingernail

water
>w. brash
>w. channel
>w. column resistor

dextrose 5% in w. (D5W, D-5-W, D_5W)
>extravascular lung w. (EVLW)
>feet of sea w. (fsw)
>w. hammer pulse
>w. lily sign
>w. retention
>w. wheel murmur

water-bottle heart

waterfall effect

water-gurgle test

Waterman bronchoscope

watermelon seeding effect

water-seal
>w.-s. chest tube
>w.-s. drainage

water-sealed spirometer

watershed
>w. infarct
>w. infarction
>w. pattern
>w. region

Waterston
>W. anastomosis
>W. anastomosis for congenital pulmonary stenosis
>W. groove
>W. operation
>W. shunt

Waterston-Cooley procedure

watertight seal

waterwheel sound

Watson
>W. heart valve holder
>W. syndrome

watt-second (WS)

wave
>A w.
>a w.
>A larger than V w.
>w. amplitude
>arterial w.
>atrial repolarization w.
>augmented V w.
>bifid P w.
>blast w.
>brain w.
>C w.
>cannon w.
>catacrotic w.
>catadicrotic w.
>constant tilt w.
>w. coronary event
>c-v systolic w.
>D w.
>deep pathologic Q w.
>delta w.
>depolarization w.
>dicrotic w.

diphasic P, T w.
duration of ECG w.
duration of P w.
E w.
early systolic w. (SE)
electrocardiographic w.
epsilon w.
E wave to A w. (E/A, E:A)
excitation w.
F w.
f w.
fibrillary w.
fibrillatory w.
flipped T w.
flutter w.
flutter-fibrillation w.'s
w. form
giant a w.
giant T w.
giant TU fusion w.
giant v w.
H w.
h w.
hyperacute T w.
inverted T w.
isolated T w.
J w.
Mayer w.
Minnesota criteria for high R w.
negative deflection that follows an
  R w. (S)
negative T, U w.
normalization of inverted T w.
notched P w.
notched S w.
NSSTT w.
Osborne (J) w.
overflow w.
P w.
palpable A w.
peaked P w.
percussion w.
peristaltic w. (PW)
polymorphic slow w.
P-on-T w.
portion of the segment between
  the end of the S wave and the
  beginning of the T w. (S-T)
posterior Q w.
postextrasystolic T w.
precordial A w.
pressure w. (PW)

prominent U w.
propagation of R w.
PRS w.
pseudonormalization of T w.
pseudo R', S w.
pulse w.
pulsed w. (PW)
Q w.
QS w.
R' w.
rapid filling w.
recoil w.
regurgitant w.
retraction w.
retrograde P w.
RF w.
S' w.
sawtooth P w.
scroll reentrant w.
seismic w.
shallow pathologic Q w.
sine w.
slow filling w.
slurred R w.
small P w.
spike w. (SW, S/W)
w. spike
spiral reentrant w.
ST w.
standardization w.
stationary arterial w.
ST-T w.
systolic reflection w.
systolic S w.
T w.
Ta w.
tall T w.
tidal w.
transient abnormal Q w. (TAQW)
U w.
undulating deflection that follows
  T w.
upright T w.
v w.
venous Corrigan w.
ventricular w.
Venturi w.
W. VM200 ventilator
x w.
X descent of the A w.
y w.
Y descent w.

NOTES

waveform
A-wave spectral velocity w.
biphasic w.
biphasic defibrillation w. (BDW)
blunted w.
CO_2 w.
dampened w.
displacement w.
distention w.
Edmark monophasic w.
E-wave spectral velocity w.
flow-delivery w.
forward pressure w.
Gurvich biphasic w.
incident pressure w.
Lown-Edmark w.
monophasic w.
monophasic defibrillation w.
  (MDW)
nonsinusoidal w.
pressure w.
quasisinusoidal w.
rectilinear biphasic w.
reentry w.
reflected pressure w.
shock w.
spectral w.
W pattern on right atrial w.
wavelength (WL)
w. of reentry
WaveMap intracoronary blood pressure measurement system
waveshape
wave-speed mechanism
WaveWire intracoronary blood pressure measurement system
wavy
w. fiber
w. respiration
waxing
w. and waning
w. and waning chest pain
w. and waning in intensity
wax-matrix technique
4-Way Long Acting Nasal Solution
WCD
wearable cardioverter-defibrillator
WCD 2000 system wearable cardioverter-defibrillator
WD
Wallerian degeneration
WDI
warfarin dose index
weakness
wean
weaning
w. index (WI)
w. protocol
terminal w.

T-piece w.
ventilator w.
wearable
w. cardioverter-defibrillator (WCD)
w. cardioverter-defibrillator device
wear-and-tear lesion
Weavenit
W. patch graft
W. prosthesis
web
esophageal w.
laryngeal w.
pulmonary arterial w.
venous w.
Weber-Christian disease
Weber experiment
Weber-Janicki cardiopulmonary exercise protocol
Weber-Osler-Rendu syndrome
web-spacer
Webster
W. halo catheter
W. orthogonal electrode catheter
Wedensky
W. effect
W. modulated signal-averaged electrocardiogram
wedge
w. angiogram
arterial w.
w. biopsy
w. excision
mediastinal w.
w. pressure (WP)
w. pressure balloon catheter
pulmonary w. (PW)
w. pulmonary angiography
pulmonary artery w. (PAW)
pulmonary capillary w. (PCW)
w. spirometer
Weeks bacillus
weeping
w. dermatitis
w. fig asthma
w. willow view
Wegener
W. granulomatosis (WG)
W. nodule
Weibel-Palade bodies
Weigert-van Gieson stain
weight
heart w. (HW)
weighted ball resistor
Weil disease
Weil-Felix reaction
Weill sign
Weinberg test
Weir method
Weiss logarithmic method

Welch
>W. Allyn Pneumocheck spirometer
>W. Allyn/Schiller AT-10 Exercise Testing system
>W. Allyn/Schiller AT-2 full-size ECG
>W. Allyn/Schiller AT-10 hospital grade ECG
>W. Allyn/Schiller AT-2*plus* full-size ECG
>W. Allyn/Schiller AT-1 three channel ECG
>W. Allyn/Schiller MS-3 pocket size ECG
>W. Allyn/Schiller SP-1 budget spirometry
>W. Allyn/Schiller SP-10 diagnostic spirometry

WelChol
Welcker method
welder's
>w. lung
>w. siderosis

welding
>spot w.

well
>pericardial w.

well-being
>Shwachman score of clinical w.-b.

well-differentiated carcinoma
Wenckebach
>W. atrioventricular block
>W. A-V block
>W. cycle
>W. cycle length
>W. disease
>W. exit block
>W. period
>W. periodicity
>W. periodicity block
>W. phenomenon
>W. sign

Werlhof disease
Werner syndrome
Wernicke aphasia
Wessex prosthetic valve
West
>W. Nile virus
>W. syndrome

Westaby tracheobronchial silicone stent
Westberg space

Westergren
>W. erythrocyte sedimentation rate
>W. method

westermani
>*Paragonimus w.*

Westermark sign
Western
>W. blot
>W. red cedar

Westminster drug-free protocol
Westrim LA
wet
>w. beriberi
>w. cough
>w. lung
>w. nebulization
>w. pleurisy
>w. rale
>w. swallow

wet-to-dry dressing
WG
>Wegener granulomatosis

wheal and flare
Wheatstone bridge
wheat weevil disease
wheeze
>asthmoid w.
>monophonic w.

wheezing
>bronchial w.
>expiratory w.

wheezy bronchitis
WHI
>Women's Health Initiative

whiff test
whip
>catheter w.

whipping
>systolic w.

Whipple disease
whippleii
whisker plot
whispered
>w. bronchophony
>w. pectoriloquy

whispering
>w. pectoriloquy
>w. resonance

Whisper Mist humidifier
whistle
>coaching w.

whistling rale

NOTES

W

white
  w. asphyxia
  w. blood cell count
  w. clot syndrome
  w. coronary thrombus
  w. light bronchoscopy (WLB)
  w. lung
  w. matter (WM)
  w. matter hyperintensity (WMHI)
  w. plaque
  w. pneumonia
  w. spot
  w. sputum
  W. system
  W. vessel sizing catheter
white-coat
  w.-c. angina
  w.-c. effect
  w.-c. hypertension
Whitfield ointment
WHO
  World Health Organization
WHO/Fredrickson classification of primary hyperlipidemia
whole
  w. blood buffer base
  w. blood cardioplegia
whole-body
  w.-b. amyloid load
  w.-b. hyperthermia
whole-grain food
Wholey
  W. Hi-Torque Floppy guidewire
  W. Hi-Torque modified J
  guidewire
  W. Hi-Torque standard guidewire
  W. wire
whoop
  precordial w.
  systolic w.
whooping
  w. cough
  w. murmur
whorling of myocardial cell
whorl motion
WHR
  waist-to-hip ratio
  WHR for upper body obesity
WI
  weaning index
Wichmann asthma
Wickwitz esophageal stricture
Widal-Abrami-Lermoyez triad
Widal test
wide
  w. complex rhythm
  w. QRS tachycardia
widely split second sound
wide-necked aneurysm

widened
  mediastinal w.
widening
  luminal w.
  mediastinal w.
  w. of pulse pressure
Wideroe test
width
  atrial pulse w.
  pulse w.
  ventricular pulse w.
Wiener filter
Wigle scale
Wigraine
Wiktor
  W. balloon expandable coronary
  stent
  W. GX coronary stent
  W. GX Hepamed coated coronary
  stent system
  W. Prime coronary stent system
Wiktor-I implantable stent
Wilders-Jongsma-van Ginneken (WJG)
Wilhelmy balance
Wilkie disease
Wilkins echocardiographic score
Wilks lambda criterion
Wilks-Schapiro test
Willebrand-Jurgens syndrome
Willett-Stampfer method
William
  W. Harvey arterial blood filter
  W. Harvey cardiotomy reservoir
  W. test
Williams
  W. phenomenon
  W. sign
  W. syndrome
  W. tracheal tone
Williams-Campbell syndrome
Williamson sign
Willis
  circle of W. (CW)
Wilms thoracoplasty
Wilson
  W. block
  W. central terminal
  W. disease
  W. lead
Wilson-Cook papillotome
Wilson-Kimmelsteil disease
Wilson-Mikity syndrome
Wilson-White method
Wilton
  W. Webster coronary sinus
  thermodilution catheter
  W. Webster thermodilution flow
  and pacing catheter

windkessel
    w. effect
    w. model
window
    acoustic w.
    aortic w.
    aorticopulmonary w.
    aortopulmonary w. (APW)
    Blackman w.
    cycle-length w.
    Hanning w.
    imaging w.
    parasternal w.
    pericardial w.
    pleuropericardial w.
    pulmonary parenchymal w.
    subxiphoid w.
    tachycardia w.
    transthoracic acoustic w.
    videothoracoscopic pericardial w.
windowed balloon
windpipe
windsock
    w. aneurysm
    w. morphology
    w. sign
winged baseplate
Winiwarter-Buerger disease
Winpred
Winslow test
Winstrol
winter
    w. bronchitis
    w. cough
    w. vomiting disease
Wintrich sign
Wintrobe sedimentation rate
wire (*See also* guidewire)
    all track w. (ATW)
    Amplatz tapered movable core w.
    Amplatz torque w.
    atrial pacing w.
    biventricular pacing w.
    catheter-guide w.
    Choice PT plus w.
    control w.
    coronary w.
    crenulated tantalum w.
    delivery w.
    dock w.
    docking w.
    Doppler velocity w.

    Eder-Puestow w.
    endocardial w.
    extraflexible w.
    flow w.
    GlideCath guide w.
    w. guide
    Hancock temporary cardiac pacing w.
    Hi-Torque balance middleweight universal guide w.
    w. holder
    w. insertion
    intracoronary Doppler flow w.
    J exchange w.
    J retention w.
    Katzen infusion w.
    Linx extension w.
    Lunderquist exchange w.
    magnet w.
    Medi-Tech w.
    w. mesh self-expandable stent
    olive-tipped Magnum w.
    pacemaker w.'s (PMW)
    Patriot moderate support guide w.
    platinum w.
    pressure guide pressure w.
    pusher w.
    Radifocus w.
    RotaWire Floppy Gold guide w.
    Stabilizer marker w.
    w. stylet
    tantalum w.
    tip-deflecting w.
    Trooper floppy moderate support guide w.
    Wholey w.
wire-loop lesion
wires
wire-wound endotracheal tube
wiring
    copper w.
    sternal w.
    w. of sternum
wiry pulse
Wiseguide guide catheter
Wiskott-Aldrich syndrome
Wizard disposable inflation device
Wizdom ST steerable guidewire
WJG
    Wilders-Jongsma-van Ginneken
    WJG pacemaker model

W

NOTES

WL
wavelength
WLB
white light bronchoscopy
WM
wall motion
white matter
WMA
wall motion abnormality
wall motion analysis
Wmax
peak work rate
WMFT
Wolf Motor Function Test
WMHI
white matter hyperintensity
WMI
wall motion index
WMSI
wall motion score index
WOB
work of breathing
Wobenzym tablet
Woillez disease
Wolff-Parkinson-White (WPW)
W.-P.-W. bypass tract
W.-P.-W. reentrant tachycardia
W.-P.-W. syndrome
Wolfina
Wolf Motor Function Test (WMFT)
Wolman disease
Womack procedure
Women's Health Initiative (WHI)
wood
W. classification
W. lamp
w. pulp worker's lung
w. pulp worker's lung disease
w. smoke
W. unit
W. units index
wooden resonance
wooden-shoe heart
Woodworth phenomenon
woody
w. edema
w. thyroiditis
Wooler-type annuloplasty
woolsorter's pneumonia
word association test (WAT)
work
w. of breathing (WOB)
w. capacity
cardiac w. (CW)
w. effect
left ventricular w. (LVW)
left ventricular stroke w. (LVSW)
w. rate
w. rate increment

w. rehabilitation
right ventricular stroke w. (RVSW)
w. status
stroke w. (SW)
w. threshold
ventricular stroke w. (VSW)
work-aggravated asthma
workhorse
w. balloon
W. percutaneous transluminal angioplasty balloon catheter
W. PTCA balloon catheter
workload
peak w.
workplace exposure
workrate
internal w.
work-related
w.-r. asthma
w.-r. bronchial hyperreactivity
worksite challenge test
workstation
EnSite 3000 electrophysiology w.
VT 1000 neonatal w.
World Health Organization (WHO)
wound
blowing w.
bullet w.
entrance w.
exit w.
gunshot w.
knife w.
stab w.
sucking chest w.
woven
w. coronary artery disease
w. Dacron catheter
w. Dacron fabric graft
w. Dacron tube graft
w. Teflon
w. Teflon prosthesis
woven-tube vascular graft prosthesis
WP
wedge pressure
WPW
Wolff-Parkinson-White
WPW syndrome
wrap
cardiac muscle w.
no-phase w.
omental w.
wrap-around ghosting artifact
wrapping
w. of abdominal aortic aneurysm
aneurysm w.
wrecking ball effect
Wright
W. peak flow
W. respirometer

W. spirometer
W. stain
Wright-Giemsa stain
Wrisberg ganglion
wrist positioning splint
WS
watt-second
WT
wall thickness

Wuchereria bancrofti
Wu-Hoak hypothesis
Wyamine Sulfate
Wycillin injection
Wylie
W. carotid artery clamp
W. endarterectomy set
W. vascular clamp
Wymox

NOTES

W

X

X depression
X depression of jugular venous pulse
X descent of the A wave
X descent of jugular venous pulse
X wave of Ohnell

x

x wave

xamoterol
xanthelasma
xanthine

x. oxidase
x. oxidase reaction

xanthogranuloma
xanthoma

eruptive x.
palmar x.
planar x.
x. regression
x. striatum palmare
x. tendinosum
tendinous x.
tuberoeruptive x.
tuberous x.

xanthomatosis
xanthomatous
Xanthomonas maltophilia
X-Cell cardiac bioprosthesis
Xcelon nylon
X-descent trough
Xe

xenon

^{127}Xe

xenon-127

^{133}Xe

xenon-133

XeCl

xenon chloride
XeCl excimer laser

XECT

xenon-enhanced computed tomography

Xeloda
xemilofiban
Xenical
xenoantibody
xenobiotic
xenodiagnosis
xenograft

Ionescu-Shiley pericardial x.
porcine x.
stentless porcine x.

xenon (Xe)

x. chloride (XeCl)
x. chloride excimer laser

x. lung ventilation imaging
x. washout technique

xenon-127 (^{127}Xe)
xenon-133 (^{133}Xe)
xenon-enhanced computed tomography (XECT)
xenopi

Mycobacterium x.
Mycoplasma x.

Xenopus

X. laevis
X. oocytes
X. tropicalis

Xenotech prosthetic valve
xenotransplant
Xeroform gauze
xerosis
xerotrachea
Xillix

X. ACCESS system
X. LIFE-Lung system

xinafoate

salmeterol x.

xipamide
xiphisternal

x. crunching sound
x. process

xiphisternum
xiphocostal
xiphodynia
xiphoid

x. angle
x. cartilage
x. process

xiphoiditis
XL

Procardia XL
Toprol XL

XLAS

X-linked aqueductal stenosis

XLCM

X-linked dilated cardiomyopathy

X-linked

X-l. aqueductal stenosis (XLAS)
X-l. dilated cardiomyopathy (XLCM)

XMI thrombectomy catheter
Xopenex inhalation solution
XO syndrome
Xpeedior t120 catheter
X-PRESS vascular closure system
XR

Dilacor XR

x-ray

babygram x-r.

X

x-ray *(continued)*
> x-r. beam filtration
> x-r. beam hardening
> chest x-r. (CX, CXR, CxR)
> x-r. cine computed tomography
> x-r. energy microprobe analysis
> x-r. generator
> Infinix DP-i vascular x-r.
> Infinix NB-i vascular x-r.
> Infinix VC-i vascular x-r.
> scanning-beam digital x-r.
> x-r. scatter collimation
> sinus x-r.
> x-r. tube

XRT
> radiotherapy

X-Scribe
> X-S. stress test
> X-S. stress testing system

X-Sizer single-use catheter system

XT
> Cartia XT

> Diltia XT
> XT radiopaque coronary stent

X-Trode stent

XXXX syndrome

XXXY syndrome

X, Y descent

xylene

Xylocaine
> X. Oral
> X. Topical Ointment
> X. Topical Solution

Xylocard

xylol pulse indicator

xylosoxidans
> *Achromobacter x.*
> *Alcaligenes x.*

X, Y, Z axis

XYZ lead system

X, Y, Z recordings

Y

Y connector
Y depression of jugular venous pulse
Y descent of jugular venous pulse
Y descent wave
Y graft
Y stenting
Y technique
Y wave pressure on right atrial catheterization

y

y wave

Yacoub and Radley-Smith classification

YAG

yttrium-aluminum-garnet
YAG laser

Yamaguchi disease

Yamasa assay kit

Yankauer

Y. bronchoscope
Y. pharyngeal speculum

Yasargil carotid clamp

Yates correction

yaws

Y-descent trough

Yeager formula

year

yellow

y. cross
y. fever

y. hepatization
Y. IRIS system
y. nail syndrome (YNS)
y. plaque
y. sputum

yellowish-green sputum

Yentl syndrome

Yersinia

Y. *enterocolitica*
Y. *pestis*
Y. *pseudotuberculosis*

Yesavage

Y. depression instrument
Y. score

YNS

yellow nail syndrome

Yodoxin

yohimbine hydrochloride

Youden index

Youlten nasal inspiratory peak flowmeter

Youman-Parlett test

Young

Y. modulus
Y. syndrome

Y-shaped

Y-s. bifurcation
Y-s. graft

YSI 4000 Telethermometer

Y-stenting

Y, Z stent

Y

Z

Z band
Z cardiac catheter
Z line
Z point pressure on left atrial catheterization
Z point pressure on right atrial catheterization
Z score weight-Z score height

zabicipril
Zaditen
zafirlukast
Zagam RespiPac
Zahn

Z. lines
pocket of Z.

Zaire subtype
zalcitabine
Zalkind lung retractor
Zanaflex
zanamivir
Zang space
Zanosar
zardaverine asthma
Zaroxolyn
Zartan
zatebradine
Zavala

Z. lung biopsy needle
Z. technique

Zebeta
zebra artifact
ZEEP

zero end-expiratory pressure

Zemuron
Zenapax
Zener diode
Zenith AAA endovascular graft system
Zenker diverticulum
Zenotech graft material
Zephrex
Zerit
zero

z. diastolic blood pressure
z. end-expiratory pressure (ZEEP)
z. end-inspiratory pressure
z. velocity line

zero-amplitude
zero-flow pressure (Pzf, ZFP)
zero-order kinetics
Zestoretic
Zestril
Zetia
ZFP

zero-flow pressure

Ziac
Ziagen
zidovudine and lamivudine
Ziehl-Neelsen stain
zigzag stent
Zilactin-L
zileuton
Zimmer antiembolism support stockings
Zimmermann arch
Zinacef injection
zinc

z. chloride
z. finger gene
z. fume fever
z. gelatin
z. protoporphyrin

Zinecard
ZIP

zoster immune plasma

Zipper antidisconnect device
zipper scar
zirconium tetrachloride
Zithromax Z-Pak
Z-Med catheter
Zocor
zofenopril
zofenoprilic acid
Zoladex Implant
Zoll

Z. NTP 1000 noninvasive pacemaker
Z. PD 1200 external defibrillator

Zollinger-Gilmore intraluminal vein stripper
zolmitriptan
zolpidem tartrate
zone

echo z.
Fraunhofer z.
Fresnel z.
H z.
Head z.
ischemic z.
midlung z.
periinfarction z.
z. 1 phenomenon
posterior upper lung z.
protective z.
slow z.
sonolucent z.
subcostal z.
subendocardial z.
tendinous z.'s of heart
z. therapy
transitional cell z.

Z

zone (*continued*)
    upper lung z.
    vascular z.
zoom
    acquisition z. (AZ)
zopolrestat
ZORprin
zoster
    herpes z.
    z. immune plasma (ZIP)
Zosyn
Z-Pak
    Zithromax Z-Pak
ZT
   Zwolle trial
Zuckerkandl bodies

Zuma guiding catheter
Zwenger test
Zwolle trial (ZT)
Zyban
Zydone
Zyflo
Zygomycetes
zygomycosis
zymogen
zymography
    substrate gel z.
Zynergy Zolution electrophysiology catheter
Zyrtec
Zyvox

Illustrations

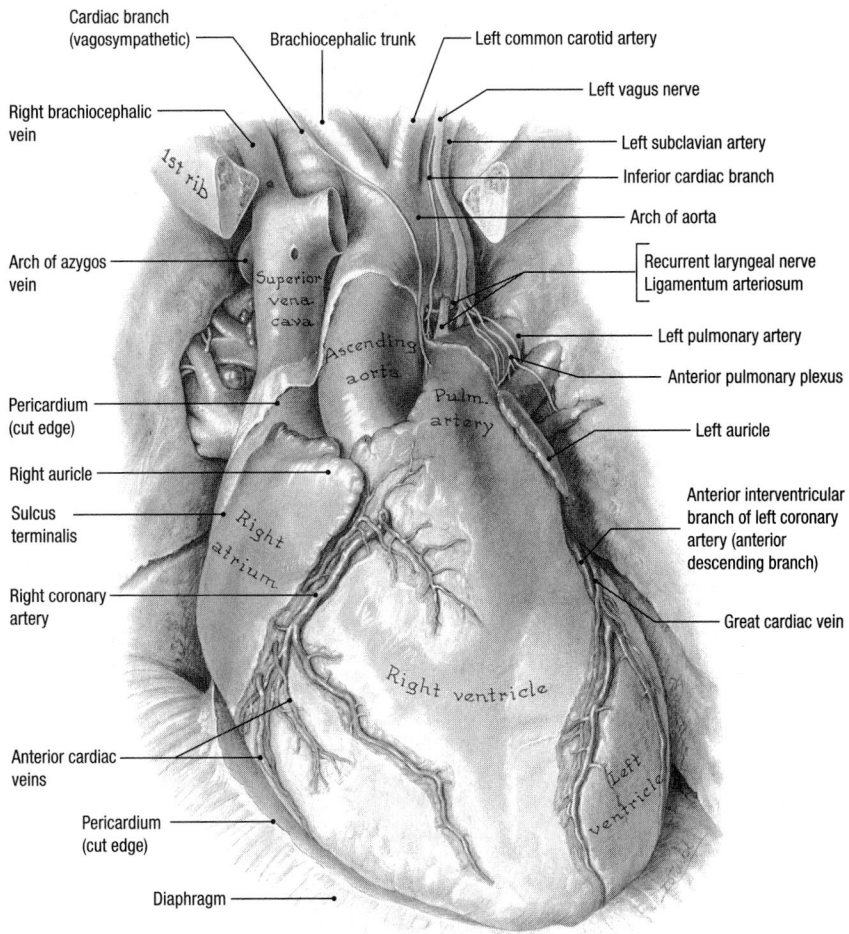

Figure 1. Sternocostal (anterior) surface of heart and great vessels in situ.

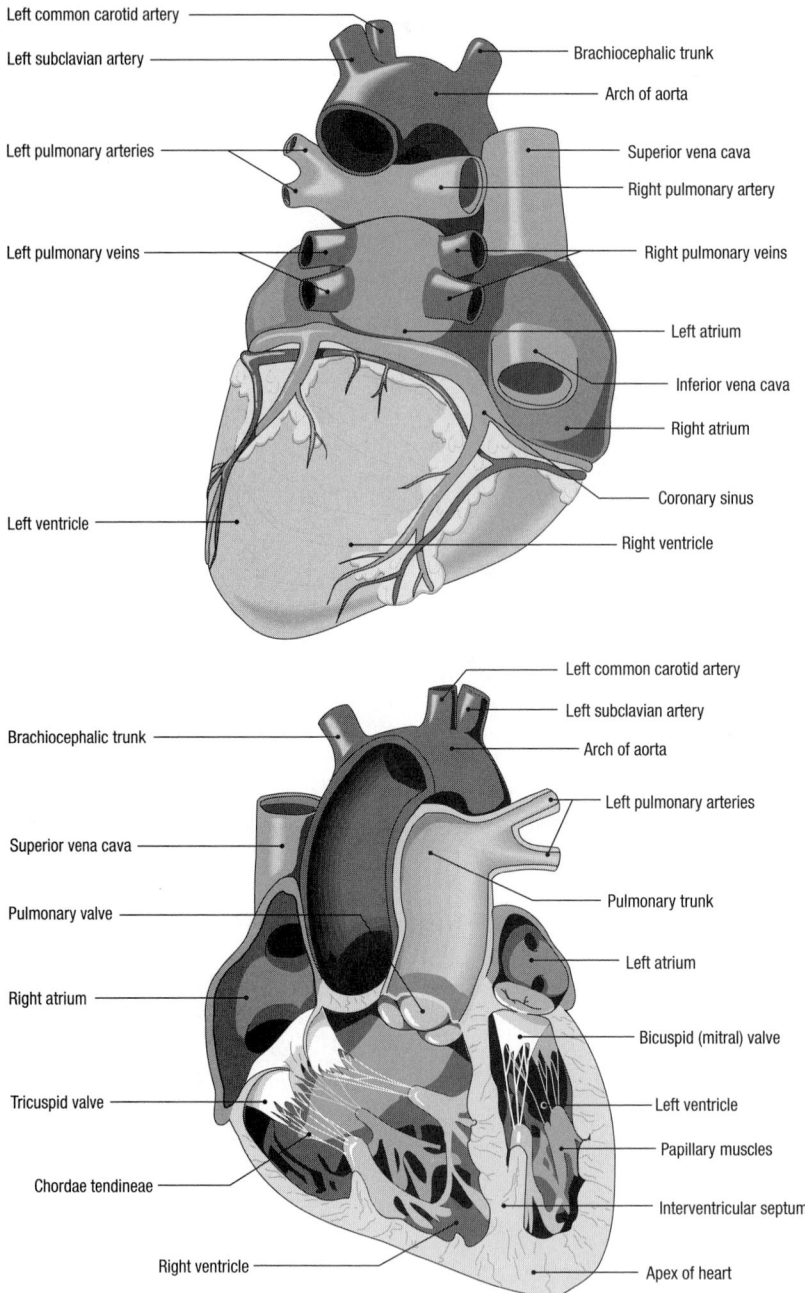

Figure 2. The relationship of the great vessels of heart. (Top) posterior view; (bottom) coronal view.

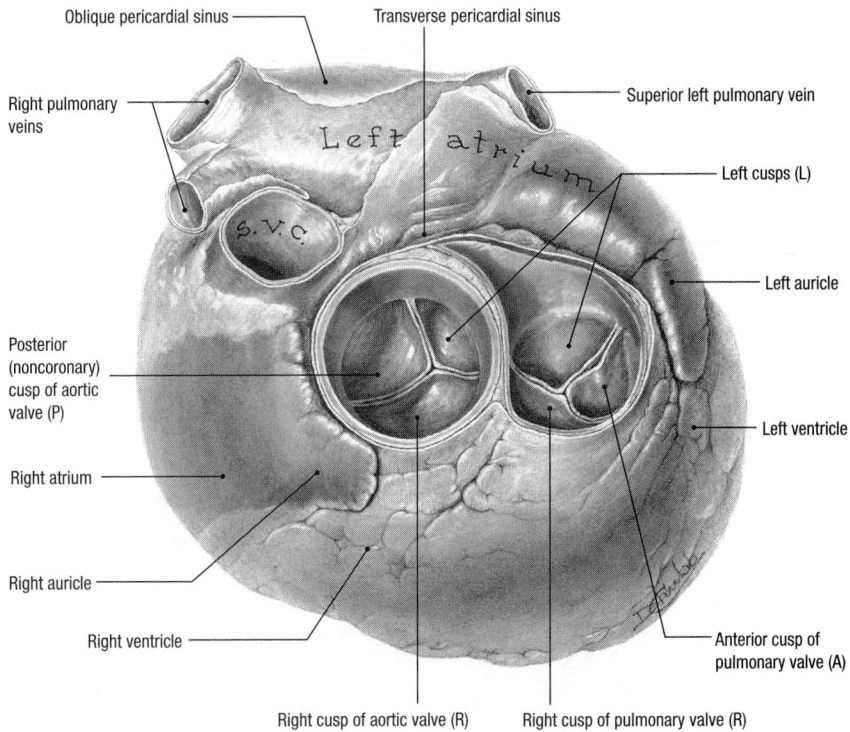

Figure 3. Excised heart, superior view.

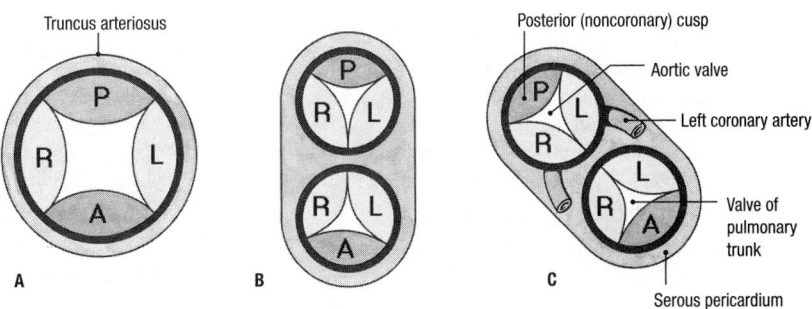

Figure 4. Pulmonary and aortic valves. The names of these cusps have a developmental origin: the truncus arteriosus with four cusps (A) splits to form two valves, each with three cusps (B). The heart undergoes partial rotation to the left on its axis, resulting in the arrangement of cusps shown in C.

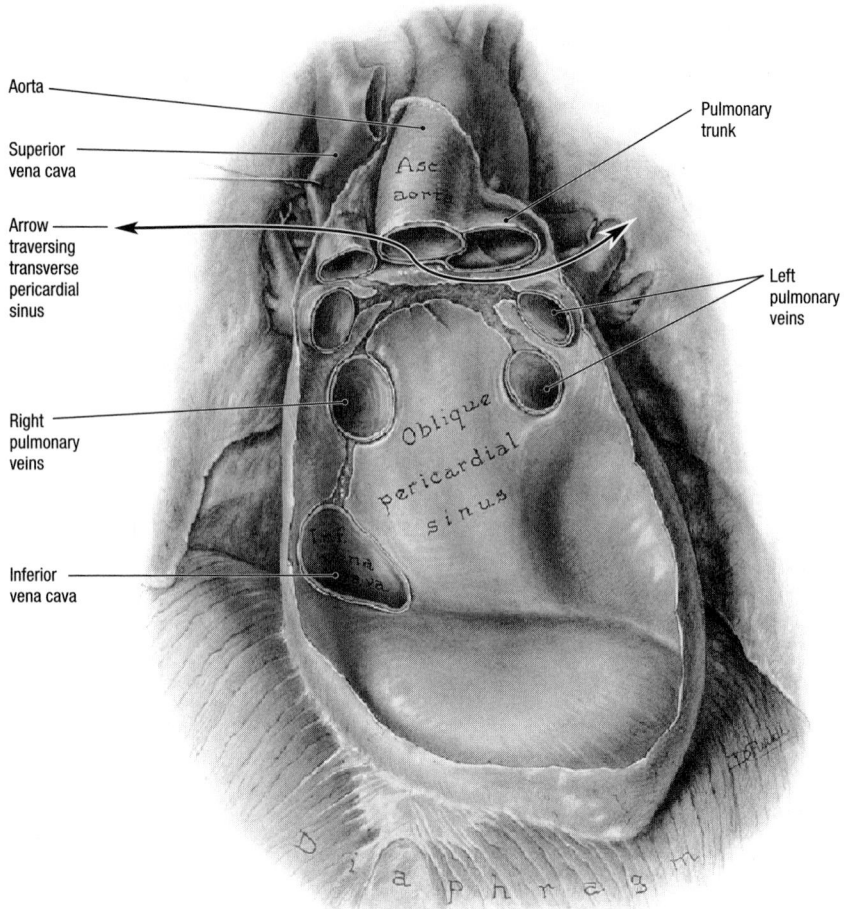

Figure 5. Interior of the pericardial sac. To remove the heart from the sac, the 8 vessels piercing it were severed. Observe that the oblique pericardial sinus is circumscribed by 5 veins and that the superior vena cava is partly inside and mostly outside the pericardium. Also observe that the peak of the pericardial sac is near the junction of the ascending aorta and the arch of the aorta. Note that the transverse pericardial sinus is bounded anteriorly by the serous pericardium covering the posterior aspect of the pulmonary trunk and ascending aorta, posteriorly by that covering the superior vena cava, and inferiorly by the visceral pericardium covering the atria of the heart.

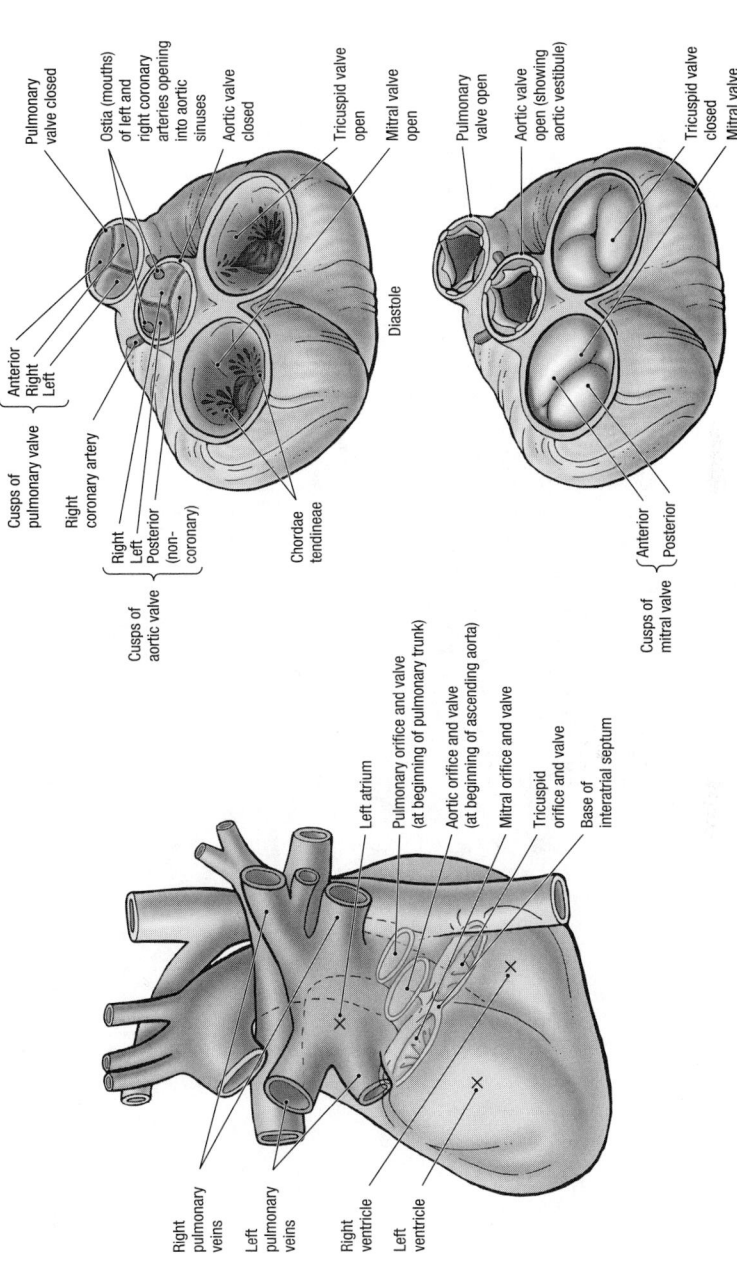

Figure 6. Valves of the heart and great vessels. At the beginning of diastole (ventricular filling), the aortic and pulmonary valves are closed; shortly thereafter, the tricuspid and mitral valves open. Shortly after systole (ventricular emptying) begins, the tricuspid and mitral valves close and the aortic and pulmonary valves open.

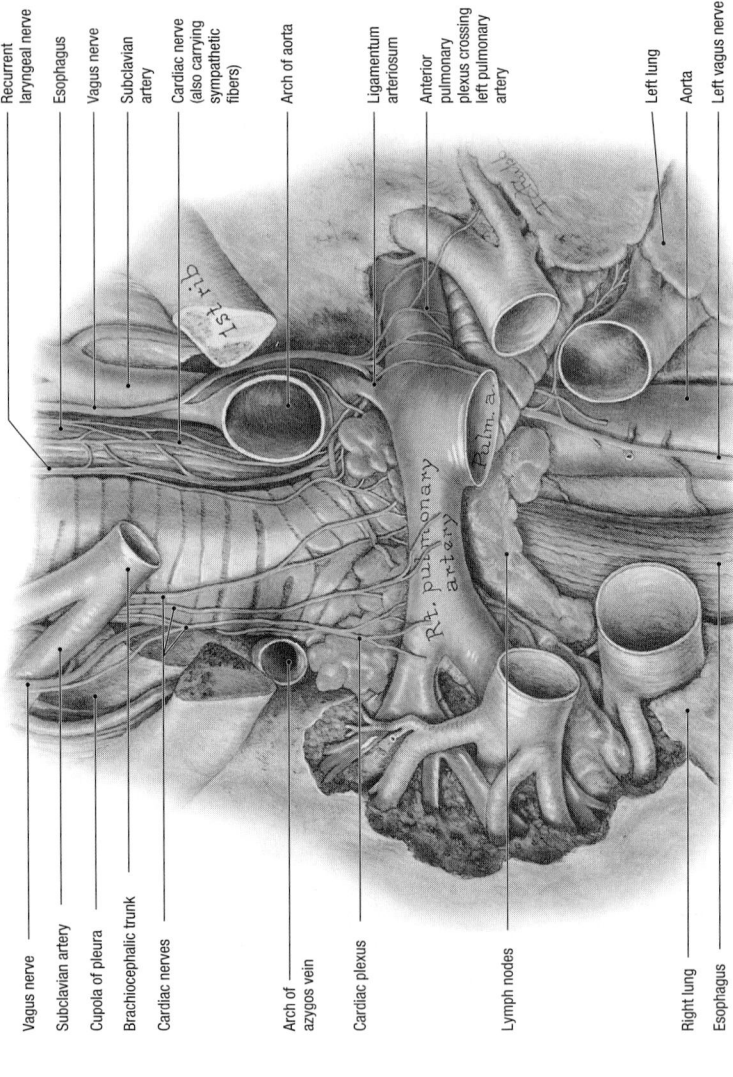

Vagus nerve

Subclavian artery

Cupola of pleura

Brachiocephalic trunk

Cardiac nerves

Arch of
azygos vein

Cardiac plexus

Lymph nodes

Right lung

Esophagus

Recurrent
laryngeal nerve

Esophagus

Vagus nerve

Subclavian
artery

Cardiac nerve
(also carrying
sympathetic
fibers)

Arch of aorta

Ligamentum
arteriosum

Anterior
pulmonary
plexus crossing
left pulmonary
artery

Left lung

Aorta

Left vagus nerve

Figure 7. Dissection of the superior mediastinum. Observe the cardiac branches of the vagus and sympathetic nerves running down the sides of the trachea and forming the cardiac plexus. Although shown lying on the trachea, the primary relationship of the cardiac plexus is to the ascending aorta and pulmonary trunks, which have been removed to expose the plexus.

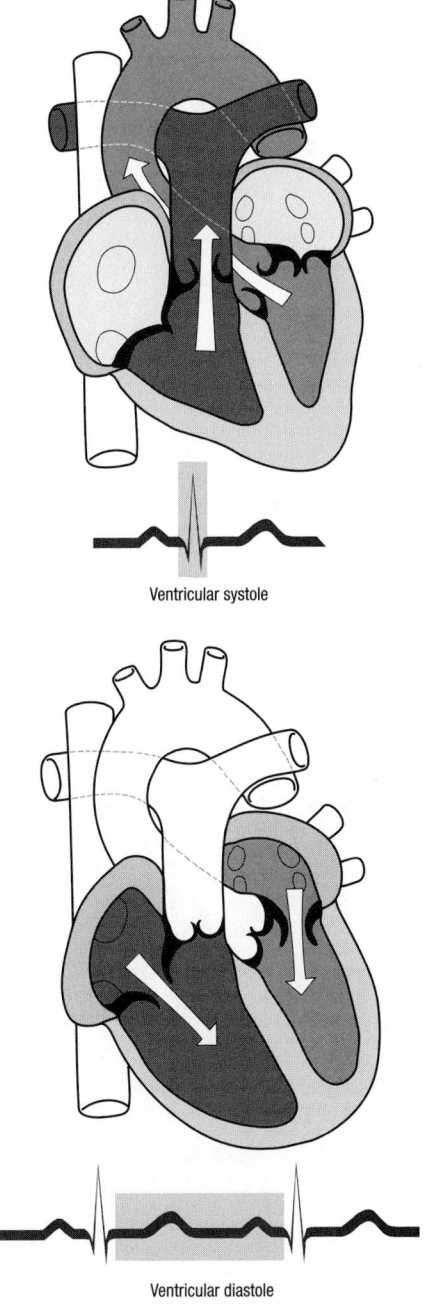

Ventricular systole

Ventricular diastole

Figure 8. The cardiac cycle.

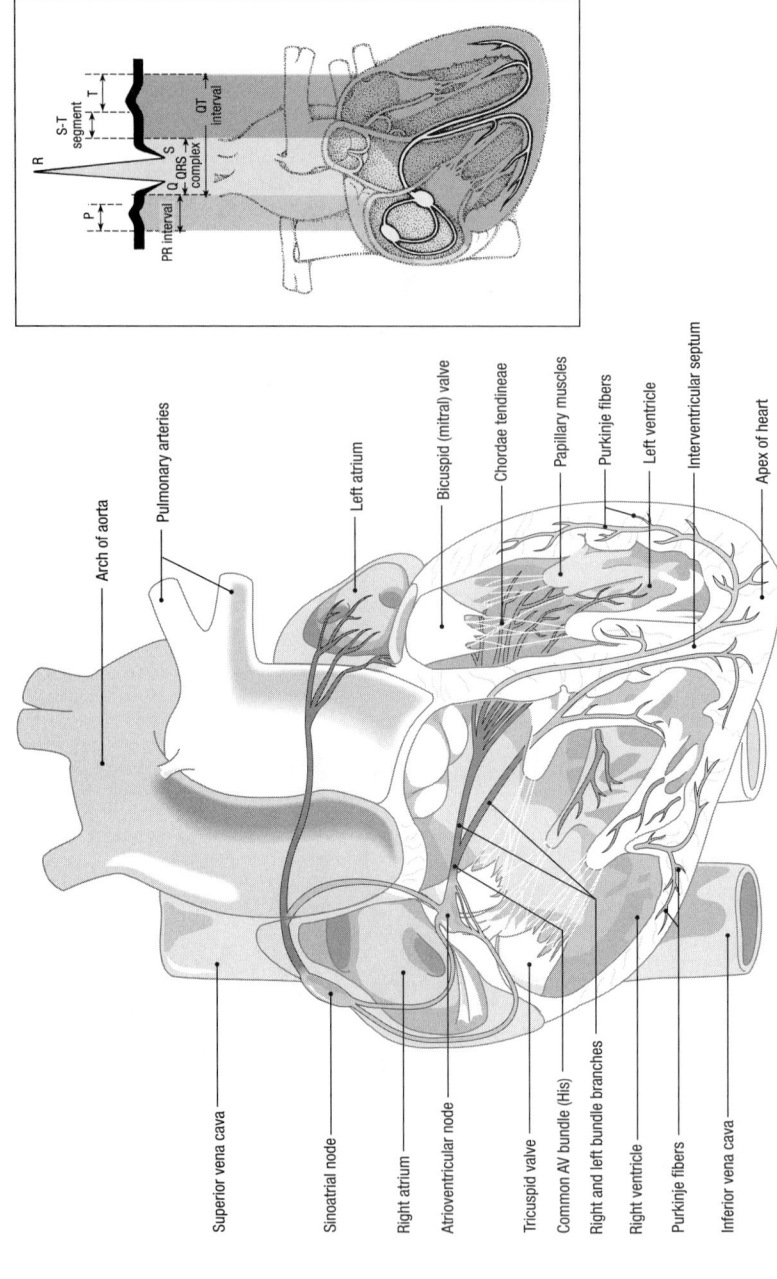

Figure 9. Conducting system of the heart. (Inset) An electrical picture of the heart is represented by positive and negative deflections on a graph labeled with the letters P, Q, R, S, and T, corresponding to the events of the cardiac cycle.

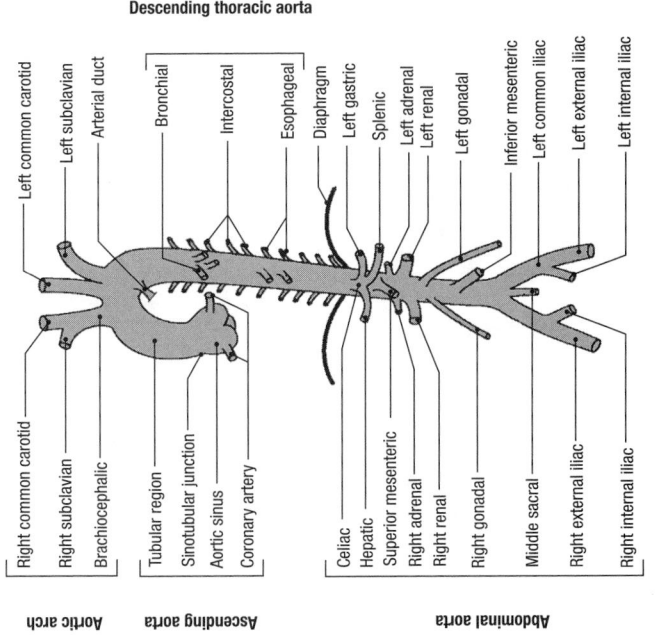

Figure 11. Systemic circulation: through the body, from the left ventricle to the right atrium.

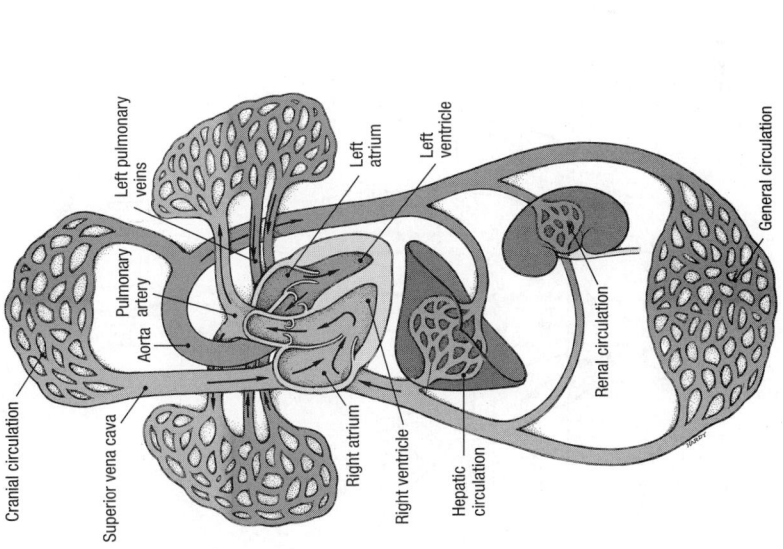

Figure 10. Pulmonary circulation: through the lungs, from the right ventricle to the left atrium.

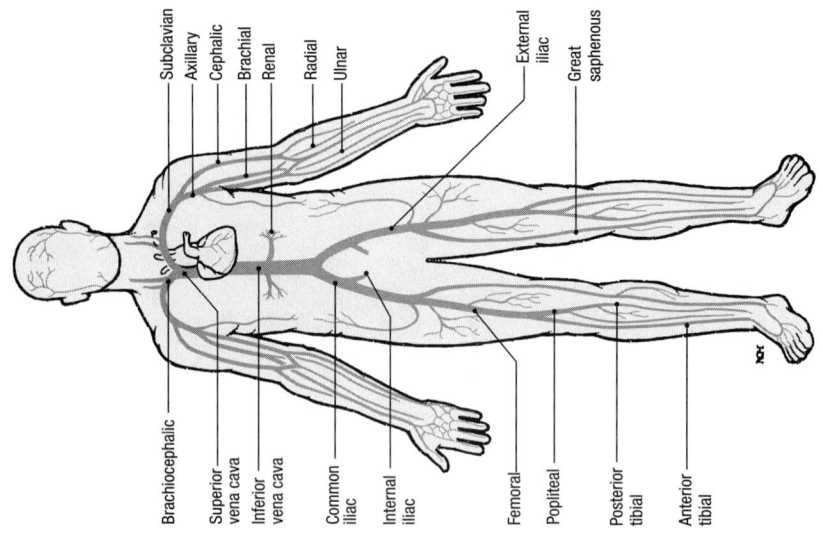

Figure 13. Major veins of the body.

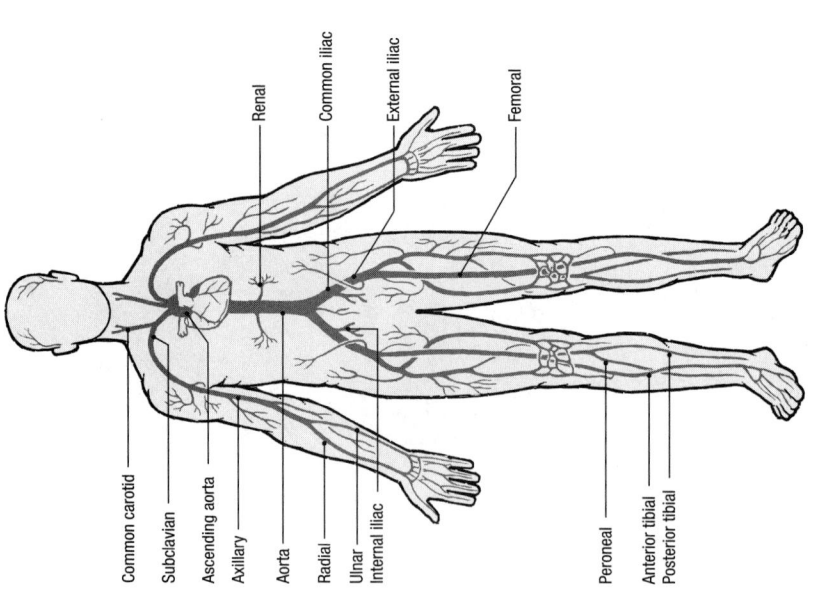

Figure 12. Major arteries of the body.

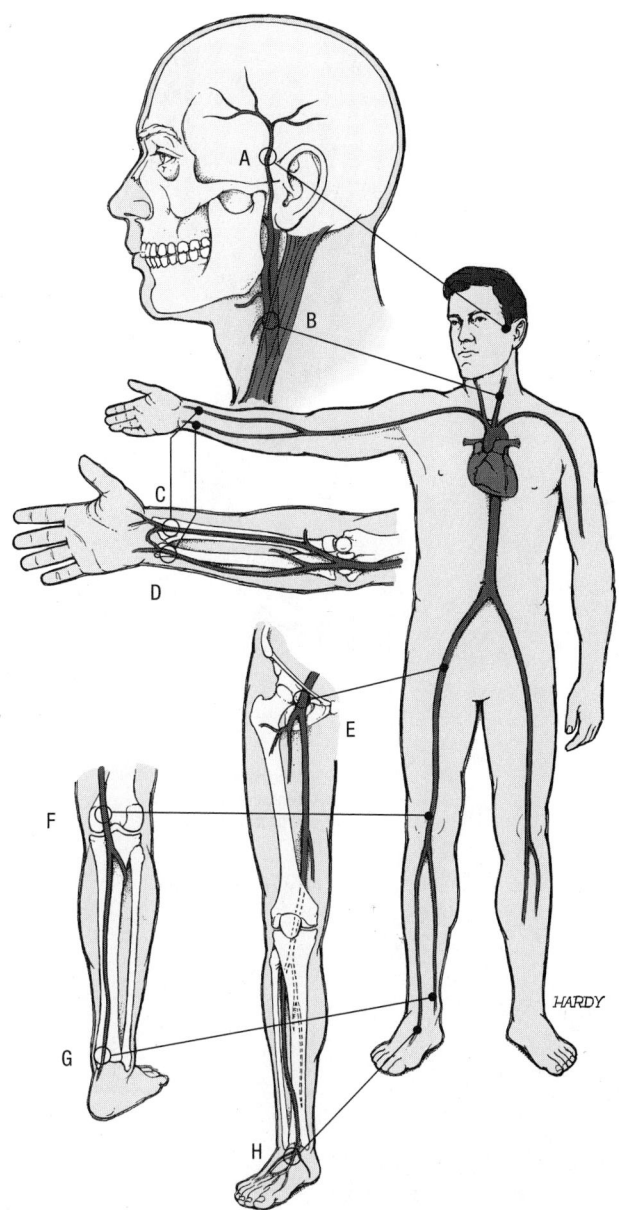

Figure 14. Peripheral pulses: (A) temporal, (B) carotid, (C) radial, (D) ulnar, (E) femoral, (F) popliteal, (G) posterior tibial, and (H) dorsalis pedis.

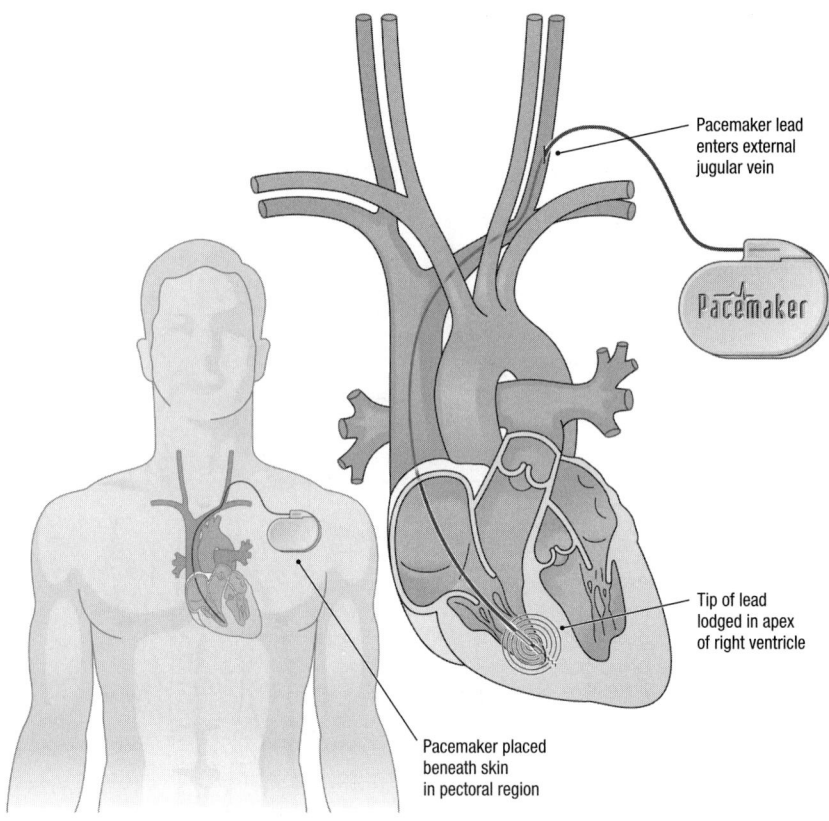

Pacemaker lead
enters external
jugular vein

Tip of lead
lodged in apex
of right ventricle

Pacemaker placed
beneath skin
in pectoral region

Figure 15. Placement of a pacemaker.

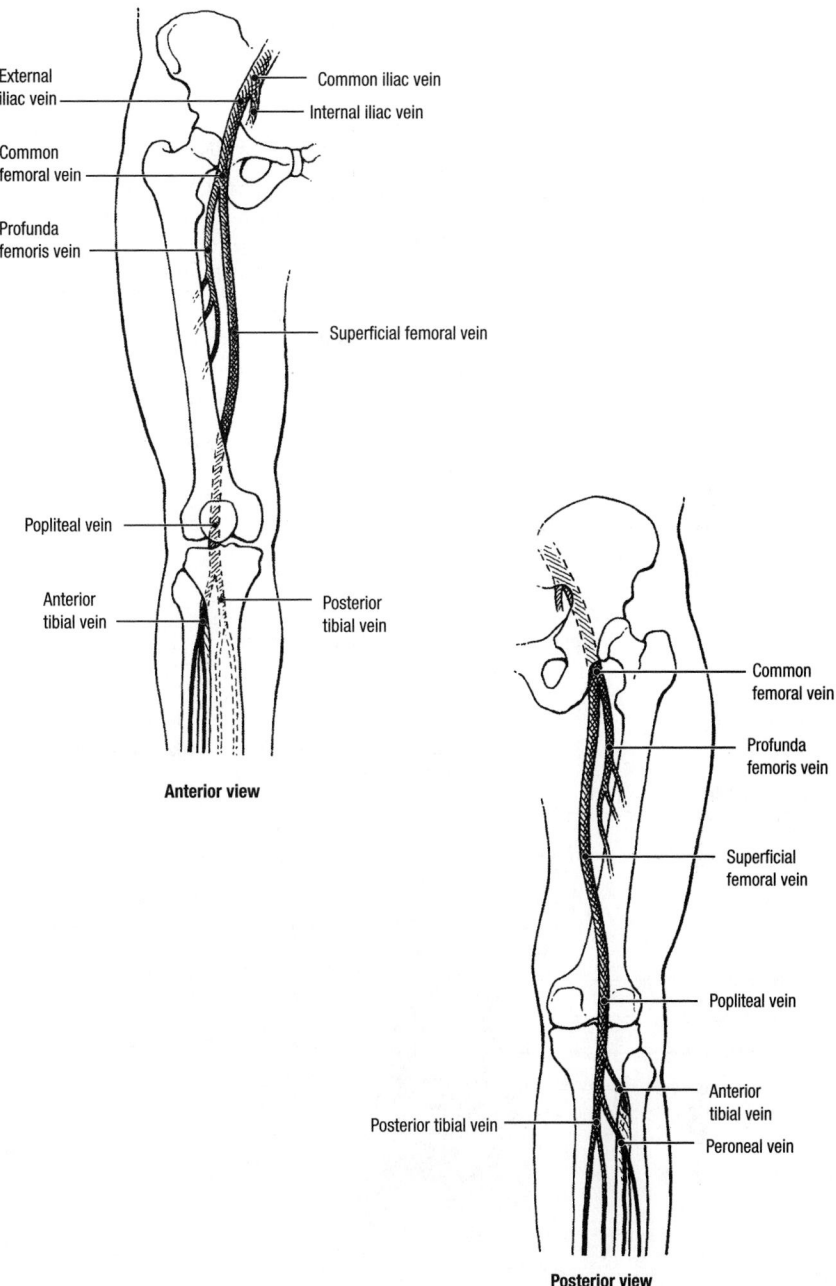

Figure 16. Anatomy of the deep venous system of the right lower limb. (Top) anterior view; (bottom) posterior view.

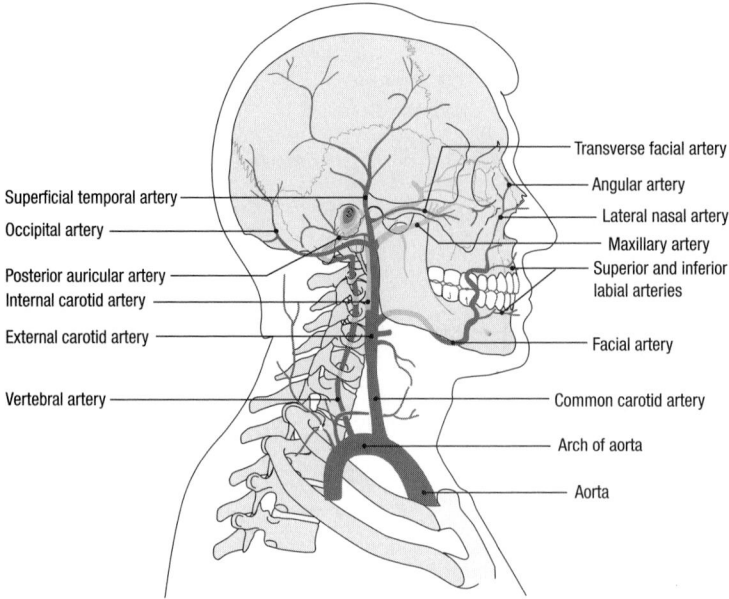

Figure 17. Arteries of the head and neck.

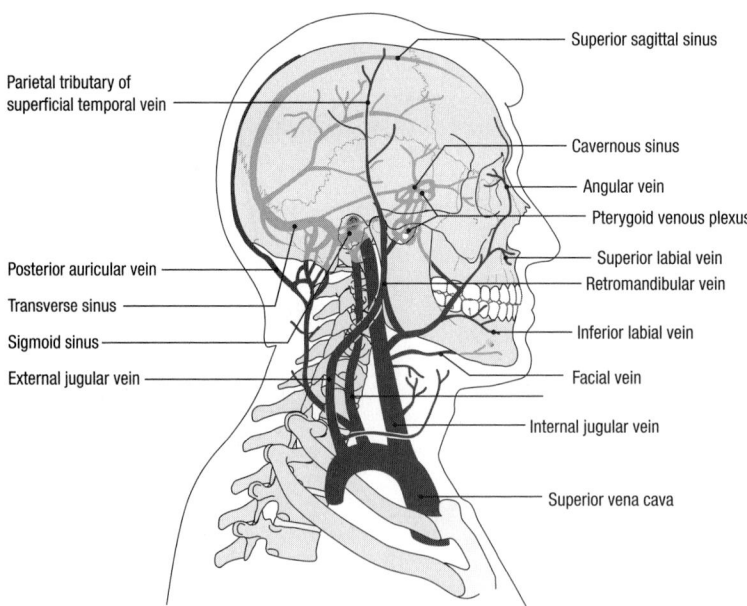

Figure 18. Veins of the head and neck.

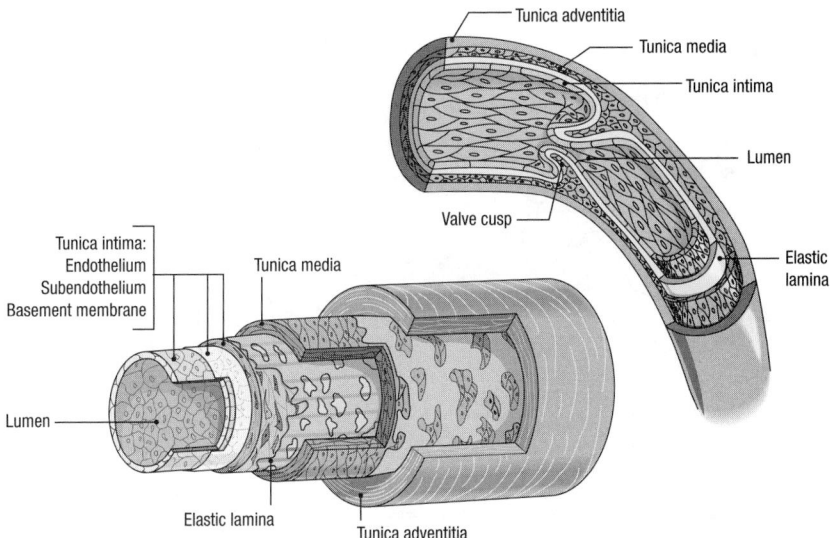

Figure 19. Structure of blood vessels. The walls of blood vessels are constructed of three concentric coats (Latin tunicae). With less muscle, veins (right) are thinner walled than their companion arteries (left) and have wide lumens (Latin lumina) that usually appear flattened in tissue sections.

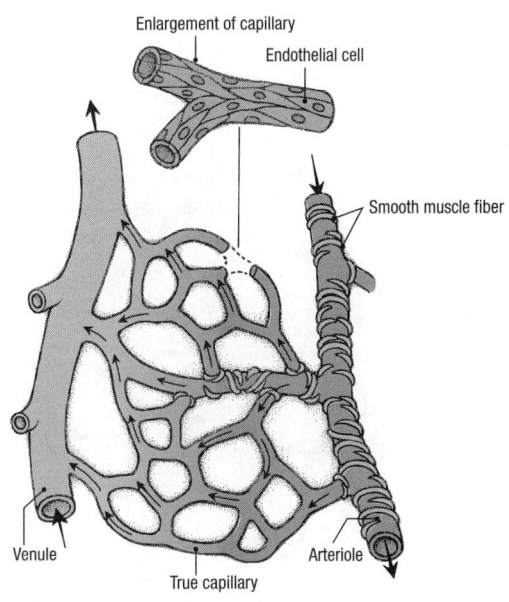

Figure 20. Capillary bed.

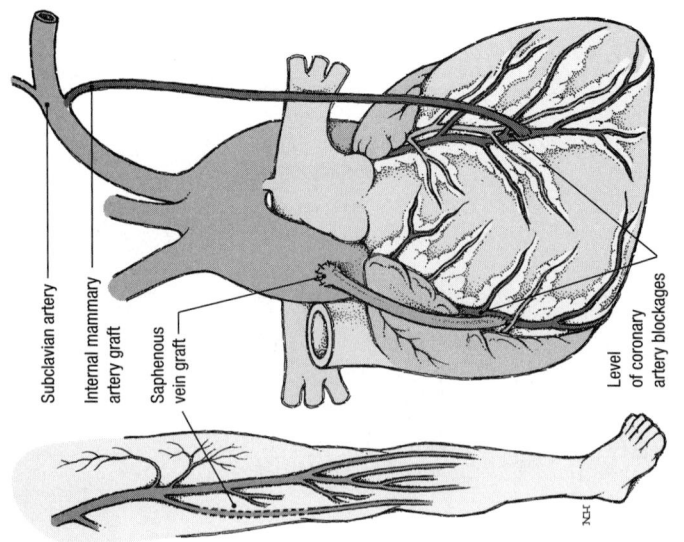

Figure 22. Aneurysm.

Subclavian artery

Internal mammary artery graft

Saphenous vein graft

Level of coronary artery blockages

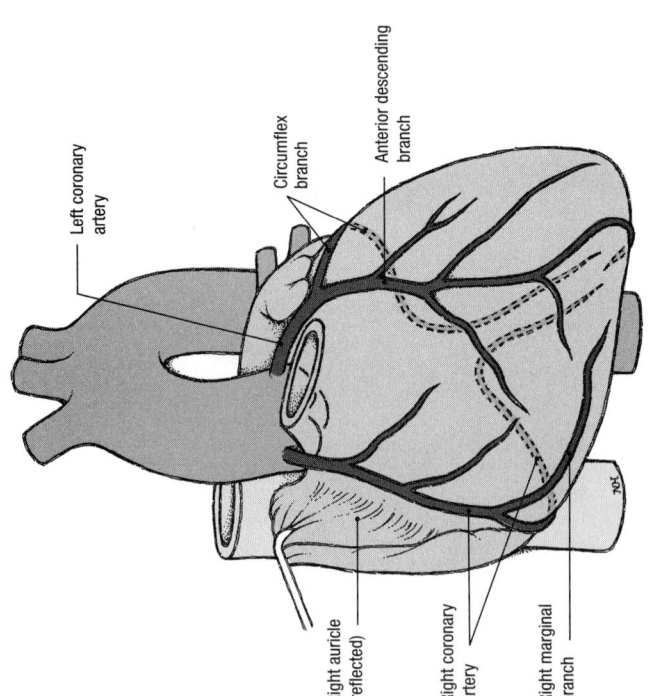

Figure 21. Coronary arteries.

Left coronary artery

Circumflex branch

Anterior descending branch

Right auricle (reflected)

Right coronary artery

Right marginal branch

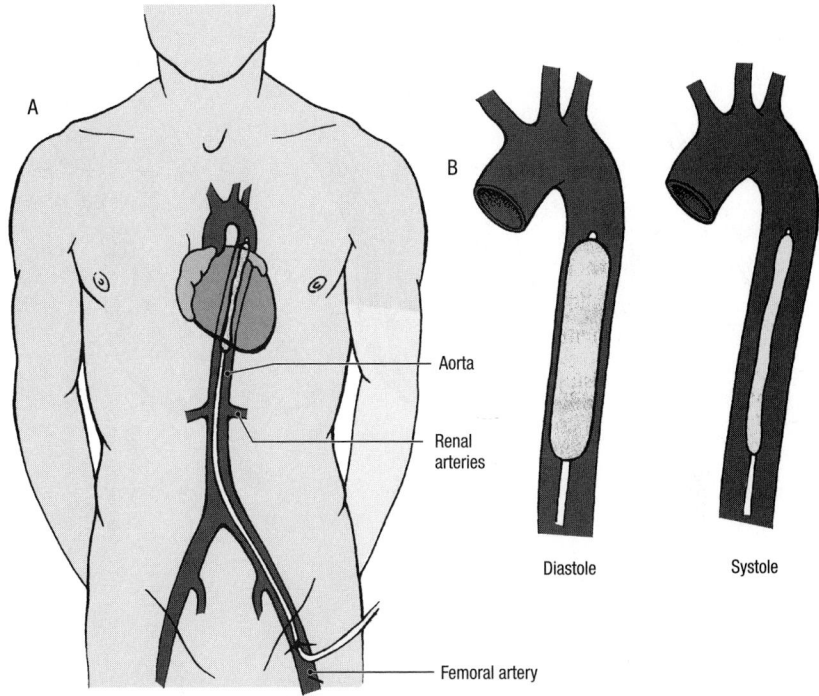

A

B

Aorta

Renal
arteries

Diastole

Systole

Femoral artery

Figure 23. Counterpulsation. (A) Introduction of the intraaortic balloon catheter via the femoral artery. (B) The intraaortic balloon pump augments diastole, resulting in increased perfusion of the coronary arteries and myocardium and a decrease in the left ventricular work load.

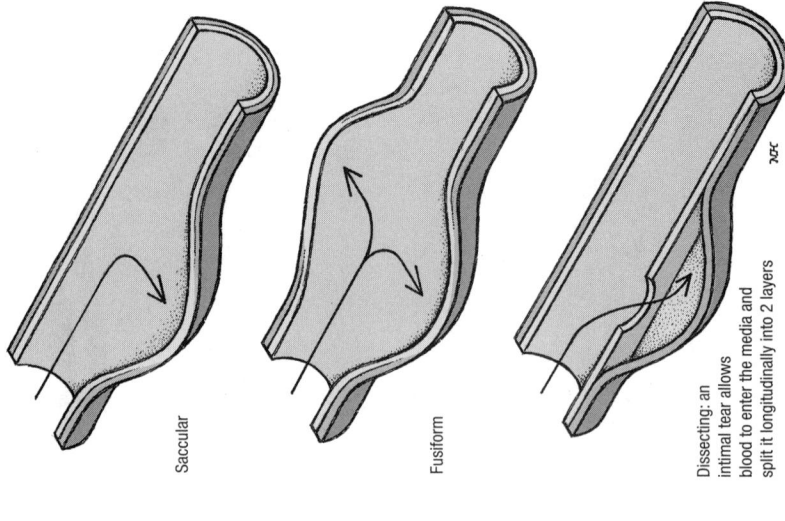

Figure 26. Aneurysm.

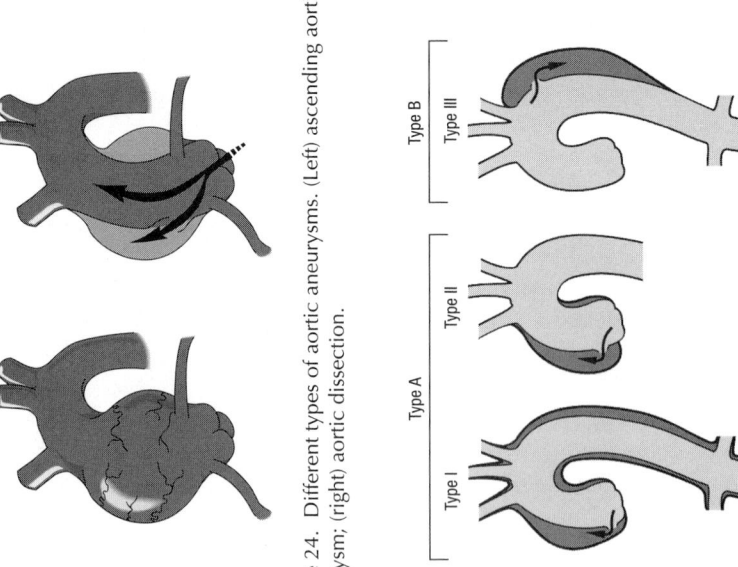

Figure 24. Different types of aortic aneurysms. (Left) ascending aortic aneurysm; (right) aortic dissection.

Figure 25. Aneurysms affecting the descending aorta: Stanford classification, Type A and Type B; deBakey classification, Types I, II, and III.

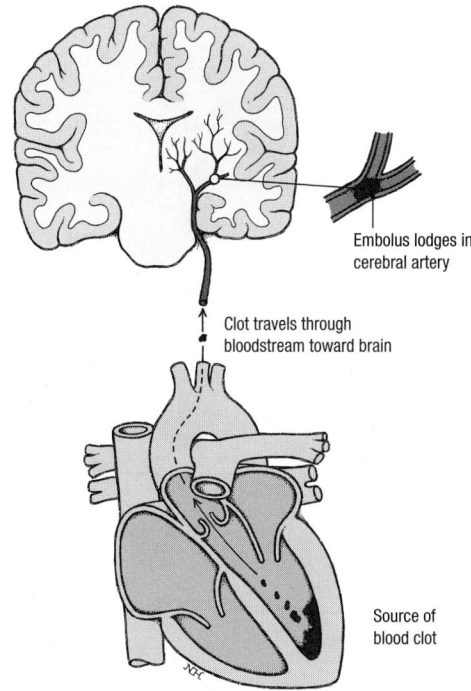

Embolus lodges in
cerebral artery

Clot travels through
bloodstream toward brain

Source of
blood clot

Figure 27. Embolism (embolus arising from a mural thrombus of the left ventricle).

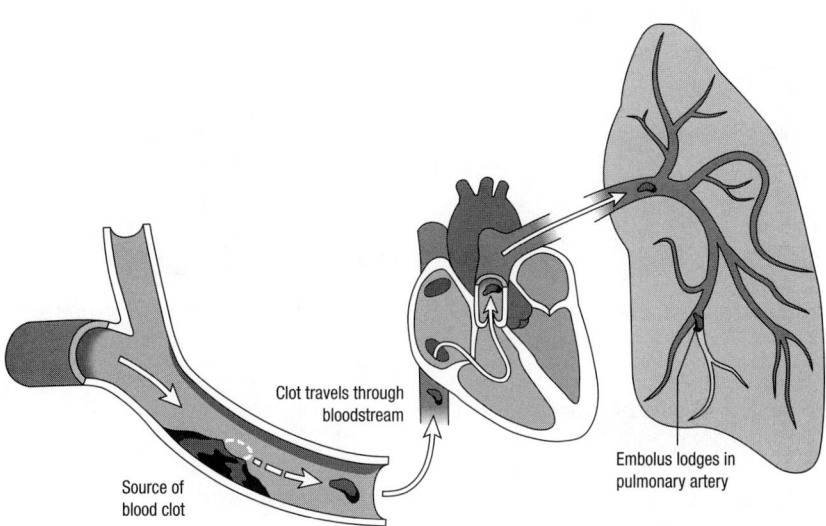

Clot travels through
bloodstream

Source of
blood clot

Embolus lodges in
pulmonary artery

Figure 28. Embolism (embolus arising from thrombus in distal vein).

A19

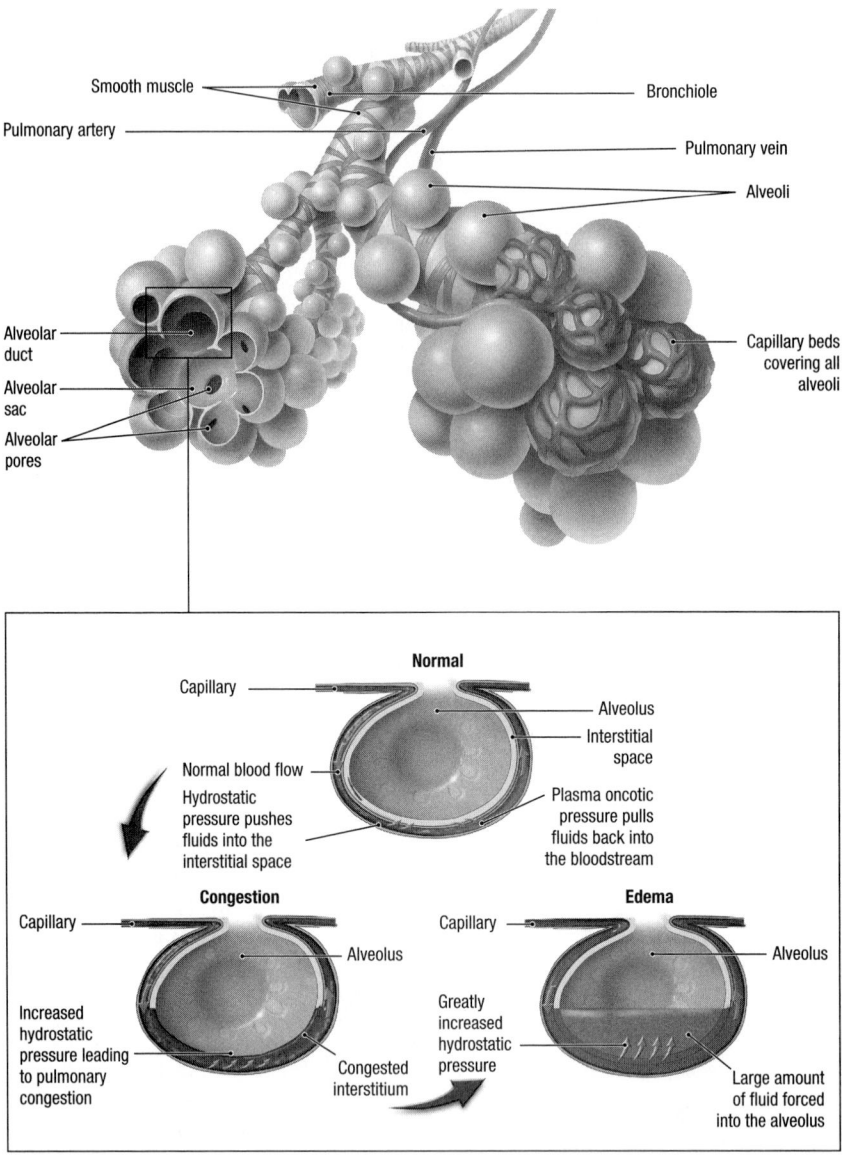

Figure 29. Normal alveoli and how pulmonary edema develops.

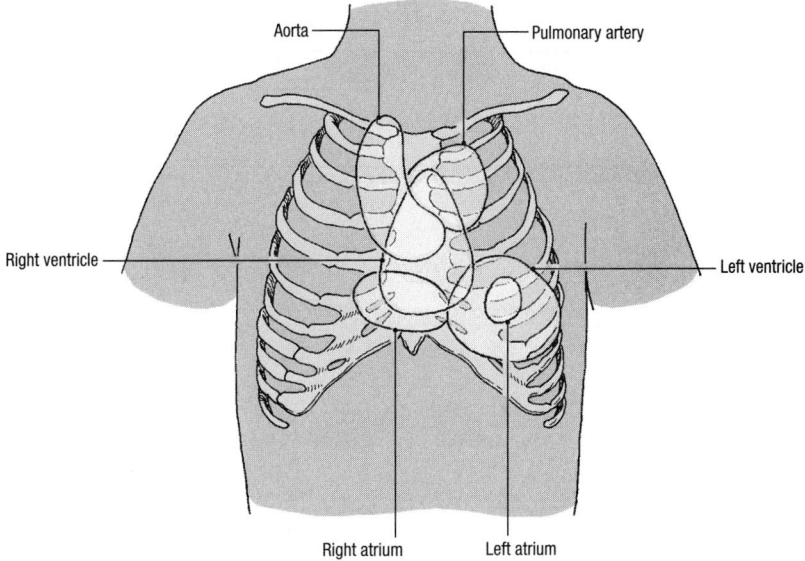

Figure 30. Auscultation points for cardiovascular structures. The sound generated by cardiovascular structures will be transmitted to areas of the chest wall that they most closely approximate.

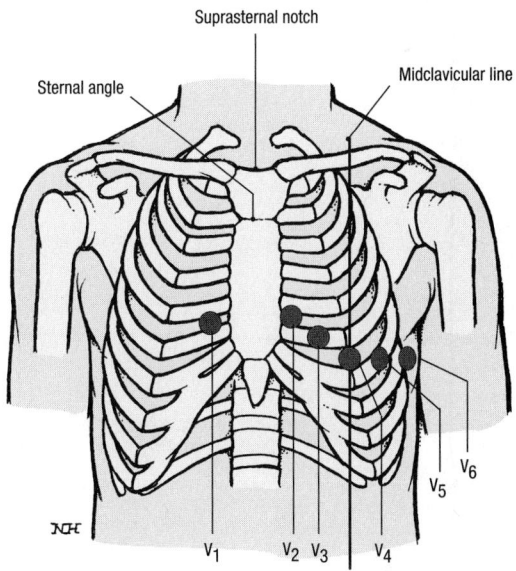

Figure 31. Electrocardiogram (ECG) lead placement: landmarks for chest lead placement.

A21

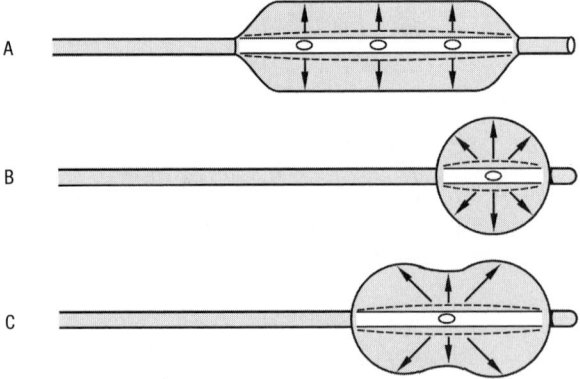

Figure 32. Three types of balloon catheters: (A) Gruentzig double-lumen dilation catheter, (B) Fogarty protrusion catheter, and (C) double-bellied balloon catheter used to expand valves.

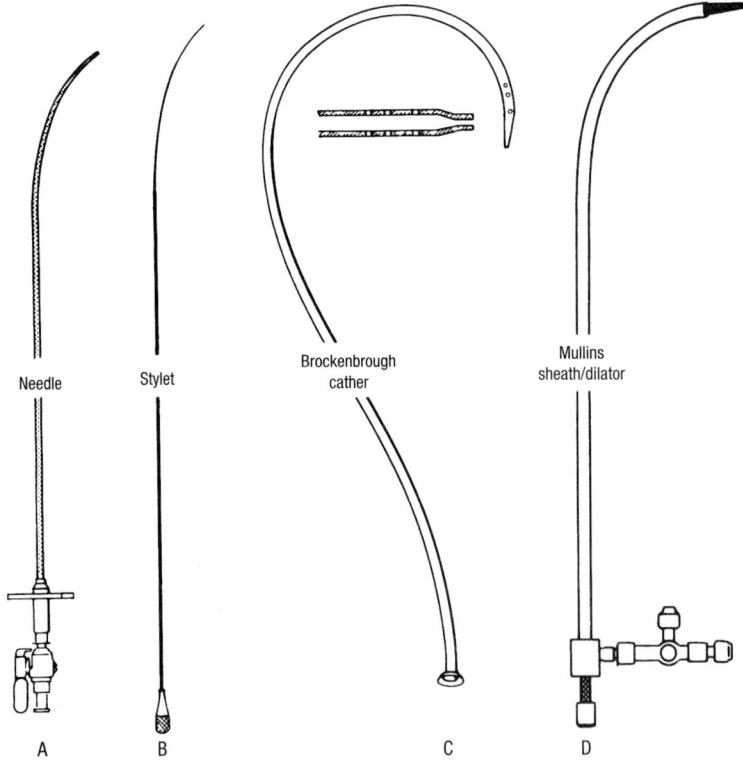

Figure 33. Equipment for transseptal puncture: (A) the Brockenbrough needle; (B) Bing stylet used in conjunction with (C) Brockenbrough catheter and (D) Mullins sheath/dilator system.

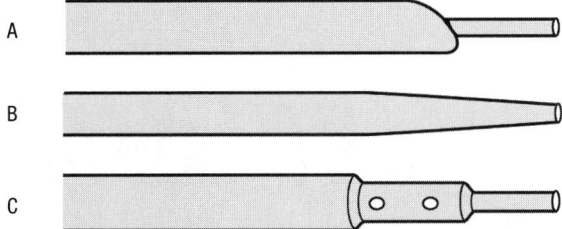

Figure 34. Catheters used to widen vessel stenosis in a stepwise manner: (A) Dotter, (B) Zeitler, and (C) Andel.

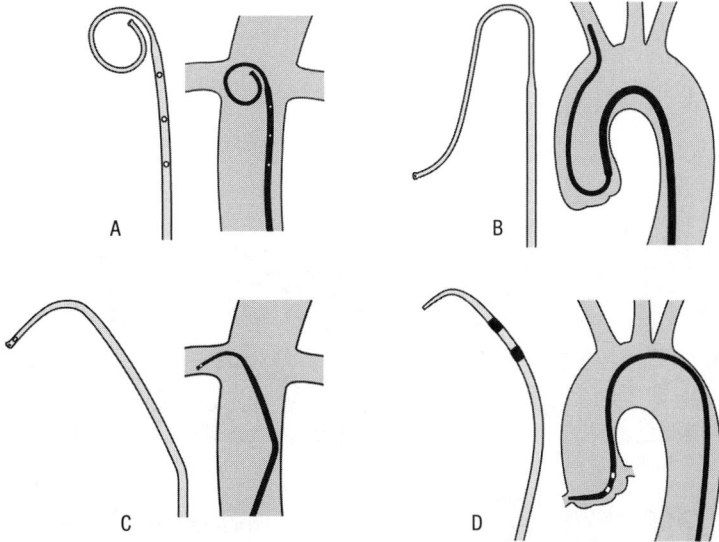

Figure 35. Various angiography catheters: (A) aorta catheter with side holes, (B) side-bending cerebral catheter (sidewinder), (C) side-bending catheter for selective viewing of visceral vessels, and (D) Judkins coronary catheter.

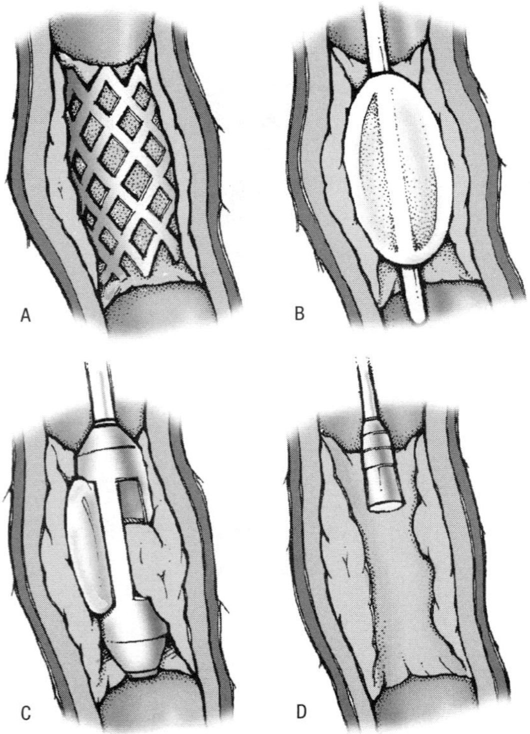

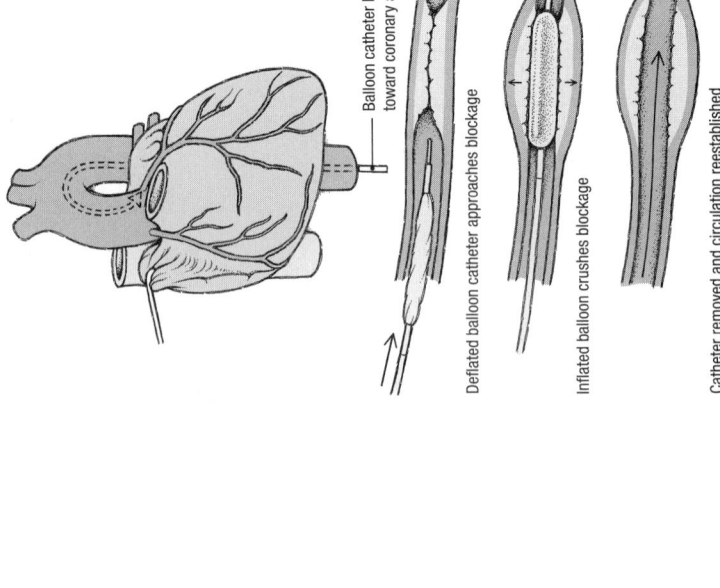

Figure 37. Percutaneous transluminal angioplasty.

Balloon catheter headed toward coronary artery

Deflated balloon catheter approaches blockage

Inflated balloon crushes blockage

Catheter removed and circulation reestablished

Figure 36. Close-up views of coronary arteries showing a variety of procedures to improve blood supply to the heart: (A) stent, (B) balloon angioplasty, (C) atherectomy, and (D) laser ablation.

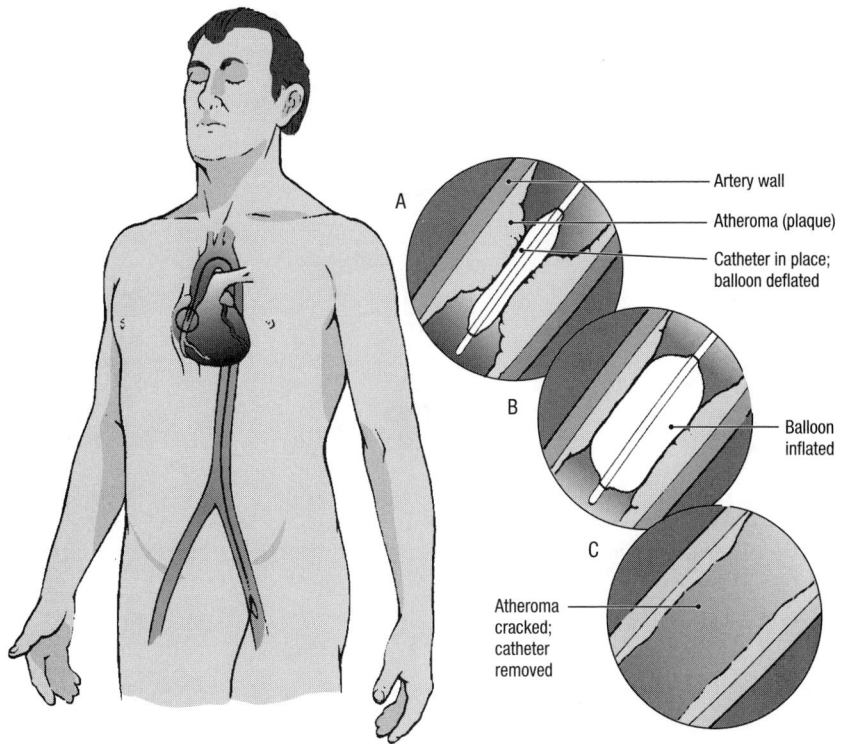

Figure 38. Percutaneous transluminal coronary angioplasty. (A) A balloon-tipped catheter is passed into the affected coronary artery and placed within the area of the atheroma (plaque). (B) The balloon is then rapidly inflated and deflated with controlled pressure. (C) After the atheroma is cracked, the catheter is removed, and blood flow improves.

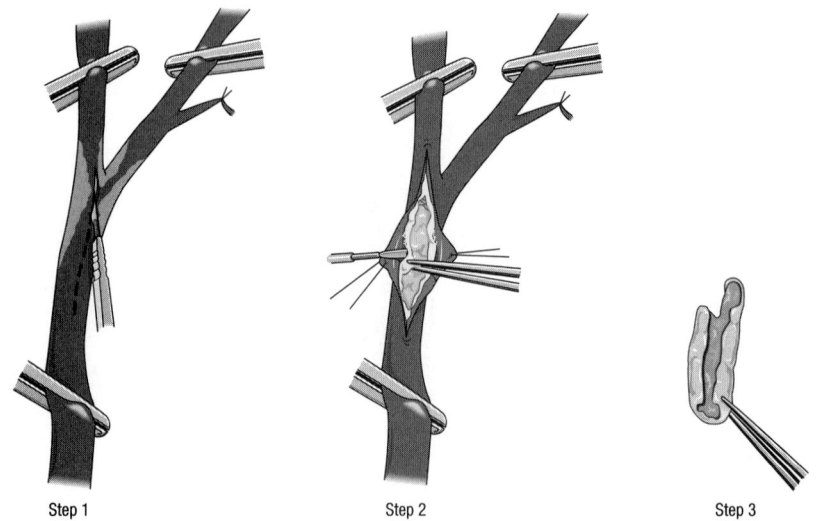

Step 1   Step 2   Step 3

Figure 39. An endarterectomy where diseased endothelium and media of an artery are removed so as to leave a smooth lining.

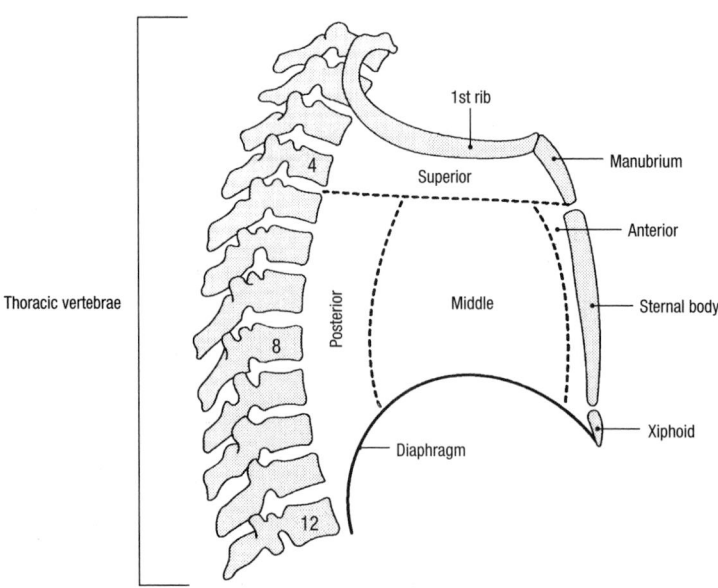

Figure 40. Mediastinum shown schematically. Viewed from a right lateral perspective, the mediastinum has four divisions: superior, posterior, middle, and anterior.

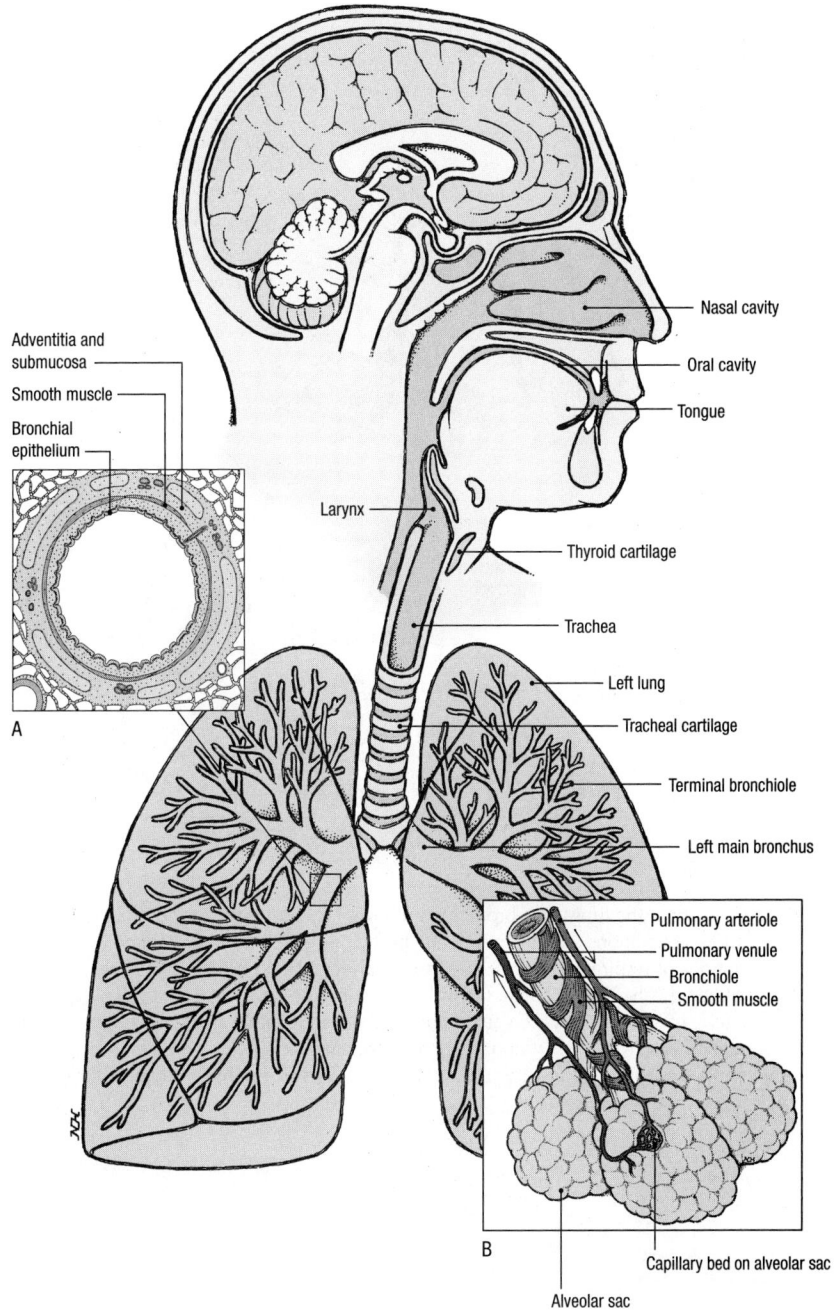

Adventitia and submucosa

Smooth muscle

Bronchial epithelium

A

Nasal cavity

Oral cavity

Tongue

Larynx

Thyroid cartilage

Trachea

Left lung

Tracheal cartilage

Terminal bronchiole

Left main bronchus

Pulmonary arteriole

Pulmonary venule

Bronchiole

Smooth muscle

B

Capillary bed on alveolar sac

Alveolar sac

Figure 41. Lungs and respiratory anatomy. (A) intrapulmonary bronchus and (B) pulmonary alveolus.

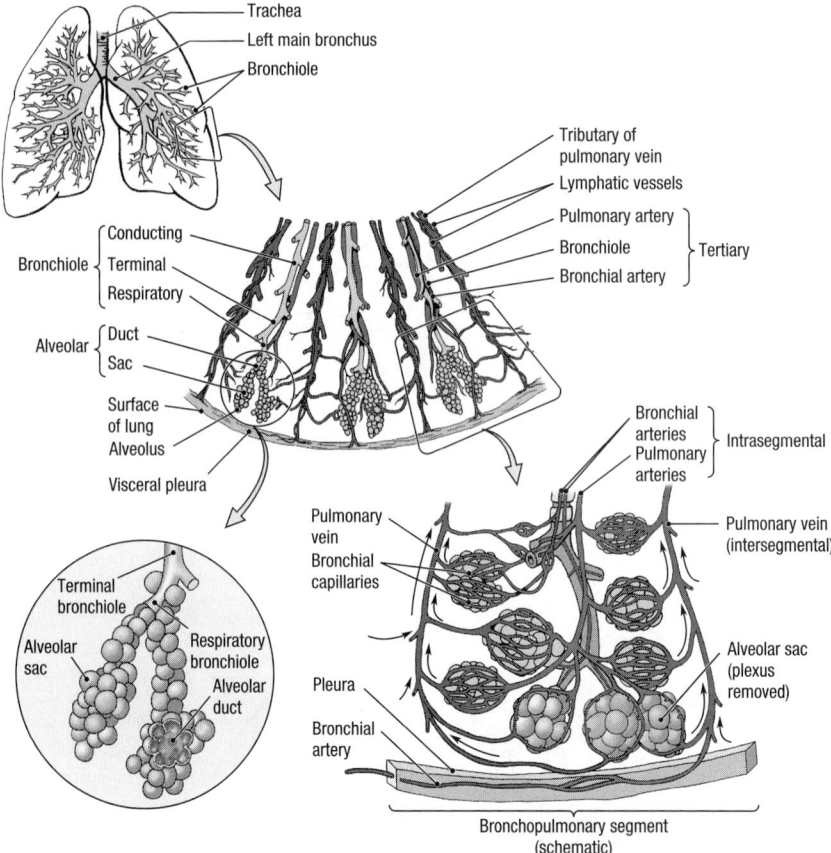

Figure 42. Structure of the lungs. The bronchopulmonary segment is the structural unit of the lung. Some 15 or more generations after the segmental bronchus, each terminal bronchiole gives rise to several generations of respiratory bronchioles, and each respiratory bronchiole gives rise to 5 or 6 alveolar sacs lined by alveoli, which are the basic structures for gas exchange. Each intrasegmental pulmonary artery, carrying poorly oxygenated blood, ends in a capillary plexus in the walls of the alveolar sacs and alveoli, where O_2 and CO_2 are exchanged. The pulmonary veins arise from the pulmonary capillaries draining toward and coursing in the septa between adjacent segments to carry well-oxygenated blood to the heart.

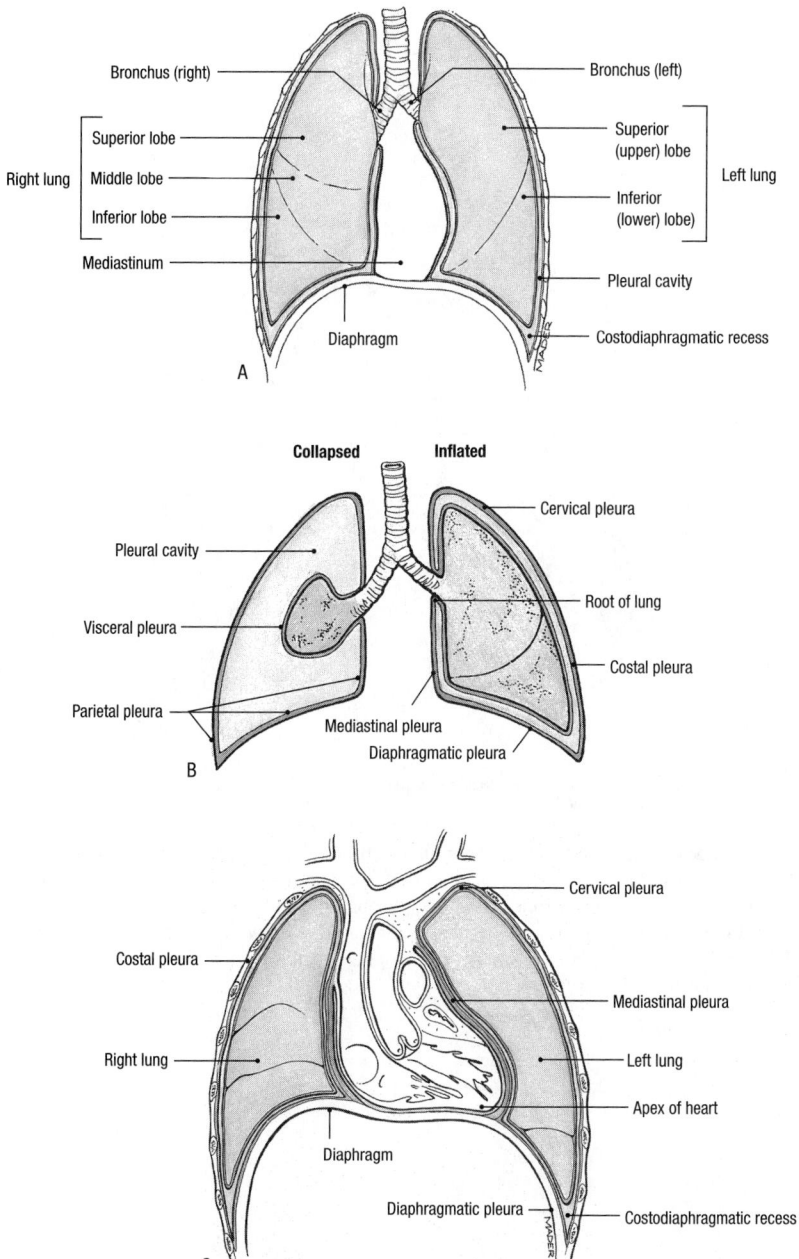

Figure 43. Respiratory system: (A) overview, (B) pleural cavity and pleura, and (C) coronal section through heart and lungs.

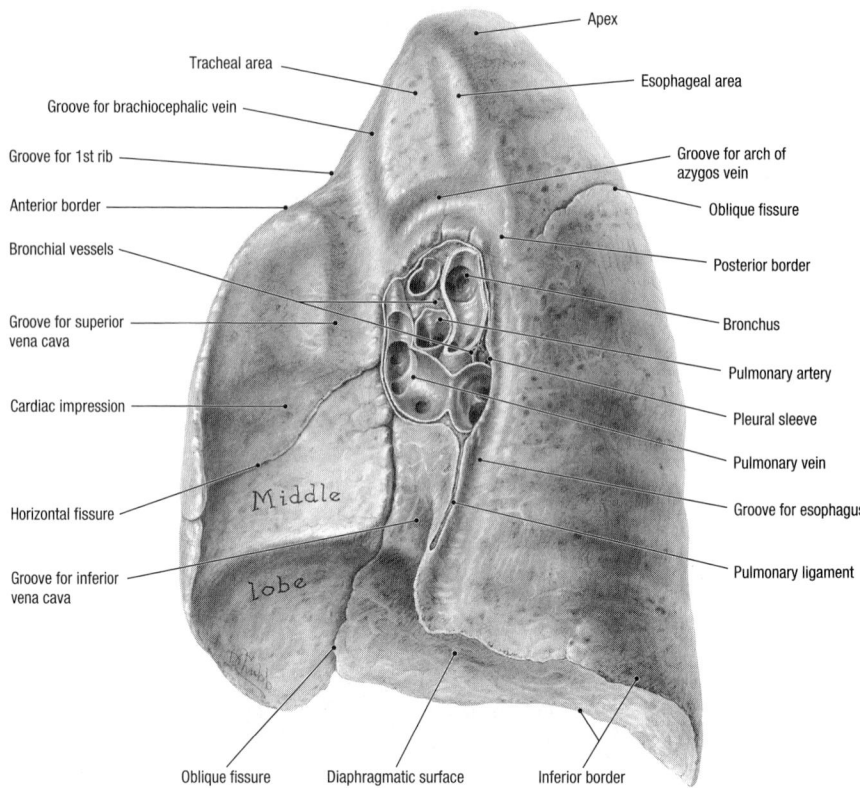

Apex

Tracheal area

Esophageal area

Groove for brachiocephalic vein

Groove for 1st rib

Groove for arch of azygos vein

Anterior border

Oblique fissure

Bronchial vessels

Posterior border

Groove for superior vena cava

Bronchus

Pulmonary artery

Cardiac impression

Pleural sleeve

Pulmonary vein

Horizontal fissure

Middle

Groove for esophagus

Groove for inferior vena cava

lobe

Pulmonary ligament

Oblique fissure   Diaphragmatic surface   Inferior border

Figure 44. Mediastinal surface of the right lung. Observe the somewhat pear-shaped depression, the hilum (doorway) of the lung near the center of this surface, containing the pulmonary vessels and bronchi that constitute the root of the lung, through which these structures (cut here) enter the lung. At the hilum, note that the pulmonary veins lie most anteriorly and inferiorly and that the bronchus is central and posteriorly placed. In the right lung, the superior lobar (eparterial) bronchus may occur superior to the pulmonary artery.

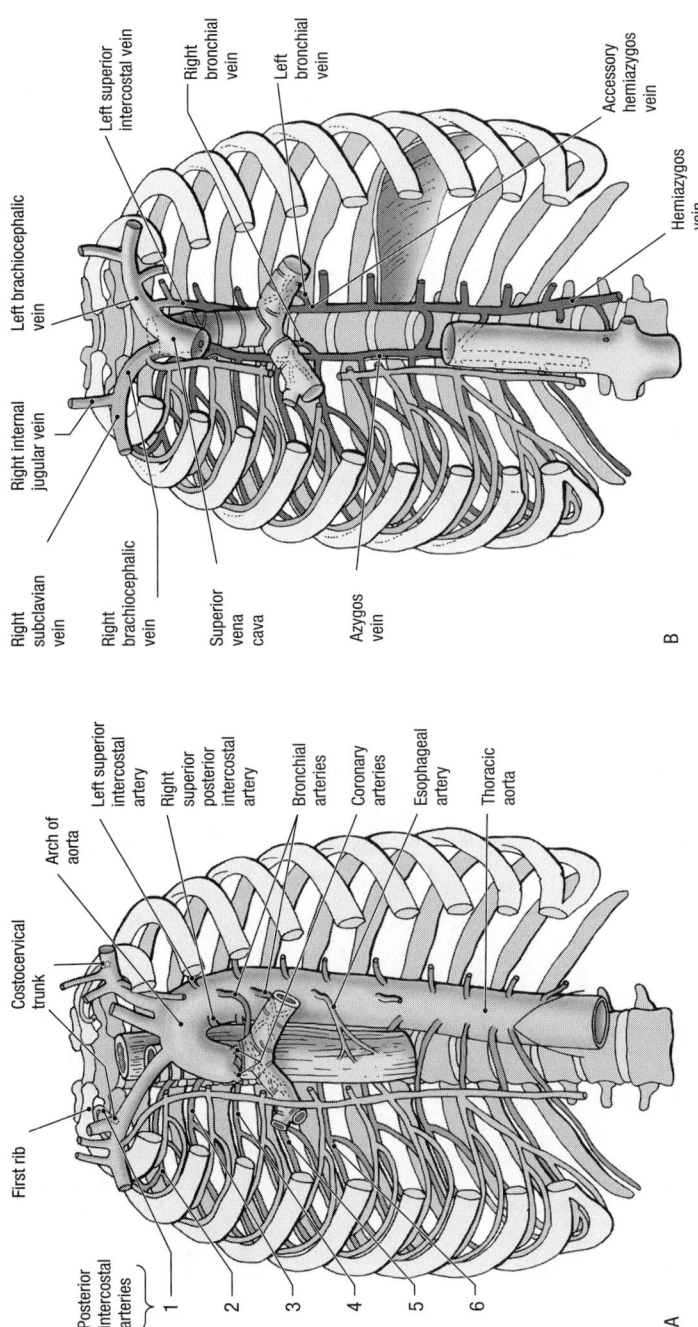

Figure 45. Bronchial arteries and veins. (A) The bronchial arteries supply blood for the nutrition of the supporting tissues of the lungs and visceral pleura. These arteries arise from the thoracic aorta but the origin of the right bronchial artery is variable. It may arise from (a) a superior posterior intercostal artery; (b) a common trunk from the thoracic aorta with the right third posterior intercostal artery; or (c) the left superior bronchial artery. (B) The bronchial veins drain some of the blood supplied to the lungs by the bronchial arteries; the rest is drained by the pulmonary veins. The right bronchial vein drains into the azygos vein and the left bronchial vein drains into the accessory hemiazygos vein or the left superior intercostal vein.

A31

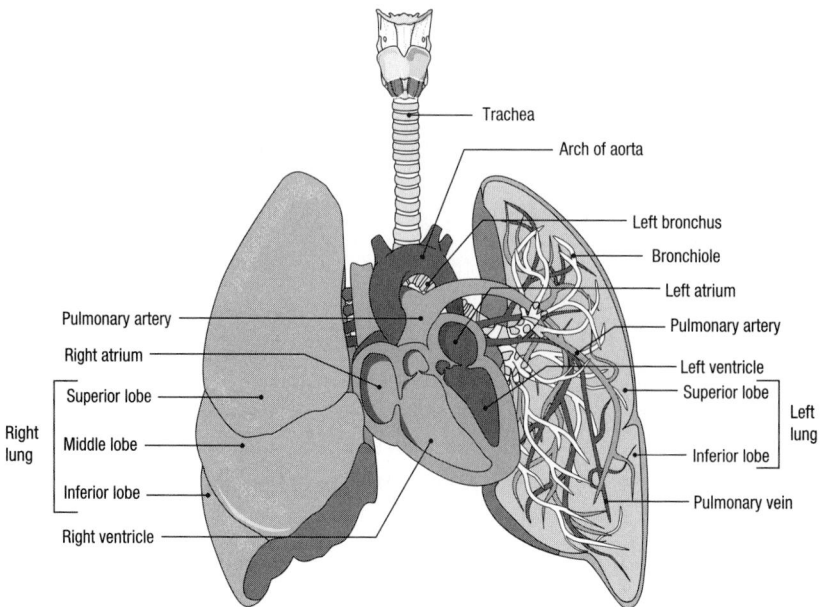

Figure 46. Cardiopulmonary system shown with cutaway of heart and left lung revealing internal anatomy.

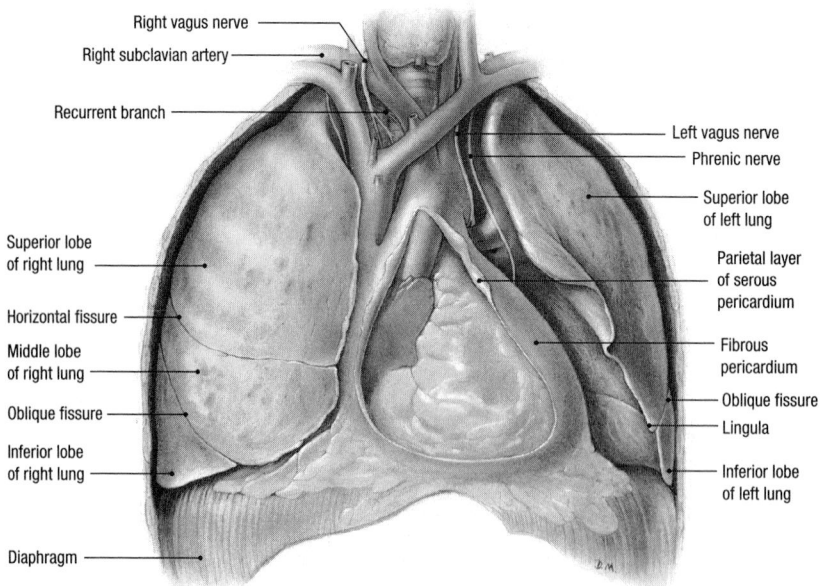

Figure 47. Thoracic contents in situ, anterior view.

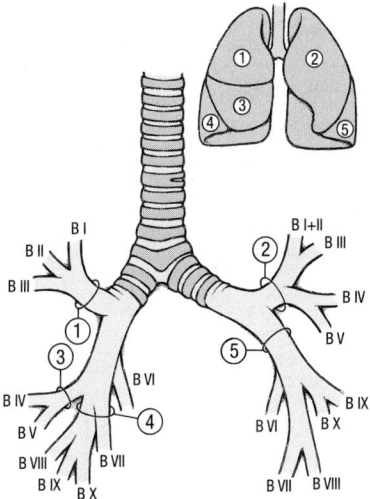

Figure 48. Segmental bronchi. Right lung: (B I) apical, (B II) posterior, (B III) anterior, (B IV) lateral, (B V) medial, (B VI) apical, (B VII) medial basal, (B VIII) anterior basal, (B IX) lateral basal, and (B X) posterior basal. Left lung: (B I+II) apicoposterior, (B III) anterior, (B IV) superior lingular, (B V) inferior lingular, (B VI) apical, (B VII) medial basal, (B VIII) anterior basal, (B IX) lateral basal, and (B X) posterior basal. Lobes of lungs supplied: (1) right superior, (2) left superior, (3) right middle, (4) right inferior, and (5) left inferior.

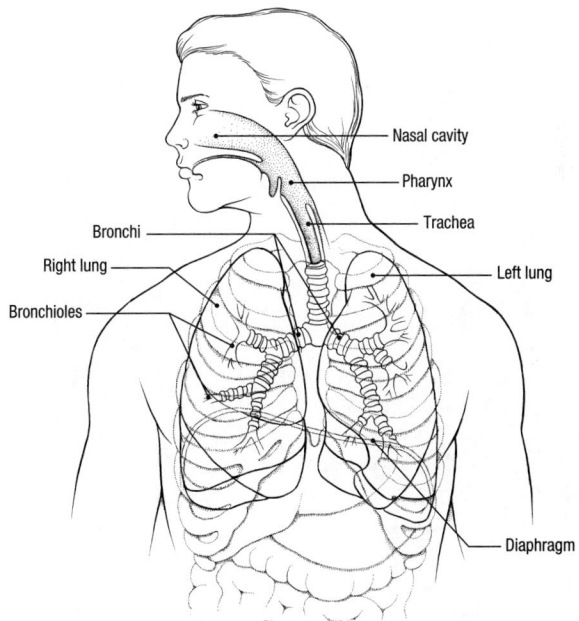

Figure 49. Anterior view of the male figure showing the main features of the respiratory system.

A33

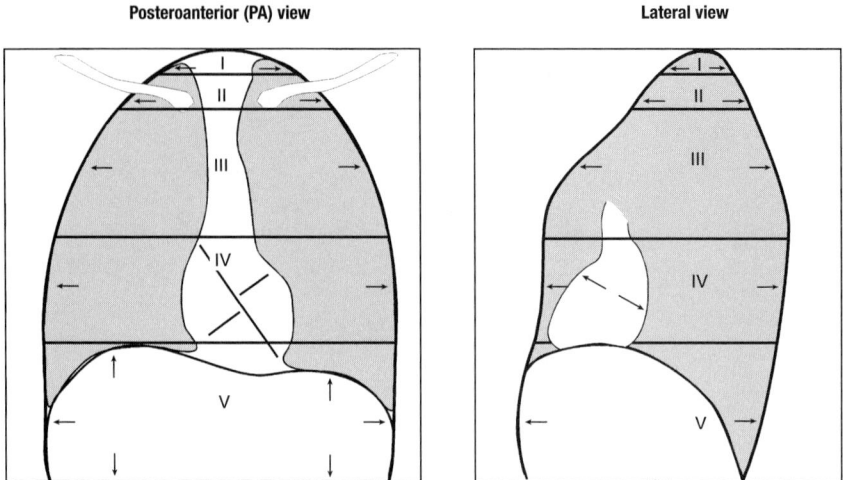

Posteroanterior (PA) view   **Lateral view**

Figure 50. Posteroanterior (PA) and lateral chest films at full inspirations are divided into five (I-V) elliptical segments for measurement of total lung capacity.

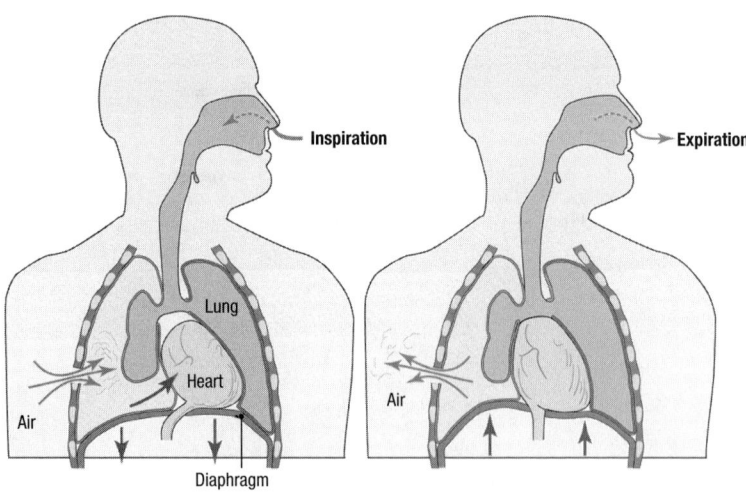

Figure 51. Left illustration shows how the heart and lungs are affected during inspiration in a person with pneumothorax. Right illustration shows how the heart and lungs are affected during expiration in a person with pneumothorax.

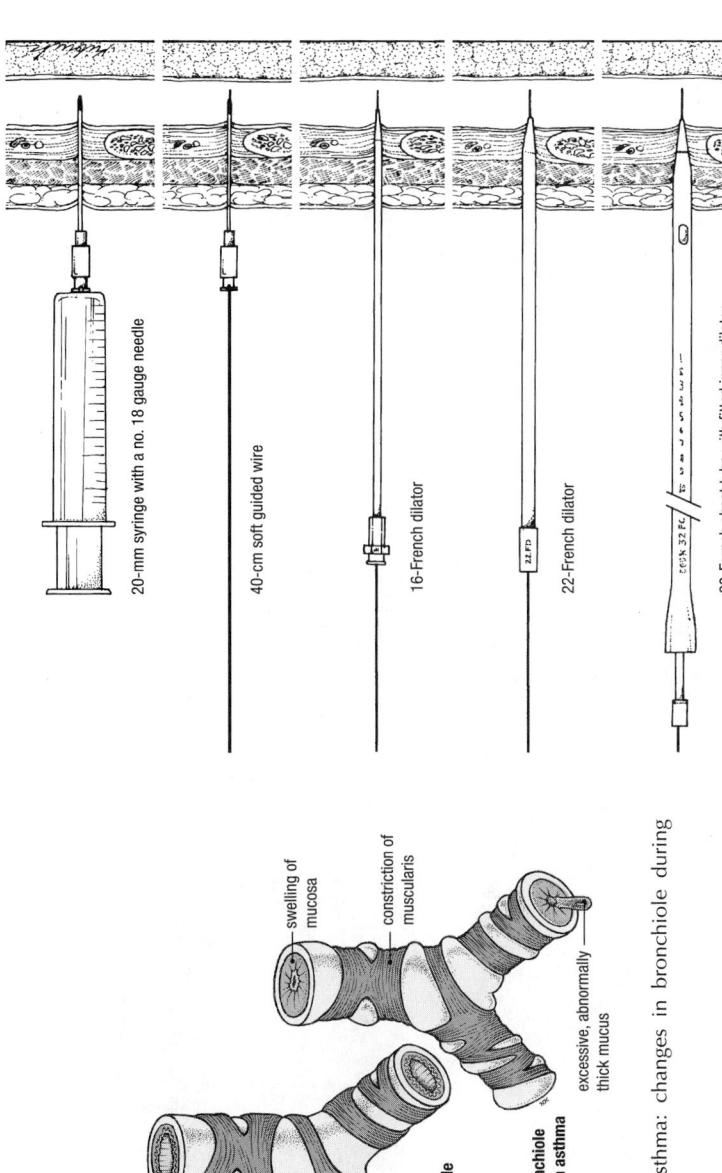

20-mm syringe with a no. 18 gauge needle

40-cm soft guided wire

16-French dilator

22-French dilator

32-French chest tube with fitted inner dilator

Figure 53. Chest tube insertion for thoracoscopy. Prior to initiating the syringe insertion, a local anesthetic is administered. Patient discomfort is minimal with use of the graduated size in dilator diameters.

swelling of mucosa

constriction of muscularis

excessive, abnormally thick mucus

normal bronchiole

bronchiole with asthma

Figure 52. Asthma: changes in bronchiole during asthma attack.

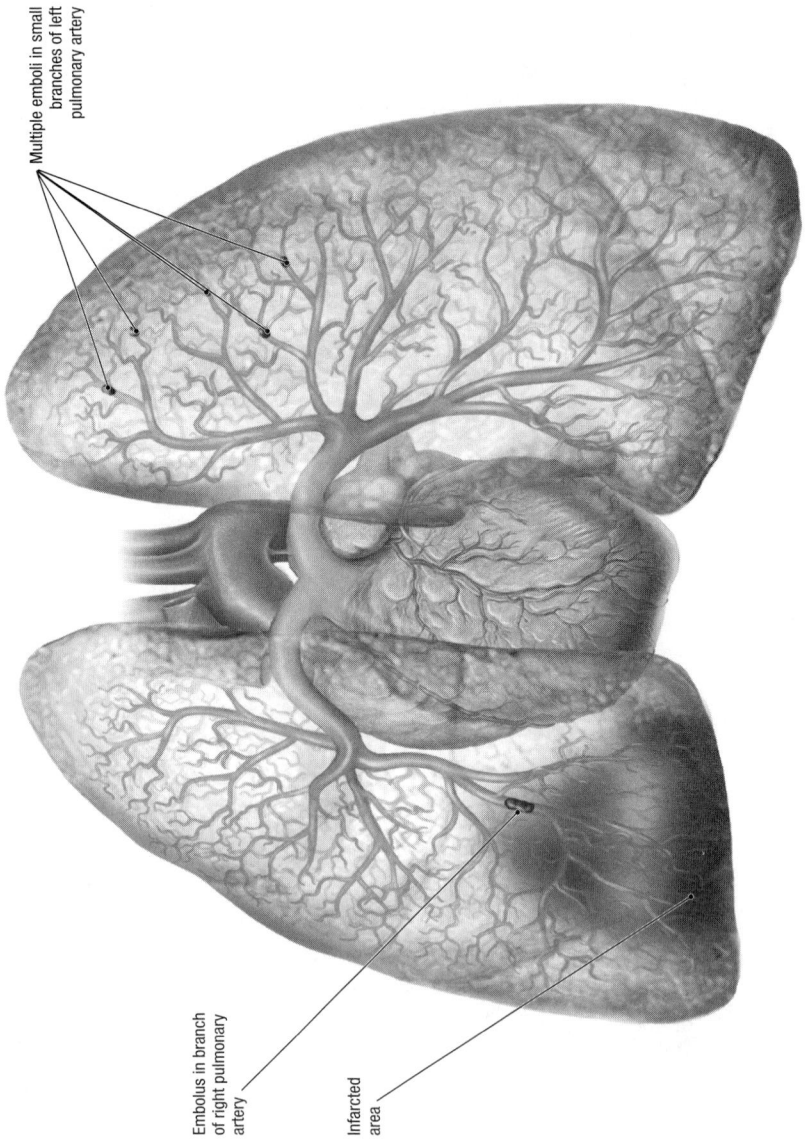

Multiple emboli in small branches of left pulmonary artery

Embolus in branch of right pulmonary artery

Infarcted area

Figure 54. Sites of pulmonary emboli.

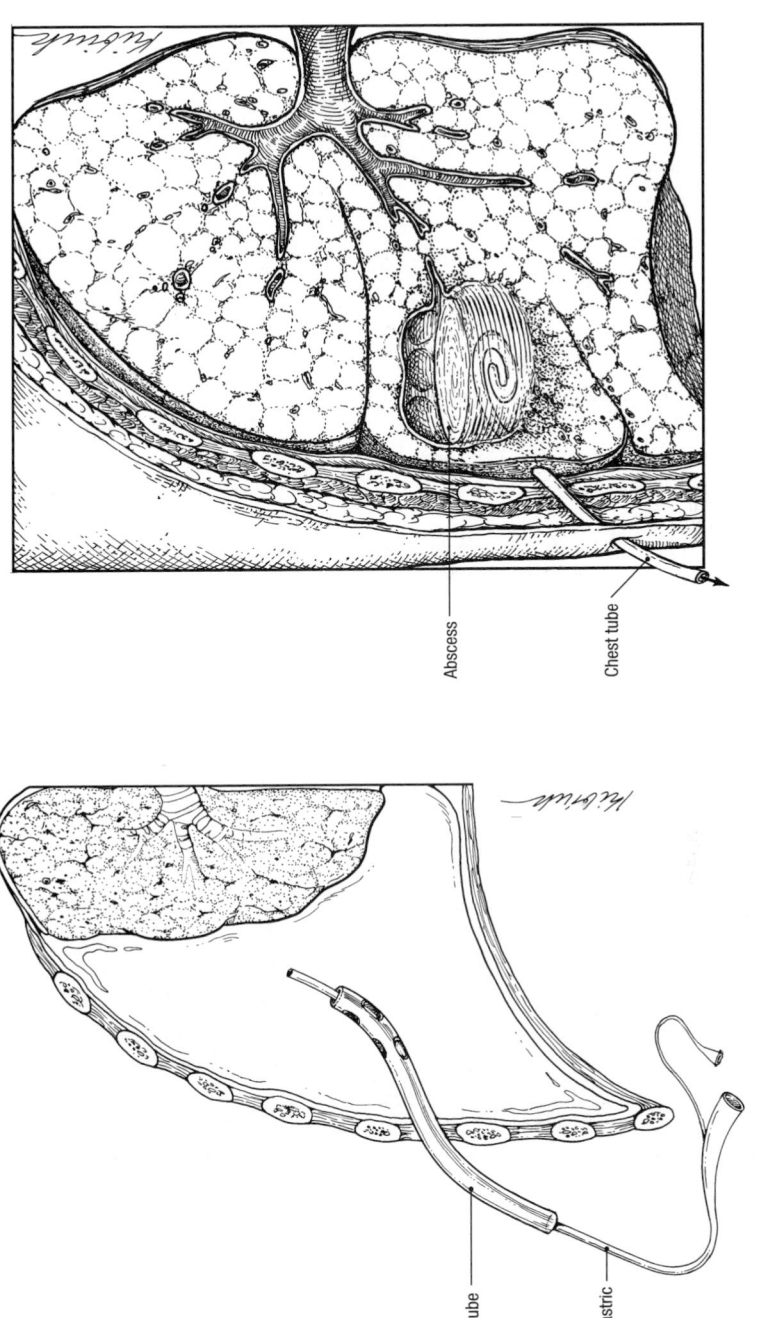

Figure 56. Chest tube placed through thoracic wall into lung in order to drain abscess.

Figure 55. Chest drainage tube can become occluded and must be replaced. Using the nasogastric tube as a guide, the new chest tube is inserted over it and into the thoracic cavity.

A37

Arterial Blood Gas Normal Lab Values

Abbreviation	Description	Normal Lab Value
AVO_2	arteriovenous oxygen	3.5 to 5.0 vol %
BE or BD	base excess or base deficit	± 3 mEq/L
CO	carbon monoxide	nonsmoker: <1.5 (arterial)
		nonsmoker: <1.5 (venous)
		smoker: 1.5 to 5 (arterial)
		smoker: 1.5 to 5 (venous)
COHb	carboxyhemoglobin	< 1.5%
ctHb	concentration of total hemoglobin in blood	males: 14.0 to 18.0 g/dL
		females: 12.0 to 16.0 g/dL
ctO_2 Hb	concentration of O_2 in hemoglobin	15 to 23 vol %
HCO_3	plasma bicarbonate; an indicator of the metabolic acid-base status	male: 23 to 29 mmol/L (arterial)
		male: 25 to 30 mmol/L (venous)
		female: 20 to 29 mmol/L (arterial)
		female: 23 to 28 mmol/L (venous)
HHb	deoxyhemoglobin	< 2.0%
MetHb	methemoglobin	< 1.5%
O_2	oxygen	15 to 23 vol % (arterial)
		15 to 23 vol % (venous)
O_2Hb	oxyhemoglobin	95 to 97 (arterial)
		40 to 70 (venous)
P_{50}	partial pressure of O2 at 50% saturation	25.0 to 29.0 mmHg
PCO_2	partial pressure (P) of carbon dioxide (CO_2)	36 to 46 mmHg (arterial)
		40 to 52 mmHg (venous)
pH	alkalinity or acidity of blood	7.35 to 7.46 (arterial)
		7.33 to 7.40 (venous)
PO_2	partial pressure (P) of oxygen (O_2)	74 to 109 mmHg (arterial)
		25 to 44 mmHg (venous)
SaO_2	percentage of available hemoglobin that is saturated (Sa) with oxygen (O_2)	94 to 100 %

Appendix 3
Pulmonary Function Terms

air trapping
airway resistance
body box plethysmography
bronchial challenge test
carbon monoxide diffusing capacity
($DLCO$, DL_{CO}, D_{CO})
ejection fraction (EF)
exercise-induced bronchospasm (EIB)
expiratory reserve volume (ERV)
flow-sensing spirometer
flow-volume loop
forced expiration
forced expiratory flow after 50% of
vital capacity has been expelled
(FEF_{50})
forced expiratory volume (FEV)
forced expiratory volume in 1 second
(FEV_1)
forced expiratory volume in 1 second to
forced vital capacity ratio
(FEV_1/FVC)
forced inspiration
forced inspiratory vital capacity (FIVC)
forced vital capacity (FVC)
fraction of inspired oxygen (FIO_2,
FiO2, FiO_2)
functional residual capacity (FRC)
helium dilution study
hyperinflation
inspiratory reserve volume (IRV)
inspiratory vital capacity (IVC)
maximal breathing capacity (MBC)
maximal expiratory flow rate (MEFR)
maximal expiratory pressure (MEP)

maximal forced expiratory flow
(FEFmax)
maximal inspiratory pressure (MIP)
maximal midexpiratory flow rate
(MMFR, MMEFR)
maximal voluntary ventilation (MVV)
mean forced expiratory flow during the
middle of forced vital capacity
($FEF_{25-75\%}$)
nitrogen washout
peak expiratory flow (PEF)
peak expiratory flow rate (PEFR)
peak flow meter
peak inspiratory flow (PIF)
plethysmography
ratio of expiratory flow to inspiratory
flow at 50% of forced vital capacity
(FEF_{50}/FIF_{50})
residual volume (RV)
residual volume determination
residual volume to total lung capacity
ratio (RV/TLC)
respiratory exchange ration (RER)
respiratory inductive plethysmography
single-breath nitrogen washout (SBN_2)
slow vital capacity (SVC)
spirogram
spirometry
static lung compliance
thoracic gas volume (V_{TG})
tidal volume (V_T)
total lung capacity (TLC)
vital capacity (VC)
volume displacement spirometer

Appendix 4
Ventilator Terms

adaptive support ventilation

airway pressure release ventilation (APRV)

artificial ventilation

assist control (AC)

assist-control ventilation (ACV)

assist-control mode ventilation

assisted ventilation

assisted mandatory ventilation (AMV)

backup ventilation (BUV)

bilevel positive airway pressure (BiPAP)

continuous-flow ventilation

continuous mandatory ventilation

continuous positive airway pressure (CPAP)

continuous positive pressure ventilation (CPPV)

continuous spontaneous ventilation (CSV)

controlled ventilation

controlled mechanical ventilation (CMV)

forced mandatory intermittent ventilation (FMIV)

fractional inspired oxygen (FIO2)

high-frequency ventilation (HFV)

high-frequency jet ventilation (HFJV)

intermittent demand ventilation (IDV)

intermittent mandatory ventilation (IMV)

intermittent mechanical ventilation (IMV)

intermittent percussion ventilation (IPV)

intermittent positive pressure ventilation (IPPV)

inverse-ratio ventilation

jet ventilation

maximal voluntary ventilation (MVV)

negative end-expiratory pressure (NEEP)

negative pressure ventilator

noninvasive mechanical ventilation

noninvasive positive pressure ventilation (NIPPV)

peak inspiratory pressure (PIP)

positive airway pressure ventilation (PAPV)

positive end-expiratory pressure (PEEP)

positive pressure ventilator

pressure support ventilation (PSV)

pressure cycled ventilator

synchronized intermittent mandatory ventilation (SIMV)

tidal volume (V_T)

time-cycled ventilator

volume-controlled ventilation (VCV)

volume-cycled ventilator

Appendix 5
Sample Reports and Dictation

ABDOMINAL AORTOGRAM: CORAL REEF AORTA

HISTORY OF PRESENT ILLNESS: This 65-year-old white female presented with a history of debilitating nausea, vomiting, and abdominal cramping following the ingestion of food.

FINDINGS: There is a filling defect in the abdominal aorta, with significant narrowing of the lumen seen on anteroposterior view of the abdominal aorta. It appears to be at the level of the renal artery origin. This is also seen on the lateral view. The superior mesenteric artery origin is markedly narrowed, and there is occlusion of the celiac origin.

DIAGNOSIS: Coral reef aorta, with mesenteric insufficiency.

CONSULTATION: PNEUMOCYSTIS CARINII PNEUMONIA

REASON FOR CONSULTATION: Rule out Pneumocystis pneumonia.

HISTORY OF PRESENT ILLNESS: This elderly Caucasian male has been on vacation, visiting his family. He is being evaluated to rule out Pneumocystis carinii pneumonia (PCP).

The patient recalls that he was in good health until around the time he was preparing to leave on vacation. At that time, he began to experience a dry, nonproductive cough, shortness of breath, dyspnea on exertion, and a low-grade fever. He has also had anorexia accompanied by an approximate 10-pound, unexplained weight loss. Because he has continued to experience symptoms, his family convinced him to seek care.

He was evaluated by his family physician, who felt that he had an atypical infection. He was given a 5-day course of Zithromax. Unfortunately, the patient failed to improve. A chest x-ray revealed bilateral interstitial and alveolar consolidation, consistent with PCP. For that reason, he was admitted to the hospital for further examination. He was started on Levaquin and Rocephin and was seen by the consulting pulmonologist.

The pulmonary consultant expressed concerns about the possibility of HIV, and appropriate serology was obtained. Today the patient was informed that his HIV status is positive, and he was placed on Septra and steroids. He is also continuing Levaquin and Rocephin.

Today the patient's primary complaints relate to his extreme shortness of breath and a dry, nonproductive cough. He does not complain about head or neck problems, nor does he have GI or GU complaints.

PAST MEDICAL AND SURGICAL HISTORY: Significant for hepatitis B and C, colon polyps, and a positive PPD test for tuberculosis. It is of interest that he cannot remember receiving treatment for the hepatitis or positive PPD. Denies history of illicit drug use. He has no history of hypertension, diabetes, or psychiatric disorder. Surgeries include tonsillectomy, appendectomy, tympanoplasty, colon polypectomy, and tendon repair on the right lower extremity following a skiing accident.

MEDICATIONS: The patient is taking Levaquin, Rocephin, and Septra.

ALLERGIES: He has no known allergies.

SOCIAL HISTORY: The patient has had a homosexual lifestyle that began in his mid teens. He has had several partners but has been sexually inactive for approximately 2 years. He does not know the status of any of his partners. He has smoked 1 pack of cigarettes per day for 45 years. He enjoys an occasional glass of wine. He is retired from his career as a retail store manager.

REVIEW OF SYSTEMS: As stated above.

PHYSICAL EXAMINATION: GENERAL: This is a rather cachectic patient, who appears to be acutely ill. He experiences mild respiratory distress as soon as he starts talking. VITAL SIGNS: Vital signs are recorded on his chart and reveal that his temperature has been as high as 103, but he is currently afebrile. HEENT: Unrevealing. Oral cavity is without thrush. BACK: Benign. PULMONARY: Chest reveals bilateral dry rales throughout. No pleural rub heard. CARDIOVASCULAR: Heart is tachycardic. S1, S2 without significant rub. There is a flow murmur of about 2/6. ABDOMEN: Bowel sounds are present. Abdomen is soft and nontender. Liver and spleen are not palpable. GENITALIA: Male genitalia normal, without a catheter. RECTAL: Rectal exam deferred. EXTREMITIES: Extremities are without unusual rash, lesion, or joint effusion. NEUROLOGIC: He is awake, alert, and oriented.

LABORATORY DATA: Potassium 3.4, sodium 136, glucose 191, BUN 10, creatine 0.7, albumin 2.5, total bilirubin 1.2. SGOT 90, SGPT 51, LDH 300, and alkaline phosphatase 6.5. White blood count 7100 and platelets 66,000. Differential reveals 87 polys, 7 bands, 5 lymphs. Arterial blood gas: pH 7.6, PCO_2 32, PO_2 46 on room air.

Chest x-ray shows diffuse changes consistent with Pneumocystis carinii pneumonia. HIV is positive. Western blot is pending.

ASSESSMENT AND PLAN: Findings on chest x-ray, the 3-week history of fever, shortness of breath, dry cough, dyspnea on exertion, elevated LDH, and HIV positive status support the diagnosis of Pneumocystis. Current treatment plan is acceptable, though the steroid dosage should be reduced because it appears that this is not a community-acquired pneumonia. Levaquin and Rocephin have been discontinued.

The patient has been counseled, including the fact that mortality can reach 15% to 20% despite best efforts, and all his questions were answered.

Thank you for the consultation. He will continue to be monitored.

CT SCAN: SUSPECTED ASBESTOSIS

INDICATIONS: Patient with history of asbestos exposure.

FINDINGS: CT exam to the chest was performed at 8-mm sections and filmed at mediastinal and lung windows, with 2-mm thin sections at the base of the left lung.

Multiple calcified pleural plaques are seen bilaterally, with bilateral pleural thickening. A 2.5 x 2.5-cm mass is noted along the posterior surface of the left lower lobe of the lung. Linear and stippled calcifications appear in the anterior aspect. Bronchovascular bundles within the vicinity of the mass appear to converge on the region.

IMPRESSION: The findings are consistent with asbestos exposure. The 2.5-cm mass at the left base is indicative of rounded atelectasis or a malignancy.

RECOMMENDATION: Recommend pulmonary consultation for consideration of percutaneous needle biopsy.

DEATH SUMMARY: COR PULMONALE

HISTORY: The patient, a 40-year-old male, was admitted through the emergency department after a syncopal episode at his place of employment. He has a history of emphysema and increasing dyspnea on exertion. He reported having intermittent night sweats and episodes of overwhelming fatigue over the past several weeks.

PHYSICAL EXAMINATION: At the time he was seen after admission, his temperature was normal at 98.6, respirations were 27 per minute, and pulse was 98 and regular. Blood pressure was 100/70. Jugular venous pressure was raised to 5 cm above the sternal angle, with prominence of the A waves. A right parasternal heave was present, and there was a loud pulmonic second heart sound. An ejection systolic murmur was heard in the pulmonary area. Pitting edema was present in the lower extremities.

X-RAY AND LABORATORY FINDINGS: Chest x-ray revealed an enlarged right ventricle, with prominent pulmonary conus. There was no obvious lung infiltrate. Pulmonary function tests revealed decreased diffusing lung capacity. There was no evidence of pulmonary embolism on ventilation/perfusion scan. Cross-sectional echocardiogram and Doppler studies revealed a significantly enlarged right atrium and ventricle with a dilated pulmonary artery and severe pericardial effusion.

Left and right cardiac catheterization revealed pulmonary hypertension with reduced cardiac output. There was also mild impairment of the left ventricle.

HOSPITAL COURSE: The patient suddenly became severely hypotensive and was transferred to the CCU for stabilization and monitoring. He received prednisolone, IV cyclophosphamide, captopril, furosemide, and plasmapheresis. He developed deep venous thrombosis for which he received warfarin.

Initially there appeared to be a somewhat overall improvement in his condition; however, on the second day in CCU he experienced cardiac arrest and, despite aggressive efforts, he was unable to be revived.

CAUSE OF DEATH: Cor pulmonale.

DISCHARGE SUMMARY: POSTTRAUMATIC AORTIC PSEUDOANEURYSM

REASON FOR ADMISSION: Posttraumatic chest discomfort.

HISTORY OF PRESENT ILLNESS: The patient is a middle-aged male who enjoyed good health until approximately 3 weeks ago when he was kicked in the area of his right chest by his horse. Following that, he experienced unremitting chest discomfort.

PHYSICAL EXAMINATIONS: His physical examination was within normal limits except for discomfort over the right chest area. See his chart for details of physical findings.

LABORATORY DATA: Laboratory values were all within normal limits.

STUDIES: Chest x-ray revealed a well-defined middle mediastinal mass. On the lateral view, the mass appeared to overlap the aorta. Rib fractures were noted on the right side. CT scan revealed a focal outpouching of the aorta with surrounding thrombus, consistent with an aortic pseudoaneurysm, most likely posttraumatic.

HOSPITAL COURSE: The patient was advised of the findings and that immediate surgical intervention was necessary to avoid possible rupture and even death. Aneurysmectomy was performed without complication, and he has done remarkably well following surgery. The patient is discharged on postoperative day 5. He is to rest at home and will be seen in my office in 2 days.

DISCHARGE MEDICATION: Tylenol Extra Strength as needed for discomfort.

ELECTROPHYSIOLOGICAL (EPS) STUDY

PROCEDURES PERFORMED
1. Comprehensive electrophysiological study.
2. With left atrial recording.
3. Venous access x2.
4. Electrocardiogram x6.
5. Conscious sedation x1 hour.
6. Pulse oximetry.

COMPLICATIONS: None.

INDICATIONS:
1. Coronary artery disease.
2. Congestive heart failure.
3. Ventricular tachycardia.
4. Palpitations.

ANESTHESIA: ASA classification class III. Conscious sedation provided by surgeon. Over a period of 1 hour, a total of 2 mg of IV Versed and 25 mcg of IV fentanyl was given. The patient was under continuous electrocardiographic, hemodynamic, pulse oximetric and clinical evaluation. His level of consciousness was assessed throughout the procedure. At the end of the procedure, he was alert and oriented with no obvious complication from the sedation.

DETAILS OF PROCEDURE: After appropriate informed consent was obtained, the patient was taken to the clinical laboratory in the fasting state. Both groins were prepared in the usual sterile fashion. Local anesthetic was applied to the skin. One 6-French and one 7-French sheath were placed in the right femoral vein. Through these sheaths, a deflectable quadripolar and a deflectable octapolar catheter were advanced to the cardiac chambers.

The quadripolar catheter was placed initially in the right ventricular (RV) apex. The octapolar catheter was placed in the coronary sinus. Ventricular pacing was performed. There was no VA conduction at 600 msec.

The octapolar catheter was then placed in the atrioventricular (AV) junction. The quadripolar catheter was then placed in the right atrium. Basic intervals were measured. Rapid atrial pacing was performed. The AV node Wenckebach cycle length was 360 msec.

Ventricular stimulation was performed with the quadripolar catheter in the right ventricular apex. The right ventricular apex effective refractory period was 400/240. Ventricular stimulation was performed. Multiple episodes of nonsustained monomorphic ventricular tachycardia, which terminated spontaneously, were documented. The catheters were removed. Hemostasis was achieved. No immediate complications were noted.

FINDINGS:
1. Sinus cycle length 1095 msec; PR interval 183 msec; QRS interval 110 msec; QT interval 439 msec; AH interval 81 msec; HV interval 56 msec. The AV node antegrade Wenckebach was 316 msec. There was no VA conduction at 600 msec.
2. Inducible monomorphic ventricular tachycardia.
3. Significant sinus node dysfunction.

RECOMMENDATIONS: Implantation of a dual-chamber implantable cardioverter-defibrillator.

ELECTROPHYSIOLOGICAL STUDY, LEFT ATRIAL RECORDING, MAPPING, AND REPEAT STIMULATION

PROCEDURES PERFORMED: Comprehensive electrophysiologic testing, left atrial recording, and repeat stimulation on isoproterenol.

MEDICATIONS: Versed 3 mg, fentanyl 100 mcg, and isoproterenol 5 mcg bolus x2.

INDICATIONS: Palpitations and near syncope and wide-complex tachycardia during exercise testing.

ASA CLASS: II

SEDATION: Conscious sedation was performed for a total of 60 minutes using Versed and fentanyl as described above. Continuous oximetric airway and heart rate monitoring as well as intermittent noninvasive blood pressure monitoring were performed throughout. At the end of the procedure, the patient was awakened from conscious sedation and returned to his room in good condition.

DETAILS OF PROCEDURE: After informed consent was obtained, the right and left femoral areas were prepped and draped in the usual sterile fashion. Then 15 mL of 1% Xylocaine was used for local anesthesia. Using a modified Seldinger technique, 6- and 7-French sheaths were inserted in the right femoral vein. Three 6-French sheaths were inserted in the left femoral vein. Under fluoroscopic guidance, a deflectable quadripolar catheter was placed in the high right atrium, deflectable octapolar was placed in the His bundle, deflectable quadripolar placed in the right ventricular apex, and deflectable decapolar was placed in the coronary sinus. Program stimulation was performed, see results below. Repeat testing was performed with isoproterenol, see results below.

At the end of the procedure, catheters were withdrawn, sheaths removed, and pressure was held tightly until hemostasis was obtained.

FINDINGS:
1. Baseline showed sinus rhythm with sinus cycle length 656, PR interval 234, QRS interval 120, AH interval 98, and HV interval 63.
2. Carotid sinus massage produced no sinus slowing.
3. Antegrade Wenckebach was 470, retrograde there was no PA conduction. AV node-ERP 600/400. Dual AV nodal physiology was not present.
4. There was no block below the His with atrial overdrive pacing.
5. There was no evidence for an accessory pathway.
6. Right ventricular apex ERP 600/240 and 400/230. Repeat testing was performed with isoproterenol with single and double premature atrial contractions as well as burst atrial pacing. Program stimulation was performed in the ventricle with up to quadruple extrastimuli at 3 drive cycle lengths in 2 right ventricular locations without production of arrhythmia.

IMPRESSION:
1. Normal sinus node.
2. Normal atrioventricular node without dual physiology.
3. Moderate His-Purkinje system disease.
4. No inducible ventricular tachycardia.

RECOMMENDATIONS:
1. Would increase Cardizem to 240 mg daily for better blood pressure control.
2. Would check outpatient event monitoring.
3. Would initiate aspirin therapy.

ELECTROPHYSIOLOGICAL STUDY, LEFT VENTRICULAR RECORDING, MAPPING, AND CENTRAL VENOGRAM

PROCEDURE: Comprehensive electrophysiologic study with left ventricular recording, mapping of the left ventricle, central venogram.

INDICATION: Congestive heart failure.

MEDICATIONS: Versed 3 mg, fentanyl 50 mcg, and Isovue as directed.

COMPLICATIONS: None.

DETAILS OF PROCEDURE: After informed consent was obtained, the patient was brought into the electrophysiologic laboratory. The patient was prepped and draped in the usual sterile fashion. Over the course of 1 hour, he was given 3 mg of Versed and 50 mcg of fentanyl. He was on continuous pulse oximetry, noninvasive blood pressure measurements, and continuous electrocardiography. His ASA classification is III. He tolerated the procedure well, was awake, alert, and oriented. Repeated measures of respiratory rate and effort, level of sedation and consciousness were maintained throughout the study, as well as hemodynamics.

Using lidocaine, skin overlying the left femoral vessel was locally anesthetized and two 6-French sheaths were placed through the right femoral vein. Deflectable quadripolar catheter was placed in the high right atrium, demonstrating underlying atrial arrhythmia. The patient has underlying complete heart block with a permanent pacemaker and HV interval could not be obtained but the catheters were then moved to the right ventricular apex, and a second catheter was used to engage the coronary sinus. With the coronary sinus engaged, mapping was performed after physically finding the os of various lateral veins. A very posterior lateral branch was found that went to the lateral aspect of the inferolateral wall out to the apex, and a high lateral branch was also found. Intraventricular pacing between left atrial wires and right ventricular wires was used to map activation times, QRS durations, and intraventricular conduction times to assist in placement of biventricular pacing tomorrow. Finally, induction of ventricular arrhythmias was performed and then a long J wire was advanced to the central circulation. A catheter was advanced to the superior vena cava and used to engage the left subclavian vein. This was advanced over the J wire, and the venogram was performed.

FINDINGS:
1. The left subclavian vein was widely patent.
2. A high left ventricular pacing site provides longer intraventricular conduction times and narrower QRS complexes with biventricular pacing versus the large inferolateral vein.
3. Easily inducible ventricular tachycardia seen.

IMPRESSION: Successful mapping of the left ventricle of biventricular pacing, inducible ventricular arrhythmias.

RECOMMENDATIONS: Implantable cardioverter-defibrillator tomorrow.

EXPLANATION OF PACEMAKER AND LEADS WITH IMPLANTATION OF ICD AND LEADS

PREOPERATIVE DIAGNOSIS: Ischemic cardiomyopathy, induced left bundle branch block, and class 3 congestive heart failure.

POSTOPERATIVE DIAGNOSIS: Ischemic cardiomyopathy, induced left bundle branch block, and class 3 congestive heart failure.

PROCEDURES:
1. Explant of dual-chamber pacemaker. This was a Guidant model 1270, serial #630955.
2. Laser extraction of 3 pacing leads. These are a Guidant 4456-203685, a Guidant 4469-304731, and a Guidant 4452-201574.
3. Coronary sinus venography.
4. Implant of coronary sinus lead. This is a Guidant model 4513, serial #401794.
5. Implant of implantable cardioverter-defibrillator Guidant lead 0157, serial #118025. The device is an H135, serial #777049.
6. Defibrillation threshold testing.

COMPLICATIONS: None.

FLUOROSCOPY TIME: 43 minutes, 30 seconds.

LASER TIME: 2 minutes 29 seconds.

DETAILS OF PROCEDURE: This gentleman with permanent atrial fibrillation, ischemic cardiomyopathy, ejection fraction (EF) 25%, and pacing-induced left bundle branch block (underlying heart rate 50 bpm), was brought to the electrophysiology (EP) laboratory in a fasting state. Informed consent was obtained prior to procedure. A radial arterial line was placed by anesthesia. The left shoulder region was prepped and draped in sterile fashion and infiltrated with 1% lidocaine solution. Access over the incision was made, and using blunt and Bovie dissection, the old generator was dissected free. The 3 leads (2 ventricular and 1 atrial) that were still in place were dissected free and exposed. Gentle traction on these leads failed to enable extraction. The first lead addressed was the atrial 4469-304731.

The lead was cut and a Spectranetics locking stylet was advanced down this lead. Traction prevented the lead from being extracted completely. The Spectranetics laser 12-French sheath was utilized, the laser was activated and the lead was easily extracted. The largest amount of scar tissue was at the level of the subclavian vein. A similar procedure was repeated on the 4452 lead, as well as the 4456 lead. Following these procedures, access to the subclavian vein was achieved twice.

Using a modified Seldinger technique, guidewires and sheaths were placed; an 8-French sheath was placed over the first guidewire and the right ventricular ICD lead was advanced to the apex. Stable pace and sense thresholds were obtained and are summarized below. The lead was secured using 0 silk.

A 9-French sheath was placed over the remaining guidewire. A hook and Rapido sheath system was advanced to the right atrium. Using contrast, the coronary sinus could not be located. An angled Glidewire was then utilized, but again the coronary sinus could not be cannulated. At this point, a deflectable quadripolar catheter was utilized to cannulate the coronary sinus through the extended hook sheath. This sheath was advanced. A balloon-tipped Swan-Ganz catheter was then advanced and coronary sinus venography was performed. A posterolateral vein was identified.

With some difficulty, the left ventricular coronary sinus lead was advanced over a Whisper wire to a posterolateral vein. Stable pacing and sensing thresholds were obtained. The lead was removed with some difficulty.

The lead was secured using 0 silk. All thresholds were then assessed and noted to be stable.

The ICD was attached and defibrillation threshold testing was performed. The results are summarized below. The ICD was positioned in the pocket, and pocket was washed with antibiotic solution and closed in 3 layers using 2-0 and 4-0 Vicryl. The patient tolerated these procedures well and was transferred to his room in stable condition.

FINDINGS: Underlying rhythm is atrial fibrillation with ventricular rate of approximately 40-50 bpm. The right ventricular R wave measured 12.4 mV, the right ventricular impedance of 50 was 608 ohms, and the right ventricular threshold of 0.5 msec was 0.6 V. The right ventricular-paced QRS complex was 234 msec.

The biventricular R wave measured 10.4 mV. The biventricular impedance of 50 was 330 ohms, and the biventricular threshold of 0.5 msec was 2.8 V. The biventricular-paced QRS complex was 168 msec.

Ventricular fibrillation was induced with shock on T and covered with a 21-joule/40-ohms countershock. The charge time was 6.7 seconds and there was 100% sensing at least sensitivity.

A 14-J and 7-J shock on T failed to induce ventricular fibrillation. A 1-J shock on T induced ventricular fibrillation and was converted with a 9-joule/41-ohms countershock. Therefore, the defibrillation threshold is ≤9 J.

The device was programmed VVIR 80-130. The VT zone is set at 175-220 bpm, and the VF zone at >220 bpm. The patient will receive adenosine triphosphate followed by 5 J, followed by 4 outputs in the VT zone and 21 J, followed by full output in the VF zone.

IMPRESSION: Successful procedures, as outlined above.

PLAN: Observation overnight. Discharge following assessment.

HISTORY AND PHYSICAL: ASBESTOSIS

CHIEF COMPLAINT: The patient is a middle-aged male who is complaining of increasing shortness of breath on exertion.

HISTORY OF PRESENT ILLNESS: The patient has always been an active individual and takes advantage of activities that require a high degree of physical involvement. For about the past year he has been preparing himself to run in a 20-mile marathon. In the past 6 weeks or so, however, he has noticed that he becomes short of breath much quicker than usual and states that he has actually become too fatigued to work out at all.

Outpatient x-ray revealed pleural calcifications along the costal margins bilaterally within the mid lung fields. Linear calcification is noted overlying the left hemidiaphragm.

PAST HISTORY: He has had several bouts of severe bronchitis and was hospitalized once with pneumonia. He was also hospitalized in the past for cholecystectomy and appendectomy.

SOCIAL HISTORY: The patient has installed insulation for a living for many years, starting in his early teens when he helped in his father's business. The patient is a non-smoker and no one in the home smokes.

FAMILY HISTORY: His mother is in her 80s and in reasonably good health. His father died of mesothelioma in his mid 60s. There are 2 brothers and 3 sisters, all in good health. He is the only one of his brothers and sisters to work in the insulation business.

REVIEW OF SYSTEMS: Negative except as noted. Eyes: Has worn glasses for several years. He denies blurred vision or difficulty seeing to drive at night. His last exam was 2 years ago. Respiratory: Notes a morning cough that produces approximately 1 teaspoon of grayish sputum.

PHYSICAL EXAMINATION: GENERAL: The patient states that he feels exhausted, but he is in good spirits. VITAL SIGNS: Within normal limits. SKIN: There are no rashes or petechiae. There is a tattoo of a motorcycle on his left upper arm and one of an eagle on his mid back. HEENT: Pupils are regular and reactive to light and accommodation. Extraocular movements are intact. NECK: Normal range of motion is noted. There is no lymphadenopathy or tenderness. Thyroid exam reveals no abnormality. CHEST: Normal symmetry with respirations. No tenderness. Crackles are heard throughout. HEART: Normal S1, S2. No rhythm abnormality is detected. ABDOMEN: The abdomen is flat and nontender. Scars are consistent with the noted surgical procedures. Bowel sounds are normal, and there are no bruits. No inguinal adenopathy. GENITALIA: Normal male genitalia. RECTAL: Not done at this time. MUSCULOSKELETAL: Range of motion is normal. No joint pain or swelling noted. NEUROLOGIC: Cranial nerves II through XII are normal.

IMPRESSION: The patient is admitted for further tests and pulmonary consultation as indicated by the history and physical examination. We are most likely dealing with asbestosis, but we need to rule out mesothelioma. A CT scan has been ordered.

ADMITTING DIAGNOSIS: Probable asbestosis.

HISTORY AND PHYSICAL: CARDIAC TAMPONADE

CHIEF COMPLAINT: Chest pain with diaphoresis.

HISTORY OF PRESENT ILLNESS: The patient is an 82-year-old white female who developed chest pain earlier today. She became diaphoretic but experienced no syncope.

PAST MEDICAL HISTORY: A dual-chamber permanent pacemaker was placed approximately a month ago because of paroxysmal atrial fibrillation and sinus node dysfunction. The patient has been in remarkably good health all her life and until her recent cardiac problems, had never been hospitalized.

MEDICATIONS: The patient is currently taking amiodarone and warfarin.

ALLERGIES: There are no known medication allergies.

FAMILY HISTORY: The patient has never been married. She is the last survivor of 8 siblings. She is a retired teacher.

PHYSICAL EXAMINATION: GENERAL: The patient is sitting up in bed. She is in obvious respiratory distress, pale, and diaphoretic. VITAL SIGNS: Blood pressure is 60 mmHg systolic; diastolic pressure is not measurable. Temperature is 99, pulse is 110, respirations 24. HEAD AND NECK: There is raised jugular venous pressure. No other abnormalities are noted. LUNGS: The lungs are clear. HEART: The heart sounds are muffled. ABDOMEN: Not examined. GENITALIA: Not examined. EXTREMITIES: There is no peripheral edema.

ASSESSMENT: Electrocardiogram on admission revealed sinus tachycardia and old left bundle branch block with no new changes. There were no abnormal findings on pacemaker interrogation. Emergency echocardiogram reveals cardiac tamponade with right atrial systolic inversion and right ventricular systolic collapse.

PLAN: She will be admitted for emergent thoracotomy and monitoring.

HISTORY AND PHYSICAL: MYOCARDIAL INFARCTION

IDENTIFICATION: The patient is a male in his mid-30s who works as a heavy equipment construction worker. He was admitted from the emergency department.

CHIEF COMPLAINT: Severe chest pain, with radiation into the left neck and down the left arm.

HISTORY OF PRESENT ILLNESS: The patient was brought to the emergency department by ambulance after awakening at approximately 4:30 a.m. with squeezing substernal chest pain that radiated into the left side of his neck and down his left arm.

The pain was associated with dyspnea and diaphoresis. He states that the pain decreased in intensity after taking 3-mg nitroglycerin sublingual that was given to him by a member of the emergency medical team. He admits to having similar chest pain about a month ago after working out at the gym. The pain subsided after resting. He did not seek medical advice following the incident. He denies episodes of tachycardia, bradycardia, orthopnea, or pedal edema.

He denied smoking when seen by me in August of last year; however, he now admits that he has smoked 2 packs of cigarettes per day for 18 years. He has attempted to quit on numerous occasions but has been unsuccessful. He rarely consumes alcohol and denies illicit drug use. The family is not attentive to a low-fat diet. He does not have a diagnosis of hypertension or diabetes. He did not follow through with his last lab work request, so there is no current cholesterol value.

PAST MEDICAL HISTORY: He has a long history of asthma. He was hospitalized in 2001 with pneumonia. He had a false-positive TB skin test in 1990 for which he was treated with Rifampin.

PAST SURGICAL HISTORY: Appendectomy in 1988, vasectomy in January 2001.

MEDICATIONS: The patient is currently on no medications.

ALLERGIES: The patient has no known medication allergies.

FAMILY HISTORY: The patient's father died at age 40 of myocardial infarction. His brother underwent bypass surgery last year at 37 years old. His mother is alive and in reasonably good health at age 70.

REVIEW OF SYSTEMS: Negative otherwise.

PHYSICAL EXAMINATION: GENERAL: The patient is lying quietly in bed. He appears anxious about his condition. VITAL SIGNS: Blood pressure 180/110, pulse 110 and steady. SKIN: He appears pale; the skin is somewhat clammy to touch. HEENT: Appears normal. CHEST: Lungs are clear to percussion and auscultation. Breath sounds are normal. HEART: There is ST elevation in leads V4, V5, and V6 on electrocardiogram. There is a harsh holosystolic murmur at the left lower sternal border, with midsystolic peak. S1 and S2 are soft. ABDOMEN: The abdomen is flat and nontender. Bowel sounds are normal, and there are no bruits. GENITALIA: Appear normal. MUSCULOSKELETAL: Tattoo on right forearm. EXTREMITIES: No extremity edema or tenderness. NEUROLOGIC: Not done at this time.

ASSESSMENT: The patient has been under considerable stress lately. His company has recently announced that they will be decreasing their workforce by approximately 20 percent. His son has recently been diagnosed with a mental disorder of some sort, possibly schizophrenia. The patient was moved to coronary care unit for close monitoring. A cardiac catheterization is ordered for this afternoon.

ADMITTING DIAGNOSIS: Myocardial infarction.

IMPLANTATION OF DUAL-CHAMBER DEFIBRILLATOR

PROCEDURE: Dual-chamber defibrillator implantation.

INDICATION: History of ventricular fibrillation.

ASA CLASSIFICATION: III

ANESTHESIA: Total intravenous anesthesia (TIVA)

ADDITIONAL CARDIOACTIVE MEDICATIONS: None.

PREOPERATIVE ANTIBIOTICS: Ancef 1 g IV piggyback.

ESTIMATED BLOOD LOSS: 10 mL.

COMPLICATIONS: Transient hypotension during lead positioning. This responded to volume and ephedrine. Because of this, however, formal defibrillator threshold (DFT) testing was postponed.

DETAILS OF PROCEDURE: After informed consent was obtained, the patient was taken to the catheterization laboratory in a fasting state. A lead remained in the left axillary vein for localization. Using a 15 blade, a 3-inch incision was made in the left shoulder. Bovie and blunt dissection were used to form a pocket in the pectoralis fascia. Using an 18-gauge needle into the floor of the pocket over the first rib, the left axillary vein was accessed on 2 separate occasions. The guidewire was inserted through the needle and advanced into the central venous system. The needles were removed and 9-French and 7-French peel-away sheaths were inserted over the wires and advanced into the central venous system. The dilators and wires were removed and a 7-French coronary pacing lead and a 9-French defibrillator leads were inserted into the appropriate sheath and advanced into the right ventricular apex and right atrium after pacing and sensing was confirmed. The patient developed hypotension, as mentioned above, requiring volume and ephedrine. Because of the concern about possible development of tamponade physiology, the remainder of the case was postponed. Otherwise, the device was empirically planted and sewn to the floor of the pocket. Both leads were secured to the pectoralis fascia, and the pocket was closed with a series of 2-0, 3-0, and 4-0 Vicryl. Benzoin and Steri-Strips were applied across the wound.

RESULTS:
1. Pacing with thresholds: Atrial threshold 2 V at 0.5 msec with impedance of 730 ohms and current of 3 mA. RV threshold 1.7 V at 0.5 msec with impedance of 1040 ohms and current of 128 mA. Threshold at 10 V did not stimulate diaphragm.
2. Signal analysis. P-wave amplitude at 5 mV, R-wave amplitude at 7 mV.
3. His induction. This was postponed because of the development of hypotension and the concern about possible tamponade physiology.
4. Serial numbers: The device was a St. Jude model V-240 Atlas DR, serial #80448. The RA lead was a St. Jude model 1688TC-5, serial #DN14254. The RV lead was a St. Jude model 1580-65, serial #RE24465.

IMPRESSION:
1. Successful insertion of a dual-chamber defibrillator system.
2. Development of hypotension.

RECOMMENDATIONS:
1. Antibiotic prophylaxis.
2. Intensive care unit monitoring.
3. Anticipate defibrillator threshold testing tomorrow to confirm adequate safety margin.

IMPLANTATION OF IMPLANTABLE CARDIOVERTER-DEFIBRILLATOR (ICD)

PROCEDURES PERFORMED:
1. Dual-chamber implantable cardioverter-defibrillator implantation.
2. Interrogation of reprogramming.
3. Fluoroscopy.
4. Superior vena cava leads x2.
5. Intracardiac atrial and ventricular pacing and recording.
6. Defibrillation threshold testing.
7. Echocardiogram x4.

COMPLICATIONS: None.

ANESTHESIA: ASA classification class III. Deep conscious sedation provided by the anesthesia service.

MEDICATIONS: Ancef 1 g IV given prior to the implantation.

DETAILS OF PROCEDURE: The patient was taken to the clinical laboratory in the fasting state. He has had documented clinical ventricular tachycardia as well as coronary artery disease and left ventricular dysfunction. During electrophysiological study, he was found to have inducible ventricular tachycardia and no reversible cause for his arrhythmia was present. He also has significant sinus node dysfunction with symptomatic bradycardia.

The left upper chest was prepared in the usual sterile fashion. Local anesthetic was applied to the skin. A 3-cm incision was performed inferior and parallel to the clavicle. Two separate punctures of the left axillary vein were performed, and the guidewire was left in place. Pocket was manufactured through a combination of sharp and blunt dissection. Good hemostasis was present.

Through the guidewire in the left axillary vein, 2 separate sheaths were placed toward the superior vena cava (SVC). The atrial and ventricular leads were advanced through each of these sheaths and placed primarily into the right atrium.

The right ventricular lead was then advanced into the right ventricular apex. After documenting satisfactory pacing parameters, the lead position was secured. The right atrial lead was then placed in the right atrial appendage. After documenting satisfactory pacing parameters, the lead position was secured with silk sutures.

Of note, after removing the sheath for the right ventricular lead, air within the pulmonary artery was noted on the fluoroscopy. The patient developed desaturation and cough. Immediately, a Swan-Ganz catheter was advanced into the pulmonary artery and the air within the pulmonary artery was aspirated. This led to complete resolution of the cough and immediate improvement in desaturations. The Swan-Ganz catheter was removed.

Good hemostasis was present in the pocket. Intracardiac atrial and ventricular pacing and recording was performed. A dual-chamber generator from St. Jude was then connected to the leads and placed in the pocket. The pocket was irrigated copiously with antibiotic solution before and after placement of the generator in the pocket. The pocket was closed in layers with 2-0 and 3-0 Vicryl. Dermabond was applied to the skin.

Defibrillation testing threshold was performed. Two separate episodes of ventricular fibrillation were induced 5 minutes apart. During the first episode, a 20-J shock was delivered, successfully restoring sinus rhythm. Charge time was 3.9 seconds with a defibrillation impedance of 42 ohms and 100% sensing when programmed to a sensitivity of 1.0 mV. For the second episode, a 15-J shock successfully restored sinus rhythm after a charge time of 2.7 seconds. Impedance was 42 ohms and again there was 100% sensing when programmed to a sensitivity of 0.3 mV. At the end of the procedure, no complications were noted and the patient recovered from the sedation well.

FINDINGS:
1. Successful implantation of a dual-chamber Epic DR, model #V235, dual-chamber pulse generator from St. Jude Medical, serial #17060.
2. Implantation of a St. Jude 1688TC, 52-cm lead in the right atrial appendage, serial #DN14249. The measured R wave was 3.1 mV with a pacing impedance of 504 ohms and an acute pacing threshold of 0.9 volts at 0.5 msec.
3. Successful implantation of St. Jude 1580, 65-cm lead in the right ventricular apex, and an acute pacing threshold of 0.8 volts at 0.5 msec.
4. Defibrillation threshold equal to or less than 15 J.

IMPRESSION: Successful implantation of a dual-chamber implantable cardioverter-defibrillator.

RECOMMENDATIONS:
1. Maximize beta blockade for the treatment of his coronary artery disease, his congestive heart failure, and to minimize the possibility of sinus tachycardia being detected as ventricular tachycardia. His clinical tachycardia had a relatively low ventricular rate; therefore, his ventricular tachycardia detection is set at 140 beats per minute.
2. Chest x-ray, antibiotics, electrocardiogram, and observation.

PACEMAKER GENERATOR REPLACEMENT

DIAGNOSIS: Tachycardia/bradycardia syndrome.

PROCEDURE: Pacemaker generator replacement.

DETAILS OF PROCEDURE: Following informed consent, the patient was brought to the catheterization lab in a postabsorptive state. Anesthesia was performed with intravenous fentanyl and Versed. Local anesthetic was infiltrated subcutaneously. The patient received prophylactic intravenous antibiotics. Local anesthetic was infiltrated subcutaneously. A #15 scalpel was used to incise the skin over the left chest. Blunt dissection requiring hemostasis was used to expose the chronically implanted generator. The chronic generator was explanted and the leads detached.

Ventricular lead showed threshold 0.7 V, resistance 600 ohms, R wave 18 mV. This is a model 1216. The atrial lead was capped due to chronic atrial fibrillation. The leads were attached to a St. Jude model 5172. Pocket was lavaged with antibiotic solution. Subcutaneous layer was closed with 3-0 Vicryl. Cutaneous layer was closed with 4-0 Vicryl. There were no apparent complications.

STRESS ECHOCARDIOGRAM

INDICATIONS: Atypical chest pain syndrome with elevated troponin levels and normal CPKs. Patient has history of hypertension. There is a strong family history of premature coronary artery disease.

MEDICATIONS: Plendil, aspirin, and p.o. nitroglycerin.

FINDINGS: Modified baseline 12-lead EKG revealed normal sinus rhythm tracing with a rightward axis.

The patient exercised for 9 minutes through stage 3 of standard Bruce protocol, achieving 10.1 METs. The exercise was terminated, as adequate level of exercise had been performed. The patient did not experience any chest pain or arm pain.

The patient's maximum heart rate was 169 beats per minute, which was 94% of the age-adjusted target heart rate. Maximum blood pressure response was 184/76.

ST-segment analysis at peak exercise did not reveal any significant ST-segment depression from baseline. No significant arrhythmias or conduction abnormalities were noted.

Echocardiographic imaging was obtained at rest and following exercise using standard parasternal long and short axis, apical, 2- and 4-chamber views. Resting color flow Doppler appeared normal.

Postexercise imaging revealed a normal global hypodynamic exercise response with no exercise-induced wall motion abnormalities noted.

CONCLUSIONS:
1. Negative electrocardiographic portion of stress echocardiogram exam for ischemia by standard criteria.
2. No chest pain or arm pain noted.
3. No high-grade arrhythmia noted.
4. Adequate exercise tolerance phase.

5. Normal echocardiographic portion of the examination with no evidence to suggest malignant underlying myocardial ischemia or recent infarction.

IMPRESSION:
1. Atypical chest pain syndrome, presumed noncardiac.
2. False-positive troponin level.

Appendix 6
Common Terms by Procedure

Abdominal Aortogram: Coral Reef Aorta
abdominal aorta
anteroposterior view (AP view)
celiac origin
coral reef aorta
filling defect
lateral view
lumen
mesenteric insufficiency
narrowing of the lumen
nausea, vomiting, and abdominal
    cramping
renal artery origin
superior mesenteric artery origin

Consultation: Pneumocystis Carinii Pneumonia
alveolar consolidation
anorexia
bilateral interstitial and alveolar
    consolidation
community-acquired pneumonia (CAP)
diffuse change
dry cough
dyspnea on exertion (DOE)
flow murmur 2/6
hepatitis B
hepatitis C
HIV positive
human immunodeficiency virus (HIV)
interstitial consolidation
Levaquin
low-grade fever
nonproductive cough
Pneumocystis carinii pneumonia
    (PCP)
positive PPD test

purified protein derivative of tuberculin
    (PPD)
pulmonologist
Rocephin
S1, S2
Septra
serology
shortness of breath (SOB)
significant rub
steroid
tachycardic
unexplained weight loss
Western blot
Zithromax

CT Scan: Suspected Asbestosis
asbestos exposure
atelectasis
base of left lung
bilateral pleural thickening
bronchovascular bundle
calcified pleural plaque
computed tomography (CT)
CT exam
left lower lobe
linear calcification
lung window
malignancy
mediastinal window
percutaneous needle biopsy
pleural plaque
pleural thickening
rounded atelectasis
stippled calcification

Death Summary: Cor Pulmonale
A wave
captopril

cardiac arrest
cardiac care unit (CCU)
cardiac catheterization (cardiac cath)
cardiac output
chest x-ray
cor pulmonale
cross-sectional echocardiogram
cyclophosphamide
decreased diffusion lung capacity
deep venous thrombosis
diffusing lung capacity
dilated pulmonary artery
Doppler study
dyspnea on exertion (DOE)
emphysema
enlarged right atrium
enlarged right ventricle
furosemide
jugular venous pressure
hypotensive
left and right cardiac catheterization
lung infiltrate
night sweats
parasternal heave
pitting edema
plasmapheresis
prednisolone
prominent pulmonary conus
pulmonary area
pulmonary artery
pulmonary conus
pericardial effusion
pulmonary embolism
pulmonary function test
pulmonary hypertension
pulmonic second heart sound
right atrium
right ventricle
second heart sound
severe pericardial effusion
systolic ejection murmur
sternal angle

ventilation/perfusion ($\dot{V}/\dot{Q}$)
ventilation/perfusion scan
warfarin

Discharge Summary: Posttraumatic Aortic Pseudoaneurysm

aneurysmectomy
aortic pseudoaneurysm
focal outpouching of the aorta
lateral view
middle mediastinal mass
outpouching of the aorta
posttraumatic chest discomfort
surgical intervention
thrombus
unremitting chest discomfort

Electrophysiological (EPS) Study

atrial-His (AH)
AH interval
American Society of Anesthesiologists (ASA)
ASA classification class III
atrial pacing
atrioventricular (AV)
AV junction
AV node
cardiac chamber
conscious sedation
coronary artery disease (CAD)
congestive heart failure (CHF)
deflectable octapolar catheter
deflectable quadripolar catheter
effective refractory period
electrocardiogram (EKG)
electrophysiological study (EPS)
fasting state
fentanyl
7-French sheath

hemodynamic
hemostasis
His-ventricular (HV)
HV interval
left atrial recording
local anesthetic
monomorphic ventricular tachycardia
nonsustained monomorphic ventricular
    tachycardia
octapolar catheter
palpitations
pulse oximetry
quadripolar catheter
PR interval
QRS interval
QT interval
rapid atrial pacing
refractory period
right atrium (RA)
right femoral vein
right ventricle (RV)
RV apex
sheath
sinus cycle length
sinus node dysfunction
usual sterile fashion
VA conduction
ventriculoatrial (VA)
venous access
ventricular apex
ventricular pacing
ventricular stimulation
ventricular tachycardia
Versed
Wenckebach cycle length

Electrophysiological Study, Left Atrial Recording, Mapping, and Repeat Stimulation

accessory pathway
atrial-His (AH)

AH interval
American Society of Anesthesiologists
    (ASA)
antegrade Wenckebach
arrhythmia
ASA class II
aspirin therapy
atrial overdrive pacing
atrioventricular (AV)
AV nodal physiology
AV node
bolus
burst atrial pacing
carotid sinus massage
comprehensive electrophysiologic
    testing
conscious sedation
continuous oximetric airway
    monitoring
coronary sinus
deflectable decapolar catheter
deflectable quadripolar catheter
deflectable octapolar catheter
drive cycle length
dual physiology
effective refractory period (ERP)
electrophysiologic testing (EPT)
event monitoring
exercise testing
femoral area
fentanyl
fluoroscopic guidance
7- French sheath
heart rate monitoring
hemostasis
high right atrium
His bundle
His-Purkinje system disease
His-ventricular (HV)
HV interval
inducible ventricular tachycardia
induction of arrhythmia

intermittent noninvasive blood pressure
    monitoring
isoproterenol
left femoral vein
local anesthesia
modified Seldinger technique
near syncope
noninvasive blood pressure monitoring
normal atrioventricular node
normal sinus node
outpatient event monitoring
PA conduction
palpitation
premature atrial contraction
PR interval
prepped and draped
program stimulation
QRS interval
repeat stimulation
right femoral vein
right ventricular apex
sinus cycle length
sinus rhythm
sinus slowing
usual sterile fashion
Versed
wide-complex tachycardia
Xylocaine

Electrophysiological Study, Left Ventricular Recording, Mapping, and Central Venogram

activation time
American Society of Anesthesiologists
    (ASA)
ASA classification
atrial arrhythmia
biventricular pacing
central circulation
central venogram
complete heart block

congestive heart failure
continuous electrocardiography
continuous pulse oximetry
coronary sinus
deflectable quadripolar catheter
electrophysiologic laboratory
electrophysiologic study (EPS)
fentanyl
6-French sheath
hemodynamics
high right atrium
HV interval
inferolateral wall
informed consent
intraventricular conduction time
intraventricular pacing
Isovue
J wire
lateral veins
left atrial wires
left femoral vessel
left subclavian vein
left ventricular pacing site
left ventricular recording
level of sedation and consciousness
lidocaine
locally anesthetized
mapping of the left ventricle
noninvasive blood pressure
    measurements
os
permanent pacemaker
posterior lateral branch
prepped and draped
QRS complex
QRS duration
respiratory rate and effort
right ventricular apex
right ventricular wire
sheath
superior vena cava (SVC)
usual sterile fashion
venogram

ventricular arrhythmia
Versed

Explanation of Pacemaker and Leads with Implantation of ICD and Leads

adenosine triphosphate
angled Glidewire
atrial fibrillation
atrial lead
balloon-tipped Swan-Ganz catheter
beats per minute (bpm)
biventricular impedance
biventricular threshold
blunt dissection
Bovie dissection
congestive heart failure (CHF)
class III congestive heart failure
contrast
coronary sinus
coronary sinus lead
coronary sinus venography
defibrillation threshold testing
dual-chamber pacemaker
ejection fraction (EF)
electrophysiology (EP)
EP lab
explant
extraction
fasting state
12-French sheath
fluoroscopy time
generator
gentle traction
Glidewire
Guidant model
guidewire
hook sheath
ICD lead
impedance
implant
implantable cardioverter-defibrillator
    (ICD)

informed consent was obtained
induced left bundle branch block
infiltrated
ischemic cardiomyopathy
laser extraction
left bundle branch block
left ventricular coronary sinus lead
1% lidocaine solution
millisecond (msec)
pace and sense thresholds
pacing and sensing thresholds
pacing-induced left bundle branch
    block
pacing lead
permanent atrial fibrillation
posterolateral vein
prepped and draped in sterile fashion
QRS complex
radial arterial line
Rapido sheath
right atrium
right ventricular impedance
right ventricular threshold
R wave
scar tissue
sheath
0 silk suture
Spectranetics laser
Spectranetics stylet
stable pace and sense thresholds
sterile fashion
subclavian vein
Swan-Ganz catheter
ventricular lead
ventricular rate
4-0 Vicryl
volt (V)
ventricular fibrillation (VF)
ventricular tachycardia (VT)
VF zone
VT zone
paced ventricle-sensed ventricle,

inhibited response, rate modulation (VVIR)
VVIR pacing

History and Physical: Asbestosis

asbestosis
costal margin
crackles
hemidiaphragm
linear calcification
mid lung field
normal S1, S2
pleural calcification
shortness of breath on exertion
short of breath

History and Physical: Cardiac Tamponade

amiodarone
bundle branch block
cardiac tamponade
chest pain
diaphoresis
diaphoretic
diastolic pressure
dual-chamber permanent pacemaker
electrocardiogram (EKG)
emergency echocardiogram
emergent thoracotomy
jugular venous pressure (JVP)
left bundle branch block
pacemaker interrogation
paroxysmal atrial fibrillation
peripheral edema
right atrial systolic inversion
right ventricular systolic collapse
sinus node dysfunction
sinus tachycardia
syncope
systolic collapse
systolic inversion

thoracotomy
warfarin

History and Physical: Myocardial Infarction

bradycardia
bypass surgery
chest pain
clear to percussion and auscultation
diaphoresis
dyspnea
EKG leads I, II, III, aVF, aVL, aVR, V1-V6
electrocardiogram
harsh holosystolic murmur
leads V4, V5, and V6
left lower sternal border
midsystolic peak
myocardial infarction
nitroglycerin sublingual
orthopnea
pedal edema
percussion and auscultation
S1, S2
severe chest pain
squeezing substernal chest pain
ST elevation
substernal chest pain
tachycardia

Implantation of Dual-Chamber Defibrillator

American Society of Anesthesiologists (ASA)
antibiotic prophylaxis
ASA classification
atrial threshold
benzoin
blunt dissection
Bovie
cardioactive medication
catheterization laboratory (cath lab)

central venous system
coronary pacing lead
defibrillation threshold (DFT)
defibrillator lead
DFT testing
dilator
dual-chamber defibrillator implantation
ephedrine
fasting state
18-gauge needle
guidewire
His induction
impedance
left axillary vein
localization
milliampere (mA)
millivolt (mV)
pacing and sensing
pectoralis fascia
peel-away sheath
piggyback
P-wave amplitude
right atrium
right ventricle (RV)
right ventricular apex
R-wave amplitude
Steri-Strips
tamponade
total intravenous anesthesia (TIVA)
transient hypotension
ventricular fibrillation
2-0 Vicryl
3-0 Vicryl
4-0 Vicryl
volt (V)

Implantation of Implantable Cardioverter- Defibrillator (ICD)

American Society of Anesthesiologists
    (ASA)
Ancef
antibiotic solution

arrhythmia
ASA classification class III
atrial and ventricular pacing
axillary vein
bradycardia
coronary artery disease (CAD)
deep conscious sedation
defibrillation impedance
defibrillation testing threshold
defibrillation threshold testing
Dermabond
desaturation
dual-chamber generator
dual-chamber implantable cardioverter-
    defibrillator
electrophysiological study (EPS)
fasting state
fluoroscopy
guidewire
hemostasis
inducible ventricular tachycardia
interrogation of reprogramming
intracardiac
left ventricular dysfunction
local anesthetic
millivolt (mV)
pacing parameter
pulmonary artery
right atrial appendage
right atrial lead
right atrium (RA)
right ventricular apex
right ventricular lead
sheath
sharp and blunt dissection
silk suture
sinus node dysfunction
St. Jude dual-chamber Epic DR pulse
    generator
superior vena cava (SVC)
Swan-Ganz catheter
usual sterile fashion

ventricular fibrillation (v-fib)
ventricular tachycardia (v-tach)
volt (V)

Pacemaker Generator Replacement

antibiotic solution
atrial lead
blunt dissection
catheterization lab (cath lab)
chronic atrial fibrillation
chronic generator
cutaneous layer
explanted
hemostasis
implanted generator
incise the skin
infiltrated
informed consent
intravenous fentanyl and Versed
local anesthetic
millivolt (mV)
pacemaker generator replacement
pocket
postabsorptive state
prophylactic intravenous
   antibiotic
R wave
#15 scalpel
St. Jude model
subcutaneous layer
subcutaneously
tachycardia/bradycardia syndrome
3-0 Vicryl
volt (V)

Stress Echocardiogram

age-adjusted target heart rate
arrhythmia
atypical chest pain syndrome
baseline 12-lead EKG

blood pressure response
Bruce protocol
2-chamber view
4-chamber view
conduction abnormality
coronary artery disease
creatine phosphokinase (CPK)
electrocardiogram (EKG)
echocardiographic imaging
elevated troponin level
exercise-induced wall motion
   abnormality
exercise response
exercise tolerance
false-positive troponin level
global hypodynamic exercise response
high-grade arrhythmia
infarction
ischemia
maximum blood pressure response
maximum heart rate
metabolic equivalent (MET)
myocardiac ischemia
normal CPKs
normal global hypodynamic exercise
   response
normal sinus rhythm
parasternal long axis view
parasternal short axis view
peak exercise
Plendil
postexercise imaging
premature coronary artery disease
resting color flow Doppler
rightward axis
standard Bruce protocol
standard criteria
stress echocardiogram
ST-segment analysis
ST-segment depression
target heart rate
wall motion abnormality

Appendix 7
Cardiology Trials and Studies

AASK
African American Study of Kidney Disease and Hypertension Pilot Study

ABACAS
adjunctive balloon angioplasty following coronary atherectomy study

ABC
Alpha Beta Canadian trial

ACAD
azithromycin coronary artery disease

ACADEMIC
azithromycin in coronary artery disease elimination of myocardial infection with chlamydia

ACCEPT
Accupril Canadian clinical evaluation and patient teaching
American College of Cardiology evaluation of preventive therapies

ACCESS
a comparison of percutaneous entry sites for coronary angioplasty
atorvastatin comparative cholesterol efficacy and safety study

ACCT
amlodipine cardiovascular community trial

ACES
alternans cardiac electrical safety study
azithromycin and coronary events study

ACHIEVE
Accupril congestive heart failure investigation and economic variable evaluation

ACP
asymptomatic cardiac ischemia pilot

ACRE
appropriateness of coronary revascularization study

ACT
angioplasty compliance trial
attacking claudication with ticlopidine study

ACTION
a coronary disease trial investigating outcome with nifedipine GITS

ACTS
American-Canadian thrombosis study

ACUTE
analysis of coronary ultrasound thrombolysis endpoints
assessment of cardioversion utilizing transesophageal echocardiography pilot study

ADAPTS
acute directional atherectomy prior to stenting

ADEG
antiarrhythmic drug evaluation group trial

ADEP
atherosclerotic disease evolution by picotamide study

ADMIRE
AMP 579 delivery for myocardial infarction reduction trial

ADMIT
arterial disease multiple intervention tria

ADOPT
Accupril decision on pharmacotherapy trial

AFASAK
atrial fibrillation aspirin anticoagulation trial

AFCAPS
Air Force coronary atherosclerosis prevention study

AFCAPS/TexCAPS
C-reactive protein substudy: Air Force/Texas coronary atherosclerosis
  prevention study

AFI
atrial fibrillation investigators study

AFIB
atrial fibrillation investigation with bidisomide trial

AFIRME
antagonist of the fibrinogen receptor after myocardial events study

AFTER
anistreplase following thrombolysis effect on reocclusion study
aspirin/anticoagulants following thrombolysis with Eminase in recurrent
  infarction study

AFTER
aspirin/anticoagulants following thrombolysis with Eminase results study

AIMS
acylated plasminogen-streptokinase activator complex intervention mortality study

AIREX
acute infarction ramipril efficacy extension study

AITIA
aspirin in transient ischemic attacks study

AITIAIS
aspirin in transient ischemic attacks Italian study

ALDUSA
aspirin low dosage in unstable angina study

ALERT
amiodarone versus lidocaine inpatient emergency resuscitation trial

ALIVE
adenosine lidocaine infarct zone viability enhancement trial
amiodarone versus lidocaine in prehospital refractory ventricular fibrillation study
azimilide postinfarction survival evaluation trial

ALL
antihypertensive and lipid lowering study

ALLHAT
antihypertensive and lipid-lowering treatment to prevent heart attack trial

AMI
argatroban in myocardial infarction study

AMICUS
Austrian multicenter isradipine cum spirapril study

AMISTAD
acute myocardial infarction study of adenosine trial

AMPI
ASPAC in acute myocardial infarction placebo controlled investigation

AMRO
Amsterdam-Rotterdam trial comparing excimer laser and percutaneous transluminal
  coronary angioplasty

AMT
adenosine scan multicenter trial

ANBP
Australian national blood pressure trial

ANS
American nimodipine study

ANTENOX
switch to oral anticoagulant from enoxaparin in treatment of acute deep venous
  thrombosis

ANZ
Australia and New Zealand heart failure collaborative study

APIS
antihypertensive patch, Italian study

APLAUD
antiplatelet useful dose trial

APPI
active Persantine in postischemic injury study

APPROACH
Alberta provincial project for outcomes assessment in coronary heart disease

APRAIS
acute phase reactions and ischemic coronary syndromes

APRAISE
antisense to prevent restenosis after intervention, stent evaluation

APRICOT
antithrombotics in the prevention of reocclusion in coronary thrombolysis trial
aspirin versus Coumadin in the prevention of reocclusion and recurrent ischemia after
  successful thrombolysis trial

APSIS
angina prognosis study in Stockholm
angina prognosis study with Isoptin and Seloken

ARCH
amiodarone reduces coronary artery bypass grafting hospitalization trial

ARCOS
Auckland region coronary or stroke study

ARCS
atherosclerosis risk in communities study

ARGAMI
argatroban compared with heparin in myocardial infarction treated with recombinant tissue
  plasminogen activator

ARIS
Anturan reinfarction Italian study

ARREST
amiodarone in out-of-hospital resuscitation of refractory sustained ventricular tachyarrhythmia

ARS
Amsterdam resuscitation study
atherogenic risk study

ART
AngioJet rapid thrombectomy catheter study

ARTIST
angioplasty versus rotational atherectomy for treatment of diffuse in-stent restenosis trial

ARTISTIC
AngioRad radiation technology for in-stent restenosis trial in coronaries

ARTS
arterial revascularization therapy study

ASAAC
acetylsalicylic acid versus anticoagulants study

ASAP
acetylsalicylic acid Persantine study
azimilide supraventricular arrhythmia program trial

ASCOT
Anglo Scandinavian cardiac outcomes trial

ASDOS
atrial septal defect occlusion system study

ASIS
American study of infarct survival
angina and silent ischemia study

ASPS
Australian Swedish pindolol study

ASSET
Anglo Scandinavian study of early thrombosis
atorvastatin simvastatin safety and efficacy trial

ASSURE
a stent versus stent ultrasound remodeling evaluation

ATACS
antithrombotic therapy in acute coronary syndromes trial

ATEST
atenolol and streptokinase trial

ATIAIS
Anturan transient ischemic attack Italian study

ATIME
Accupril titration intervention management interval management evaluation

ATLANTIC
angina treatment, lasers and normal therapy in comparison

ATLAST
antiplatelet therapy versus Lovenox plus antiplatelet therapy for patients with increased risk
  of stent thrombosis
aspirin/ticlopidine versus low-molecular weight heparin/aspirin/ticlopidine stent trial

ATMA
amiodarone trials meta analysis

ATRAMI
autonomic tone and reflexes after myocardial infarction trial

ATTMH
Australian therapeutic trial of mild hypertension

AWESOME
angina with extremely serious operative mortality evaluation

BAATAF
Boston area anticoagulation trial for atrial fibrillation

BACUS
balloon angioplasty compliance ultrasound study

BADE
bioimpedance as an adjunct to dobutamine echocardiography study

BAHAMA
Baragwanath hypertension ambulatory blood pressure monitoring
  multiarm study

BARASTER
balloon angioplasty versus rotational atherectomy for stent restenosis

BASC
blood pressure in acute stroke collaboration

BBPP
beta-blocker pooling project

BCAPS
beta-blocker cholesterol-lowering asymptomatic plaque study

BCSP
Bavarian cholesterol screening project

BENESTENT
Belgian-Netherlands stent study

BEPS
Belgian Eminase prehospital study

BERT
beta energy restenosis trial

BESMART
BeStent in small arteries study

BESS
Berlin pacemaker study on syncope

BESSAMI
Berlin stent study in acute myocardial infarction

BEST
Beta-Cath system trial
Medtronic BeStent coronary stent versus Palmaz-Schatz coronary stent

BHACAS
beating heart against cardioplegic arrest studies

BHS
Bogalusa heart study
Brisighella heart study

BIGMAC
Beaumont interventional group, Mevacor, ACE inhibitor, colchicine restenosis trial
bidirectional gantry multiarray coil study

BIOMACS
biochemical markers of acute coronary syndromes study

BIP
bezafibrate infarction prevention study

BIRD
bolus versus infusion Rescupase development study

BLASP
Barbados low-dose aspirin study in pregnancy

BMS
Belfast metoprolol study

BNS
Belfast nifedipine study

BOILER
balloon occlusive intravascular lysis enhanced recanalization strategy study

BOSS
balloon optimization versus stent study

BPEG
British packing and electrophysiology group study

BPSMC
blood pressure study in Mexican children

BRESUS
British hospital resuscitation study

BRH
British regional heart study

BRHS
British regional heart study

BRITE II
beta radiation to reduce in-stent restenosis II

CAASET
Canadian amlodipine and atenolol stress echo trial

CABADAS
prevention of coronary artery bypass graft occlusion by aspirin, dipyridamole and
  acenocoumarol study

CACTIS
comparison of aspirin with clopidogrel or ticlopidine in stents
  trial

CADHYP
coronary artery disease in hypertension study

CADRES
coronary artery descriptors and restenosis project

CAFA
Canadian atrial fibrillation anticoagulation study

CAFE
coronary artery flow evaluation

CAMCAT
Canadian multicenter clentiazem angina trial

CAPARES
coronary angioplasty amlodipine in restenosis trial

CAPAS
cutting balloon angioplasty versus plain old balloon angioplasty
  randomized study

CAPE
circadian antiischemia program in Europe

CAPITOL
captopril postinfarction tolerance trial

CAPP
captopril prevention project study
concerted action polyp prevention

CAPPHY
captopril primary prevention in hypertension study

CAPPP
captopril prevention project

CAPRICORN
carvedilol postinfarct survival controlled evaluation

CAPTIN
captopril before reperfusion in acute myocardial infarction
captopril plus tissue plasminogen activator following acute myocardial infarction

CARDIAC
cardiovascular disease and alimentary comparison study

CARD PORT
cardiac arrhythmia and risk of death patient outcome research team

CARE
carvedilol arthrectomy restenosis trial
cholesterol and recurrent events study

CARMEN
carvedilol angiotensin converting enzyme inhibitors remodeling mild heart failure evaluation

CARPORT
coronary artery restenosis prevention on repeated thromboxane A2-receptor antagonism study

CARS
coronary artery regression study
Coumadin aspirin reinfarction study

CART
colchicine angioplasty restenosis trial

CASCO
calcium sensitization in congestive heart failure

CASH
cardiac arrest study, Hamburg
consensus action on salt and hypertension

CASIS
Canadian amlodipine/atenolol in silent ischemia study

CASIS
coronary artery stent implantation study
coronary artery surgery study

CASSIS
Czech and Slovak spirapril intervention study

CASTEL
cardiovascular study in the elderly

CASTOR
coronary angioscopic study of restenosis

CAT
cardiomyopathy trial
Chinese angiotensin converting enzyme inhibitor in acute myocardial infarction trial
coronary angioplasty trial

CATCH
child and adolescent trial for cardiovascular heath
community action to control high blood pressure

CAVA
coronary atherectomy versus angioplasty study

CCCCP
comprehensive cardiovascular community control program

CCHAT
Canadian Cozaar, Hyzaar and amlodipine trial

CCHD
Caerphilly collaborative heart disease study

CCHP
Corpus Christi heart project

CCHS
Copenhagen city heart study

CCP
cooperative cardiovascular project

CCRT
cardiac catheter reuse trial

CCS
Chinese cardiac study

CCT
Chinese captopril trial

CDP
coronary drug project

CDPAS
coronary disease prevention with aspirin study
coronary drug project aspirin study

CEDARS
comprehensive evaluation of defibrillators and resuscitative shock study

CEI-AMI
converting enzymes inhibitor in the treatment of acute myocardial infarction

CELL
cost effectiveness of lipid lowering study

CERT
cardiovascular event reduction trial

CESAR
centralised European studies in angina research

CESARZ
clinical European studies in angina and revascularization

CESNA
comparative efficacy and safety of nisoldipine and amlodipine in hypertension

CESNA II
comparative efficacy and safety of nisoldipine and amlodipine in hypertension with ischemic heart disease

CHAD
cholesterol hypertension and diabetes study

CHAMP
cardiac hospitalization atherosclerosis management program

CHANGE
chronic heart failure and graded exercise study

CHARM
candesartan in heart failure assessment in reduction of mortality

CHEAPER
confirmation that heparin is an alternative to promote early reperfusion in acute myocardial infarction study

CHEER
chest pain evaluation in emergency room trial

CHEPER
chest pain evaluation registry study

CHF-IES
congestive heart failure, Italian epidemiological study

CHIP
coronary health improvement project

CHOICE
caring for hypertension on initiation cost and effectiveness study
congestive heart failure mortality investigation on carvedilol's efficacy

CHOICES
coronary heart disease, osteoporosis interventions, and community evaluation studies

CHRISTMAS
carvedilol hibernation reversible ischemia trial: marker of success

CHS
cardiovascular health study
Charleston heart study
Congenital Heart Surgeons Society study
Copenhagen city heart study
coronary heart study

CIAIT
Chinese infarction angiotensin converting enzyme inhibitor trial

CIDS
Canadian internal defibrillator study

CIS
coronary intervention study

CITTS
central Illinois thrombolytic therapy study

CLASP
collaborative low-dose aspirin study in pregnancy

CLASSICS
clopidogrel aspirin stent interventional cooperative study

CLEOPAD
clopidogrel in peripheral artery disease study

CLIP
cholesterol-lowering intervention program

CLOT
clinical perspectives on lysis of thrombi study

COAT
cooperative Osaka adenosine trial

COBRA
comparison of balloon versus rotational angioplasty

COLTS
coronary observational long-term study

COMET
carvedilol or metoprolol European trial
carvedilol or metoprolol evaluation trial

COMMIT
comprehensive multidisciplinary interventional trial for regression of coronary
  heart disease

CONSENSUS
cooperative north Scandinavian enalapril survival study

CONVINCE
controlled onset verapamil investigation for cardiovascular endpoints study

COPERNICUS
carvedilol prospective randomized cumulative survival trial

CORGENE
coronary disease and angiotensin converting enzyme I/D genotype study

CORIS
coronary risk factor study

CORRECT
complete versus restrictive revascularization by coronary angioplasty trial

CORSICA
chronic occlusion revascularization with stent implantation versus coronary angioplasty
study

CORTES
Clivarin assessment of regression of thrombosis efficacy and safety study

COST
cardiac output study technology

COTAIM
continuation of trial antihypertensive interventions and management

COURAGE
clinical outcomes using revascularization versus aggressive strategies
clinical outcomes utilization revascularization and aggressive drug evaluation

COURT
contrast media utilization in high risk percutaneous transluminal coronary
angioplasty trial

CPAS
Canadian Prinivil atenolol study

CPEP
Chicago coronary prevention evaluation program

CPHRP
coronary prevention and hypertension research project

C-PORT
cardiovascular patient outcomes research team trial

CPPT
coronary primary prevention trial

CPRG
coronary prevention research group

CRAC
compliance-related angioplasty complications study

CRAF
Canadian registry of atrial fibrillation

CRAFT
catheterization rescue angioplasty following thrombolysis trial
controlled randomized atrial fibrillation trial

CREATE
cholesterol research education and treatment evaluation

CREDO
clopidogrel reduction of events during extended observation study

CREW
coronary regression with estrogen in women study

CRIS
calcium antagonist reinfarction Italian study

CRISP
cholesterol reduction in seniors program pilot study

CRIYFS
cardiovascular risk in young Finns study

CRUISE
can routine ultrasound influent stent expansion study

CRUSADE
coronary reserve utilization for stent angiography Doppler endpoint study
coronary revascularization ultrasound angioplasty device trial

CSCHDS
Caerphilly and Speedwell collaborative heart disease studies

CSGTEI
collaborative study group trial on the effect of irbesartan

C-SMART
cardiomyoplasty skeletal muscle assist randomized trial

CTA
committee on thrombolytic agents

CTAF
Canadian trial of atrial fibrillation

CTOPP
Canadian trial of physiological pacing

CTRD
cardiac transplant research database

CTS
collaborative transplant study

CTSP
cooperative triglyceride standardization program

CUBA
cutting balloon versus conventional balloon angioplasty study

CURE
clopidogrel in unstable anginal to prevent recurrent ischemic events trial
Columbia University restenosis elimination trial

CVIR
cardiovascular information registry

CYCAZAREM
cyclophosphamide versus azathioprine during remission of systemic vasculitis trial

DAAF
digoxin in acute atrial fibrillation study

DAIS
diabetes atherosclerosis intervention study

DAMAD
diabetic microangiopathy modification with aspirin versus dipyridamole

DANAMI
Danish multicenter study of acute myocardial infarction

DAPPAF
dual-site atrial pacing for prevention of atrial fibrillation trial

DART
diet and reinfarction trial
dilation versus ablation revascularization trial

DATA
diltiazem as adjunctive therapy to Activase study

DATOS
diet and antismoking trial of Oslo study

DAVIT
Danish verapamil infarction trial

DBLE
double bolus lytic efficacy trial

DDDD-CAT
drug delivery device dispatch in coronary angioplasty trial

DEBATE
Doppler endpoints balloon angioplasty trial, Europe

DEER
diet and exercise in elevated risk trial

DEFIBRILAT
defibrillator as bridge to later transplantation study

DELIVER
The RX ACHIEVE drug-eluting coronary stent system in the treatment of patients with de novo native coronary lesions

DES
Danish enoxaparin study

DESIRE
debulking and stenting in restenosis elimination trial

DESTINI
Doppler endpoint stent international investigation
Duke University clinical cardiology study elective stent trial: a cost containment initiative

DHAOS
Dutch hypertension and offspring study

DHCCP
Department of Health and Social Security hypertension care computing project

DHFS
diet, heart feasibility study

DIAMOND
Danish investigation of arrhythmia and mortality on dofetilide

DIAMOND-CHF
Danish investigation of arrhythmia and mortality on dofetilide in congestive heart failure

DIAMOND-MI
Danish investigation of arrhythmia and mortality on dofetilide in myocardial infarction

DiDi
diltiazem in dilated cardiomyopathy trial

DIGAF
digoxin in atrial fibrillation study

DIGAMI
diabetes mellitus, insulin glucose infusion in acute myocardial infarction

DIG-CAPTOPRIL
Canadian digoxin captopril study

DILCACOMP
diltiazem captopril comparative study

DILDURANG
diltiazem duration in angina study

DILPLACOMP
diltiazem placebo comparative trial

DIMT
Dutch ibopamine multicenter trial

DIRECT
direct myocardial revascularization in regeneration of endomyocardial channels trial

DIRS
Dutch invasive reperfusion study

DISH
dietary intervention study of hypertension

DISTRESS
dispatch stent restenosis study

DOMIOS
determinants of myocardial infarction onset study

DOUBLE
double bolus lytic efficacy trial

DOUBTLESS
Doppler and ultrasound-guided balloon therapeutics for coronary lesions study

DRS
diltiazem reinfarction study

DUCCS
Duke University clinical cardiology study

DUTCH-TIA
Dutch transient ischemic attack study

DVT
Danish verapamil trial

EAFT
European atrial fibrillation trial

EAGAR
estrogen and graft atherosclerosis research trial

EARS
European atherosclerosis research study

EAS
Edinburgh artery study

EASI
European antiplatelet stent investigation

EAST
Emory angioplasty versus surgery trial

ECAA
European concerted action on anticoagulation study

ECAP
European concerted action project

ECAT
European concerted action on thrombosis and disabilities study

ECAT AP
European concerted action on thrombosis: angina pectoris study

ECCE
effects of captopril on cardiopulmonary exercise study

ECSG
European cooperative study group

ECSS
European coronary surgery study

EDIC
echocardiography dobutamine international cooperative study

EDIT
early defibrillator implantation trial
early diabetes intervention trial

EDRES
effects of debulking on restenosis trial

EFERF
enalapril felodipine extended release factorial study

EFICAT
ejection fraction in carvedilol-treated transplant candidates study

EFS
European Fraxiparine study

EHVT
Edinburgh heart valve trial

EIHDW
evaluation of ischemic heart disease in women study

EIS
European infarction study

ELAT
embolism in left atrial thrombi study

ELCA
excimer laser coronary angioplasty registry

ELHE
evaluation of losartan in hemodialysis study

ELITE
evaluation of losartan in the elderly study

ELSA
European lacidipine study on atherosclerosis
European longitudinal study on aging

ELVD
exercise in left ventricular dysfunction trial

ELVD-CHF
exercise in left ventricular dysfunction and chronic heart failure trial

EMIAT
European myocardial infarction amiodarone trial
European myocardial infarction arrhythmia trial

EMIP
European myocardial infarction project

EMIP-FR
European myocardial infarction project, free radicals

EMP
European myocardial infarction project

EMPAR
enoxaparin MaxEPA prevention of angioplasty restenosis study

EMPIRE
economics of myocardial perfusion imaging in Europe study

ENASA
enoxaparin and/or aspirin in unstable angina trial

ENCORE
evaluation of nifedipine and cerivastatin on recovery of endothelial function trial

ENDPT
evaluation of Doppler parameters during percutaneous transluminal coronary angioplasty

ENOXART
enoxaparin in arterial surgery study

ENRICAD
enhancing recovery in coronary heart disease trial

ENRICHD
enhancing recovery in coronary heart disease patients trial

ENTICES
enoxaparin and ticlopidine after elective stenting study

EPIC
echocardiography Persantine international cooperative study
echo Persantine Italian cooperative study
evaluation of 7E3 for the prevention of ischemic complications

EPIDS
early postmyocardial infarction intravenous dipyridamole study

EPILOG
evaluation of percutaneous transluminal coronary angioplasty to improve long-term outcome with abciximab glycoprotein IIb/IIIa blockade trial

EPISTENT
Epilog stent trial

EPRCSS
European prospective randomized coronary surgery study

EQUIPP
evaluation of quinapril in primary practice trial

ERA
estrogen replacement in atherosclerosis study

ERACI II
Argentine randomized trial of percutaneous transluminal coronary angioplasty versus coronary artery bypass surgery in multivessel disease II

ERNST
European resuscitation nimodipine study

ESBY
electrical stimulation versus coronary artery bypass study

ESCALAT, ESCALATE
efegatran and streptokinase to canalize arteries like accelerated tissue plasminogen activator study

ESCOBAR
emergency stenting compared to conventional balloon angioplasty randomized trial

ESETCID
European study of epidemiology and treatment of cardiac inflammatory diseases

ESMIR
echocardiographic selection of patients for mitral regurgitation study

ESPRIM
European study prevention research of infarct with molsidomine

ESPRIT
European study of the prevention of reocclusion after initial thrombolysis

ESSENCE
efficacy safety subcutaneous enoxaparin in non-Q wave coronary events study

ESSEX
European Scimed stent experience

ESVEM
electrophysiologic study versus electrocardiographic monitoring

EURAMIC
European community multicenter study on antioxidants, myocardial infarction and breast cancer

EURID
European Registry for Implantable Cardioverter Defibrillators

EURO-ART
European AngioJet rapid thrombectomy study

EUROCARE
European carvedilol restenosis trial

EUROCARDI
European concerted action for the rapid diagnosis of myocardial infarction

EURO-DIRECT
European direct myocardial revascularization in regeneration of endomyocardial channels trial

EUROPA
European trial of reduction of cardiac events with perindopril in stable coronary artery disease

EUROSCOP
European Registry Society study of chronic obstructive pulmonary diseases

EUROWINTER
European study on cold exposure and winter mortality from ischemic heart disease

EVADE
experience with left ventricular assist device with exercise trial

EWGCP
European working group on cardiac pacing

EWPHE
European working party on hypertension in the elderly

EWR
European Wallstent registry

EXACTO
excimer laser angioplasty in coronary total occlusion

EXCEL
expanded clinical evaluation of lovastatin trial

EXCITE
evaluation of oral xemilofiban in controlling thrombotic events

EXPAPS
Exeter primary angioplasty pilot study

EXTRA
evaluation of XT stent for restenosis of native arteries

FACET
flosequinan angiotensin converting enzyme inhibitor trial
fosinopril versus amlodipine cardiovascular events trial

FACIT
folate after coronary intervention trial

FACTS
functional angiometric correlation with thallium scintigraphy trial

DAMIS
fosinopril in acute myocardial infarction study

FANTASTIC
full anticoagulation versus aspirin ticlopidine after stent implantation study
full anticoagulation versus ticlopidine plus aspirin after stent implantation study

FAP
fibrinolytics versus primary angioplasty trial

FAPIS
flecainide and propafenone Italian study

FAPS
felodipine atherosclerosis prevention study
French aortic plaque study

FASTEST
femoral artery stent study

FAST-MI
field ambulance study of thrombolysis in myocardial infarction

FATIMA
Fraxiparin anticoagulant therapy in myocardial infarction study in Amsterdam

FATS
familial atherosclerosis treatment study

FEMINA
felodipine ER and metoprolol in the treatment of angina pectoris

FEST
fosinopril efficacy/safety trial
fosinopril on exercise tolerance study

FHRS
familial hypercholesterolemia regression study

FHS
family heart study
Framingham heart study

FIG
flosequinan investigator group

FINESS
first international new intravascular rigid-flex endovascular stent study

FINMONICA
Finnish monitoring trends and determinants in cardiovascular diseases

FINRISK
Finland cardiovascular risk study

FIRST
Flolan international randomized survival trial

FISH
Finnish isradipine study in hypertension

FLARE
fluvastatin angioplasty restenosis trial

FLEQUIN
flecainide compared to oral quinidine study

FLUENT
fluvastatin long-term extension trial

FMS
Fragmin multicenter study

FMT
Fragmin multicenter trial

FORECAST
fractional flow reserve or relative fractional velocity reserve evaluation of coronary artery
  stenosis versus thallium

FORT
fish oil restenosis trial

FOS
Framingham offspring study

FOSS
Framingham offspring, spouse study

FRAMI
Fragmin in acute myocardial infarction study

FRAXIDIS
Fraxiparine in posthospital discharge study

FRAXIS
Fraxiparine in ischemic syndromes study

FRAXODI
Fraxiparine once daily injection study

FRESCO
Florence randomized elective stenting in acute coronary occlusion study

FRIC
Fragmin in unstable coronary artery disease trial

FRISC
fast revascularization during instability in coronary artery disease
Fragmin during instability in coronary artery disease trial

FRISC II
Fragmin and/or revascularization during instability in coronary artery disease trial

FROG
French Rotablator group study

FROST
French optimal stenting trial

FTC
fibrinolysis trialists collaboration

FTT
fibrinolytic therapy trialist collaboration

GABI
German angioplasty bypass intervention trial
German angioplasty bypass surgery investigation

GAMIS
German-Austrian myocardial infarction study

GARS
German-Austrian reinfarction study

GCP
German cardiovascular prevention study

GDCMS
German dilated cardiomyopathy study

GEART
gemfibrozil atherosclerosis regression trial

GELIA
German experience with low-intensity anticoagulation

GIPSI
gradual inflation at optimum pressure versus stent implantation study

GISSI
Grupo Italiano per lo Studio della Streptochinasi Nell'infarto Miocardico

GMT
Göteborg metoprolol trial

GR II
Gianturco Roubin second-generation coronary stent trial

GRACE
Gianturco Roubin stent in acute closure evaluation

GRAMI
Gianturco Roubin second-generation coronary stent in acute coronary infarction

GRASP
Glaxo restenosis and symptoms project

GREAT
Grampian region early anistreplase trial

GRECO
German recanalization of coronary occlusion trial
German recombinant plasminogen activator study

GUARANTEE
global unstable angina registry and treatment evaluation

GUIDE
guidance by ultrasound imaging for decision endpoints trial

GUIDE II
guidance by ultrasound imaging for decision endpoints II trial

GUSTO-I
global utilization of streptokinase and tissue plasminogen activator for occluded coronary arteries trial

GUSTO-IIa
global use of strategies to open occluded arteries

GUSTO-IIb
global use of strategies to open occluded arteries in acute coronary syndromes trial

GUSTO-III
global use of strategies to open occluded coronary arteries trial

GUSTO-IV
global use of streptokinase and tissue plasminogen activator for occluded arteries trial

HAL
heart attacks in London study

HALF
homocysteine, atherosclerosis, lipid and familial hypercholesterolemia study

HALT
hypertension and lipid trial

HALT MI
Hu23F2G anti-adhesion to limit cytotoxic injury following acute myocardial infarction study

HAMIT
heparin in acute myocardial infarction trial

HANE
hydrochlorothiazide, atenolol, nitrendipine, enalapril study

HAPI
heparin as an alternative to promote patency in acute myocardial infarction study

HAPORT
heart attack patient outcome research team study

HAPPHY
heart attack primary prevention in hypertension

HAROLD
hypertension and ambulatory recording in the old

HARP
Harvard atherosclerosis reversibility project

HART
heparin-aspirin reperfusion trial
hypertension audit of risk factor therapy study

HART II
heparin and reperfusion therapies study

HAS
Hirulog angioplasty study, hypertensive arteriosclerotic

HASI
Hirulog angioplasty study investigators

HATS
HDL-atherosclerosis treatment study

HDDRISC
heart disease and diabetes risk indicators in a screened cohort study

HDES
Heidelberg diet and exercise study

HDFP
hypertension detection and followup program

HDS
hypertension in diabetes study

HEART
hyperlipidemia, epidemiology, atherosclerosis risk factor trial
hypertension and ambulatory recording Venetia study

HELP
heart European leaders panel study

HELPS
hypertension, exercise and lifestyle programs for seniors study

HELVETICA
hirudin in European restenosis prevention trial versus heparin treatment in percutaneous transluminal coronary angioplasty

HEMOSTAT
hemostasis with Prostar XL versus Angio-Seal after coronary intervention trial

HEP
hypertension in elderly persons trial

HERO
Hirulog early reperfusion/occlusion study

HEROICS
how effective are revascularization options in cardiogenic shock trial

HERS
heart and estrogen-progestin replacement study

HHP
Honolulu heart program

HHS
Helsinki heart study
Honolulu heart study

HIC
heart information center

HINT
Holland Interuniverisity nifedipine/metoprolol trial

HIPOS
hypertension in pregnancy, offspring study

HIPS
heparin delivery with InfusaSleeve catheter prior to stent implantation study
heparin infusion prior to stenting study

HIRMIT
high-risk myocardial ischemia trial

HIS
Hungarian isradipine study

HIT
high-density lipoprotein cholesterol intervention trial
hirudin for the improvement of thrombolysis study

A95

HIT-SK
hirudin for the improvement of thrombolysis with streptokinase

HOCAP
hypertrophic obstructive cardiomyopathy ablation pacing study

HOPE
health outcomes prevention evaluation
hypertensive old people in Edinburgh study

HOT
hypertension optimal treatment study

HOT MI
hyperbaric oxygen and thrombolysis in myocardial infarction study

HPT
hypertension prevention trial

Hy-C
hydralazine versus captopril trial

HYNON
hypertension non-drug treatment cooperative study

HYPPOS
hypertensive population survey

HYPREN
hypertension under prazosin and enalapril study

HYSTENOX
enoxaparin following hysterectomy study

HYVET
hypertension in the very elderly trial

IAMA
infection in atherosclerosis and use of macrolide antibiotics study

IAP
international atherosclerosis project

IARG
international anticoagulant review group study

ICARIS
intervention cardiology risk stratification study

ICIN
intracoronary streptokinase trial of the Interuniversity Cardiology Institute of the
   Netherlands

IDCS
idiopathic dilated cardiomyopathy study

IDHS
Indian diet heart study

IDHPORT
ischemic heart disease patient outcomes research team

IDHSDP
ischemic heart disease shared decision making program

IIHD
Israeli ischemic heart disease study

IIUK
intraoperative intraarterial urokinase study

ILRCFS
Iowa lipid research clinics family study

IMAGE
international metoprolol/nifedipine anginal exercise trial
international multicenter angina exercise study
international multicenter aprotinin graft patency experience trial

IMEP
investigation in menopausal women of the effect of estradiol and progesterone on
   cardiovascular risk factors

IMPACT
Integrilin to minimize platelet aggregation and prevent coronary thrombosis trial
international mexiletine and placebo antiarrhythmia coronary trial

IMPACT-II
Integrilin to minimize plate aggregation and coronary thrombosis trial

IMPACT-AMI
Integrilin to minimize plate aggregation and coronary thrombosis, acute myocardial
   infarction trial

IMPACT-stent
Integrilin to minimize plate aggregation and coronary thrombosis in stenting trial

IMPRESS
intramural low molecular weight heparin for prevention of restenosis study

IMPROVED
is introduction of mycophenolate mofetil and reduction of cyclosporine valuable in renal
   dysfunction after heart transplantation study

IN-CHF
Italian network congestive heart failure

INDANA
individual data analysis of antihypertensive intervention trials

INJECT
international joint efficacy comparison of thrombolytics trial

INLINIS
Ireland-Netherlands lisinopril, nifedipine study

INROAD
in-stent restenosis optimal angioplasty device trial

INSIGHT
international nifedipine study intervention as a goal in hypertension treatment

INSPIRE
increasing participation in cardiac rehabilitation
intravascular ultrasound study predictor of restenosis trial

INTACT
international nifedipine trial on antiatherosclerotic therapy

INTEGRITI
Integrilin and tenecteplase in acute myocardial infarction study

INTERCEPT
incomplete infarction trial of European research collaborators evaluating prognosis post-thrombolysis

INTERMAP
international study of macronutrients and blood pressure

INTERSALT
international study of salt and blood pressure

INTIMA
infusion of tissue plasminogen activator in myocardial infarction at the acute phase study

In-TIME
intravenous lanoteplase for treating infarcting myocardium early trial

INTRO-AMI
Integrilin and reduced dose of thrombolysis in acute myocardial infarction

INVEST
international verapamil SR/trandolapril study

IPPHS
international primary pulmonary hypertension study

IPPPSH
international prospective primary prevention study in hypertension

IRAD
International Registry of Aortic Dissection

IRAS
insulin resistance atherosclerosis study

IRBOT
oral glycoprotein IIb/IIIa receptor blockade to inhibit thrombosis trial

IRIS
Isostent for reperfusion intervention study

IRS
invasive reperfusion study

ISAM
intravenous streptokinase in acute myocardial infarction trial

ISAR
intracoronary stenting and antithrombotic regimen trial

ISCAB
Israeli coronary artery bypass study

ISCOAT
Italian study on complications of oral anticoagulant therapy

ISHT
international society for heart transplantation registry

ISIS
international study of infarct survival

ITPASMT
international tissue plasminogen activator/streptokinase mortality trial

ITS
Israeli thrombolytic survey

IVUS/QCA
intravascular ultrasound quantitative coronary angiography study

JIMI
Japanese intervention trial in myocardial infarction

JLRCPS
Jerusalem lipid research clinic prevalence study

JNC-V
Fifth Report of the Joint National Committee on Detection, Evaluation and Treatment of
  High Blood Pressure

JNC-VI
Sixth Report of the Joint National Committee on Detection, Evaluation and Treatment of
  High Blood Pressure

KAMI
Koch acute myocardial infarction study

KAMIT
Kentucky acute myocardial infarction trial

KAPS
Kuopio atherosclerosis prevention study

KAT
Kuopio angioplasty gene transfer trial

KIHD
Kuopio ischemic heart disease risk factor study

KISS
Kobe idiopathic cardiomyopathy survival study

KUMIS
Kumamoto University myocardial infarction study

KYSMI
Kyoto Shiga myocardial infarction study

LAPIS
late potentials in myocardial infarction study

LARA
low-dose aspirin trial on restenosis after angioplasty

LARS
laser angioplasty in restenosed stents trial

LASAR
local alcohol and stent against restenosis trial

LASTLHY
Latin American study of lacidipine in hypertension

LATE
late assessment of thrombolytic efficacy trial

LAVA
laser angioplasty versus angioplasty
Leiden artificial valves and anticoagulation study

LBS
Lübeck blood pressure study

L-CAPS
low-density lipoprotein coronary atherosclerosis prospective study

LCAS
lipoprotein and coronary atherosclerosis study

LEET
low-energy Endotak trial

LET
losartan effectiveness and tolerability study

LHIPS
local heparin infusion prestenting trial

LHS
losartan hemodynamic study

LHT
lifestyle heart trial

LIFE
losartan intervention for endpoint reduction in hypertension trial

LIHPS
local delivery of heparin in stenting for suboptimal result or threatened closure post-
percutaneous transluminal coronary angioplasty using the local med InfusaSleeve

LIMIT
Leicester intravenous magnesium intervention trial

LIMIT-AMI
double blind, placebo controlled, multicenter angiographic trial of rhuMAb CD18 in acute
myocardial infarction

LIMITS
Liquaemin in myocardial infarction during thrombolysis with
saruplase trial

LIPID
long-term intervention with pravastatin in ischemic disease trial

LIPS
Lescol intervention prevention study

LISA
Lescol in severe atherosclerosis trial

LIT
Leiden intervention trial with vegetarian diet for coronary atherosclerosis
Lopressor intervention trial

LIVE
left ventricular hypertrophy indapamide versus enalapril trial

LOMIR-MCT-IL
Lomir (isradipine) multicenter study in Israel

LOT
long-term outcome after thrombolysis study

LPS
lovastatin pravastatin study

LRC-CDPT
lipid research clinics coronary drugs project trial

LRC-CPPT
lipid research clinics coronary primary prevention trial

LRC-MFS
lipid research clinics mortality followup study

LRT
lovastatin restenosis trial

L-TAP
lipid treatment assessment project

MAAS
multicenter antiatherosclerosis study
multicenter antiatheroma study

MABIS
Munich and Berlin infarction study

MACAS
Marburg cardiomyopathy study

MADAM
moexipril as antihypertensive drug after menopause study

MADIT/CES
multicenter automatic defibrillator implantation trial
  cost/effectiveness study

MAGIC
magnesium in cardiac arrest trial
magnesium in coronaries trial

MAGICA
magnesium in cardiac arrhythmia trial

MAJIC
Mayo Japan investigation on chronic total occlusion

MAPHY
metoprolol atherosclerosis prevention in hypertension study

MAPPET
management strategy and prognosis of pulmonary embolism trial

MAPS
multivessel angioplasty prognosis study

MARCATOR
multicenter American research trial with cilazapril after angioplasty to prevent transluminal
  coronary obstruction and restenosis

MARISA
monotherapy assessment of ranolazine in stable angina trial

MARS
monitored atherosclerosis regression study

MASS
medicine, angioplasty or surgery study

MAST
managing anticoagulation services trial

MATE
medicine versus angiography for thrombolytic exclusions trial

MATH
modern approach to treatment of hypertension study

MATTIS
multicenter aspirin and ticlopidine trials after intracoronary stenting

MAVERIC
Midlands trial of empirical amiodarone versus electrophysiological guided intervention and cardioverter implant in ventricular arrhythmias

MBVT
Munich and Berlin trial for sustained ventricular tachyarrhythmias

MCBIT
Munich coronary bypass intervention trial

MCS
Minnesota coronary survey

MCSDT
Minnesota coronary survey dietary trial

McSPI
multicenter study of perioperative ischemia

MDC
metoprolol in dilated cardiomyopathy trial
multicenter dilated cardiomyopathy trial

MDIPT
multicenter diltiazem postinfarction trial

MEADOW
method alternative, distal occlusion and washout in saphenous vein graft study

MEHP
metoprolol in elderly hypertensive patients study

MELODHY
metoprolol low dose in hypertension study

MENTOR
Medtronic Wiktor Hepamed stent trial

MERCATOR
multicenter European research trial with cilazapril after angioplasty to prevent transluminal
  coronary obstruction and restenosis

MERIT-HF
metoprolol controlled-release randomized intervention trial in heart failure

MEXIS
metoprolol and xamoterol infarction study

M-HART
Montreal heart attack readjustment trial

M-HEART
multihospital eastern Atlantic restenosis trial

MHFT
Munich mild heart failure trial

MHHP
Minnesota heart health program

MHHS
Minnesota heart health survey

MHS
Minnesota heart survey

MIAMI
metoprolol in acute myocardial infarction study

MICOL
multicenter Italian study of cholesterol

MICRO-HOPE
microalbuminuria, cardiovascular and renal outcomes, heart outcomes prevention evaluation

MICS
myocardial infarction cost study

MIDAS
multicenter isradipine diuretic atherosclerosis study
myocardial infarction data acquisition system study

MILIS
multicenter investigation of the limitations of infarct size

MIMS
migraine and myocardial ischemia study

MINT
myocardial infarction with Novastan and tissue plasminogen activator study

MIOS
myocardial infarction onset study

MIRACL
myocardial ischemia reduction with aggressive cholesterol lowering study

MIRRACLE
myocardial infarction risk recognition and conversion of life-threatening events into
  survival trial

MIRSA
multicenter international randomized study of angina pectoris

MiSAD
Milan study on atherosclerosis and diabetes

MISNES
multicenter Italian study on neonatal electrocardiography and sudden infant death
  syndrome

MIST
mibefradil ischemia suppression trial
multicenter isradipine salt trial

MITI
myocardial infarction triage and intervention project

MITRA
maximal individual therapy in acute myocardial infarction

MLCCHF
multicenter lisinopril captopril congestive heart failure study

MMIRG
multicenter myocardial ischemia research group

MMTT
multicenter myocarditis treatment trial

MOCHA
multicenter oral carvedilol in heart failure assessment

MONICA
monitoring trends and determinants in cardiovascular diseases

MOST
mode selection trial in sinus node dysfunction

M-PATHY
multicenter pacing therapy for hypertrophic cardiomyopathy
multicenter study of pacing therapy for hypertrophic cardiomyopathy

MPIP
multicenter postinfarction program

MPPCD
multifactorial primary prevention of cardiovascular diseases

MPRG
multicenter postinfarction research group

MRC/BHF
medical research council, British Heart Foundation protection study

MRFIT
multiple risk factor intervention trial

MR-PET
magnetic resonance versus positron emission tomography for detection of myocardial viability study

MSHT
Mount Sinai hypertension trial

MSMI
multicenter study of myocardial ischemia

MSSMI
multicenter study of silent myocardial ischemia

MTT
myocarditis treatment trial

MUSCAT
MUSIC criteria for stent implantation using the controlled angioplasty technology catheter

MUSIC
multicenter ultrasound during stent implantation in coronary arteries study
multicenter ultrasound stent in coronary artery disease study
multicentre ultrasound study in coronaries

MUST
multicenter stent study

MUST
multicenter stents ticlopidine study
multicenter ultrasound study with Ticlid

MUST-EECP
multicenter study of enhanced external counterpulsation

MUSTIC
multisite stimulation in cardiac insufficiency
multisite stimulation in cardiomyopathy

MUSTT
multicenter unstable tachycardia trial
multicenter unsustained tachycardia trial

NACI
new applications for coronary interventions registry
new approaches to coronary interventions registry

NACI DCA
new approaches to coronary interventions registry directional coronary
atherectomy study

NAMIS
nifedipine angina myocardial infarction study

N-CAP
nifedipine gastrointestinal therapeutic system circadian antiischemic program

NDHS
national diet-heart study

NEAT
neurohumoral effects in acute myocardial infarction of trandolapril study

NEET
Nordic enalapril exercise trial

NEWDILTIL
new diltiazem versus Tildiem study

NEXT
new European XT stent registry

NHAAP
national heart attack alert program

NHBPCC
national high blood pressure coordinating committee

NHBPEP
national high blood pressure education program

NHLBI II
national heart, lung and blood institute type II coronary intervention study

NHLBI-ICD
National Heart, Lung and Blood Institute implantable cardioverter defibrillator trial

NHLBI-PTCA
National Heart, Lung and Blood Institute percutaneous transluminal coronary angioplasty
registry

NHLBITS
National Heart, Lung and Blood Institute twin study

NHP
national hypertension project (Egypt)

NHS-1
first natural history study of congenital heart defects

NHS-2
second natural history study of congenital heart defects

NICOLE
nisoldipine in coronary artery disease in Leuven

NIHS
National Institute of Hypertension Studies

NIR
new intravascular rigid stent trial

NNLIT
north Norwegian lidocaine intervention trial

NNMT
Norwegian nifedipine multicenter trial

NORDIL
Nordic diltiazem study

NOWIS
North Wurttemberg infarction study

NPHDO
nadroparin posthopsital discharge in orthopedy study

NPHS
Northwick Park heart study

NRICR
national registry of inhospital cardiopulmonary resuscitation

NUAPS
national unstable angina pectoris study

OARS
optimal atherectomy restenosis study

OASIS
organization to assess strategies for ischemic syndromes

OAT
Ochanomizu aspirin trial
open artery trial

OCBAS
optimal coronary balloon angioplasty versus stent trial
optimal coronary balloon angioplasty with provisional stenting versus primary stent trial

OCS
Oxford cholesterol study

OD-1
organ disease 1 coronary atherosclerosis multicenter study

ODES
Oslo diet and exercise study

OHS
Oslo hypertension study

OHT
Oslo heart trial

OIS
Olso ischemia study

OPTICUS
optimization with intracoronary ultrasound to reduce stent restenosis trial

OPTIMAAL
optimal trial in myocardial infarction with angiotensin II antagonist losartan

OPTIME
outcomes of a prospective trial of intravenous milrinone for exacerbations

OPTIME CHF
outcomes of a prospective trial of intravenous milrinone for exacerbations of chronic heart failure

OPUS
orbofiban in patients with unstable coronary syndromes study

OSCAR
olive oil, safflower oil, canola oil and rapeseed oil dietary study

OSDAT
Oslo study diet and antismoking trial

OSIRIS
optimization study of infarct reperfusion investigated by ST monitoring

OSTI
optimal stent implantation trial

OUTCLAS
outpatient coronary low profile angioplasty study

OXMIS
Oxford myocardial infarction incidence study

PA3
atrial pacing periablation for paroxysmal atrial fibrillation trial

PAC-A-TACH
pacemaker atrial tachycardia trial

PACCO
pulmonary artery catheterization and clinical outcomes study

PACCS
prospective army coronary calcium study

PACE
pacing and clinical electrophysiology
prevention with low-dose aspirin of cardiovascular diseases in the elderly study

PACIFIC
potential angina class improvement from intramyocardial channels

PACK
prevention of atherosclerotic complications with ketanserin study

PACT
plasminogen activator angioplasty compatibility trial
plasminogen activator coronary angioplasty trial
prehospital application of coronary thrombolysis study
prospective acute coronary syndrome trial
prourokinase in acute coronary thrombosis study

PAD-I
public access defibrillation I trial

PAFAC
prevention of atrial fibrillation after cardioversion study

PAFIT
paroxysmal atrial fibrillation Italian trial

PAFT
propafenone atrial fibrillation trial

PAIMS
plasminogen activator Italian multicenter study

PAIS
pravastatin in acute ischemic syndromes study

PAIVS
pulmonary atresia with intact ventricular septum collaborative study

PAMI
primary angioplasty in myocardial infarction trial

PAMI-No SOS
primary angioplasty in myocardial infarction with no surgery on site

PARADIGM
platelet aggregation receptor antagonist dose investigation for perfusion gain in myocardial
  infarction study

PARADISE
platelet IIb/IIIa antagonism for the reduction of acute coronary events dose investigation and
  safety evaluation study

PARAGON
platelet IIb/IIIa antagonism for the reduction of acute coronary events in a global
  organization network study

PARAT
prevention of arterial restenosis angiographic trial

PARIS
Persantine and aspirin reinfarction study
effect of ACE inhibitors on angiographic restenosis from PARIS investigators

PARK
postangioplasty restenosis ketanserin study
prevention of angioplasty reocclusion with ketanserin

PART
prevention of atherosclerosis with ramipril therapy trial
probucol angioplasty restenosis trial

PART-1
predictors of atherosclerosis risk and thrombosis trial

PART-2
predictors of atherosclerosis risk and thrombosis trial

PAS
Paragon (stent) elective or acute stent trial
Polish amiodarone study

PASE
pacemaker selection in the elderly trial

PASS
practical applicability of saruplase study
prehospital applicability of saruplase study

PASTA
percutaneous ambulatory stent trial
primary angioplasty versus stent implantation in acute myocardial infarction trial

PAD
Polish amiodarone trial

PATAF
prevention of arterial thromboembolism in nonvalvular atrial fibrillation study
primary prevention of arterial thromboembolic processes in atrial fibrillation trial

PATE
pravastatin antiatherosclerosis trial in the elderly

PATENT
prourokinase and tissue plasminogen activator enhancement of thrombolysis trial

PATHS
prevention and treatment of hypertension study

PATS
poststroke antihypertensive treatment study
prehospital administration of tissue plasminogen activator study

P2C2 HIV
pediatric pulmonary and cardiac complications of vertically transmitted HIV infection study

PCMR
pediatric cardiomyopathy registry

PCS
prevention of coronary atherosclerosis study

PDAY
pathological determinants of atherosclerosis in youth study

PDAY/RFEHA
pathobiological determinants of atherosclerosis in youth/risk factors in early human atherogenesis study

PEACH
physiologic evaluation after coronary hyperemia trial

PECTE
pulmonary embolism Colfarit trial in the elderly

PEGASUS
percutaneous endarterectomy, the goal of atherectomy successfully guided by ultrasound trial

PEPP
pregnancy exposures and preeclampsia prevention project

PERFEXT
perfusion, performance, exercise trial

PERM
prospective evaluation of perfusion markers study

PHARM
pharmacist in heart failure: assessment, recommendation and monitoring study

PHASE
prehospital arrest survival evaluation

PHHP
Pawtucket heart health program

PHYLLIS
plaque hypertension lipid-lowering Italian study

PICO
pimobendan in congestive heart failure study

PICS
pacing in cardiomyopathy study

PICTURE
post-intracoronary treatment ultrasound results evaluation study

PIG
Polaris investigator group

PILOT
Polish intramural low molecular weight heparin outpatient stent trial
preliminary investigation of local therapy

PIOPED
prospective investigation of pulmonary embolism diagnosis data base

PISA-PED
prospective investigative study of acute pulmonary embolism diagnosis

PLAC
pravastatin limitation in atherosclerosis in the coronary arteries study

PLAC-2
pravastatin, lipids and atherosclerosis in the carotid arteries study

PLEXES
pacing lead explant with excimer sheath study

PLM
prevention of mortality with low-molecular weight heparin in medical patients study

PLOSA
physiologic low-stress angioplasty trial

PLS
postsurgery Logiparin study

PMNSG
pravastatin multinational study group

PMS
pravastatin multinational study

POEM
patency, outcomes and economics of MIDCAB grafting

POLISH
Polish investigators to evaluate the effect of amiodarone on mortality after myocardial
  infarction

Pol-MONICA
Polish monitoring trends and determinants in cardiovascular diseases study

POLONIA
Polish-American local Lovenox-NIR stent assessment study

POSCH
program on surgical control of hyperlipidemia

POSSUM
physiological and operative severity score for the enumeration of morbidity and mortality study

POST
predictors and outcomes of stent thrombosis study

POST-CABG
postcoronary artery bypass graft study

PPP
prospective pravastatin pooling project

PPS
Paris prospective study

PQRST
probucol quantitative regression Swedish trial

PRACTICAL
placebo-controlled randomized ACE inhibition comparative trial in cardiac infarction and
left ventricular function

PRAGUE
primary angioplasty after transfer of patients from general community hospitals to
catheterization units with or without emergency thrombolytic infusion study

PRAISE
prospective randomized amlodipine survival evaluation

PREDICT
prospective randomized evaluation of diltiazem CD trial

PREFACE
pravastatin-related effects following angioplasty on coronary endothelium study

PREFER
patient randomized to either femoral or radial catheterization

PREMIS
prehospital myocardial infarction study

PRESERVE
prospective randomized enalapril study evaluating regression of ventricular enlargement

PREVENT
proliferation reduction using vascular energy trial
prospective randomized evaluation of the vascular effects of Norvasc trial

PRIDE

platelet aggregation and receptor occupancy with Integrilin-A dynamic evaluation study
primary implantable defibrillator study

PRIME

promotion of reperfusion by inhibition of thrombin during myocardial infarction evaluation
  study
promotion of reperfusion in myocardial infarction evolution study
prospective randomized ibopamine mortality evaluation study
prospective randomized study of ibopamine on mortality and efficacy in heart failure

PRIMI

prourokinase in myocardial infarction trial

PRISAM

primary stenting for acute myocardial infarction

PRISM

platelet receptor inhibition in ischemic syndrome management study

PRISM-PLUS

platelet receptor inhibition in ischemic syndrome management in patients limited by
  unstable signs and symptoms study

PROBE

prospective, randomized, open blinded endpoint trial
prospective randomized, open trial with blinded endpoint evaluation

PROCAM

prospective cardiovascular Münster study

PROMISE

prospective randomized milrinone survival evaluation study

PROSPECT

Proscar safety plus efficacy Canadian two-year study

PROSPER

prospective study of pravastatin in the elderly at risk

PROTECT

prospective reinfarction in the thrombolytic era Cardizem-CD trial

PROVED

prospective randomized study of ventricular failure and the efficacy of
  digoxin

PSAAMI

primary stenting versus angioplasty in acute myocardial infarction trial

PSTAF

pilsicainide suppression trial of atrial fibrillation

PURSUIT
platelet glycoprotein IIb/IIIa underpinning the receptor for suppression of unstable ischemia trial
platelet glycoprotein IIb/IIIa in unstable angina, receptor suppression using Integrilin therapy

QCS
Quebec cardiovascular study

QHFT
quinapril heart failure trial

QOLHS
quality of life hypertension study

QUADS
quinapril Australian dosing study

QUASAR
quinapril antiischemia and symptoms of angina reduction trial

QUEXTRA
quantitative exercise testing and angiography study

QUIET
quinapril ischemic event trial

RAAMI
randomized angiographic trial of alteplase in myocardial infarction
rapid administration of alteplase in myocardial infarction trial

RAAS
randomized angiotensin II receptor antagonist, angiotensin-converting enzyme inhibitor study

RACE
ramipril cardioprotective evaluation trial
rapid amplification of complementary deoxyribonucleic acid ends
rapid assessment of cardiac enzymes

RADIANCE
randomized assessment of digoxin on inhibitors of angiotensin-converting enzyme study

RAFT
recurrent atrial fibrillation trial
Rythmol-SR atrial fibrillation trial

RALES
randomized aldactone evaluation study investigators

RaMI
Ravenna myocardial infarction trial

RAMIT
Ravenna myocardial infarction trial

RAPID
recombinant plasminogen activator angiographic phase II international dose finding study
regional Arizona prehospital infarction diagnosis study
reteplase angiographic patency international dose-ranging study

RAPT
ridogrel versus aspirin potency trial

RAVES
reduced anticoagulation in saphenous vein graft stent trial
reduced anticoagulation vein graft study

REACH
research on endothelin antagonism in chronic heart failure
resource utilization in congestive heart failure study

RECREATE
rescue of closed arteries treated by stent for threatened or abrupt closure study

REDUCE
randomized double-blind unfractionated heparin and placebo-controlled multicenter trial
restenosis reduction by cutting balloon evaluation study

REFLECT-1
randomized evaluation of flosequinan on exercise tolerance, initial efficacy trial

REFLECT-2
randomized evaluation of flosequinan on exercise tolerance, dose response study

REFLEX
randomized evaluation of flosequinan on exercise tolerance study
restenosis rates with flexible GFX stents study

REFSA
randomized European femoral stent versus angioplasty trial

RENEWAL
randomized trial of endoluminal reconstruction using the NIR stent or Wallstent in
  angioplasty of long segment disease

REPAIR
reperfusion in acute infarction, Rotterdam study

RES
reproducibility echocardiography study

RESCUE
randomized evaluation of salvage angioplasty with combined utilization of endpoints trial

RESIST
restenosis after intravascular ultrasound-guided stenting study

REST
restenosis stent trial

RESTORE
randomized efficacy study of tirofiban for outcomes and restenosis trial

RETA
registry for the endovascular treatment of aneurysms

RIGHT
cerivastatin gemfibrozil hyperlipidemia treatment study

RISC
research group on instability in coronary artery disease study

RITA
randomized intervention treatment of angina (UK)

RITED
Italian registry of echo-dobutamine tests

ROBUST
recanalization of occluded bypass graft with prolonged urokinase infusion site trial

ROCKET
regionally organized cardiac key European trial

ROMIO
rule out myocardial infarct observation study

ROSETTA
routine versus selective exercise treadmill test after angioplasty trial

ROSTER
rotational atherectomy versus balloon angioplasty for in-stent restenosis trial

ROTASTENT
rotational atherectomy with adjunctive stenting trial

RS
Reykjavik study

RUTH
raloxifene use for the heart study

4S
Scandinavian simvastatin survival study group

SABER
stent-assisted balloon angioplasty and its effects on restenosis study

SAFE-PACE
syncope and falls in the elderly, role of pacemaker study

SAFIRE-D
symptomatic atrial fibrillation investigation and randomized evaluation of dofetilide study

SAGES
signal-averaged electrocardiographic study

SAHCS
streptokinase, aspirin, heparin collaborative study

SAHS
San Antonio heart study

SALAD
surgery versus angioplasty for proximal left anterior descending coronary artery stenosis trial

SALT
Swedish aspirin in low dose trial

SALTS
strategic alternatives with ticlopidine in stenting study

SAMI
streptokinase and angioplasty in myocardial infarction trial
streptokinase in acute myocardial infarction study

SAMII
survey of acute myocardial ischemia and infarction study

SAMIT
streptokinase and angioplasty myocardial infarction trial

SAMPLE
study on ambulatory monitoring of pressure and lisinopril evaluation

SAPAT
Swedish angina pectoris aspirin trial

SAPPHIRE
Stanford Asian Pacific program in hypertension and insulin resistance

SAPS
San Antonio Rotablator study

SAS
Scandinavian Angiopeptin study

SAT
saruplase alteplase study

SATE
safety antiarrhythmic trial evaluation

SAVE
survival and ventricular enlargement trial

SCAMP
Stanford coronary artery monitoring project

SCAT
simvastatin and enalapril coronary atherosclerosis trial

SCD-HeFT
sudden cardiac death in heart failure

SCD-HeFT
trial of prophylactic amiodarone versus implantable defibrillator therapy

SCIV
subcutaneous versus intravenous heparin in deep venous thrombosis study

SCORES
stent comparative restenosis trial

SCRIP
Stanford coronary risk intervention project

SCRIPPS
Scripps coronary radiation to inhibit proliferation poststenting trial

SEARCH
study of the effectiveness of additional reductions of cholesterol and homocysteine

SECURE
study to evaluate carotid ultrasound changes in patients treated with ramipril and vitamin E

SELCA
smooth excimer laser coronary angioplasty study

SENDCAP
St. Mary's Ealing, Northwick Park diabetes cardiovascular prevention study

SEQOL
substudy of economics and quality of life

SESAM
study in Europe of saruplase and alteplase in myocardial infarction

SHARE
study of heart assessment and risk in ethnic groups

SHARP
Scottish heart and arterial disease risk prevention program
subcutaneous heparin in angioplasty restenosis prevention trial

SHAVE
steerable housing for atherovascular excision

SHEP
systolic hypertension in the elderly program

SHHS
Scottish heart health study
sleep heart health study

SHIPS
Shiga pravastatin study

SHOCK
should we emergently revascularize occluded coronaries for cardiogenic shock, international
  randomized trial

SHOT
shunt occlusion trial

SHP
Skaraborg hypertension project

SHS
strong heart study

SHVRC
Shiley heart valve research center project

SIAM
streptokinase in acute myocardial infarction study

SICCO
stenting in chronic coronary occlusion study

SIHDSPS
Stockholm ischemic heart disease secondary prevention study

SIMA
stenting versus internal mammary artery for single left anterior descending arterial lesion
  trial

SIPS
strategy for intracoronary ultrasound-guided percutaneous transluminal coronary angioplasty
  and stenting trial

SISA
stenting in small arteries trial

SISAMI
silent ischemia in survivors of acute myocardial infarction study

SISH
stage I systolic hypertension in the elderly study

SISTEMI
Southern Italian study on thrombolysis early in myocardial infarction

SKDAMI
streptokinase plus desmopressin in acute myocardial infarction study

SKHYDIP
Skara hypertension and diabetes project

SMART
self-measurement for assessment of the response to trandolapril study
study of medicine versus angioplasty reperfusion trial
study of Microstent's ability to limit restenosis trial

SMARTT
serum markers, acute myocardial infarction and rapid treatment trial

SMASH
Swiss multicenter evaluation of early angioplasty for shock

SMILE
survival of myocardial infarction, long-term evaluation study

SMISS
silent myocardial ischemia stress study

SMS
simvastatin multicenter study

SMT
Stockholm metoprolol trial

SNAP
study of nitroglycerin and chest pain

SNaP
study of sodium and blood pressure

SNAPE
study of nicorandil in angina pectoris in the elderly

SOAR
safety of orbofiban in acute coronary research study

SOCIAIDS
study of cardiac involvement in acquired immunodeficiency syndrome

SOCRATES
study of coronary revascularization and therapeutic evaluations

SOLD
stenting after optimal lesion debulking trial

SOLVD
studies of left ventricular dysfunction

SoS
stent or surgery study

SPACTO
stent versus percutaneous angioplasty in chronic total occlusion trial

SPAF TEE
stroke prevention in atrial fibrillation, transesophageal echo study

SPICE
study of patients intolerant to converting enzyme inhibitors

SPICED TEAS
study of pacemakers and implantable cardioverter defibrillator triggering by electronic article
  surveillance devices

SPINAF
stroke prevention in nonrheumatic atrial fibrillation study

SPIR
study of perioperative ischemia research

SPIRIT
salvage from perindopril in reperfused infarction trial
stroke prevention in reversible ischemia trial

SPORT
stent implantation postrotational atherectomy trial

SPRINT
secondary prevention of reinfarction Israeli nifedipine trial

SPRS
sixty plus reinfarction study

SPRT
sixty plus reinfarction trial

STAMI
stenting for acute myocardial infarction study

STAMP
systemic thrombolysis in acute myocardial infarction with prourokinase and urokinase trial

STARS
stent anticoagulation regimen study
stent antithrombolytic regimen study
stent anticoagulation restenosis study
St. Thomas atherosclerosis regression study

START
saruplase and taprostene acute reocclusion trial
St. Thomas atherosclerosis regression trial
stent versus angioplasty restenosis trial
stent versus directional coronary atherectomy randomized trial

STAT
stent thrombosis after ticlopidine study

STATRS
stent antithrombotic regimen study

STENT-BY
stent versus bypass surgery for vessels undergoing abrupt closure trial

STENTIM
stenting in acute myocardial infarction study

STENT PAMI
stent primary angioplasty for myocardial infarction

STEP
study of taprostene in elective percutaneous transluminal coronary angioplasty

STEPHY
Starnberg trial on epidemiology of parkinsonism and hypertension in the elderly

STEPS
significance of transesophageal electrocardiographic findings in prevention of stroke study

STEREO
stents and ReoPro trial

STIMIS
study of time intervals in myocardial ischemic syndromes

STIMS
Swedish ticlodipine multicenter study

STONE
Shanghai trial of nifedipine in the elderly

STOP
shunt thrombotic occlusion prevention by picotamide study
stenting for total occlusion and restenosis prevention study
study of hypertension in the elderly (Sweden)
Swedish trial in old patients with hypertension

STOP 2
Swedish trial in old patients with hypertension 2

STOP-AF
systematic trial of pacing to prevent atrial fibrillation

STOP-hypertension
Swedish trial in older patients with hypertension

STRATAS
study to determine Rotablator and transluminal angioplasty strategy

STRESS
stent restenosis study

STRETCH
symptom tolerability response to exercise trial of candesartan cilexetil in patients with heart failure

STRIP
special Turku coronary risk factor intervention project

SURE
serial ultrasound analysis of restenosis study

SUSHI
stent use is superior for hospitalized infarction patients study

SUTAMI
saruplase and urokinase in the treatment of acute myocardial infarction trial

SVTS
sotalol ventricular tachycardia study

SWEET
square wave endurance exercise trial

SWISH
Swedish isradipine study in hypertension

SWISSI
Swiss interventional study in silent ischemia

SYMPHONY
sibrafiban versus aspirin to yield maximum protection from ischemic heart events postacute coronary syndromes trial

SYST-CHINA
systolic hypertension in elderly Chinese trial

SYST-EUR
systolic hypertension in Europeans study

TACS
thrombolysis and angioplasty in cardiogenic shock study

TACT
ticlopidine angioplasty coronary trial
ticlopidine versus placebo for prevention of acute closure after angioplasty trial

TACTICS
thrombolysis and counterpulsation to improve cardiogenic shock survival trial

TACTICS-TIMI 18
treat angina with Aggrastat and determine cost of therapy with an invasive or conservative strategy, thrombolysis in myocardial infarction trial

TAIM
trial of antihypertensive intervention and management

TAM
total atherosclerosis management study

TAMI
thrombolysis and angioplasty in myocardial infarction study

TARGET
do tirofiban and ReoPro give similar efficacy trial

TASC
trial of angioplasty and stents in Canada

TASH
transcoronary ablation of septum hypertrophy study

TASMAN
thrombolysis anticoagulant study, Mediterranean, Australia, New Zealand

TASS
ticlopidine aspirin stroke study

TASTE
ticlopidine aspirin stent evaluation

TAUSA
thrombolysis and angioplasty in unstable angina trial

TAXUS II
paclitaxel-eluting stent study

TCG
thromboprophylaxis collaborative group

TCI
to come in (open heart surgery program at Cleveland Clinic)

TEAHAT
thrombolysis early in acute heart attack trial

TEAM
thrombolytic trial of Eminase in acute myocardial infarction

TECBEST
transluminal extraction catheter before stent study

TECSS
the European coronary surgery study

TEST
timolol, encainide, sotalol trial

THAMES
Tenormin in hypertension and myocardial ischemia epidemiological study

THAT
thrombolysis in acute myocardial infarction trial

THIS
tissue plasminogen activator heparin interaction study

THS
Tromso heart study
Turkish heart study

TIBBS
total ischemic burden bisoprolol study

TIBET
total ischemic burden European trial

TICO
thrombolysis in coronary occlusion study

TIG
thrombosis interest group study

TIM
triflusal in myocardial infarction study

TIME
treatment of infarcting myocardium early trial

TIMED
trials to investigate morning versus evening dosing
  (nisoldipine in hypertension)

TIMI IIIA
thrombolysis in myocardial ischemia trial

TIMI IIIB
thrombolysis in myocardial infarction trial

TIMI-7
thrombin inhibition in myocardial ischemia trial

TIMI-9
thrombolysis and thrombin inhibition in myocardial infarction trial

TIMIKO
thrombolysis in myocardial infarction in Korea study

TIMS
tertatolol international multicentre study

TIPE
thrombolysis in pulmonary embolism study

TIPS
transjugular intrahepatic portacaval shunt study

TOAT
the open artery trial

TOCC
total occlusion of coronary arteries, chronic study

TOHP
trial of hypertension prevention

TOLC
treatment of low-density lipoprotein-bound cholesterol study

TOMHS
treatment of mild hypertension study

TOMIIS
total occlusion postmyocardial infarction intervention study

TOP
thrombolysis in old patients study

TOPAS
thrombolysis or peripheral artery surgery study

TOPLIT
transluminal extraction catheter or percutaneous transluminal coronary angioplasty in
  thrombus study

TOPS
thrombolysis in old patients study
treatment of postthrombolytic stenosis study

TOSCA
total occlusion study in Canada

TOTAL
total occlusion trial with angioplasty by using laser guidewire

TPASK
tissue plasminogen activator versus streptokinase trial

TPAT
tissue plasminogen activator, Toronto trial

TPI
thrombolytic predictive instrument project

TRACE
trandolapril cardiac evaluation trial

TRANDA
trandolapril Andalusian study

TRANSFAIR
transfatty acids in food in Europe study

TRAP
twin reversed arterial perfusion study

TRAPIST
trapidil versus placebo to prevent in-stent intimal hyperplasia study

TREAT
tranilast restenosis following angioplasty trial

TRENT
trial of early nifedipine treatment of acute myocardial infarction

TRIC
thrombolysis with recombinant tissue plasminogen activator during instability in coronary artery disease trial

TRIM
thrombin inhibition in myocardial ischemia study

TRIMM
triggers and mechanisms of myocardial infarction study

TROPHY
treatment effects of lisinopril versus hydrochlorothiazide in obese patients with hypertension trial
treatment of obese patients with hypertension trial
trial of preventing hypertension

TTOPP
thrombolytic therapy in older patient population study

TUCC
tissue plasminogen activator/urokinase comparison in China study

TUGMI
Tsukuba University group for myocardial infarction

TWISTER
trial of within-stent treatment of endoluminal restenosis

UCARE, U-CARE
unexplained cardiac arrest registry of Europe

UD-AHF
UD-CG 115 BS in acute heart failure study

UKCSG
United Kingdom collaborative study group (timolol trial)

UKHAS
United Kingdom heart attack study

UKHEART
United Kingdom heart failure evaluation and assessment of risk trial

UK in USA
urokinase in unstable angina study

UKNCSPAIVS
United Kingdom national collaborative study of pulmonary atresia with intact ventricular septum

UKPACE
United Kingdom pacing and cardiovascular events study
United Kingdom pacing and clinical events study

UKSAT
United Kingdom small aneurysm trial

UK-TIA
United Kingdom transient ischemic attack (aspirin trial)

UKTSSA
United Kingdom transplant support service authority

ULTIMA
unprotected left main trunk intervention multicenter assessment

ULTRA
utilizing GFX 2.5 stent in small diameter arteries

UNASEM
unstable angina study using Eminase

UNRPCA
use of nicardipine to retard the progression of coronary atherosclerosis trial

UNSA
unstable angina study

UPET
urokinase pulmonary embolism trial

UPSIZE
ultrasound-controlled percutaneous transluminal coronary angioplasty with optimal balloon
  size study

URALMI
urokinase and alteplase in myocardial infarction study

USPET
urokinase streptokinase pulmonary embolism trial

UTOPIA
utilization of platelet inhibition in angina trial

VACA
valvuloplasty and angioplasty in congenital anomalies registry

VA-HIT
Veterans Affairs high-density lipoprotein intervention trial

Val-HeFT
valsartan heart failure trial

Val-HeFT Echocardiographic Study
valsartan benefits left ventricular structure and function in heart failure

VALIANT
valsartan in acute myocardial infarction study

VALUE
valsartan antihypertensive long-term use evaluation

VAS
verapamil angioplasty study

VASD
vascular access service database

VASPNAF
Veterans Administration stroke prevention in nonrheumatic atrial
  fibrillation study

VEGAS
vein graft AngioJet study

VERDI
verapamil versus diuretics trial

VERDICT
verapamil digoxin cardioversion trial

VHAS
verapamil in hypertension atherosclerosis study

V-HeFT
vasodilator heart failure trial
Veterans Administration heart failure trial

VIGOUR
virtual coordinating center for global collaborative cardiovascular research

VITA
Vicenza thrombophilia and atherosclerosis project

VOTE
value of transesophageal echocardiography study

VPS
vasovagal pacemaker study

VT-MASS
metoprolol and sotalol for sustained ventricular tachycardia study

WAAT
warfarin plus aspirin versus aspirin trial

WACS
women's atherosclerosis cardiovascular study

WAFUS
warfarin anticoagulation followup study

WALLSTENT-CABG
Wallstent European study on stenting for coronary artery bypass grafts

WARF
Wisconsin alumni research foundation

WARIS
warfarin reinfarction study

WARIS II
warfarin-aspirin reinfarction study, Norwegian

WASH
warfarin-aspirin study of heart failure

WATCH
warfarin antiplatelet trial in chronic heart failure
Worcester-area trial for counseling in hyperlipidemia

WCUS
Wiktor stent and cutting balloon angioplasty study

WELL-HART
women's estrogen/progestin and lipid-lowering hormone atherosclerosis
  regression trial

WEST
Western European stent trial

WHAS
women's heart attack study

WHAT
Worcester heart attack trial

WHO-ISH
World Health Organization/internation society of hypertension survey

WHS
women's health study

WHT
women's heart trial

WIN
Wallstent in native vessel study

WINS
Wallstent in saphenous vein grafts study

WISE
women's ischemic syndrome evaluation

WOLF
work, lipids, fibrinogen study

WOOFS
warfarin optimized outpatient followup study

WOSCOPS
prevention of coronary heart disease with pravastatin in men with hypercholesterolemia:
  West of Scotland coronary prevention study

WTH
women take heart project

WWICT
Western Washington intracoronary streptokinase trial

WWISK
Western Washington intracoronary streptokinase trial

WWIST
Western Washington intravenous streptokinase trial

WWIV
Western Washington intravascular streptokinase trial

WWIVSK
Western Washington intravenous streptokinase trial

WWSIMIT
Western Washington streptokinase in myocardial infarction trials

XAD
external atrial defibrillation trial

X-TRACT
X-Sizer for treatment of thrombus and atherosclerosis in coronary
  interventions trial

YCT
YMCA cardiac therapy program

YCVDS
Yugoslavia cardiovascular disease study

ZWOLLE
primary coronary angioplasty compared with intravenous streptokinase

AMERICAN HEART ASSOCIATION
SCIENTIFIC SESSIONS 2003 TRIALS

PAD
public access defibrillation trial

PRIMO-CABG
pexelizumab for the reduction of infarction and mortality in coronary artery bypass graft
  surgery

PAPABEAR
prophylactic amiodarone for the prevention of arrhythmias that begin early after
revascularization

PREVEND IT
prevention of renal and vascular endstage disease intervention trial

VALIANT
valsartan in acute myocardial infarction trial

ACUTE CORONARY SYNDROME
Antiplatelet Agent
   Aggrastat® [US/Can]
   eptifibatide
   Integrilin® [US/Can]
   tirofiban

ADAMS-STOKES SYNDROME
Adrenergic Agonist Agent
   Adrenalin® Chloride [US/Can]
   epinephrine
   isoproterenol
   Isuprel® [US]

ALVEOLAR PROTEINOSIS
Expectorant
   potassium iodide
   SSKI® [US]

ANESTHESIA (GENERAL)
Barbiturate
   Brevital® Sodium [US/Can]
   methohexital
General Anesthetic
   Amidate® [US/Can]
   desflurane
   Diprivan® [US/Can]
   enflurane
   Ethrane® [US]
   etomidate
   Forane® [US/Can]
   halothane
   isoflurane
   Ketalar® [US/Can]
   ketamine
   methoxyflurane
   Penthrane® [US/Can]
   propofol
   sevoflurane
   Sevorane AF™ [Can]
   Suprane® [US/Can]
   Ultane® [US]

ANESTHESIA (LOCAL)
Local Anesthetic
   Alcaine® [US/Can]
   Americaine® Anesthetic Lubricant [US]
   Americaine® [US-OTC]
   Ametop™ [Can]
   Anbesol® Baby [US/Can]
   Anbesol® Maximum Strength [US-OTC]
   Anbesol® [US-OTC]
   Anestacon® [US]
   Anusol® [US-OTC]
   Babee® Teething® [US-OTC]
   benzocaine
   benzocaine, butyl aminobenzoate, tetracaine, benzalkonium chloride
   benzocaine, gelatin, pectin, sodium carboxymethylcellulose
   Benzodent® [US-OTC]
   bupivacaine
   Carbocaine® [US/Can]
   Cepacol® Anesthetic Troches [US-OTC]
   Cepacol® Mouthwash/Gargle [US-OTC]
   Cetacaine® [US]
   cetylpyridinium
   cetylpyridinium and benzocaine
   Chiggerex® [US-OTC]
   Chiggertox® [US-OTC]
   chloroprocaine
   Citanest® Forte [Can]
   Citanest® Plain [US/Can]
   cocaine

Cylex® [US-OTC]
Dermaflex® Gel [US]
Detane® [US-OTC]
dibucaine
Diocaine® [Can]
Duranest® [US/Can]
Dyclone® [US]
dyclonine
ELA-Max® [US-OTC]
ethyl chloride
ethyl chloride and
    dichlorotetrafluoroethane
etidocaine
Fleet® Pain Relief [US-OTC]
Fluoracaine® [US]
Fluro-Ethyl® Aerosol [US]
Foille® Medicated First Aid
    [US-OTC]
Foille® Plus [US-OTC]
Foille® [US-OTC]
HDA® Toothache [US-OTC]
hexylresorcinol
Hurricaine® [US]
Isocaine® HCl [US]
Itch-X® [US-OTC]
lidocaine
lidocaine and epinephrine
Lidodan™ [Can]
Lidoderm® [US/Can]
LidoPen® Auto-Injector
    [US]
Marcaine® Spinal [US]
Marcaine® [US/Can]
mepivacaine
Mycinettes® [US-OTC]
Naropin™ [US/Can]
Nesacaine®-CE [Can]
Nesacaine®-MPF [US]
Nesacaine® [US]
Novocain® [US/Can]
Nupercainal® [US-OTC]
Ophthetic® [US]
Orabase®-B [US-OTC]

Orabase® With Benzocaine
    [US-OTC]
Orajel® Baby Nighttime
    [US-OTC]
Orajel® Baby [US-OTC]
Orajel® Maximum Strength
    [US-OTC]
Orajel® [US-OTC]
Orasol® [US-OTC]
Parcaine® [US]
Phicon® [US-OTC]
Polocaine® [US/Can]
Pontocaine® [US/Can]
Pontocaine® With Dextrose [US]
PrameGel® [US-OTC]
pramoxine
Prax® [US-OTC]
prilocaine
procaine
ProctoFoam® NS [US-OTC]
proparacaine
proparacaine and fluorescein
ropivacaine
Sensorcaine®-MPF [US]
Sensorcaine® [US/Can]
Solarcaine® Aloe Extra Burn Relief
    [US-OTC]
Solarcaine® [US-OTC]
Sucrets® Sore Throat [US-OTC]
Sucrets® [US-OTC]
tetracaine
tetracaine and dextrose
Trocaine® [US-OTC]
Tronolane® [US-OTC]
Tronothane® [US-OTC]
Xylocaine® [US/Can]
Xylocaine® With Epinephrine
    [US/Can]
Xylocard® [Can]
Zilactin® Baby [US/Can]
Zilactin®-B [US/Can]
Zilactin® [Can]
Zilactin-L® [US-OTC]

Local Anesthetic, Amide Derivative
 Chirocaine® [US/Can]
 levobupivacaine
Local Anesthetic, Injectable
 Chirocaine® [US/Can]
 levobupivacaine

ANGINA PECTORIS

Beta-Adrenergic Blocker
 acebutolol
 Alti-Nadolol [Can]
 Apo-Acebutolol [Can]
 Apo®-Atenol [Can]
 Apo®-Metoprolol [Can]
 Apo®-Nadol [Can]
 Apo®-Propranolol [Can]
 atenolol
 Betaloc® [Can]
 Betaloc® Durules®
 carvedilol
 Coreg® [US/Can]
 Corgard® [US/Can]
 Gen-Acebutolol [Can]
 Gen-Atenolol [Can]
 Gen-Metoprolol [Can]
 Inderal® LA [US/Can]
 Inderal® [US/Can]
 Lopressor® [US/Can]
 metoprolol
 Monitan® [Can]
 nadolol
 Novo-Acebutolol [Can]
 Novo-Atenol [Can]
 Novo-Metoprolol [Can]
 Novo-Nadolol [Can]
 Nu-Acebutolol [Can]
 Nu-Atenol
 Nu-Metop [Can]
 Nu-Propranolol [Can]
 PMS-Atenolol [Can]
 PMS-Metoprolol [Can]
 propranolol
 Rhotral [Can]

 Rhoxal-atenolol [Can]
 Sectral® [US/Can]
 Tenolin [Can]
 Tenormin® [US/Can]
 Toprol-XL® [US/Can]
Calcium Channel Blocker
 Adalat® CC [US]
 Adalat® XL® [Can]
 Alti-Diltiazem [Can]
 Alti-Diltiazem CD [Can]
 Alti-Verapamil [Can]
 amlodipine
 Apo®-Diltiaz [Can]
 Apo®-Diltiaz CD [Can]
 Apo®-Diltiaz SR [Can]
 Apo®-Nifed [Can]
 Apo®-Nifed PA [Can]
 Apo®-Verap [Can]
 bepridil
 Calan® SR [US]
 Calan® [US/Can]
 Cardene® IV [US]
 Cardene® SR [US]
 Cardene® [US]
 Cardizem® CD [US/Can]
 Cardizem® SR [US/Can]
 Cardizem® [US/Can]
 Cartia® XT [US]
 Chronovera® [Can]
 Covera® [Can]
 Covera-HS® [US]
 Dilacor® XR [US]
 Diltia® XT [US]
 diltiazem
 felodipine
 Gen-Diltiazem [Can]
 Gen-Verapamil [Can]
 Gen-Verapamil SR [Can]
 Isoptin® SR [US/Can]
 Isoptin® [US/Can]
 nicardipine
 Nifedical™ XL [US]
 nifedipine

Norvasc® [US/Can]
Novo-Diltazem [Can]
Novo-Diltazem SR [Can]
Novo-Nifedin [Can]
Novo-Veramil [Can]
Novo-Veramil SR [Can]
Nu-Diltiaz [Can]
Nu-Diltiaz-CD [Can]
Nu-Nifed [Can]
Nu-Verap [Can]
Plendil® [US/Can]
Procardia® [US/Can]
Procardia XL® [US]
Renedil® [Can]
Rhoxal-diltiazem SR [Can]
Syn-Diltiazem® [Can]
Tiazac® [US/Can]
Vascor® [US/Can]
verapamil
Verelan® PM [US]
Verelan® [US]
Vasodilator
amyl nitrite
Apo®-Dipyridamole FC [Can]
Apo®-ISDN [Can]
Cedocard®-SR [Can]
Dilatrate®-SR [US]
dipyridamole
Imdur® [US/Can]
Ismo® [US]
Isordil® [US]
isosorbide dinitrate
isosorbide mononitrate
Minitran™ [US/Can]
Monoket® [US]
Nitrek® [US]
Nitro-Bid® Ointment [US]
Nitro-Dur® [US/Can]
Nitrogard® [US]
nitroglycerin
Nitrolingual® [US]
Nitrol® [US/Can]
Nitrong® SR [Can]

NitroQuick® [US]
Nitrostat® [US/Can]
Nitro-Tab® [US]
NitroTime® [US]
Novo-Dipiradol [Can]
Persantine® [US/Can]
Transderm-Nitro® [Can]

ANGIOEDEMA (HEREDITARY)
Anabolic Steroid
stanozolol
Winstrol® [US]
Androgen
Cyclomen® [Can]
danazol
Danocrine® [US/Can]

ARRHYTHMIA
Adrenergic Agonist Agent
isoproterenol
Isuprel® [US]
phenylephrine
Antiarrhythmic Agent, Class I
Ethmozine® [US/Can]
moricizine
Antiarrhythmic Agent, Class I-A
Apo®-Procainamide [Can]
Apo®-Quinidine [Can]
disopyramide
Norpace® CR [US]
Norpace® [US/Can]
procainamide
Procanbid® [US]
Procan™ SR [Can]
Pronestyl-SR® [US/Can]
Pronestyl® [US/Can]
Quinaglute® Dura-Tabs® [US]
Quinidex® Extentabs® [US]
quinidine
Rythmodan® [Can]
Rythmodan®-LA [Can]
Antiarrhythmic Agent, Class I-B

lidocaine
mexiletine
Mexitil® [US/Can]
Novo-Mexiletine [Can]
phenytoin
tocainide
Tonocard® [US]
Xylocaine® [US/Can]
Xylocard® [Can]
Antiarrhythmic Agent, Class I-C
flecainide
propafenone
Rythmol® [US/Can]
Tambocor™ [US/Can]
Antiarrhythmic Agent, Class II
acebutolol
Alti-Sotalol [Can]
Apo-Acebutolol [Can]
Apo®-Propranolol [Can]
Apo®-Sotalol [Can]
Betapace AF™ [US/Can]
Betapace® [US]
Brevibloc® [US/Can]
esmolol
Gen-Acebutolol [Can]
Gen-Sotalol [Can]
Inderal® LA [US/Can]
Inderal® [US/Can]
Monitan® [Can]
Novo-Acebutolol [Can]
Novo-Sotalol [Can]
Nu-Acebutolol [Can]
Nu-Propranolol [Can]
Nu-Sotalol [Can]
PMS-Sotalol [Can]
propranolol
Rho®-Sotalol [Can]
Rhotral [Can]
Sectral® [US/Can]
Sorine™ [US]
Sotacor®
sotalol
Antiarrhythmic Agent, Class III

Alti-Amiodarone [Can]
Alti-Sotalol [Can]
amiodarone
Apo®-Sotalol [Can]
Betapace AF™ [US/Can]
Betapace® [US]
bretylium
Cordarone® [US/Can]
Corvert® [US]
dofetilide
Gen-Amiodarone [Can]
Gen-Sotalol [Can]
ibutilide
Novo-Amiodarone [Can]
Novo-Sotalol [Can]
Nu-Sotalol [Can]
Pacerone® [US]
PMS-Sotalol [Can]
Rho®-Sotalol [Can]
Sorine™ [US]
Sotacor®
sotalol
Tikosyn™ [US/Can]
Antiarrhythmic Agent, Class IV
Alti-Verapamil [Can]
Apo®-Verap [Can]
Calan® SR [US]
Calan® [US/Can]
Chronovera® [Can]
Covera® [Can]
Covera-HS® [US]
Gen-Verapamil [Can]
Gen-Verapamil SR [Can]
Isoptin® SR [US/Can]
Isoptin® [US/Can]
Novo-Veramil [Can]
Novo-Veramil SR [Can]
Nu-Verap [Can]
verapamil
Verelan® PM [US]
Verelan® [US]
Antiarrhythmic Agent, Miscellaneous
Adenocard® [US/Can]

Adenoscan® [US]
adenosine
Digitek® [US]
digoxin
Lanoxicaps® [US/Can]
Lanoxin® Pediatric [US]
Lanoxin® [US/Can]
Anticholinergic Agent
atropine
Calcium Channel Blocker
Alti-Diltiazem [Can]
Alti-Diltiazem CD [Can]
Apo®-Diltiaz [Can]
Apo®-Diltiaz CD [Can]
Apo®-Diltiaz SR [Can]
Cardizem® CD [US/Can]
Cardizem® SR [US/Can]
Cardizem® [US/Can]
Cartia® XT [US]
Dilacor® XR [US]
Diltia® XT [US]
diltiazem
Gen-Diltiazem [Can]
Novo-Diltazem [Can]
Novo-Diltazem SR [Can]
Nu-Diltiaz [Can]
Nu-Diltiaz-CD [Can]
Rhoxal-diltiazem SR [Can]
Syn-Diltiazem® [Can]
Tiazac® [US/Can]
Cholinergic Agent
edrophonium
Enlon® [US/Can]
Reversol® [US]
Tensilon® [US]
Theophylline Derivative
aminophylline
Phyllocontin®-350 [Can]
Phyllocontin® [Can]

ASCITES

Diuretic, Loop
Apo®-Furosemide [Can]

bumetanide
Bumex® [US/Can]
Burinex® [Can]
Demadex® [US]
Edecrin® [US/Can]
ethacrynic acid
Furocot® [US]
furosemide
Lasix® Special [Can]
Lasix® [US/Can]
torsemide
Diuretic, Miscellaneous
Apo®-Chlorthalidone [Can]
Apo®-Indapamide [Can]
chlorthalidone
Gen-Indapamide [Can]
indapamide
Lozide® [Can]
Lozol® [US/Can]
metolazone
Mykrox® [US/Can]
Novo-Indapamide [Can]
Nu-Indapamide [Can]
PMS-Indapamide [Can]
Thalitone® [US]
Zaroxolyn® [US/Can]
Diuretic, Potassium Sparing
Aldactone® [US/Can]
Novo-Spiroton [Can]
spironolactone
Diuretic, Thiazide
Apo®-Hydro [Can]
Aquacot® [US]
Aquatensen® [US/Can]
Aquazide H® [US]
bendroflumethiazide
chlorothiazide
Diuril® [US/Can]
Enduron® [US/Can]
Ezide® [US]
hydrochlorothiazide
Hydrocot® [US]
HydroDIURIL® [US/Can]

Metatensin® [Can]
methyclothiazide
Microzide™ [US]
Naqua® [US/Can]
Naturetin® [US]
Oretic® [US]
polythiazide
Renese® [US]
Trichlorex® [Can]
trichlormethiazide
Zide® [US]

ASPERGILLOSIS
Antifungal Agent
Abelcet® [US/Can]
Amphocin® [US]
Amphotec® [US]
amphotericin B cholesteryl sulfate
complex
amphotericin B (conventional)
amphotericin B lipid complex
Ancobon® [US/Can]
flucytosine
Fungizone® [US/Can]
VFEND® [US]
voriconazole
Antifungal Agent, Systemic
AmBisome® [US/Can]
amphotericin B liposomal
Cancidas® [US]
caspofungin

ASTHMA
Adrenal Corticosteroid
Alti-Beclomethasone [Can]
Alti-Dexamethasone [Can]
Apo®-Beclomethasone [Can]
Azmacort® [US]
beclomethasone
Decadron®-LA [US]
Decadron® [US/Can]
Decaject-LA® [US]
Decaject® [US]
dexamethasone (systemic)

Dexasone® L.A. [US]
Dexasone® [US/Can]
Dexone® LA [US]
Dexone® [US]
Flovent® Rotadisk® [US]
Flovent® [US]
fluticasone (oral inhalation)
Gen-Beclo [Can]
Hexadrol® [US/Can]
Nu-Beclomethasone [Can]
PMS-Dexamethasone [Can]
Propaderm® [Can]
QVAR™ [US/Can]
Rivanase AQ [Can]
triamcinolone (inhalation, oral)
Vanceril® [US/Can]
Adrenergic Agonist Agent
AccuNeb™ [US]
Adrenalin® Chloride [US/Can]
albuterol
Alti-Salbutamol [Can]
Alupent® [US]
Apo®-Salvent [Can]
bitolterol
Brethine® [US]
Bricanyl® [Can]
Bronchial Mist® [US]
ephedrine
epinephrine
isoetharine
isoproterenol
Isuprel® [US]
Levophed® [US/Can]
Maxair™ Autohaler™ [US]
Maxair™ [US]
metaproterenol
norepinephrine
Novo-Salmol [Can]
pirbuterol
Pretz-D® [US-OTC]
Primatene® Mist [US-OTC]
Proventil® HFA [US]
Proventil® Repetabs® [US]

Proventil® [US]
salmeterol
Serevent® Diskus® [US]
Serevent® [US/Can]
terbutaline
Tornalate® [US/Can]
Vaponefrin® [Can]
Ventolin® HFA [US]
Ventolin® [US]
Volmax® [US]
Anticholinergic Agent
   Alti-Ipratropium [Can]
   Apo®-Ipravent [Can]
   Atrovent® [US/Can]
   Gen-Ipratropium [Can]
   ipratropium
   Novo-Ipramide [Can]
   Nu-Ipratropium [Can]
   PMS-Ipratropium [Can]
Beta-2 Adrenergic Agonist Agent
   Advair™ Diskus® [US/Can]
   Berotec® [Can]
   fenoterol (Canada only)
   fluticasone and salmeterol
   Foradil® Aerolizer™ [US/Can]
   formoterol
Corticosteroid, Inhalant
   Advair™ Diskus® [US/Can]
   fluticasone and salmeterol
Leukotriene Receptor Antagonist
   Accolate® [US/Can]
   montelukast
   Singulair® [US/Can]
   zafirlukast
5-Lipoxygenase Inhibitor
   zileuton
   Zyflo™ [US]
Mast Cell Stabilizer
   Apo®-Cromolyn [Can]
   cromolyn sodium
   Intal® [US/Can]
   nedocromil (inhalation)
   Nu-Cromolyn [Can]

Tilade® [US/Can]
Theophylline Derivative
   Aerolate III® [US]
   Aerolate JR® [US]
   Aerolate SR® [US]
   aminophylline
   Apo®-Theo LA [Can]
   Choledyl SA® [US]
   Dilor® [US/Can]
   dyphylline
   Elixophyllin® GG [US]
   Elixophyllin® [US]
   Lufyllin® [US/Can]
   Neoasma® [US]
   Novo-Theophyl SR [Can]
   oxtriphylline
   Phyllocontin®-350 [Can]
   Phyllocontin® [Can]
   Quibron®-T/SR [US/Can]
   Quibron®-T [US]
   Quibron® [US]
   Slo-Phyllin® [US]
   Theo-24® [US]
   Theochron® [US]
   Theocon® [US]
   Theo-Dur® [US/Can]
   Theolair™ [US/Can]
   Theolate® [US]
   Theomar® GG [US]
   theophylline
   theophylline and guaifenesin
   T-Phyl® [US]
   Uniphyl® [US/Can]

ASTHMA (CORTICOSTEROID-DEPENDENT)
Macrolide (Antibiotic)
   Tao® [US]
   troleandomycin

ASTHMA (DIAGNOSTIC)
Diagnostic Agent

methacholine
Provocholine® [US/Can]

ATELECTASIS
Expectorant
  potassium iodide
  SSKI® [US]
Mucolytic Agent
  acetylcysteine
  Acys-5® [US]
  Mucomyst® [US/Can]
  Parvolex® [Can]

BACTERIAL ENDOCARDITIS (PROPHYLAXIS)
Aminoglycoside (Antibiotic)
  Alcomicin® [Can]
  Diogent® [Can]
  Garamycin® [US/Can]
  Garatec [Can]
  Gentak® [US]
  gentamicin
Antibiotic, Miscellaneous
  Alti-Clindamycin [Can]
  Cleocin HCl® [US]
  Cleocin Pediatric® [US]
  Cleocin Phosphate® [US]
  Cleocin® [US]
  Clindagel™ [US]
  clindamycin
  Dalacin® C [Can]
  Vancocin® [US/Can]
  Vancoled® [US]
  vancomycin
Cephalosporin (First Generation)
  Apo®-Cefadroxil [Can]
  Apo®-Cephalex [Can]
  Biocef® [US]
  cefadroxil
  cephalexin
  Duricef® [US/Can]
  Keflex® [US]

Keftab® [US/Can]
Novo-Cefadroxil [Can]
Novo-Lexin® [Can]
Nu-Cephalex® [Can]
Macrolide (Antibiotic)
  azithromycin
  Biaxin® [US/Can]
  Biaxin® XL [US]
  clarithromycin
  Zithromax® [US/Can]
  Z-PAK® [US/Can]
Penicillin
  amoxicillin
  Amoxicot® [US]
  Amoxil® [US/Can]
  ampicillin
  Apo®-Amoxi [Can]
  Apo®-Ampi [Can]
  Apo®-Pen VK [Can]
  Gen-Amoxicillin [Can]
  Lin-Amox [Can]
  Marcillin® [US]
  Moxilin® [US]
  Nadopen-V® [Can]
  Novamoxin® [Can]
  Novo-Ampicillin [Can]
  Novo-Pen-VK® [Can]
  Nu-Amoxi [Can]
  Nu-Ampi [Can]
  Nu-Pen-VK® [Can]
  penicillin V potassium
  Principen® [US]
  PVF® K [Can]
  Suspen® [US]
  Trimox® [US]
  Truxcillin® [US]
  Veetids® [US]
  Wymox® [US]

BLASTOMYCOSIS
Antifungal Agent
  Apo®-Ketoconazole [Can]
  itraconazole

ketoconazole
Nizoral® [US/Can]
Novo-Ketoconazole [Can]
Sporanox® [US/Can]

BRONCHIECTASIS

Adrenergic Agonist Agent
AccuNeb™ [US]
Adrenalin® Chloride [US/Can]
albuterol
Alti-Salbutamol [Can]
Alupent® [US]
Apo®-Salvent [Can]
Brethine® [US]
Bricanyl® [Can]
Bronchial Mist® [US]
ephedrine
epinephrine
isoproterenol
Isuprel® [US]
metaproterenol
Novo-Salmol [Can]
Pretz-D® [US-OTC]
Primatene® Mist [US-OTC]
Proventil® HFA [US]
Proventil® Repetabs® [US]
Proventil® [US]
terbutaline
Vaponefrin® [Can]
Ventolin® HFA [US]
Ventolin® [US]
Volmax® [US]
Mucolytic Agent
acetylcysteine
Acys-5® [US]
Mucomyst® [US/Can]
Parvolex® [Can]

BRONCHIOLITIS

Antiviral Agent
Rebetol® [US]
ribavirin
Virazole® [US/Can]

BRONCHITIS

Adrenergic Agonist Agent
AccuNeb™ [US]
Adrenalin® Chloride [US/Can]
albuterol
Alti-Salbutamol [Can]
Apo®-Salvent [Can]
bitolterol
Bronchial Mist® [US]
ephedrine
epinephrine
isoetharine
isoproterenol
Isuprel® [US]
Novo-Salmol [Can]
Primatene® Mist [US-OTC]
Proventil® HFA [US]
Proventil® Repetabs® [US]
Proventil® [US]
Tornalate® [US/Can]
Vaponefrin® [Can]
Ventolin® HFA [US]
Ventolin® [US]
Volmax® [US]
Antibiotic, Cephalosporin
cefditoren
Spectracef™ [US]
Antibiotic, Quinolone
ABC Pack™ (Avelox®) [US]
Avelox® [US/Can]
moxifloxacin
trovafloxacin
Trovan® [US/Can]
Cephalosporin (Third Generation)
cefdinir
Omnicef® [US/Can]
Mucolytic Agent
acetylcysteine
Acys-5® [US]
Mucomyst® [US/Can]
Parvolex® [Can]
Theophylline Derivative
Aerolate III® [US]

Aerolate JR® [US]
Aerolate SR® [US]
aminophylline
Apo®-Theo LA [Can]
Choledyl SA® [US]
Dilor® [US/Can]
dyphylline
Elixophyllin® GG [US]
Elixophyllin® [US]
Lufyllin® [US/Can]
Neoasma® [US]
Novo-Theophyl SR [Can]
oxtriphylline
Phyllocontin®-350 [Can]
Phyllocontin® [Can]
Quibron®-T/SR [US/Can]
Quibron®-T [US]
Quibron® [US]
Slo-Phyllin® [US]
Theo-24® [US]
Theochron® [US]
Theocon® [US]
Theo-Dur® [US/Can]
Theolair™ [US/Can]
Theolate® [US]
Theomar® GG [US]
theophylline
theophylline and guaifenesin
T-Phyl® [US]
Uniphyl® [US/Can]

BRONCHOSPASM

Adrenergic Agonist Agent
AccuNeb™ [US]
Adrenalin® Chloride [US/Can]
albuterol
Alti-Salbutamol [Can]
Alupent® [US]
Apo®-Salvent [Can]
bitolterol
Brethine® [US]
Bricanyl® [Can]
Bronchial Mist® [US]

ephedrine
epinephrine
isoetharine
isoproterenol
Isuprel® [US]
levalbuterol
Maxair™ Autohaler™
    [US]
Maxair™ [US]
metaproterenol
Novo-Salmol [Can]
pirbuterol
Pretz-D® [US-OTC]
Primatene® Mist [US-OTC]
Proventil® HFA [US]
Proventil® Repetabs® [US]
Proventil® [US]
salmeterol
Serevent® Diskus® [US]
Serevent® [US/Can]
terbutaline
Tornalate® [US/Can]
Vaponefrin® [Can]
Ventolin® HFA [US]
Ventolin® [US]
Volmax® [US]
Xopenex™ [US/Can]
Anticholinergic Agent
atropine
Beta-2 Adrenergic Agonist Agent
Foradil® Aerolizer™
    [US/Can]
formoterol
levalbuterol
Xopenex™ [US/Can]
Bronchodilator
levalbuterol
Xopenex™ [US/Can]
Mast Cell Stabilizer
Apo®-Cromolyn [Can]
cromolyn sodium
Intal® [US/Can]
Nu-Cromolyn [Can]

CACHEXIA
Progestin
Apo®-Megestrol [Can]
Lin-Megestrol [Can]
Megace® OS
Megace® [US/Can]
megestrol acetate
Nu-Megestrol [Can]

CARDIAC DECOMPENSATION
Adrenergic Agonist Agent
dobutamine
Dobutrex® [US/Can]

CARDIOGENIC SHOCK
Adrenergic Agonist Agent
dobutamine
Dobutrex® [US/Can]
dopamine
Intropin® [Can]
Cardiac Glycoside
Digitek® [US]
digoxin
Lanoxicaps® [US/Can]
Lanoxin® Pediatric [US]
Lanoxin® [US/Can]
CARDIOMYOPATHY
Cardiovascular Agent, Other
dexrazoxane
Zinecard® [US/Can]

CEREBROVASCULAR ACCIDENT (CVA)
Antiplatelet Agent
Alti-Ticlopidine [Can]
Apo®-ASA [Can]
Apo®-Ticlopidine [Can]
Asaphen [Can]
Asaphen E.C. [Can]
aspirin
Bayer® Aspirin Regimen Adult Low
Strength [US-OTC]
Bayer® Aspirin Regimen Adult Low
Strength with Calcium
[US-OTC]
Ecotrin® Low Adult Strength
[US-OTC]
Entrophen® [Can]
Gen-Ticlopidine [Can]
Halfprin® [US-OTC]
Novasen [Can]
Nu-Ticlopidine [Can]
Rhoxal-ticlopidine [Can]
Ticlid® [US/Can]
ticlopidine
Fibrinolytic Agent
Activase® rt-PA [Can]
Activase® [US]
alteplase
Cathflo™ Activase®
[US]

CHRONIC OBSTRUCTIVE PULMONARY DISEASE (COPD)
Adrenergic Agonist Agent
AccuNeb™ [US]
albuterol
Alti-Salbutamol [Can]
Alupent® [US]
Apo®-Salvent [Can]
isoproterenol
Isuprel® [US]
metaproterenol
Novo-Salmol [Can]
Proventil® HFA [US]
Proventil® Repetabs®
[US]
Proventil® [US]
Ventolin® HFA [US]
Ventolin® [US]
Volmax® [US]
Anticholinergic Agent
Alti-Ipratropium [Can]
Apo®-Ipravent [Can]

Atrovent® [US/Can]
Gen-Ipratropium [Can]
ipratropium
Novo-Ipramide [Can]
Nu-Ipratropium [Can]
PMS-Ipratropium [Can]
Bronchodilator
Combivent® [US/Can]
DuoNeb™ [US]
ipratropium and albuterol
Expectorant
potassium iodide
SSKI® [US]
Theophylline Derivative
Aerolate III® [US]
Aerolate JR® [US]
Aerolate SR® [US]
aminophylline
Apo®-Theo LA [Can]
Dilor® [US/Can]
dyphylline
Elixophyllin® GG [US]
Elixophyllin® [US]
Lufyllin® [US/Can]
Neoasma® [US]
Novo-Theophyl SR [Can]
Phyllocontin®-350 [Can]
Phyllocontin® [Can]
Quibron®-T/SR [US/Can]
Quibron®-T [US]
Quibron® [US]
Slo-Phyllin® [US]
Theo-24® [US]
Theochron® [US]
Theocon® [US]
Theo-Dur® [US/Can]
Theolair™ [US/Can]
Theolate® [US]
Theomar® GG [US]
theophylline
theophylline and guaifenesin
T-Phyl® [US]
Uniphyl® [US/Can]

COCCIDIOIDOMYCOSIS
Antifungal Agent
Apo®-Ketoconazole [Can]
ketoconazole
Nizoral® A-D [US-OTC]
Nizoral® [US/Can]
Novo-Ketoconazole [Can]

CONGESTIVE HEART FAILURE
Adrenergic Agonist Agent
dopamine
inamrinone
Intropin® [Can]
Alpha-Adrenergic Blocking Agent
Alti-Prazosin [Can]
Apo®-Prazo [Can]
Minipress® [US/Can]
Novo-Prazin [Can]
Nu-Prazo [Can]
prazosin
Angiotensin-Converting Enzyme
    (ACE) Inhibitor
Accupril® [US/Can]
Altace™ [US/Can]
Alti-Captopril [Can]
Apo®-Capto [Can]
Apo®-Lisinopril [Can]
Capoten® [US/Can]
captopril
cilazapril (Canada only)
enalapril
fosinopril
Gen-Captopril [Can]
Inhibace® [Can]
lisinopril
Mavik® [US/Can]
Monopril® [US/Can]
Novo-Captopril [Can]
Nu-Capto® [Can]
PMS-Captopril® [Can]
Prinivil® [US/Can]
quinapril

ramipril
trandolapril
Vasotec® IV [US/Can]
Vasotec® [US/Can]
Zestril® [US/Can]
Beta-Adrenergic Blocker
carvedilol
Coreg® [US/Can]
Calcium Channel Blocker
bepridil
Vascor® [US/Can]
Cardiac Glycoside
Digitek® [US]
digoxin
Lanoxicaps® [US/Can]
Lanoxin® Pediatric [US]
Lanoxin® [US/Can]
Cardiovascular Agent, Other
milrinone
Primacor® [US/Can]
Diuretic, Loop
Apo®-Furosemide [Can]
bumetanide
Bumex® [US/Can]
Burinex® [Can]
Demadex® [US]
Furocot® [US]
furosemide
Lasix® Special [Can]
Lasix® [US/Can]
torsemide
Diuretic, Potassium Sparing
amiloride
Dyrenium® [US/Can]
Midamor® [US/Can]
triamterene
Vasodilator
Apo®-Hydralazine [Can]
Apresoline® [US/Can]
hydralazine
Minitran™ [US/Can]
Nitrek® [US]
Nitro-Bid® Ointment [US]

Nitro-Dur® [US/Can]
Nitrogard® [US]
nitroglycerin
Nitrolingual® [US]
Nitrol® [US/Can]
Nitrong® SR [Can]
Nitropress® [US]
nitroprusside
NitroQuick® [US]
Nitrostat® [US/Can]
Nitro-Tab® [US]
NitroTime® [US]
Novo-Hylazin [Can]
Nu-Hydral [Can]
Transderm-Nitro® [Can]

COUGH

Antihistamine
Acot-Tussin® Allergy [US-OTC]
diphenhydramine
Dytuss® [US-OTC]
Truxadryl® [US-OTC]
Tusstat® [US-OTC]
Antihistamine/Antitussive
hydrocodone and chlorpheniramine
Phenergan® With Codeine [US]
Promatussin® DM [Can]
promethazine and codeine
promethazine and dextromethorphan
Tussionex® [US]
Antihistamine/Decongestant/Antitussive
Andehist DM NR Drops [US]
Aprodine® w/C [US]
Carbaxefed DM RF [US]
carbinoxamine, pseudoephedrine,
    dextromethorphan
Cerose-DM® [US-OTC]
chlorpheniramine, ephedrine,
    phenylephrine, carbetapentane
chlorpheniramine, phenylephrine,
    codeine
chlorpheniramine, phenylephrine,
    dextromethorphan

chlorpheniramine, pseudoephedrine,
  codeine
CoActifed® [Can]
Decohistine® DH [US]
Dihistine® DH [US]
Pediacof® [US]
Pedituss® [US]
promethazine, phenylephrine,
  codeine
Rentamine® [US-OTC]
Rondec®-DM Drops [US]
Ryna-C® [US]
Rynatuss® Pediatric Suspension
  [US-OTC]
Rynatuss® [US-OTC]
Triacin-C® [US]
triprolidine, pseudoephedrine,
  codeine
Antihistamine/Decongestant
  Combination
Allerest® Maximum Strength
  [US-OTC]
chlorpheniramine and
  pseudoephedrine
Chlor-Trimeton®
  Allergy/Decongestant [US-OTC]
Codimal-LA® Half [US-OTC]
Codimal-LA® [US-OTC]
Deconamine® SR [US-OTC]
Deconamine® [US-OTC]
Hayfebrol® [US-OTC]
Histalet® [US-OTC]
Rhinosyn-PD® [US-OTC]
Rhinosyn® [US-OTC]
Ryna® [US-OTC]
Sudafed® Cold & Allergy
  [US-OTC]
Antitussive
Benylin® Pediatric [US-OTC]
benzonatate
codeine
Creo-Terpin® [US-OTC]
Delsym® [US-OTC]

dextromethorphan
Hold® DM [US-OTC]
Hycodan® [US]
Hycomine® Compound [US]
hydrocodone and homatropine
hydrocodone, chlorpheniramine,
  phenylephrine, acetaminophen,
  caffeine
Hydromet® [US]
Hydropane® [US]
Hydrotropine® [US]
Pertussin® CS [US-OTC]
Pertussin® ES [US-OTC]
Robitussin® Cough Calmers
  [US-OTC]
Robitussin® Pediatric [US-OTC]
Scot-Tussin DM® Cough Chasers
  [US-OTC]
Silphen DM® [US-OTC]
St. Joseph® Cough Suppressant
  [US-OTC]
Tessalon® Perles [US/Can]
Trocal® [US-OTC]
Tussigon® [US]
Vicks Formula 44® Pediatric
  Formula [US-OTC]
Vicks Formula 44® [US-OTC]
Antitussive/Decongestant
Balminil DM D [Can]
Benylin® DM-D [Can]
Children's Sudafed® Cough & Cold
  [US-OTC]
Koffex DM-D [Can]
Novahistex® DM Decongestant
  [Can]
Novahistine® DM Decongestant
  [Can]
pseudoephedrine and
  dextromethorphan
Robitussin® Childrens Cough &
  Cold [Can]
Robitussin® Maximum Strength
  Cough & Cold [US-OTC]

Robitussin® Pediatric Cough & Cold
[US-OTC]
Vicks® 44D Cough & Head
Congestion [US-OTC]
Antitussive/Decongestant/Expectorant
Benylin® 3.3 mg-D-E [Can]
Calmylin with Codeine [Can]
Cheratussin DAC [US]
Codafed® Expectorant [US]
Codafed® Pediatric Expectorant
[US]
Dihistine® Expectorant [US]
Duratuss® HD [US]
guaifenesin, pseudoephedrine,
codeine
Guiatuss™ DAC® [US]
Halotussin® DAC [US]
hydrocodone, pseudoephedrine,
guaifenesin
Hydro-Tussin™ HD [US]
Hydro-Tussin™ XP [US]
Mytussin® DAC [US]
Nucofed® Expectorant [US]
Nucofed® Pediatric Expectorant
[US]
Nucotuss® [US]
Pancof®-XP [US]
Su-Tuss®-HD [US]
Tussend® Expectorant [US]
Antitussive/Expectorant
Aquatab® DM [US]
Balminil DM E [Can]
Benylin® DM-E [Can]
Benylin® Expectorant [US-OTC]
Brontex® [US]
Cheracol® D [US-OTC]
Cheracol® Plus [US-OTC]
Cheracol® [US]
Codiclear® DH [US]
Diabetic Tussin® DM Maximum
Strength [US-OTC]
Diabetic Tussin® DM [US-OTC]
Duratuss® DM [US]

Fenesin™ DM [US]
Gani-Tuss® NR [US]
Genatuss DM® [US-OTC]
guaifenesin and codeine
guaifenesin and dextromethorphan
Guaifenex® DM [US]
Guaituss AC® [US]
Guiatuss-DM® [US-OTC]
Humibid® DM [US]
Hycotuss® Expectorant Liquid [US]
hydrocodone and guaifenesin
Hydro-Tussin™ DM [US]
Koffex DM-Expectorant
Kolephrin® GG/DM [US-OTC]
Kwelcof® [US]
Mytussin® AC [US]
Mytussin® DM [US-OTC]
Respa® DM [US]
Robafen® AC [US]
Robitussin® DM [US/Can]
Robitussin® Sugar Free Cough [US-
OTC]
Romilar® AC [US]
Safe Tussin® 30 [US-OTC]
Silexin® [US-OTC]
Tolu-Sed® DM [US-OTC]
Touro® DM [US]
Tussi-Organidin® DM NR [US]
Tussi-Organidin® NR [US]
Tussi-Organidin® S-NR [US]
Vicks® 44E [US-OTC]
Vicks® Pediatric Formula 44E [US-
OTC]
Vicodin Tuss™ [US]
Cold Preparation
acetaminophen, dextromethorphan,
pseudoephedrine
Alka-Seltzer® Plus Flu Liqui-Gels®
[US-OTC]
Aquatab® C [US]
Balminil DM + Decongestant +
Expectorant [Can]
Benylin® DM-D-E [Can]

Comtrex® Non-Drowsy Cough and
Cold [US-OTC]
Contac® Cough, Cold and Flu Day
& Night™ [Can]
Contac® Severe Cold and Flu/Non-
Drowsy [US-OTC]
guaifenesin, pseudoephedrine,
dextromethorphan
Guiatuss™ CF [US]
Infants' Tylenol® Cold Plus Cough
Concentrated Drops [US-OTC]
Koffex DM + Decongestant +
Expectorant [Can]
Maxifed® DM [US]
Novahistex® DM Decongestant
Expectorant [Can]
Novahistine® DM Decongestant
Expectorant [Can]
PanMist®-DM [US]
Robitussin® Cold and Congestion
[US-OTC]
Robitussin® Cough and Cold Infant
[US-OTC]
Sudafed® Cold & Cough Extra
Strength [Can]
Sudafed® Severe Cold [US-OTC]
Thera-Flu® Non-Drowsy Flu, Cold
and Cough [US-OTC]
Touro™ CC [US]
Triaminic® Sore Throat Formula
[US-OTC]
Tylenol® Cold [Can]
Tylenol® Cold Non-Drowsy
[US-OTC]
Tylenol® Flu Non-Drowsy
Maximum Strength [US-OTC]
Vicks® DayQuil® Cold and Flu
Non-Drowsy [US-OTC]
Cough and Cold Combination
Detussin® Liquid [US]
Histussin D® Liquid [US]
hydrocodone and pseudoephedrine
Expectorant

Amibid LA [US]
Balminil Expectorant [Can]
Benylin® E Extra Strength [Can]
Diabetic Tussin® EX [US-OTC]
Duratuss-G® [US]
Fenesin™ [US]
Glytuss® [US-OTC]
guaifenesin
Guaifenex® G [US]
Guaifenex® LA [US]
Guiatuss® [US-OTC]
Humibid® L.A. [US]
Humibid® Pediatric [US]
Hytuss-2X® [US-OTC]
Hytuss® [US-OTC]
Koffex Expectorant [Can]
Liquibid® 1200 [US]
Liquibid® [US]
Mucinex™ [US-OTC]
Organidin® NR [US]
Phanasin [US-OTC]
Respa-GF® [US]
Robitussin® [US/Can]
Scot-Tussin® Sugar Free
Expectorant [US-OTC]
Touro Ex® [US]

CRYPTOCOCCOSIS

Antifungal Agent
Abelcet® [US/Can]
Amphocin® [US]
Amphotec® [US]
amphotericin B cholesteryl sulfate
complex
amphotericin B (conventional)
amphotericin B lipid complex
Ancobon® [US/Can]
Apo®-Fluconazole [Can]
Diflucan® [US/Can]
fluconazole
flucytosine
Fungizone® [US/Can]
itraconazole

Sporanox® [US/Can]
Antifungal Agent, Systemic
  AmBisome® [US/Can]
  amphotericin B liposomal

CYSTIC FIBROSIS

Enzyme
  dornase alfa
  Pulmozyme® [US/Can]

DUCTUS ARTERIOSUS (CLOSURE)

Nonsteroidal Antiinflammatory Drug
    (NSAID)
  Indocin® IV [US]
  indomethacin

DUCTUS ARTERIOSUS (TEMPORARY MAINTENANCE OF PATENCY)

Prostaglandin
  alprostadil
  Prostin VR Pediatric® [US/Can]

EDEMA

Antihypertensive Agent, Combination
  Aldactazide® [US/Can]
  Aldoril® [US]
  Apo®-Methazide [Can]
  Apo®-Triazide [Can]
  atenolol and chlorthalidone
  benazepril and hydrochlorothiazide
  Capozide® [US/Can]
  captopril and hydrochlorothiazide
  clonidine and chlorthalidone
  Combipres® [US]
  Dyazide® [US]
  enalapril and hydrochlorothiazide
  Enduronyl® Forte [US/Can]
  Enduronyl® [US/Can]
  hydralazine and
    hydrochlorothiazide

  hydralazine, hydrochlorothiazide,
    reserpine
  Hydra-Zide® [US]
  hydrochlorothiazide and
    spironolactone
  hydrochlorothiazide and triamterene
  Hyserp® [US]
  Hyzaar® [US/Can]
  Inderide® LA [US]
  Inderide® [US]
  lisinopril and hydrochlorothiazide
  losartan and hydrochlorothiazide
  Lotensin® HCT [US]
  Maxzide® [US]
  methyclothiazide and deserpidine
  methyldopa and hydrochlorothiazide
  Minizide® [US]
  Novo-Spirozine [Can]
  Novo-Triamzide [Can]
  Nu-Triazide [Can]
  prazosin and polythiazide
  Prinzide® [US/Can]
  propranolol and hydrochlorothiazide
  Tenoretic® [US/Can]
  Vaseretic® [US/Can]
  Zestoretic® [US/Can]
Diuretic, Combination
  amiloride and hydrochlorothiazide
  Apo®-Amilzide [Can]
  Moduret® [Can]
  Moduretic® [US/Can]
  Novamilor [Can]
  Nu-Amilzide [Can]
Diuretic, Loop
  Apo®-Furosemide [Can]
  bumetanide
  Bumex® [US/Can]
  Burinex® [Can]
  Demadex® [US]
  Edecrin® [US/Can]
  ethacrynic acid
  Furocot® [US]
  furosemide

Lasix® Special [Can]
Lasix® [US/Can]
torsemide
Diuretic, Miscellaneous
Apo®-Chlorthalidone [Can]
Apo®-Indapamide [Can]
caffeine and sodium benzoate
chlorthalidone
Gen-Indapamide [Can]
indapamide
Lozide® [Can]
Lozol® [US/Can]
metolazone
Mykrox® [US/Can]
Novo-Indapamide [Can]
Nu-Indapamide [Can]
PMS-Indapamide [Can]
Thalitone® [US]
Zaroxolyn® [US/Can]
Diuretic, Osmotic
mannitol
Osmitrol® [US/Can]
Resectisol® Irrigation Solution [US]
Diuretic, Potassium Sparing
Aldactone® [US/Can]
amiloride
Dyrenium® [US/Can]
Midamor® [US/Can]
Novo-Spiroton [Can]
spironolactone
triamterene
Diuretic, Thiazide
Apo®-Hydro [Can]
Aquacot® [US]
Aquatensen® [US/Can]
Aquazide H® [US]
bendroflumethiazide
chlorothiazide
Diuril® [US/Can]
Enduron® [US/Can]
Ezide® [US]
hydrochlorothiazide
Hydrocot® [US]

HydroDIURIL® [US/Can]
Metatensin® [Can]
methyclothiazide
Microzide™ [US]
Naqua® [US/Can]
Naturetin® [US]
Oretic® [US]
polythiazide
Renese® [US]
Trichlorex® [Can]
trichlormethiazide
Zide® [US]

EMBOLISM

Anticoagulant (Other)
Coumadin® [US/Can]
dicumarol
enoxaparin
Hepalean® [Can]
Hepalean® Leo [Can]
Hepalean®-LOK [Can]
heparin
Hep-Lock® [US]
Innohep® [US/Can]
Lovenox® [US/Can]
Taro-Warfarin [Can]
tinzaparin
warfarin
Antiplatelet Agent
Apo®-ASA [Can]
Apo®-Dipyridamole FC [Can]
Asaphen [Can]
Asaphen E.C. [Can]
aspirin
Bayer® Aspirin Regimen Adult Low
    Strength [US-OTC]
Bayer® Aspirin Regimen Adult Low
    Strength with Calcium
    [US-OTC]
dipyridamole
Ecotrin® Low Adult Strength
    [US-OTC]
Halfprin® [US-OTC]

Novo-Dipiradol [Can]
Persantine® [US/Can]
Fibrinolytic Agent
Abbokinase® [US]
Activase® rt-PA [Can]
Activase® [US]
alteplase
Retavase® [US/Can]
reteplase
Streptase® [US/Can]
streptokinase
urokinase

EMPHYSEMA
Adrenergic Agonist Agent
AccuNeb™ [US]
Adrenalin® Chloride [US/Can]
albuterol
Alti-Salbutamol [Can]
Alupent® [US]
Apo®-Salvent [Can]
bitolterol
Brethine® [US]
Bricanyl® [Can]
Bronchial Mist® [US]
ephedrine
epinephrine
isoproterenol
Isuprel® [US]
metaproterenol
Novo-Salmol [Can]
Primatene® Mist [US-OTC]
Proventil® HFA [US]
Proventil® Repetabs® [US]
Proventil® [US]
terbutaline
Tornalate® [US/Can]
Vaponefrin® [Can]
Ventolin® HFA [US]
Ventolin® [US]
Volmax® [US]
Anticholinergic Agent
Alti-Ipratropium [Can]

Apo®-Ipravent [Can]
Atrovent® [US/Can]
Gen-Ipratropium [Can]
ipratropium
Novo-Ipramide [Can]
Nu-Ipratropium [Can]
PMS-Ipratropium [Can]
Expectorant
potassium iodide
SSKI® [US]
Mucolytic Agent
acetylcysteine
Acys-5® [US]
Mucomyst® [US/Can]
Parvolex® [Can]
Theophylline Derivative
Aerolate III® [US]
Aerolate JR® [US]
Aerolate SR® [US]
aminophylline
Apo®-Theo LA [Can]
Choledyl SA® [US]
Dilor® [US/Can]
dyphylline
Elixophyllin® GG [US]
Elixophyllin® [US]
Lufyllin® [US/Can]
Neoasma® [US]
Novo-Theophyl SR [Can]
oxtriphylline
Phyllocontin®-350 [Can]
Phyllocontin® [Can]
Quibron®-T/SR [US/Can]
Quibron®-T [US]
Quibron® [US]
Slo-Phyllin® [US]
Theo-24® [US]
Theochron® [US]
Theocon® [US]
Theo-Dur® [US/Can]
Theolair™ [US/Can]
Theolate® [US]
Theomar® GG [US]

theophylline
theophylline and guaifenesin
T-Phyl® [US]
Uniphyl® [US/Can]

ENDOCARDITIS TREATMENT
Aminoglycoside (Antibiotic)
  Alcomicin® [Can]
  amikacin
  Amikin® [US/Can]
  Diogent® [Can]
  Garamycin® [US/Can]
  Garatec [Can]
  gentamicin
  Nebcin® [US/Can]
  PMS-Tobramycin [Can]
  tobramycin
  Tobrex® [US/Can]
  Tomycine™ [Can]
Antibiotic, Miscellaneous
  Vancocin® [US/Can]
  Vancoled® [US]
  vancomycin
Antibiotic, Penicillin
  pivampicillin (Canada only)
  Pondocillin® [Can]
Antifungal Agent
  Amphocin® [US]
  amphotericin B (conventional)
  Fungizone® [US/Can]
Cephalosporin (First Generation)
  Ancef® [US/Can]
  Cefadyl® [US/Can]
  cefazolin
  cephalothin
  cephapirin
  Ceporacin® [Can]
  Kefzol® [US/Can]
Penicillin
  ampicillin
  Apo®-Ampi [Can]
  Marcillin® [US]

nafcillin
Novo-Ampicillin [Can]
Nu-Ampi [Can]
oxacillin
penicillin G (parenteral/aqueous)
Pfizerpen® [US/Can]
Principen® [US]
Quinolone
  ciprofloxacin
  Cipro® [US/Can]

FEBRILE NEUTROPENIA
Quinolone
  ciprofloxacin
  Cipro® [US/Can]

FEVER
Antipyretic
  Abenol® [Can]
  Acephen® [US-OTC]
  acetaminophen
  Advil® Children's [US-OTC]
  Advil® Infants' Concentrated Drops [US-OTC]
  Advil® Junior [US-OTC]
  Advil® [US/Can]
  Aleve® [US-OTC]
  Amigesic® [US/Can]
  Anaprox® DS [US/Can]
  Anaprox® [US/Can]
  Apo®-Acetaminophen [Can]
  Apo®-ASA [Can]
  Apo®-Ibuprofen [Can]
  Apo®-Napro-Na [Can]
  Apo®-Napro-Na DS [Can]
  Apo®-Naproxen [Can]
  Apo®-Naproxen SR [Can]
  Argesic®-SA [US]
  Asaphen [Can]
  Asaphen E.C. [Can]
  Ascriptin® Enteric [US-OTC]
  Ascriptin® Extra Strength [US-OTC]
  Ascriptin® [US-OTC]

Aspercin Extra [US-OTC]
Aspercin [US-OTC]
aspirin
Aspirin Free Anacin® Maximum
  Strength [US-OTC]
Atasol® [Can]
Bayer® Aspirin Extra Strength
  [US-OTC]
Bayer® Aspirin Regimen Regular
  Strength [US-OTC]
Bayer® Aspirin [US-OTC]
Bayer® Plus Extra Strength [US-
  OTC]
Bufferin® Extra Strength [US-OTC]
Bufferin® [US-OTC]
Cetafen Extra® [US-OTC]
Cetafen® [US-OTC]
Disalcid® [US]
Easprin® [US]
EC-Naprosyn® [US]
Ecotrin® Maximum Strength
  [US-OTC]
Ecotrin® [US-OTC]
Entrophen® [Can]
Feverall® [US-OTC]
Genapap® Children [US-OTC]
Genapap® Extra Strength [US-OTC]
Genapap® Infant [US-OTC]
Genapap® [US-OTC]
Genebs® Extra Strength [US-OTC]
Genebs® [US-OTC]
Gen-Naproxen EC [Can]
Genpril® [US-OTC]
ibuprofen
Ibu-Tab® [US]
Infantaire [US-OTC]
I-Prin [US-OTC]
Liquiprin® for Children [US-OTC]
Mapap® Children's [US-OTC]
Mapap® Extra Strength [US-OTC]
Mapap® Infants [US-OTC]
Mapap® [US-OTC]
Menadol® [US-OTC]

Mono-Gesic® [US]
Motrin® Children's [US/Can]
Motrin® IB [US/Can]
Motrin® Infants' [US-OTC]
Motrin® Junior Strength [US-OTC]
Motrin® [US/Can]
Naprelan® [US]
Naprosyn® [US/Can]
naproxen
Naxen® [Can]
Novasen [Can]
Novo-Naprox [Can]
Novo-Naprox Sodium [Can]
Novo-Naprox Sodium DS [Can]
Novo-Naprox SR [Can]
Novo-Profen® [Can]
Nu-Ibuprofen [Can]
Nu-Naprox [Can]
Pediatrix [Can]
Redutemp® [US-OTC]
Riva-Naproxen [Can]
Salflex® [US/Can]
salsalate
Silapap® Children's [US-OTC]
Silapap® Infants [US-OTC]
sodium salicylate
Sureprin 81™ [US-OTC]
Synflex® [Can]
Synflex® DS [Can]
Tempra® [Can]
Tylenol® Children's [US-OTC]
Tylenol® Extra Strength [US-OTC]
Tylenol® Infants [US-OTC]
Tylenol® Junior Strength
  [US-OTC]
Tylenol® [US/Can]
Valorin Extra [US-OTC]
Valorin [US-OTC]
ZORprin® [US]

FIBROCYSTIC DISEASE
Vitamin, Fat Soluble
  Amino-Opti-E® [US-OTC]

Aquasol E® [US-OTC]
E-Complex-600® [US-OTC]
E-Vitamin® [US-OTC]
vitamin E
Vita-Plus® E Softgels® [US-OTC]
Vitec® [US-OTC]
Vite E® Creme [US-OTC]

FIBROMYOSITIS

Antidepressant, Tricyclic (Tertiary
    Amine)
amitriptyline
Apo®-Amitriptyline [Can]
Elavil® [US/Can]
Vanatrip® [US]

GRAM-NEGATIVE INFECTION

Aminoglycoside (Antibiotic)
    AKTob® [US]
    Alcomicin® [Can]
    amikacin
    Amikin® [US/Can]
    Diogent® [Can]
    Garamycin® [US/Can]
    Garatec [Can]
    Genoptic® [US]
    Gentacidin® [US]
    Gentak® [US]
    gentamicin
    kanamycin
    Kantrex® [US/Can]
    Nebcin® [US/Can]
    PMS-Tobramycin [Can]
    TOBI™ [US/Can]
    tobramycin
    Tobrex® [US/Can]
    Tomycine™ [Can]
Antibiotic, Carbapenem
    ertapenem
    Invanz™ [US]
Antibiotic, Miscellaneous
    Apo®-Nitrofurantoin [Can]

Azactam® [US/Can]
aztreonam
colistimethate
Coly-Mycin® M [US/Can]
Furadantin® [US]
Macrobid® [US/Can]
Macrodantin® [US/Can]
nitrofurantoin
Novo-Furantoin [Can]
Antibiotic, Penicillin
    pivampicillin (Canada only)
    Pondocillin® [Can]
Antibiotic, Quinolone
    gatifloxacin
    Levaquin® [US/Can]
    levofloxacin
    Tequin® [US/Can]
Carbapenem (Antibiotic)
    imipenem and cilastatin
    meropenem
    Merrem® IV [US/Can]
    Primaxin® [US/Can]
Cephalosporin (First Generation)
    Ancef® [US/Can]
    Apo®-Cefadroxil [Can]
    Apo®-Cephalex [Can]
    Biocef® [US]
    cefadroxil
    Cefadyl® [US/Can]
    cefazolin
    cephalexin
    cephalothin
    cephapirin
    cephradine
    Ceporacin® [Can]
    Duricef® [US/Can]
    Keflex® [US]
    Keftab® [US/Can]
    Kefzol® [US/Can]
    Novo-Cefadroxil [Can]
    Novo-Lexin® [Can]
    Nu-Cephalex® [Can]
    Velosef® [US]

Cephalosporin (Second Generation)
Apo®-Cefaclor [Can]
Ceclor® CD [US]
Ceclor® [US/Can]
cefaclor
cefamandole
Cefotan® [US/Can]
cefotetan
cefoxitin
cefpodoxime
cefprozil
Ceftin® [US/Can]
cefuroxime
Cefzil® [US/Can]
Kefurox® [US/Can]
Mandol® [US]
Mefoxin® [US/Can]
Novo-Cefaclor [Can]
Nu-Cefaclor [Can]
PMS-Cefaclor [Can]
Vantin® [US/Can]
Zinacef® [US/Can]
Cephalosporin (Third Generation)
Cedax® [US]
cefixime
Cefizox® [US/Can]
Cefobid® [US/Can]
cefoperazone
cefotaxime
ceftazidime
ceftibuten
ceftizoxime
ceftriaxone
Ceptaz® [US/Can]
Claforan® [US/Can]
Fortaz® [US/Can]
Rocephin® [US/Can]
Suprax® [US/Can]
Tazicef® [US]
Tazidime® [US/Can]
Cephalosporin (Fourth Generation)
cefepime
Maxipime® [US/Can]

Genitourinary Irrigant
neomycin and polymyxin B
Neosporin® GU Irrigant [US/Can]
Macrolide (Antibiotic)
Apo®-Erythro Base [Can]
Apo®-Erythro E-C [Can]
Apo®-Erythro-ES [Can]
Apo®-Erythro-S [Can]
azithromycin
Biaxin® [US/Can]
Biaxin® XL [US]
clarithromycin
Diomycin® [Can]
dirithromycin
Dynabac® [US]
E.E.S.® [US/Can]
Erybid™ [Can]
Eryc® [US/Can]
EryPed® [US]
Ery-Tab® [US]
Erythrocin® [US/Can]
erythromycin and sulfisoxazole
erythromycin (systemic)
Eryzole® [US]
Lincocin® [US/Can]
lincomycin
Lincorex® [US]
Nu-Erythromycin-S [Can]
PCE® [US/Can]
Pediazole® [US/Can]
PMS-Erythromycin [Can]
Tao® [US]
troleandomycin
Zithromax® [US/Can]
Z-PAK® [US/Can]
Penicillin
amoxicillin
amoxicillin and clavulanate
potassium
Amoxicot® [US]
Amoxil® [US/Can]
ampicillin
ampicillin and sulbactam

Apo®-Amoxi [Can]
Apo®-Ampi [Can]
Apo®-Pen VK [Can]
Augmentin ES-600™ [US]
Augmentin® [US/Can]
Bicillin® C-R 900/300 [US]
Bicillin® C-R [US]
Bicillin® L-A [US]
carbenicillin
Clavulin® [Can]
Gen-Amoxicillin [Can]
Geocillin® [US]
Lin-Amox [Can]
Marcillin® [US]
Moxilin® [US]
Nadopen-V® [Can]
Novamoxin® [Can]
Novo-Ampicillin [Can]
Novo-Pen-VK® [Can]
Nu-Amoxi [Can]
Nu-Ampi [Can]
Nu-Pen-VK® [Can]
penicillin G benzathine
penicillin G benzathine and procaine
    combined
penicillin G procaine
penicillin V potassium
Permapen® [US]
piperacillin
piperacillin and tazobactam sodium
Pipracil® [US/Can]
Principen® [US]
PVF® K [Can]
Suspen® [US]
Tazocin® [Can]
ticarcillin
ticarcillin and clavulanate
    potassium
Ticar® [US]
Timentin® [US/Can]
Trimox® [US]
Truxcillin® [US]
Unasyn® [US/Can]

Veetids® [US]
Wycillin® [US/Can]
Wymox® [US]
Zosyn® [US]
Quinolone
Apo®-Norflox [Can]
Apo®-Oflox [Can]
Cinobac® [US/Can]
cinoxacin
ciprofloxacin
Cipro® [US/Can]
Floxin® [US/Can]
lomefloxacin
Maxaquin® [US]
nalidixic acid
NegGram® [US/Can]
norfloxacin
Noroxin® [US/Can]
Novo-Norfloxacin [Can]
Ocuflox® [US/Can]
ofloxacin
Riva-Norfloxacin [Can]
sparfloxacin
Zagam® [US]
Sulfonamide
Apo®-Sulfatrim [Can]
Bactrim™ DS [US]
Bactrim™ [US]
erythromycin and sulfisoxazole
Eryzole® [US]
Gantrisin® Pediatric Suspension
    [US]
Novo-Trimel [Can]
Novo-Trimel D.S. [Can]
Nu-Cotrimox® [Can]
Pediazole® [US/Can]
Septra® DS [US/Can]
Septra® [US/Can]
sulfadiazine
sulfamethoxazole and trimethoprim
Sulfatrim® DS [US]
Sulfatrim® [US]
sulfisoxazole

sulfisoxazole and phenazopyridine
    Sulfizole® [Can]
    Truxazole® [US]
Tetracycline Derivative
    Adoxa™ [US]
    Alti-Minocycline [Can]
    Apo®-Doxy [Can]
    Apo®-Doxy Tabs [Can]
    Apo®-Minocycline [Can]
    Apo®-Tetra [Can]
    Brodspec® [US]
    Doryx® [US]
    Doxy-100™ [US]
    Doxycin [Can]
    doxycycline
    Doxytec [Can]
    Dynacin® [US]
    EmTet® [US]
    Gen-Minocycline [Can]
    Minocin® [US/Can]
    minocycline
    Monodox® [US]
    Novo-Doxylin [Can]
    Novo-Minocycline [Can]
    Novo-Tetra [Can]
    Nu-Doxycycline [Can]
    Nu-Tetra [Can]
    oxytetracycline
    Periostat® [US]
    Rhoxal-Minocycline [Can]
    Sumycin® [US]
    Terramycin® IM [US/Can]
    tetracycline
    Vibramycin® [US]
    Vibra-Tabs® [US/Can]
    Wesmycin® [US]

HEART BLOCK

Adrenergic Agonist Agent
    Adrenalin® Chloride [US/Can]
    epinephrine
    isoproterenol
    Isuprel® [US]

HAEMOPHILUS INFLUENZAE

Toxoid
diphtheria, tetanus toxoids, acellular
        pertussis vaccine and
        Haemophilus type B
conjugate vaccine
    TriHIBit® [US]
Vaccine, Inactivated Bacteria
    ActHIB® [US/Can]
diphtheria, tetanus toxoids, acellular
        pertussis vaccine and
        Haemophilus type B
conjugate vaccine
    Haemophilus type B conjugate
        vaccine
    HibTITER® [US]
    PedvaxHIB® [US/Can]
    TriHIBit® [US]
Vaccine, Inactivated Virus
    Comvax® [US]
    Haemophilus type B conjugate and
        hepatitis B vaccine

HISTOPLASMOSIS

Antifungal Agent
    Amphocin® [US]
    amphotericin B
      (conventional)
    Apo®-Ketoconazole [Can]
    Fungizone® [US/Can]
    itraconazole
    ketoconazole
    Nizoral® A-D [US-OTC]
    Nizoral® [US/Can]
    Novo-Ketoconazole [Can]
    Sporanox® [US/Can]

HYPERTENSION (ARTERIAL)

Beta-Adrenergic Blocker
    Levatol® [US/Can]
    penbutolol

HYPERTENSION (CEREBRAL)

Barbiturate
    Pentothal® Sodium [US/Can]
    thiopental
Diuretic, Osmotic
    mannitol
    urea

HYPERTENSION (CORONARY)

Vasodilator
    nitroglycerin
    Nitrol® [US/Can]

HYPERTENSION (EMERGENCY)

Antihypertensive Agent
    Corlopam® [US/Can]
    fenoldopam

HYPERTROPHIC CARDIOMYOPATHY

Calcium Channel Blocker
    Adalat® CC [US]
    Adalat® XL® [Can]
    Apo®-Nifed [Can]
    Apo®-Nifed PA [Can]
    Nifedical™ XL [US]
    nifedipine
    Novo-Nifedin [Can]
    Nu-Nifed [Can]
    Procardia® [US/Can]
    Procardia XL® [US]

HYPOTENSION

Adrenergic Agonist Agent
    Adrenalin® Chloride [US/Can]
    dopamine
    ephedrine
    epinephrine
    Intropin® [Can]
    isoproterenol
    Isuprel® [US]
    Levophed® [US/Can]
    mephentermine
    metaraminol
    norepinephrine
    Wyamine® Sulfate [US]

HYPOTENSION (ORTHOSTATIC)

Adrenergic Agonist Agent
    ephedrine
    phenylephrine
Alpha-Adrenergic Agonist
    Amatine® [Can]
    midodrine
    ProAmatine [US]
Central Nervous System Stimulant,
    Nonamphetamine
    Concerta™ [US]
    Metadate® CD [US]
    Metadate™ ER [US]
    Methylin™ ER [US]
    Methylin™ [US]
    methylphenidate
    PMS-Methylphenidate [Can]
    Riphenidate [Can]
    Ritalin® LA [US]
    Ritalin-SR® [US/Can]
    Ritalin® [US/Can]

HYPOXIC RESPIRATORY FAILURE

Vasodilator, Pulmonary
    INOmax® [US/Can]
    nitric oxide

INFLAMMATION (NONRHEUMATIC)

Adrenal Corticosteroid
    Acthar® [US]
    A-HydroCort® [US/Can]
    Alti-Dexamethasone [Can]
    A-methaPred® [US]

Apo®-Prednisone [Can]
Aristocort® Forte Injection [US]
Aristocort® Intralesional Injection
  [US]
Aristocort® Tablet [US/Can]
Aristospan® Intra-articular Injection
  [US/Can]
Aristospan® Intralesional Injection
  [US/Can]
Betaject™ [Can]
betamethasone (systemic)
Betnesol® [Can]
Celestone® Phosphate [US]
Celestone® Soluspan® [US/Can]
Celestone® [US]
Cel-U-Jec® [US]
Cortef® [US/Can]
corticotropin
cortisone acetate
Cortone® [Can]
Decadron®-LA [US]
Decadron® [US/Can]
Decaject-LA® [US]
Decaject® [US]
Delta-Cortef® [US]
Deltasone® [US]
Depo-Medrol® [US/Can]
Depopred® [US]
dexamethasone (systemic)
Dexasone® L.A. [US]
Dexasone® [US/Can]
Dexone® LA [US]
Dexone® [US]
Hexadrol® [US/Can]
H.P. Acthar® Gel [US]
hydrocortisone (systemic)
Hydrocortone® Acetate [US]
Kenalog® Injection [US/Can]
Key-Pred-SP® [US]
Key-Pred® [US]
Medrol® Tablet [US/Can]
methylprednisolone
Meticorten® [US]

Orapred™ [US]
Pediapred® [US/Can]
PMS-Dexamethasone [Can]
Prednicot® [US]
prednisolone (systemic)
Prednisol® TBA [US]
prednisone
Prelone® [US]
Solu-Cortef® [US/Can]
Solu-Medrol® [US/Can]
Solurex L.A.® [US]
Sterapred® DS [US]
Sterapred® [US]
Tac™-3 Injection [US]
Triam-A® Injection [US]
triamcinolone (systemic)
Triam Forte® Injection [US]
Winpred™ [Can]

ISCHEMIA

Blood Viscosity Reducer Agent
  Albert® Pentoxifylline [Can]
  Apo®-Pentoxifylline SR [Can]
  Nu-Pentoxifylline SR [Can]
  pentoxifylline
  Trental® [US/Can]
Platelet Aggregation Inhibitor
  abciximab
  ReoPro® [US/Can]
Vasodilator
  ethaverine
  Ethavex-100® [US]
  Papacon® [US]
  papaverine
  Para-Time S.R.® [US]
  Pavacot® [US]

LUNG SURFACTANT

Lung Surfactant
  beractant
  colfosceril palmitate
  Exosurf® Neonatal™ [US/Can]
  Survanta® [US/Can]

MALIGNANT EFFUSION
Antineoplastic Agent
Thioplex® [US]
thiotepa

MITRAL VALVE PROLAPSE
Beta-Adrenergic Blocker
Apo®-Propranolol [Can]
Inderal® LA [US/Can]
Inderal® [US/Can]
Nu-Propranolol [Can]
propranolol

MYCOBACTERIUM AVIUM-INTRACELLULARE
Antibiotic, Aminoglycoside
streptomycin
Antibiotic, Miscellaneous
Mycobutin® [US/Can]
rifabutin
Rifadin® [US/Can]
rifampin
Rimactane® [US]
Rofact™ [Can]
Antimycobacterial Agent
ethambutol
Etibi® [Can]
Myambutol® [US]
Antitubercular Agent
streptomycin
Carbapenem (Antibiotic)
imipenem and cilastatin
meropenem
Merrem® IV [US/Can]
Primaxin® [US/Can]
Leprostatic Agent
clofazimine
Lamprene® [US/Can]
Macrolide (Antibiotic)
azithromycin
Biaxin® [US/Can]
Biaxin® XL [US]
clarithromycin

Zithromax® [US/Can]
Z-PAK® [US/Can]
Quinolone
ciprofloxacin
Cipro® [US/Can]

MYCOSIS (FUNGOIDES)
Psoralen
methoxsalen
8-MOP® [US/Can]
Oxsoralen® Lotion [US/Can]
Oxsoralen-Ultra® [US/Can]
Ultramop™ [Can]
Uvadex® [US/Can]

MYOCARDIAL INFARCTION
Anticoagulant (Other)
Coumadin® [US/Can]
enoxaparin
Hepalean® [Can]
Hepalean® Leo [Can]
Hepalean®-LOK [Can]
heparin
Hep-Lock® [US]
Lovenox® [US/Can]
Taro-Warfarin [Can]
warfarin
Antiplatelet Agent
Apo®-ASA [Can]
Apo®-Dipyridamole FC [Can]
aspirin
Bayer® Aspirin Regimen Adult Low Strength [US-OTC]
Bayer® Aspirin Regimen Adult Low Strength with Calcium [US-OTC]
clopidogrel
dipyridamole
Ecotrin® Low Adult Strength [US-OTC]
Halfprin® [US-OTC]
Persantine® [US/Can]
Plavix® [US/Can]

Beta-Adrenergic Blocker
Alti-Nadolol [Can]
Apo®-Atenol [Can]
Apo®-Metoprolol [Can]
Apo®-Nadol [Can]
Apo®-Propranolol [Can]
Apo®-Timol [Can]
Apo®-Timop [Can]
atenolol
Betaloc® [Can]
Betaloc® Durules®
Betimol® [US]
Blocadren® [US]
Corgard® [US/Can]
Gen-Atenolol [Can]
Gen-Metoprolol [Can]
Gen-Timolol [Can]
Inderal® LA [US/Can]
Inderal® [US/Can]
Lopressor® [US/Can]
metoprolol
nadolol
Novo-Atenol [Can]
Novo-Metoprolol [Can]
Novo-Nadolol [Can]
Nu-Atenol
Nu-Metop [Can]
Nu-Propranolol [Can]
Nu-Timolol [Can]
Phoxal-timolol [Can]
PMS-Atenolol [Can]
PMS-Metoprolol [Can]
PMS-Timolol [Can]
propranolol
Rhoxal-atenolol [Can]
Tenolin [Can]
Tenormin® [US/Can]
Tim-AK [Can]
timolol
Timoptic® OcuDose® [US]
Timoptic® [US/Can]
Timoptic-XE® [US/Can]
Toprol-XL® [US/Can]

Fibrinolytic Agent
Activase® rt-PA [Can]
Activase® [US]
alteplase
Retavase® [US/Can]
reteplase
Streptase® [US/Can]
streptokinase
Thrombolytic Agent
tenecteplase
TNKase™ [US]

MYOCARDIAL REINFARCTION

Antiplatelet Agent
Aggrenox® [US/Can]
Apo®-ASA [Can]
Apo®-Dipyridamole FC [Can]
Asaphen [Can]
Asaphen E.C. [Can]
aspirin
Bayer® Aspirin Regimen
Adult Low Strength [US-OTC]
Bayer® Aspirin Regimen
Adult Low Strength with Calcium
[US-OTC]
Bayer® Aspirin [US-OTC]
dipyridamole
dipyridamole and aspirin
Ecotrin® Low Adult Strength
[US-OTC]
Halfprin® [US-OTC]
Persantine® [US/Can]
Sureprin 81™ [US-OTC]
Beta-Adrenergic Blocker
Apo®-Metoprolol [Can]
Apo®-Propranolol [Can]
Apo®-Timol [Can]
Apo®-Timop [Can]
Betaloc® [Can]
Betaloc® Durules®
Betimol® [US]
Blocadren® [US]

Gen-Metoprolol [Can]
Gen-Timolol [Can]
Inderal® LA [US/Can]
Inderal® [US/Can]
Lopressor® [US/Can]
metoprolol
Novo-Metoprolol [Can]
Nu-Metop [Can]
Nu-Propranolol [Can]
Nu-Timolol [Can]
Phoxal-timolol [Can]
PMS-Metoprolol [Can]
PMS-Timolol [Can]
propranolol
Tim-AK [Can]
timolol
Timoptic® OcuDose®
    [US]
Timoptic® [US/Can]
Timoptic-XE® [US/Can]
Toprol-XL® [US/Can]

ORGAN REJECTION
Immunosuppressant Agent
    daclizumab
    Zenapax® [US/Can]

ORGAN TRANSPLANT
Immunosuppressant Agent
    basiliximab
    CellCept® [US/Can]
    cyclosporine
    Gengraf™ [US]
    muromonab-CD3
    mycophenolate
    Neoral® [US/Can]
    Orthoclone OKT® 3
        [US/Can]
    Prograf® [US/Can]
    Protopic® [US]
    Rapamune® [US/Can]
    Sandimmune® [US/Can]
    Simulect® [US/Can]

sirolimus
tacrolimus

PAIN
Analgesic, Miscellaneous
    acetaminophen and tramadol
    Ultracet™ [US]
Analgesic, Narcotic
    acetaminophen and codeine
    Actiq® [US/Can]
    alfentanil
    Alfenta® [US/Can]
    Anexsia® [US]
    aspirin and codeine
    Astramorph™ PF [US]
    Avinza™ [US]
    Bancap HC® [US]
    belladonna and opium
    B&O Supprettes® [US]
    Buprenex® [US/Can]
    buprenorphine
    butalbital compound and codeine
    butorphanol
    Capital® and Codeine [US]
    codeine
    Co-Gesic® [US]
    Coryphen® Codeine [Can]
    Darvocet-N® 50 [US/Can]
    Darvocet-N® 100 [US/Can]
    Darvon® Compound-65 [US]
    Darvon-N® Tablet [US/Can]
    Darvon® [US]
    Demerol® [US/Can]
    DHC Plus® [US]
    DHC® [US]
    dihydrocodeine compound
    Dilaudid-5® [US]
    Dilaudid-HP-Plus® [Can]
    Dilaudid-HP® [US/Can]
    Dilaudid® [US/Can]
    Dilaudid-XP® [Can]
    Dolacet® [US]
    Dolophine® [US/Can]

droperidol and fentanyl
Duragesic® [US/Can]
Duramorph® [US]
Empirin® With Codeine [US]
Empracet®-30 [Can]
Empracet®-60 [Can]
Emtec-30 [Can]
Endocet® [US/Can]
Endodan® [US/Can]
fentanyl
Fiorinal®-C 1/2 [Can]
Fiorinal®-C 1/4 [Can]
Fiorinal® With Codeine [US]
Hydrocet® [US]
hydrocodone and acetaminophen
hydrocodone and aspirin
hydrocodone and ibuprofen
Hydrogesic® [US]
Hydromorph Contin® [Can]
hydromorphone
Infumorph® [US]
Innovar® [US]
Kadian® [US/Can]
Lenoltec [Can]
Levo-Dromoran® [US]
levorphanol
Lorcet® 10/650 [US]
Lorcet®-HD [US]
Lorcet® Plus [US]
Lortab® ASA [US]
Lortab® [US]
Margesic® H [US]
Mepergan® [US]
meperidine
meperidine and promethazine
Meperitab® [US]
M-Eslon® [Can]
Metadol™ [Can]
methadone
Methadose® [US/Can]
Morphine HP® [Can]
morphine sulfate
M.O.S.-Sulfate® [Can]

MS Contin® [US/Can]
MSIR® [US/Can]
nalbuphine
Norco® [US]
Nubain® [US/Can]
Numorphan® [US/Can]
opium tincture
Oramorph SR® [US/Can]
Oxycodan® [Can]
oxycodone
oxycodone and acetaminophen
oxycodone and aspirin
OxyContin® [US/Can]
Oxydose™ [US]
OxyFast® [US]
OxyIR® [US/Can]
oxymorphone
paregoric
PC-Cap® [US]
pentazocine
pentazocine compound
Percocet® 2.5/325 [US]
Percocet® 5/325 [US]
Percocet® 7.5/325 [US]
Percocet® 7.5/500 [US]
Percocet® 10/325 [US]
Percocet® 10/650 [US]
Percodan®-Demi® [Can]
Percodan® [US/Can]
Phenaphen® With Codeine [US]
PMS-Hydromorphone [Can]
Pronap-100® [US]
propoxyphene
propoxyphene and acetaminophen
propoxyphene and aspirin
remifentanil
RMS® [US]
Roxanol 100® [US]
Roxanol®-T [US]
Roxanol® [US]
Roxicet® 5/500 [US]
Roxicet® [US]
Roxicodone™ Intensol™ [US]

Roxicodone™ [US]
Stadol® NS [US/Can]
Stadol® [US]
Stagesic® [US]
Statex® [Can]
Sublimaze® [US]
sufentanil
Sufenta® [US/Can]
Supeudol® [Can]
Synalgos®-DC [US]
642® Tablet [Can]
Talacen® [US]
Talwin® Compound [US]
Talwin® NX [US]
Talwin® [US/Can]
Tecnal C 1/2 [Can]
Tecnal C 1/4 [Can]
T-Gesic® [US]
Triatec-8 [Can]
Triatec-30 [Can]
Triatec-Strong [Can]
Tylenol® with Codeine [US/Can]
Tylox® [US]
Ultiva™ [US/Can]
Vicodin® ES [US]
Vicodin® HP [US]
Vicodin® [US]
Vicoprofen® [US/Can]
Zydone® [US]
Analgesic, Nonnarcotic
Abenol® [Can]
Acephen® [US-OTC]
acetaminophen
acetaminophen and diphenhydramine
acetaminophen and
    phenyltoloxamine
acetaminophen and tramadol
acetaminophen, aspirin, and caffeine
Acular® PF [US]
Acular® [US/Can]
Advil® Children's [US-OTC]
Advil® Infants' Concentrated Drops
    [US-OTC]

Advil® Junior [US-OTC]
Advil® Migraine [US-OTC]
Advil® [US/Can]
Aleve® [US-OTC]
Alti-Flurbiprofen [Can]
Alti-Piroxicam [Can]
Amigesic® [US/Can]
Anacin® PM Aspirin Free [US-OTC]
Anaprox® DS [US/Can]
Anaprox® [US/Can]
Ansaid® Oral [US/Can]
Apo®-Acetaminophen [Can]
Apo®-ASA [Can]
Apo®-Diclo [Can]
Apo®-Diclo SR [Can]
Apo®-Diflunisal [Can]
Apo®-Etodolac [Can]
Apo®-Flurbiprofen [Can]
Apo®-Ibuprofen [Can]
Apo®-Indomethacin [Can]
Apo®-Keto [Can]
Apo®-Keto-E [Can]
Apo®-Ketorolac [Can]
Apo®-Keto SR [Can]
Apo®-Mefenamic [Can]
Apo®-Nabumetone [Can]
Apo®-Napro-Na [Can]
Apo®-Napro-Na DS [Can]
Apo®-Naproxen [Can]
Apo®-Naproxen SR [Can]
Apo®-Piroxicam [Can]
Apo®-Sulin [Can]
Argesic®-SA [US]
Arthropan® [US-OTC]
Asaphen [Can]
Asaphen E.C. [Can]
Ascriptin® Arthritis Pain [US-OTC]
Ascriptin® Enteric [US-OTC]
Ascriptin® Extra Strength [US-OTC]
Ascriptin® [US-OTC]
Aspercin Extra [US-OTC]
Aspercin [US-OTC]
Aspergum® [US-OTC]

aspirin
Aspirin Free Anacin® Maximum
    Strength [US-OTC]
Atasol® [Can]
Bayer® Aspirin Extra Strength
    [US-OTC]
Bayer® Aspirin Regimen Adult Low
    Strength [US-OTC]
Bayer® Aspirin Regimen Adult Low
    Strength with Calcium [US-OTC]
Bayer® Aspirin Regimen Children's
    [US-OTC]
Bayer® Aspirin Regimen Regular
    Strength [US-OTC]
Bayer® Aspirin [US-OTC]
Bayer® Plus Extra Strength
    [US-OTC]
Brexidol® 20 [Can]
Bufferin® Arthritis Strength
    [US-OTC]
Bufferin® Extra Strength [US-OTC]
Bufferin® [US-OTC]
Cataflam® [US/Can]
Cetafen Extra® [US-OTC]
Cetafen® [US-OTC]
choline magnesium trisalicylate
choline salicylate
Clinoril® [US]
Daypro™ [US/Can]
diclofenac
Diclotec [Can]
diflunisal
Disalcid® [US]
Dolobid® [US]
Easprin® [US]
EC-Naprosyn® [US]
Ecotrin® Low Adult Strength
    [US-OTC]
Ecotrin® Maximum Strength
    [US-OTC]
Ecotrin® [US-OTC]
Entrophen® [Can]
etodolac

Excedrin® Extra Strength [US-OTC]
Excedrin® Migraine [US-OTC]
Excedrin® P.M. [US-OTC]
Feldene® [US/Can]
fenoprofen
Feverall® [US-OTC]
flurbiprofen
Froben® [Can]
Froben-SR® [Can]
Genaced [US-OTC]
Genapap® Children [US-OTC]
Genapap® Extra Strength [US-OTC]
Genapap® Infant [US-OTC]
Genapap® [US-OTC]
Genebs® Extra Strength [US-OTC]
Genebs® [US-OTC]
Genesec® [US-OTC]
Gen-Etodolac [Can]
Gen-Naproxen EC [Can]
Gen-Piroxicam [Can]
Genpril® [US-OTC]
Goody's® Extra Strength Headache
    Powder [US-OTC]
Goody's PM® Powder [US-OTC]
Halfprin® [US-OTC]
Haltran® [US-OTC]
ibuprofen
Ibu-Tab® [US]
Indocid® [Can]
Indocid® P.D.A. [Can]
Indocin® IV [US]
Indocin® SR [US]
Indocin® [US]
Indo-Lemmon [Can]
indomethacin
Indotec [Can]
Infantaire [US-OTC]
I-Prin [US-OTC]
ketoprofen
ketorolac
Legatrin PM® [US-OTC]
Liquiprin® for Children [US-OTC]
Lodine® [US/Can]

Lodine® XL [US]
Mapap® Children's [US-OTC]
Mapap® Extra Strength [US-OTC]
Mapap® Infants [US-OTC]
Mapap® [US-OTC]
meclofenamate
mefenamic acid
Menadol® [US-OTC]
Midol® Maximum Strength Cramp
    Formula [US-OTC]
Mono-Gesic® [US]
Motrin® Children's [US/Can]
Motrin® IB [US/Can]
Motrin® Infants' [US-OTC]
Motrin® Junior Strength [US-OTC]
Motrin® Migraine Pain [US-OTC]
Motrin® [US/Can]
nabumetone
Nalfon® [US/Can]
Naprelan® [US]
Naprosyn® [US/Can]
naproxen
Naxen® [Can]
Norgesic™ Forte [US/Can]
Norgesic™ [US/Can]
Novasen [Can]
Novo-Difenac® [Can]
Novo-Difenac-K [Can]
Novo-Difenac® SR [Can]
Novo-Diflunisal [Can]
Novo-Flurprofen [Can]
Novo-Keto [Can]
Novo-Keto-EC [Can]
Novo-Ketorolac [Can]
Novo-Methacin [Can]
Novo-Naprox [Can]
Novo-Naprox Sodium [Can]
Novo-Naprox Sodium DS [Can]
Novo-Naprox SR [Can]
Novo-Pirocam® [Can]
Novo-Profen® [Can]
Novo-Sundac [Can]
Nu-Diclo [Can]

Nu-Diclo-SR [Can]
Nu-Diflunisal [Can]
Nu-Flurprofen [Can]
Nu-Ibuprofen [Can]
Nu-Indo [Can]
Nu-Ketoprofen [Can]
Nu-Ketoprofen-E [Can]
Nu-Mefenamic [Can]
Nu-Naprox [Can]
Nu-Pirox [Can]
Nu-Sundac [Can]
Ocufen® Ophthalmic [US/Can]
Orafen [Can]
orphenadrine, aspirin, and caffeine
Orphengesic Forte [US]
Orphengesic [US]
Orudis® KT [US-OTC]
Orudis® SR [Can]
Oruvail® [US/Can]
oxaprozin
Pediatrix [Can]
Percogesic® [US-OTC]
Pexicam® [Can]
Phenylgesic® [US-OTC]
piroxicam
piroxicam and cyclodextrin
    (Canada only)
PMS-Diclofenac [Can]
PMS-Diclofenac SR [Can]
PMS-Mefenamic Acid [Can]
Ponstan® [Can]
Ponstel® [US/Can]
Redutemp® [US-OTC]
Relafen® [US/Can]
Rhodacine® [Can]
Rhodis™ [Can]
Rhodis-EC™ [Can]
Rhodis SR™ [Can]
Riva-Diclofenac [Can]
Riva-Diclofenac-K [Can]
Riva-Naproxen [Can]
Salflex® [US/Can]
salsalate

Silapap® Children's [US-OTC]
Silapap® Infants [US-OTC]
sodium salicylate
Solaraze™ [US]
St. Joseph® Pain Reliever [US-OTC]
sulindac
Sureprin 81™ [US-OTC]
Synflex® [Can]
Synflex® DS [Can]
Teejel® [Can]
Tempra® [Can]
Tolectin® DS [US]
Tolectin® [US/Can]
tolmetin
Toradol® [US/Can]
tramadol
Tricosal® [US]
Trilisate® [US/Can]
Tylenol® Arthritis Pain [US-OTC]
Tylenol® Children's [US-OTC]
Tylenol® Extra Strength [US-OTC]
Tylenol® Infants [US-OTC]
Tylenol® Junior Strength [US-OTC]
Tylenol® PM Extra Strength [US-OTC]
Tylenol® Severe Allergy [US-OTC]
Tylenol® Sore Throat [US-OTC]
Tylenol® [US/Can]
Ultracet™ [US]
Ultram® [US/Can]
Utradol™ [Can]
Valorin Extra [US-OTC]
Valorin [US-OTC]
Vanquish® Extra Strength Pain Reliever [US-OTC]
Voltaren Rapide® [Can]
Voltaren® [US/Can]
Voltaren®-XR [US]
Voltare Ophtha® [Can]
ZORprin® [US]
Decongestant/Analgesic

Advil® Cold & Sinus Caplets [US-OTC]
Advil® Cold & Sinus Tablet [Can]
Dristan® Sinus Caplets [US]
Dristan® Sinus Tablet [Can]
pseudoephedrine and ibuprofen
Local Anesthetic
Alcaine® [US/Can]
Diocaine® [Can]
ethyl chloride
ethyl chloride and dichlorotetrafluoroethane
Fluro-Ethyl® Aerosol [US]
Ophthetic® [US]
Parcaine® [US]
proparacaine
Neuroleptic Agent
Apo®-Methoprazine [Can]
methotrimeprazine (Canada only)
Novo-Meprazine [Can]
Nozinan® [Can]
Nonsteroidal Antiinflammatory Drug (NSAID)
Backache Pain Relief Extra Strength [US]
Doan's®, Original [US-OTC]
Extra Strength Doan's® [US-OTC]
Keygesic-10® [US]
magnesium salicylate
Mobidin® [US]
Momentum® [US-OTC]
Nonsteroidal Antiinflammatory Drug (NSAID), COX-2 Selective
rofecoxib
Vioxx® [US/Can]
Nonsteroidal Antiinflammatory Drug (NSAID), Oral
floctafenine (Canada only)
Idarac® [Can]

PERSISTENT PULMONARY VASOCONSTRICTION
Alpha-Adrenergic Blocking Agent

Priscoline® [US]
tolazoline

PNEUMONIA
Aminoglycoside (Antibiotic)
AKTob® [US]
Alcomicin® [Can]
amikacin
Amikin® [US/Can]
Diogent® [Can]
Garamycin® [US/Can]
Garatec [Can]
Gentacidin® [US]
Gentak® [US]
gentamicin
Nebcin® [US/Can]
PMS-Tobramycin [Can]
tobramycin
Tobrex® [US/Can]
Tomycine™ [Can]
Antibiotic, Carbapenem
ertapenem
Invanz™ [US]
Antibiotic, Miscellaneous
Alti-Clindamycin [Can]
Azactam® [US/Can]
aztreonam
Cleocin HCl® [US]
Cleocin Pediatric® [US]
Cleocin Phosphate® [US]
Cleocin® [US]
clindamycin
Dalacin® C [Can]
Vancocin® [US/Can]
Vancoled® [US]
vancomycin
Antibiotic, Penicillin
pivampicillin (Canada only)
Pondocillin® [Can]
Antibiotic, Quinolone
gatifloxacin
Levaquin® [US/Can]
levofloxacin

Tequin® [US/Can]
Carbapenem (Antibiotic)
imipenem and cilastatin
meropenem
Merrem® IV [US/Can]
Primaxin® [US/Can]
Cephalosporin (First Generation)
Ancef® [US/Can]
Apo®-Cefadroxil [Can]
Apo®-Cephalex [Can]
Biocef® [US]
cefadroxil
Cefadyl® [US/Can]
cefazolin
cephalexin
cephalothin
cephapirin
cephradine
Ceporacin® [Can]
Duricef® [US/Can]
Keflex® [US]
Keftab® [US/Can]
Kefzol® [US/Can]
Novo-Cefadroxil [Can]
Novo-Lexin® [Can]
Nu-Cephalex® [Can]
Velosef® [US]
Cephalosporin (Second Generation)
Cefotan® [US/Can]
cefotetan
cefoxitin
cefpodoxime
cefprozil
Ceftin® [US/Can]
cefuroxime
Cefzil® [US/Can]
Kefurox® [US/Can]
Mefoxin® [US/Can]
Vantin® [US/Can]
Zinacef® [US/Can]
Cephalosporin (Third Generation)
cefdinir
cefixime

Cefizox® [US/Can]
Cefobid® [US/Can]
cefoperazone
cefotaxime
ceftazidime
ceftizoxime
ceftriaxone
Ceptaz® [US/Can]
Claforan® [US/Can]
Fortaz® [US/Can]
Omnicef® [US/Can]
Rocephin® [US/Can]
Suprax® [US/Can]
Tazicef® [US]
Tazidime® [US/Can]
Cephalosporin (Fourth Generation)
cefepime
Maxipime® [US/Can]
Macrolide (Antibiotic)
Apo®-Erythro Base [Can]
Apo®-Erythro E-C [Can]
Apo®-Erythro-ES [Can]
Apo®-Erythro-S [Can]
azithromycin
Biaxin® [US/Can]
Biaxin® XL [US]
clarithromycin
Diomycin® [Can]
dirithromycin
Dynabac® [US]
E.E.S.® [US/Can]
Erybid™ [Can]
Eryc® [US/Can]
EryPed® [US]
Ery-Tab® [US]
Erythrocin® [US/Can]
erythromycin (systemic)
Nu-Erythromycin-S [Can]
PCE® [US/Can]
PMS-Erythromycin [Can]
Zithromax® [US/Can]
Z-PAK® [US/Can]
Penicillin

amoxicillin
amoxicillin and clavulanate
  potassium
Amoxicot® [US]
Amoxil® [US/Can]
ampicillin
ampicillin and sulbactam
Apo®-Amoxi [Can]
Apo®-Ampi [Can]
Apo®-Cloxi [Can]
Apo®-Pen VK [Can]
Augmentin ES-600™ [US]
Augmentin® [US/Can]
Bicillin® C-R 900/300 [US]
Bicillin® C-R [US]
Bicillin® L-A [US]
carbenicillin
Clavulin® [Can]
cloxacillin
dicloxacillin
Dynapen® [US]
Gen-Amoxicillin [Can]
Geocillin® [US]
Lin-Amox [Can]
Marcillin® [US]
Moxilin® [US]
Nadopen-V® [Can]
nafcillin
Novamoxin® [Can]
Novo-Ampicillin [Can]
Novo-Cloxin [Can]
Novo-Pen-VK® [Can]
Nu-Amoxi [Can]
Nu-Ampi [Can]
Nu-Cloxi® [Can]
Nu-Pen-VK® [Can]
oxacillin
penicillin G benzathine
penicillin G benzathine and procaine
  combined
penicillin G (parenteral/aqueous)
penicillin G procaine
penicillin V potassium

Permapen® [US]
Pfizerpen® [US/Can]
piperacillin
piperacillin and tazobactam sodium
Pipracil® [US/Can]
Principen® [US]
PVF® K [Can]
Suspen® [US]
Tazocin® [Can]
ticarcillin
ticarcillin and clavulanate potassium
Ticar® [US]
Timentin® [US/Can]
Trimox® [US]
Truxcillin® [US]
Unasyn® [US/Can]
Veetids® [US]
Wycillin® [US/Can]
Wymox® [US]
Zosyn® [US]
Quinolone
Apo®-Oflox [Can]
ciprofloxacin
Cipro® [US/Can]
Floxin® [US/Can]
lomefloxacin
Maxaquin® [US]
ofloxacin
sparfloxacin
Zagam® [US]
Sulfonamide
Apo®-Sulfatrim [Can]
Bactrim™ DS [US]
Bactrim™ [US]
Novo-Trimel [Can]
Novo-Trimel D.S. [Can]
Nu-Cotrimox® [Can]
Septra® DS [US/Can]
Septra® [US/Can]
sulfamethoxazole and trimethoprim
Sulfatrim® DS [US]
Sulfatrim® [US]
Vaccine

pneumococcal conjugate vaccine
(7-valent)
Prevnar™ [US]
Vaccine, Inactivated Bacteria
Pneumo 23™ [Can]
pneumococcal vaccine
Pneumovax® 23 [US/Can]
Pnu-Imune® 23 [US]

PNEUMONIA, COMMUNITY-ACQUIRED
Antibiotic, Quinolone
ABC Pack™ (Avelox®) [US]
Avelox® [US/Can]
moxifloxacin

PRIMARY PULMONARY HYPERTENSION (PPH)
Platelet Inhibitor
epoprostenol
Flolan® [US/Can]

PULMONARY ARTERY HYPERTENSION (PAH)
Endothelin Antagonist
bosentan
Tracleer™ [US]
Vasodilator
Remodulin™ [US]
treprostinil

PULMONARY EMBOLISM
Anticoagulant (Other)
Coumadin® [US/Can]
dicumarol
enoxaparin
Hepalean® [Can]
Hepalean® Leo [Can]
Hepalean®-LOK [Can]
heparin
Hep-Lock® [US]
Lovenox® [US/Can]
Taro-Warfarin [Can]

warfarin
Fibrinolytic Agent
   Abbokinase® [US]
   Activase® rt-PA [Can]
   Activase® [US]
   alteplase
   Streptase® [US/Can]
   streptokinase
   urokinase
Low Molecular Weight Heparin
   Fraxiparine™ [Can]
   nadroparin (Canada only)

PULMONARY TUBERCULOSIS

Antitubercular Agent
   Priftin® [US/Can]
   rifapentine

RESPIRATORY DISORDERS

Adrenal Corticosteroid
   Acthar® [US]
   A-HydroCort® [US/Can]
   Alti-Dexamethasone [Can]
   A-methaPred® [US]
   Apo®-Prednisone [Can]
   Aristocort® Forte Injection [US]
   Aristocort® Intralesional Injection [US]
   Aristocort® Tablet [US/Can]
   Aristospan® Intra-articular Injection [US/Can]
   Aristospan® Intralesional Injection [US/Can]
   Azmacort® [US]
   Betaject™ [Can]
   betamethasone (systemic)
   Betnesol® [Can]
   Celestone® Phosphate [US]
   Celestone® Soluspan® [US/Can]
   Celestone® [US]
   Cel-U-Jec® [US]
   Cortef® [US/Can]

corticotropin
cortisone acetate
Cortone® [Can]
Decadron®-LA [US]
Decadron® [US/Can]
Decaject-LA® [US]
Decaject® [US]
Delta-Cortef® [US]
Deltasone® [US]
Depo-Medrol® [US/Can]
Depopred® [US]
Dexacort® Phosphate in Respihaler® [US]
dexamethasone (oral inhalation)
dexamethasone (systemic)
Dexasone® L.A. [US]
Dexasone® [US/Can]
Dexone® LA [US]
Dexone® [US]
Hexadrol® [US/Can]
H.P. Acthar® Gel [US]
hydrocortisone (systemic)
Hydrocortone® Acetate [US]
Kenalog® Injection [US/Can]
Key-Pred-SP® [US]
Key-Pred® [US]
Medrol® Tablet [US/Can]
methylprednisolone
Meticorten® [US]
Orapred™ [US]
Pediapred® [US/Can]
PMS-Dexamethasone [Can]
Prednicot® [US]
prednisolone (systemic)
Prednisol® TBA [US]
prednisone
Prelone® [US]
Solu-Cortef® [US/Can]
Solu-Medrol® [US/Can]
Solurex L.A.® [US]
Sterapred® DS [US]
Sterapred® [US]
Tac™-3 Injection [US]

Triam-A® Injection [US]
triamcinolone (inhalation, oral)
triamcinolone (systemic)
Triam Forte® Injection [US]
Winpred™ [Can]

RESPIRATORY DISTRESS SYNDROME (RDS)
Lung Surfactant
    beractant
    calfactant
    colfosceril palmitate
    Curosurf® [US/Can]
    Exosurf® Neonatal™ [US/Can]
    Infasurf® [US]
    poractant alfa
    Survanta® [US/Can]

RESPIRATORY SYNCYTIAL VIRUS (RSV)
Antiviral Agent
    Rebetol® [US]
    ribavirin
    Virazole® [US/Can]
Immune Globulin
    RespiGam™ [US]
    respiratory syncytial virus immune
        globulin (intravenous)
Monoclonal Antibody
    palivizumab
    Synagis® [US]

RESPIRATORY TRACT INFECTION
Aminoglycoside (Antibiotic)
    AKTob® [US]
    Alcomicin® [Can]
    Diogent® [Can]
    Garamycin® [US/Can]
    Garatec [Can]
    Gentacidin® [US]
    Gentak® [US]
    gentamicin

Nebcin® [US/Can]
PMS-Tobramycin [Can]
tobramycin
Tobrex® [US/Can]
Tomycine™ [Can]
Antibiotic, Carbacephem
    Lorabid™ [US/Can]
    loracarbef
Antibiotic, Macrolide
    Rovamycine® [Can]
    spiramycin (Canada only)
Antibiotic, Miscellaneous
    Alti-Clindamycin [Can]
    Azactam® [US/Can]
    aztreonam
    Cleocin HCl® [US]
    Cleocin Pediatric® [US]
    Cleocin Phosphate® [US]
    Cleocin® [US]
    clindamycin
    Dalacin® C [Can]
Antibiotic, Penicillin
    pivampicillin (Canada only)
    Pondocillin® [Can]
Antibiotic, Quinolone
    gatifloxacin
    Levaquin® [US/Can]
    levofloxacin
    Quixin™ Ophthalmic [US]
    Tequin® [US/Can]
Cephalosporin (First Generation)
    Ancef® [US/Can]
    Apo®-Cefadroxil [Can]
    Apo®-Cephalex [Can]
    Biocef® [US]
    cefadroxil
    Cefadyl® [US/Can]
    cefazolin
    cephalexin
    cephalothin
    cephapirin
    cephradine
    Ceporacin® [Can]

Duricef® [US/Can]
Keflex® [US]
Keftab® [US/Can]
Kefzol® [US/Can]
Novo-Cefadroxil [Can]
Novo-Lexin® [Can]
Nu-Cephalex® [Can]
Velosef® [US]
Cephalosporin (Second Generation)
Apo®-Cefaclor [Can]
Ceclor® CD [US]
Ceclor® [US/Can]
cefaclor
cefamandole
Cefotan® [US/Can]
cefotetan
cefoxitin
cefpodoxime
cefprozil
Ceftin® [US/Can]
cefuroxime
Cefzil® [US/Can]
Kefurox® [US/Can]
Mandol® [US]
Mefoxin® [US/Can]
Novo-Cefaclor [Can]
Nu-Cefaclor [Can]
PMS-Cefaclor [Can]
Vantin® [US/Can]
Zinacef® [US/Can]
Cephalosporin (Third Generation)
Cedax® [US]
cefixime
Cefizox® [US/Can]
Cefobid® [US/Can]
cefoperazone
cefotaxime
ceftazidime
ceftibuten
ceftizoxime
ceftriaxone
Ceptaz® [US/Can]
Claforan® [US/Can]

Fortaz® [US/Can]
Rocephin® [US/Can]
Suprax® [US/Can]
Tazicef® [US]
Tazidime® [US/Can]
Cephalosporin (Fourth Generation)
cefepime
Maxipime® [US/Can]
Macrolide (Antibiotic)
Apo®-Erythro Base [Can]
Apo®-Erythro E-C [Can]
Apo®-Erythro-ES [Can]
Apo®-Erythro-S [Can]
azithromycin
Biaxin® [US/Can]
Biaxin® XL [US]
clarithromycin
Diomycin® [Can]
dirithromycin
Dynabac® [US]
E.E.S.® [US/Can]
Erybid™ [Can]
Eryc® [US/Can]
EryPed® [US]
Ery-Tab® [US]
Erythrocin® [US/Can]
erythromycin and sulfisoxazole
erythromycin (systemic)
Eryzole® [US]
Nu-Erythromycin-S [Can]
PCE® [US/Can]
Pediazole® [US/Can]
PMS-Erythromycin [Can]
Zithromax® [US/Can]
Z-PAK® [US/Can]
Penicillin
amoxicillin
amoxicillin and clavulanate
potassium
Amoxicot® [US]
Amoxil® [US/Can]
ampicillin
ampicillin and sulbactam

Apo®-Amoxi [Can]
Apo®-Ampi [Can]
Apo®-Cloxi [Can]
Apo®-Pen VK [Can]
Augmentin ES-600™ [US]
Augmentin® [US/Can]
Bicillin® C-R 900/300 [US]
Bicillin® C-R [US]
Bicillin® L-A [US]
carbenicillin
Clavulin® [Can]
cloxacillin
dicloxacillin
Dynapen® [US]
Gen-Amoxicillin [Can]
Geocillin® [US]
Lin-Amox [Can]
Marcillin® [US]
Moxilin® [US]
Nadopen-V® [Can]
nafcillin
Novamoxin® [Can]
Novo-Ampicillin [Can]
Novo-Cloxin [Can]
Novo-Pen-VK® [Can]
Nu-Amoxi [Can]
Nu-Ampi [Can]
Nu-Cloxi® [Can]
Nu-Pen-VK® [Can]
oxacillin
penicillin G benzathine
penicillin G benzathine and procaine
   combined
penicillin G (parenteral/aqueous)
penicillin G procaine
penicillin V potassium
Permapen® [US]
Pfizerpen® [US/Can]
piperacillin
piperacillin and tazobactam sodium
Pipracil® [US/Can]
Principen® [US]
PVF® K [Can]

Suspen® [US]
Tazocin® [Can]
ticarcillin
ticarcillin and clavulanate potassium
Ticar® [US]
Timentin® [US/Can]
Trimox® [US]
Truxcillin® [US]
Unasyn® [US/Can]
Veetids® [US]
Wycillin® [US/Can]
Wymox® [US]
Zosyn® [US]
Quinolone
   Apo®-Oflox [Can]
   ciprofloxacin
   Cipro® [US/Can]
   Floxin® [US/Can]
   lomefloxacin
   Maxaquin® [US]
   ofloxacin
   sparfloxacin
   Zagam® [US]
Sulfonamide
   erythromycin and sulfisoxazole
   Eryzole® [US]
   Pediazole® [US/Can]

SARCOIDOSIS
Corticosteroid, Topical
   Aclovate® [US]
   Acticort® [US]
   Aeroseb-HC® [US]
   Ala-Cort® [US]
   Ala-Scalp® [US]
   alclometasone
   Alphatrex® [US]
   amcinonide
   Aquacort® [Can]
   Aristocort® A Topical [US]
   Aristocort® Topical [US/Can]
   Bactine® Hydrocortisone [US-OTC]
   Betaderm® [Can]

Betamethacot® [US]
betamethasone (topical)
Betatrex® [US]
Beta-Val® [US]
Betnovate® [Can]
CaldeCORT® Anti-Itch Spray [US]
CaldeCORT® [US-OTC]
Capex™ [US/Can]
Carmol-HC® [US]
Celestoderm®-EV/2 [Can]
Celestoderm®-V [Can]
Cetacort®
clobetasol
Clocort® Maximum Strength
    [US-OTC]
clocortolone
Cloderm® [US/Can]
Cordran® SP [US]
Cordran® [US/Can]
Cormax® [US]
CortaGel® [US-OTC]
Cortaid® Maximum Strength
    [US-OTC]
Cortaid® with Aloe [US-OTC]
Cort-Dome® [US]
Cortizone®-5 [US-OTC]
Cortizone®-10 [US-OTC]
Cortoderm [Can]
Cutivate™ [US]
Cyclocort® [US/Can]
Del-Beta® [US]
Delcort® [US]
Dermacort® [US]
Dermarest Dricort® [US]
Derma-Smoothe/FS® [US/Can]
Dermatop® [US]
Dermolate® [US-OTC]
Dermovate® [Can]
Dermtex® HC with Aloe
    [US-OTC]
Desocort® [Can]
desonide
DesOwen® [US]

desoximetasone
diflorasone
Diprolene® AF [US]
Diprolene® [US/Can]
Diprosone® [US/Can]
Ectosone [Can]
Eldecort® [US]
Elocon® [US/Can]
fluocinolone
fluocinonide
Fluoderm [Can]
flurandrenolide
fluticasone (topical)
Gen-Clobetasol [Can]
Gynecort® [US-OTC]
halcinonide
halobetasol
Halog®-E [US]
Halog® [US/Can]
Hi-Cor-1.0® [US]
Hi-Cor-2.5® [US]
Hyderm [Can]
hydrocortisone (topical)
Hydrocort® [US]
Hydro-Tex® [US-OTC]
Hytone® [US]
Kenalog® in Orabase® [US/Can]
Kenalog® Topical [US/Can]
LactiCare-HC® [US]
Lanacort® [US-OTC]
Lidemol® [Can]
Lidex-E® [US]
Lidex® [US/Can]
Locoid® [US/Can]
Luxiq™ [US]
Lyderm® [Can]
Lydonide [Can]
Maxiflor® [US]
Maxivate® [US]
mometasone furoate
Nasonex® [US/Can]
Novo-Clobetasol [Can]
Nutracort® [US]

Olux™ [US]
Orabase® HCA [US]
Penecort® [US]
  prednicarbate
  Prevex® [Can]
  Prevex® HC [Can]
  Psorcon™ E [US]
  Psorcon™ [US/Can]
  Qualisone® [US]
  Sarna® HC [Can]
  Scalpicin® [US]
  S-T Cort® [US]
  Synacort® [US]
  Synalar® [US/Can]
  Taro-Desoximetasone [Can]
  Taro-Sone® [Can]
  Tegrin®-HC [US-OTC]
  Temovate® [US]
  Texacort® [US]
  Tiamol® [Can]
  Ti-U-Lac® H [Can]
  Topicort®-LP [US]
  Topicort® [US/Can]
  Topilene® [Can]
  Topisone®
  Topsyn® [Can]
  Triacet™ Topical [US]
Oracort [Can]
  Triaderm [Can]
  triamcinolone (topical)
  Tridesilon® [US]
  U-Cort™ [US]
  Ultravate™ [US/Can]
  urea and hydrocortisone
  Uremol® HC [Can]
  Valisone® Scalp Lotion [Can]
  Westcort® [US/Can]

SKELETAL MUSCLE RELAXANT (SURGICAL)
Skeletal Muscle Relaxant
  Anectine® Chloride [US]
  Anectine® Flo-Pack® [US]

Arduan® [US/Can]
atracurium
cisatracurium
doxacurium
Nimbex® [US/Can]
Norcuron® [US/Can]
Nuromax® [US/Can]
pancuronium
pipecuronium
Quelicin® [US/Can]
rocuronium
succinylcholine
Tracrium® [US]
vecuronium
Zemuron® [US/Can]

SMOKING CESSATION
Antidepressant, Monoamine Oxidase
    Inhibitor
  Alti-Moclobemide [Can]
  Apo®-Moclobemide [Can]
  Manerix® [Can]
  moclobemide (Canada only)
  Novo-Moclobemide [Can]
  Nu-Moclobemide [Can]
Smoking Deterrent
  Habitrol® [Can]
  Nicoderm® [Can]
  NicoDerm® CQ® [US-OTC]
  Nicorette® [US/Can]
  nicotine
  Nicotrol® Inhaler [US]
  Nicotrol® NS [US]
  Nicotrol® Patch [US/Can]

STROKE
Antiplatelet Agent
  Alti-Ticlopidine [Can]
  Apo®-ASA [Can]
  Apo®-Ticlopidine [Can]
  Asaphen [Can]
  Asaphen E.C. [Can]
  aspirin

Bayer® Aspirin Regimen Adult Low
   Strength [US-OTC]
Bayer® Aspirin Regimen Adult Low
   Strength with Calcium [US-OTC]
Ecotrin® Low Adult Strength
   [US-OTC]
Halfprin® [US-OTC]
Nu-Ticlopidine [Can]
Sureprin 81™ [US-OTC]
Ticlid® [US/Can]
ticlopidine
Fibrinolytic Agent
   Activase® rt-PA [Can]
   Activase® [US]
   alteplase
Skeletal Muscle Relaxant
   Dantrium® [US/Can]
   dantrolene

SYNCOPE

Adrenergic Agonist Agent
   Adrenalin® Chloride [US/Can]
   epinephrine
   isoproterenol
   Isuprel® [US]
Respiratory Stimulant
   ammonia spirit (aromatic)
   Aromatic Ammonia Aspirols® [US]

THROMBOLYTIC THERAPY

Anticoagulant (Other)
   anisindione
   Coumadin® [US/Can]
   dalteparin
   dicumarol
   enoxaparin
   Fragmin® [US/Can]
   Hepalean® [Can]
   Hepalean® Leo [Can]
   Hepalean®-LOK [Can]
   heparin
   Hep-Lock® [US]
   Innohep® [US/Can]

Lovenox® [US/Can]
Miradon® [US]
Taro-Warfarin [Can]
tinzaparin
warfarin
Fibrinolytic Agent
   Abbokinase® [US]
   Activase® rt-PA [Can]
   Activase® [US]
   alteplase
   Retavase® [US/Can]
   reteplase
   Streptase® [US/Can]
   streptokinase
   urokinase

THROMBOSIS (ARTERIAL)

Fibrinolytic Agent
   Streptase® [US/Can]
   streptokinase

TOPICAL ANESTHESIA

Local Anesthetic
   Americaine® Anesthetic Lubricant
      [US]
   Americaine® [US-OTC]
   Ametop™ [Can]
   Anbesol® Baby [US/Can]
   Anbesol® Maximum Strength
      [US-OTC]
   Anbesol® [US-OTC]
   Anestacon® [US]
   Babee® Teething® [US-OTC]
   benzocaine
   Benzodent® [US-OTC]
   Chiggerex® [US-OTC]
   Chiggertox® [US-OTC]
   Citanest® Forte [Can]
   Citanest® Plain [US/Can]
   cocaine
   Cylex® [US-OTC]
   Dermaflex® Gel [US]
   Detane® [US-OTC]

ELA-Max® [US-OTC]
ethyl chloride
ethyl chloride and
  dichlorotetrafluoroethane
Fleet® Pain Relief [US-OTC]
Fluro-Ethyl® Aerosol [US]
Foille® Medicated First Aid
  [US-OTC]
Foille® Plus [US-OTC]
Foille® [US-OTC]
HDA® Toothache [US-OTC]
Hurricaine® [US]
Itch-X® [US-OTC]
lidocaine
Lidodan™ [Can]
Lidoderm® [US/Can]
LidoPen® Auto-Injector [US]
Mycinettes® [US-OTC]
Orabase®-B [US-OTC]
Orajel® Baby Nighttime [US-OTC]
Orajel® Baby [US-OTC]
Orajel® Maximum Strength
  [US-OTC]
Orajel® [US-OTC]
Orasol® [US-OTC]
Phicon® [US-OTC]
Pontocaine® [US/Can]
PrameGel® [US-OTC]
pramoxine
Prax® [US-OTC]
prilocaine
ProctoFoam® NS [US-OTC]
Solarcaine® Aloe Extra Burn Relief
  [US-OTC]
Solarcaine® [US-OTC]
tetracaine
Trocaine® [US-OTC]
Tronolane® [US-OTC]
Tronothane® [US-OTC]
Xylocaine® [US/Can]
Xylocard® [Can]
Zilactin® Baby [US/Can]
Zilactin®-B [US/Can]

Zilactin® [Can]
Zilactin-L® [US-OTC]

TRANSIENT ISCHEMIC ATTACK (TIA)

Anticoagulant (Other)
  enoxaparin
  Hepalean® [Can]
  Hepalean® Leo [Can]
  Hepalean®-LOK [Can]
  heparin
  Hep-Lock® [US]
  Lovenox® [US/Can]
Antiplatelet Agent
  aspirin
  Bayer® Aspirin Regimen Adult Low
    Strength [US-OTC]
  Bayer® Aspirin Regimen Adult Low
    Strength with Calcium [US-OTC]
  Ecotrin® Low Adult Strength
    [US-OTC]
  Halfprin® [US-OTC]
  Sureprin 81™ [US-OTC]

TUBERCULOSIS

Antibiotic, Aminoglycoside
  streptomycin
Antibiotic, Miscellaneous
  Capastat® Sulfate [US]
  capreomycin
  cycloserine
  Rifadin® [US/Can]
  Rifamate® [US/Can]
  rifampin
  rifampin and isoniazid
  rifampin, isoniazid, and
    pyrazinamide
  Rifater® [US/Can]
  Rimactane® [US]
  Rofact™ [Can]
  Seromycin® Pulvules® [US]
Antimycobacterial Agent
  ethambutol

ethionamide
Etibi® [Can]
Myambutol® [US]
Trecator®-SC [US/Can]
Antitubercular Agent
isoniazid
Isotamine® [Can]
Nydrazid® [US]
PMS-Isoniazid [Can]
pyrazinamide
streptomycin
Tebrazid™ [Can]
Biological Response Modulator
BCG vaccine
ImmuCyst® [Can]
Oncotice™ [Can]
Pacis™ [Can]
TheraCys® [US]

TICE® BCG [US]
Nonsteroidal Antiinflammatory Drug
(NSAID)
aminosalicylate sodium
Nemasol® Sodium [Can]

TUBERCULOSIS (DIAGNOSTIC)
Diagnostic Agent
Aplisol® [US]
Tine Test PPD [US]
tuberculin tests
Tubersol® [US]

VASCULAR DISORDER
Vasodilator
isoxsuprine
Vasodilan® [US]